Clinical Neuropsychology
Study Guide and Board Review

Clinical Neuropsychology Study Guide and Board Review

SECOND EDITION

Editors

Kirk J. Stucky, PsyD, ABPP-CN, RP
Michael W. Kirkwood, PhD, ABPP-CN
Jacobus Donders, PhD, ABPP-CN, RP

Managing Editor

Christine D. Liff, PhD

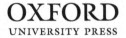
OXFORD
UNIVERSITY PRESS

OXFORD
UNIVERSITY PRESS

Oxford University Press is a department of the University of Oxford. It furthers
the University's objective of excellence in research, scholarship, and education
by publishing worldwide. Oxford is a registered trade mark of Oxford University
Press in the UK and certain other countries.

Published in the United States of America by Oxford University Press
198 Madison Avenue, New York, NY 10016, United States of America.

Library of Congress Cataloging-in-Publication Data
Names: Stucky, Kirk J., editor. | Kirkwood, Michael W., editor. |
Donders, Jacobus, editor..
Title: Clinical neuropsychology study guide and board review / editors,
Kirk J. Stucky, PsyD, ABPP-CN, RP, Michael W. Kirkwood, PhD,
ABPP-CN, Jacobus Donders, PhD, ABPP-CN, RP; managing editor,
Christine D. Liff, PhD
Description: Second edition. | New York, NY : Oxford University Press, 2020. |
Includes bibliographical references and index.
Identifiers: LCCN 2019038637 (print) | LCCN 2019038638 (ebook) |
ISBN 9780190690021 (paperback) | ISBN 9780190690045 (epub) |
ISBN 9780190690038
Subjects: LCSH: Clinical neuropsychology—Certification—Study guides. |
Clinical neuropsychology—Examinations, questions, etc. |
Clinical psychologists—Certification—Study guides.
Classification: LCC RC386.6.N48 C5278 2020 (print) |
LCC RC386.6.N48 (ebook) | DDC 616.80076—dc23
LC record available at https://lccn.loc.gov/2019038637
LC ebook record available at https://lccn.loc.gov/2019038638

9 8 7 6

Printed by LSC Communications, United States of America

For Mary, who managed to be tenaciously supportive during the formation of yet another collection of words that has very little to do with being a dutiful husband. And to all students of neuroscience, whatever their level of experience and whatever their needs.

Kirk J. Stucky

For Jane Holmes Bernstein, Keith Yeates, Scott Grewe, and Warren Rosen, who at each stage of my training, with their own inimitable styles, taught me how to be a neuropsychologist.

Michael W. Kirkwood

For all my former postdoctoral residents who have made me proud by successfully completing the board-certification process in clinical neuropsychology.

Jacobus Donders

For my son, Evan, who has been my biggest champion and who fills my heart every day. And to my mentors, colleagues, and students, who have enriched my professional development.

Christine D. Liff

About the Editors

Kirk J. Stucky obtained his PsyD from Florida Tech in 1995. He completed his internship at Union Memorial Hospital in Baltimore, Maryland, and his residency at Hurley Medical Center in Flint, Michigan. He is the current chair of the Department of Behavioral Health at Hurley Medical Center and an assistant professor for the Michigan State University College of Human Medicine, Department of Medicine. Being board certified in rehabilitation psychology and clinical neuropsychology, he has been dedicated to advancing the interests of both specialties including the development of integrated training standards and exploring new opportunities for advanced hospital practice. As a program director, he has had the privilege of supervising postdoctoral residents for 24 years and mentoring a talented cadre of psychologists who have successfully obtained board certification in clinical neuropsychology, rehabilitation psychology, and health psychology. During that time, he has developed, modified, and improved various study and professional development materials, some of which are included in this study guide.

Michael W. Kirkwood obtained his PhD from DePaul University in 1998. He completed his internship at Nationwide Children's Hospital in Columbus, Ohio, and his postdoctoral fellowship at Boston Children's Hospital. He is Director of the Rehabilitation Psychology & Neuropsychology Program at Children's Hospital Colorado in Aurora, Colorado, and Professor in the Department of Physical Medicine and Rehabilitation at the University of Colorado School of Medicine. He is a pediatric neuropsychologist, board-certified in clinical neuropsychology and subspecialty-certified in pediatric neuropsychology by the American Board of Professional Psychology. He has been involved in the supervision of innumerable neuropsychology students and trainees over the last 20 years and has helped mentor many neuropsychologists through the board certification process. He was a founding member and leader of the BRAIN support group and key contributor to the development of many available study materials through BRAIN. He co-authored the Oxford published volume *Board Certification in Clinical Neuropsychology: A Guide to Becoming ABPP/ABCN Certified Without Sacrificing Your Sanity* and served as co-editor of the second edition of the *AACN Study Guide for Board Certification in Clinical Neuropsychology*.

Jacobus Donders obtained his PhD from the University of Windsor in 1988. He completed his internship at Henry Ford Hospital in Detroit, Michigan, and his residency at the University of Michigan in Ann Arbor, Michigan. He is currently the chief psychologist at Mary Free Bed Rehabilitation Hospital in Grand Rapids, Michigan. Dr. Donders is board-certified by the American Board of Professional Psychology in both clinical neuropsychology (including subspecialty certification in pediatric clinical neuropsychology) and rehabilitation psychology. He has served on multiple editorial and professional executive boards, has authored or co-authored more than 100 publications in peer-reviewed journals, and has co-edited five books. He is a fellow of the National Academy of Neuropsychology and of Divisions 40 (Clinical Neuropsychology) and 22 (Rehabilitation Psychology) of the American Psychological Association.

Managing Editor **Christine D. Liff** completed her internship at Cincinnati VA Medical Center, and obtained her PhD from the University of North Texas in 2003. She completed pre- and post-doctoral clinical training at the University of Texas Southwestern Medical Center, Terrell State Hospital, Pate Rehabilitation, and Detroit Medical Center. She is currently director of the Neuropsychology Practicum Program at Michigan Neurology Associates, where she has had the opportunity to supervise master- and doctoral-level psychology students, and is also a member of the Program Committee for the Michigan Psychological Association. She assisted with the initial creation of select topic pages for the Be Ready for ABPP In Neuropsychology (BRAIN) website. Her main research interests include validity of neuropsychological test instruments, neuropsychological malingering, and assessment of multiple sclerosis and Alzheimer's disease.

Contents

CONTENTS

CONTENTS

List of Tables, Figures, and Boxes

Tables

Figures

Boxes

Preface and Acknowledgments

Seven years have passed since we sent the first edition of the *Clinical Neuropsychology Study Guide and Board Review* off to the publisher. During the years that followed, it was gratifying to know that the book was generally quite well received by ABCN candidates and the professional community at large. In this second edition, we added three new chapters and generated enough questions to seed four full-length practice exams. Furthermore, every chapter has been thoroughly reviewed and revised. A special effort was made to update references when possible but also to retain seminal papers that we and the authors believed were important for neuropsychologists, both young and old, to know and understand.

As with the first edition, the completion of this book was inevitably a herculean effort, requiring participation from a wide range of individuals. However, we would like to first thank those who took the time to provide us with honest feedback and constructive criticism about the first edition. Thoughtful comments, both favorable and unfavorable, from many readers at different career phases and with varying expectations have helped shape this second edition.

Retaining the best of the first edition while expanding upon and improving the depth of coverage required substantial effort from the authors, who are all widely recognized experts in neuropsychology and very busy professionals. As editors, we greatly appreciated their efforts and collaboration, as well as their knowledge, expertise, and dedication to the field of clinical neuropsychology and board certification.

We also would like to recognize a few individuals in particular for their support. Dr. Christine Liff acted as the managing editor for both volumes and coauthor of several chapters. Dr. Liff has selflessly contributed her talents and helped in all matters, large and small, pertaining to this book. Her meticulous eye for detail has ensured a level of quality that we hope readers will appreciate.

Jennifer Godlesky MLIS, library manager at Hurley Medical Center, relentlessly searched for and diligently verified innumerable citations used throughout the text. Joan Bossert, at Oxford, encouraged us to work on and publish this second edition a bit ahead of our original timeline. Throughout the process, these people have been supportive and responsive, and helped us maintain a "big picture" perspective in producing such a large volume. Finally, gratitude to our loved ones who have graciously accepted our time away from other responsibilities and provided so much support in the process.

Contributors

Kenneth M. Adams, PhD, ABPP (CN, CL)
Professor
Department of Psychiatry
Neuropsychology Program
Medical School
Professor
Department of Psychology
School of Literature, Science and the Arts
University of Michigan
Ann Arbor, MI

Mark T. Barisa, PhD, ABPP-CN
Independent Practice
Performance Neuropsychology
Frisco/Dallas, TX

Russell M. Bauer, PhD, ABPP-CN
Preeminence Term Professor
Director
Doctoral Program in Clinical Psychology
Department of Clinical & Health Psychology
University of Florida
Director
Brain Rehabilitation Research Center of
    Excellence (151)
Malcom Randall Veterans Administration
    Medical Center
Gainesville, FL

Katherine Baum, PhD, ABPP-CN
Pediatric Neuropsychologist
Department of Child and Adolescent Psychiatry and
    Behavioral Sciences
Children's Hospital of Philadelphia
Philadelphia, PA

Hilary C. Bertisch, PhD, ABPP-CN
Clinical Assistant Professor of Rehabilitation Medicine
Associate Director
Postdoctoral Fellowship in Rehabilitation Research
Department of Psychology
Rusk Institute of Rehabilitation Medicine
New York, NY

Robert M. Bilder, PhD, ABPP-CN
Michael E. Tennenbaum Family Distinguished
    Professor and Chief of Psychology
Department of Psychiatry and Biobehavioral Sciences
UCLA David Geffen School of Medicine
Department of Psychology
UCLA College of Letters and Science
Jane & Terry Semel Institute for Neuroscience and
    Human Behavior at UCLA
Stewart & Lynda Resnick Neuropsychiatric Hospital
    at UCLA
Los Angeles, CA

Richard Boada, PhD, ABPP-CN
Clinical Neuropsychologist
Division of Neurology
Children's Hospital Colorado
Associate Professor of Pediatrics and Neurology
University of Colorado School of Medicine
Aurora, CO

Doug Bodin, PhD, ABPP-CN
Neuropsychologist
Department of Pediatric Psychology and
    Neuropsychology
Nationwide Children's Hospital
Associate Professor of Clinical Pediatrics
The Ohio State University
Columbus, OH

Shane S. Bush, PhD, ABPP (CN, CP, GP, RP)
Psychologist
Long Island Neuropsychology, P.C.
Lake Ronkonkoma, NY
Department of Psychology
University of Alabama
Tuscaloosa, AL
VA New York Harbor Healthcare System
Stony Brook, NY

Desiree Byrd, PhD, ABPP-CN
Assistant Professor of Neurology and Psychiatry
Mt. Sinai School of Medicine
New York, NY
Associate Professor of Psychology
City University of New York, Queens College
Flushing, NY

Dominic A. Carone, PhD, ABPP-CN
Neuropsychologist and Clinical Associate Professor
Physical Medicine and Rehabilitation, and
    Psychiatry
Coordinator of Neuropsychology Assessment Program
State University of New York
Upstate Medical University
Syracuse, NY

Christine Clancy, PhD, ABPP-CN
Pediatric Neuropsychologist
Division of Rehabilitation Psychology
Seattle Children's Hospital
Seattle, WA

Amy K. Connery, PsyD, ABPP-CN
Assistant Clinical Professor
Department of Physical Medicine and Rehabilitation
University of Colorado Denver School of Medicine
Children's Hospital Colorado
Aurora, CO

C. Munro Cullum, PhD, ABPP-CN
Professor of Psychiatry, Neurology, and Neurological
    Surgery
Pamela Blumenthal Distinguished Professor of
    Clinical Psychology
Vice Chair and Chief
Division of Psychology
University of Texas Southwestern Medical Center
Dallas, TX

Sid Dickson, PhD, ABPP-CN
Clinical Neuropsychologist
Baylor Scott & White Institute for Rehabilitation
Frisco, TX

Jacobus Donders, PhD, ABPP (CN, RP)
Chief Psychologist
Mary Free Bed Rehabilitation Hospital
Grand Rapids, MI

Deborah Fein, PhD, ABPP-CN
University of Connecticut Board of Trustees
    Distinguished Professor
Department of Psychological Services
Department of Pediatrics
University of Connecticut
Storrs, CT

Jack M. Fletcher, PhD, ABPP-CN
Chair
Department of Psychology
Interim Associate Vice President for Research
    Administration
University of Houston
Houston, TX

Daryl Fujii, PhD, ABPP-CN
Clinical Neuropsychologist
Veteran's Administration Pacific Island Health
    Care System
Community Living Center
Honolulu, HI

William Garmoe, PhD, ABPP-CN
Director of Psychology
MedStar National Rehabilitation Network
Associate Professor
Clinical Rehabilitation Medicine
Clinical Neurology
Georgetown University School of Medicine
Washington, DC

Leslie S. Gaynor, MS
Doctoral Program in Clinical Psychology
Department of Clinical & Health Psychology
University of Florida
Gainesville, FL

Manfred F. Greiffenstein, PhD, ABPP (CN, F)
Psychological Systems, Inc.
Royal Oak, MI

Leslie M. Guidotti Breting, PhD, ABPP-CN
Senior Clinician Educator
Department of Psychiatry and Behavioral Sciences
NorthShore University HealthSystem
Evanston, IL
University of Chicago, Pritzker School of Medicine
Chicago, IL

Kathleen Y. Haaland, PhD, ABPP-CN
Professor of Psychiatry and Behavioral
  Sciences
University of New Mexico School of Medicine
Albuquerque, NM

Lana Harder, PhD, ABPP-CN
Clinical Manager
Neuropsychology Service
Neuropsychology Training Director
Children's Medical Center, Dallas
Associate Professor of Psychiatry
Associate Professor of Neurology and
  Neurotherapeutics
University of Texas Southwestern Medical Center
Dallas, TX

Nancy Hebben, PhD, ABPP-CN
Independent Practice
Newton, MA
Assistant Professor in Psychology, Part-time
Department of Psychiatry
Harvard Medical School
Boston, MA
Cambridge Health Alliance
Cambridge, MA

Robin C. Hilsabeck, PhD, ABPP-CN
Associate Professor
Department of Neurology
Dell Medical School
The University of Texas (UT) at Austin
Comprehensive Memory Center
Mulva Clinic for the Neurosciences
UT Health Austin
Austin, TX

Jennifer L. Huffman, PhD, ABPP-CN
Owner
Huffman Psychology, PLLC
East Lansing, MI

Jennifer Janusz, PsyD, ABPP-CN
Associate Professor
Department of Pediatrics and Neurology
University of Colorado School of Medicine
Program Director
Neurofibromatosis Program
Children's Hospital Colorado
Aurora, CO

Amy M. Jimenez, PhD
Assistant Research Psychologist
Department of Psychiatry and Biobehavioral Sciences
University of California, Los Angeles
Desert Pacific MIRECC
VA Greater Los Angeles Healthcare System
Los Angeles, CA

Tedd Judd, PhD, ABPP-CN
Certified Hispanic Mental Health Specialist
Cross-Cultural Specialist
Neuropsychologial and Psychoeducational Services
Universidad del Valle de Guatemala
Bellingham, WA

Vidyulata Kamath, PhD, ABPP-CN
Assistant Professor
Division of Medical Psychology
Department of Psychiatry and Behavioral Sciences
The Johns Hopkins University School of Medicine
Baltimore, MD

John W. Kirk, PsyD, ABPP-CN
Lecturer
School of Education and Human Development
University of Colorado Denver
Denver, Colorado
Kirk Neurobehavioral Health
Louisville, CO

Michael W. Kirkwood, PhD, ABPP-CN
Director of Rehabilitation Psychology and
  Neuropsychology
Department of Rehabilitation Medicine
Children's Hospital Colorado
Professor of Physical Medicine & Rehabilitation
University of Colorado School of Medicine
Aurora, CO

Lauren Krivitzky, PhD, ABPP-CN
Department of Child and Adolescent Psychiatry and
  Behavioral Sciences
Director of Fellowship and Externship Training
The Children's Hospital of Philadelphia
Associate Professor
Department of Psychiatry
Perelman School of Medicine
University of Pennsylvania
Philadelphia, PA

Laura Lacritz, PhD, ABPP-CN
Professor of Psychiatry, and Neurology and
    Neurotherapeutics
Director
Neuropsychology Clinic
University of Texas Southwestern Medical Center
Dallas, TX

Greg J. Lamberty, PhD, ABPP-CN
Psychology Supervisor and Program Manager
Neuropsychological and Psychological Assessment
Clinic (NPAC)
Clinical Neuropsychology Training Director
Minneapolis Veteran's Administration Health
    Care System
University of Minnesota Medical School
Minneapolis, MN

Glenn J. Larrabee, PhD, ABPP-CN
Neuropsychologist
Independent Practice
Sarasota, FL

Jennifer C. G. Larson, PhD, ABPP-CN
Assistant Clinical Professor
Department of Physical Medicine and Rehabilitation
University of Michigan
Ann Arbor, MI

Christine D. Liff, PhD
Independent Practice
Director
Neuropsychology Practicum Program
Michigan Neurology Associates, P.C.
St. Clair Shores, MI

William S. MacAllister, PhD, ABPP-CN
Neuropsychologist
Neurosciences Program
Alberta Children's Hospital
Alberta Children's Hospital Research Institute (ACHRI)
Calgary, Alberta, CA

E. Mark Mahone, PhD, ABPP-CN
Vice President
Neuropsychology & Related Services
Director
Intellectual and Developmental Disabilities
Research Center
Kennedy Krieger Institute
Professor of Psychiatry and Behavioral Sciences
Johns Hopkins University School of Medicine
Baltimore, MD

Robert L. Mapou, PhD, ABPP-CN
Independent Practice
Oceanside Neuropsychology
Lewes, DE
Center for Assessment and Treatment
Chevy Case, MD

Eileen M. Martin, PhD, ABPP-CN
Professor of Psychiatry
College of Medicine
Rush University Medical Center
Chicago, IL

Yuka K. Matsuzawa, PsyD, ABPP-CN
Senior Psychologist and Clinical Instructor
Department of Psychology
Rusk Institute of Rehabilitation Medicine
New York, NY

Michelle Mattingly, PhD, ABPP-CN
Departments of Psychiatry and Behavioral
    Neurosciences, and Neurology
Morsani College of Medicine
University of South Florida
Tampa, FL

Emily C. Maxwell, PhD
Pediatric Neuropsychology Bugher Fellow
Division of Neurology
Instructor
Department of Pediatrics
University of Colorado School of Medicine
Aurora, CO

Mary-Ellen Meadows, PhD, ABPP-CN
Clinical Director of the Division of
    Neuropsychology
Department of Neurology
Brigham and Women's Hospital
Clinical Neuropsychologist
Dana Farber Cancer Institute
Assistant Professor of Psychology (Psychiatry)
Harvard Medical School
Boston, MA

Scott R. Millis, PhD, ABPP (CN, CL, RP) CStat, PStat
Professor
Department of Physical Medicine &
    Rehabilitation
Wayne State University School of Medicine
Detroit, MI

Paul J. Moberg, PhD, ABPP-CN
Professor of Neuropsychology
Departments of Psychiatry, Neurology and
    Otorhinolaryngology: Head & Neck Surgery
Perelman School of Medicine
University of Pennsylvania
Philadelphia, PA

Donna Morere, PhD
Professor
Department of Psychology
Gallaudet University
Washington, DC

Joel E. Morgan, PhD, ABPP-CN
Independent Practice
Morristown, NJ

Nathaniel W. Nelson, PhD, ABPP-CN
Associate Professor
Graduate School of Professional Psychology
University of St. Thomas
Minneapolis, MN

Summar Reslan, PhD
Associate Director of Training
Department of Rehabilitation Psychology and
    Neuropsychology
Detroit Medical Center
Rehabilitation Institute of Michigan
Clinical Assistant Professor
Department of Physical Medicine and Rehabilitation
Wayne State University School of Medicine
Detroit, MI

Celiane Rey-Casserly, PhD, ABPP-CN
Director
Center for Neuropsychology
Boston Children's Hospital
Assistant Professor of Psychology (Psychiatry)
Harvard Medical School
Boston, MA

Joseph H. Ricker, PhD, ABPP (CN, RP)
Professor of Rehabilitation Medicine
Psychiatry and Radiology
New York University School of Medicine
Director
Department of Psychology
Rusk Institute of Rehabilitation Medicine
New York, NY

Eric Rinehardt, PhD, ABPP-CN
Assistant Professor
Department of Psychiatry and Behavioral
    Neurosciences, and Neurology
Morsani College of Medicine
University of South Florida
Tampa, FL

Lynn A. Schaefer, PhD, ABPP-CN
Director of Neuropsychology
Department of Physical Medicine and Rehabilitation
Nassau University Medical Center
East Meadow, NY
Clinical Associate Professor
Physical Medicine and Rehabilitation
Stony Brook Medicine
Stony Brook, NY
Clinical Associate Professor in Psychiatry
NYIT College of Osteopathic Medicine
Old Westbury, NY

Mike R. Schoenberg, PhD, ABPP-CN
Chief
Neuropsychology Division
Professor
Department of Neurosurgery and Brain Repair
Morsani College of Medicine
University of South Florida
Tampa, FL

James G. Scott, PhD, ABPP-CN
Professor and Vice Chair
Department of Psychiatry and Behavioral Sciences
University of Oklahoma Health Sciences Center
College of Medicine
Oklahoma City, OK

Tara V. Spevack, PhD, ABPP-CN
Independent Practice
St. Louis, MO

Kirk J. Stucky, PsyD, ABPP (CN, RP)
Chair
Department of Behavioral Health
Assistant Professor
Michigan State University
Program Director
Postdoctoral Fellowship Program
Rehabilitation Psychology
Hurley Medical Center
Flint, MI

Jerry J. Sweet, PhD, ABPP-CN
Director
Neuropsychology Service
Head
Psychology Division
Vice Chair
Psychiatry & Behavioral Sciences
NorthShore University HealthSystem
Evanston, IL
Senior Clinician Educator
Psychiatry & Behavioral Neuroscience
University of Chicago, Pritzker School of Medicine
Chicago, IL

Andrew A. Swihart, PhD, ABPP-CN
Professor of Psychology
Saginaw Valley State University
University Center, MI

Eva Troyb, PhD
Pediatric Neuropsychologist
EASTCONN Regional Education Service Center
Psychological and Behavioral Consultation Services
Columbia, CT

Wendy A. VanVoorst, PhD, ABPP-CN
Staff Neuropsychologist
Neuropsychological and Psychological Assessment
    Clinic (NPAC)
Minneapolis VA Health Care System
Minneapolis, MN

Brigid Waldron-Perrine, PhD, ABPP-CN
Clinical Associate Director
Department of Outpatient Neurological Rehabilitation
    (Med Rehab)
Department of Physical Medicine and Rehabilitation
Michigan Medicine
Ann Arbor, MI
Clinical Assistant Professor
Department of Physical Medicine and Rehabilitation
Wayne State University School of Medicine
Detroit, MI

Michael Westerveld, PhD, ABPP-CN
Director
AdventHealth Neuropsychology-Orlando
Orlando, FL

Dixie J. Woolston, PhD
Senior Associate Consultant
Psychiatry and Psychology
Mayo Clinic
Scottsdale, AZ

Keith Owen Yeates, PhD, ABPP-CN
Ronald and Irene Ward Chair in Pediatric Brain Injury
Professor and Head
Department of Psychology
Adjunct Professor
Departments of Pediatrics and Clinical Neurosciences
Lead
Integrated Concussion Research Program
University of Calgary
Calgary, Alberta, CA

CONTRIBUTORS

Clinical Neuropsychology
Study Guide and Board Review

1   Introduction

Kirk J. Stucky, Michael W. Kirkwood, and Jacobus Donders

The first edition of the *Clinical Neuropsychology Study Guide & Board Review* was well received by the international neuropsychology community. This was in large part due to high-caliber contributions from numerous authors who were willing to commit their time and expertise to the project. As a consequence of this success, in this second edition, we have included four 125-question mock exams and three new chapters as well as expanded coverage of specific areas that we were unable to include in the first volume.

Like the first edition, this book's primary purpose is to promote the pursuit of board certification by providing a comprehensive study guide with sample questions that are specifically designed to help individuals prepare for the ABCN written examination. The first author of each chapter is an ABCN-certified neuropsychologist (i.e., an expert who passed the exam during their own journey toward ABCN certification). Essentially, the book contains a summary of the information that graduates of a two-year postdoctoral fellowship in clinical neuropsychology are expected to be familiar with. We also asked authors to include information that was especially relevant to the performance of entry-level board-certified neuropsychologists in an everyday practice setting and information that, if not known by an examinee, could likely result in harm to the public or profession.

This volume differs from existing textbooks in that it has been designed from the outset to cover material in a manner that is likely to be welcomed by those studying for the exam. The format is much less dense than a textbook, with generous use of bullets, numbering, tables, and other means that allow for summarizing information and highlighting important points. For ease of study, the chapters are written in an outline-type format that remains consistent across all chapters and includes additional material specifically designed to assist those preparing for the written exam. In each chapter, the terms in italics refer readers to a "relevant definitions" section, which provides further explanation. The multiple-choice questions in each chapter and the mock exams (which cover the entire range of chapters) are paired with answers and explanations that often emphasize critical teaching points. Because the editorial team wanted to provide a guide that was easy to both read and study, we dealt with citations in a manner different from traditional textbooks and more similar to licensing exam materials and board review study guides in medicine. We felt that outlines and study materials that were broken up with numerous citations would not be user-friendly for the purpose of studying for the written exam. Thus, at the end of each chapter, a short, manageable list of recommended readings is provided to encourage further study and assist with exam preparation. Some of the recommended readings include work authored by some of the chapter authors. This was unavoidable due to the fact that they were specifically recruited because of their prominence in particular subject areas.

Readers familiar with the first edition will notice that for some chapters much of the original content remains similar, although authors did address the following when updating their chapter:

1. Review additional research, updates, and practice changes since 2013.
2. Update so that the majority of chapter references fall within the last ten years (2008–2018) while retaining references to seminal articles, chapters, or books when appropriate.

3. Continued use of charts, figures, diagrams, and illustrations to facilitate study and memorization.

4. A minimum of ten new questions for each chapter with an increased emphasis on applied content (in line with the current ABCN written exam).

5. When appropriate, additional coverage of lifespan/developmental issues. This includes discussion of how pediatric versus adult onset differs in terms of etiology, correlates, clinical manifestations, and later-in-life outcomes.

6. When appropriate, additional coverage of cultural and diversity considerations.

7. When appropriate, expanded discussion of evidence-based practice.

In addition to exam preparation, this book can also be used as a teaching tool for graduate students and trainees at various levels. Of course, this volume in no way replaces the formal education and training necessary to become competent in clinical neuropsychology, consistent with the Houston Conference guidelines. This book is only one of many possible board preparation resources, and reviewing the information contained herein in no way guarantees success on the exam. Furthermore, the fact that some chapter authors serve or have served in ABCN or AACN leadership roles should not be construed as providing special advantage in preparing for the ABCN written exam. Other texts and information sources relevant to neuropsychology, many of them cited in this book, should be included in the study process. The sample test items in this book were not derived from and will never be included in the actual ABCN written examination item pool. Thus, completing the sample items should also not be viewed as sufficient or necessary to successfully complete the ABCN written examination.

This volume is intended to be a complementary resource to the text *Board Certification in Clinical Neuropsychology: A Guide to Becoming ABPP/ABCN Certified Without Sacrificing Your Sanity (Second Edition)*, by Armstrong, Beebe, Hilsabeck, and Kirkwood (2019), which provides practical tips and excellent advice on how to prepare for and successfully complete the entire board certification process. Unlike the Armstrong et al. book, this study guide focuses exclusively on content material relevant to the written exam. The current volume is also meant to complement the many valuable resources available through BRAIN (Be Ready for ABPP in Neuropsychology), which we continue to strongly recommend. BRAIN is a peer-support network of neuropsychologists that has compiled a multitude of resources to support completion of the board certification process including topic outlines, flash cards, mock exams, and sample study schedules. All of these resources are available through BRAIN's freely accessible website (https://brainaacn.org/). The primary differences between the current volume and the BRAIN materials are that the current volume focuses on content material more exclusively, and the content coverage is provided by leading experts in the field, whereas the BRAIN materials are more expansive and were created primarily by neuropsychologists preparing for the exam.

Like other board review books, this volume is not a comprehensive review that addresses every aspect of clinical neuropsychology necessary for daily practice. Controversial areas or cutting-edge research and future directions for the field are not discussed as those topics are not likely to be on the exam. The book is divided into three sections, which are briefly described later: Section I: Foundations of Clinical Neuropsychology; Section II: Fundamentals of Assessment; and Section III: Disorders and Conditions. Each section was prepared with the assumption that readers are familiar with information and concepts presented in standard neuropsychology textbooks. We also assumed that readers are planning to supplement their study with review of additional materials, including readings that are recommended throughout this volume. Thus, this text should be primarily used as a guide to inform and organize a candidate's preparation for the exam.

Section I: Foundations of Clinical Neuropsychology

Section I focuses on bedrock topics that are essential to competent everyday practice for all clinical neuropsychologists regardless of specialty. Chapter 3 reviews important theories in neuropsychology, cognitive science, and neuroscience, and their relevance to practice today. Functional neuroanatomy is reviewed in Chapter 4, which highlights central neuroanatomical, neurophysiological, and neurochemistry principles and information. Chapter 5 summarizes the domains of cognitive function and associated classic neurobehavioral syndromes (e.g., aphasia, amnesia, apraxia, agnosia). Chapter 6 covers commonly used tests and procedures in neurology. Outlines and critical teaching points regarding the neurologic examination, electroencephalogram (EEG), computed tomography (CT), magnetic resonance imaging (MRI), and functional radiology are provided. This section closes with Chapter 7, a new chapter that focuses on ethical issues commonly encountered in the practice of clinical neuropsychology.

Section II: Fundamentals of Assessment

This section emphasizes various aspects of assessment at both conceptual and applied levels. Chapter 8 reviews psychometrics, test design, and essential statistics. Fundamental concepts are reviewed, such as test construction, reliability, validity, sensitivity, and specificity. This chapter also highlights the psychometric properties of commonly used tests in clinical neuropsychology and the relevance of understanding the difference between tests with normal versus non-normal distributions. Chapter 9 discusses test administration and interpretation in more depth, including topics such as decision theory, the impact of demographic and cultural factors on test performance, the importance of prevalence rates in test score interpretation, estimation of premorbid functioning, and measuring change over time. Personality and mood assessment in neuropsychology are covered in Chapter 10, highlighting important concepts such as the use of score modifiers in neurologic populations. Chapter 11 is a new addition and covers multicultural issues in neuropsychological assessment, while Chapter 12, also new, reviews symptom and performance validity testing.

Section III: Disorders and Conditions

The final section contains the most chapters because it covers the majority of cerebral diseases and conditions commonly seen by neuropsychologists. Section III is divided into subsections that cover common developmental, medical, and psychiatric conditions that affect central nervous system functioning. Each chapter contains an outline including the neuropathology, epidemiology, presentation, clinical course, common neuropsychological assessment findings, and treatment considerations. An emphasis is placed on how these disorders can affect neuropsychological and psychological functioning across the lifespan. The section on psychiatric conditions also includes discussion regarding how psychiatric and neurological disorders can mimic each other and/or coexist.

One Final Note

The field of neuroscience continues to evolve, and, over time, some of the information in this study guide will become dated and some websites listed may change. The editors and authors of this guide have made efforts to provide information that is as accurate and timely as possible. However, like other board review books, this volume is not a comprehensive summary that addresses every single aspect of clinical neuropsychology necessary for daily practice. Additionally, considering the depth and breadth of coverage attempted in this volume, we anticipate that users will identify alternative ways to present, relay, or summarize information. Although we have been committed to accuracy, there may be minor typographical errors or mistakes that were missed in the editing process. We certainly welcome constructive criticism and feedback intended to improve future versions. We also hope that you consider proposing alternative multiple-choice questions, which we request be accompanied by a recent peer-reviewed reference. If you have suggestions for future questions or how this volume could be improved, please feel free to contact a member of the editorial team.

Best wishes in your preparation for the written exam!

Kirk J. Stucky, PsyD, ABPP-CN, RP
Chair, Department of Behavioral Health
Assistant Professor, Michigan State University
Program Director, Postdoctoral Fellowship Program, Rehabilitation Psychology
Hurley Medical Center
1 Hurley Plaza
Flint, MI 48503
kstucky2@hurleymc.com

Michael W. Kirkwood, PhD, ABPP-CN
Director, Rehabilitation Psychology and Neuropsychology
Professor, University of Colorado School of Medicine
Department of Physical Medicine & Rehabilitation
Children's Hospital Colorado
13123 E. 16th Avenue
Aurora, CO 80045
Michael.Kirkwood@childrenscolorado.org

Jacobus Donders, PhD, ABPP-CN, RP
Chief Psychologist
Mary Free Bed Rehabilitation Hospital
235 Wealthy, S.E.
Grand Rapids, MI 49503
Jacobus.Donders@maryfreebed.com

Christine D. Liff, PhD
Director, Neuropsychology Practicum Program
Michigan Neurology Associates
19699 East 8 Mile Road
St. Clair Shores, MI 48080
Christinpy@aol.com

References

Armstrong, K., Beebe, D. W., Hilsabeck, R. C., & Kirkwood, M. W. (2019). *Board certification in clinical neuropsychology: A guide to becoming ABPP/ABCN certified without sacrificing your sanity* (2nd ed.). New York, NY: Oxford University Press.
Be Ready for ABPP In Neuropsychology (BRAIN) website at https://brainaacn.org/

2 How to Prepare for the Written Exam

Kirk J. Stucky

The written portion of the American Board of Clinical Neuropsychology (ABCN) examination is administered electronically at a freestanding testing center in North America four times a year, each during a two-week window. Once the Credential Review process has been passed, a candidate can register for the examination through the ABCN website. Qualified neuropsychologists with disabilities can request reasonable accommodations for the examination by contacting the Board in writing no later than the deadline for submitting required application materials.

The exam consists of 125 multiple-choice questions that have a single best answer. The exam contains 25 "pre-test" items that are included for data collection/test development purposes and do not count toward the final score. However, examinees are masked to which questions are "pre-test" and which count toward the final score. This is a criterion-based examination in which the passing standard is established on the basis of formal psychometric criteria. Examinees have up to two and a half hours to complete the test. Every few years the exam is revised to ensure that it remains current with advancements in the field. Over the years, the exam has shifted from item formats requiring rote memorization to formats requiring more applied clinical knowledge. This study guide should help you to become familiar with the typical question design and format. Questions on the exam cover the foundational and functional/practice core knowledge bases for neuropsychologists identified by Section VI of the Houston Conference guidelines: General Psychology (including statistics and methodology), Clinical Psychology, Psychopathology, Neuroanatomy/Neuropathology, Brain–Behavior Relationships, and the professional practice of Clinical Neuropsychology. Questions may also cover factual, historical, practice, and/or professional issues, including ethics. All of these domains are covered in this study guide and should provide you with a good idea of what you need to review in more depth.

Preparing in Advance

Your training and experiences during graduate school, internship, and residency form the foundation upon which advanced clinical knowledge and expertise are accumulated. Thus, preparation for the written examination starts at the very beginning of training in clinical neuropsychology. For all those interested in taking the written exam, a number of preparatory suggestions are offered in this chapter.

First, set reasonable expectations about the amount of time and effort needed to complete this task. If you are still on internship or just entering residency, you do not need to start intense studying. Instead, make a point of reading articles and books recommended by your supervisors or knowledgeable colleagues. Develop your organizational skills, ability to plan, and advanced learning strategies. Set small accomplishable goals each month. Write notes in this book as you learn. The clinical training and regular study habits formed and reinforced during your training years are critical experiences that should help tremendously not only in your preparation for the examination but for your professional development more generally as well.

Second, this book is an excellent resource for brushing up on important board-relevant information before the exam, but it cannot take the place of more comprehensive books in clinical neuropsychology. Thorough study of standard textbooks (some listed in this chapter) is essential to developing a basic neuropsychological knowledge base. Many have found it helpful to select one or two good textbooks (e.g., Morgan & Ricker, 2018; Heilman & Valenstein, 2012, Schoenberg & Scott, 2011) and supplement these with specific outstanding chapters or articles from additional sources. Furthermore, most clinicians will read about medical or neurologic conditions they are seeing for the first time. Some learn best by carving out time for additional reading when they encounter a patient with a specific condition, even if they are somewhat familiar with it. In the early stages of training, some supervisors recommend reading about at least one patient's condition each work week. Of course, supervisors will also provide personalized guidance to focus study and maximize the training experience.

Current Resources

This book is intended to complement other available resources that are updated periodically on the ABCN website. In line with this goal, we have intentionally avoided rewriting too much of what has been written elsewhere and instead recommend that you utilize some or all of these materials during your preparation.

First, additional exam information and resources are available at https://theabcn.org/resources/. This website contains more detailed information regarding the mentorship program, information about the BRAIN (Be Ready for ABPP In Neuropsychology) group, and the ABCN candidate manual. A wealth of information about how to prepare for the exam is also available in the text, *Board Certification in Clinical Neuropsychology: A Guide to Becoming ABPP/ABCN Certified without Sacrificing Your Sanity (2nd ed.)*, by Armstrong, Beebe, Hilsabeck, and Kirkwood (2019). In addition, if you do not have easy access to an ABCN-boarded neuropsychologist to help you prepare for the written exam, the Mentorship program and the BRAIN group are available to assist you in finding such support.

Second, although this study guide does not provide specific, detailed chapters on basic neuroscience, a stand-alone chapter in functional neuroanatomy and essential neurochemistry is provided (Chapter 4). Furthermore, functional neuroanatomy concepts critical to competence in neuropsychology are woven into relevant chapters. Chapter 4 also provides a list of suggested books, neuroanatomy programs, and online resources to assist with exam preparation. It is important to bear in mind that the written exam is designed to assess the candidate's integrative knowledge and their ability to apply it clinically. Thus, detailed understanding or rote memorization of minute neuroanatomic structures is not nearly as important as an integrative understanding of brain–behavior relations in the day-to-day practice of clinical neuropsychology.

Third, throughout this study guide, each chapter recommends a short list of books, book chapters, and articles to assist in studying for the exam. We strongly encourage you to review some of these additional materials to augment your unique background and knowledge base as needed. It is important to identify the areas you are less familiar with and dedicate additional time to studying them. For example, if you are especially experienced or specialized in the evaluation of seniors, your background knowledge and the review materials in this book may be sufficient for exam preparation. In contrast, you may want to dedicate extra time to reading the recommended supplemental materials for pediatric topics with which you are less familiar.

Fourth, update and expand your personal library. You no doubt have a large number of texts already sagging your bookshelves or hundreds of PDFs clogging your hard drive. We have listed ten books that we personally believe should be on the shelf of any neuropsychologist, regardless of specialty. Mind you, we have intentionally limited ourselves to ten books, recognizing that it is neither practical nor possible to read a mountain of books cover to cover in preparation for this exam. We also recognize that we have left off many excellent texts and resources that could aid you in pursuit of board certification. However, many candidates have found these texts especially valuable in their preparation, and they have been repeatedly referenced by the various authors in this guide, which speaks to their overall utility and practical value. Also note that the BRAIN website includes some other useful texts.

Clinical Neuropsychology

Blumenfeld, H. (2010). *Neuroanatomy through clinical cases* (2nd ed.). Sunderland, MA: Sinauer Associates.

Donders, J., & Hunter, S. (Eds.). (2018). *Neuropsychological conditions across the lifespan.* Cambridge, UK: Cambridge University Press.

Heilman K. M., & Valenstein, E. (Eds.). (2012). *Clinical neuropsychology* (5th ed.). New York, NY: Oxford University Press.

Kolb, B., & Whishaw, I. Q. (2015). *Fundamentals of human neuropsychology* (7th ed.). New York, NY: Worth Publishers.

Morgan, J. E., & Ricker, J. H. (Eds.). (2018). *Textbook of clinical neuropsychology* (2nd ed.). New York, NY: Taylor and Francis.

Schoenberg, M. R., & Scott, J. G. (Eds). (2011). *The little black book of neuropsychology: A syndrome-based approach.* New York, NY: Springer.

Strauss, E., Sherman, E., & Spreen, O. (in press). *A compendium of neuropsychological tests: Administration, norms, and commentary* (4th ed.). New York, NY: Oxford University Press.

Geriatric Neuropsychology

McPherson, S., & Koltai, D. (2018). *A practical guide to geriatric neuropsychology.* New York, NY: Oxford University Press.

Pediatric Neuropsychology

Baron, I. S. (2018). *Neuropsychological evaluation of the child* (2nd ed.). New York, NY: Oxford University Press.

Beauchamp, M. H., Ris, M. D., Taylor, H. G., Peterson, R. L., & Yeates, K. O. (Eds.) (in press). *Pediatric neuropsychology: Research, theory, and practice* (3rd ed.). New York, NY: Guilford Press.

How to Use This Book

This book provides a balance between topic areas in pediatric, adult, and geriatric neuropsychology. Each chapter provides an up-to-date practical outline and questions that should help you brush up on familiar information while identifying areas of relative strength or weakness while preparing for the exam. For topics you feel confident about and do not anticipate a need for detailed study, consider first taking the multiple-choice questions at the end of those chapters. This can serve as an informal self-assessment tool to help you prioritize what areas you may wish to study more aggressively. For topics in which you find the material challenging or sample questions difficult, supplement study of the chapter with the recommended readings.

- *Sections 1 and 2 (Chapters 3 through 12)* These sections are complementary, and it may be helpful to study them as a unit due to the fact that some of the subject matter overlaps. Foundational knowledge and competencies in clinical neuropsychology are covered in these chapters. Additionally, responsible ethical practice and sensitivity to cultural issues is expected of all clinicians and is also covered on the written exam. In this Study Guide these important topic areas are specifically addressed in two new chapters (Chapter 7, Ethics in Clinical Neuropsychology, and Chapter 11, Cultural and Disability Issues in Neuropsychological Assessment). Of note, advanced knowledge regarding ethics will also be assessed in the oral examination. Thus, once you pass the written exam, study for the oral examination should include additional and careful preparation in ethics and other applied practice topics.

- *Section 3 (Chapters 13 through 37)* The disorders and conditions chapters are designed to be studied alone. Order of review/study is not important. You may want to focus on less familiar topics first, so that you have time to return to studying them several times before the exam.

- *Appendices A through H (Full-Length Examinations)* The four 125-question mock exams at the end of this book contain extra questions created by chapter authors and are designed to provide readers with a simulated test experience. Considering this, it may be advisable to take the practice tests after you have spent sufficient time studying and believe you are close to taking the formal exam. The questions were designed to mimic the same style and level of difficulty of real exam questions. However, none of the questions in this book were sanctioned by ABCN or drawn from the actual exam item pool, so your performance on these questions may be better or worse than your performance on the ABCN exam. In addition to increasing your familiarity with the exam format, the questions at the end of each chapter and in the mock exams should also allow you to identify areas in which you may need more review.

The Science of Study

Throughout the course of your academic and professional career, you have undoubtedly come to appreciate how you learn best. Unlike many doctoral-level clinicians, you also have a very unique and specialized understanding of brain-behavior relationships. Nonetheless, we have summarized some scientifically backed principles about effective learning that may be of assistance in using the current volume and more broadly preparing for the written exam.

Massed Versus Distributed Practice If you are like most college graduates, you have probably crammed for more than one exam in your academic career. This strategy is unlikely to be successful for the written exam. Distributed practice and spaced review will easily outperform massed practice. Thus, creating a reasonable study schedule and distributing your efforts across at least several months should maximize your retention of information. Sample study schedules are also provided on the BRAIN website. Additionally, although cramming might work in the short run, it does not have much value in regard to long-term retention, conceptualization, and/or critical thinking. Exam questions often require you to integrate your knowledge of multiple concepts or facts to determine the correct answer. Questions will not ask you to simply regurgitate a random fact, but you will likely need to use your knowledge of terms and facts to answer more complex questions.

Active Versus Passive Learning When people use active rather than passive learning strategies, comprehension and retention improve. Active approaches include creating outlines, flashcards, and detailed notes while you read. Additionally, the process of writing and thinking about what is being read typically results in the creation of personally tailored study materials that can be used later. Consequently, we strongly encourage you to take detailed notes and use the book margins in this volume to write comments or personalize mnemonics. If something does not look right or seems wrong, look it up, take the time to research your questions. The process of investigation will seal the memory more effectively than just accepting the information as presented.

Error-Free or Errorless Learning This concept is often applied to teaching individuals with severe memory impairment, but it has applications for advanced learners as well. If you are taking sample tests in this book or others, and find that you are guessing a great deal or often getting questions wrong, it is most likely a red flag that you need to read or reread the material in more depth. Similarly, if you cannot clearly discuss, teach to another, or answer basic questions about a topic, more in-depth studying is also likely indicated.

Chunking Break material into smaller chunks and use the principle of vanishing cues. For example, when learning the basal ganglia structures, start with learning to name all of them from memory, then proceed to identifying their location and function, then add recall of which disorders commonly involve damage to that structure, and finally focus on how such damage leads to specific syndromes (e.g., Parkinson's vs. Huntington's). This process of stepwise memorization will, for most people, outperform efforts to memorize detailed information about a concept or brain structure before you have retained bedrock or basic information.

Salience We tend to more easily remember information that is salient (i.e., personally relevant). Many clinicians report that they are able to retain specific neuroanatomical concepts and facts because they had a particular patient with related issues. Also, most salient information is delivered through multiple sensory modalities simultaneously, which further increases the odds of retention. Not surprisingly, your current patients and clinical cases are excellent sources for this type of learning. Consider taking the time to look up more specific details on your patient's conditions, current workup, and treatment. Review the neuroanatomic, neurophysiologic, and neuropsychological issues relevant to the case with supervisors, mentors, and colleagues. All of these efforts should not only lead to better patient care but also increase the odds that you will retain the information over time.

Test-Taking Strategies

Some candidates have failed the exam despite having the requisite knowledge and clinical skill necessary to pass. This is sometimes related to a limited ability to understand and interpret questions properly. In fact, many test takers have accidentally answered a question too quickly, failing to recognize words that modified the question. Some refer to the skill of understanding the subtleties in questions as "boardsmanship." You probably already have a fair amount of experience with multiple choice exams, but some tips are worth restating. The Armstrong et al. book (2019) provides some helpful test-taking strategies as well.

1. It is generally wise to start with the first question and proceed sequentially, answering the easier questions first and tagging those questions that will require more time or careful thought. This strategy will allow you to get a sense of the entire exam quickly before spending too much time on any one individual question. Also, by answering easy questions first, some candidates are able to build up momentum and confidence. Furthermore, the process of taking the exam often decreases anxiety, and sometimes subsequent questions provide information that assists retrieval of concepts relevant to a previous question.

2. Keep track of your time. You have two and a half hours to answer 125 questions so there is adequate time to read each one carefully. There is no need to rush or force yourself to respond quickly. Track your time and make sure that you are halfway or more than halfway through the test after one hour has passed.

3. All questions in which you know the answer quickly should be answered first, but make sure you read the question right the first time. Always spend adequate time on apparently easy questions to make certain that you are answering correctly; careless mistakes on easy questions happen more often than you think. Read the final sentence in the question several times to make sure you understand how to answer. Read each option thoroughly and to the end, because sometimes a response is only partially correct.

4. Be cautious of answers with overly restrictive words (e.g., always, never, must, almost). Answers that contain absolute statements are often incorrect. Watch closely for qualifiers such as "next," "initially," or "immediately."

5. Try to think of the correct answer before reading the options. If your answer is not among the choices, you may have misinterpreted the question or read too quickly.

6. Rule out answers that you know are wrong to increase your odds of selecting the correct answer. Be cautious about overthinking a question. The exam will ask you to critically think about common neuropsychological issues and general knowledge as opposed to esoteric topics or rare conditions.

7. For particularly difficult questions:

    (a) Cover the options, read the stem, and try to answer. Select the option that most closely matches your answer.

    (b) Read the stem with each option. Treat each option as a true-false question and choose the "most true."

    (c) In lengthy questions, look for the salient points. In confusing or (in your opinion) poorly worded questions, note them and come back to them later at the end of the test.

    (d) For options that look alike, carefully choose what you view as the best response. Remember that you are looking for the best answer, not one that must be true all of the time, in all cases, and without exception.

    (e) Options that contain qualifiers are often more inclusive and thus more likely to be correct.

    (f) If you are really stuck and unsure, always guess. There is no penalty for guessing incorrectly.

After the Exam

After the exam, please remember that you are bound by oath not to discuss specific examination content.

If you pass, do not wait too long before thinking about and preparing your practice samples. If you do not have ready access to another board certified neuropsychologist, consider taking advantage of the AACN mentoring program. Additionally, the Armstrong et al. guide (2019) provides detailed information on preparing practice samples and can be an invaluable resource in completing the next step. *The Neuropsychology Fact-Finding Casebook: A Training Resource* (Stucky & Bush, 2017) also contains information that may help in preparation for the fact-finding portion of the oral exam.

There are a variety of reasons why a competent neuropsychologist might not pass the written exam, including insufficient preparation, stress, and anxiety. If you do not pass on your first or second attempt, we are hopeful that you will still recognize personal and professional gains from your preparation. You most certainly know more now than you did at the beginning of the process, which should be of considerable benefit to your patients. Furthermore, the exam experience will no doubt give you some idea as to what you need to focus on for the next test. If you did not take advantage of the various resources listed in this chapter, reassess your strategy. Many successful candidates have had positive experiences through a BRAIN study group and/or mentor. In addition to this book, these various resources can help you to narrow down and identify what you need to work on to be more successful next time. It is also important to remember that you can take the written examination up to three times but the entire certification process must be completed within seven years of the date on your credential review decision letter. Thus, if you do not pass do not wait too long before planning out a strategy and timeline for retaking the exam.

References

Armstrong, K., Beebe, D., Hilsabeck, R., & Kirkwood, M. (2019). *Board certification in clinical neuropsychology: A guide to becoming ABPP/ABCN certified without sacrificing your sanity* (2nd ed.). New York, NY: Oxford University Press.

Stucky, K. J., & Bush, S. (2017). *The neuropsychology fact-finding casebook: A training resource.* New York, NY: Oxford University Press.

Websites

https://theabcn.org/becoming-certified/
https://theabcn.org/exam-schedule

Section I Foundations of Clinical Neuropsychology

3 Important Theories in Neuropsychology: A Historical Perspective

Manfred F. Greiffenstein and Joel E. Morgan

Introduction

The history of science provides remarkable insight into the factual discoveries of the world and of our human experience. This chapter presents some of the historical underpinnings of the discipline of neuropsychology, the emergence of ideas and discovery of facts, with prominent figures drawn from neurology, medicine, and philosophy, among other disciplines. The names of these important figures, as well as the eras in which they lived and worked, will not be on ABCN exams. Rather, this chapter sets the stage for the development of the profession and its evolution from academia to the clinic.

As this book is largely intended for a specialized audience of doctoral-level neuropsychologists pursuing board certification, it stands to reason that readers have knowledge of *brain–behavior relationships*. Recall that there was a time in the past, however, when brain and its relationship to human behavior were largely unknown. Prior to the 1860s, a doctor might wonder why his patient with stroke could no longer speak or why a railroadman's behavior changed so radically after he survived a serious penetrating head injury.

A scientific theory attempts to explain phenomena that are not understood. A theory is important for attempting to understand data (behavior), orienting the clinician to what is essential about a case, selecting assessment methods, and making predictions from scores. There is no such thing as an atheoretical approach. Your preference for one test over another means you have a theory—in this case, a theory about assessment of function. All theories begin with premises or intuitions about the cause of phenomena. These are assumptions that you accept as true to advance the reasoning process. When assumptions are later disproved, the theory has to be modified or discarded. Like all science, the entire field of clinical neuropsychology concerns evaluating hypotheses about a patient's functioning.

As the reader will see, theories in neuropsychology have their historical roots in other, related disciplines—especially anatomy (neuroanatomy), neurology, and philosophy. Neuropsychology's "theories" deal with an effort to understand "*brain-behavior relationships*," a phrase commonly used to define the discipline itself. Of course, some theories evolve into undisputable facts, while others are simply wrong.

Domain-Specific ("Localization") Theory Versus Domain-General ("Generalist") Theory

There are two dominant paradigms concerning cerebral functional organization that underlie neuropsychology and behavioral neurology. From a historical perspective, these paradigms should be viewed dynamically as relatively competing views, rising and falling in influence historically. Yet more contemporary views would suggest more of a peaceful semi-coexistence. As an example of semi-coexistence of these views, take the concept of intelligence (*g*), which posits a general, overarching, cognitive function, largely thought to be a *whole-brain* phenomenon. Yet, neuropsychologists clearly recognize that intelligence tests are made up of various cognitive tasks, assessing essentially discrete, or loosely related, functions—many of which have identified brain regions associated with them—the *modular/localization view*.

Cerebral Localization Theory

Also termed "domain-specificity," cerebral localization theory is the dominant paradigm that permeates modern clinical neuropsychology. This may seem obvious now, but the idea that brain zones subserved specific cognitive tasks was dismissed for decades at a time and did not become dominant until the early 1960s. Aphasia is the paradigmatic clinical example of brain modularity because of its frequency, symptom salience, and clear neuroanatomical underpinnings. Domain-specificity theory states that:

- The brain has a modular organization.
- Each module is a specialized processor devoted to one task, or function (e.g., expressive speech, facial recognition).
- Each specialized processor is reliably associated with specific zones in the brain (the [usually] left inferior frontal gyrus in the case of expressive speech, and the inferior temporal lobes and fusiform gyri in the case of facial recognition).

Domain-General Theory

Domain-general theory is a countervailing view. Popular synonyms for this school of thought include holistic, generalist, and "field" approaches. The term "organismic" was popularized by Kurt Goldstein in the 1930s. The catch-all "organic brain syndrome" is the paradigmatic clinical case. A variant of the generalist view, proposed by both John Hughlings Jackson and Lev Vygotsky, is that mental activity is hierarchical, with higher and lower levels. Although the levels were never detailed, the core premise of the generalist theory is that mental function is not reducible to specific anatomic locations in the brain—that the brain works in a wholistic sense. With this statement, the contrast with localization theory becomes obvious. Domain-general theory states that:

- The brain has only one or a few fundamental properties, such as general learning and reasoning capacity, a position also favored by behaviorists and anthropologists.
- Any mental act or function requires the entire brain working in concert.
- Long-term memory is distributed around the brain.
- Symptoms are in part the expression of the undamaged part of the brain.
- Only motor and sensory functions are localized, not higher cognitive functions. Brain tissue has *equipotentiality*: any brain area can do what any other brain area can do for perception; only sensory and motor function are specialized.
- The observed variety of organic syndromes is explained by either lesion size, lesion "intensity," or the combination of the fundamental cognitive deficit (whatever it is) with a specific motor-sensory impairment.

Key Figures in the Prominence of Localization

- Franz Gall (from about 1796) proposed that personality traits were localized and predictable by studying variations ("prominences") in skull contour by palpating the skull. This practice of "phrenology" (the term was coined by Spurzheim) was the major tenet of Faculty Psychology, now the subject of derision. Nevertheless, the movement represented two important conceptual breakthroughs: (a) the materialist view of the brain as subject to scientific scrutiny and (b) mental modularity/localization (of personality traits or "faculties," rather than cognitive functions, in this view).

- French neurologist Paul Pierre Broca (mid 1800s), a founder of the idea of cerebral dominance, observed that (a) acquired language loss was reliably associated with left-brain strokes in most patients and (b) loss of expressive speech and syntactic sentence structure was associated with left frontal strokes. This led to Broca's now famous dictum, "nous parlons avec l'hémisphère gauche"—i.e., "we speak with the left hemisphere." Somewhat later, Broca discovered that some left-handed people apparently had language in the right hemisphere. This eventually led to the realization of the crossed relationship between hand dominance and cerebral language representation.

- German neurologist Carl Wernicke (mid to late 1800s) further correlated types of aphasia with cerebral anatomy, observing that (a) auditory comprehension (receptive language) but not fluency (expressive language) was impaired by left hemisphere posterior lesions and (b) disconnection explained why some left subcortical, i.e., white matter, lesions affected language repetition but not comprehension (i.e., conduction aphasia due to damage to the arcuate fasciculus).

- Joseph Dejerine (late 1800s) described two forms of reading loss or "alexia" associated with either (a) direct destruction of left angular and supramarginal gyrus of the left brain or (b) disconnection of visual input to an intact memory center.

- Anticipating evolutionary psychology, William James (late 1800s) proposed that the brain evolved to contain dozens and perhaps hundreds of "instincts."

- Hugo Liepmann (late 19th–early 20th century) showed that left parietal lesions affected skilled movement in both hands, even when language was intact (ideomotor praxis).

- Alexander Luria (1930s–1970s) systematized the modular geography of the entire brain based on inferences from clinical cases consisting mostly of Russian soldiers with brain injuries. Unlike his contemporary Vygotsky, Luria suggested prototypical bedside tasks for each module, tasks still used today.

Key Figures in the Generalist Vein

Localization theory fell into disfavor in the 1920s. Domain-general theory became influential, even well into modern scientific times, because the theory fit well with political progressivism and its scientific partners, behaviorism and cultural anthropology. Resistance to treating the human mind as subject to biological laws was long rooted in politics, religion, and philosophy (e.g., Cartesian dualism). Further inhibition was imposed in reaction to Nazi biological reductionism. The central idea of domain-general theory is that experience and culture facultatively shape the mind as a whole, whereas biology plays little role ("nurture over nature"). Key developments and figures included:

- German Gestalt psychologists such as Wolfgang Kohler, studying visual perception, illustrated how the brain transformed separate parts into a new whole, such that the individual parts lost their distinct identity, and were "transformed" into a new perceptual whole (i.e., "the whole is greater than the mere sum of its parts"). The essence of Gestalt theory was that the whole brain, working in concert, plays a central role in human experience.

- The influence of American behaviorists such as John B. Watson (early 1900s) and B. F. Skinner (1930–1960s) maintained that the brain had only a general capacity to learn.

- British neurologist John Hughlings Jackson (1870–1890s) argued that mental functions are hierarchical, not localized. He proposed that only two types of deficits were caused by cerebral damage: positive symptoms that represent the disinhibited expression of lower centers (like the brainstem) when removed from higher cortical control, and negative symptoms that represent the loss of function when the superordinate functions are impaired. Essentially, this was a regression theory of brain damage.

- The regression theory of Lev Vygotsky (1920–1930s) also asserted that brain damage causes regression to earlier developmental stages. Consistent with Marxist orthodoxy, he argued that (a) mental function evolves steadily through the internal representation of social experience only, and (b) inner speech is the domain-general processor that directs all goal-directed behaviors.

- The work of physiological psychologist Karl Lashley (1920–1950) revealed a group effect for lesion size, not localization in rat brain lesion studies. For example, he reported in 1948 that primate frontal lesions caused no greater deficit in conditional learning (now termed "flexibility") than did nonfrontal lesions.

- Neurologist Kurt Goldstein (1930s–1950s) argued that "loss of abstract attitude" (reasoning) was the fundamental defect in any type of brain damage. He used his famous patient Schneider (*Schn.* in print) to prove that a small occipital lesion resulted in many deficits that were thought to have localization elsewhere.

Domain-General Approach Fades

Domain-general theory could not cope with (a) the voluminous empirical data clearly linking function to discrete anatomical sites from the human brain lesion literature and (b) internal inconsistencies. Key developments dooming the generalist view included:

- In a famous 1950 essay, Karl Lashley implied domain-general theory was an intellectual dead-end because his methods forced him to the absurd conclusion that memory could not be located in the brain.

- Evidence developed that Goldstein and Gelb's famous patient *Schn.* may have malingered diffuse impairments. Later independent examinations showed that he had no visual complaints, interacted with the visual world normally in his everyday life, and acted differently when tested than when unobtrusively observed. An independent review of his skull x-ray and electroencephalogram failed to show any compelling biomarkers that he had even sustained occipital lobe injury during World War I.

- Norman Geschwind pointed out that Goldstein's insights were indistinguishable from those of the classical localizationists.

- "Regression theories" were illogical because they implied that children must act like adults with brain-damage. To the contrary, children are capable of extraordinary feats of memory and learning, with rapid language acquisition being the best example.

Modern Evidence Favoring Domain-Specificity

Brain modularity prevailed by the early 1960s and continues to be strengthened by compelling evidence from functional neuroimaging. Single-case and group studies, too many to be reviewed here, proved cerebral localization of function in adults beyond reasonable dispute. Landmark studies include:

- The famous case of HM, who suffered dense amnesia due to bilateral hippocampal damage (1953), clearly linking function (anterograde memory) to specific neuroanatomy.
- The split-brain studies of Sperry and Gazzaniga (early 1960s), who proved that qualitatively different forms of information (verbal, visual) were specifically encoded with either the right or left hemispheres (i.e., the lateralization of material-specific memory); this delivered a particularly fatal blow to the domain-general theory.
- Ralph Reitan's 1964 demonstration that single tests of "organicity" were poor at classifying persons with brain damage. Instead, patterns of performance, pathognomonic signs, and interrelationships of different test scores, as well as a composite score that represented the battery average (Impairment Index), improved prediction and understanding.
- Norman Geschwind's catalogue of disconnection syndromes, which proved that small lesions that interrupt subcortical pathways to specific brain zones still result in striking specific impairment (e.g., alexia without agraphia).
- Brenda Milner's team (1980s–1990s), who found that large excisions of prefrontal tissue cause impairment in executive functions such as shifting of strategy, without any generalized intellectual decline (essentially dissociating general intellect, *g*, from executive function).
- The finding that right-brain strokes were more likely to cause hemifield inattention than were left-brain strokes, proving a role for what was referred to as "reality monitoring" in the right hemisphere.
- The finding that inferior temporal lobe lesions in the fusiform gyrus cause prosopagnosia, the inability to recognize familiar faces, with retained ability to detect faces.
- The results of frontal lobotomies and leukotomies, popular in the 1940s to 1950s, which resulted primarily in affective and personality changes.
- Hans Lukas Teuber (1955) coined the concept "double dissociation" as an important standard of proof in neuropsychology. An example of double dissociation occurs when a lesion in brain zone A impairs verbal memory but not visual memory, but a lesion in zone B weakens or impairs visual memory but not verbal learning. Used in conjunction with neuropsychological, neuropathological, and neuroimaging results, the observation of double dissociation has allowed neuroscience to draw inferences regarding the localization of certain cognitive functions.

Current Theoretical Status

Domain-specific theory still has problems to resolve.

- The "executive problem": How are domain-specific modules integrated to inform the production system that makes decisions and initiates complex actions, which constitutes most of human activity?
- Some neuropsychologists and cognitive scientists argue that a domain-general processor is still necessary to coordinate modules and resolve conflicts when more than one module is triggered by a circumstance.
- Some even propose multiple domain-general processors, such as "verbal processing" in the left brain and "spatial processing" in the right.
- Because of Alexander Luria's influence, the prefrontal lobes are viewed as playing a major role in coordination of specialized processors in the posterior brain. However, Luria's views on the frontal lobes have not been reliably validated.

Practice Implications

The implications that follow from the two views are good examples of why theory is important.

- According to domain-general theory, damage to any location in the brain should cause at least one or several fundamental cognitive deficits. Therefore, one need only design a single neuropsychological test that best captures that fundamental deficit. The result was single "organicity" measures such as the Bender Visual-Motor Gestalt Test, the Weigl Colour-Form Sorting Test, and the Symbol Digit Modalities Test. Carrying the notion of "organicity" to its absurd conclusion, it erroneously postulates abnormality of the *whole-brain* even with a discrete, localized lesion.

- Conversely, domain-specificity predicts that lesion location is critical because discrete cognitive functions (e.g., visual memory) are subserved by particular brain regions (e.g., right mesial temporal lobe) and assessment requires a battery of tests measuring narrowly defined functions. Hence, there needs to be a battery of narrowly focused measures. Examples from the Iowa-Benton Battery include the Auditory Verbal Learning Test, the Benton Facial Recognition Test, the Multilingual Aphasia Examination (which includes word list generation measures), and the Judgment of Line Orientation Test.

Macrolevel Theory: Cerebral Laterality

Cerebral laterality is a middle theory, a hybrid of domain-specificity and domain-generality. Cerebral laterality proposes two domain-general processors rather than one, in which the two halves of our brain are organized differently and control qualitatively different (but still broad) classes of behavior. Laterality theory goes under other names, including "cerebral asymmetry" and "hemispheric specialization."

Historically, right-left functional differences have been studied since the observations of Broca. The paradigmatic evidence for lateral organization was based mostly on the association of left-brain lesions with speech and language disorders, collectively termed the aphasias. Liepmann coined the term "apraxia" to describe disorders of skilled movement and hand gesture, also associated with left-brain lesions. Because aphasia and apraxia (two, of the three, classical "cortical signs"—along with agnosia) became the focus of so much behavioral neurology, the left brain was long identified as the "dominant hemisphere."

It was not until the late 1950s that the nonverbal-perceptual functions of the right brain were appreciated, and the historical label of "nondominant hemisphere" eventually dropped. A watershed event was the 1961 Interhemispheric Relations and Cerebral Dominance Conference held in Baltimore. The proceedings were published in a book by Vernon Mountcastle (1962). In this book, the nonverbal perceptual functions of the right brain were compiled and appreciated. It was further recommended that the term "dominant" refer only to specialized functions, not to an entire hemisphere. For example, the "language-dominant brain" replaced "the dominant left brain." The second watershed event was the split-brain research of Michael Gazzaniga, Roger Sperry,* and colleagues (1980s and 1990s). Patients whose corpus callosum was surgically cut (to control seizure spread) represented natural experiments that allowed neuropsychologists to study processing in isolated hemispheres.

*As a scientific historical note, Roger Sperry won the 1981 Nobel Prize in Physiology or Medicine for his split-brain research (along with Hubel and Wiesel). He was the only psychologist to have done so.

Key Evidence

Besides the experience with aphasia, much additional evidence supports the idea that right-left brain division describes qualitatively different mental processes. For example, considerable weight is placed on dichotic listening studies that show a right ear advantage for verbal stimuli. The right auditory nerve has its strongest connection with the left brain, and vice versa. Persons tracking two different sets of auditory stimuli presented separately to the ears do a better job of identifying sounds to the right ear than to the left. Split-brain studies show that the right hemisphere is better than the left at:

- translating a three-dimensional object into its unfolded equivalent
- discriminating nonsense shapes from each other
- remembering designs (object recognition) and locations (spatial recognition)
- making similarity judgments among designs
- recognizing and processing faces

Unilateral lesion cases suggest the following specializations:

- The right hemisphere plays a key role in regulating arousal and attention by acting as a literal "sentinel": Focal right parietal lesions often cause left-sided hemispatial inattention (i.e., neglect), but left-brain lesions typically do not cause contralateral neglect.
- The right hemisphere places negative valence on stimuli whereas the left hemisphere places positive valence: Right-sided lesions are often associated with euphoria and focal left lesions with dysphoria, in a sense inhibiting, disabling the natural hemispheric emotional valence tendencies.
- Prosodic aspects of speech (e.g., tone, inflection, and cadence) are more affected by right-brain lesions.

Practical Implications

The rejection of the terms "dominant and nondominant" now requires a test battery that is divided roughly equally between tasks that draw on the specializations of the two brain halves. Conversely, batteries that only emphasize verbal functions would be inappropriate. Many omnibus IQ tests roughly capture hemispheric specialization (e.g., the Wechsler IQ series measures both verbal and perceptual reasoning). Neuropsychological screening measures typically do not capture verbal and nonverbal functions. The Folstein Mini Mental State Examination, for example, is biased toward verbal measures.

Caveats and Current Status

Facts we can state with confidence include:

- For the vast majority of adults, the left hemisphere specializes for speech/language, phonetic analysis (i.e., reading), and hand gestures (praxis). However, it remains unclear how these specializations unfold developmentally in infants and children.
- Language (sans speech) is not limited to the left hemisphere. The right hemisphere has semantic knowledge, although the extent of that knowledge is still debated.

Yet cerebral asymmetry theory has its problems.

- One problem is oversimplification with domain-general labels, leading to popular myths. For example, left-right processing styles have been dichotomized respectively as:
  - Local-Global
  - Analytic-Holistic
  - High-Low Spatial Frequencies
  - Categorical-Metric
  - Logical-Intuitive

- These labels do not easily fit empirical facts. For example, syllables presented to isolated left brains are globally encoded into a speech code, but sequentially encoded letter-by-letter in the right brain. This is opposite to the prediction of the "right global, left analytic-sequential" dichotomy. This implies that there is no single characterization of hemispheric differences; that is, a domain-general approach is problematic.

- It remains possible that a correct domain-general characterization has so far escaped consideration.

- Left-right differences may be more quantitative than qualitative. For example, the much touted "right ear advantage" during dichotic listening is actually not that strongly associated with the left brain. A meta-analysis (Speaks et al., 1982) showed that fewer than 50% of studies showed a significant right-ear left-hemisphere advantage.

- Gazzaniga's most recent dichotomy is compelling and of heuristic value: The Right-Left Brain Reporter-Interpreter distinction. The right hemisphere seems to document facts in a concrete fashion, and the left hemisphere interprets those facts by weaving a connecting narrative. When acting in isolation, the left hemisphere produces delusions.

Macro-Level Theory: Two-Streams Hypothesis (Dorsal and Ventral Systems)

Some argue that right-left cerebral organization is overly simplified and has achieved more popular than factual status. Animal and human lesion research suggests that top-down organization is a better way to anatomically subdivide the brain. The *two-streams hypothesis* describes two qualitatively different cognitive systems that stream sensory input to the perceptual and production systems. Key terms and findings include:

- The dorsal ("top") brain refers roughly to structures above the horizontal plane formed by the Sylvian fissure. The dorsal brain includes the parietal lobes and dorsolateral prefrontal cortex. The dorsal system is concerned with processing and storage of the spatial features of information, such as where something is located either in space or in an event sequence. This is commonly referred to as the "where system," i.e., spatial location.

- The ventral ("bottom") brain refers to structures below the Sylvian plane, for example, the inferotemporal cortex. The ventral portion of the posterior cortex extracts object information, such as shape, color, and identity. The ventral system is commonly referred to as the "what system," i.e., the nature of the object.

- This top-bottom organization is carried forward into the action system of the frontal lobe: The dorsal frontal zone determines how action is carried out. The ventral frontal lobes make decisions about causal relations between objects and actions, but do not carry out actions.

- Landmark studies and findings supportive of the top-bottom view include:

  - Pohl (1973) integrated decades of primate research to prove distinct functions can be organized into a ventral-dorsal scheme, such as egocentric versus allocentric perception.

  - Ungerledier and Mishkin (1982) lesioned primate inferotemporal cortex and found not only object discrimination deficits but also the inability to relearn spatial location tasks following parietal lobe lesions.

- Goldman-Rakic and colleagues (1980s–1990s) showed dorsal-ventral organization in monkey frontal lobes: dorsolateral areas serve spatial working memory and ventrolateral areas serve object working memory.

- People with Balint syndrome (identified in 1909; bilateral superior occipital-parietal lesions) have difficulty reaching for objects directly, but can recognize them (i.e., optic ataxia).

- Borst, Thomson, and Kosslyn's (2011) recent meta-analysis showed a strong association between dorsal activation/damage and grouped data for (a) spatial relations and (b) movement detection. Ventral activation/damage was associated with parallel processing performance.

Automatic Versus Controlled Processing

Separate from task content, neuropsychology requires awareness of task demands as informative of diagnostic questions. Task demands correlate roughly with task difficulty. The two key concepts are automatic and controlled processing, and most tests have both components to varying degrees.

- *Automaticity* Refers to behavioral routines that are carried out quickly, effortlessly, accurately, and with little forethought. A popular synonym from clinical jargon is "overlearned." Examples include basic mental addition or reciting math facts, digits forward, speaking and formulating sentences, recognizing written words, greetings and helping responses in social settings, and motor skills such as riding a bicycle. Individuals with normal reading skills (those without a reading disorder) for example, are said to read automatically, effortlessly. Poor readers typically do not read effortlessly.

- *Effortful Processing* Refers to mental operations carried out with effort, planning, and careful attention to proximate conditions. Synonyms are "effortful" and "online." Examples include striking out all the letter A's preceded by the letter X in a novel cancellation task, reciting digits backward, driving to an unfamiliar location, remembering what you did last Tuesday, and learning a new work skill.

Important Facts

- Much of human behavior is composed of automatic response patterns that are triggered by common contexts.

- Automaticity can be seen in any neurobehavioral domain, including language, motor skills, psychomotor speed, and even some forms of problem solving. Many automatic responses are perceptual-motor biases built into the brain by evolution. For example, localizing sound during sensory-perceptual testing is not learned.

- Automatic response patterns, termed the "habit system," likely have a neuroanatomical base. There is compelling evidence that subcortical areas, particularly the basal ganglia, form an integrated habit system with respect to motor skills.

- Evidence for a separate neurobiological substrate is a double dissociation: preserved pursuit-rotor learning in patients with Korsakoff amnesia, patients who have no motor impairment (no basal ganglia damage), versus impaired motor learning in patients with subcortical disease (e.g., Huntington's).

Practice Implications

In general, effortful ("online") tasks are more sensitive to brain injury or dysfunction than are tasks calling on automatic response systems. For this reason, dividing or subdividing tasks into automatic and effortful processing informs clinical neuropsychological diagnosis in the following important ways:

- Automatized mental operations are usually captured by easy tasks or by more difficult tasks dependent on premorbid learning history.

- Measures saturated with automaticity (e.g., retrieval of old information) are often used as a control measure ("yardstick") to determine whether a patient has cognitively deteriorated. The basis for this practice is the historically consistent finding that some functions are well-preserved even in the face of serious brain insult. A classic example is David Wechsler's finding that IQ subtests are differentially affected by brain damage; diagnosis is based on comparing subtests that "hold" and "don't hold" against documented brain disease. For example, in general, Vocabulary holds up better against brain disease than does Block Design.

- Unless there is conduction aphasia, digit span forward is better preserved than backward, it is more automatic, while digits backward is more effortful.

- Performance on automatic tasks can also inform questions about deficit validity in adults. Errors or slow completion times on effortless tasks raise suspicions about deficit simulation, task engagement, in the absence of aphasia or subcortical disease. Adult examples include difficulties with:
  - reciting the alphabet
  - reading a simple sentence
  - completing Trailmaking Test, Part A (if hemispatial neglect has been ruled out)
  - repeating a short string of digits forward
  - reproducing the Rey 15-Item Memory Test
  - simple mental arithmetic

Brain Reserve Hypothesis and Cognitive Reserve Hypothesis

The brain reserve hypothesis (BRH) and cognitive reserve hypothesis (CRH) are related but different concepts that overlap but are not simply interchangeable. The central premise of both theories is that increased reserve can be protective against the onset of dementia or the long-term impact of acquired brain injury. The BRH (also referred to as cerebral reserve) refers to a brain's ability to absorb insult and potentially recover. This is often described as a "passive threshold model" because it hinges primarily on the brain's physical health prior to insult or disease onset. The BRH states that a critical threshold of brain cell loss must be crossed before a deficit achieves clinical expression in symptoms or test score abnormalities. Those with "brain matter to spare" (more brain cells or denser synaptic networks) are less likely to show observed deficits, despite documented brain disease. A variant of this theory is the CRH, which states that education and enriched experience can increase cerebral reserve and are relatively protective against the expression of symptoms following brain disease or injury. Higher cognitive reserve does not prevent dementia or impairments following traumatic brain injury (TBI) or other neurological conditions, but it can modify the functional and clinical expression of such conditions. Thus, CRH is an "efficiency model" because it refers to the mind's resistance to brain damage due to the presence of more efficient synaptic networks or preexisting cognitive abilities. Some research on environmental enrichment and brain development has supported the idea that there are modifiable variables that can enhance synaptic networks and provide a buffer against the impact of brain compromise on mental abilities. Quality of education, healthy lifestyle variables, and learning history are good examples (see also Chapter 29, Traumatic Brain Injury).

Key Facts and Findings

- The CRH was developed to explain the disagreement between diseases (objective brain damage) versus illness (the felt experience of the patient) in neuropsychology.

- The theory was stimulated by findings in the dementia field when an imperfect correlation was observed between brain abnormalities at autopsy and scores on cognitive screens such as the Folstein Mini-Mental State when the patient lived.

- Landmark studies evoking or testing CRH notions include:

  - Sisters of Notre Dame prospective dementia study—Nuns with limited literacy showed dementia signs at earlier ages than did more literate (and presumably more intelligent) nuns. Essays written to the Pope (prior to convent admission) were scored as to complexity as a proxy for verbal intelligence (Snowden et al., 1996).

  - Bigio et al. (2002) showed lower synaptic count in early as compared to late dementia onset.

  - Stern (2002) showed that level of education, talents/skills, and life achievements were associated with later onset of Alzheimer's disease.

Current Status

A number of predictions can be made from the BRH and CRH:

- The BRH would predict that persons with remote TBIs should experience earlier or more frequent age-related declines in function than uninjured persons matched for age. One population-based study found no increased risk for Alzheimer dementia in a large TBI sample, but found age of onset eight years earlier than in controls. Severity of initial TBI has to be a factor under BRH. Some cross-sectional studies find the more severe the TBI, the greater the incremental risk.

- The BRH and CRH research produces mixed results. Some report no association between age-related memory decline and quantified intracranial volume; others found a significant association but also found association with education.

- Enriched experience (education and occupation, for example) and synaptic organization are intertwined, making it difficult to evaluate each factor separately.

Executive Function Theory

As described in the section on cerebral localization theory, an important problem remains: what coordinates specific cognitive activities in complex behavior, and where in the brain is this carried out? Executive function theory (EFT) is an attempt to supply an answer. According to EFT, one or more general-purpose processors control domain-specific (specialized) mental operations to guide attention and action. Different sets of control processes have been proposed, with different localization. Some EFTs propose a single controller, others a family of semi-general-purpose controllers.

Examples

By illustration but not exclusion, the proposed control processes include:

- Alan Baddeley (1970s–1980s) argued for a single *central executive*, a mental process that regulates ("manipulates" in his terms) the content of two domain-specific short-term memory stores (phonological loop and visuospatial sketchpad). The combination of this single control mechanism and the two "slave" operations constitutes "working memory," although some critics point out that this is indistinguishable from other views on short-term memory.

- Akira Miyake's (2000) factor analysis proposes three general-purpose mechanisms: shifting, inhibiting, and "updating" (monitoring in other terms). These are latent variables that underlie most commonly used neuropsychological measures of "frontal system functioning."

- Donald Norman and Timothy Shallice's supervisory attentional system (SAS; circa 1986). These cognitive psychologists relied on the automatic-controlled distinction (see previous section) to identify situations that are novel and require "attentional" control for an optimal adaptive response. Examples are hazards, poorly practiced responses, decision-making, and "troubleshooting." They proposed only one mechanism: inhibition of a prepotent response, meaning effort to suppress the perceptual-motor patterns ("schema" in their terms) that are typically evoked. Two criticisms include (a) no situation is truly novel; a situation is hazardous only because we recognize it as dangerous (implying familiarity), and (b) the SAS model only refers to ordinary learning.

Relevant Definitions

Automaticity Refers to automatic processing; automatic in the sense that a function does not require a good deal of cognitive effort. Take a normal, good reader for example, who does not have to struggle over reading a word—it comes effortlessly—*automatically*. On the other hand, **Effortful Processing** is not automatic, and requires greater cognitive effort. A reader with dyslexia is said to show effortful reading.

Brain–Behavior Relationship Refers to the role the brain plays with regard to human behavior, including cognition, emotion, sensory-motor, and related abilities. Largely due to the discovery that discrete brain regions underlie specific cognitive, motor and other functions, i.e., localization theory, the term has largely become synonymous with neuropsychology.

Central Executive Alan Baddeley's term for the system responsible for the control and regulation of cognitive processes. Largely related to prefrontal brain regions, the central executive helps to regulate attention, working memory, and memory. The related concept of **Executive Functions** refers to the regulatory mechanisms responsible for higher-level human functions involved in organization, reasoning, flexibility, initiation, and related skills, and is largely subserved by prefrontal regions and networks.

Equipotentiality Karl Lashley's theory that an intact brain region can carry out the functions of damaged brain regions. Lashley thought that the brain has the capacity to transfer "functional memory" from the damaged brain region to the intact region.

Modular/Localization View Research into brain functions has shown that discrete brain regions are responsible for specific mental and behavioral functions, i.e., different parts of the brain do different things. Expressive speech, for example, is governed by Broca's area in the left frontal lobe (usually), Brodmann's areas 44 and 45.

Two-Streams Hypothesis As visual information leaves the occipital lobe, it follows two main streams or paths: the dorsal stream and the ventral stream. The dorsal stream is associated with an object's spatial location and is referred to as the "where stream." The ventral stream is associated with an object's identity and is referred to as the "what stream." The dual stream processing system has been identified for auditory information as well.

Whole-Brain Refers to domain-general theory and states that the whole brain acts in concert to produce functions. The Gestalt psychologists, for example, believed that visual perception was a whole-brain phenomenon, essentially transforming discrete visual images into a larger/greater whole. Domain-general theory has been largely supplanted by the factual basis of localization.

Important Theories and Constructs Questions

NOTE: Questions 5, 12, and 68 on the First Full-Length Practice Examination, Questions 7, 19, and 62 on the Second Full-Length Practice Examination, Questions 9 and 37 on the Third Full-Length Practice Examination, and Questions 2 and 72 on the Fourth Full-Length Practice Examination are from this chapter.

1. Which brain zone is commonly viewed as a domain-general control processor?
   - (a) pericallosal region
   - (b) temporal lobes
   - (c) parietal lobes
   - (d) prefrontal region

2. Cerebral reserve theory began with what observation?
   - (a) Some patients with Alzheimer brain changes did not show dementia when living.
   - (b) Brain dendrite counts during adolescence predicted reading level in older adulthood.
   - (c) Persons with higher gray to white matter ratios recover more quickly from brain injuries.
   - (d) Males have larger brains than females and recover more quickly from stroke of equal severity.

3. Which of the following both refer to executive control processes?
   - (a) updating and phonological looping
   - (b) facial recognition and expression
   - (c) contextual shifting and updating
   - (d) grammatical and lexical access

4. Which of the following dichotomies has been used to describe right-left cerebral lateralization?
   - (a) emotional-pedantic
   - (b) nonverbal-verbal
   - (c) metric-linear
   - (d) parietal-temporal

5. Split-brain research revealed a number of new insights about the corpus callosum (CC) including which one of the following?
   - (a) The CC is inert in and by itself, it does little if the anterior commissure is not also active.
   - (b) Right and left hemispheres continued to communicate even with disconnected CC.
   - (c) Right and left hemispheres never communicate with each other, with or without the CC.
   - (d) Splitting the CC resulted in failure of the hemispheres to communicate or be aware of each other.

6. Alexia without agraphia is a neurobehavioral phenomenon best understood to be an example of ____.
   - (a) equipotentiality
   - (b) dorsal versus ventral stream processing
   - (c) localization theory
   - (d) domain-general theory

7. Why was the term "dominant hemisphere" dropped as a descriptor of left-brain functions?

    (a) The specializations of the right hemisphere were finally appreciated.

    (b) The right hemisphere is equally efficient in inferential aspects of speech.

    (c) Dominant was considered a pejorative term; too sexist and elitist.

    (d) Left lesions proved less disruptive of daily function than right ones.

8. The concept of intelligence, *g*, is an example of which theory?

    (a) Gestalt theory

    (b) domain-general theory

    (c) global-local theory

    (d) localization theory

9. Domain-general theory ____.

    (a) has been supplanted by localization theory

    (b) is partially accepted today

    (c) is completely misunderstood

    (d) remains ascendant today

10. That many specific functions have been associated with discrete brain regions is an example of ____.

    (a) lateralization

    (b) double dissociation

    (c) domain-specific, localization theory

    (d) brain reserve

Important Theories and Constructs Answers

1. **D—prefrontal region**   *The bilateral prefrontal areas do not seem to serve any specific motor or sensory modality. Instead, the prefrontal areas seem to integrate many different sensory inputs from both the external world (e.g., sight and sound) and the internal world (hormonal and proprioceptive stimuli) and then choose the motor program most appropriate to the information. Persons with frontal lesions do have problems with shifting attention and updating critical information.*

    Reference: Luria, A. (1973). *The working brain.* New York, NY: Basic Books.

2. **A—Some patients with Alzheimer brain changes did not show dementia when living.**   *Correlation of mental status scores with postmortem findings in dementia.*

    Reference: Katzman, R., Terry, R., DeTeresa, R., Brown, T., Davies, P., Fuld, P., . . . Peck. A. (1988). Clinical, pathological, and neurochemical changes in dementia: A subgroup with preserved mental status and numerous neocortical plaques. *Annals of Neurology, 23*, 138–144.

3. **C—contextual shifting and updating**   *These functions are generally agreed upon executive processes.*

    Reference: Miyake, A., Friedman, N. P., Emerson, M. J., Witzki, A. H., & Howerter, A. (2000). The unity and diversity of executive functions and their contributions to complex "frontal lobe" tasks: A latent variable analysis. *Cognitive Psychology, 41*, 49–100.

4. **B—nonverbal-verbal**   *For the vast majority of individuals, the left hemisphere is specific for verbal skills, while the right hemisphere is specific for nonverbal/visuospatial skills. A small percentage of left handers may have the opposite pattern.*

    Reference: Gazzaniga, M. S. (1998). The split-brain revisited. *Scientific American*, July, 50–55. http://www.utdallas.edu/~otoole/CGS/R5.pdf

5. **D—Splitting the CC resulted in failure of the hemispheres to communicate or be aware of each other.** *Sperry discovered that severing the corpus callosum resulted in failure of the hemispheres to be aware of each other and communicate with each other.*

   Reference: https://www.nobelprize.org/prizes/medicine/1981/sperry/article/

6. **C—localization theory** *Alexia without agraphia is a disconnection syndrome, typically resultant from a lesion in the splenium of the corpus callosum disconnecting the posterior language area in the parietal lobe (angular gyrus/supramarginal gyrus) from the left hemisphere motor area in the frontal lobe. These, and related disorders, speak clearly to localization of brain functions.*

   Reference: Lezak, M. D., Howieson, D. B., Bigler, E. D. & Tranel, D. (2012). *Neuropsychological assessment* (5th ed.). New York, NY: Oxford, pp. 348–349.

7. **A—The specializations of the right hemisphere were finally appreciated.** *Nonverbal perceptual functions became a focus of research and were found dominant in the right brain for some tasks. Alternative terms were proposed for the left side, such as "language-dominant brain."*

   Reference: Levy, J. (2000). Hemispheric functions. In A. Kazdin (Ed.), *Encyclopedia of psychology* (pp. 113–115). Washington DC: APA and Oxford University Press.

8. **B—domain-general theory** *In its original conception, Spearman's g (Spearman, 1927) referred to a general, overarching factor of intelligence, thought to be a product of the entire brain. However, the typical individual intelligence test (Wechsler scales, for example) is composed of discrete subtests assessing specific cognitive functions, that are understood to be subserved by particular brain regions. Modern conceptualizations of intelligence are therefore more representative of domain-specific/localization notions, while the concept of g is an implicit overall abstraction representing the putative combinative quality of the individual, discrete functions.*

   Reference: Sternberg, R. J. & Sternberg, K. (2016). *Cognitive psychology* (7th ed.). New York, NY: Wadsworth.

9. **A—has been supplanted by localization theory** *Modern neuropsychology understands the indisputable fact that localization theory predominates brain–behavior relationships. As time goes on, we learn more and more about the specificity of brain regions and associated functions. Nevertheless, domain-general notions are embedded in our culture colloquially, as in "talent," "artistic," and "intelligent," among others.*

   Reference: Gazzaniga, M. S. (2014). *Human: Tales from both sides of the brain.* New York, NY: Harper Collins.

10. **C—domain-specific, localization theory** *The voluminous literature concerning the relationship between specific brain regions and functions is the cornerstone of modern brain science.*

    References:
    (a) Blumenfeld, H. (2018). *Neuroanatomy through clinical cases* (2nd ed.). New York, NY: Oxford University Press/ Sinauer Associates.
    (b) Morgan, J. E., & Ricker, J. H. (Eds.), (2018). *Textbook of clinical neuropsychology* (2nd ed.). New York, NY: Routledge.

Recommended Readings

Borst, G., Thompson, W. L., & Kosslyn, S. M. (2011). Understanding the dorsal and ventral systems of the human cerebral cortex. *American Psychologist, 66,* 624–632.

Catani, M., & Mesulam, M. (2008). What is a disconnection syndrome? *Cortex, 44,* 1–3.

Gazzaniga, M. S. (1998). The split-brain revisited. *Scientific American*, July, 50–55. http://www.utdallas.edu/~otoole/CGS/R5.pdf

Levy, J. (2000). Hemispheric functions. In A. Kazdin (Ed.), *Encyclopedia of psychology* (pp. 113–115). Washington DC: APA and Oxford University Press.

Lezak, M., Howieson, D. B., & Loring, D. W. (2004). The behavioral geography of the brain. In M. Lezak, D. B. Howieson, & D. W. Loring (Eds.), *Neuropsychological assessment* (4th ed., pp. 35–85). New York, NY: Oxford.

Luria, A. R. (1973). *The working brain.* New York, NY: Basic Books.

Speaks, C., Niccum, N., & Carney, E. (1982). Statistical properties of responses to dichotic listening with CV nonsense syllables. *Journal of the Acoustical Society of America*, *72*(4), 1185–1194.

4 Functional Neuroanatomy and Essential Neuropharmacology

Russell M. Bauer and Leslie S. Gaynor

Introduction

Basic knowledge of functional neuroanatomy and neurochemistry is a critical tool in the toolbox of the competent neuropsychologist. Together with knowledge of clinical syndromes and the principles and practices of neuropsychological assessment, such knowledge not only provides information needed for proper differential diagnosis but also allows neuropsychologists to predict the nature of cognitive impairments expected in patients with localized lesions and to plan their assessments accordingly. The process of integrating anatomic knowledge and understanding of behavioral and cognitive syndromes is a fundamental step in neuropsychological assessment known as *anatomico-clinical correlation*. This chapter reviews key aspects of functional neuroanatomy and neurochemistry essential for the practicing neuropsychologist and focuses on cortical and subcortical function, organized by functional domain. We forego a detailed description of basic motor and sensory systems, focusing instead on higher cortical functions. This chapter is designed to point the way to more directed and in-depth study because a comprehensive review of these vast topics would far exceed space limitations. Excellent, clinically oriented neuroanatomy texts are available (Blumenfeld, 2010; Mendoza & Foundas, 2008) and should be part of every neuropsychologist's library. In addition, several excellent websites, some of which provide interactive experiences, are available and listed at the end of "Recommended Readings." Chapter 5, Domains of Neuropsychological Function and Related Neurobehavioral Disorders, provides more detail regarding cognitive domains that map generally onto the anatomic systems described here. A broad command of clinical-anatomic correlation will enhance the neuropsychologist's ability to relate neuropsychological findings to underlying brain abnormalities. For the written examination and day-to-day clinical practice an understanding of functionally relevant systems is most important, which, in most instances, is not further enhanced by rote memorization of minutiae.

General Organizational Principles

Divisions and Directions

The human nervous system is composed of the central nervous system (CNS; brain and spinal cord) and the peripheral nervous system (everything else). The brain itself is divided into three main components:

- The forebrain (cerebral hemispheres and diencephalon)
- The midbrain
- The hindbrain (comprised of the medulla, pons, and cerebellum, which together form a connection between the brain and spinal cord)

In discussing the relative location of structures and orientation of fiber tracks, the following planes of section and directional terms are used. The "front-back" direction is denoted by the distinction between "ventral" (literally, toward the "belly") and "dorsal," whereas the "up-down" direction is represented by the "rostral/superior"–"caudal/inferior" dimension. The reader should note that, in the human nervous system, these planes take a 90-degree turn above the spinal cord. Thus, "ventral/dorsal" means "toward the front/back" in the cord, but is synonymous with "inferior/superior" in the brain. Similarly, "rostral/caudal" means "toward the head/toes" in the cord, but denotes "anterior/posterior" in the brain. The neuropsychologist should be familiar with major planes of section in the nervous system because these are also used in diagnostic imaging studies. The "horizontal" (or axial) plane is parallel to the floor. The "coronal" plane is perpendicular to the floor and cuts across the brain in approximately the plane that would connect the two ears (think of wearing a "corona" or "crown"). The "sagittal" plane, also perpendicular to the ground, from forehead to occiput, is much like the plane assumed by an archer shooting an arrow with a bow.

Cortical Organization and Laminar Structure

The brain is comprised of gray matter (cell bodies of neurons) and white matter (mostly myelinated axons). Basic synaptic communication takes place in the gray matter, whereas the white matter tracts provide communication among cortical areas and between cortical and subcortical structures over longer distances. It is important to recognize that distinct clinical syndromes (disconnection syndromes) arise from damage to white matter pathways when functional brain regions are deprived of inputs and outputs through white matter damage.

A fundamental distinction can be made between "unimodal" cortex, which processes information pertaining to a specific sensory modality, and "polymodal" cortex, which processes information received from disparate modalities through afferent connections. While unimodal cortex plays a prominent role in perception, polymodal cortex is critically involved in higher-order *conceptual* processes that are less dependent on concrete sensory information than on abstract features extracted from multiple inputs. Examples of polymodal cortex include the convergence zones of the anterior temporal lobe and inferior parietal lobule.

The cerebral hemispheres are divided into "lobes," defined both by their functional proclivities and by architectural boundaries. Each cortical region has further subdivisions that have important functional implications. For example, the frontal lobe can be further subdivided into:

- The *orbitofrontal/ventromedial region*, important for emotional regulation, reward monitoring, and personality; damage to the orbitofrontal sector produces disinhibition, whereas damage to the ventromedial sector results in disordered reward/punishment processing and problems marking perceptual or learning experiences with reward value and emotional significance.

- The *dorsolateral region*, important in a broad range of cognitive-executive functions; damage produces dysexecutive syndromes, impairments in working memory, and poor attentional control of behavior.

- The *dorsomedial region*, important for intentional and behavioral activation; extensive damage to this region produces striking impairments in initiated behavior including *akinetic mutism*, in which the person is alert and awake (not comatose) but cannot move or speak.

The temporal lobes can be divided roughly into three regions:

- The *temporal polar cortical areas*, a polymodal convergence zone important for intersensory integration and semantic memory.

- The **ventral temporal areas**, important for object recognition and discrimination; bilateral damage can produce object or face agnosia.
- The **posterior temporal region**, comprised of the middle and superior temporal sulci, which contains the primary auditory areas and Wernicke's area in the language-dominant hemisphere, important for language comprehension, and prosodic comprehension in the homologous non-dominant hemisphere.

The parietal lobe can be divided into three regions:

- The **superior parietal lobe**, important for sensory–motor integration, body schema, and spatial processing.
- The **temporoparietal junction**, important for phonological and sound-based processing; language comprehension (left) and music comprehension (right).
- The **inferior parietal lobule**, important for complex spatial attention, integration of tactile sensation, and self-awareness.

The occipital lobe contains the primary visual cortex (surrounding the calcarine fissure) and the visual association cortex. Complete damage to the primary visual cortex produces cortical blindness or (rarely) phenomena of Anton's syndrome (denial of cortical blindness) or blindsight (detection of unconsciously perceived stimuli in the blind field). Partial damage produces visual field defects that reflect the region of visual cortex damaged. The occipital lobe is also the origin of the two main visual-cortical pathways:

- The **ventral visual pathway**, connecting occipital and temporal lobe; important for object and face recognition, item-based memory, and complex visual discrimination.
- The **dorsal visual pathway**, connecting the occipital and parietal lobes via the superior temporal sulcus; important for spatial vision and visuomotor integration.

An important feature of the neocortex is its six-layer laminar structure, which distinguishes it from limbic cortex (archicortex), which has only three. Each of the six layers has distinct input–output connections and, when examining any cortical region, evaluation of the region's laminar structure provides important clues regarding that region's function by elucidating other brain regions to which it is preferentially connected. So, for example, portions of dorsolateral prefrontal cortex (DLPFC) are characterized by a proportionally large layer IV, which predominantly contains inputs from the thalamus; other regions are comprised of large layers II and III, containing *cortico-cortical connections*. These facts provide clues to the functions of the DLPFC, which, in performing complex abstract reasoning and problem-solving tasks, depends upon modulatory input that engages and disengages areas of cortex (the role played by input from subcortical re-entrant circuits that include the thalamus) as well as rich associations among adjacent and nonadjacent cortical regions for processing task demands (the role played by *cortico-cortical connections*). In general, the functions of many areas can be understood in terms of the friends they keep; that is, their connections to other cortical and subcortical regions.

Functional Specialization and Modularity

In his classic study of regional anatomy, Brodmann parsed the cortex into 52 distinct regions based on microscopic cytoarchitectonic features. Many of these regions have become associated with identified cognitive functions (e.g., area 44 in the language-dominant hemisphere is Broca's area, important for planning of articulatory speech movements, whereas area 21 in the inferotemporal region is important for auditory processing). More precise characterization of these functionally specialized regions has become possible through advanced structural and functional neuroimaging techniques. The concept of modular/specialized brain systems is critical for understanding normal function and for understanding how focal brain disease or injury can sometimes produce impairments in highly selective neuropsychological functions.

A critical concept regarding how functionally specialized areas are organized to support cognitive function is the notion of a *functional system*—an interconnected group of cortical and subcortical structures that each contributes important components of a complex behavior or skill. Complex behaviors such as memory or language can be impaired by damage to the processors themselves or by damage to their connecting fibers. When damage affects a specific processor, the resulting deficit reflects a loss of that processor's contribution to the complex behaviors supported by the system. When damage affects the interconnections among processors, a *disconnection syndrome* results. Disconnection syndromes occur when fiber damage causes functional processors to lose their ability to coordinate or communicate in performing a complex task or behavior.

Neuroanatomy of Vision

Retinal ganglion cells in each eye send their axons into the optic nerve, which projects posteriorly and comes together at the optic chiasm, where the optic tracts originate. The majority of optic tract fibers terminate in the lateral geniculate nucleus (LGN) of the thalamus, which then projects to the primary visual cortex in *Brodmann area* (BA) 17 ("striate cortex") in the occipital pole. This "geniculostriate" pathway is critical to visual discrimination and form perception. A small proportion of fibers bypasses the LGN and terminates in the pretectal area and superior colliculus, forming the "extrageniculate" or "extrastriate" visual pathway. Pretectal and collicular fibers then project to broad areas of parietal and frontal association cortex (including frontal eye fields, BA 8) via relays in the pulvinar nucleus of the thalamus. This "tectopulvinar" system subserves the pupillary light reflex, attention-directed eye movements, and general orientation to visual stimuli and is more sensitive to movement than to form.

The cortical representation of vision is the product of complex parallel processing of multiple, anatomically separate visual input "channels" that compute form, motion, and color. The fact that these "channels" are anatomically distinct means that form, motion, and color processing can be selectively impaired in focal brain disease.

A general "dorsal-ventral" dimension in human vision can be appreciated in projections from the visual cortex to nearby cortical structures. The "dorsal" pathway, which projects to parieto-occipital association cortex, preferentially processes spatial information and is likely involved in visuomotor interaction (e.g., reaching, manipulating objects) in the environment, whereas the "ventral" pathway, which projects to occipitotemporal association cortex and thereafter to anterior portions of inferotemporal cortex, processes structural and feature-based information important for the analysis and recognition of visual form such as faces and objects. Neuropsychologists recognize that more dorsally placed lesions produce impairments in spatial perception, attention, and visuomotor processing (e.g., hemispatial neglect, impaired visual reaching, etc.), whereas more ventrally placed lesions produce perceptual disturbances and, in severe forms, disorders of recognition of familiar objects and/or faces, known as agnosias. When the disorder results from impairment in processing basic visual elements of objects (e.g., shape, contour, depth), the disorder is *apperceptive* in nature. When the recognition disorder results from relating a well-perceived stimulus to stored representations based on prior experience with the stimulus, it is referred to as an *associative* agnosia. Apperceptive agnosias result from extensive damage to visual association areas, while associative agnosias may involve less extensive or disconnecting lesions in the regions between association cortex and memory.

Neuroanatomy of Memory

Severe disorders of memory (the so-called amnesic syndrome) can result from focal damage to the medial temporal lobes, the medial diencephalon, or the *basal forebrain (BF)*. An understanding of the underlying circuitry provides a basis for considering these three regions not as discrete entities, but as parts of an integrated, distributed memory system.

Temporal Lobe Structures

The Hippocampus and Parahippocampal Region

The hippocampus is a phylogenetically ancient cortical structure consisting of the dentate gyrus, the sectors of Ammon's horn (cornu Ammonis [CA] 1–4), and the subiculum. The primary internal connections of the hippocampus comprise what is known as the *trisynaptic circuit* (entorhinal cortex → dentate granule cells [synapse 1] → CA3 via mossy fibers [synapse 2] → CA1 via Schaffer collaterals [synapse 3]). CA1 neurons project to the subiculum, which is the major source of direct hippocampal cortical efferent projections. The subiculum projects back to the entorhinal cortex, completing the circuit. Although the circuit described is unidirectional, non-human primate and rodent studies have revealed bidirectional reciprocal connections between the hippocampus, the entorhinal cortex, and other extrahippocampal structures.

The primary cortical inputs into the hippocampus are depicted in Figure 4.1. Most hippocampal cortical connections are with the adjacent parahippocampal region, which includes rhinal (entorhinal and perirhinal) cortex, pre- and parasubicular cortex, and parahippocampal cortex. The perirhinal cortex and parahippocampal cortex receive a majority of the cortical input to the temporal lobe memory circuit. These connections come from *unimodal* and heteromodal association cortices, and information from both sources of input is combined into 3D representations of experienced stimuli. The apparent simplicity of the unidirectional downstream medial temporal lobe pathway has given rise to two contrasting views about the function of this system. First, the perirhinal and parahippocampal cortex appear to receive input from separable cortical regions, such that the perirhinal cortex receives more anterior temporal "non-spatial" information and the parahippocampal cortex receives more posterior medial "spatial" information. According to one view, these two "streams" provide separate inputs to the hippocampus,

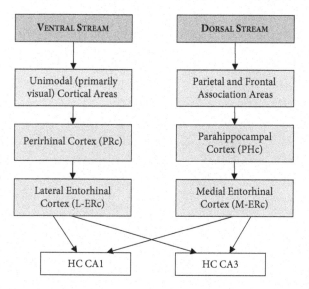

FIGURE 4.1 Segregated Cortical Inputs to Hippocampus

which then "binds" them together to form an episode. However, recent findings suggest that input from the parahippocampal cortex to the perirhinal cortex, as well as present "spatial" and "non-spatial" cortical connections to both the perirhinal and parahippocampal cortices, allows both structures access to non-spatial and spatial information from the cortex prior to their interaction with the hippocampus.

More posteriorly, the entorhinal cortex receives most information from the cortex indirectly through input from the perirhinal and parahippocampal cortices, although some direct connections have been identified. The entorhinal cortex is divided into anterior-lateral and posterior-medial parts, in which the anterior/lateral entorhinal cortex receives a majority of its input from the perirhinal cortex and "non-spatial" cortical regions and the posterior/medial medial entorhinal cortex (or medial entorhinal cortex) receives a majority of its input from the parahippocampal cortex and "spatial" cortical regions. The posterior medial entorhinal cortex evidences greater spatial-specific function compared to the anterior lateral entorhinal cortex due to the presence of grid cells, which encode for spatial location in the environment, and communicate with the place cells of the hippocampus.

Complex and dense reciprocal interconnections between the many structures belonging to the temporal lobe memory system suggest that non-spatial and spatial information co-mingles prior to reaching the hippocampus, and that perhaps a network model better explains the function of these structures in daily memory encoding.

There are three main subcortical projections from the hippocampus to structures outside of the temporal lobe memory circuit, two of which involve the fornix, which divides into two pathways at the anterior commissure:

- Fibers from CA1, CA3, and the subiculum project in the precommissural fornix to the lateral septal nucleus.
- Subicular projections travel in the postcommissural fornix and terminate on the mammillary bodies or the anterior nucleus of the thalamus.
- The hippocampus also projects to the amygdala, nucleus accumbens, other regions of the BF, and ventromedial hypothalamus.

The hippocampal → postcommissural fornix → mammillary body projection was part of the "circuit" described by Papez, in 1937, to explain how the hypothalamus and cortex coordinate emotion–cognition interaction. The remaining part of the circuit, which has since been referred to as the *medial limbic circuit*, involves a projection from the mammillary bodies to the anterior thalamic nucleus and subsequent thalamic projections to the cingulate gyrus and cingulate projections, via the cingulate bundle or cingulum, which extend back to the hippocampus. This circuit, and its partner, the *lateral limbic circuit*, are depicted in Figure 4.2.

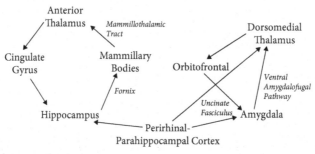

FIGURE 4.2 Medial and Lateral Limbic Circuits

The Amygdala

The amygdala is situated immediately anterior to the hippocampus, deep to the periamygdaloid and perirhinal cortices in the temporal lobe. It has two main parts: a large basolateral group of nuclei (which connect to limbic system, association cortex, and dorsomedial thalamic nucleus) and a smaller corticomedial segment, which has extensive connections with BF, hypothalamus, and brainstem. The anatomic connections of amygdala and *hippocampus* are alike in the following ways:

- both are strongly interconnected with frontal and temporal limbic cortex.
- both have indirect access to polymodal neocortical association areas.
- both project to BF and hypothalamus.
- both connect directly with each other.

But there are also striking anatomic differences:

- the amygdala derives from paleocortex and is related to the BF and ventral striatum, whereas the hippocampus is archicortical and is more closely related to the neocortex.
- the amygdala projects to dorsomedial thalamus, whereas the hippocampus projects primarily to mammillary bodies of the hypothalamus.
- the amygdala relates to different portions of the BF (bed nucleus of the stria terminalis) than does the hippocampus (septal region).
- cholinergic inputs to the amygdala (nucleus basalis of Meynert [nbM]) are different from that of the hippocampus (diagonal band of Broca).
- unlike the hippocampus, the amygdala has strong connections with brainstem autonomic centers (nucleus of the solitary tract), providing a direct pathway for limbic–autonomic interaction.

Thus, in contrast to Papez's *medial limbic circuit*, the amygdala participates in a *lateral limbic circuit*: amygdala → dorsomedial nucleus of the thalamus → orbitofrontal cortex → uncinate fasciculus → amygdala, as depicted in Figure 4.2.

The Anatomical Basis of Temporal Lobe Amnesia

Since the landmark description by Scoville and Milner of H. M. in 1957, an explosion of interest in the neuroanatomy of memory occurred among human and animal researchers. In Scoville and Milner's series, removal of the uncus and amygdala (in one patient) caused no memory loss, but more posterior resections involving the hippocampus and parahippocampal gyrus produced amnesia that was more severe with more extensive resections. Scoville and Milner concluded that amnesia would not occur unless the surgery extended far enough back to involve the hippocampus.

The *two-system theory of amnesia* forms a core principle of understanding memory disorders from a functional systems perspective, and explains how amnesia can be caused by several different lesion profiles. The basic principle is that amnesia occurs when both the *lateral* and *medial limbic circuit* are damaged (this principle explains most diencephalic and BF amnesias as well). Thus, for example, lesions that interrupt both the fornix (disrupting Papez's circuit) and the ventral amygdalofugal pathways (disrupting the lateral circuit) cause severe amnesia, whereas lesions restricted to either pathway alone cause less severe memory disturbance. Many other combinations on this general theme are possible and have been documented in the literature.

Lesions that affect either the posteromedial or anteromedial aspect of the thalamus cause little memory disturbance; but severe amnesia, comparable to that associated with medial temporal ablations, occurs when both anterior and posterior medial thalamic regions are involved. Finally, lesions that affect the frontal projections of both Papez's circuit (anterior cingulate gyrus) and the lateral circuit (ventromedial frontal lobe) produce greater memory loss than lesions of either alone. Six decades of primate lesion studies suggest (1) that structures within each memory system are highly interdependent, since damage to different parts of each system can cause apparently equivalent deficits; and (2) that each system can, to a large extent, carry on the function of the other, since lesions affecting only one system result in memory loss that is far less severe than if both systems are damaged.

More recently, it has been shown that collateral damage to the perirhinal cortex was responsible for the memory deficits seen after amygdala lesions, and, in fact, extensive lesions of the perirhinal and parahippocampal cortices produce an amnesia equivalent to or worse than that produced by impairment of the two circuits described earlier, even when the hippocampus and amygdala are spared. This means that the perirhinal/parahippocampal cortex contributes to memory in its own right. Because both the amygdala and the perirhinal/parahippocampal cortex project to dorsomedial thalamus, the dual-system theory can be easily modified by substituting "perirhinal/parahippocampal cortex" for "amygdala" in Figure 4.2.

An extensive literature, a detailed review of which is beyond the scope of this chapter, documents memory disturbances as a result of damage to other specific elements of this complex limbic circuitry, including the fornix, mammillary bodies, the anterior thalamic nuclei, and the retrosplenial cortex.

In summary, we can reach four conclusions about the temporal lobe and amnesia:

- Damage to cortical and subcortical structures within the temporal lobe, whether focal or extensive, can result in amnesia.

- Amnesia most likely results from damage to both the hippocampally based *medial limbic circuit* and the amygdala-based *lateral limbic circuit*.

- Damage to individual elements of these circuits can all result in amnesia, provided that both circuits are damaged.

- The hippocampus appears critical for episodic memory, whereas the amygdala appears more directly involved in emotional aspects of cognition, including emotional memory and assigning emotional significance to stimuli.

Thalamus

The thalamus is important as a sensory relay nucleus but also has critical functions in higher cognitive processes including alertness, behavioral activation, and memory. It is comprised of a number of nuclear groups separated in the ventral-dorsal and anterior-posterior planes by a system of myelinated fiber tracks called the internal medullary lamina (IML). It is within the IML that memory-relevant fibers of the mammillothalamic tract and the ventral amygdalofugal pathways travel on their way to their terminations in the anterior and dorsomedial thalamic nuclei, respectively.

Amnesia has traditionally been associated with dorsomedial thalamic lesions, as shown by studies of tumors in the walls of the third ventricle and of Wernicke-Korsakoff disease. However, more recent research suggests that thalamic amnesia best correlates with lesions affecting the IML and mammillothalamic tract. More posterior lesions that involve portions of the dorsomedial nucleus but spare the IML and mammillothalamic tract are not associated with amnesia. The modified dual-pathway theory described earlier suggests that severe and lasting amnesia requires disruption of both the *medial* and *lateral limbic circuits*.

Alternative explanations of thalamic amnesia suggest a role for the midline thalamic nuclei. These nuclei have connections with the hippocampus and are consistently damaged in patients with

Wernicke-Korsakoff disease. Aside from impairing connections to the hippocampus, thalamic lesions may disconnect thalamic connections with the frontal lobes. It has also been proposed that restricted thalamic lesions in Wernicke-Korsakoff disease might disconnect dorsomedial-frontal connections important for imposing cognitive structure on semantic memories resident in posterior cortex.

Basal Forebrain

The third major region essential for normal human memory function is the BF. The BF is at the junction of the diencephalon and the cerebral hemispheres and has the following components: the septal area, diagonal band of Broca, nucleus accumbens septi, olfactory tubercle, substantia innominata (containing the nucleus basalis of Meynert), bed nucleus of the stria terminalis, and preoptic area. It has been known for many years that some patients develop memory loss after hemorrhage from aneurysms of the anterior communicating artery, and it is now thought that damage to cholinergic neurons in the BF (which project to both the medial and *lateral limbic circuits*) may be responsible.

Most BF lesions reported in human cases of amnesia have been large and probably affect all or many of the aforementioned structures. Often, they also involve areas outside the BF, such as the orbitofrontal and ventromedial frontal cortices and the caudate nucleus. It may be that severe memory loss involves damage in addition to BF, but occasional case reports of very small lesions suggest otherwise, and it is important to remember that, in the case of BF, lesion size may not be as critical as whether the lesion is situated to produce a cholinergic disconnection with memory-relevant structures in the diencephalic and medial temporal lobe memory systems. Although the cholinergic hypothesis has been popular, other neurotransmitter pathways (e.g., dopamine) may be of importance, and their contribution to memory remains to be elucidated.

Summary of the Anatomy of Memory

Earlier conceptions that memory was a localized function subserved by a specific structure such as the hippocampus or dorsomedial thalamus have given way to the view that memory is a distributed function of the human brain. The bulk of the evidence suggests that the distributed system contains two functionally and anatomically integrated circuits, the medial one involving the hippocampus and the lateral one involving the amygdala. Amnesia is associated with medial temporal, thalamic, BF, and parahippocampal gyrus damage, to the extent that such damage either directly or indirectly impairs the functional integrity of these systems. Most existing evidence suggests that functional impairment of more than one circuit is necessary for dense amnesia to occur. Less severe forms of memory disturbance can result from more restricted lesions that do not impair both circuits. A summary diagram of the neuroanatomy of memory, depicting potential lesion scenarios in temporal lobe, diencephalic, and BF amnesia, is given in Figure 4.3.

Neuroanatomy of Language

The neuroanatomy of language, like that of memory, is distributed throughout many brain regions. The left hemisphere is dominant for language in more than 95% of right-handers and in more than 60–70% of left-handers. We touch on only the key structures involved in classic language functions here; the reader is referred to other more in-depth analyses of language-relevant brain regions (Goodglass, 1993) (see also Chapter 5, Domains of Neuropsychological Function and Related Neurobehavioral Disorders, and Chapter 26, Stroke).

The two regions implicated in Broca's and Wernicke's seminal cases lie adjacent to the Sylvian fissure separating the temporal and frontal lobes, and subsequent analyses of language disorders associated with these and associated regions have led to the concept of "perisylvian" aphasias. The key structures

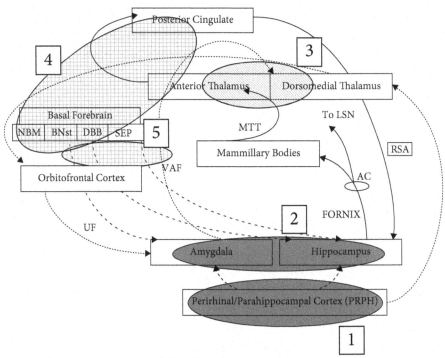

FIGURE 4.3 Integrated Memory Circuits with Possible Lesion Scenarios

NOTE: Medial (Papez) circuit depicted by solid arrows; lateral circuit depicted by dotted arrows; basal forebrain connections depicted by dashed arrows. Key: NBM = Nucleus Basalis of Meynert; BNst = Bed Nucleus of the Stria Terminalis; DBB = Diagonal Band of Broca; SEP = Septal nucleus; VAF = Ventral amygdalofugal pathway; MTT = Mammillothalamic tract; AC = anterior commissure; LSN = Lateral septal nucleus; RSA = Retrosplenial area.

Lesion Scenarios: [1] Extensive damage to perirhinal-parahippocampal cortex produces severe amnesia as in Zola-Morgan et al., 1989b; [2] Lesion involves both amygdala and hippocampus and their connections to thalamus, as in Mishkin, 1982; [3] Lesion is situated in the anterior thalamus and damages both the ventral amygdalofugal pathway (from amygdala to dorsomedial thalamus) and the mammillothalamic tract (from mammillary bodies to anterior thalamus); [4] large hemorrhagic lesion of basal forebrain from aneurysmic rupture/repair damages elements of the medial circuit (cingulate cortex, and connections from thalamus), and lateral circuit (connections and cortical targets of fibers from dorsomedial thalamus); [5] smaller, neurochemical lesion affecting cholinergic input from basal forebrain to medial and lateral limbic circuits. Adapted from Bauer (2008), used with permission.

involved in the perisylvian language system are depicted in Figure 4.4 and Table 4.1, which summarize the key clinical characteristics and underlying anatomy responsible for major perisylvian language syndromes.

The initial perceptual steps of language processing enable phonological (sound-based) sequences to be identified and comprehended as words (Wernicke's area and adjacent *Brodmann areas* 37, 39, and 40). Damage to these regions produces a fluent aphasia (because motor-articulatory regions in the frontal lobe are intact) characterized primarily by a disturbance in comprehension (e.g., Wernicke's aphasia). Articulation of speech sounds and production of words and sentences depends on a variety of regions, including the face area of the primary motor cortex, but begins in Broca's area, which plans and activates sequences of speech sounds. Damage to this region produces a nonfluent aphasia with relatively intact comprehension, known as Broca's aphasia or its variants. Repetition of language requires that the phonological representations generated by processing in Wernicke's area be converted to motor-articulatory sequences and utterances in Broca's area. The two regions are connected by a large subcortical white matter pathway, the arcuate fasciculus, which is volumetrically larger in the left hemisphere than in the right. Damage restricted to the arcuate fasciculus produces a disproportionate deficit in repetition, with relative sparing of comprehension and fluency, a syndrome known as conduction aphasia. Although

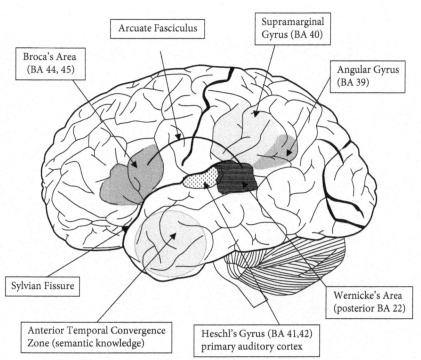

FIGURE 4.4 Perisylvian Language Areas

disconnection of the arcuate fasciculus is the classic interpretation of this syndrome, recent work suggests that the anatomic substrate may be somewhat more complex.

Although these three key perisylvian regions are critical to basic language abilities, they do not function in isolation and perform their functions only by extensive connections with other cortical regions. There are extensive reciprocal connections with broad areas of visual, auditory, and motor cortex that enable functions key to language processing and that provide the substrate for understanding meaning, processing visual language stimuli (reading), performing meaningful actions (praxis), selecting morphemes for use in speech, establishing the intention to communicate, and using language pragmatically in everyday life. For example, Broca's area connects with other frontal lobe regions, including the prefrontal, premotor, and supplementary motor areas, and intact interconnections among these regions appear necessary for processing syntax and grammatical structure of language. Wernicke's area connects reciprocally with the supramarginal and angular gyri in the parietal lobe, a system important not only for language comprehension but also for writing and for mapping sounds to meaning (lexical semantics). Connections with specific visual areas in the inferior temporal lobe critical to the recognition of word forms is one part of the substrate for grapheme-phoneme conversion, key to reading ability. Callosal connections enable the language-nondominant hemisphere to participate in the language-processing network, thus integrating linguistic processing with prosodic information communicating the emotional aspects of speech.

Prosody is defined as the use of tone, pitch, rhythm, and other vocal intonation patterns to convey both meaning (e.g., marking a question vs. an exclamation) and emotion (e.g., marking specific states such as anger, sadness, or mirth) in language. Prosody is primarily processed in the right hemisphere, where focal lesions can produce prosodic syndromes (aprosodias) that bear striking similarity to their contralateral language-based counterparts. For example, damage to the inferior right frontal lobe produces a deficit in expressing emotional prosody in speech that is analogous to Broca's aphasia, while posterior temporal-parietal lesions produce a deficit in prosody comprehension with fluent production, akin to Wernicke's aphasia.

TABLE 4.1 Localization and Characteristics of Aphasic Syndromes

Syndrome	Symptom	Deficit	Lesion Location
Broca's Aphasia	↓speech production; sparse, halting speech, missing function words, syntactic deficits, right hemiparesis (often)	Impaired speech planning and production	Posterior aspect of third frontal convolution (damage to adjacent motor fibers may produce right hemiparesis)
Wernicke's Aphasia	↓ auditory comprehension, fluent speech, paraphasias, poor repetition and naming, may have right homonymous hemianopia	Impaired representation of the sound structure of words	Posterior half of the superior (first) temporal gyrus (geniculostriate white matter damage may produce right homonymous hemianopia)
Anomic Aphasia	↓single word production, marked for common nouns; repetition and comprehension relatively intact	Impaired storage or access to lexicon	Inferior parietal lobe or connections within perisylvian language areas; many other forms of aphasia evolve to anomia in recovery
Transcortical Motor Aphasia	Disturbed spontaneous speech similar to Broca's; relatively preserved repetition and comprehension	Disconnection between conceptual word/ sentence representations in perisylvian region and motor speech areas	Deep white matter tracts connecting BA to parietal lobe; usually caused by anterior watershed infarcts
Transcortical Sensory Aphasia	Disturbance in word comprehension with relatively intact repetition	Disturbed activation of word meanings despite normal recognition of auditorily presented words	White matter tracts connecting parietal and temporal lobe; usually caused by posterior watershed infarcts
Conduction Aphasia	Disturbance of repetition and spontaneous speech, phonemic paraphasia	Disconnection between sound patterns and speech production mechanisms	Arcuate fasciculus; connections between Broca's and Wernicke's areas

An understanding of cortico-cortical language connections is critical for understanding several rare but classic syndromes affecting the person's ability to use language in important everyday tasks (see also Chapter 5, Domains of Neuropsychological Function and Related Neurobehavioral Disorders, and Chapter 26, Stroke). In these cases, the damaged area involved the left visual cortex, thus producing a right homonymous hemianopia, and extended anteriorly to affect interhemispheric crossing fibers in the splenium of the corpus callosum. These lesions prevented information that was appropriately perceived in the right hemisphere/left visual field from accessing the perisylvian language areas in the left hemisphere. This lesion produces the classic syndromes of alexia without agraphia (the inability to read in the context of spared writing ability), color "agnosia" (or, more properly, color naming disturbances), and optic aphasia. In optic aphasia, the patient cannot name a visually apprehended object but can demonstrate its use, presumably because more anterior callosal fibers connecting the intact visual areas to left hemisphere praxis mechanisms are intact. Similarly, the syndrome of "pure word deafness," in which the patient cannot understand language but can identify nonverbal sounds such as a chirping bird or jingling keys, results from white matter disconnection of fibers from left and right auditory receptive areas (Heschl's gyrus, BA 41, 42 in each hemisphere) from Wernicke's area in the left hemisphere.

Neuroanatomy of Frontal/Executive Skills

The frontal lobes are widely regarded as critical to high-level executive functions, a class of ability that is most highly developed in humans but which is represented to varying degrees in nonhuman primates. The frontal lobes are phylogenetically the youngest regions of the brain and are the last to fully develop and interconnect with other brain regions in ontogeny. Insight into the anatomic systems in which the frontal lobes participate can be gained by considering the following facts:

- Vast regions of the DLPFC have large granular layers (layer IV), suggesting strong and broadly distributed interactions with subcortical networks involving the thalamus.

- Architectonically, frontal cortex also contains regions with large layers II and III, suggesting the presence of extensive cortico-cortical connectivity.

These facts suggest that frontal regions participate in extensive cortico-cortical networks, interacting with parietal lobe systems involved in attention, proprioception, and visuomotor interaction with the environment, and with temporal lobe memory and emotional systems. They also participate in reciprocal circuits involving the basal ganglia and thalamus. Such interactions allow modulation and volitional control to be exerted on perceptual, emotional, and action systems toward the completion of goal-directed action.

Frontal-Subcortical Interactions: Cortico-Striatal-Pallidal-Thalamo-Cortical Loops

The frontal lobes participate extensively in cortical-subcortical networks involved in behavioral activation and selection. These networks allow for the flexible selection and activation of cortical regions necessary to perform cognitive work. This overall process has been referred to as "selective engagement." When summoning up the name of a familiar friend, cortical regions involved in storage and retrieval of personal names, together with regions involved in formulating and executing the motor program that gives rise to the spoken name, must be engaged while other regions that engage competing activities must be inhibited. Selective engagement involves a key aspect of frontal lobe anatomy that is embodied in the concept of a *cortical-striatal-pallidal-thalamo-cortical loop*. The basic architecture, described first in a seminal paper by Alexander, Delong, and Strick (1986), is depicted in Figure 4.5, and the key loops relevant to cognition are described in Table 4.2. Each loop reflects functional specialization for different cognitive/emotional domains; each loop differs in its origin in particular regions of frontal lobe, and each involves different target nuclei in the striatum, pallidum, and thalamus, although the basic architecture is the same in all loops. The special role played by basal ganglia structures in modulating the activity of thalamic and cortical components of these re-entrant loops is critical.

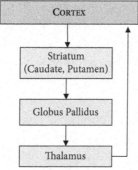

FIGURE 4.5 Core Architecture of Subcortical Loops in Frontal Lobe

TABLE 4.2 Cortico-Striatal-Pallidal-Thalamo-Cortical Loops Most Relevant to Cognition

Channel	Orbitofrontal	Anterior Cingulate/ Limbic	Dorsolateral Prefrontal	Oculomotor	Motor
Cortical Input	Lateral orbitofrontal, temporal cortex, anterior cingulate	Temporal cortex, hippocampus, amygdala	Posterior parietal, premotor	Posterior parietal, prefrontal	Somatosensory motor premotor
Striatal Input Target	Ventro-medial caudate (head)	Nucleus accumbens, ventral striatum	Caudate head	Caudate body	Putamen
Output Nucleus	GPi, SNr	Ventral pallidum, GPi; SNr	GPi, SNr	GPi, SNr	GPi, SNr
Thalamic Target	MD, VA	MD, VA	VA, MD	VA, MD	VL, VA
Cortical Target	Orbitofrontal cortex	Anterior cingulate, orbitofrontal cortex	Prefrontal cortex	Frontal eye fields	SMA, premotor, primary motor
Presumed Function	Response- reward learning	Emotion regulation	Executive functions	Eye movement subserving cognition	Motor control

NOTE: GPi = globus pallidus, internal segment; SNr = substantia nigra pars reticulata; VL = ventrolateral, VA = ventral anterior; MD = mediodorsal. Note that each loop projects to slightly different sub-regions of GPi and SNr, in the globus pallidus and to subcomponents of VA, MD, and VA in the thalamus. Adapted from Alexander, et al. (1986) and Blumenfeld (2010).

Frontal Lobe Attentional Mechanisms

A key aspect of attention is that it must be volitionally utilized in the service of ongoing goals, plans, and cognitive demands that evolve over time. Basic perceptual mechanisms of object-based and spatial attention are thus dependent on a complex frontoparietal network. "Top-down" attention requires interaction with frontal lobe regions involved in volitional deployment of attention and in establishing behavioral priorities in the face of conflicting demands. Posner and Rothbart (2007) indicate that there are three interconnected systems for attention: one for orienting to stimuli, one for alerting, and one for executive aspects of attention. Orienting refers to the tuning of perceptual systems to incoming stimuli so that relevant information from sensory input can be selected for further processing. It is primarily dependent on acetylcholine and involves a functional system consisting of the superior colliculus, pulvinar thalamic nucleus, posterior temporoparietal cortex, and a region within the frontal lobes known as the frontal eye fields (BA 8, involved in volitional control of eye movements). Alerting is a state of sensitivity to incoming stimuli. It is modulated by norepinephrine and depends primarily on ascending sensory inputs from the thalamus. Executive attention involves monitoring and resolving conflicts among thoughts, feelings, and behaviors. It is primarily dependent on dopamine and involves key structures including the anterior cingulate cortex and DLPFC.

Interactions between frontal lobe and posterior perceptual systems intricately balance attentional deployment and sensory tuning to result in the selection of appropriate stimuli for further processing. Sensory signals arrive at frontal and parietal cortices, having been preprocessed by superior colliculi and pulvinar, providing "bottom-up" information that is biased toward salient environmental stimuli. In turn, top-down biases from parietal lobe (which provides visuomotor frames of reference) and frontal lobe (which provides the substrate for working memory and goal setting) are transmitted to colliculi, pulvinar, and frontal eye fields, such that any complex attentional act is a combination of bottom-up and top-down influences. Evidence suggests that a dorsal frontoparietal system forms the cortical substrate of top-down attention, whereas a more ventral frontoparietal system is involved in target detection in the sensory environment.

Frontal Lobes and Working Memory

The seminal neuroscientific work establishing the neural substrate for working memory was conducted by Goldman-Rakic, who, through an elegant series of primate studies, showed that functionally separate working memory subsystems exist in DLPFC. These studies reveal populations of neurons that are silent during stimulation or response execution, but are selectively active during the delay period of working memory tasks and thus responsible for keeping information "active" or "on-line" during this time. Neuronal subpopulations in the dorsal prefrontal cortex (arcuate sulcus; *Brodmann area* 46) code spatial information, whereas others in the ventral prefrontal cortex (inferior prefrontal convexity; *Brodmann area* 12) are selectively active during object working memory tasks.

Key anatomic facts concerning working memory can be summarized as follows:

- A dorsal (spatial)–ventral (object-based) distinction appears to exist in frontal working memory systems just as it does in posterior cortex.
- Dorsal components of the frontal working memory system are preferentially connected to structures in the dorsal visual stream and vice-versa.

Some researchers argue that the dorsal–ventral distinction reflects domain-specificity (spatial- vs. object-based), whereas others argue for process-specificity. The latter view that ventral regions are preferentially activated when the task requires sequential organization and storage (e.g., as in forward digit span), while more dorsal regions are activated when the task additionally requires mental manipulation and reorganization (e.g., as in letter-number sequencing). Although the anatomic facts are clear, ongoing work is needed to decide between these alternatives, and there appears to be evidence supporting both domain- and process-specific views.

Basics of Neurotransmitter Projection Systems and Function

Neurochemical projection systems provide widespread innervations of many of the functional brain systems already described, and a basic understanding of neurotransmitter systems is essential in understanding basic neuronal function, neurochemical relationships among different brain systems, and in appreciating how psychopharmacological interventions designed to affect neurotransmitter activity might affect cognition. We have already discussed key contributions of acetylcholine to regions subserving memory; other neurotransmitter systems have similar relationships with other domains of neurocognitive function. This treatment is necessarily cursory and brief. We will not attempt a review of the basics of neural transmission, nor will the effects of specific drugs be discussed beyond the most cursory detail. The reader is referred to the classic text by Stahl (2008) for a comprehensive and readable review of this fascinating field. Blumenfeld (2010) also briefly describes the anatomic localization of ascending neurotransmitter systems, and we rely heavily on his excellent summary in the section that follows (see Table 4.3).

TABLE 4.3 Major Neurotransmitter Systems of the Brain

Transmitter	Origin	Projection	Role	Cognitive Relevance
Acetylcholine	Pontomesencephalic region	Intralaminar nucleus of thalamus	Indirect excitation of thalamo-cortical projection	Attention, memory, regulation of thalamic output
	Basal forebrain; Nucleus basalis of Meynert (nbM); medial septum (MS); nucleus of the diagonal band (nDB)	Widespread cortical (nbM); hippocampus (MS, nDB)	Excitation/facilitation	Attention, learning, memory
Norepinephrine/Noradrenaline	Locus coeruleus	Widespread cortical	Excitation/facilitation	Attentional shifting; arousal
	Lateral tegmental area	Widespread cortical	Excitation/facilitation	Mood; sleep-wake cycle
Serotonin	Rostral raphe	Forebrain (thalamus, basal ganglia, cortex)	Post-synaptic inhibition	Mood Arousal
	Dorsal raphe	Cerebellum, medulla, spinal cord	Post-synaptic inhibition	Pain, respiration, temperature, motor control
Dopamine	Mesostriatal; substantia nigra pars compacta (SNpc)	Striatum (caudate and putamen)	Mixed	Motor regulation; thalamic gating
	Mesolimbic; ventral tegmental area (VTA)	Medial temporal lobe, amygdala, cingulate gyrus, nucleus accumbens	Mixed	Memory, reward systems
	Mesocortical; VTA	Cortical/frontal lobe	Mixed	Executive function, working memory, "top-down" attention, motor initiation
	Tubero-infundibular; Hypothalamus	Pituitary gland	Excitation/facilitation	Lactation, menstruation, sexual behavior
GABA	Widely distributed	Widely distributed	Inhibitory	Broad neuromodulatory functions
Glutamate	Widely distributed	Widely distributed	Post-synaptic excitation	Broad excitatory functions

Acetylcholine

Acetylcholine is the primary efferent neurotransmitter of the peripheral nervous system and plays a more limited neuromodulatory role in the CNS. Cholinergic neurons are found primarily in two regions:

- The pontomesencephalic region
- The nuclear groups of the BF

The former group of neurons project primarily to the intralaminar nuclei of the thalamus, providing modulatory input, then to widespread areas of cortex. These neurons generally incite cortical arousal through indirect projections from thalamus to cortex. The neurons arising from the BF (nucleus basalis of Meynert) project to widespread cortical regions. Cholinergic input to the hippocampus is provided by projections from the medial septal nuclei and the nucleus of the diagonal band. In the CNS, acetylcholine acts to facilitate cortical activity subserving memory, attention, and other higher cognitive processes. Two subclasses of acetylcholine-containing receptors (muscarinic and nicotinic) have been described. Muscarinic receptors mediate the main cognitive effects attributed to cholinergic pathways, with measurable effects on attention, learning, and short-term memory. Nicotinic receptors trigger rapid neural and neuromuscular transmission within the sympathetic and parasympathetic nervous system and at the neuromuscular junction. Drugs with strong anticholinergic properties (e.g., antihistamines, first-generation antipsychotics, and tricyclic antidepressants) thus may exert negative effects on cognitive performance in these areas, particularly when administered to the elderly or others with reduced cognitive and or cerebral reserve.

Norepinephrine (Noradrenaline)

Adrenergic neurons exist primarily in the locus coeruleus and lateral tegmental area of the pons and medulla. Ascending projections from these regions innervate the entire cerebral cortex and can be inhibitory or excitatory. These projections can facilitate cortical activity associated with attentional shifting. Norepinephrine (NE), sometimes described as a "stress hormone," plays a role in modulating sleep-wake cycles, attention, and mood and may have a role in modulating pain. Its role in neuropsychiatric disorders such as depression, bipolar disorder, and in anxiety disorders such as obsessive-compulsive disorder (OCD) is well established. Cholinergic and serotonergic activation can inhibit NE neurotransmission. Drugs commonly prescribed for ADHD (methylphenidate [Ritalin, Concerta], amphetamine/dextroamphetamine [Adderall]) increase levels of NE and dopamine, whereas atomoxetine (Strattera) is a specific norepinephrine reuptake inhibitor that only affects NE.

Serotonin

Neurons containing serotonin are found in the raphe nuclei of the midbrain, pons, and medulla. The rostral raphe projects to the entire forebrain, including the thalamus, cortex, and basal ganglia. Such projections play a role in several psychiatric syndromes including anxiety, depression, OCD, aggressive behavior, and certain eating disorders. The dorsal raphe projects to the cerebellum, medulla, and spinal cord, regulating pain, breathing, temperature regulation, and motor control. Serotonin neurotransmission is quite complex, with at least four categories of receptor, each with further varieties (Stahl, 2008). Drugs affecting serotonin metabolism are commonly prescribed for depression, generalized anxiety, and social phobia. Some (e.g., fluoxetine [Prozac], sertraline [Zoloft]) are serotonin-specific reuptake inhibitors, whereas others (e.g., venlafaxine [Effexor]) effect reuptake inhibition in the serotonergic and noradrenergic system. These drugs may be used in combination with serotonin 2A antagonists (e.g., trazodone [Desyrel], mirtazapine [Remeron]), or other agents to treat refractory depression.

Dopamine

Dopamine-containing neurons exist primarily in the substantia nigra pars compacta (SNpc) and in the ventral tegmental area. The projection system for dopamine is in some ways more complex than for other neurotransmitters and is generally organized into three separate subsystems. The mesostriatal system arises from SNpc and projects to the striatum (caudate and putamen). This is the pathway implicated in Parkinson's disease, and dysfunction here can produce disabling motor and nonmotor symptoms. The mesolimbic pathway originates in the ventral tegmental area and projects to the medial temporal lobe, amygdala, cingulate gyrus, and nucleus accumbens. This pathway also plays a key role in reward functions and has been implicated in addictive behavior. Overactivity of this pathway has been associated with the positive symptoms of schizophrenia, such as delusions and hallucinations, which respond well to dopamine-serotonin 2A antagonist drugs (e.g., clozapine [Clozaril], quetiapine [Seroquel], risperidone [Risperdal]). The mesocortical system arises mainly from the ventral tegmental area and projects primarily to cortical regions of the frontal lobe. This system plays a key role in executive functions, working memory, top-down attention, and initiation of motor activity. Dysfunction in this system can produce some of the negative symptoms of schizophrenia, as well as dysexecutive syndrome and bradykinesia.

Other Neurotransmitters

Many other pathways in addition to those mentioned here may play a role in alertness, cognition, mood regulation, memory, and other functions. Stahl (2008) lists 63 molecules that have proven or putative action as neurotransmitters in the brain, including pituitary peptides, circulating hormones, hypothalamic-releasing hormones, amino acids, opioid peptides, and other classes. In this regard, it is important to recognize that knowledge of chemical neurotransmission is a rapidly evolving field.

- *Gamma-aminobutyric acid (GABA)* Although most of the previously described molecules are excitatory or facilitatory of cortical function, GABA is one key inhibitory transmitter of significant importance to memory, anxiety/arousal, and neuromodulation. GABA-ergic neurons participate in short- and long-range inhibitory projections that innervate many of the same areas as other neurotransmitters and provide counteracting inhibitory input. The balance of GABA-ergic influences, together with the action of other neurotransmitters, is a key basis of neuromodulation. It is generally believed that certain GABA-ergic neurons located in the reticular nucleus of the thalamus may be critical for gating thalamocortical interactions and for regulating sleep and arousal. Similarly, GABA-ergic neurons in the BF regulate attentional shifting and alternation between response–reinforcement contingencies. Many antianxiety drugs act to enhance GABA-ergic neurotransmission, thus offsetting abnormally strong excitatory influences in these disorders.

- *Glutamate* The most abundant excitatory neurotransmitter in the brain, glutamate is widely distributed and plays a key role in learning and memory, and the glutamatergic NMDA receptor is implicated in processes of long-term potentiation and *synaptic plasticity/neurogenesis*, keys to the development of new experience-dependent memories. The CNS has well-developed mechanisms for rapid removal of glutamate from the synapse because excess glutamatergic activity can lead to *excitotoxicity* and cell death, and it is part of the ischemic cascade that has been implicated in stroke and in neurodegenerative diseases such as Alzheimer disease (AD) and amyotrophic lateral sclerosis (ALS). Memantine (Namenda), an N-methyl-D-aspartate (NMDA) receptor antagonist, is widely prescribed for the treatment of AD. It may seem paradoxical that antagonizing a receptor that is important in learning and long-term potentiation (LTP) would be of benefit in AD. NMDA receptor antagonists may be able to enhance cognition by selectively inhibiting pathological aspects of glutamatergic activation while preserving the physiological activation of NMDA receptors, thus restoring LTP.

Essential Neuropharmacology

This very brief review of the major neurochemical projection systems should give the reader some idea of how abnormal or imbalanced neurotransmission might affect certain domains of cognitive function. For example, reductions in dopaminergic neurotransmission in the mesostriatal and mesocortical systems can be seen as key players in producing both motor and nonmotor aspects of Parkinson's disease, whereas disruptions in cholinergic neurotransmission due to damage to the basal ganglia can affect widespread cortical and limbic projections of these systems, producing characteristic neurobehavioral syndromes such as amnesia, dysexecutive syndromes, and frontally mediated confabulation.

Although most neuropsychologists do not prescribe medications, competent practice requires a working knowledge of neurochemical–neurocognitive relationships, including basic knowledge of the effects of common medications on these systems. As described earlier, many drugs prescribed by neurologists and psychiatrists are used explicitly for their expected impact on neurotransmission and behavior. However, many medications prescribed for the treatment of systemic illness have side effects with measurable neurobehavioral implications. For example, many common medications used for treatment of hypertension, cardiac arrhythmia, glaucoma, and migraine have broad effects on β-adrenergic function that may or may not be part and parcel of their intended mechanism of action. Antihistamines may produce sedation and cognitive inefficiency through their effects on cholinergic and serotonergic systems. Benzodiazepines, when used to treat insomnia and other sleep disturbances, can affect daytime cognition, including memory and psychomotor speed by potentiating $GABA_A$ function. Understanding the downstream effects of common medications provides the competent neuropsychologist with alternative hypotheses that must be considered in conceptualizing the individual patient's profile of abilities and deficits. Achieving a simultaneous understanding of anatomico-clinical and neuropharmacological effects on neurobehavioral function, even in the most common diseases we encounter, is undoubtedly a complex and ill-defined area of neuropsychological practice and certainly one in which continuing education in neuropharmacology, biological psychiatry, and neuroanatomy is essential for maintenance of competency as the field evolves.

Relevant Definitions

Akinetic mutism A neurologic condition resulting from bilateral medial frontal lobe injury in which the patient does not move or speak but remains aware of ongoing events. It can be seen in stroke syndromes, tumors of the olfactory groove, and in the final stage of certain neurodegenerative diseases.

Anatomico-clinical correlation The experimental or clinical method of establishing direct associations between anatomic damage to the brain and sensory, motor, emotional, or cognitive impairments. Such associations can be established through careful case analysis or experimental study and involve the use of both neuropsychological methods and techniques for characterizing and localizing lesions. The core knowledge base of clinical neuropsychology depends in part on precise anatomico-clinical correlations.

Basal forebrain (BF) A group of structures located in the vicinity of the ventromedial frontal lobe, anterior to the caudate and putamen. Comprised of the nucleus basalis, diagonal band of Broca, substantia innominata, and medial septal nuclei, it is the major source of cholinergic input throughout the brain. Damage to the BF is associated with profound memory loss with confabulation, the latter of which is likely associated with neighboring frontal lobe damage.

Brodmann areas A region of cortex defined by its cytoarchitectonics (cellular structure and organization). Fifty-two separate areas were described in this way by Brodmann in 1909 and have been refined through clinical and basic neuroscience research ever since. The Brodmann system remains the most frequently cited, widely known, and generally useful system of cortical organization today.

Cortico-cortical connections In general, depictions of white matter connections within the brain adopt the form of "from (region)–to (region)." Thus, cortico-cortical connections begin in one region of cortex and end in another. Practically any connection can be depicted in this way. Cortico-striatal connections project from a region of cortex to the striatum (caudate and putamen). Thalamo-cortical projections start in the thalamus and project to cortex. The route of a complex pathway can be similarly depicted, as in a cortico-striatal-pallidal-thalamo-cortical loop. Fiber tracts can also be identified by reference to particular structures in which they are found or to the functions they perform. For example, "commissural" fibers are found in the anterior commissure and corpus callosum, where they cross the midline and connect homologous areas in the right and left hemisphere. "Association" fibers are short cortico-cortical connections linking primary sensory areas with their surrounding association cortices.

Cortico-striatal-pallidal-thalamo-cortical loop An essential feature of cortical-subcortical interaction in a variety of cognitive domains. Cortical activity is modulated by connections from cortex, through inhibitory and excitatory structures in the basal forebrain and thalamus, and back to cortex as a way of engaging a cortical region needed for task performance or of inhibiting another region whose function would interfere with processing or compete for output. The process of activating cortical regions for task performance is known as selective engagement.

Disconnection theory A prominent anatomico-clinical theory in neuropsychology which describes certain neurobehavioral syndromes as the result of damage to white matter connections as opposed to cortical processors. The resulting syndrome occurs because two or more normally functioning processors are incapable of cooperating in performing a complex task because their connections have been severed. Prominent disconnection syndromes include alexia without agraphia, optic aphasia, and impaired naming of objects in the left hemispace due to callosal disconnection of the right hemisphere from left-hemisphere language regions.

Dorsal/ventral visual systems After being processed in primary visual area and unimodal visual association cortex, visual information takes two distinct routes in interacting with other, more anterior cortical regions. A ventral route courses through the inferior temporal lobe and is important for form and object identification. A dorsal route courses through the superior temporal cortex and parietal lobe and is important for spatial processing and visuomotor interaction. The "two visual systems" concept is highly influential in contemporary neuroscience and accounts for a variety of neuropsychological syndromes, including visual agnosia, spatial neglect, and attentional dysfunction. The "dorsal-ventral" distinction also appears in other anatomic regions, including working memory systems in the frontal lobe, suggesting that this anatomic feature of brain organization may have widespread functional implications.

Excitotoxicity A pathological process by which nerve cells are damaged or destroyed by excessive stimulation by neurotransmitters such as glutamate. It is thought to be a key factor in the CNS response to spinal cord injury, traumatic brain injury, and neurodegenerative disease. It may also be involved in CNS injury after medical events such as hypoglycemia and status epilepticus.

Lateral limbic circuit One of two limbic circuits subserving memory in the medial temporal lobe, diencephalon, and frontal lobe. The circuit is as follows: Amygdala → dorsomedial thalamic nucleus (via amygdalofugal pathway) → orbitofrontal lobe → amygdala (via uncinate fasciculus). It must be damaged along with the medial limbic circuit for dense amnesia to occur.

Medial limbic circuit (Papez circuit) This circuit, described by Papez in 1938 in the context of emotion, is one of two limbic circuits subserving memory in the medial temporal lobe and diencephalon. The circuit is as follows: Hippocampus → mammillary bodies (via the fornix) → anterior thalamic nucleus (via the mammillothalamic tract) → cingulate gyrus → hippocampus (via cingulum and parahippocampal cortex). It must be damaged along with the lateral limbic circuit for dense amnesia to occur.

Neurogenesis The birth and proliferation of new neurons, most active during pre- and perinatal development. In certain regions of the brain (e.g., dentate gyrus of the hippocampus), neurogenesis continues into adulthood and is thought to be a critical basis for the formation of new memories and for experience-dependent neuroplasticity.

Neuroplasticity/synaptic plasticity Changes in neural pathways and synapses due to changes in behavior, environment, or neurochemical processes. Neuroplasticity is critical to normal development of CNS-dependent abilities and is critical to recovery from brain damage. The concept of the brain as a "plastic" organ has replaced earlier conceptualizations that no further structural development or repair was possible after a certain point in development and is an important idea in contemporary advancements in recovery of function, neurorehabilitation, and neural repair. The concept of "experience-dependent neuroplasticity" refers to changes that result from exposure to enriched environments, behavioral practice, or other environmental stimulation.

Trisynaptic circuit The pattern of synaptic transmission within the hippocampus, which describes three linearly organized synapses. The circuit is as follows: Entorhinal cortex → dentate gyrus (DG) via the perforant path (synapse 1), DG → CA3 via mossy fibers (synapse 2), CA3 → CA1 via Schaffer collaterals (synapse 3). Although a simple and easily comprehended pathway, recent anatomic work has found many complexities to this presumed structure and has questioned whether it appropriately represents the actual pathway by which information is transmitted and processed within the hippocampus, or whether the function of the medial temporal lobe memory system is the result of densely reciprocal interconnections between and within structures.

Two-system theory of amnesia The contemporary viewpoint that argues that the necessary and sufficient lesion producing human amnesia involves damage to two limbic circuits, one (medial) involving the hippocampus, and the other (lateral) involving the amygdala. According to this view, dense amnesia occurs only when both circuits are damaged, whereas less severe memory impairment may occur with partial damage. This theory provides an integrative account of how and why amnesia can be produced by lesions to the medial temporal lobe, diencephalon, and basal forebrain structures.

Unimodal/polymodal cortex Cortex devoted to processing information within a specific sensory modality (vision, audition, tactile). Thus, for example, areas 17–19 are unimodal visual cortex. Unimodal association cortices, located adjacent to primary sensory areas, eventually project to regions of cortex that integrate information from multiple modalities, enabling more complex modes of thought including semantic processing. These convergence regions are referred to as heteromodal or supramodal because the nature of their processing utilizes and develops representations that go beyond simple sensory input channels.

Functional Neuroanatomy and Essential Neuropharmacology Questions

NOTE: Questions 1, 43, 88 and 123 on the First Full-Length Practice Examination, Questions 10, 44, 70, and 108 on the Second Full-Length Practice Examination, Questions 17, 65, 97, and 124 on the Third Full-Length Practice Examination, and Questions 20, 49, 78, and 100 on the Fourth Full-Length Practice Examination are from this chapter.

FOUNDATIONS

1. You are looking at a slice of a brain scan that is oriented so that it depicts one hemisphere with the frontal lobe on the left of the scan and the occipital lobe on the right. You are looking at a _____.

    (a) coronal slice

    (b) sagittal slice

    (c) horizontal slice

    (d) vertical slice

2. The parietal lobe is _____ to the temporal lobe.

    (a) lateral

    (b) ventral

    (c) caudal

    (d) dorsal

3. A patient with a lesion of the ventral occipitotemporal area is most likely to experience an impairment in _____.

    (a) auditory comprehension

    (b) visuospatial skills

    (c) face recognition

    (d) writing ability

4. Which of the following is a cortical region directly implicated in episodic memory processing?

    (a) hippocampus

    (b) perirhinal cortex

    (c) preoptic area

    (d) lateral tegmental area

5. Which of the following structures is not part of the diencephalon?

    (a) hypothalamus

    (b) epithalamus

    (c) extended amygdala

    (d) subthalamus

6. The classic interpretation of conduction aphasia is that it involves damage to the _____, thus disconnecting Broca's and Wernicke's areas.

    (a) arcuate fasciculus

    (b) supramarginal gyrus

    (c) cortical watershed areas

    (d) Heschl's gyrus

7. Regions that appear important for mapping sounds to meaning in language include _____.

    (a) the inferior temporoparietal region and hippocampus

    (b) the supramarginal and angular gyri

    (c) Heschl's gyrus and anterior temporal pole

    (d) the supplementary motor area and dorsolateral prefrontal cortex (DLPFC)

8. Dysfunction of the mesolimbic dopamine pathway has been associated with _____.

    (a) negative symptoms of schizophrenia

    (b) bradykinesia

    (c) impaired reward functioning

    (d) nonfluent aphasia

9. Which of the following statements about glutamate is false?

    (a) It is the most abundant excitatory neurotransmitter in the brain.

    (b) It inhibits the formation of new memories.

    (c) Too much glutamate can cause excitotoxicity and cell death.

    (d) Glutamate has been implicated in stroke and Alzheimer's disease.

10. In the brain (above the spinal cord), "ventral" means the same as ____.

    (a) anterior   (c) inferior

    (b) posterior   (d) superior

11. A piece of cortex with a very large layer IV most likely ____.

    (a) contains many cholinergic neurons   (c) is from a sensory region

    (b) is from the primary motor area   (d) is in the basal ganglia

12. Which of the following is not part of the basal forebrain?

    (a) septal area   (c) substantia innominata

    (b) dorsomedial nucleus   (d) red nucleus of the stria terminalis

13. Fluent aphasia results from lesions in the ____.

    (a) anterior inferior left frontal lobe   (c) left dorsolateral prefrontal cortex

    (b) inferior left occipitotemporal junction (d) posterior left temporal lobe

14. Bilateral damage to the DLPFC produces ____.

    (a) akinetic mutism   (c) disinhibited emotion and personality

    (b) a disorder of executive attention   (d) apathy

15. Lesions in the superior (dorsal) aspects of the DLPFC produce deficits in ____.

    (a) object-based working memory   (c) storage capacity of working memory

    (b) spatial working memory   (d) object recognition

Functional Neuroanatomy and Essential Neuropharmacology Answers

1. **B—sagittal slice** *The scan is described such that you are looking at the brain from the side. As described, the cut must be sagittal, perpendicular to the ground and running in a rostral-caudal (anterior-posterior) plane.*

   Reference: Blumenfeld, H. (2010). *Neuroanatomy through clinical cases* (2nd ed., p. 17). Sunderland, MA: Sinauer Associates.

2. **D—dorsal** *Dorsal means "toward the back" in the spinal cord, but above the brainstem, the neuraxis undergoes a 90-degree bend such that its meaning in the brain is essentially "superior" or" upper." Caudal means "toward the front," or "anterior" in the brain. Thus, dorsal is the only possible answer to this question.*

   Reference: Blumenfeld, H. (2010). *Neuroanatomy through clinical cases* (2nd ed., p. 17). Sunderland, MA: Sinauer Associates.

3. **C—face recognition** *The ventral occipitotemporal area refers to that region of cortex at the border between visual association area and posterior temporal lobe. Reference to the "ventral" portion of this region means that it is part of the ventral visual pathway, which is important for object, face, and form/shape recognition.*

References:
(a) Bauer, R. (2012). Agnosia. In K. Heilman & E. Valenstein (Eds.), *Clinical neuropsychology* (5th ed.). New York, NY: Oxford University Press.
(b) Ungerleider, L. G., & Mishkin, M. (1982). Two cortical visual systems. In D. Ingle, A. Milner, & R. Mansfield (Eds.), *Analysis of visual behavior* (pp. 549–586). Cambridge: MIT Press.

4. **B—perirhinal cortex** *The perirhinal cortex is on the basolateral temporal lobe surface and is one of the neocortical regions that project to the hippocampal memory system. It, along with the parahippocampal cortex, was implicated in memory in a second-generation animal model proposed after Mishkin by Zola-Morgan and colleagues. The hippocampus cannot be the correct answer because it is not a cortical structure.*

Reference: Zola-Morgan, S., Squire, L., Amaral, D., & Suzuki, W. (1989). Lesions of perirhinal and parahippocampal cortex that spare the amygdala and hippocampal formation produce severe memory impairment. *Journal of Neuroscience, 9,* 4355–4370.

5. **C—extended amygdala** *All structures within the diencephalon end with "thalamus" so the extended amygdala is the only possible answer.*

Reference: Mendoza, J., & Foundas, A. (2008). *Clinical neuroanatomy: A neurobehavioral approach.* New York, NY: Springer Science and Business.

6. **A—arcuate fasciculus** *Conduction aphasia involves a disruption of repetition with relatively spared verbal comprehension and verbal fluency. The classic interpretation is a disconnection between Broca's and Wernicke's areas, both of which are relatively intact.*

References:
(a) Benson, D. (1979). *Aphasia, alexia, and agraphia.* New York, NY: Churchill Livingstone.
(b) Benson, D., & Geschwind, N. (1985). Aphasia and related disorders: A clinical approach. In M.-M. Mesulam (Ed.), *Principles of behavioral neurology.* Philadelphia, PA: F.A. Davis.

7. **B—the supramarginal and angular gyri** *These cortical regions provide an interface between Wernicke's area and polymodal cortical areas that process meaning/semantics.*

References:
(a) Benson, D. (1979). *Aphasia, alexia, and agraphia.* New York, NY: Churchill Livingstone.
(b) Benson, D., & Geschwind, N. (1985). Aphasia and related disorders: A clinical approach. In M. M. Mesulam (Ed.), *Principles of behavioral neurology.* Philadelphia: F.A. Davis.

8. **C—impaired reward functioning** *Mesolimbic dopamine depletion has been associated with impaired reward functioning and overactivation of this system has been associated with* positive, not negative *symptoms of schizophrenia. Bradyphrenia is associated with impairment in mesostriatal, not mesolimbic, dopamine. Nonfluent aphasia is not specifically associated with the dopaminergic systems* per se.

Reference: Stahl, S. (2008). *Essential psychopharmacology: Neuroscientific basis and practical applications.* Cambridge, UK: Cambridge University Press.

9. **B—It inhibits the formation of new memories.** *Glutamatergic activity stimulates, rather than inhibits, new memory formation.*

Reference: Riedel, G., Platt, B., & Micheau, J. (2003). Glutamate receptor function in learning and memory. *Behavioral Brain Research, 140,* 1–47.

10. **C—inferior** *The planes of section take a 90-degree turn above the spinal cord, such that what is "ventral" (toward the front) in the lower body is now "inferior" (toward the bottom) in the brain.*

    Reference: Blumenfeld (2010). *Neuroanatomy through clinical cases* (2nd ed.). Sunderland, MA: Sinauer Associates.

11. **C—is from a sensory region** *Of all the alternatives listed, alternative C is most likely. A large Layer IV indicates extensive input from the thalamus, which would not be characteristic of cholinergic neurons generally and would not be characteristic of neurons in the motor strip or basal ganglia.*

    Reference: Blumenfeld, H. (2010). *Neuroanatomy through clinical cases* (2nd ed., pp. 29–30). Sunderland, MA: Sinauer Associates.

12. **B—dorsomedial nucleus** *The dorsomedial nucleus is part of the thalamus, not the basal forebrain. All of the other structures are part of the basal forebrain.*

    Reference: Botly, L. C. P., Baxter, M. G., & DeRosa, E. (2009). Basal forebrain and memory. In L. R. Squire (Ed.). *Encyclopedia of neuroscience* (pp. 47–52). Amsterdam, NL: Elsevier.

13. **D—posterior left temporal lobe** *Posterior lesions are associated with fluent aphasic syndromes. All of the other alternative lesions would either (a) not produce an aphasia, or (b) would produce a nonfluent aphasic syndrome.*

    Reference: Goodglass, H. (1993). *Understanding aphasia.* New York, NY: Academic Press.

14. **B—a disorder of executive attention** *Apathy and akinetic mutism would be produced by lesions to the medial sector of the frontal lobe, while disinhibition would be produced by orbitofrontal lesions. Top-down (executive) attention is the only alternative associated with DLPFC function.*

    Reference: Stuss, D. T. (2011). Functions of the frontal lobes: relation to executive functions. *Journal of the International Neuropsychological Society, 17,* 759–765.

15. **B—spatial working memory** *The text describes how working memory may be organized in a way similar to posterior cortex in terms of spatial vs. object-based processing. More dorsal lesions in DLPFC tend to produce problems in spatial, as opposed to object-based working memory, just as lesions in dorsal parietal lobe tend to produce disorders dominated by spatial dysfunction.*

    Reference: Goldman-Rakic, P. S. (1996). Regional and cellular fractionation of working memory. *Proceedings of the National Academy of Sciences of the United States of America, 93,* 13473–13480.

Recommended Readings

Alexander, G. E., DeLong, M. R., & Strick, P. L. (1986). Parallel organization of functionally segregated circuits linking basal ganglia and cortex. *Annual Review of Neuroscience, 9,* 357–381.

Bauer, R. M., & Asken, B. (2018). The three amnesias. In J. E. Morgan & J. H. Ricker (Eds.), *Textbook of clinical neuropsychology* (pp. 678–700). New York, NY: Psychology Press.

Blumenfeld, H. (2018). *Neuroanatomy through clinical cases* (2nd ed.). Sunderland, MA: Sinauer Associates.

Burke, S. N., Gaynor, L. S., Barnes, C. A., Bauer, R. M., Bizon, J. L., Roberson, E. D., & Ryan, L. (2018). Shared functions of perirhinal and parahippocampal cortices: Implications for cognitive aging. *Trends in Neurosciences, 41,* 349–359.

Mendoza, J., & Foundas, A. (2008). *Clinical neuroanatomy: A neurobehavioral approach.* New York, NY: Springer Science and Business.

Mishkin, M. (1982). A memory system in the monkey. *Philosophical Transactions of the Royal Society of London, 298*, 85–95.

Papez, J. (1937). A proposed mechanism of emotion. *Archives of Neurology and Psychiatry, 39*, 725–743.

Posner, M. I., & Rothbart, M. K. (2007). Research on attention networks as a model for the integration of psychological science. *Annual Review of Psychology, 58*, 1–23.

Stahl, S. M. (2008). *Stahl's essential psychopharmacology: Neuroscientific basis and practical applications.* Cambridge, UK: Cambridge University Press.

Websites

http://www.g2conline.org/2022 This is the G2C whole brain sponsored by Cold Spring Harbor Laboratories. It has links to cognition in addition to rotatable three-dimensional depictions of various brain structures.

http://library.med.utah.edu/kw/hyperbrain/syllabus/index.html Contains 14 chapters and diagrams, a glossary, quizzes, and practical exams.

https://pathology.duke.edu/files/neuroanat/nawr_index.html Numerous diagrams and brief descriptions of overall organization.

http://sig.biostr.washington.edu/projects/da/ This is the University of Washington's digital anatomist project. The diagrams are not the most graphically sophisticated, but there is a lot of explanation to go with them, making this a very useful site.

Blumenfeld's (2010) *Neuroanatomy through clinical cases* also offers extensive online material with purchase of the book.

5 Domains of Neuropsychological Function and Related Neurobehavioral Disorders

Lynn A. Schaefer and Nancy Hebben

Introduction

Neuropsychological evaluation requires the use of standardized instruments to assess cognitive functioning and behavior. Cognition comprises the mental processes associated with the awareness, acquisition, storage and retrieval, mental organization, comprehension, and communication of information. These neuropsychological processes can be organized into specific major domains presented here as intelligence, attention/concentration and processing speed, language, visuospatial, memory, executive functions, sensorimotor, and emotional/neuropsychiatric. Review of these domains reveals various models and neurobehavioral syndromes that are useful in characterizing the functioning of a patient and in understanding any associated pathology. Many standard test instruments measure more than one functional domain, and some disorders are associated with dysfunction within more than one domain. Where relevant, primary brain structures related to each domain and/or associated disorders are discussed here, but Chapter 4, Functional Neuroanatomy and Essential Neuropharmacology, covers functional neuroanatomy essentials in more depth.

Section 1: Intelligence

Definition

Although intelligence can be viewed as innate general cognitive functioning or capability, no unitary definition exists, and no unitary view as to how it should be measured predominates. Subsumed under intelligence are descriptions including, but not limited to, the ability to problem solve, think rationally but also abstractly, adapt to circumstances, act in a goal-directed manner, reason, learn, and comprehend. Correspondingly, various models of intelligence posit different types of intelligence, and various tests of intelligence have been developed or interpreted in accordance with these models. In his creation of the Wechsler intelligence scales, Wechsler was greatly influenced by Spearman's (1904) general-factor theory that states all abilities share a general factor, or *g* factor, in common, and a global IQ can summarize all abilities. The most contemporary and currently influential model of intelligence is the Cattell-Horn-Carroll (CHC) (1993) model, which was empirically derived via factor analysis and represents the combination of Cattell's and Horn's *Gf-Gc* (i.e., *fluid intelligence* and *crystallized intelligence*) theory and Carroll's Three-Stratum Theory. It is a top-down hierarchical model that posits multiple distinct intelligences; eight relatively broad intelligences, such as *Gf* and *Gc*; and approximately 70 other relatively narrow or specific abilities. Since its introduction, it has greatly influenced newer versions of the Wechsler scales and other tests, such as the Stanford-Binet and the Woodcock-Johnson. The most commonly used IQ tests focus on generating a single IQ score specifying how much overall *g* a person has, while at the same time permitting identification of the specific abilities making up that *g* (see also Chapter 9, Test Administration, Interpretation, and Issues in Assessment).

In addition to definitions of intelligence stressing linguistic, logical-mathematical, and spatial intelligence, other definitions of intelligence include consideration of noncognitive factors. One, in particular, is emotional intelligence, which is generally viewed as the ability to perceive, process, understand, and control emotion in oneself and others. Another is the concept of Theory of Mind, which is the ability to make inferences about other people's intentions, motivations, and emotional states. In an effort to integrate these concepts Howard Gardner (1983, 1999) put forward a theory of multiple intelligences that includes linguistic, logical-mathematical, and spatial, but also includes musical, bodily-kinesthetic, naturalistic, interpersonal, and intrapersonal. These latter areas of ability are not generally captured by commonly used intelligence tests. There are other theories of intelligence that propose that intellect consists of different components, for example, Robert Sternberg's (1985) triarchic theory of intelligence is another influential model.

Associated Disorders

Intellectual Disability

Intellectual disability is a developmental disorder with onset before age 18 requiring a substantially subnormal IQ (i.e., approximately $\geq$ 2 standard deviations below the mean), reflecting limitations in general intellectual functioning, combined with significant deficits in two or more adaptive skills (see also Chapter 13, Intellectual Disability).

Dementia

By definition, dementia is a syndrome (i.e., a set of signs and symptoms) that stems from a disease or medical condition involving a decline in or loss of general cognitive ability or multiple areas of cognitive impairment of sufficient severity to impair social and/or occupational functioning. Performances on tests of general intelligence decline as dementia advances; in cases of Alzheimer's disease (AD), decline in IQ may not be evident until the middle stages (see also Chapter 30, Mild Cognitive Impairment and Alzheimer's Disease; Chapter 31, Vascular Cognitive Impairment; Chapter 32, Frontotemporal Dementias; and Chapter 33, Movement Disorders).

Savantism

This is a very rare syndrome in which individuals with an intellectual disability or autism spectrum disorder (see also Chapter 14, Autism Spectrum Disorder) have one or more specific or narrow remarkable talents that exist in stark contrast to their intellectual disability. The cause or causes of savant syndrome are unknown but may be congenital or acquired as a result of central nervous system (CNS) disease or injury. Savant syndrome is associated with autism spectrum disorders, as well as other psychological disorders and CNS injuries/diseases. It is approximately six times more common in males than females. Savant skills most commonly involve exceptional memory, but can also involve exceptional calculation, calendar knowledge, artistic, and/or language abilities.

Section 2: Attention/Concentration and Processing Speed

Definition

Multiple models of attention currently exist (e.g., spotlight, filter, capacity, automatic vs. effortful, top-down vs. bottom-up, etc.), each with strengths and weaknesses (see also Chapter 3, Important Theories in Neuropsychology: A Historical Perspective). In general, attention refers to the process whereby individuals receive and subsequently process incoming information. It is closely associated with perception, executive functioning and memory, particularly working memory (which is dependent on attention but is not synonymous). Working memory refers to the form of processed information before it is sent to short-term memory (see also the section "Memory" later in this chapter), whereby information that is being actively maintained or rehearsed can be retained for up to several minutes. If something is passively received (i.e., attention span) but not rehearsed or manipulated, it is lost.

Attention has a number of subtypes (see Table 5.1). One that is frequently used interchangeably with attention is concentration, which is the ability to sustain attention over time or to mentally manipulate information. Although there is no pure test of attention, given its overlap with executive functioning, memory, and processing speed, examples of tests targeting each subtype of attention are provided (some tests measure more than one subtype as well).

TABLE 5.1 Types of Attention

Types of Attention		Example of Test Used
Simple	Voluntary; capacity; attention to information that is lost if not rehearsed	Digit Span; Corsi blocks
Focused	Ability to allocate and direct attention that is dependent on capacity	Digit Symbol Coding
Selective	Process by which one chooses some information from amidst other surrounding information or distractors	Cancellation
Sustained (Vigilance / Concentration)	Maintaining attention over a period of time	Continuous Performance Test
Alternating	Shifting one's attention back and forth between tasks	Trail Making B
Divided	Concentrating on more than one task at a time or multiple aspects within a task, referred to as multi-tasking by some in the lay public	Paced Auditory Serial Addition Test

Although there are a number of neurobiological models of attention, the one by Posner and Petersen (2012) is most salient for the exam. This model divides attention into two major areas: posterior and anterior networks. The posterior network has to do with orienting and shifting attention. The anterior system serves as the detection subsystem (or executive attention subsystem) and involves detecting stimuli either from sensory events or from memory. The two networks also interconnect, allowing for completion of multiple aspects of a task, such as both the orienting and detection of a stimulus. A third area, the alerting network (subserved by the ascending reticular activating system [ARAS]), can influence both anterior and posterior networks, operating at high or low levels of arousal (see Table 5.2).

Processing speed is the speed at which mental activities are performed and is a prominent feature of the brain's cognitive efficiency, affecting attention as well as other higher-order cognitive processes. Processing speed is dependent on neural transmission and integrity and volume of white matter making up cortico-cortical connections. Other brain areas affecting processing speed include basal ganglia, frontal regions (especially dorsolateral prefrontal), and the cerebellum. Example of tests measuring processing speed include Coding and PASAT.

TABLE 5.2 Brain Structures Relevant to Attention

Attention: Relevant Brain Structures	Function
Ascending Reticular Activating System (ARAS)	Arousal and attention
Anterior Cingulate (and Limbic System)	Determines saliency of stimuli and associated emotion/motivation
Prefrontal	Response selection, control, sustained attention, focus, switching, searching, and alternating attention
Orbitofrontal	Inhibition of responses; sustained attention
Dorsolateral Frontal	Initiation of responses; sustained attention; shifting attention
Medial Frontal	Motivation; consistency of responding; focused attention
Thalamus	Sensory relay between subcortical areas and the cortex. Various nuclei play a role in specific attentional functions.
• **Pulvinar Nuclei**	Extracting information from the target location and filtering distractors
• **Superior Colliculus**	Shifting attention; eye movements
• **Inferior Colliculus**	Orientation to auditory stimuli
Inferior and Posterior Parietal	Underlies disengagement from a stimulus and the representation of space; damage is associated with hemispatial inattention/neglect
Right Hemisphere	Spatial attention; appreciation of the gestalt; associated with hemispatial inattention/neglect

Associated Disorders

Attentional difficulties are the most common type of cognitive impairment following brain injury or illness because the white matter tracts and structures subsuming these functions are diffusely represented throughout the brain. Not surprisingly, problems with aspects of attention are often cited as "memory problems" among patients and collaterals, even when memory storage is proved to be intact. Below are some examples of specific disorders affecting attention.

Delirium

Delirium is a disorder marked by waxing and waning deficits in attention, often including increased distractibility, poor awareness, and persistent confusion. The primary attentional processes affected are span and arousal (see also Chapter 27, Delirium and Disorders of Consciousness).

Attention-Deficit/Hyperactivity Disorder (ADHD)

By definition, ADHD is a developmental disorder characterized by inattention, impulsivity, and sometimes hyperactivity. The executive aspects of attention (i.e., self-regulation) as well as sustained attention are primarily affected in ADHD (see also Chapter 16, Attention-Deficit/Hyperactivity Disorder).

Hemispatial Inattention (a.k.a. Neglect)

Hemispatial inattention is characterized by impairment in awareness of visual (and other) stimuli on the side contralateral to a brain lesion and is not the result of a primary sensory deficit. Associated features can include anosognosia or denial of illness, extinction of stimuli, and asomatognosia, or denial of body part (see somatagnosias, discussed later in this chapter). The underlying pathology is most commonly associated with lesions in the temporal-parietal region but is not exclusive to this region. Usually the left side of space is affected as a result of a right-hemisphere lesion, but the right side of space can be affected with left-hemisphere lesions. The type of attention affected is spatial focused attention and selective attention.

- *Sensory Neglect* An acquired inattention or unawareness to part (typically half) of space; as in hemineglect, it is contralateral to the lesion.
- *Motor Neglect* Involves a failure to respond or initiate movement (akinesia) to stimuli in contralateral space.
- *Combined Sensory-Motor Neglect* Involves both ignoring stimuli and performing fewer movements in contralateral space.

Traumatic Brain Injury (TBI)

Moderate to severe TBI often results in reduced arousal, poor attentional capacity, distractibility, impairments in executive aspects of attention, and reduced information-processing speed. Concussion can also temporarily affect working memory, attention, and processing speed (see also Chapter 29, Traumatic Brain Injury).

Other Disorders and Factors Affecting Attention

Depression and anxiety, fatigue and lack of sleep/sleep disorders, low or poor arousal, environmental factors (i.e., noise, etc.), and medications are all non-neurological factors that can negatively influence attentional processes. Reduced motivation or effort is another factor that can affect attention. Factors affecting processing speed include those already mentioned, as well as conditions that diffusely impact various brain structures and white matter integrity (e.g., multiple sclerosis, TBI, vascular cognitive impairment, Parkinson's disease).

Section 3: Language

Definition

Human language is a system of communication involving a formal symbolic scheme reliant on *phonology* and rules of *syntax* to express lexical or semantic meaning (i.e., using words). The components of language competence comprise four areas: *phonology, syntax, semantics*, and *pragmatics*. Language is distinct from speech in that the latter is the physical oral expression of language. At its most basic, language can be seen as comprising expressive and receptive functions, with expressive language controlled by anterior brain regions and receptive language by posterior brain regions of the dominant hemisphere. Despite evidence that the right hemisphere mediates some language function (e.g., prosodic aspects), it is the left hemisphere in humans that mediates or performs most language function related to *semantics* and syntactics.

Aphasia

Aphasia is an acquired loss or impairment of language following brain damage or disease that comprises a family of clinically diverse disorders that affect the ability to communicate by oral or written language or both (see Table 5.3). Developmental language disorders such as dyslexia, apraxia of speech, and *dysarthria* are not aphasic disorders.

TABLE 5.3 Essential Facts about Aphasia

Aphasia: Essential Information	
Syndromes	Each type of aphasia reflects a collection of clinical findings, not a specific disease entity
Neuropathology	Occurs with any type of neuropathology capable of producing structural alterations in cortical and subcortical language areas; type of syndrome is determined by brain part affected, not by the etiology
Etiology	Primary etiology is stroke (as many as 40% of patients after stroke have some degree of aphasia); other potential etiologies include neoplasm, intracranial tumor and infection, traumatic injury and other brain diseases affecting language areas, including neurodegenerative diseases, such as frontotemporal dementia (see also Chapter 32, Frontotemporal Dementias)
Exclusions	Speech disturbances, such as *dysarthria, dysphonia,* and apraxia of speech are not necessarily evidence of aphasia but can be seen in some acquired language disorders.

There are, of course, competing models of language disruption, including the localizationist, associationistic/connectionistic, and cognitive models. Broca's discovery relating motoric type aphasia to a lesion in the left hemisphere and Wernicke's discovery relating sensory aphasia (i.e., loss of memory for words) to the left temporal lobe led to various schematic models localizing language and language pathology to particular centers in the brain. One localizationist model by Lichtheim involves a rather complex scheme of five interrelated cortical and subcortical areas proposed to underlie language processing: these include centers for movement patterns of oral speech, for word sounds, for the movement patterns of writing, for written words, and for forming concepts or ideas to be expressed.

Language disturbances can also occur, however, as a result of destruction of connections or associations between verbal labels and thoughts, objects, or incidents. Geschwind reintroduced this connectionistic approach theorizing that disorders of aphasia, apraxia, and agnosia were really "disconnexion syndromes" or disorders as a result of lesions interrupting the transfer of information from one neural region to another. Finally, reacting against the ideas that aphasia solely involved a deficit in language and that language was actually localized in specific areas of the brain, many theorists put forth models that posited cognitive factors, such as abstract reasoning, as playing a role in aphasia and that impairment in patients with aphasia is not wholly attributable to just language impairment, but also impairment in other cognitive domains.

Assessment of Aphasia

The different syndromes of aphasia are distinguished best by language symptoms, such as fluency versus nonfluency, auditory comprehension, and the ability to repeat, and, to a lesser extent, by agrammatism and disturbances in reading and writing. Diagnosis and localization of the different syndromes can be accomplished with an examination that includes evaluation of both expressive and receptive language, including spontaneous or conversational speech, repetition, auditory comprehension, word finding, reading and writing, and naming (see Tables 5.4 and 5.5).

- *Spontaneous Speech* Can be elicited through simple conversation while interviewing a patient or taking a medical history or by asking for a description of a picture, such as the Cookie Theft picture in the Boston Diagnostic Aphasia Examination, 3rd Edition (BDAE-3). Two specific areas must be addressed: form and content.

  - *Form of Speech* Refers to whether a patient's speech is fluent or nonfluent and is examined by looking at the effort required to produce speech, the rate of speech, and the melody and the length of phrases.

- In *fluent aphasic speech* (e.g., Wernicke's, transcortical sensory), verbal output is normal, with normal phrase length (more than five or six words between pauses) and with no apparent articulatory difficulty and normal melody, although the speech may be non-meaningful with paraphasic errors (i.e., word or sound substitutions) evident.

- In *nonfluent aphasic speech* (e.g., Broca's, transcortical motor), verbal output is diminished with decreased phrase length (less than three or four words between pauses), laborious articulation, and poor rhythm. Impaired speech initiation and impairment in production of grammatical sequences is also common.

- **Content of Speech** Refers to word choice and *syntax* and the presence or absence of paraphasic errors in spontaneous speech.

  - In *fluent aphasic syndromes*, word output itself is likely to be normal, but in terms of content may not be informative or convey meaning (i.e., "empty").

  - In *nonfluent aphasic syndromes*, the critical word or words needed to convey meaning can be present but may not be in the correct order and or with the correct grammatical structure. Agrammatism, resulting in an appearance of "telegraphic" speech, can be seen.

- **Comprehension of Spoken and Written Language** can be assessed by questions and commands that increase in complexity and examine comprehension of individual words, category-specific information (e.g., letters, colors, body parts), and meaning imparted from *syntax* and word order. The standard auditory comprehension section of the BDAE-3, for example, is comprised of tests of basic word discrimination; one-, two-, and then three-step commands; and complex ideational material. To examine comprehension, the examiner must first establish that the patient has a controllable output channel in which to indicate their response, even if it is limited to pointing or yes/no answers. Comprehension difficulties can be of two types: syntactic and lexical/semantic.

  - Lesions involving anterior speech areas can result in disturbed comprehension of phonological (syntactic) information used to construct word names.

  - Lesions in posterior language areas more often result in disturbed comprehension of the sequencing of meaningful word sounds to convey meaning (lexical/semantic).

- **Repetition** is easily tested by beginning with single, simple words then multisyllabic words, followed by short sentences and longer sentences, increasing in complexity. Establishing whether or not repetition is intact is important because the ability to repeat typically indicates that the perisylvian language centers are functional.

- **Naming** problems or **anomia** (the terms "anomia" and "dysnomia" can be used interchangeably) can be present in all types of aphasia syndromes and can involve problems naming an object, color, and body part or finding a specific word in spontaneous speech. Word-finding difficulties can be evident in spontaneous speech when a patient pauses to search for a word or uses too many words to describe something better described in fewer words (i.e., *circumlocution*), or it can be elicited by presenting a stimulus and asking the patient to name it. Anomia can occur with many of the aphasic syndromes and is, therefore, not generally useful for localization, but distinctions between anterior and posterior aphasic syndromes can often be made because patients with nonfluent syndromes may have difficulty with naming as a result of initiation or production problems, whereas patients with fluent syndromes may have difficulty as a result of selection problems or an inability to find the right word.

- *Reading* aloud and reading silently for comprehension should each be tested separately. Examination of reading should begin with single letters and digits, then words and sentences of increasing length and complexity. When the patient does not have expressive language available, the ability to understand what is read can be tested by allowing the patient to match words to pictures. All aphasic syndromes that include severe impairment of auditory language—with the exception of pure word deafness—are almost always also associated with an acquired impairment of reading or alexia. Alexia can be seen in aphasias of all kinds and it can be seen in isolation, in which case it can be important for localization. That alexia can be seen in isolation without other features of aphasia, including agraphia, suggests that the brain has evolved specific areas required for reading that are separate from other language areas.

- *Writing* can be tested by asking the patient to write single letters and digits, then words and multidigit numbers, and then sentences of increasing length and complexity. Writing tasks can involve both writing to dictation and writing based on visual input such as pictures. *Agraphia* is loss of the ability to write. Pure agraphia is rare; it is usually seen in combination with alexia or aphasia. Generally, because of the close relationship between writing and oral language ability, a patient's writing will be disordered comparable to the disorder in the patient's speech.

TABLE 5.4 Comparison of Fluent Versus Nonfluent Speech

Patient with a Fluent Aphasia Describing the BDAE Cookie Theft Picture	
Doctor	I'd like you to tell me about this picture.
Patient	That's a boy playing there. The woman she's fixing the faring splashing the thing there. A family, the two children and her evidently.
Doctor	(points to woman on right) What is she doing there?
Patient	(returns attention to the children on left) Well, they're fighting two of them the two of them are fighting each other. Pool pooling cutting other and he was kind of playing too. So she broke the broke the way a mix there just kind of playing. It wasn't heavy hard. It was very hammy like, just like kids, you know like do.
Doctor	What's happening here?
Patient	Well, of course, he fell off the gas there. He fell off. He was supposed to help the boy and the she tried to helping the boy. She wasn't missing very good. No, she wasn't no. Kind of rough speak.
Patient with a Nonfluent Aphasia Describing the BDAE Cookie Theft Picture	
Doctor	What can you tell me about this picture?
Patient	Girl. Aid, aid. Falling down. Girl. Dishes, dishes. Sink, sink.
Doctor	What's happening at the sink?
Patient	Spill down, yea.
Doctor	Very good, right. What is it that's spilling down?
Patient	Ah . . .
Doctor	Is it milk?
Patient	No, no.
Doctor	It's not milk, it's . . . it's . . . ?
Patient	Floor.
Doctor	(introduces a phonemic cue) Wa . . .
Patient	Water, water.

TABLE 5.5 Distinguishing Language Characteristics of the Major Aphasic Syndromes

Aphasic Syndrome	Spontaneous Speech	Comprehension	Repetition	Naming	Reading	Writing
Broca's	Nonfluent	Intact	Impaired	Limited	Limited	Impaired similar to speech
Wernicke's	Fluent	Impaired	Impaired	Impaired	Impaired	Impaired
Conduction	Fluent	Intact	Impaired	Impaired	Intact	Impaired
Global	Nonfluent	Impaired	Impaired	Impaired	Impaired	Impaired
Anomic	Fluent, empty	Intact	Intact	Impaired	Intact	Impoverished content
Subcortical	Fluent or nonfluent	Intact	Intact	Impaired	Intact or impaired	Intact or impaired
Transcortical Motor	Nonfluent	Intact	Intact	Limited	Intact	Impaired
Transcortical Sensory	Fluent, echolalic	Impaired	Intact	Impaired	Impaired	Impaired
Transcortical Mixed	Nonfluent, echolalic	Impaired	Intact	Impaired	Impaired	Impaired

Associated Disorders

Aphasic Syndromes

In adults, each aphasic syndrome can be localized within the brain and language areas by the various clinical characteristics of the language disorder. Nonfluent aphasias are associated with dysfunction within anterior language centers, whereas fluent aphasias involve dysfunction of posterior language areas. Aphasic disorders without repetition difficulties are located in the borderzone language areas; aphasic disorders with repetition difficulties are located in the perisylvian areas. There are few pure syndromes: all patients with aphasia vary in their presentation but usually one syndrome better describes the clinical status of a patient than do the others (see Figure 5.1 and Table 5.6). Most improvement in language function will occur in the first few months after injury and the extent and persistence of deficits is directly related to the size and location of the lesion. Strokes isolated to the cortex tend to have better outcomes than strokes that include deeper structures and the white matter pathways that connect them because strokes affecting cortex are less disruptive of the multiple systems needed for normal language. Strokes that affect both cortical and subcortical structures tend to have the poorest functional outcomes.

- *Perisylvian Aphasia Syndromes* Structures and the area around the Sylvian fissure are important in language. The hallmark of perisylvian aphasia syndromes is impaired repetition.
    - *Nonfluent syndromes*:
        - *Broca's aphasia* (also known as motor, expressive, and anterior aphasia) is characterized by strikingly nonfluent verbal output that is sparse, effortful, dysarthric, dysprosodic, of

short-phrase length, and agrammatic, with poor repetition in the context of relatively spared auditory comprehension for content. Writing is usually impaired commensurate with speech. Naming is often impaired, but contextual and phonemic cues can aid retrieval. Singing can be preserved as well as emotionally charged language (e.g., swear words, overlearned expressions). Prognosis for recovery is good if the lesion involves only cortex and/or if there is no associated right hemiparesis. If the lesion extends from the cortex deep into the basal ganglia and internal capsule, then the aphasia is likely to be permanent.

- *Fluent syndromes*:
  - *Wernicke's aphasia* (also known as sensory, receptive, and posterior aphasia) is best characterized by fluent verbal output with normal word count and phrase length and difficulty in word finding, along with significantly impaired auditory comprehension and poor repetition. Speech can often be described as empty or nonsensical because there can be long syntactic strings replete with paraphasic errors, neologisms, and *circumlocutions*.
  - *Conduction aphasia* (also known as associative aphasia) is characterized by impaired repetition in the context of relatively fluent speech and relatively well-preserved auditory comprehension. *Literal paraphasias*, word-finding difficulties, and severely impaired writing are common. Naming ability is limited by paraphasias, and reading aloud is severely disturbed, whereas reading comprehension may be normal.

- *Extrasylvian Aphasia Syndromes* Aphasic syndromes involving the borderzone region are known as transcortical aphasia syndromes. In these syndromes, the ability to repeat spoken language is preserved in the face of distinct language impairment.

  - *Nonfluent syndromes*:
    - *Transcortical motor aphasia (TMA)* is an anterior borderzone-related aphasia resembling Broca's aphasia except for the normal or near normal ability to repeat. It is characterized by preservation of the ability to repeat spoken language in the face of impoverished speech and writing. Comprehension is intact, but verbal output is nonfluent.
    - *Mixed transcortical aphasia (MTA)* combines the motor and sensory forms of this disorder and resembles global aphasia, except for preservation of the ability to repeat spoken language. It usually involves extensive borderzone damage. Usually the patient is nonfluent. Common causes include hypoxic brain injury due to decreased cerebral circulation, as in cardiac arrest, carbon monoxide poisoning, or in some cases temporary occlusion/stenosis of the carotid artery.

  - *Fluent syndromes*:
    - *Transcortical sensory aphasia (TSA)* is a posterior borderzone-related aphasia resembling Wernicke's aphasia, but characterized by preservation of the ability to repeat spoken language in the absence of intact auditory comprehension or meaningful expression and, like MTA, can feature echolalia. It features a significant comprehension disorder, fluent and paraphasic output, and good repetition ability. Heard language is processed, allowing for repetition, but cannot be interpreted.

- *Nonlocalizing Aphasia Syndromes*
  - *Anomic aphasia* is a syndrome in which the primary problem is one of difficulty with word finding, causing multiple pauses, frequent *circumlocution*, and a somewhat stumbling verbal output in the face of intact repetition and comprehension. Reading and writing are often disturbed. This is a common residual disorder following improvement from other types of aphasia.
  - *Global aphasia* involves severe disturbances in all major language functions and is usually the result of an occlusion early in the middle cerebral artery (MCA) vascular tree. As a result, large sections of the language-dominant hemisphere are impacted.
- *Subcortical Aphasia Syndrome* refers to language disorders that may arise from lesions to the striatum, internal capsule, or thalamus. These aphasias may share some of the characteristics of the cortical aphasias already described and may be fluent or nonfluent. When the causative lesion is entirely subcortical, then the prognosis for recovery is good, although some residual speech impairment may be evident. However, if there is also cortical involvement the aphasia is likely to persist.
- *Alexia* refers to the inability to read unrelated to simple sensory or motor problems.
  - *Alexia without agraphia* or pure word blindness is a rare disorder involving selective loss of the ability to read configurations of letters without a comparable disturbance in the ability to write and without other significant language disturbances. In this disorder, the patient retains the ability to write, but cannot read his or her own writing.
  - *Alexia with agraphia* combines the specific loss of the ability to read with the specific loss of the ability to produce written language in spite of intact manual motor abilities. Speech and comprehension may be intact, but an anomia may be present.
- *Pure Word Deafness* This disorder is rare and involves the loss of auditory comprehension of speech. Patients with this disorder react to speech sounds as though they are deaf. They are able to speak, read, and write, but are unable to repeat.

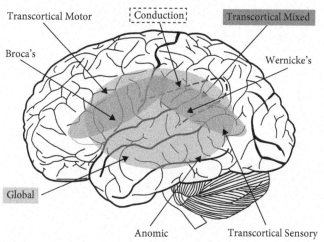

FIGURE 5.1 Classic Neuroanatomical Localization of Aphasic Syndromes

TABLE 5.6 Neuroanatomical Findings and Possible Associated Features of the Aphasic Syndromes

Aphasic Syndromes		Neuroanatomical Findings	Possible Associated Features
Perisylvian	Broca's	Frontal operculum in the dominant hemisphere or posterior portion of the inferior frontal gyrus of the left hemisphere, including the third frontal convolution of the left hemisphere and subcortical white matter extending posteriorly to the inferior portion of the motor strip	Common right hemiparesis (arm more affected than leg), right facial droop
	Wernicke's	Posterior superior portion of the left temporal lobe or the auditory association cortex adjacent to Heschl's gyrus of the primary cortical auditory center	Occasional superior quadrantopsia
	Conduction	Considered a disconnection syndrome because of damage to the arcuate fasciculus, thus disconnecting Broca's area from Wernicke's area, but the syndrome can also occur with damage to the posterior superior aspect of the left temporal lobe, supramarginal gyrus, or deep parietal matter.	Common hemisensory defect and cortical sensory loss
	Global	Involves the entire perisylvian region in a typical middle cerebral artery pattern but may be caused by two separate noncontiguous lesions affecting Broca's and Wernicke's areas and excluding primary motor cortices.	Common right hemiplegia and right hemisensory defect
	Anomic	No specific location for the pathology, but it often involves the angular gyrus in the dominant hemisphere and disconnection between Wernicke's area and intrasensory input areas in the parietal, temporal, and occipital lobes	Rare
Extrasylvian	Transcortical Motor	Usually anterior to Broca's area, often in the supplementary motor area of the dominant hemisphere or in the frontal tissues between that region and the dominant hemisphere operculum.	Occasional right hemiparesis
	Transcortical Sensory	Usually at the junction of parietal, temporal, and occipital regions in the angular gyrus in the dominant parietal region, sparing Wernicke's area	Common hemisensory defect; uncommon right hemiparesis
	Transcortical Mixed	Essentially isolation or disconnection of the speech area; involves the entire vascular borderzone area in both the frontal and parietal zones	Common right hemiparesis and hemisensory defect
Alexia	Without Agraphia	Considered a disconnection syndrome isolating higher order visual systems from the language systems; involves the left occipital area and corresponding inferior portion of the left side of the splenium of the corpus callosum	Color anomia, trouble spelling and comprehending spelling, bilateral right visual field hemianopsia
	With Agraphia	Involves lesions in the posterior margin of the parietal lobe (i.e., the angular gyrus)	Common right hemiparesis and hemisensory defect
Word Deafness		Appears to involve damage to both temporal lobes with destruction of Heschl's gyrus on the left and the white matter tract connecting it to the auditory association area on the right	None specific

Nonlanguage Auditory Processing Syndromes

Auditory agnosias are a form of agnosia that manifests in a disturbed capacity to recognize the nature of formerly familiar nonverbal acoustic stimuli despite intact hearing and intact ability to recognize verbal stimuli (i.e., speech). Specific localization for the pathology of auditory agnosia is uncertain beyond involvement of auditory cortex of the right temporal and/or bilateral temporal lobes.

- *Auditory Agnosias*
  - *Agnosia for Sounds* involves an inability to recognize the meaning of nonverbal environmental sounds (e.g., the sound of a train or the bark of a dog). It is often associated with disorders of pure word deafness. These disorders are usually associated with bilateral lesions in the primary auditory cortex located within the temporal plane, especially the structures around Heschl's gyrus.
  - *Agnosia for Music* Also known as amusia, is an inability to recognize the meaning of musical sounds. Deficits can range from an inability to appreciate or understand rhythm to an inability to understand musical sounds as anything more than noise. This disorder is rare and is associated with lesions in the right or bilateral temporal lobes.

- *Aprosodias*
  - Disorders of *prosody* indicate that the nondominant hemisphere does contribute some important input to language in the form of paraverbal communication. There are two types of aprosodia. The first is expressive aprosodia, characterized by an inability to properly convey the inflection and tonal quality of emotion, such that speech often has a robotic quality. The pathology here typically involves the area contralateral to Broca's area. The second is receptive aprosodia, characterized by difficulty interpreting emotional *prosody*, rhythm, pitch, stress, intonation, and so on and manifested in an inability to recognize sarcasm, cynicism, jokes, and other idiomatic forms of speech. The pathology is often due to dysfunction in regions contralateral to Wernicke's area.

Section 4: Visuoperceptual, Visuospatial, and Visuoconstructional

Definition

This cognitive domain is comprised of the abilities to perceive, localize, process, identify, interpret, and manipulate visual information including objects, colors, faces, forms, and figures. It is well established that the two main streams of higher order visual processing are analyzing the form or the "what" of visual stimuli and analyzing the localization or the "where" of visual stimuli. This double dissociation of "what" versus "where" is evident in case studies of patients with disturbed recognition of objects but intact spatial abilities, and vice-versa, and it implies two different cortical pathways in humans (see Table 5.7). A third stream, which is often referred to as the superior temporal sulcus system has also been proposed. This system is also known as the "specialized movement" stream and involves the analysis of objects and body parts in motion.

TABLE 5.7 Two Streams of Visual Processing

Two Streams of Visual Processing	"What"	"Where"
Pathway	Ventral	Dorsal
Processing	Identifying the form of visual stimuli in terms of colors, objects, faces, and letters	Spatial relationships: locating and analysis of objects in space
Neuroanatomical Findings	Projects to occipital-temporal association cortex, connecting striate, prestriate, and inferior temporal regions	Projects to parietal-occipital association cortex, connecting striate, prestriate, and inferior parietal regions
Associated Disorders	Visual Agnosias	Spatial Analysis/Processing Impairments
Example of Test Measures	• Hooper Visual Organization Test • Picture Completion	• Judgment of Line Orientation • Block Design

Associated Disorders

Visual Agnosias

Agnosia is an acquired disorder, caused by brain disease or injury, resulting in an inability to recognize formerly familiar objects. The visual agnosias involve a disturbance of visual perceptual function concerning the identification and recognition of objects, faces, or their representation; and meaningful or meaningless forms, colors, and spatial information. The disturbance is not the result of a deficit in vision, attention, naming, or lack of familiarity with the object.

- *Visual Object Agnosia* involves the inability to visually recognize and appreciate the meaning or character of an object. Although patients with visual agnosia may be able to describe features of the object, such as its color or shape, they are unable to recognize what the object is. Two forms have been posited: apperceptive agnosia and associative agnosia (see Table 5.8).

  - *Apperceptive agnosia* is the inability to perceive visual objects. Patients are unable to copy or draw objects. They cannot match similar objects or sort object categories. It is presumed to result from a disruption in object recognition during visual perception.

TABLE 5.8 Neuroanatomical Findings Associated with the Visual Agnosias

Visual Agnosias	Neuroanatomical Findings
Visual Object Agnosia	Typically left occipital lesions with extension into subcortical white matter, but also bilateral lesions involving peristriate angular gyrus and the lingual and fusiform lobules: • *Apperceptive agnosia*—Usually diffuse • *Associative agnosia*—Likely a disconnect between areas important in visual perception and areas important in language function
Prosopagnosia	Usually bilateral and involves the inferior occipital-temporal junction or inferior parietal-occipital area, but when unilateral, typically in the right hemisphere involving the inferior longitudinal fasciculus and splenium of the corpus callosum
Color Agnosia	Usually involves the left or bilateral occipital-temporal areas

- *Associative agnosia* is the inability to recognize visual objects. Although they are unable to name or demonstrate how to use objects these patients can match and draw objects accurately. It results from a disruption in object recognition because of an inability to access stored information regarding the meaning of the object.

- *Prosopagnosia* refers to an inability to recognize, identify, or revisualize holistic face representations of familiar or unfamiliar people. Individuals with prosopagnosia instead rely on other personal details, such as speech or manner of walking, to recognize familiar people. Prosopagnosia is more often genetic or developmental but can result from acquired brain injury typically involving bilateral lesions in ventral/inferior occipital-temporal areas (i.e., the fusiform gyrus). The developmental form of prosopagnosia is not necessarily associated with other developmental conditions. Spontaneous recovery has been seen in acquired prosopagnosia. It is viewed as an associative agnosia, wherein the patient is unable to recognize faces because of an inability to access stored information about the face. Unilateral lesions generally produce less prominent deficits in the ability to recognize faces than bilateral lesions.

- *Color Agnosia* involves an inability to recognize colors even though the ability to discriminate between colors is intact.

Spatial Analysis/Processing

Impairments in spatial processing can include difficulties locating objects in space, difficulty discriminating between complex visual stimuli, and difficulty constructing simple and complex shapes (see Table 5.9).

- *Constructional Apraxia* involves loss or impairment of the ability to carry out purposeful movements, as is required in an apraxia, but it is really a visuospatial disorder that signals an inability to construct shapes and geometric designs and to assemble block arrangements. The term "constructional apraxia" is sometimes misused and is better characterized as a visuoconstructional or visuospatial impairment than an actual problem with motor planning.

- *Dressing Apraxia* is considered a form of constructional apraxia because it involves, in part at least, difficulty localizing objects in space. It refers to an isolated disturbance in dressing ability but may present as part of a hemispatial neglect syndrome.

TABLE 5.9 Neuroanatomical Findings Associated with Disorders in Spatial Analysis and Processing

Disorders in Spatial Analysis/Processing	Neuroanatomical Findings
Location of Objects in Space	Typically located in either unilateral or bilateral occipital parietal junction
Spatial Analysis	Typically located in the posterior right hemisphere
Constructional Apraxia	Usually involves both frontal and parietal systems and may result from either left or right hemisphere damage, but is most likely to result from right parietal lesions and bilateral parietal lobe lesions
Dressing Apraxia	Usually implies a lesion in the right parietal-occipital region
Achromatopsia	Can be both unilateral and bilateral, involving posterior medial regions and the calcarine cortex more on the left than the right
Spatial Acalculia	Generally subsumed by the right parietal lobe

- *Achromatopsia* refers to impairment in color perception, such that patients cannot see colors. Their world is black and white. Typically this is associated with occipital-temporal lesions and is usually restricted to a hemifield or quadrant.

- *Spatial Acalculia* Although acalculia is not always spatially based, in some cases of acalculia, the acquired deficit in calculation ability results from spatial confusion, that is, difficulty processing the spatial aspects of written problems (e.g., confusing the columns within problems). This is most often associated with right hemisphere lesions.

Section 5: Memory

Definition

Memory refers to the complex process of encoding, retaining, and retrieving information. Learning is highly dependent on various aspects of attention in that information cannot be initially attained or encoded if the individual does not perceive or process. Memory and learning are critical drivers in the process of behavioral change. Like attention, memory is diffusely represented, subsumed/coordinated by various brain structures, and comprised of multiple types (see Table 5.10), as well as of various models, such as the information processing and multistorage models.

Associated Disorders

Amnestic Disorders

By definition, an amnestic disorder is an isolated loss of memory without loss of any other cognitive functions. Declarative (explicit) memory is affected, whereas procedural (implicit) memory is not (see also the section "Neuroanatomy of Memory" in Chapter 4, Functional Neuroanatomy and Essential Neuropharmacology).

- *Retrograde Amnesia* is amnesia for events prior to an accident, illness, or event; it is typically temporally graded, whereby events immediately before are lost, whereas more remote memories remain intact. Ribot's Law states that the oldest memories are the most resistant to amnesia. Studies have underscored an association between severity of retrograde amnesia and extent of hippocampal pathology.

- *Anterograde Amnesia* is an inability to learn or encode new information or form new memories. It is often referred to as an inability to form continuous memories.

  - *Post-Traumatic Amnesia (PTA)* is a type of anterograde amnesia that typically results from acquired brain injury but can also occur during other conditions and acutely impact brain function (e.g., delirium). The length of PTA is one of the best indicators/predictors of TBI severity/long term outcome.

- *Functional Amnesia* (psychogenic amnesia, including fugue) is believed to have a psychiatric etiology, rather than one caused by physical injury. Anterograde amnesia is rare. Retrograde amnesia can include personal identity and/or be limited to autobiographical memory. It is often triggered by an emotionally traumatic event.

- *Infantile Amnesia* is failure to recall autobiographical information from early childhood years; thought to be a normal part of development.

TABLE 5.10 Types of Memory

Memory: Essential Terms		
Information Processing Model	**Encoding**	Active organization or manipulation of incoming stimuli, such as through rehearsal and repetition
	Storage	Transfer of transient memory to where it can be made more permanent
	Consolidation	Process by which encoded information undergoes a series of processes that render the memory representations progressively more stable and permanent
	Retrieval	The ability to access previously stored information; by way of cues. "tip of the tongue phenomenon"
3-Stage Model	**Sensory Memory**	Holds information only 1–2 seconds for "iconic" (visual) and 3–4 seconds for "echoic" (auditory)
	Short-Term Memory	Limited capacity of 7 +/- 2 items (Ebbinghaus); temporary store whereby information can be held for up to several minutes; often equated with working memory and attention
	Long-Term Memory	A more permanent memory store where information is stored by way of consolidation or learning. It requires the hippocampus where structural change takes place due to long-term potentiation (LTP). Not as chronologically old as remote memory
	Remote Memory	Old memories, which are thought to be more stable or resilient to damage and disease than recent memory
Types of Memory	**Declarative Memory** (Explicit)	Memory system concerned with the conscious retrieval or recognition of contextually related information or episodes
	Semantic Memory	Knowledge of facts; not time dependent
	Episodic Memory	Knowledge of temporal events; autobiographical
	Prospective Memory	Remembering to do something at a particular time in the future. It is a process that also involves executive abilities and frontal systems. Declines with age.
	Non-Declarative Memory (Implicit or Procedural)	A memory system that is responsible for skills, procedures, habits, and classically conditioned responses and takes place largely without awareness
	Source Memory	Knowledge of where and when something was learned; related to episodic memory
	Metamemory	Knowledge of one's own memory
Retrieval	**Free Recall**	Remembering information independent of cues
	Recognition	Remembering information with the aid of stimuli; easier than recall.
Types of Interference	**Retroactive Interference**	A process by which recently learned information interferes with the ability to remember previously learned information
	Proactive Interference	A process by which previously learned information interferes with new or current learning

- *Transient Global Amnesia* has an etiology usually due to hypoperfusion of medial temporal or diencephalic areas, and resultant disconnection of lateral and medial limbic circuits. However, causes are often unclear and can include strategic infarction (e.g., perirhinal/parahippocampal cortex), migraine, and can also occur after electroconvulsive therapy (ECT). This is an acute-onset memory loss that typically lasts for less than ten hours (but can last days) and results in profound anterograde amnesia and variable retrograde amnesia. The person usually remains alert and oriented to self. Confabulation is common.

- *Anoxia/Hypoxia* Damage to the medial temporal lobe, particularly area CA1 of the hippocampus (part of the medial limbic circuit), may result from an anoxic injury, with consequential memory loss. However, when the lateral limbic circuit is affected as well, memory loss is more severe with a consequence of dense amnesia (typically, a pronounced anterograde amnesia). In some cases, the amnesia is profound but in others memory performance improves with retrieval cues. Unlike other amnestic disorders, insight may be preserved and confabulation is not often present (see also the section "Neuroanatomy of Memory" in Chapter 4, Functional Neuroanatomy and Essential Neuropharmacology; Chapter 28, Hypoxic and Ischemic Brain Injury).

- *ACoA (Anterior Communicating Artery) Aneurysm* Rupture of an aneurysm of the ACoA often results in basal forebrain, striatal, and frontal system damage, as well as disruption of cholinergic neurons that project to both medial and lateral limbic circuits. This, in turn, causes a "frontal amnesia" characterized by confabulation, attentional problems, disorientation, some apathy/lack of insight, sensitivity to proactive interference and variable retrograde amnesia (see also Chapter 25, Stroke).

- *Wernicke-Korsakoff's Syndrome* occurs as a result of chronic alcohol use and thiamine deficiency. Korsakoff's syndrome involves a diencephalic amnesia that results in both anterograde and retrograde amnesia (loss of remote memory), proactive interference, temporal order impairment, confabulation, and poor insight. It is also associated with gait ataxia, oculomotor palsy, and encephalopathy (see also Chapter 36, Substance Use Disorders).

- *Herpes Encephalopathy* is an infection caused by the herpes virus which preferentially affects the medial and inferior temporal lobes and the amygdala. Often, this initially results in amnesia, aphasia, and agnosia (See also Chapter 27, Delirium and Disorders of Consciousness).

- *Surgical Ablation* Historically, extensive bilateral medial temporal resection for intractable epilepsy (e.g., patient H. M.) has resulted in severe anterograde amnesia, due to hippocampal/parahippocampal (medial circuit) as well as amygdala (lateral circuit) damage. Unlike some of the other disorders listed here, many patients have preserved insight and are not prone to confabulation (see also the section "Neuroanatomy of Memory" in Chapter 4, Functional Neuroanatomy and Essential Neuropharmacology).

- *Posterior Cerebral Artery (PCA) Stroke* The brain regions affected, and the resulting amnesia, depends on the laterality of the lesion; however, the pathology involves medial temporal and posterior occipital lobes. Associated cognitive deficits also include visual deficits, hemianopic alexia, color agnosia, and object agnosia (see Table 5.11 and Chapter 26, Stroke).

TABLE 5.11 Distinguishing Characteristics of the Amnesias

Etiology	Brain Region	Amnesia	Insight	Confabulation
Transient Global Amnesia	Medial temporal; diencephalic	Profound anterograde; variable retrograde	Present	Rare
Anoxia/Hypoxia	Medial temporal	Anterograde	Present	Rare
ACoA	Frontal; basal forebrain	Frontal	Maybe	Often
Wernicke-Korsakoff's	Diencephalic	Anterograde and Retrograde	No	Often
Herpes Encephalopathy	Medial temporal	Severe retrograde	Present	Rare
PCA Infarct	Medial temporal	Depends on laterality	Present	Rare

Dementia

Whereas AD affects memory encoding, patients with dementia impacting frontal-subcortical systems (i.e., vascular dementia, multiple sclerosis, Parkinson's disease, etc.) typically display retrieval difficulties and thus often benefit from recognition cueing (see Table 5.12; Chapter 30, Mild Cognitive Impairment and Alzheimer's Disease; Chapter 31, Vascular Cognitive Impairment; Chapter 32, Frontotemporal Dementias; and Chapter 33, Movement Disorders).

TABLE 5.12 Brain Systems, Underlying Structures, and Disorders Associated with Memory

Relevant Brain Systems	Brain Structures	Associated Disorders
Hippocampal Pathway (or Papez circuit)	• Entorhinal cortex • Fornix • Mammillary bodies • Mammillothalamic tract • Cingulate cortex	• Hypoxia and Anoxia
Amygdaloid Pathway	• Amygdala • Dorsal medial thalamus • Dorsomedial cortex	• Herpes encephalitis • PTSD
Diencephalon	• Anterior nucleus of the thalamus • Dorsomedial nucleus of the thalamus • Fornix • Mammillary bodies	• Korsakoff's • CVA
Basal Forebrain	• Medial septal nucleus • Diagonal band of Broca • Nucleus Basalis of Meynert	• Affected in AD • ACoA aneurysm
Cortex	• Medial and anterior temporal lobe • Frontal lobe (see basal forebrain)	• Surgical ablation • TBI • Herpes • Anoxia/Hypoxia

NOTE: ACoA, anterior communicating artery; PTSD, posttraumatic stress disorder; TBI, traumatic brain injury

Section 6: Executive Functions

Definition

Executive functioning is a multifaceted construct, with a great deal of overlap with attention, memory, language, emotional functioning, and personality, as well as social functioning. Executive functioning enables individuals to engage in independent, purposeful behavior. Although often included in a chapter entitled "the frontal lobes," executive functioning actually involves multiple systems and connections with other cortical and subcortical areas. Like attention, multiple models of executive functioning exist. One of the more commonly known is the three-syndrome model (Cummings, 1993), in which particular deficits result from damage to three discrete areas:

- *Dorsolateral Prefrontal Syndrome* (dysexecutive syndrome) Characterized by poor problem solving, word-list generation, organization, sequencing, *abulia*/amotivation ("pseudo depression"), and sometimes perseveration.

- *Orbitofrontal Syndrome* (inferior/ventral frontal syndrome) Characterized by emotional lability, impulsivity, disinhibition, childishness, personality change, and distractibility.

- *Medial Frontal/Cingulate Syndrome* Characterized by decreased initiation and indifference, but can also have amnesia, incontinence, and leg weakness. Cummings also identified the motor circuit (supplementary motor area) and oculomotor circuit (frontal eye fields).

It is important to emphasize that executive functioning is intimately linked to the coordination of emotional/social and cognitive functioning. The structures responsible for reasoning and emotion are both activated when someone has to make a judgment about an emotional situation (i.e., interpretation of facial expression, *prosody*, humor, etc.) or must use emotion to prioritize a decision (i.e., what to pay attention to first). Patients, particularly those with right-hemisphere damage, often experience difficulties interpreting or using these signals (see Table 5.13).

Associated Disorders

Dementias

Both cortical (e.g., frontotemporal dementia, Lewy body dementia) and frontal-subcortical dementias (e.g., Parkinson's disease, Huntington's disease) often present with executive dysfunction. The former dementias sometimes present with reduplicative paramnesia or Capgras syndrome; the latter, because of their frontal-subcortical circuit involvement, involve personality change and or depression (see also Chapter 30, Mild Cognitive Impairment and Alzheimer's Disease; Chapter 31, Vascular Cognitive Impairment; Chapter 32, Frontotemporal Dementias; and Chapter 33, Movement Disorders).

Acquired or Traumatic Brain Injury

Diffuse frontal system and diencephalic damage can result in confabulation and decreased awareness (see also Chapter 29, Traumatic Brain Injury). Depending on where the damage is, patients can present with dysexecutive symptoms and/or personality change (e.g., Phineas Gage).

TABLE 5.13 Symptoms Commonly Associated with Disorders Involving Executive Systems

Symptoms Associated with Executive System Disorders	Definition	Brain System Damaged
Motor sequencing	Performing tasks in a specific order	• Prefrontal • Dorsolateral prefrontal area
Poor directed attention	Ability to allocate and direct attention	• Prefrontal • Frontal eye fields
Poor working memory	Information that is actively maintained or rehearsed, that can be retained for up to several minutes	• Dorsolateral prefrontal area
Perseveration	Uncontrolled repetition of a response	• Dorsolateral prefrontal area
Failure to maintain response set	Inability to maintain a task after it has been acquired; due to distractibility	• Prefrontal
Poor reasoning	Abstract reasoning, judgment	• Dorsolateral prefrontal area
Abulia	Lacking in initiation / motivation / concern	• Dorsolateral prefrontal area; also basal ganglia and anterior cingulate (medial frontal)
Poor planning/ organization	Inefficient planning and/or organization (involves prioritizing and goal-setting)	• Dorsolateral prefrontal area • Orbitofrontal area
Impulsivity	Acting on impulse, without thought	• Orbitofrontal area
Emotional lability (see Emotional/ Neuropsychiatric)	Inability to control emotions	• Orbitofrontal area
Utilization behavior/ environmental dependency (stimulus-bound behavior)	When patients tend to respond to whatever stimuli are at hand, even when inappropriate	• Orbitofrontal area • Mesial frontal • Anterior cingulate
Witzelsucht	Inappropriate jocularity	• Orbitofrontal area
Disinhibition	Inability to inhibit, or control, a response or behavior, regardless of its appropriateness	• Orbitofrontal area • Anterior cingulate
Apathy/akinetic mutism	Inability to speak or move	• Anterior cingulate
Depression	The left frontal lobe is thought to underlie positive emotional valence so that, with injury, depression results	• Left frontal
Reduplicative paramnesia	Feeling that a place has been duplicated	• Right posterior parietal • Frontal
Capgras syndrome	Feeling that a person has been duplicated or is an imposter	• Right temporal • Bilateral frontal
Anosognosia	Unawareness of deficit; different than denial in that there is often limited defensiveness and the lack of awareness is not related to psychological denial or avoidance	• May result from diffuse brain injury and focal damage to frontal, posterior parietal (i.e., Wernicke's), and right hemisphere regions

Addiction/Impulse Control Disorders

Impaired executive functioning, particularly inhibitory control and working memory, has been implicated in some impulse control disorders (ICDs). For example, ICDs (i.e., binge eating disorder, pathological gambling, etc.) have been observed in approximately 40% of Parkinson's patients undergoing dopaminergic treatment, resulting in impaired fronto-striatal (sub-thalamic nucleus) and cingulo-frontal connections associated with compulsive repetition. Children with Prader Willi syndrome also exhibit hyperphagia and obesity, secondary to hyperactivation in limbic reward circuitry (amygdala) and hypoactivation in cortical inhibitory regions.

Focal Lesions Affecting Frontal Circuits and Systems

Brain tumors and strategic vascular lesions can also compromise frontal systems and lead to executive dysfunction (see also Chapter 25, Cancers; and Chapter 26, Stroke). Please also refer to the discussion of AcoA aneurysm in the "Memory" section earlier in this chapter.

Section 7: Sensorimotor

Definition

Combined in this domain are functions related to somatosensory abilities and body orientation, along with motor abilities, including lateralized problems in speed and dexterity, as well as loss of the ability to carry out purposeful movements.

Associated Disorders

Finger Agnosia

Finger agnosia refers to loss of the ability to name or identify the fingers of one's own hand(s) or the fingers of the hand(s) of another person. Disordered finger recognition, along with acalculia (discussed earlier in this chapter), right–left disorientation (discussed next), and agraphia (discussed later in this section) comprise the four parts of Gerstmann syndrome. Finger agnosia is a special case of autotopagnosia, wherein one loses the ability to identify the parts of one's body to command or imitation.

Right–Left Disorientation

Right–left disorientation involves an inability or loss of the ability to identify the right and left sides of one's own body and the right and left sides of the body of another person. Like finger agnosia, right–left disorientation is a special case of autotopagnosia, wherein one loses the ability to identify the parts of one's body to command or imitation (see Table 5.14).

Somatagnosias

Somatagnosias refer to disturbances in the general feeling pertaining to the existence of one's body or recognition of one's body schema. Disorders here typically result from parietal lobe system dysfunction.

- *Astereognosia* involves loss or acquired impairment in one's ability to recognize the nature of an object by tactual ability or other physical features, such as size and shape.
- *Asomatognosia* is an acquired disturbance in the knowledge or sense of one's own body and bodily condition (see hemispatial inattention discussed earlier in this chapter).

TABLE 5.14 Neuroanatomical Findings Associated with the Somatosensory Disorders

Somatosensory Disorders	Neuroanatomical Findings
Finger Agnosia	Can result from a lesion in the left inferior parietal lobe, in particular, the angular gyrus
Right-Left Disorientation	Can result from a lesion of the left inferior parietal lobe, especially the angular gyrus
Astereognosia	Usually unilateral and typically associated with lesions of the posterior parietal region and rolandic gyri
Asomatognosia	Can be seen as a result of lesions in the bilateral parietal lobes, a unilateral lesion in the right inferior parietal region bordering the interparietal sulcus, the supramarginal gyrus, and the angular gyrus, or a unilateral lesion involving the dominant parietal lobe, especially in the region of the angular gyrus

Apraxia

Apraxia is an impairment of the ability to carry out previously learned purposeful, skilled movements despite normal primary motor skills and normal comprehension of the act to be performed. Apraxia:

- cannot be explained by weakness, incoordination, sensory loss, impaired concentration, inattention, or intellectual impairment;

- can appear as an isolated disorder, but its common association with aphasic syndromes makes it difficult to differentiate from impaired comprehension;

- can manifest in relation to focal lesions, progressive dementing disorders, and stroke; and

- is frequently associated with anosognosia (see hemispatial inattention discussed earlier in this chapter), so patients may be unaware of their apraxic deficits, and patients with apraxia often have right hemiparesis, so they may mistake their apraxic deficits with difficulty moving the affected limb.

Examination for apraxia should include pantomime of object use and tests designed to evaluate transitive movements (i.e., those done as a goal-directed movement with an object) and intransitive movements (i.e., those done without a specific goal and without use of an object, like hand gestures), as well as the ability to carry out serial acts (e.g., pretending to prepare a cup of tea or light a pipe) (see Table 5.15).

TABLE 5.15 Neuroanatomical Findings Associated with Disorders of Apraxia

Disorders of Apraxia	Neuroanatomical Findings
Frequently associated with lesions in or near the language zone of the left hemisphere, but can be the result of bilateral lesions. Localizes generally to the left inferior parietal lobule (sensory area), and frontal lobe systems, particularly the premotor cortex, supplementary motor area, and frontal convexity, and—as a result of disconnection—the corpus callosum	
Apraxia of Speech	Not specific to one location, as apraxia of speech can occur in multiple conditions that do not necessarily share anatomical substrates.
Ideational Apraxia	Has been associated with bilateral, nonfocal lesions and with left hemisphere lesions, especially the posterior temporal-parietal junction
Ideomotor Apraxia	Usually involves lesions in the left inferior parietal lobe or supplementary motor area or a lesion in the corpus callosum
Limb-Kinetic Apraxia	Unlike other apraxic disorders, appears to be the result of lesions in the pyramidal motor system

- *Apraxia of Speech* is not a language disorder but involves impairment in planning the movements necessary for speech production. Both the acquired version and the childhood version (i.e., childhood apraxia of speech) can be manifest in inconsistent articulation errors and difficulty with correct articulatory placement. Apraxia of speech is a disorder of the planning and organization of articulatory movement, in contrast to *dysarthria*, which is a disorder of motor coordination. In the childhood version, a defining characteristic is often the child's ability to pronounce single words or words in series (e.g., ABCs, numbers) but in conversation/volitional speech dysprosodic rhythm and poor articulation are apparent.

- *Buccofacial Apraxia* involves difficulty performing voluntary skilled motor movements of the face, tongue, lips, and cheeks on command. Measures to assess intransitive buccofacial gestures might include puffing out the cheeks and sticking out the tongue; measures to assess transitive buccofacial gestures might include pretending to suck on a straw or sniff a flower.

- *Gait Apraxia* refers to a loss of the normal capacity to use the legs appropriately for the act of walking, in spite of the ability to demonstrate correctly the use of the legs for the act of walking when lying flat.

- *Ideational Apraxia* is a loss of the ability to plan and execute complex gestures, as though one has lost the "idea" behind the gesture or use of a tool even though knowledge about the use of the tool is unaffected. It involves problems in motor planning and is manifest in errors in sequencing the necessary actions for a task (e.g., lighting a pipe before putting in the tobacco). Assessment of serial acts is important in identifying this disorder.

- *Ideomotor Apraxia* refers to loss of the ability to perform or pantomime transitive or intransitive gestures on command and to imitate, although spontaneous production of the gesture may remain intact. It involves difficulty making believe one is using a tool and is manifest in tool use and gestures. During pantomime, patients with ideomotor apraxia will often use a body part as if it were an object (e.g., their hand as a "comb"). Measures to assess intransitive limb gestures might include waving or saluting, whereas those that assess transitive limb gestures might include pretending to use a comb or scissors.

- *Limb-Kinetic Apraxia* involves an inability to precisely move one's hands or legs, but it is not viewed as related to skilled movement because there is no apparent inability to select or sequence motor movements, and it is present with pantomime, imitation, and the use of objects. It affects goal-directed transitive movements more than simple intransitive gestures, is more often asymmetric than symmetric, and affects distal more than proximal movement.

Agraphia

A language disorder frequently associated with aphasia and alexia, as discussed earlier in this chapter, agraphia can also be related primarily to motoric and spatial deficits. Agraphia refers to the inability to write despite intact sensory and motor skills. Agraphic writing disorders can include writing impairments due to impaired sensory feedback, impaired written production secondary to errors of omission, or motor/sensory deficits, impaired letter formation, and impaired writing as a result of spatial deficits manifested in problems such as poor spacing and poor use of the space.

Section 8: Emotional/Neuropsychiatric

Definition

Brain injury and/or dysfunction often results in neuropsychiatric symptoms, such as those involving emotional dysregulation and changes in personality. These neuropsychiatric issues can be due to the

TABLE 5.16 Emotional Symptoms Commonly Associated with Neurological Disorders

Emotional Symptoms	Definition	Relevant Brain System Damaged
Anosodiaphoria	Disorder wherein patients are aware that they have impairments (e.g., paralysis), yet show no emotional concern or distress about it; neglect also often present. This is in contrast to la belle indifference, which is lack of concern for symptoms/disability secondary to conversion disorder.	Right parietal or frontal systems
Alexithymia	An inability to understand, process, or describe one's own emotions	Right hemisphere, particularly amygdala; also insula, anterior cingulate, and fusiform gyrus
Emotional Lability	Fluctuations of emotion and/or increased emotional reactivity	Orbitofrontal area Limbic system
Rumination	Obsessively going over a thought or problem in an unproductive way	Subgenual prefrontal cortex
Pseudobulbar Affect	Type of emotional lability; extreme involuntary emotional responses (i.e., tearful crying, excessive laughing) to mild stimulation	Due to pseudobulbar palsy, or damage to the upper motor neuron corticobulbar tract and connections to the cerebellum

direct impact of the injury or disease, emotional adjustment issues, or a combination of the two. For example, incidence rates of depression are quite high in various neurologic conditions such as Huntington's disease, multiple sclerosis, and left cerebrovascular accident (CVA). This is due to the complex interplay between physiologic dysregulation, chemical changes (in neurotransmitters; medication effects), and the biopsychosocial consequences of disability.

Similarly, individuals with chronic psychiatric disorders also often have cognitive deficits, in addition to behavioral and emotional changes. Examples include schizophrenia and bipolar disorder (see also Chapter 34, Mood Disorders: Depression, Mania, and Anxiety; and Chapter 35, Schizophrenia Spectrum and Other Psychotic Disorders). Thus, the so-called organic and functional really are one and the same. Further, patients with various psychiatric disorders can present with speech and language problems, for example, fluent but unintelligible speech or alternatively sparse verbal output, either of which could be mistaken for a fluent aphasia or a nonfluent aphasia, respectively. The opposite can also occur: a patient with a Wernicke's aphasia could be mistaken for a patient with the "word salad" of schizophrenia. Understanding the distinguishing language characteristics of the major aphasic syndromes and their associated features is crucial in differentiating psychiatric disorders from aphasic disorders.

Although they are often contrasted, emotion and reason are inseparable; they are intertwined and mutually dependent in a healthy brain (see the work of Damasio & Carvalho (2013); see also the "Executive Functions" section earlier in this chapter). Multiple neuroanatomical regions have long been considered important in emotional regulation, including frontal lobe systems (particularly orbitofrontal and left frontal), the right hemisphere, and limbic areas such as the amygdala and septum. The cerebellum has also recently been implicated in emotional and affective processing and regulation (see Table 5.16).

Relevant Definitions

Abulia Passive behavior wherein one exhibits little spontaneous activity and markedly delayed responses and tends to speak briefly or softly. In the extreme the patient may be immobile, akinetic, and mute, but will continue to appear awake, sitting with their eyes open.

Circumlocution The purposeful substitution of multiple words or descriptions for a word or other words that the patient is unable to find. This manifests as talking around word-finding difficulties, rather than using specific words. These are not considered paraphasic errors, and circumlocution is not the equivalent of tangentiality.

Crystallized Intelligence (Gc) This refers to the breadth and depth of knowledge and understanding that is acquired through learning, education, experience, and acculturation; it is often resistant to the effects of aging and neurologic injury or illness.

Dysarthria A speech disorder involving difficulty in articulation. Not an aphasia or language disorder although sometimes confused with them. Patients with dysarthria are able to read and write normally which readily differentiates them from patients with expressive aphasia.

Dysphonia A speech disorder involving difficulty in vocalization.

Fluid Intelligence (Gf) This refers to the ability to reason, adapt, solve problems, form concepts, and understand relationships in unfamiliar or novel circumstances. Unlike Gc, it is more susceptible to the effects of aging, injury, and illness.

Literal (or Phonemic) Paraphasias The substitution or the rearrangement of sounds or syllables in otherwise correct words (e.g., fig instead of pig).

Phonology The underlying speech sounds in a language and the rules governing the production of speech sounds.

Pragmatics The context in which the words are used.

Prosody An element of speech that contributes to the conveyance of meaning through rhythm, stress, pitch, loudness, tempo, and intonation. It can indicate the basic structure of a sentence, the emotional content, or the main point in an utterance.

Semantics The meanings of words and the rules governing the use of words. It is the sequencing of meaningful words sounds to convey meaning.

Semantic Paraphasias The substitution of a correct word or phrase for another semantically related word or phrase (e.g., dog instead of cat). Semantic paraphasias in the form of multi-word paraphasic errors or "paragrammatism" is one feature that differentiates the syndrome of Wernicke's aphasia from other fluent aphasic syndromes.

Syntax The rules governing the structure of phrases and sentences.

Verbal Paraphasias The substitution of one correct word for another. Some substitutions may have no obvious semantic relationship with the correct word, while others involve substitution of a correct word or phrase for another semantically related word or phrase. Sometimes paraphasias take the form of neologisms (e.g., "zoctor" for doctor).

Domains of Neuropsychological Function Questions

NOTE: Questions 11, 51, 71, 99, and 117 on the First Full-Length Practice Examination; Questions 1, 36, 76, 99, and 115 on the Second Full-Length Practice Examination; Questions 3, 48, 74, 90, and 103 on the Third Full-Length Practice Examination; and Questions 10, 61, 86, 104, and 123 on the Fourth Full-Length Practice Examination are from this chapter.

1. A cancellation task with a single target would be a valid measure of ____.

   (a) divided attention

   (b) selective attention

   (c) attention span

   (d) sustained attention

2. The patient is a 72-year-old man who sustained a thrombotic stroke of the left middle cerebral artery three months ago. Examination now reveals significant word-finding difficulty but otherwise grammatically accurate, fluent, and well-formed speech and intact repetition. His speech lacks substantive words and there are frequent circumlocutions. The most likely type of aphasia is ____.

   (a) anomic aphasia

   (b) Wernicke's aphasia

   (c) conduction aphasia

   (d) Broca's aphasia

3. In the case described in question #2 above, where was the patient's lesion likely to have been?

   (a) extrasylvian area

   (b) Broca's area

   (c) Wernicke's area

   (d) arcuate fasciculus

4. In acquired prosopagnosia, ____.

   (a) the damage is likely to involve dorsal frontal areas

   (b) there is often an inability to recognize colors

   (c) the damage is likely to involve dorsal parietal areas

   (d) spontaneous recovery has been documented in some cases

5. You are consulted to see a 79-year-old, right-handed gentleman who sustained a right thalamic stroke. While preparing your doctoral intern for the initial assessment what might you provide in terms of education? He may ____.

   (a) not be able to speak fluently.

   (b) engage in inappropriate behavior.

   (c) not express emotions.

   (d) be inappropriately jocular.

6. On examination, you find that a patient picks up a toothbrush and the toothpaste and tries to put the toothpaste on the toothbrush without taking off the cap. This could be an example of ____.

   (a) constructional apraxia

   (b) ideomotor apraxia

   (c) ideational apraxia

   (d) buccofacial apraxia

7. Your patient presents with nonfluent, sparse language and symptoms of apathy. To differentiate this condition as an aphasia syndrome from a primary psychiatric disorder, you would want to first evaluate for the presence of ____.

   (a) paraphasic errors

   (b) suicidal ideation

   (c) anosognosia

   (d) motor or sensory deficits

8. Which brain area plays a key role in motivating selective attention toward a salient stimulus?

   (a) inferior parietal

   (b) basal forebrain

   (c) dorsolateral frontal

   (d) anterior cingulate

9. Posner and Petersen's attentional model would predict difficulty with ____ as a result of damage to the ascending reticular activating system (ARAS).

   (a) alerting

   (b) detection

   (c) orienting

   (d) shifting

10. Classification of aphasia is based primarily on which three parts of the language assessment?

    (a) fluency, repetition, prosody

    (b) fluency, comprehension, naming

    (c) fluency, comprehension, repetition

    (d) comprehension, naming, repetition

11. Which of the following is not a symptom of Gerstmann's syndrome?

    (a) agraphia

    (b) acalculia

    (c) alexia

    (d) finger agnosia

12. Intact spatial abilities, but disturbed recognition of objects implies disruption in the _____ pathway.

    (a) dorsal

    (b) mesial

    (c) ventral

    (d) rostral

13. Which of the following might you see with damage to the dorsolateral frontal lobe?

    (a) emotional lability

    (b) Witzelsucht

    (c) abulia

    (d) lack of empathy

14. A 5-year-old boy demonstrates delayed language, parallel play, and an obsession with electrical outlets, but can recite the day of the week of any date. He most likely demonstrates _____.

    (a) aphasia

    (b) Obsessive-Compulsive Disorder

    (c) savantism

    (d) Schizophrenia

15. You are called to evaluate a patient in the hospital with a history of alcohol abuse who tried to elope from his assisted living facility by climbing a tree two days ago. Upon admission, his toxicology screen was negative. Testing indicated poor orientation and attention, fair memory, and poor reasoning. Your tentative diagnosis is _____.

    (a) Korsakoff dementia

    (b) transient global amnesia

    (c) delirium

    (d) transient ischemic attack

Domains of Neuropsychological Function Answers

1. **B—selective attention** *Selective attention is the choosing of a target from amidst distractors. Divided attention is concentrating on two or more tasks simultaneously. Attention span is similar to capacity. Sustained attention is maintaining attention over a period of time.*

    Reference: Loring, D. W. (2015). *INS dictionary of neuropsychology and clinical neurosciences* (2nd ed.). New York, NY: Oxford University Press.

2. **A—anomic aphasia** *The characteristics of an anomic aphasia are fluent speech and intact comprehension and repetition but impaired naming. The patient appears to recognize objects but cannot come up with their name. They may be able to describe concepts they are trying to express but cannot come up with the specific name; for example, they might say, "The animal with a mane that lives in the jungle and roars," but they cannot say, "lion."*

    References:
    (a) Caplan, D. (2012). Aphasic syndromes. In K. M. Heilman & E. Valenstein (Eds.), *Clinical neuropsychology* (5th ed., pp. 22–41). New York, NY: Oxford University Press.
    (b) Gazzaniga, M. S., Ivry, R. B., & Mangun, G. R. (2014). *Cognitive neuroscience: The biology of the mind* (4th ed.). New York, NY: W. W. Norton & Co.

(c) Schoenberg, M. R., & Scott, J. G. (2011). Aphasia syndromes. In M. R. Schoenberg & J. G. Scott (Eds.), *The little black book of neuropsychology: A syndrome-based approach*. New York, NY: Springer.

3. **A—extrasylvian area** *The extrasylvian lesion effectively isolates the parts of the brain needed for the interpretation of language from the parts of the brain that merely connect the interpretation of speech sounds or phonology to speech production. Repetition is intact because speech sounds can be directly mapped into speech articulation without using the parts of the brain necessary for comprehension of speech.*

Reference: Caplan, D. (2012). Aphasic syndromes. In K. M. Heilman & E. Valenstein (Eds.), *Clinical neuropsychology* (5th ed., pp. 22–41). New York, NY: Oxford University Press.

4. **D—spontaneous recovery has been documented in some cases** There is also preliminary evidence of possible treatments for both acquired and developmental prosopagnosia.

Reference: DeGutis, J. M., Chiu, C., Grosso, M. E., & Cohan, S. (2014). Face processing improvements in prosopagnosia: Successes and failures over the last 50 years. *Frontiers in Human Neuroscience, 8*(561). Retrieved from 10.3389/fnhum.2014.00561

5. **C—not express emotions** *His right-sided CVA likely eliminates the possibility of an expressive aphasia. B and D are indicative of orbitofrontal damage. Right hemisphere lesions can result in aprosodias and other conditions which impact an individual's ability to express emotion.*

Reference: Patel, S., Oishi, K., Wright, A., Sutherland-Foggio, H., Saxena, S., Sheppard, S. M., & Hillis, A. E. (2018). Right hemisphere regions critical for expression of emotion through prosody. *Frontiers in Neuroscience, 9*(224). Retrieved from 10.3389/fneur.2018.00224

6. **C—ideational apraxia** *This limb apraxia is characterized by difficulty correctly sequencing motor movements.*

References:
(a) Loring, D. W. (2015). *INS dictionary of neuropsychology and clinical neurosciences* (2nd ed.). New York, NY: Oxford University Press.
(b) Scott, J. G., & Schoenberg, M. R. (2011). Deficits in visuospatial/visuoconstructional skills and motor praxis. In M. R. Schoenberg & J.G. Scott (Eds.), *The little black book of neuropsychology: A syndrome-based approach*. New York, NY: Springer.

7. **D—motor or sensory deficits** *Psychiatric conditions are rarely associated with focal motor or sensory neurologic symptoms, whereas hemiparesis is not uncommon in Broca's aphasia. While language errors can occur in acute psychosis as well as anosognosia but in these instances orientation will often remain intact and it is unlikely there will be a focal motor or sensory disorder.*

Reference: Schoenberg, M. R., & Scott, J. G. (2011). Aphasia syndromes. In M. R. Schoenberg & J. G. Scott (Eds.), *The little black book of neuropsychology: A syndrome-based approach*. New York, NY: Springer.

8. **D—anterior cingulate** *Motivation and saliency involve executive systems such as the anterior cingulate (limbic).*

Reference: Blumenfeld, H. (Ed.). (2010). *Neuroanatomy through clinical cases* (2nd ed.). Sunderland, MA: Sinauer Associates, Inc.

9. **A—alerting** *Orienting and shifting, according to Posner and Petersen's model, involves the posterior network; detection is the anterior network; alerting and arousal involve the ARAS.*

Reference: Petersen, S. E., & Posner, M. I. (2012). The attention system of the human brain: 20 years after. *Annual Review of Neuroscience, 35*, 73–89.

10. **C—fluency, comprehension, repetition** *Fluent versus nonfluent speech localizes anterior from posterior aphasic syndromes; impairment in comprehension distinguishes Wernicke's from conduction aphasia; and the ability to repeat implies that perisylvian language areas are intact.*

References:

(a) Caplan, D. (2012). Aphasic syndromes. In K. M. Heilman & E. Valenstein (Eds.), *Clinical neuropsychology* (5th ed., pp. 22–41). New York, NY: Oxford University Press.

(b) Gazzaniga, M. S., Ivry, R. B., & Mangun, G. R. (2014). *Cognitive neuroscience: The biology of the mind* (4th ed.). New York, NY: W. W. Norton & Co.

(c) Schoenberg, M. R., & Scott, J. G. (2011). Aphasia syndromes. In M. R. Schoenberg & J. G. Scott (Eds.), *The little black book of neuropsychology: A syndrome-based approach.* New York, NY: Springer.

11. **C—alexia** *The four components of Gerstmann's syndrome are finger agnosia, acalculia, right-left disorientation, and agraphia.*

References:

(a) Croslett, H. B. (2012). Acquired dyslexia. In K. M. Heilman & E. Valenstein (Eds.), *Clinical neuropsychology* (5th ed.). New York, NY: Oxford University Press.

(b) Gazzaniga, M. S., Ivry, R. B., & Mangun, G. R. (2014). *Cognitive neuroscience: The biology of the mind* (4th ed.). New York, NY: W. W. Norton & Co.

12. **C—ventral** *The ventral pathway is the "what" pathway; its disruption would affect recognition of objects. The dorsal pathway, in contrast, is the "where" pathway, which affects spatial perception.*

Reference: Farah, M. J., & Epstein, R. A. (2012). Disorders of visual-spatial perception and cognition. In K. M. Heilman & E. Valenstein (Eds.), *Clinical neuropsychology* (5th ed.). New York, NY: Oxford University Press.

13. **C—abulia** *Emotional lability, lack of empathy, and Witzelsucht would more likely be seen with orbitofrontal damage.*

Reference: Loring, D. W. (2015). *INS dictionary of neuropsychology and clinical neurosciences* (2nd ed.). New York, NY: Oxford University Press.

14. **C—savantism** *The patient described has autistic spectrum disorder, which has some association with savantism.*

Reference: Baron-Cohen, S., Ashwin, E., Ashwin, C., Tavassoli, T., & Chakrabarti, B. (2009). Talent in autism: Hyper-systemizing, hyper-attention to detail and sensory hypersensitivity. *Philosophical Transaction of the Royal Society B: Biological Sciences, 364,* 1385–1391.

15. **C—delirium** *The patient's fair memory eliminates Korsakoff's and TGA; his poor orientation and attention are consistent with delirium. Symptoms following a true TIA would resolve quickly on the same day, which is not the case here.*

Reference: Smith, G. E., & Bondi, M. W. (2013). *Mild cognitive impairment and dementia: Definitions, diagnosis, and treatment.* New York, NY: Oxford University Press.

Recommended Readings

Damasio, A., & Carvalho, G. B. (2013). The nature of feelings: Evolutionary and neurobiological origins. *Nature Reviews Neuroscience, 14*(2), 143–152.

Goodglass, H., with the collaboration of Kaplan, E., & Barresi, B. (2001). *The assessment of aphasia and related disorders* (3rd ed.). Baltimore, MD: Lippincott, Williams & Wilkins.

Grant, I., & Adams, K. M. (Eds.). (2009). *Neuropsychological assessment of neuropsychiatric and neuromedical disorders* (3rd ed.). New York, NY: Oxford University Press.

Heilman, K. M., & Valenstein, E. (Eds.). (2012). *Clinical neuropsychology* (5th ed.). New York, NY: Oxford University Press.

Loring, D. W. (Ed.). (2015). *INS dictionary of neuropsychology and clinical neurosciences* (2nd ed.). New York, NY: Oxford University Press.

Morgan, J. E., & Ricker, J. H. (Eds.). (2018). *Textbook of clinical neuropsychology* (2nd ed.). New York, NY: Routledge.

Schoenberg, M. R., & Scott, J. G. (Eds.). (2011). *The little black book of neuropsychology: A syndrome-based approach.* New York, NY: Springer.

6   The Neurologic Examination, Radiologic and Other Diagnostic Studies

Yuka K. Matsuzawa, Hilary C. Bertisch, and Joseph H. Ricker

Introduction

Neuropsychologists often review documents from medical providers including results of neurological examinations, radiologic tests, or various medical tests. Such findings provide valuable information to facilitate interpretation of neuropsychological data. Therefore, a basic understanding of such studies is beneficial in order to generate hypotheses and recommendations.

The Neurological Examination

Findings from a neurological examination often include cranial nerve functioning, sensorimotor findings, *reflexes*, gait, coordination, and mental status. Results can serve as supplemental data to be examined in conjunction with neuropsychological data to affirm hypotheses as well as to raise awareness of discrepancies.

Examination of the Cranial Nerves

In total, there are twelve cranial nerves that originate from the brain stem (medulla, pons, and midbrain). They are often grouped based on sensory functions (I, II, VIII), motor functions (III, IV, VI, XI, XII), and mixed functions (V, VII, IX, X). Furthermore, there are some cranial nerves often examined in conjunction as functional units (e.g., cranial nerves IX and X to assess gag reflex) and for syndromes (e.g., III-IV-VI nerve palsy).

- *Olfactory Nerve (CN I)* The olfactory nerve projects from the olfactory regions to the midbrain. The function of CN I is smell, which is the only uncrossed sense. Each nostril is tested independently by occluding one nostril and asking the patient to identify a fragrance (e.g., coffee). Olfactory loss (anosmia) can occur with subfrontal masses (e.g., tumors, abscesses), trauma particularly to the orbitofrontal region where nerves penetrate the cribriform plate of the ethmoid, and viral infections due to damage to the olfactory neuroepithelium.

- *Optic Nerve (CN II)* The optic nerve projects from the retina to the midbrain. The function of CN II is vision. The two optic nerves, one from each eye, meet and form the optic chiasm. Abnormality in the optic chiasm often causes loss of visual temporal fields (*bitemporal hemianopsia*). Visual fields are assessed by having the patient look directly at the examiner's eye and identify finger motion in the periphery. Postchiasmic lesions can result in loss of half of a contralateral visual hemifield on the same side in both eyes (*homonymous hemianopsia*). Prechiasmic lesions can result in monocular blindness. Involvement of the optic radiations in the posterior temporal lobe (Meyer's loop) can result in loss of a superior quadrant visual field on the contralateral side (*homonymous* superior *quadrantanopsia*). Involvement of the optic radiations in the parietal lobe can result in loss of an inferior quadrant visual field on the contralateral side (*homonymous* inferior *quadrantanopsia*).

- *Oculomotor Nerve (CN III)* The oculomotor nerve originates from the midbrain and projects to all extraocular muscles (EOM) except for oblique and lateral rectus muscles. CN III is assessed by observing eye movements and by shining a light into the pupil. CN III is responsible for eye movements medially (adduction), superiorly, and inferiorly. Additional CN III functions include pupil constriction due to parasympathetic fibers to the pupillary constrictor muscles. Compression of CN III from aneurysms or uncal herniation can result in a fixed and dilated pupil ("*blown pupil*"). Significant pupillary constriction ("pinpoint pupil") can suggest pontine involvement or drug overdose (e.g., morphine).

- *Trochlear Nerve (CN IV) and Abducens Nerve (CN VI)* The trochlear nerve originates from the midbrain and projects to the superior oblique muscle. The abducens nerve originates from the pons, and projects to the lateral rectus muscle. CN IV and VI functions are evaluated by observing vertical and lateral eye movements. Compression of CN IV can occur with cerebellar tumors or damage due to shear injury from head trauma and produces vertical *diplopia* (*suppression* of the eye). Compression of CN VI can occur with elevated intracranial pressure and produces horizontal *diplopia* (failure to adduct).

- *Trigeminal Nerve (CN V)* The trigeminal nerve originates from the pons and innervates the upper, middle, and lower portions of the face via the ophthalmic, maxillary, and mandibular divisions respectively. CN V functions to provide sensory innervation to the face, nasal sinuses, mouth, and anterior two thirds of the tongue and controls muscles of mastication. The ophthalmic division supplies the *afferent* limb of the corneal reflex. CN V functioning is tested by assessing facial sensation, corneal *reflexes*, and jaw jerk *reflexes*.

- *Facial Nerve (CN VII)* The facial nerve originates from the lower pons and upper medulla. The main function of CN VII is to control muscles of facial expression. Additional CN VII functions include parasympathetic (tears and salivation), visceral sensory (taste) and general somatosensory functions. As inputs above the CN VII nucleus are bilaterally represented, unilateral *upper motor neuron* (UMN) lesions spare the forehead. Facial droop following stroke involves the mouth/lower face sparing the forehead and involvement of the forehead implies lesion of CN VII. On the other hand, *lower motor neuron* (LMN) lesions result in contralateral forehead denervation. CN VII function is assessed by looking for asymmetry in spontaneous facial expressions.

- *Vestibulocochlear Nerve (CN VIII)* Vestibulocochlear nerve projects from the auditory canal to the pontomedullary junction. CN VIII is responsible for auditory and *vestibular* functions. Auditory function is tested by the Rinne test, in which a vibrating tuning fork is placed just outside each ear to assess air conduction and on the forehead or mastoid to assess bone conduction. In normal hearing, air conduction is greater than bone conduction. In sensorineuronal hearing loss caused by CN VIII dysfunction, air conduction remains greater than bone conduction and sound lateralizes to the normal ear. Conductive hearing loss caused by external auditory canal or middle ear abnormalities is detected when bone conduction is better than air conduction. *Vestibular* functions are tested with the Dix-Hallpike maneuver, which can differentiate peripheral from central causes of vertigo. The examiner supports the patient's head as they lie back on the exam table and the head is rotated. Vertigo with *nystagmus* suggests CN VIII dysfunction.

- *Glossopharyngeal Nerve (CN IX)* This nerve stems from the medulla and projects to the pharynx, middle ear, and posterior tongue. General somatic sensory functions of the CN IX include the sensation of touch, pain, and temperature. CN IX is evaluated by inducing a gag reflex, typically by touching the uvula. Unilateral nerve dysfunction results in retraction to the stronger side.

- *Vagus Nerve (CN X)* Originates in the medulla and provides parasympathetic innervation to the heart, lungs, and digestive tract. The brachial motor component controls pharyngeal and upper esophageal muscles (swallowing and gag reflex) and larynx muscles (voice box). In addition, CN X provides somatic and visceral sensory functions. CN X and CN IX in conjunction mediates the gag reflex and therefore are tested together.

- *Spinal Accessory Nerve (CN XI)* This nerve stems from the spinal cord rather than the brainstem to the sternocleidomastoid muscle and trapezius. Cranial Nerve XI is often tested by having the patient shrug their shoulders. Dysfunction is indicated on the lower side when the shrug is asymmetric.

- *Hypoglossal Nerve (CN XII)* Originates in the medulla and innervates the tongue muscles. Lesions of the hypoglossal nucleus or nerve cause ipsilateral tongue weakness. Assessment of CN XII is conducted by examining the tongue protruded. The tongue will deviate toward the side of the lesion. In addition, subtle dysarthria may be noted with CN XII lesions, particularly when asked to repeat challenging phrases, such as "Methodist Episcopal."

Examination of Motor Function

The motor exam includes components such as observational findings, muscle tone, and strength testing. Upon observation, abnormal movements ranging from lack of movement (*akinesia*), slow writhing like movement (*athetosis*), irregularly timed excessive jerky movements (*chorea*), and extreme choreiform movement (*ballismus*) are noted. To assess muscle tone abnormalities (resistance to passive movement), patients passively move each limb at several joints for examination of the presence of resistance or rigidity. Examination of motor functions can also assist with differentiating UMN versus LMN lesions. UMNs include projections from the cortex to spinal cord (corticospinal tract) including the part that crosses (decussates) in the medulla (pyramidal tract). LMNs include projections from the brainstem and spinal cord, via motor nerves to innervate skeletal muscle. Hyperreflexia, and increased tone can be indicative of UMN lesions. On the other hand, atrophy, fasciculations, and hyporeflexia can be indicative of LMN lesions. UMN problems are also indicated if a "pronator drift" is observed. This is when the hand or arm that is extended with palms facing upward begin to rotate into pronation when the patient is standing with feet together. Muscle strength is rated on an ordinal scale from 0 (no visible muscle contraction) to 5 (normal strength). Testing muscles that represent specific nerves and nerve root innervations can assist in localization.

Examination of Sensory Functioning

An examination of cutaneous sensory topography is useful in understanding the findings of neurologic examinations. Sensory dermatomes are referred to by the anatomic level of the spinal cord from which the innervating nerve root emerges (i.e., C, cervical; T, thoracic; L, lumbar; and S, Sacral) and by a number representing the specific vertebra at which they emerge (e.g., "L5"). Pattern of sensory loss can assist to localize lesions to particular nerves, nerve roots, spinal cord regions, brainstem, thalamus, or cortex. Sensory modalities tested include light touch (tested with cotton swab or light finger touch), pain (using a sterile safety pin), temperature (using a cool piece of metal), vibration (using a tuning fork), and position (by minimally moving a digit and asking the patient to identify direction of movement).

Neuropsychologists are more likely to utilize standardized measures (e.g., the Reitan-Klove Sensory-Perceptual Exam or the Benton Laboratory tests) to assess cortical sensation or higher-order aspects of sensation such as stereognosis, *graphesthesia*, and sensory extinction. During a clinical neurological examination, these same functions are often evaluated in a nonstandardized manner. For example, *graphesthesia* is assessed by having patients close their eyes and identify letters or numbers traced on the palm of their hand. Stereognosis is examined by having patients identify various objects by touch using one hand and with eyes closed. Intact primary sensation with agraphesthesia or astereognosis suggests lesion in the contralateral sensory cortex. Extinction is assessed by first establishing intact primary bilateral sensation followed by assessing the patient's ability to detect alternating unilateral and bilateral stimulation. Intact primary sensation and inability to detect unilateral input during simultaneous stimulation suggest contralateral parietal lobe dysfunction.

Examination of Gait and Coordination

Many systems, including cerebellar functions, can disrupt gait and coordination. Gait abnormalities are described as spastic, scissored, steppage, parkinsonian, or ataxic. More specifically, spastic gait suggests spastic hemiparesis and is when the affected leg swings in an arc motion ("circumduct"). Scissored gait suggests corticospinal dysfunction and is when gait appears stiff and the thigh crosses over in front of the other thigh. Steppage gait results when a foot or both feet are weak resulting in "foot drop." Parkinsonian gait usually entails short or shuffling steps in which the individual often has difficulty starting or stopping. The person is often stooped over and arm swing can be reduced. Ataxic gait is unsteady and wide based and suggests cerebellar dysfunction. Turning is completed with difficulty.

Coordination abnormalities, often termed ataxia, can be associated with cerebellar disorders. Cerebellar functions in the upper extremities are examined by having patients alternately touch their nose and the examiner's finger as well as by switching hand movements from palm facing up to palm facing down. Inaccuracy in doing so is referred to as *dysmetria* and *dysdiadochokinesia* respectively and suggests ipsilateral cerebellar hemispheric dysfunction. Cerebellar functions in the lower extremities are examined by the heel-shin-test in which the patient lies on their back and lifts the heel of their foot and moves it in a straight line along their opposite shin up to the knee. In the Romberg test, patients are asked to stand with their feet together and close their eyes. The "Romberg sign" is when unsteadiness occurs within several seconds of closing the eyes. With the eyes open, truncal stability is maintained by vision, *proprioception* and *vestibular* senses providing input to the cerebellum. With eyes closed and visual input removed, instability suggests poor *proprioception* due to posterior column dysfunction. With eyes open, instability suggests more severe proprioceptive or *vestibular* dysfunction or midline cerebellar lesion.

Examination of Reflexes

Deep tendon reflexes (DTRs) evaluate *afferent* (i.e., carrying neural impulses to CNS) and *efferent* (carrying neural impulses from the CNS) functioning. DTRs are assessed with a single brisk tap from a reflex hammer directly on the skin of the tendon. Increased *reflexes* ("hyperactive") is observed with corticospinal dysfunction, and decreased or absent *reflexes* with peripheral nerves or nerve roots dysfunction. Grading of DTRs is from 0 to 5+ with 1+, 2+, or 3+ being normal unless they are asymmetric or discrepant between the arms and legs. *Reflexes* rated as 0, 4+, or 5+ are usually considered abnormal. Dysfunction of corticospinal tracts can lead to *long-tract signs*, which may be seen, for example, in normal pressure hydrocephalus, and include hyperactive *deep tendon reflexes, clonus*, and *spasticity* (i.e., increased muscle tone or resistance to stretching). Corticospinal system dysfunction is often tested by elicitation of the *Babinski sign* or the "extensor plantar response" when the handle of a reflex hammer is scraped on the lateral surface of the foot from the heel upward and across the ball of the foot toward the big toe. The *Babinski sign* is present when there is fanning of the toes and upward flexion of the big toe and is associated in UMN dysfunction in adults (The *Babinski sign* is normal in children up to about one year old). The Wartenberg's sign consists of involuntary abduction of the fifth digit and can be caused by *upper motor neuron* disorders.

Examination of Mental Status

While neuropsychologists complete detailed psychometric evaluation of cognitive domains, physicians usually conduct brief screens of mental status to evaluate global brain function. More specifically, they may begin by assessing level of alertness, attention, and cooperation followed by orientation. Subsequently, limbic system function (memory), dominant usually left hemisphere function (language), left parietal function (Gerstmann's syndrome), right parietal function (neglect and praxis), and frontal function (sequencing, logic, abstraction) are examined. Furthermore, the examiner asks questions to determine presence of delusions, hallucinations, and mood. To assess the above domains, physicians mostly engage in nonstandardized methods judged by impressions rather than norms. At times, standardized methods are implemented such as utilizing the Folstein Mini Mental Status Examination (MMSE) or the Montreal Cognitive Assessment (MoCA). While the MMSE is often utilized, it de-emphasizes working memory and executive functions and often lacks sensitivity with regard to a variety of conditions/symptoms involving frontal-subcortical systems (e.g., Parkinson's disease, multiple sclerosis, traumatic brain injury [TBI]). It is important to note that scoring below cutoff is clinically significant but "within normal limits" may not reflect the patient's true neurocognitive status. In other words a normal score on a screening instrument does not always indicate intact cognitive function.

Over the years, physicians have begun to incorporate computerized tests to assess for specific diagnosis (e.g., evaluation of ADHD or concussion) as well as for a wide range of cognitive functions or diagnoses. Neuropsychologists should be familiar with the psychometric properties of these tests. See Bauer et al. (2012) under "Recommended Readings" for a review of this topic. In addition, in line with technological advances, neuropsychologists should be aware of the benefits of integrating technology while also considering the potential issues. See Miller and Barr (2017) under "Recommended Readings" for review.

Neuroimaging Studies: Structural Imaging

Prior to neuroimaging techniques, lesions and disorders of the nervous system were diagnosed and localized by clinical neurologic examination. Neuroimaging has allowed direct visualization of structural abnormalities and localization. Further, advances in imaging techniques are increasingly sensitive to the detailed visualization of nervous system structure.

Conventional Skull X-Rays

Conventional skull x-rays are used in rapid examination of skull injuries or abnormalities. Computerized tomography (CT) was developed directly from conventional x-ray technology and may be more useful in characterizing skull fractures and other defects.

Computed Tomography (CT)

In CT, the x-ray beam is rotated around the patient's head to take many different views, which are digitally reconstructed. As the rays travel through the head, they are absorbed to different degrees based on density. Greatest absorption occurs for the densest structures (hyperdense) such as bone, freshly congealed blood, or other calcifications to intermediate density (isodense) such as brain tissue and CSF to less dense materials (hypodense) such as air and fat. On CT hyperdense structures are lighter in color and hypodense structures are darker on a monochromatic scale.

The primary advantage of CT is the ability to detect gross abnormalities. Therefore, CTs are useful for detecting skull fractures, hemorrhage, and mass effect, making it the modality of first choice in acute care. On the other hand, CT is less effective at detecting white matter changes (e.g., plaques in MS, microvascular ischemic changes) or refined differential diagnosis (e.g., tumor or other mass). Intravenous contrast can be used to enhance CT in patients with brain tumors, arteriovenous malformations (AVMs), aneurysms, cerebral abscesses, chronic isodense subdural hematomas, or infarctions. Risks associated with CT are exposure to small amounts of ionizing radiation and allergic reactions to the iodine-based contrast media.

Magnetic Resonance Imaging (MRI)

MRI is used to generate high-resolution anatomic images of brain structure. In MRI specific radiofrequency pulses generate an electromagnetic reaction of hydrogen protons in water molecules. When the pulses are stopped, the protons return to their original alignment, resulting in emission of electrical signals that are detected by the scanner and can be reconstructed by computer to produce an image. The physical behavior of water molecules in brain tissue can be further characterized by two time constants ("T1" and "T2"). T1 scans demonstrate greater anatomic detail but less tissue contrast, whereas T2 scans have enhanced contrast and are more sensitive to detecting damaged versus intact tissue, making them useful for lesion identification. For example, in T2 scans, intact white matter appears gray and plaques associated with MS or lesions associated with axonal injury will appear much brighter (i.e., demonstrating increased or "high" signal intensity). CSF also appears "brighter" on T2 scans, thus facilitating the identification of cavitated lesions, such as lacunar infarcts. An additional clinical MRI sequence, fluid-attenuated inversion recovery (FLAIR), allows for the representation of even greater contrast between normal and pathological tissue. There are also IV-injected paramagnetic contrast media (e.g., gadolinium) for detection of blood-brain barrier perturbations, cerebral blood flow, infection, or inflammation. As technology advances, there are additional radiologic techniques that are increasingly becoming available and affordable, which may ultimately lead to changes in acute assessment. For example, fast magnetic resonance imaging (fsMRI) sequences, single-shot spin echo images have replaced CT scans for many conditions (e.g., hydrocephalus, macrocephaly).

Benefits of MRI include highly detailed images of brain anatomy, both of cell-rich areas and the fibers that connect them. Therefore, in contrast to CT, it is the method of choice for detection of low-contrast or small lesions (e.g., MS, AVM, low-grade astrocytoma). Unlike CT, MRI does not use ionizing radiation, allowing repeat use for adults and children. While there are minimal risks associated with MRIs, it can be noisy and can produce claustrophobia in some individuals. Furthermore individuals with implanted devices or residual metal fragments from accidents may be unable to have an MRI.

Diffusion-Weighted MRI

Diffusion-weighted imaging (DWI), a variant of MRI, is a method of using diffusion of water molecules to generate contrast in MR images. DWI has been well established in stroke imaging, white matter diseases, and oncology. While conventional imaging focused on anatomical information, DWI allows collection of information about molecular activity and cellular function. For example, DWI can detect stroke during the first few hours of onset prior to detectability on standard MRI as it can discriminate cytotoxic edema (more likely in stroke) from vasogenic edema (associated with other cerebral lesions or events). It is often utilized with perfusion MRI, which outlines salvageable areas of ischemia and has clinical implications with regard to the use of thrombolytic agents and differentiation of acute versus chronic stroke. DWI is also sensitive to microstructural changes and can detect abnormalities such as white matter disease prior to changes observed on conventional imaging.

Perfusion-Weighted MRI

Perfusion-weighted MRI allows the clinican to infer how blood travels through the brain's vasculature through the use of a contrast medium or an endogenous blood flow marker. Hemodynamic parameters commonly measured include cerebral blood volume (CBV), cerebral blood flow (CBF), mean transit time (MTT), and Time to peak of the tissue response (T max). In primary cerebral perfusion disorders such as ischemic stroke and transient ischemic attack, perfusion imaging allows more detailed understanding of the cerebral vasculature's response to changes in perfusion pressure by examination of regional CBV, CBF, MTT, and T max. Perfusion imaging is increasingly utilized in the diagnosis and imaging of brain tumors which exhibit unusual diffusion due to mass effect, modulated metabolism, and pathological leakage across the blood-brain barrier. Perfusion imaging of brain tumors typically focuses on evaluation of CBV and blood flow and is often combined with conventional MRI images in order to characterize brain tumors, select optimal treatment strategies as well as monitoring effects of treatment.

Susceptibility-Weighted Imaging (SWI)

SWI is an MRI sequence that can detect the unique magnetic susceptibility differences between various tissues or background. SWI is particularly sensitive to detecting small amounts of blood products and calcium, which may be undetectable with other MRI sequences. Therefore, SWI can be useful for very small lesions, increasing the ability to detect more subtle TBIs as well as microhemorrhages in cerebral amyloid angiopathy.

Diffusion Tensor Imaging (DTI)

DTI is an MRI method to examine white matter integrity and white matter tracts by detecting the directional movements of water molecules. Movement of water molecules in nerve fibers follows the tract's orientation, a property referred to as anisotropy. DTI generates a fractional anisotropy (FA) value, which is usually higher in very organized densely myelinated regions of the brain (e.g., corpus callosum and pyramidal tracts). Less organized, less myelinated, or state of edema, injury, or inflammation can produce lower FA values. There is much ongoing research to advance the diagnosis and treatment of conditions (e.g., axonal degeneration due to MS, fiber distortion due to tumors, fiber damage due to TBI or stroke) using DTI. The Human Connectome Project is one such large-scale study involving a consortium of research centers (Toga et al., 2012). DTI has the potential to be utilized in the evaluation of the pediatric population whose white matter tracts mature during early life then degenerate with aging.

Magnetic Resonance Spectroscopy (MRS)

MRS is an MRI method to localize and characterize brain-based biomarkers. As in other MRI-based techniques, the biophysics involves altering the radiofrequency used for aligning hydrogen protons. In addition, MRS can image endogenous biological markers such as creatinine (Cre), an acid that assists with cell energy, and n-acetyl aspartate (NAA), a brain metabolite found in neurons and glia. Further, MRS can image glutamate (Glu), a major excitatory neurotransmitter, and choline (Cho), a precursor molecule for acetylcholine. Therefore, MRS can detect brain-cell loss in degenerative diseases such as Alzheimer's disease (AD) and demyelinating diseases such as MS.

Magnetic Resonance Angiography (MRA)

MRA is a technique to generate images of arteries (and less commonly veins) for the purpose of evaluating stenosis, occlusions, and aneurysms. Advantages of MRA include the noninvasive nature of the examination compared to catheter angiography and no exposure to ionizing radiation such as with CT angiography. Disadvantages include poorer spatial resolution, less sensitivity to vessels with slower blood flow, and lengthier procedure time than CT angiography. While current techniques allow visualization of AVMs and aneurysms greater than 3 mm in diameter, conventional angiography remains the "gold standard."

Neuroimaging Studies: Functional Imaging

Advances from static to dynamic brain imaging techniques have allowed investigation of changes in brain activity by measuring changes in blood flow and oxygen. There are two broad categories of functional imaging: "resting" or "activated." In resting paradigms, images are acquired during nonactivated or static conditions. Of note, there are multiple brain networks that are active despite a non-task-engaged state. Activation paradigms involve acquisition of images during engagement in a cognitive or motor task.

Single-Photon Emission Computed Tomography (SPECT)

SPECT examines regional changes in cerebral activity or brain chemistry through the use and detection of tracer flow or receptor-binding isotopes. SPECT has mostly been utilized to study regional blood flow (rCBF), which is correlated with brain activity. Radioisotopes are absorbed by glia and remain in greater concentration in more active regions of the brain. As they undergo decay, they emit radioactive particles, which are detected to generate a computerized reconstruction. SPECT markers (as well as PET markers) have been developed for specific types of neuropathology such as beta amyloid and tau. The advantages of SPECT are that it is generally more widely available due to less extensive technological and technical requirements than PET or fMRI. Furthermore, the radiotracers used for SPECT are stable enough that an on-site chemist or cyclotron is often not needed.

Positron Emission Tomography (PET)

Positron Emission Tomography (PET) is also a radioisotope-based technology, which examines glucose utilization with radioisotopes. PET examines metabolic activity in brain cells engaged in cognitive tasks. PET imaging utilizes intravenous tracers such as ^{18}F-flurodeoxyglucose (FDG) and Oxygen-15 to characterize resting regional brain metabolism. PET can be useful in the differential diagnosis of dementia due to differing patterns of abnormal cerebral metabolism. For example, in AD, PET imaging typically reveals bilaterally reduced regional glucose metabolism in the posterior temporoparietal cortices in addition to anterior and mesial temporal lobes. In FTD, PET imaging shows hypometabolism mostly in the frontal and anterior temporal cortices. In addition, in vivo imaging of amyloid-beta with PET can assist in diagnosis of AD. However, it should be noted that while biomarkers like amyloid levels are specific to etiology, they do not associate well with disease burden. Combined PET and CT or MRI are now commercially available typically for very specific diagnostic questions such as tumor characterization. The computer reconstructed color-coded image is based on glucose uptake with regions of high blood flow typically depicted as bright red and yellow. The advantages of PET include greater spatial resolution than SPECT. Limitations of PET include the expense of the procedure, which requires an on-site chemist and cyclotron.

Functional Magnetic Resonance Imaging (fMRI)

fMRI examines regional changes in brain activity. Neural activity is associated with blood flow to that region and the localized surplus of oxyhemoglobin relative to deoxyhemoglobin results in signal intensity referred to as the blood oxygen level dependent (BOLD) effect. Use of fMRI for clinical purposes has been limited mostly to presurgical mapping for epilepsy surgeries and tumor resections. The advantages of fMRI are that the procedure utilizes the natural physical responses to high-strength magnetism and therefore no exogenous tracers, radioisotopes, or contrast agents are necessary. Furthermore, fMRI resolution is superior to that of SPECT and PET. Disadvantages include technical limitations such as difficulties when applying group findings to individual cases and in reliably executing fMRI experiments.

Electrophysiological Studies

Neural transmission is an electrophysiological process and there are several methods in which activity is measured and recorded.

Electroencephalography (EEG)

EEG is electrophysiologically based technology to monitor brain electrical activity along the scalp. Voltage fluctuations within neurons of the brain closest to the skull are recorded. Since the signal produced by each neuron is quite small, the EEG signal recorded is the sum of rhythmical activity of thousands of neurons. The primary clinical application of EEG is to differentiate epileptic seizures from other types of events (e.g., nonepileptic seizures, fainting, or subcortical disorders). Secondary clinical applications of EEG include diagnosis of coma, determination of brain death, polysomnography, and monitoring anesthesia depth. Furthermore, certain neurologic disorders produce characteristic although nonspecific EEG abnormalities to aid in diagnostic suggestion, establishment or support. For example, repetitive slow wave complexes over temporal lobe (unilateral or bilateral) in patients with acute cerebral function disturbance suggests a diagnosis of herpes simplex encephalitis. An application of EEG referred to as quantitative EEG (QEEG) uses digital signal analysis to obtain continuous monitoring and quantification across several wave frequencies (i.e., amounts of alpha, beta, delta, and theta activity in a complex waveform).

The EEG waveforms are classified according to frequency, amplitude, and shape as well as the scalp regions from which they are recorded. The most common classifications of waveform frequencies are as follows:

- *Alpha* waves (i.e., 8–12 Hz waveforms) are observed in all age groups although more commonly in adults. Alpha amplitude manifests when the patient is relaxed with eyes closed and ablated by eye opening. They occur bilaterally in the posterior regions, being higher in amplitude on the dominant side. Frontal alpha consisting of alpha activity over anterior head regions may be related to drugs, anesthesia, or following arousal from sleep.

- *Beta* waves (i.e., 12–30 Hz) are observed in all age groups. Beta is the dominant rhythm in patients who are alert, anxious, or have their eyes open. They are usually seen in symmetrical distribution and is most evident frontally. Beta activity is enhanced by sedating drugs such as benzodiazepines and barbiturates thought to be caused by a compensatory mechanism that allows for behavioral activation despite sedation.

- *Theta* waves (i.e., 4–7 Hz) are observed in children and during sleep at any age. They may be transiently observed during normal wakefulness but are more prominent during drowsiness.

- *Delta* waves (i.e., up to 4 Hz) are observed during sleep across all age groups and are normally the dominant rhythm in infants. They are observed more frontally in adults and posteriorly in children. Both theta and delta activity may occur in generalized distribution with diffuse disorders or metabolic encephalopathy.

Evoked Potentials (EPs)

EP procedure involves the noninvasive stimulation of *afferent* pathways. Electrophysiologic responses of the nervous system to various stimuli such as visual, auditory, and somatosensory are measured with EEG. Visual EP tests conduction of visual pathways by presenting a fixed visual pattern (e.g., checkerboard array) to each eye and recording electrical activity. The most clinically relevant component is the P100 response. Prolongation of latency of this EP may indicate optic nerve dysfunction, ischemic disturbance, or demyelinating disease, often confirmed by additional laboratory testing. Auditory EP is assessed by administering repetitive clicks to each ear. Somatosensory EP may be elicited using mechanical or brief electrical stimulation to the skin. EP studies are frequently used to detect and localize lesions in the CNS such as in MS as well as other CNS disorders such as acquired immunodeficiency syndrome (AIDS) and neurosyphilis. EP studies have also been used to assess prognosis after CNS trauma or hypoxia and to assist during intraoperative monitoring.

Electromyography (EMG) and Nerve Conduction Studies

EMG involves the recording of electrical activity in specific muscles as well as peripheral nerves. During a needle EMG, a needle electrode is inserted into the muscle and a nerve conduction study utilizes electrodes taped to the skin to measure specific waveforms generated in the presence of certain pathologies (e.g., following traumatic denervation or in degenerative disorders of the spinal cord.)

Magnetoencephalography and Magnetic Source Imaging (MEG/MSI)

MEG technology detects minute magnetic fields generated by neuronal activity. When a neuronal synapse becomes active, there is current flow across membranes that can be recorded. A MEG scanner allows participants to be seated upright, which differs from SPECT and PET scans. Advantages of MEG include greater ease of recording due to detectors placed in a helmet rather than with EEG, where detectors are applied individually and interconnected. A disadvantage of MEG is that it is not widely available and physical facilities must be specially constructed to support its use.

Invasive Examination Procedures

Cerebral Arteriography

Cerebral arteriography (also "angiography") involves the injection of an iodine-based contrast into the cerebrovasculature via a catheter inserted into the femoral or brachial artery and threaded up the aortic arch. It provides excellent characterization of AVMs, aneurysms, and cerebral venous sinus thrombosis. It is also useful for differential diagnosis of tumors that produce a "stain" or "blush" as a result of neovascularization. Interventional techniques such as coil embolization of aneurysms are performed with cerebral arteriography. Complications include stroke, an allergic reaction to the contrast, and thrombosis or embolism formation.

Intracarotid Sodium Amobarbital Procedure

This procedure (referred to as "Wada testing," named for its developer, Juhn Wada) involves injecting sodium amobarbital into the cerebrovasculature via an angiographically guided catheter to produce a brief period of anesthesia of the ipsilateral hemisphere. Testing of various functions such as language, memory, movement is conducted to determine capabilities of one hemisphere while the other is anesthetized. Testing is performed for presurgical candidates with epilepsy to determine hemispheric dominance for language and potential postoperative cognitive losses.

Computed Tomographic Angiography (CTA)

CTA is a technique utilized to visualize arterial and venous vessels. This requires a combination of intravenous injection of radiocontrast and CT scanning. It is used to produce highly detailed three-dimensional renderings of the relationship between vasculature and anatomy. This feature can assist in the evaluation of conditions such as carotid stenosis, intra and extracranial atherosclerosis, and aneurysms. The advantage of CTA is the acquisition of high-quality images in 5–10 seconds that are useful for diagnosis and follow-up of cerebrovascular diseases. Furthermore, images are less likely to be impacted by patient movement in comparison to MR angiography. Disadvantages include reduced sensitivity for aneurysms less than 3 mm, and it may not reveal plaque ulceration or disease of small vessels.

Lumbar Puncture

Lumbar puncture (LP, or spinal tap) provides direct access to the subarachnoid space to obtain samples of CSF, measure CSF pressure, or to remove CSF. The patient is often in a lying or seated position, and a needle is inserted below the spinal cord to avoid contact (usually between L4 or L5 intervertebral space). The CSF fluid is inspected visually and microscopically for blood or bacteria to assess for infectious or inflammatory disorders, sub-arachnoid hemorrhage and abnormalities of intracranial pressure that affect CSF. Lumbar puncture also allows detection of biomarkers. For instance, levels of tau in CSF is utilized as a biomarker for AD. Moreover, a decreased CSF phosphor-tau 181 to total tau ratio (p/t-tau ratio) has been suggested to be useful in identification in frontotemporal lobar degeneration with TDP-43 inclusions (FTLD-TDP) and for amyotrophic lateral sclerosis.

Relevant Definitions

Afferent Carrying neural impulses to the CNS.

Akinesia Lack of movement.

Athetosis Slow writhing-like movement.

Blown pupil A pupil that is dilated and unresponsive to changes in light.

Babinski sign Fanning of the toes and upward flexion of the big toe. Also referred to as the "extensor plantar response."

Ballismus Extreme choreiform movement.

Bitemporal hemianopsia Loss of visual temporal fields often due to abnormality in the optic chiasm.

Chorea Irregularly timed excessive jerky movements.

Clonus Repetitive, involuntary vibratory movements.

Deep tendon reflexes Muscular contractions that occur in response to the stretching of a muscle.

Diplopia The experience of double vision.

Dysdiadochokinesia Impaired ability to smoothly alternate hand movements.

Dysmetria Inaccurate range of movement during motion-based activities.

Efferent Carrying neural impulses away from the nervous system.

Graphesthesia The ability to identify letters or numbers traced on the skin.

Hemianopsia The loss of a visual hemifield.

Homonymous On the same side (e.g., homonymous hemianopsia).

Long-tract signs Neurologic signs related to upper motor neuron lesions, including hyperactive deep tendon reflexes, clonus, and spasticity.

Lower motor neuron (LMN) Motor neuron that originate in the anterior horn of the spinal cord. The motor cranial nerve nuclei are also classified as lower motor neurons.

Nystagmus Rapid involuntary eye movements, which may be lateral, vertical, rotational, or mixed.

Proprioception Perception of one's body position in space, based on sensory input from the muscles and tendons.

Quadrantanopsia Loss of one quadrant of the visual field.

Reflexes An involuntary response to a stimulus.

Spasticity Increased muscle tone or increased resistance to stretching.

Suppression The unilateral diminution of sensory input perception in the presence of bilateral stimulation.

Upper motor neuron (UMN) Neurons that originate from the cerebral primary motor cortex (i.e., the precentral gyrus) or from certain brainstem nuclei (e.g., the rubrospinal tract from the red nucleus).

Vestibular Referring to the sense of balance.

The Neurologic Examination, Radiologic, and Other Diagnostic Studies Questions

NOTE: Questions 36, 81, and 124 on the First Full-Length Practice Examination, Questions 24, 38, 45, 116, and 117 on the Second Full-Length Practice Examination, Questions 12, 54, 104, and 121 on the Third Full-Length Practice Examination, and Questions 16, 54, 89, and 124 on the Fourth Full-Length Practice Examination are from this chapter.

1. You evaluated a patient with a traumatic brain injury who demonstrated relative weakness on tests of visuospatial function. Based on his self-report as well as behavioral observations, you suspect oculomotor difficulties that underlie his performance. Which cranial nerves associated with eye movement may be involved?

    (a) an implausible visual defect

    (b) cranial nerves II, III, IV, VI

    (c) cranial nerves III, IV, VI

    (d) cranial nerves VIII, IX, X

2. Your patient sustained a traumatic brain injury, resulting in a fixed and dilated ("blown") pupil. This is typically associated with dysfunction or injury to which cranial nerve?

    (a) II

    (b) III

    (c) IV

    (d) VI

3. Your review of medical records for a new patient suggests damage to the trigeminal nerve. You would expect this individual to have symptoms associated with ____.

    (a) neither sensory nor motor functions of the face or jaw

    (b) only sensory functions of the face and jaw

    (c) only motor functions of the face and jaw

    (d) both sensory and motor functions of the face and jaw

4. Your patient who sustained a cerebrovascular accident is experiencing difficulties with swallowing, including her gag reflex. You would expect to see testing of _____ during her neurological evaluation, as this pair of nerves elicits a gag reflex when tested together.

    (a) cranial nerves IX, X

    (b) cranial nerves VII, X

    (c) cranial nerves VII, IX

    (d) cranial nerves V, VI

5. A patient with a known upper motor neuron lesion is asked to stand with her feet together and arms held palms up and extended at shoulder level as part of her neurological examination. She is unable to maintain the position, and her left arm slowly turns toward a palm-down position. She is exhibiting a _____, which suggests _____ dysfunction.

    (a) Hoffmann reflex; contralateral pyramidal tract

    (b) Romberg sign; ipsilateral cerebellar

    (c) pronator drift; contralateral pyramidal tract

    (d) Wartenberg sign; ipsilateral cerebellar

6. When evaluating a patient with chronic alcoholism, impairment in the ability to perform alternating hand movements, referred to as _____ suggests cerebellar dysfunction _____ to the more affected side.

    (a) dysmetria; ipsilateral

    (b) dysdiadochokinesia; ipsilateral

    (c) dysmetria; contralateral

    (d) dysdiadochokinesia; contralateral

7. You are looking at medical records of a patient who was admitted to the emergency department due to acute head trauma. Which type of imaging will have been completed upon admission?

    (a) magnetic resonance imaging

    (b) single photon emission tomography

    (c) computed tomography

    (d) diffusion tensor imaging

8. You are interested in determining white matter integrity of a patient with multiple sclerosis. Therefore, diffusion tensor imaging is utilized in which the primary dependent variable is _____.

    (a) diffuse axonal injury (DAI)

    (b) blood oxygen level dependent response (BOLD)

    (c) cerebral metabolic rate of glucose metabolism (CMRGlu)

    (d) fractional anisotropy (FA)

9. In the absence of neurological disorders such as epilepsy, electroencephalographic alpha activity is typically _____ during relaxation and _____ during mental activity.

    (a) increased; disappears

    (b) decreased; increased

    (c) never present; increased

    (d) present; unknown

10. The EEG signal represents _____.

    (a) real-time activity of individual neurons

    (b) the summation of activity from thousands to millions of neurons

    (c) normal background activity and epileptiform spikes

    (d) activity from only those neurons immediately beneath each electrode

11. A patient with an extensive cardiac history presents for neuropsychological assessment following a stroke. As part of her record, which scan would most likely have been explicitly conducted as a method of evaluating possible occlusions and aneurysms during her initial inpatient admission?

    (a) computed tomography
    (b) diffusion tensor imaging
    (c) magnetic resonance imaging
    (d) magnetic resonance angiography

12. Your patient who presents after a stroke is describing a neuroimaging procedure he underwent as part of an examination. Which of the following is considered most sensitive to acute infarcts within the first 24 hours?

    (a) functional magnetic resonance imaging
    (b) diffusion tensor imaging
    (c) diffusion weighted MRI (DWI)
    (d) tau spectroscopy

13. You receive records regarding neuroimaging that was conducted to characterize the brain tumor of your patient. The report references hypermetabolism of glucose in select regions. The kind of imaging that was most likely conducted is _____.

    (a) positron emission tomography
    (b) functional magnetic resonance imaging
    (c) electroencephalography
    (d) perfusion weighted MRI

14. You receive records regarding studies that were conducted to characterize the seizures of your patient with a likely epilepsy diagnosis, and to distinguish them from nonepileptic seizures, syncope, and other subcortical disorders. The report most likely describes the results of _____.

    (a) computed tomography
    (b) magnetic resonance angiography
    (c) diffusion tensor imaging
    (d) electroencephalography

15. The results of an electroencephalography (EEG) report that you receive describe waveforms that are associated with drowsiness, possibly associated with your patient's use of sedatives. The waveform frequencies are most likely to be consistent with _____.

    (a) alpha waves
    (b) beta waves
    (c) theta waves
    (d) delta waves

The Neurologic Examination, Radiologic, and Other Diagnostic Studies Answers

1. **C—cranial nerves III, IV, VI**   *Each of these nerves projects to extraocular muscles involved in eye movement. Cranial nerve II only carries visual information. Cranial nerve VIII can be involved in nystagmus, but IX and X have no role in eye movement.*

   References:
   (a) Blumenfeld, H. (2011). *Neuroanatomy through clinical cases* (2nd ed.). Sunderland, MA: Sinauer Associates.
   (b) Goldberg, S. (2017). *The four-minute neurological exam* (2nd ed.). Miami, FL: MedMaster.
   (c) Simon, R. P., Aminoff, M., & Greenberg, D. A. (2018). *Clinical neurology* (10th ed.). New York, NY: Lange Medical Books/McGraw-Hill Education.

2. **B—III**   *Cranial nerve III (oculomotor) specifically mediates the parasympathetic (constricting) ciliary response of the eye. Mechanical damage to CN III interferes with pupil constriction, but sympathetic function remains and the dilation function remains.*

References:
(a) Blumenfeld, H. (2011). *Neuroanatomy through clinical cases* (2nd ed.). Sunderland, MA: Sinauer Associates.
(b) Goldberg, S. (2017). *The four-minute neurological exam* (2nd ed.). Miami, FL: MedMaster.
(c) Simon, R. P., Aminoff, M., & Greenberg, D. A. (2018). *Clinical neurology* (10th ed.). New York, NY: Lange Medical Books/McGraw-Hill Education.

3. **D—both sensory and motor functions of the face and jaw**   *The trigeminal is a mixed cranial nerve and has both sensory and motor capacities.*

References:
(a) Blumenfeld, H. (2011). *Neuroanatomy through clinical cases* (2nd ed.). Sunderland, MA: Sinauer Associates.
(b) Goldberg, S. (2017). *The four-minute neurological exam* (2nd ed.). Miami, FL: MedMaster.
(c) Simon, R. P., Aminoff, M., & Greenberg, D. A. (2018). *Clinical neurology* (10th ed.). New York, NY: Lange Medical Books/McGraw-Hill Education.

4. **A—cranial nerves IX, X**   *The glossopharyngeal and vagus nerves co-mediate the gag reflex. Cranial nerve VII is involved in swallowing and coughing, but only at the level of the neck muscles, not the pharynx. Cranial nerve V mediates face and jaw sensorimotor functions. Cranial nerve VI is ocular.*

References:
(a) Blumenfeld, H. (2011). *Neuroanatomy through clinical cases* (2nd ed.). Sunderland, MA: Sinauer Associates.
(b) Goldberg, S. (2017). *The four-minute neurological exam* (2nd ed.). Miami, FL: MedMaster.
(c) Simon, R. P., Aminoff, M., & Greenberg, D. A. (2018). *Clinical neurology* (10th ed.). New York, NY: Lange Medical Books/McGraw-Hill Education.

5. **C—pronator drift; contralateral pyramidal tract**   *The example described is classic pronator drift, which localizes to contralateral pyramidal tracts. Wartenberg and Hoffmann signs do not involve standing. A Romberg sign refers to sway when standing, but no upper extremity signs.*

References:
(a) Blumenfeld, H. (2011). *Neuroanatomy through clinical cases* (2nd ed.). Sunderland, MA: Sinauer Associates.
(b) Goldberg, S. (2017). *The four-minute neurological exam* (2nd ed.). Miami, FL: MedMaster.
(c) Simon, R. P., Aminoff, M., & Greenberg, D. A. (2018). *Clinical neurology* (10th ed.). New York, NY: Lange Medical Books/McGraw-Hill Education.

6. **B—dysdiadochokinesia; ipsilateral**   *Dysdiadochokinesia refers to an impairment in alternating motor coordination. Dysmetria refers to unilateral movement. Cerebellar output is always ipsilateral, thus contralateral dysfunction is not a feasible response.*

References:
(a) Blumenfeld, H. (2011). *Neuroanatomy through clinical cases* (2nd ed.). Sunderland, MA: Sinauer Associates.
(b) Goldberg, S. (2017). *The four-minute neurological exam* (2nd ed.). Miami, FL: MedMaster.
(c) Simon, R. P., Aminoff, M., & Greenberg, D. A. (2018). *Clinical neurology* (10th ed.). New York, NY: Lange Medical Books/McGraw-Hill Education.

7. **C—computed tomography**   *CT is the imaging modality of choice in acute trauma. Although MRI has better resolution, high field magnetization is unsafe for many trauma patients because of external stabilizers or cardiac leads. Single proton emission CT remains investigational in head trauma, as does DTI. In addition, traumatic axonal injury takes days or weeks to become detectable with DTI.*

Reference: Kurth, S., & Bigler, E. D. (2008). Structural neuroimaging in clinical neuropsychology. In J. E. Morgan & J. H. Ricker (Eds.), Textbook of clinical neuropsychology (pp. 783–839). New York, NY: Psychology Press/Taylor & Francis Publishing.

8. **D—fractional anisotropy (FA)**   *Fractional anisotropy is the primary dependent variable in DTI. Diffusion tensor imaging may be used to characterize DAI, but it is not a specific DTI*

index. The BOLD response is elicited in blood flow-based technologies such as fMRI. Cerebral metabolic rate of glucose metabolism (CMRGlu) is only measured with PET.

Reference: Kurth, S., & Bigler, E.D. (2008). Structural neuroimaging in clinical neuropsychology. In J. E. Morgan & J. H. Ricker (Eds.), *Textbook of clinical neuropsychology* (pp. 783–839). New York, NY: Psychology Press/Taylor & Francis Publishing.

9. **A—increased; disappears** *Electroencephalographic alpha activity has been consistently demonstrated to increase with relaxation and disappear when persons engage in mental activity (**e.g.,** mental arithmetic). It is not specific to sleep.*

Reference: Kolb, B., & Whishaw, I. Q. (2015). *Fundamentals of human neuropsychology* (7th ed.). New York, NY: Worth Publishers.

10. **B—the summation of activity from thousands to millions of neurons** *The EEG signal represents the summation of many relatively large areas of neurons. Although it is time-linked, it does not equate to single-neuron recording, nor is it specific to epileptiform activity.*

Reference: Kolb, B., & Whishaw, I. Q. (2015). *Fundamentals of human neuropsychology* (7th ed.). New York, NY: Worth Publishers.

11. **D—magnetic resonance angiography (MRA)** *MRA is a technique to generate images of arteries (and less commonly veins) for the purpose of evaluating stenosis, occlusions, and aneurysms. Conventional skull x-rays, MRI, and CT scans are typically used as gross methods of assessing abnormalities such as skull injuries, and diffusion tensor imaging is most commonly used in research to examine white matter integrity and white matter tracts.*

Reference: Ricker, J. H., & Arenth, P. M. (2018). Functional and molecular neuroimaging in clinical neuropsychology. In J. E. Morgan & J. H. Ricker (Eds.), *Textbook of clinical neuropsychology* (2nd ed., pp. 373). New York, NY: Psychology Press/Taylor & Francis Publishing.

12. **C—diffusion weighted MRI (DWI)** *DWI is a variant of MRI that provides information on a microcellular level. Among other conditions, DWI has been well established and is more precise for ischemic damage detection than standard CT or MRI. Of the choices above, fMRI and DTI are generally implemented within the context of research studies rather than clinical examinations, and tau spectroscopy is not typically a scan of choice for stroke.*

Reference: Cullum, C. M., Rossetti, H. C., Festa, J. R., Haaland, K. Y., & Lacritz, L. H. (2018). Cerebrovascular disease. In J. E. Morgan & J. H. Ricker (Eds.), *Textbook of clinical neuropsychology* (2nd ed., p. 387). New York, NY: Psychology Press/Taylor & Francis Publishing.

13. **A—positron emission tomography** *PET is the only option that examines glucose utilization with radioisotopes and provides computer reconstructed color-coded images based on glucose uptake with regions of high blood flow. Combined PET and CT or MRI are now commercially available typically for very specific diagnostic questions such as tumor characterization. fMRI examines neural activity by assessing blood flow to specific brain regions and the localized surplus of oxyhemoglobin relative to deoxyhemoglobin. EEG monitors brain electrical activity along the scalp through fluctuations in voltage. Perfusion-weighted MRI allows one to infer how blood travels through the brain's vasculature through the use of a contrast medium or an endogenous blood flow marker.*

Reference: Ricker, J. H., & Arenth, P. M. (2018). Functional and molecular neuroimaging in clinical neuropsychology. In J. E. Morgan & J. H. Ricker (Eds.), *Textbook of clinical neuropsychology* (2nd ed., pp. 111–123). New York, NY: Psychology Press/Taylor & Francis Publishing.

14. **D—electroencephalography** *The primary clinical application of EEG is to differentiate epileptic seizures from other types of events (**e.g.,** nonepileptic seizures, fainting, or subcortical disorders). CT is generally used to assess gross abnormalities, and magnetic resonance angiography is a technique to generate images of arteries (and less commonly veins) for the purpose of evaluating stenosis, occlusions, and aneurysms. Diffusion tensor imaging is most commonly used in research to examine white matter integrity and white matter tracts.*

Reference: Kolb, B., & Whishaw, I. Q. (2015). Fundamentals of human neuropsychology (7th ed.). New York, NY: Worth Publishers.

15. **B—beta waves** *Beta is the dominant rhythm in patients who are alert, anxious, or have their eyes open. However, beta activity is also enhanced by sedating drugs such as benzodiazepines and barbiturates. This is thought to be caused by a compensatory mechanism that allows for behavioral activation despite sedation. Alpha amplitude manifests when the patient is relaxed with eyes closed, theta waves are prominent during drowsiness but can be observed during wakefulness, and delta waves are typically observed during sleep. The best answer is therefore "B."*

Reference: Kolb, B., & Whishaw, I. Q. (2015). *Fundamentals of human neuropsychology* (7th ed.). New York, NY: Worth Publishers.

Recommended Readings

Bauer, R. M., Iverson, G. L., Cernich, A. N., Binder, L. M., Ruff, R. M., & Naugle, R. I. (2012). Computerized neuropsychological assessment devices: Joint position paper of the American Academy of Clinical Neuropsychology and the National Academy of Neuropsychology. *The Clinical Neuropsychologist, 26*(2), 177–196.

Blumenfeld, H. (2011). *Neuroanatomy through clinical cases* (2nd ed.). Sunderland, MA: Sinauer Associates, Inc.

Cullum, C. M., Rossetti, H. C., Festa, J. R., Haaland, K. Y., & Lacritz, L. H. (2018). Cerebrovascular disease. In J. E. Morgan & J. H. Ricker (Eds.), *Textbook of clinical neuropsychology* (2nd ed., p. 387). New York, NY: Psychology Press/Taylor & Francis Publishing.

Goldberg, S. (2014). *Clinical neuroanatomy made ridiculously simple* (5th ed.) (Interactive Edition). Miami, FL: MedMaster.

Goldberg, S. (2017). *The four-minute neurologic exam* (2nd ed.). Miami, FL: MedMaster.

Kolb, B., & Whishaw, I. Q. (2015). *Fundamentals of human neuropsychology* (7th ed.). New York, NY: Worth Publishers.

Kurth, S., & Bigler, E. D. (2008). Structural neuroimaging in clinical neuropsychology. In J. E. Morgan & J. H. Ricker (Eds.), *Textbook of clinical neuropsychology* (pp. 783–839). New York, NY: Psychology Press/Taylor & Francis Publishing.

Miller, J. B., & Barr, W. B. (2017). The technology crisis in neuropsychology. *Archives of Clinical Neuropsychology, 32*, 541–554.

Ricker, J. H., & Arenth, P. M. (2018). Functional neuroimaging in clinical neuropsychology. In J. E. Morgan & J. H. Ricker (Eds.), *Textbook of clinical neuropsychology* (2nd ed., pp. 111–123). New York, NY: Psychology Press/Taylor & Francis Publishing.

Simon, R. P., Aminoff, M., & Greenberg, D. A. (2018). *Clinical neurology* (10th ed.). New York, NY: Lange Medical Books/McGraw-Hill Education.

Toga, A. W., Clark, K. A., Thompson, P. M., Shattuck, D. W., & Van Horn, J. D. (2012). Mapping the human connectome. *Neurosurgery 71*(1), 1–5.

7   Ethics in Clinical Neuropsychology

Shane S. Bush and Kirk J. Stucky

Introduction

The ability to provide effective neuropsychological services requires a fundamental understanding of relevant ethical issues and an investment in designing and maintaining practices that are consistent with high ethical standards. Ethical competence is an essential aspect of clinical competence and serves as a foundation for sound clinical decision-making. Ethical principles and guidelines, reflecting the shared values of the profession, should drive clinical practice rather than only being resources that practitioners turn to when confronting dilemmas. This chapter outlines an approach to ethical decision-making and describes 12 ethical issues that are particularly relevant to, and can become sources of conflict in, the practice of clinical neuropsychology.

Ethical dilemmas typically involve complex and unique issues that are not specifically addressed in ethics codes. Generally speaking, ethical dilemmas often involve conflicts between (1) different parties in which one or more has a specific ethical or professional duty, (2) two or more ethical principles or standards, (3) ethical requirements and an individual's morals or values, or (4) ethical principles and the law. Given that coverage of all potential ethical issues in clinical practice is beyond the scope of this chapter, efforts have been made to summarize and consolidate essential information with which neuropsychologists should be intimately familiar.

The Ethical Decision-Making Process

Ethical decision-making, like clinical decision-making, tends to be most efficient and effective when practitioners follow a systematic process. Most clinical decisions in neuropsychology are not made simply by hearing about nonspecific presenting problems or looking at a patient. Rather, the clinician uses a systematic, multimethod approach to gather information and empirical data and then integrates that information with knowledge gained from the scientific literature and experience to arrive at evidence-based conclusions. Similarly, a structured approach to ethical decision-making that involves consideration of multiple sources of information facilitates sound ethical decisions.

Positive Ethics and the 4 A's of Ethical Practice

Enforceable ethical standards and most risk management techniques provide the ethical floor or minimum acceptable level of ethical behavior that allows practitioners to avoid ethical misconduct. In contrast, positive ethics refers to the pursuit of ethical ideals or the highest standards of ethical practice (Knapp, VandeCreek, & Fingerhut, 2017). The pursuit of ethical ideals often requires more time and resources than is necessary for compliance with remedial ethics, but it allows practitioners to consider the underlying moral principles and to integrate shared professional values with personal ideals.

Consistent with positive ethics, the development of ethical practices should be a proactive process rather than a reaction to an ethically challenging situation, although reaction to challenges and dilemmas may be necessary at times. The "Four A's of Ethical Practice" provide a framework for thinking about one's approach to ethical practice. Bush (2009) described the importance of (a) **anticipating** and preparing for ethical issues and challenges commonly encountered in specific practice contexts, (b) **avoiding** ethical misconduct, (c) **addressing** ethical challenges when they are anticipated or encountered, and (d) **aspiring** to the highest standards of ethical practice. Being mindful of the four A's of ethical practice promotes appropriate professional practices and the modeling of ethical behavior for students and trainees, other psychologists and neuropsychologists, and interdisciplinary colleagues (Bush, 2018).

An Ethical Decision-Making Model

The answer to the question "What should I do?" is often best generated at the end of a decision-making process. A structured model promotes systematic ethical decision-making, thus providing neuropsychologists a method for making sound ethical choices. Ethics scholars have provided a variety of models, typically with overlapping features but differing numbers of steps. Bush, Allen, and Molinari (2017) offered a model with a seven-letter mnemonic that may facilitate its retention and recall. The mnemonic **CORE OPT** can help neuropsychologists understand the ethical issues and possible solutions and select a correct option. The model consists of the following steps:

(a) *C*larify the ethical issue, distinguishing it from clinical, legal, or other professional issues;

(b) identify the *O*bligations owed the relevant stakeholders;

(c) identify and review or consult ethical, legal, and professional *R*esources;

(d) *E*xamine one's own personal beliefs and values and the potential impact of each on the decision-making process;

(e) consider the possible *O*ptions, including solutions and their consequences,

(f) *P*ut the plan into practice, and

(g) *T*ake stock, evaluate the outcome, and revise as needed.

Resources

An essential step in the ethical decision-making process involves identifying and reviewing published ethical, legal, and professional resources and consulting colleagues who are particularly knowledgeable about ethical issues. Sources of related information include the following: (a) ethics codes; (b) *Code of Conduct* of the Association of State and Provincial Psychology Boards; (c) jurisdictional laws; (d) publications and position papers of professional organizations; (e) scholarly works, such as books, articles, and chapters; (f) ethics committees; (g) professional liability insurance carriers; (h) institutional guidelines and resources; (i) continuing education workshops and other presentations; and (j) colleagues.

Among the various published resources, the *Ethical Principles of Psychologists and Code of Conduct* of the American Psychological Association (APA, 2017) is a primary resource for practitioners in the United States, with the Canadian Psychological Association and the psychological associations in other countries providing ethics codes to govern the professional behavior of their members. Its Ethical Standards are enforceable rules of professional conduct for APA members and those practicing in states which have adopted some or all of the APA Ethics Code for their rules governing the professional behavior of psychologists. Ethics codes are by necessity fairly general in their guidance so that they can be applied across psychological activities and specialties. Because of this, additional aspirational guidelines or informational papers are published by APA and some specialty-specific organizations.

Numerous professional guidelines and position papers are available to neuropsychologists to inform specific aspects of practice and professional behavior. Bush (2018) identified thirty-three position statements or educational papers published by various neuropsychological organizations from 1999 to 2018. The American Academy of Clinical Neuropsychology (AACN) and National Academy of Neuropsychology (NAN) are the primary organizations that have provided position papers that are specifically relevant to neuropsychologists, although in recent years multiple organizations have collaborated in the drafting and publication of such papers. Related professional organizations also provide valuable position statements or educational information to help guide neuropsychologists in the pursuit of high standards of ethical practice. Most of these papers are accessible on the websites of the organizations that authored or endorsed them. Some of the topics that are reviewed in the next section of this chapter have been addressed by position papers. In preparation for the ABCN written and oral exams, neuropsychologists should be familiar with these position papers and be able to explain how they apply or adhere to those guidelines in day-to-day practice.

Common Sources of Ethical Conflict

The development of ethical practices and the ability to successfully address ethical challenges require an understanding of the ethical issues that are most likely to become sources of conflict. Although any ethical issue can become problematic, some are more likely than others to pose problems for members of a given specialty. Bush (2018) identified the following 12 ethical issues that seem to be among the most common sources of ethical or professional contention for neuropsychologists.

Professional Competence

Proper training, acquisition of necessary competencies, and the ability to properly apply knowledge and skills is required for ethical neuropsychological practice. Foundational and functional competence must be established in order for the practitioner to provide services that benefit and do not harm patients (Lamberty & Nelson, 2012). Professional competence is also an ethical requirement according to the APA Ethics Code. Ethical Standard 2.01 (Boundaries of Competence) section (a) states, "Psychologists provide services, teach, and conduct research with populations and in areas only within the boundaries of their competence, based on their education, training, supervised experience, consultation, study, or professional experience" (p. 4). Thus, incompetent practice *is* unethical practice. This point is emphasized because some colleagues have suggested that another's actions were not unethical but rather simply reflected incompetence. Such an argument does not make sense when it is understood that competence itself is an ethical requirement.

Although board certification in neuropsychology is not currently required, it, along with specialty-specific licensure required in some jurisdictions, provides the clearest evidence of competence in neuropsychology. Of course, board certification does not imply competence in all aspects or subspecialties of the profession, and it does not indicate that competence has been maintained over time. When career paths within neuropsychology change, competence must be achieved in the new areas of practice. Additionally, as the profession evolves, neuropsychologists must "undertake ongoing efforts to develop and maintain their competence" (Ethical Standard 2.03, Maintaining Competence; APA, 2017).

A brief comment on subspecialty practice in neuropsychology is also warranted. Specifically geriatric, pediatric, rehabilitation, and forensic neuropsychology and other subspecialties have unique training requirements and competencies. Board certification in clinical neuropsychology does not automatically imply competence in all subspecialties. In fact, many board-certified neuropsychologists focus on one subspecialty and, in line with ethical practice, refer to other providers when asked to render services that

TABLE 7.1 Common Sources of Ethical Conflict in Clinical Neuropsychology with Corresponding APA Ethical Standards

Ethical Issue	APA Ethical Standard
Professional Competence	2.01 Boundaries of Competence 2.03 Maintaining Competence
Roles/Relationships (Dual/Multiple)	3.05 Multiple Relationships 3.06 Conflict of Interest
Test Security / Release of Raw Test Data	9.04 Release of Test Data 9.11 Maintaining Test Security
Third-Party Observers	9.02 Use of Assessments 9.11 Maintaining Test Security
Confidentiality	4.01 Maintaining Confidentiality 4.02 Discussing the Limits of Confidentiality
Assessment (Methods, Norms)	2.04 Bases for Scientific and Professional Judgments 9.01 Bases for Assessments 9.02 Use of Assessments 9.06 Interpreting Assessment Results
Conflicts Between Ethics and Law	1.02 Conflicts between Ethics and Law, Regulations, or Other Governing Legal Authority 1.03 Conflicts Between Ethics and Organizational Demands
False or Deceptive Statements	5.01 Avoidance of False or Deceptive Statements
Objectivity	3.06 Conflict of Interest
Cooperation with Other Professionals	3.09 Cooperation with Other Professionals
Third-Party Requests for Services/ Informed Consent	3.07 Third-Party Requests for Services 3.11 Psychological Services Delivered to, or Through, Organizations 3.10 Informed Consent 9.03 Informed Consent in Assessments
Recordkeeping and Fees	6.01 Documentation of Professional and Scientific Work and Maintenance of Records 6.04 Fees and Financial Arrangements

NOTE: From Bush, S. S. (2018). *Ethical decision making in clinical neuropsychology (2nd ed.).* New York, NY: Oxford University Press. Used with permission of Oxford University Press.

do not fall within their scope of practice. Presently, pediatric neuropsychology is the only subspecialty certification available through the American Board of Professional Psychology, although additional subspecialties are likely to be formally recognized in the future.

Roles and Relationships

Neuropsychologists in many contexts, such as those working with pediatric or geriatric populations or those in rehabilitation or forensic contexts, commonly interact with persons other than the patient or examinee while providing services. In such circumstances, neuropsychologists appropriately rely on family members, colleagues, and others for valuable information about the patient. Interviewing collateral sources of information is typically an important aspect of forensic evaluations as well. Problems arise when neuropsychologists have a professional relationship with a person and also have another role with the same person or a closely associated person (or promises to enter into such a relationship in the future), and the multiple relationships would reasonably be expected to cause harm or exploitation (Ethical Standard 3.05, Multiple Relationships).

Much of the concern about relationships in neuropsychological practice can be found in medicolegal or forensic contexts in which a practitioner assumes both treating and forensic roles. In such situations, there is a high likelihood that having both roles will impact the practitioner's objectivity and thus ability to contribute to just legal decisions. Taking on such dual professional roles also has the potential to adversely affect the patient's treatment and, by extension, well-being. Ethical Standard 3.06 (Conflict of Interest), states, "Psychologists refrain from taking on a professional role when personal, scientific, professional, legal, financial, or other interests or relationships could reasonably be expected to (1) impair their objectivity, competence, or effectiveness in performing their functions as psychologists or (2) expose the person or organization with whom the professional relationship exists to harm or exploitation" (p. 6). All involved parties are best served when reasonably foreseeable roles, relationships, expectations, and limitations to services are clearly established and agreed upon at the outset of the professional relationship.

Test Security/Release of Raw Test Data

Threats to the security of psychological and neuropsychological tests threaten the usefulness of the tests to measure constructs of interest, such as memory. Exposure of a patient to test materials prior to an evaluation can impact the validity of the results for that patient, particularly if not known and taken into account by the clinician, as occurs in a re-evaluation. Widespread dissemination of test materials can invalidate the measure for an unknown number of persons, leading to inappropriate conclusions and various harmful outcomes that can result from inaccurate or flawed conclusions. The APA Ethics Code addresses this issue in two Standards (9.11 & 9.04). Ethical Standard 9.11 (Maintaining Test Security) defines test materials as "manuals, instruments, protocols, and test questions or stimuli" (p. 13). This Ethical Standard requires practitioners to "make reasonable efforts to maintain the integrity and security of test materials and other assessment techniques consistent with law and contractual obligations" (p. 13). Ethical Standard 9.04 (Release of Test Data) defines test data as "raw and scaled scores, client/patient responses to test questions or stimuli, and psychologists' notes and recordings concerning client/patient statements and behavior during an examination. Those portions of test materials that include client/patient responses are included in the definition of *test data*" (p. 12). According to this standard, practitioners must, having obtained an appropriate release from the patient, provide the test data to the patient or anyone specified by the patient unless doing so is likely to subject someone to substantial harm or result in the data being misused or misrepresented. Although this standard promotes the patient's autonomy, there are problems with its application.

The primary problem with the Ethics Code's requirements is that for many commonly used neuropsychological measures it is impossible in practice to separate test materials and data as the Code attempts to do. According to the Code, test stimuli, such as word lists or complex designs, are to be protected, but the patient's responses, including the same word lists and complex figures, must be released. The word list that the neuropsychologist reads to the patient is to be protected, but the same word list repeated back to the neuropsychologist must be released. These dual requirements result in an irreconcilable bind for the practitioner. As a result, neuropsychological professional organizations (Attix et al., 2007, National Academy of Neuropsychology, 2000a, 2000b) have provided clarifying guidance to help neuropsychologists negotiate the competing values of protecting the usefulness of the tools of the trade while also respecting patient autonomy and the importance of appropriate disclosure of the information in some situations. Jurisdictional laws, including copyright laws, and agreements between test publisher and purchaser also need to be considered. Further description of appropriate responses to requests for test materials and raw test data is beyond the scope of this chapter, but readers should see the sources cited here or the summaries provided in other resources (e.g., Bush, 2018).

Third-Party Observers

Requests are made in some neuropsychology practice contexts to have an observer present during an evaluation (e.g., parent, attorney, spouse). The presence of a third party most commonly occurs in forensic and pediatric contexts. In forensic contexts, the party that has not retained the neuropsychologist may want an observer to ensure that an appropriate evaluation is performed, and possibly to attempt to advise the examinee about responses to interview questions or to intimidate the neuropsychologist. With pediatric patients, it may be the wish of the child or a parent to have a parent present during the evaluation, typically to help alleviate the child's anxiety or manage difficult behavior. Primary problems with having a third party present during neuropsychological testing involve test security and the impact of the observer on the test-taker's performance. There is a noteworthy body of literature demonstrating that the mere presence of a third party, including a parent or recording device, affects the examinee's performance (Howe & McCaffrey, 2010). Thus, the presence of a third party can invalidate the results, potentially leading to unhelpful or unfair outcomes. Neuropsychological professional organizations have taken the position that, with few exceptions (e.g., training, interpreters), having a third party present during neuropsychological testing should be avoided.

Confidentiality

Effective psychotherapy is dependent upon patients being able to express their innermost thoughts and feeling, which most patients are only comfortable doing if they know that the therapist will keep the information in confidence and protect their privacy. In contrast, the results of the vast majority of neuropsychological evaluations are intended to be shared with others, rather than, or in addition to, the person being evaluated. Before beginning the evaluation, it is essential that examinees, or their designated representatives, understand what information will be shared and who the anticipated recipients of the information will be. The ethical mandate to maintain *confidentiality* is described in Ethical Standard 4.01 (Maintaining Confidentiality) and reflects the underlying ethical principle of respect for patient autonomy, which in the APA Ethics Code is subsumed under General Principle E (Respect for People's Rights and Dignity). The requirement to explain the limits of confidentiality exists in Ethical Standard 4.02, and the permissible disclosures, such as with appropriate consent or as mandated by law, are identified in Ethical Standard 4.05.

While it is important to arrive at a mutual understanding of privacy and confidentiality issues at the outset of the service or as soon thereafter as possible, it may also be necessary to revisit the issue at later points. For example, if a patient who was evaluated for purposes of differential diagnosis and treatment later decides to pursue litigation for the injury that reportedly resulted in the neuropsychological problems, the patient should be informed that the information will likely be requested by both parties in the legal matter and ultimately could end up in the public domain. The patient would then be in a position to make an informed decision about whether to engage in litigation. In the interests of privacy, all sensitive personal information shared by the patient need not be included in the neuropsychological report if it is irrelevant to the goals of the evaluation and does not advance the understanding of the patient's neuropsychological functioning.

Privilege is a narrower concept than confidentiality that relieves neuropsychologists from having to testify in court about information conveyed by patients. By "invoking privilege," patients prevent treating neuropsychologists from releasing records or testifying about sensitive personal information shared in the context of the professional relationship. By "waiving privilege," patients allow treating neuropsychologists to release records or testify in legal proceedings. Thus, privilege is held by competent adult patients and is invoked or waived as they choose. Significant limitations regarding privacy, confidentiality, and privilege exist in forensic contexts; neuropsychologists should be aware of the requirements that exist in the jurisdictions in which they practice.

Assessment Measures

There are many tests and procedures from which neuropsychologists can choose to measure constructs of interest and facilitate an understanding of patients. Selecting the specific measures and norms to use for a given patient based on an understanding of the evidence bases supporting the use of various measures with diverse patient populations reflects ethical practice (Ethical Standards 2.04 (Bases for Scientific and Professional Judgments and 9.01, Bases for Assessments). The methods and procedures selected should be sufficient to support the statements or conclusions generated about the neuropsychological characteristics of the patient (Ethical Standard, 9.01). It is important to note that while tests that are obsolete and not useful for a given case should not be used (Ethical Standard 9.08), publication of a new test or new edition or version of a test does not automatically render prior tests obsolete (Bush et al., 2018). The newer test may or may not be preferable for a given patient. As with test selection, use of assessment instruments should be an evidence-based endeavor (Ethical Standard 9.02, Use of Assessments).

Sometimes, typically due to sensory or motor limitations, tests or the testing environment may need to be adapted to meet the needs of the patient. For example, to understand the visuoconstructional ability of a patient with hemiparesis of the dominant side, the patient may need to perform tasks with the nondominant hand. Such decisions to modify tests or test administration, as well as the interpretation of the results, should be based on evidence of the usefulness of the technique. Interpretation also takes into account other characteristics of the person being assessed, such as cultural and linguistic differences, age, and education, as well as any situational factors that could affect the clinician's judgments or the accuracy of their interpretations (Ethical Standard 9.06, Interpreting Assessment Results). Any significant limitations in the interpretations should be described.

Conflicts Between Ethics and Law

Ethical requirements are often consistent with jurisdictional laws, both of which represent shared societal values. For example, both professional ethics and mental health law reflect the importance of confidentiality and the right of competent adults to make decisions about how their personal information is used. Ethics and law also both allow for, or require, confidentiality to be breached to warn others of, or protect them from, harm. However, in some instances ethics and laws conflict with each other. For example, the Ethics Code requires clinicians to provide copies of test data (including test materials that include patient responses) to the patient or anyone else specified by the patient (Ethical Standard 9.04), whereas copyright law prohibits the copying of test materials. Additionally, under the Health Insurance Portability and Accountability Act (HIPAA) regulations patients may actually have a right to access raw data if they press the issue despite being informed of test security concerns. When such conflicts between ethics and law, regulations, or other governing legal authority occur, clinicians are to make known their commitment to the Ethics Code and strive to resolve the matter in a manner consistent with professional ethics (Ethical Standard 1.02).

Sometimes, however, adherence to the law may be a more appropriate course of action; certainly the consequences for the practitioner can be more severe for violating laws than violating an ethical standard. Attempts at resolution typically occur through the provision of education to the parties involved. The 2002 version of the Ethics Code addressed the clinician's options for situations in which attempts at education are unsuccessful by stating, "If the conflict is unresolvable via such means, psychologists may adhere to the requirements of the law, regulations, or other governing legal authority." However, this statement was deleted in 2010 when amendments were added to the Code, because the statement had been used by some to justify or defend apparent abuses of human rights. Nevertheless, for some situations in which the stakes are not quite as high as abuse of human rights, the prior guideline still seems appropriate. In some work situations, the conflict is not between ethics and law but between ethics and organizational requirements. The position of the Ethics Code is the same in both situations.

False or Deceptive Public Statements

The Ethics Code (Ethical Standard 5.01, Avoidance of False or Deceptive Statements) defines public statements as including but not being limited to the following: "paid or unpaid advertising, product endorsements, grant applications, licensing applications, other credentialing applications, brochures, printed matter, directory listings, personal resumes or curricula vitae, or comments for use in media such as print or electronic transmission, statements in legal proceedings, lectures and public oral presentations, and published materials" (p. 8). Practitioners must not knowingly provide false, deceptive, or fraudulent statements about any professional matters in any of those forums or documents. Although the list does not include neuropsychological reports, to the extent that statements made in reports may be used in legal proceedings, such statements would be included. Additionally, General Principle C (Integrity) encourages accuracy, honesty, and truthfulness in all professional activities. "Puffery" in the context of one's credentials, such as listing "board certification eligible" or "Ph.D. (candidate)" in one's materials, can also be misleading to members of the public who do not understand such distinctions.

Although any neuropsychologist can inadvertently misspeak or otherwise be incorrect or inaccurate, incentive for intentionally providing misleading information seems to be greatest in forensic practice. For example, rigidly advocating for an opinion about a professional issue (e.g., a causal link between a remote event and a current symptom constellation) that is counter to a large empirical evidence base when the opinion favors the retaining party in a legal matter may reflect an intentionally deceptive statement, or a lack of professional competence, either of which would be ethically problematic.

Objectivity

Human beings are subject to a variety of biases, and neuropsychologists are no exception. Potential threats to objectivity are most obvious in forensic contexts, but many exist in clinical contexts as well. For example, based on information obtained in the initial telephone contact from a patient or patient's family member or obtained during the clinical interview, neuropsychologists begin to generate hypotheses about the nature of the patient's problems. Once initial impressions are established, there is a risk that subsequent information will be interpreted through that lens and that unintentional efforts will be made to confirm the initial impressions (i.e., confirmation bias), rather than interpret the data in an evidence-based manner. The opinions of neuropsychologists may also be affected by personal opinions about individual and diversity characteristics of the patient, such as age, gender, gender identity, race, ethnicity, culture, national origin, religion, sexual orientation, disability, language, and socioeconomic status. Effective, ethical neuropsychologists strive to identify such threats to objectivity and to take them into account in the interpretation of assessment results and conceptualization of the patient (Ethical Standards 9.06, Interpreting Assessment Results).

Objectivity and effectiveness can also be compromised when neuropsychologists take on competing roles, such as treating doctor and forensic examiner or providing clinical services to someone with whom the clinician has a personal or other professional relationship. Adopting competing roles can bias opinions and have potentially harmful results and in most cases should be avoided (Ethical Standard 3.06, Conflict of Interest). Exceptions might include rural settings or emergencies, and in those situations considerable attention should be given to maximizing objectivity.

Cooperation with Other Professionals

Neuropsychologists commonly practice in interdisciplinary contexts in which interaction with colleagues from other disciplines as well as within the same specialty facilitates patient care. Establishing and maintaining positive working relationships with other professionals tends to enhance neuropsychological and other healthcare services through the exchange of information about patients and is consistent with ethical practice (Ethical Standard 3.09, Cooperation with Other Professionals). Failure to cooperate with other professionals, which includes but is not necessarily limited to neuropsychology colleagues and other healthcare professionals, can interfere with the provision of appropriate services, resources, or benefits. For example, a neuropsychologist who receives an appropriately authorized release of information form and a request for a copy of a report but does not respond in a reasonably prompt manner is, in most circumstances, acting in an unprofessional and unethical manner that may provide unnecessary delays in care, administrative decisions, or other matters for which the report is important.

Third-Party Requests for Services and Informed Consent

Neuropsychologists commonly evaluate patients or forensic examinees at the request of a third party, such as a healthcare professional, family member, attorney, school official, or an administrative system (e.g., Veterans Affairs, Social Security Disability). Compared to patients who pursue healthcare or mental health services for their own information and well-being, there are unique ethical implications for services provided at the request of a third party. Such ethical issues include roles, confidentiality, and consent. Specifically, the neuropsychologist should clarify with all parties at the outset of the services the nature of the relationships with each party, including the nature and objectives of the services, the role of the neuropsychologist, who the identified client is, the anticipated uses of the information, who will have access to information, and limits to confidentiality (Ethical Standards 3.07, Third-Party Requests for Services, and 3.11, Psychological Services Delivered to or Through Organizations). Such information should be conveyed in a tactful manner and using language that the examinee and other participants can understand. After being duly informed about these issues, competent adults should be asked to consent to such services. For those not legally capable of providing informed consent, the information should be conveyed and their assent sought, with consent provided by a surrogate decision-maker (Ethical Standard 3.10, Informed Consent). In assessment situations in which consent is implied (e.g., routine organizational activity) or mandated by law or governmental regulations, neuropsychologists describe the process as is done with other types of evaluations and seek the examinee's assent, with an understanding by the examinee of the probable consequences of not participating in the planned services (Ethical Standard 9.03, Informed Consent in Assessments). In those instances in which a surrogate decision-maker is not legally required, permitted, or available, the neuropsychologist should be mindful of the importance of promoting and protecting the person's rights and welfare.

Recordkeeping and Fees

Because the neuropsychological work product is often a written report, neuropsychologists understand the importance of documenting clinical encounters. Some neuropsychologists, particularly those working in institutional settings, may be less attuned to the need to document the informed consent process and the specific details that payors and oversight bodies might consider important (e.g., start and stop times of face-to-face contact with the examinee). Neuropsychologists also vary in the information contained in reports, some including raw test scores with standardized scores, and some reporting no specific scores at all. Patients and neuropsychology colleagues are best served when documentation includes sufficient information for informed readers to (a) understand the process, evidence, and reasoning that led to the conclusions and (b) facilitate additional services or a re-evaluation at a later time. The documentation should also meet institutional and billing requirements and be in compliance with relevant laws (e.g., confidentiality) (Ethical Standard 6.01, Documentation of Professional and Scientific Work and Maintenance of Records).

The manner in which neuropsychologists handle fees and billing varies substantially according to the practice setting. Some neuropsychologists in independent practice handle all details of all fees and billing, including detailed discussions with patients or other retaining parties, whereas other practitioners, particularly those in some institutional settings, have no involvement with establishing fees or billing for services other than coding the services that were provided, listing the number of units, and providing a diagnosis. In general, clinicians have a responsibility to discuss fees and billing arrangements with the patient or other responsible party and reach an agreement as early in the professional relationship as possible (Ethical Standard 6.04, Fees and Financial Arrangements). Fees must be consistent with law and represented truthfully, with any anticipated limitations to services based on financial issues discussed as soon as possible. Clinicians may withhold an examinee's or patient's records for nonpayment unless the records are needed for emergency treatment (Ethical Standard 6.03). Clients should understand what they will be getting for their time and money; they need to understand that they will be getting evidence-based conclusions that may or may not support their desired outcome. See APA's 2007 Record Keeping Guidelines for additional information.

An Additional Issue of Emerging Interest

In addition to the previous sections, which covered issues that have been identified as common sources of ethical conflict for neuropsychologists, neuropsychologists are increasingly becoming interested in what is known as neuroethics. "Neuroethics studies the social, legal, ethical and policy implications of advances in neuroscience" (The International Neuroscience Society; www.neuroethicssociety.org). The overlap of neuropsychology, technology, and ethics has been discussed in the professional literature since at least 1990, with the specific topic of neuroethics raised by a neuropsychologist (Bush) at a conference more than a decade ago. The issue has become increasingly important and addressed by scholars in recent years because of the dramatic, technology-infused advances in the neurosciences and their clinical applications. Bush (2018a) noted, "Understanding the ethical implications of such exciting developments is needed to help keep patient welfare at the forefront of the efforts of innovators. Neuropsychological ethics should guide the innovation efforts, rather than react to them" (pp. 124–125).

While promising developments are underway and becoming available, there can be a temptation for practitioners to rapidly adopt and use new neuroscience technologies to facilitate their practices. The primary ethical concern is that the use of new tests or treatments may occur before their safety and usefulness are adequately established, potentially placing the patient at risk for harm without being in a position to make a fully informed decision about participating. APA General Principles A (*Beneficence* and Nonmaleficence) and E (Respect for Peoples Rights and Dignity, which includes respect for autonomy) are of particular relevance in this context. See Bush (2018a) for additional information on this topic.

Relevant Definitions

Beneficence An ethical obligation to take action to advance the welfare of others. Beneficence encompasses the promotion of the rights and health of others, as well as defense of the rights of others and the prevention of harm.

Confidentiality A subset of privacy that represents the responsibility of the practitioner not to disclose information shared by the patient in the professional relationship.

Expert Witness A forensic examiner retained for the purpose of developing an expert opinion to be offered in court on a psycholegal matter. In contrast to the fact witness role of the clinical provider, the forensic expert role requires review of all materials and completion of all procedures upon which to base an opinion sufficient to withstand rigorous peer and judicial scrutiny.

Fact Witness A clinician providing testimony about the facts of the clinical evaluation, including diagnostic impressions, and treatment services. In the clinical/treatment role, the neuropsychologist may be required to provide records to, and/or testify before, the court on a legal matter in which the neuropsychological functioning or treatment of a patient may be relevant to the court. The treating clinician must limit opinion to that for which adequate data has been gathered and typically refrain from offering opinion on the ultimate psycholegal issue before the court.

Neuroethics The study of the social, legal, ethical, and policy implications of advances in neuroscience.

Nonmaleficence An ethical obligation for clinicians to do no harm.

Positive Ethics The pursuit of ethical ideals or the highest standards of ethical practice.

Privacy Freedom from unauthorized intrusion into one's life, including one's thoughts, feelings, beliefs, and experiences. Privacy, a core societal value, is based on the individual's right to self-determination and to be protected from harm. The U.S. Supreme Court has recognized privacy as a constitutional right. An individual's healthcare information is protected by these privacy laws and they in turn have a right to that information under HIPPA. The healthcare provider is legally and ethically obligated to protect that information as well.

Privilege A narrower concept than confidentiality that relieves neuropsychologists from having to testify in court about information conveyed by patients. Privilege can be invoked or waived by competent adults and emancipated minors not legally mandated to undergo a neuropsychological evaluation.

Ethics in Neuropsychology Questions

NOTE: Questions 26, 65, and 100 on the First Full-Length Practice Examination, Questions 2, 42, and 90 on the Second Full-Length Practice Examination, Questions 5, 53, and 83 on the Third Full-Length Practice Examination, and Questions 3 and 25 on the Fourth Full-Length Practice Examination are from this chapter.

1. You are at your outpatient clinic when two attorneys arrive and provide proper identification indicating that they are members of a federal law enforcement agency. They tell you that they are in the process of an important investigation regarding one of your patients and need to see the chart immediately. You initially refuse but they inform you that you are interfering with a federal investigation and will be prosecuted if you do not cooperate. What should you do?

    (a) Give them the chart but remain in the room while they review it.

    (b) Give them the chart but do not allow them to copy any records.

    (c) Ask them to sign a release of information so you are absolved of responsibility.

    (d) Refuse to provide access without a release of information from the patient or a court order.

2. Which of the following most accurately describes ownership of the healthcare record?

    (a) The record is entirely the property of the patient and can be fully released with his or her permission.

    (b) The record is entirely the property of the healthcare provider and can be released with a court order.

    (c) The information is the patient's property and the physical or electronic record is the property of the healthcare provider.

    (d) The information is the property of the healthcare provider and the physical or electronic record is the property of the patient.

3. You are evaluating an 8-year-old boy to determine if he has a learning disability and/or attention-deficit/hyperactivity disorder. He has a history of oppositional defiant disorder and, according to the mother and teacher, he has been caught lying on multiple occasions. The patient displays low average intelligence, impulsivity, and low average to extremely low scores on measures of executive function. During the course of the evaluation, he shows you a large bruise on his rib cage and states that his mother's boyfriend punched him yesterday. He asks you not to tell his mother. What do you do?

   (a) Question the child in more detail, recognizing that his self-report may be false.

   (b) Privately inform the patient's mother and inquire regarding possible abuse.

   (c) Report the abuse to child protective services immediately and inform the mother.

   (d) Complete the evaluation and privately discuss during feedback with the mother.

4. Dr. Apple is studying a new memory test he recently developed. To assess concurrent validity he starts to include this test in all of the outpatient assessments at his private practice. Which of the following is most accurate concerning Dr. Apple's use of the new memory test?

   (a) Institutional review board approval (IRB) is not necessary.

   (b) Informed consent is required but billing for the new test is not appropriate.

   (c) Informed consent is not required because he is still giving a standard battery.

   (d) It is inappropriate to study a new test under such conditions.

5. You are the principal investigator of a new intellectual assessment measure and in the process of finalizing a research article for publication. The test publisher provided major funding for the study. Which of the following is the most accurate statement regarding authorship of the publication?

   (a) Accepting money from the company prohibits you from being listed as an author.

   (b) The funding sources have no impact on publication requirements.

   (c) If the IRB determines no evidence of bias, you can be listed as an author.

   (d) There are no restrictions on authorship if you disclose the financial relationship.

6. You have been asked to give grand rounds at your hospital. A rehabilitation program you frequently refer to is sponsoring your talk. In exchange for your lecture, you are being offered $1,000. What should you do?

   (a) Accept the money but request independent review of the presentation in advance.

   (b) Refuse the money and reveal the professional relationship to the audience.

   (c) Accept the money but reveal the relationship and honorarium to the audience.

   (d) Refuse the money but ask the sponsor to donate it to your hospital.

7. An 87-year-old gentleman drives to your office but clearly displays visuospatial impairments and does not appear to have appropriate prescription glasses. He gets lost coming back from the bathroom, stumbles several times, and is unable to complete written forms. At the end of the appointment he plans to drive home. What do you do first?

   (a) Assist the patient in identifying alternative means of transportation.

   (b) Report the patient as a driver of concern to the state as per regulations.

(c) Do not allow the patient to leave and contact law enforcement.

(d) Wait until more detailed neuropsychological evaluation can be done.

8. You are in the first year of a new job at a prominent medical center. You notice that the medical director periodically comes to work with alcohol on his breath and exhibits some abnormal behavior while on patient care rounds and team conferences. No one except you seems to notice. What should you do first?

(a) Talk with your staff and colleagues about options.

(b) Write a letter to the physician regarding your concern.

(c) Inform the director's supervisor as soon as possible.

(d) Report the physician to the licensing board.

9. Several well-designed research studies are published in respected professional journals indicating that memory test A is superior to memory test B in evaluating patients with suspected dementia. Furthermore, memory test B is shown to result in a high number of false negative results. Dr. Bean has been using memory test B for years and remains confident in its utility in dementia assessments. Additionally, memory test A is rather expensive and Dr. Bean does not have the time or desire to learn this new assessment measure. What can be said regarding this decision?

(a) It is unethical, but not illegal in clinical practice.

(b) It is non-evidence-based but it is not unethical.

(c) It is defensible if other tests in the battery are valid.

(d) It is clinically inappropriate and unethical to use old tests.

10. Dr. Apple has completed a neuropsychological assessment of a 13-year-old girl who had a brain tumor removed three months ago. The evaluation was requested to assist with school reentry planning. After three weeks, Dr. Apple has not received formal healthcare records despite multiple requests, but she feels that the information is important to include in the report. The parents are requesting completion of the report as soon as possible without those records because they cannot start school reentry and other treatments without the evaluation. What should Dr. Apple do?

(a) Don't complete the report until the records arrive but give feedback.

(b) Write the report after three months even if the records don't arrive.

(c) Write the report and indicate that healthcare records were not available.

(d) Don't write the report unless the school and parents demand it.

11. You specialize in geriatric assessment. An 80-year-old woman arrives for an initial intake but is confused regarding the reason for referral. She explains that she has a sizable estate and that some of her children do not get along. The family infighting has been very stressful for her and she has been considering a change in her trust. After 45 minutes, you have sufficient reason to believe that she is in the early stages of a progressive dementia. It is also probable that your examination will reveal cognitive impairments and capacity limitations that might lead you to recommend some level of supervision, monitoring, or even guardianship. How should you proceed first?

(a) Contact the referral source and explain that the patient cannot give informed consent for the procedure.

(b) Inform the patient of your concerns and how assessment and differential diagnosis could impact her.

(c) Inform the patient that your evaluation could likely result in a recommendation for guardianship and loss of personal freedom.

(d) This is beyond your scope of practice, refer the patient to an attorney and forensic neuropsychologist.

12. One of your patients requests a copy of his entire record, including all raw data from his recent neuropsychological assessment. If the patient insists despite your attempts to dissuade them, which of the following represents the best option?

(a) Do not provide the raw data, but provide a detailed test score summary sheet including computer generated test score summaries.

(b) Provide the raw data, but black out the test questions and identifying information on all protocols.

(c) Do not provide the raw data, but give a copy of the position paper on test security.

(d) Provide the raw data, but have them sign a legal document promising that they will not share the information with anyone else.

13. You are in the process of evaluating a 14-year-old. The parents are requesting a second opinion regarding another psychologist's diagnosis of learning disability one year ago. The other psychologist used a bachelor's level psychometrician to administer and score psychological measures. The report also indicates that the psychometrician wrote the report but that it was reviewed and approved by the doctoral level psychologist. What should you do?

(a) Report the psychologist to the state ethics board.

(b) Report the psychologist to the licensing board.

(c) Indicate in your report that the evaluation was improper.

(d) Call the psychologist and discuss your concerns.

14. You are evaluating a patient who sustained a mild TBI and comminuted femur fracture in a car accident one year ago. Her husband was killed in the accident as well. She reports nightmares and flashbacks from seeing his body. Additionally, during the course of your evaluation she discloses a significant pre-accident history of physical and sexual abuse. Test results, history, and interview are highly suggestive of untreated PTSD before the accident but now worsened as a consequence of all she has been through. You write this in the report, but the patient asks you to take out her past abuse history because she does not want her physician to know and also thinks the auto insurance company may use the information to deny coverage. You are convinced that her past history is important in understanding her current condition and informing treatment recommendations. What is the ethically appropriate thing to do?

(a) Leave the report as is and explain to the patient that you are obligated to be truthful regardless of impact.

(b) Leave the information in but work with the patient on more acceptable or palatable wording that discloses her abuse history.

(c) Respect the patient's right to privacy and remove the abuse history; focus on the accident and its consequences.

(d) Consult with your professional ethics committee before giving the report to anyone including the patient.

15. You are evaluating a 14-year-old non-emancipated minor for a suspected learning disorder. In the middle of your assessment the teenager discloses that he has been periodically using cannabis and alcohol with his friends after school. He asks you not to inform his parents or teachers as he does not want to lose his friends or get into trouble. He insists that the substance use is just for fun and that it is not affecting him negatively. He also maintains that a lot of kids at school are doing it. What are you required to do?

(a) Tell the patient that you have to inform his parents.

(b) Maintain confidentiality until you are able to thoroughly assess the patient.

(c) Inform the parents privately but do not include the substance abuse information in the report.

(d) Refer the patient for substance abuse counseling but do not inform the parents.

Ethics in Neuropsychology Answers

1. **D—Refuse to provide access without a release of information from the patient or a court order.** *You cannot release the patient's healthcare record unless there is a signed release from the patient or there is a court order. This applies no matter who is asking. If the agents have a court order for the records, they have a right to the information. However, in such circumstances it would be appropriate to inform the patient and consult with legal counsel. Although the physical healthcare record is the property of the psychologist and/or health care facility, the healthcare information is the property of the patient. Patients, like all United States citizens, have a constitutional right against illegal search and seizure of their property.*

General Principles and Ethical Standards: B, E; 4.01 and 4.04

Reference: Bush, S. S., Grote, C., Johnson-Greene, D., & Macartney-Filgate, M. (2008). A panel interview on the ethical practice of neuropsychology. *The Clinical Neuropsychologist, 22,* 321-344

2. **C—The information is the patient's property and the physical or electronic record is the property of the healthcare provider.** *A healthcare provider can provide copies of the healthcare record to the patient and others with a proper release but the physical record is the property of the psychologist, clinic, or healthcare organization. Therefore, the original record must always remain with the provider of care. The information in the record is protected health information and the property of the patient, which is why the patient is entitled to access their chart. In neuropsychology practice a complicating factor is the requirement to maintain test security and thus requests for the entire record results in a conflict between two standards.*

General Principles and Ethical Standards: B, E; 4.01, 6.01, 6.02, 9.08

Reference: Bush, S. S. (2007). *Ethical decision making in clinical neuropsychology.* New York, NY: Oxford University Press.

3. **B—Privately inform the patient's mother and inquire regarding possible abuse.** *While it certainly would be appropriate to interview the child in more depth, it would not be appropriate to complete the evaluation and wait until feedback to discuss the matter further. In the case of a child or a vulnerable adult, the psychologist must act to protect the patient. In this case, you have input from two independent sources who both give you reason for concern. Depending on the mother's response to inquiry and results of further evaluation, a formal report to child protective services may or may not be appropriate. You have the right and responsibility to report suspected abuse over the objections of a parent or caregiver. Although the legal requirements for reporting*

suspected abuse are not identical in all states, the ethical requirement that psychologists can re-
lease confidential information to protect people from harm is clear and uncompromising.

General Principles and Ethical Standards: A, B, E; 4.01, 4.02, 4.04, 4.05

References:
(a) Fennell, E. B. (2005). Ethical challenges in pediatric neuropsychology, part I. In S. S. Bush (Ed.), *A casebook of ethical challenges in neuropsychology* (pp. 133–136). New York, NY: Psychology Press.
(b) Goldberg, A. L. (2005). Ethical challenges in pediatric neuropsychology, part II. In S. S. Bush (Ed.), *A casebook of ethical challenges in neuropsychology* (pp. 137–144). New York, NY: Psychology Press.

4. **B—Informed consent is required but billing for the new test is not appropriate.** *Even if the standard battery is still administered, the patient is entitled to know that a study is being conducted and that experimental tests are being used. Furthermore, the patient should be informed of the foreseeable risks and benefits of participating and should be given the option not to participate, and their decision to forgo the study should not impact services in any fashion. Furthermore, the patient should not be billed for the time spent taking this test. In any healthcare organization, IRB approval would certainly be required in such a case. For research conducted in a private practice a formal informed consent process must be established to safeguard patient/subject rights. There are also IRB-type reviews available for private researchers, and these resources should be utilized or at least strongly considered.*

General Principles and Ethical Standards: B, C, E; 8.01, 8.02, 8.05, 9.02, 9.03

Reference: Johnson-Green, D., and the NAN Policy & Planning Committee (2005). Informed consent in clinical neuropsychology practice: Official statement of the National Academy of Neuropsychology. *Archives of Clinical Neuropsychology, 20,* 335–340.

5. **D—There are no restrictions on authorship if you disclose the financial relationship.** *There is no automatic ethical concern with grant- or industry-sponsored research. Also, financial support from an outside agency does not limit you as an author as long as you disclose all of your affiliations with the party and any potential conflict of interest. There is an absolute requirement to reveal financial or business affiliations at the time of publication for all authors. You must also reveal support even if the payments are made by a third party such as the hospital or medical school. The key issue is not whether you or your institution accepted money but being transparent about the financial connections which could lead to bias.*

General Principles and Ethical Standards: B, C, D; 8.01, 8.10, 8.12

References:
(a) Thompson, L. L. (2005). Ethical challenges in neuropsychological research, part I. In S. S. Bush (Ed.), *A casebook of ethical challenges in neuropsychology* (pp. 201–208). New York, NY: Psychology Press.
(b) van Gorp, W. G. (2005). Ethical challenges in neuropsychological research, part II. In S. S. Bush (Ed.), *A casebook of ethical challenges in neuropsychology* (pp. 209–212). New York, NY: Psychology Press.

6. **C—Accept the money but reveal the relationship and honorarium to the audience.** *Sponsorship of speakers in educational forms is acceptable as long as there is no sponsor expectation of control or undue influence over the presentation content. In other words, clinicians should not actively advocate or advertise for the sponsor while giving the audience an impression of objectivity. Speakers have a mandatory responsibility to disclose all financial relations with sponsors or products. This disclosure allows the audience to judge for itself whether there is undue influence. There is no requirement to donate speaker fees to charity. There is no ethical requirement for prior review of your presentation by an independent party.*

General Principles and Ethical Standards: B, C; 3.05, 3.06, 3.07

7. **A—Assist the patient in identifying alternative means of transportation.** *This vignette clearly outlines a situation in which the patient is potentially at high risk for endangering himself or others by continuing to drive. Although neuropsychological evaluation is typically not sufficient to determine driving ability, in this case there are multiple indications that the patient should not be driving; thus, the psychologist has an obligation to protect the patient and innocent third parties. The most appropriate initial course of action is to try to work with the patient on a reasonable solution, but, if that fails, contacting someone in a position to protect the patient is often a logical next step. It should be noted that state laws vary regarding the psychologist's obligations or ability to contact law enforcement and/or the Department of Motor Vehicles (DMV) in such circumstances.*

General Principles and Ethical Standards: A, B, D, E; 4.01, 4.02, 4.05

Reference: Bush, S. S., & Martin, T. A. (2008). Confidentiality in neuropsychological practice. In A. M. Horton, Jr., & D. Wedding (Eds.), *The neuropsychology handbook* (3rd ed., pp. 517–532). New York, NY: Springer Publishing Co.

8. **C—Inform the director's supervisor as soon as possible.** *Reports of clinician impairment should first go to supervisory personnel. In this case the director's supervisor is the best option listed. If this is unsuccessful or not applicable, then reporting to the state licensing board might be appropriate. Initially talking to colleagues is not sufficient because they do not supervise or oversee the potentially impaired physician. Although discussion of unethical conduct directly with a colleague is often the appropriate first step, just writing a letter is not sufficient. For example, even if the physician promised to stop the behavior, you have no guarantee this will indeed occur and that patients will be protected. Also, if the physician denies or rejects your approach, you still must report the behavior. Similar to reporting abuse, if you are aware of something that can impact patient safety or well-being and do not report it, then you potentially become liable for any harm to a patient.*

General Principles and Ethical Standards: B, C, E; 1.03, 1.04, 1.05, 1.07

Reference: Deidan, C., & Bush, S. (2002). Addressing perceived ethical violations by colleagues. In S. S. Bush & M. L. Drexler (Eds.), *Ethical issues in clinical neuropsychology* (pp. 281–305). Lisse, NL: Swets & Zeitlinger Publishers.

9. **A—It is unethical, but not illegal in clinical practice.** *Incompetent or non-evidence-based practice is unethical practice. In this vignette the psychologist has chosen to ignore the scientific evidence in preference for personal convenience. Consequently patient care is compromised. Although Dr. Bean would not likely be prosecuted for this practice, it is certainly unethical. Also, it is not inappropriate or unethical to use older tests if they still have known utility or value. In fact, newer tests are not automatically superior to older tests which may often, initially, have stronger scientific support.*

General Principles and Ethical Standards: A, B, C, D; 9.01, 9.02, 9.08

Reference: Bush, S. S., Sweet, J. J., Bianchini, K. J., Johnson-Greene, D., Dean, P. M., & Schoenberg, M. R. (2018). Deciding to adopt revisions and new psychological and neuropsychological tests: Official position of the Neuropsychology Inter-Organizational Practice Committee. *The Clinical Neuropsychologist, 32*, 319–325.

10. **C—Write the report and indicate that healthcare records were not available.** *The timely completion of assessments and reports can become an ethical matter. In clinical circumstances such as the one above it should be the highest priority to make decisions that are in the best interest of the patient. In some contexts these priorities supersede but do not preclude the requirement to verify the accuracy of claims regarding past and present history. Delays caused by waiting on healthcare records can interfere with the primary responsibility of the neuropsychologist to render expeditious diagnostic decisions and treatment recommendations. In this case not writing*

the report will likely cause delays in the patient's treatment and education. Additionally, in circumstances such as this the treating doctor can easily indicate in the report that opinions may be subject to change or that an addendum may be forthcoming if or when additional records arrive. The neuropsychologist should certainly comment regarding any information that is missing and the implications that its absence has for the conclusions and recommendations. In some cases failure to temper conclusions in the absence of relevant information could potentially result in erroneous opinions, but this vignette does not outline such concerns.

General Principles and Ethical Standards: A, B; 9.06, 9.09

References:

(a) Bush, S. S., & MacAllister, W. S. (2010). Ethical and legal guidelines for pediatric neuropsychologists. In A. S. Davis (Ed.), *Handbook of pediatric neuropsychology* (pp. 1005–1016). New York, NY: Springer Publishing Co.

(b) McSweeny, A. J., & Naugle, R. I. (2002). Competence and appropriate use of neuropsychological assessments and interventions. In S. Bush & M. Drexler (Eds.), *Ethical issues in clinical neuropsychology* (pp. 23–37). Lisse, NL: Swets & Zeitlinger Publishers.

11. **B—Inform the patient of your concerns and how assessment and differential diagnosis could impact her.** *Ideally, informed consent is a shared decision-making process between the patient and their provider. Neuropsychologists should make explicit the need for informed consent when conducting any assessment. However, fully informed consent may be difficult or impossible to obtain from patients with moderate to severe cognitive impairments. There are situations in which some patients would choose not to undergo an evaluation if they fully understood that certain results could limit or jeopardize their decision-making rights. Answer D is not optimal as it is untactful, indicates a "likely" outcome that cannot be stated with confidence before assessment, and may prevent the patient from obtaining an evaluation that could ultimately help them. In this scenario a reasonable attempt should be made to provide an explanation as to the purpose of the evaluation, the risks and benefits, the roles of all parties involved, the type and nature of the procedures used, and the limits of confidentiality.*

General Principles and Ethical Standards: A, B, C, E; 2.01, 9.02, 9.03

References:

(a) Bush, S. S. (2012). Ethical considerations in the psychological evaluation and treatment of older adults. In S. Knapp (Ed.), *Handbook of ethics in psychology* (pp. 15-28). Washington, DC: American Psychological Association.

(b) Johnson-Green, D., and the NAN Policy & Planning Committee (2005). Informed consent in clinical neuropsychology practice: Official statement of the National Academy of Neuropsychology. *Archives of Clinical Neuropsychology, 20,* 335–340.

12. **A—Do not provide the raw data, but provide a detailed test score summary sheet including computer-generated test score summaries.** *This vignette entails a conflict between the psychologist's duty to maintain test security and the patient's right to their healthcare information. The Code requires psychologists to safeguard test materials (e.g., test questions or stimuli) but also requires that test data (including client/patient responses to test questions or stimuli) be released to anyone specified by the patient. In this vignette, the neuropsychologist, understanding the challenges inherent in these two ethical requirements, wants to be helpful to the patient while maintaining a commitment to test security. The neuropsychologist believes that providing the detailed summary sheet and related materials will satisfy both interests. In other circumstances it would be appropriate to release all raw data to another psychologist whether or not they are a clinical neuropsychologist. This decision can be defended as all psychologists are bound by ethics to safeguard test security and practice within the boundaries of their own competence. Note: The American Academy of Clinical Neuropsychology and the National Academy of Neuropsychology have position papers regarding how to respond to requests and/or subpoenas for records and raw*

data. In this case, if needed upon further pressing from the patient, it can be explained that it is the neuropsychologist's policy, consistent with multiple professional guidelines, to only release raw test data to other psychologists, unless provided with a court order.

General Principles and Ethical Standards: B, C, D, E; 9.04, 9.11

References:

(a) Attix, D. K., Donders, J., Johnson-Greene, D., Grote, C. L., Harris, J. G., & Bauer, R. M. (2007). Disclosure of neuropsychological test data: Official position of Division 40 (Clinical Neuropsychology) of the American Psychological Association, Association of Postdoctoral Programs in Clinical Neuropsychology, and American Academy of Clinical Neuropsychology. *The clinical neuropsychologist, 21*, 232–238.

(b) Bush, S. S., Rapp, D. L., & Ferber, P. S. (2010). Maximizing test security in forensic neuropsychology. In A. M. Horton, Jr., & L. C. Hartlage (Eds.), *Handbook of forensic neuropsychology* (2nd ed., pp. 177–195). New York, NY: Springer Publishing Co.

13. **D—Call the psychologist and discuss your concerns.** *The use of psychometricians is commonplace and acceptable in neuropsychology practice in most jurisdictions, although their educational requirements vary. However, asking or directing those same individuals to write reports on the basis of those assessments is not. This falls under the ethical standards regarding the supervision of, and delegation of work to, students, colleagues, and others. Referral to the licensing board is not appropriate as there is no direct evidence that patient safety is a concern or that something illegal or unethical is occurring. In this scenario you could and likely should call the psychologist first to discuss your concerns.*

General Principles and Ethical Standards: B, C, D; 1.04, 1.05, 1.07, 2.01, 2.05, 9.09

References:

(a) American Academy of Clinical Neuropsychology. (1999). Policy on the use of non-doctoral-level personnel in conducting clinical neuropsychological evaluations. *The Clinical Neuropsychologist, 13*(4), 385.

(b) Deidan, C., & Bush, S. (2002). Addressing perceived ethical violations by colleagues. In S. S. Bush & M. L. Drexler (Eds.), *Ethical issues in clinical neuropsychology* (pp. 281–305). Lisse, NL: Swets & Zeitlinger Publishers.

14. **B—Leave the information in but work with the patient on more acceptable or palatable wording that discloses her abuse history.** *The conflict here is between confidentiality, truthfulness, integrity, and respect for patient rights and dignity. By not disclosing the abuse history, future providers may not fully understand factors contributing to her symptoms. In some situations if specific sensitive information is not pertinent to the test interpretation, diagnosis, or recommendations, it is likely appropriate to leave it out of the report entirely, but this is not the case in this vignette. The neuropsychologist has a professional obligation to reveal all information that informs their opinion. Also, if that information is pivotal, it cannot and should not be withheld in the report because it would potentially be misleading. In situations like this it is certainly appropriate to work with the patient on an acceptable compromise as long as it does not result in deceptive or misleading statements and does not compromise the clinician's integrity. Finally, it is easy to imagine destructive consequences from inclusion of detailed sensitive information, and the psychologist must remain mindful of appropriate disclosure, always thinking of the patient's best interests in the short and long term.*

General Principles and Ethical Standards: A, B, C, E; 4.04, 4.05

References:

(a) Ameis, A., Zasler, N. D., Martelli, M. F., & Bush, S. S. (2006). Ethical issues in clinicolegal practice. In N. D. Zasler, D. Katz, & R. Zafonte (Eds.), *Brain injury medicine: Principles and practice* (pp. 1163–1182). New York, NY: Demos Medical Publishing.

(b) Bush, S. S. (2005). Introduction to ethical issues in forensic neuropsychology. *Journal of Forensic Neuropsychology, 4*(3), 1–9.

15. A—Tell the patient that you have to inform his parents. *The presence of substance use could certainly impact school performance and might in fact be a primary concern as opposed to the suspected learning disorder. Thus, it would be inappropriate to leave this information out of a report especially since it will most certainly be taken into consideration when formulating an opinion. Furthermore, the patient is a minor and the parents are entitled to know if their child is at risk. The clinician would want to be as tactful as possible in explaining this to the teenager in hopes that the discussion would lead to meaningful and healthy change without negatively impacting the patient's willingness to follow through on recommendations.*

General Principles and Ethical Standards: A, B, C, E; 4.04, 4.05

Reference: Knapp, S. J., VandeCreek, L. D., & Fingerhut, R. (2017). *Practical ethics for psychologists: A positive approach* (3rd ed.). Washington, DC: American Psychological Association.

Recommended Readings

American Academy of Clinical Neuropsychology. (2007). Practice guidelines for neuropsychological assessment and consultation. *The Clinical Neuropsychologist, 21*, 209–231.

American Educational Research Association, American Psychological Association, & National Council on Measurement in Education. (2014). *Standards for educational and psychological testing.* Washington, DC: American Psychiatric Publishing.

American Psychological Association. (2017). *Ethical principles of psychologists and code of conduct.* Retrieved from www.apa.org/ethics/code/index.aspx.

Attix, D. K., Donders, J., Johnson-Greene, D., Grote, C. L., Harris, J. G., & Bauer, R. M. (2007). Disclosure of neuropsychological test data: Official position of Division 40 (Clinical Neuropsychology) of the American Psychological Association, Association of Postdoctoral Programs in Clinical Neuropsychology, and American Academy of Clinical Neuropsychology. *The clinical neuropsychologist, 21*, 232–238.

Beauchamp, T. L., & Childress, A. F. (2013). *Principles of biomedical ethics* (7th ed.). New York, NY: Oxford University Press.

Bush, S. S. (2009). *Geriatric mental health ethics: A casebook.* New York, NY: Springer Publishing Company.

Bush, S. S. (2018). *Ethical decision making in clinical neuropsychology* (2nd ed.). New York, NY: Oxford University Press.

Bush, S. S. (2018). Ethical practice of clinical neuropsychology. In J. H. Ricker & J. E. Morgan (Eds.), *Textbook of clinical neuropsychology* (2nd ed., pp. 1000–1006). New York, NY: Psychology Press.

Bush, S. S., Allen, R. S., & Molinari, V. A. (2017). *Ethical practice in geropsychology.* Washington, DC: American Psychological Association.

Bush, S. S., Sweet, J. J., Bianchini, K. J., Johnson-Greene, D., Dean, P. M., & Schoenberg, M. R. (2018). Deciding to adopt revisions and new psychological and neuropsychological tests: Official position of the Neuropsychology Inter-Organizational Practice Committee. *The Clinical Neuropsychologist, 32*, 319–325.

Howe, L. L. S., & McCaffrey, R. J. (2010). Third party observation during neuropsychological evaluation: An update on the literature, practical advice for practitioners, and future directions. *The Clinical Neuropsychologist, 24*, 518–537.

Knapp, S. J., VandeCreek, L. D., & Fingerhut, R. (2017). *Practical ethics for psychologists: A positive approach* (3rd ed.). Washington, DC: American Psychological Association.

Lamberty, G. J., & Nelson, N. W. (2012). *Specialty competencies in clinical neuropsychology.* New York, NY: Oxford University Press.

National Academy of Neuropsychology. (2000a). Test security: Official statement of the National Academy of Neuropsychology. *Archives of Clinical Neuropsychology, 15*, 383–386.

National Academy of Neuropsychology. (2000b). Handling requests to release test data, recording and/or reproductions of test data. *Official statement of the National Academy of Neuropsychology.* Retrieved from http://www.nanonline.org/paio/secappend.shtm.

Section II Fundamentals of Assessment

8 Psychometrics, Test Design, and Essential Statistics

Brigid Waldron-Perrine, Summar Reslan, and Kenneth M. Adams, with assistance from Scott R. Millis

Introduction

Clinical neuropsychology's central tools in the characterization of brain-behavior relationships are psychological and neuropsychological tests. The understanding of the science of testing is essential to the realization of its power as an objective basis for decisions regarding neuropsychological issues. This chapter is divided into five sections relevant to clinical neuropsychologists: fundamentals-theory, foundations-distributions, test construction, test evaluation, and test interpretation.

Section I: Fundamentals—Theory

Classical Test Theory: Descriptive and Inferential Statistics

- Any obtained test score X for an individual consists of a true score (T) and a random error component (E). The random errors around the true score have a *normal distribution* and have a mean over infinite trials of 0. The standard deviation (SD) of the random errors around the true score is termed the *standard error of measurement*.

- The ratio of the variance of true scores divided by the variance of the observed scores provides an estimate of the reliability of a measure. However, not all error in tests is random. Some of the error is systematic and the various contributions of attribute and history variables are not well addressed by classical test theory.

Descriptive Statistics

- Descriptive statistics quantitatively describe the main features of a collection of data. The most widely generated measures are for central tendency (mean, median, mode, and interquartile range) and variability (SD, variance). The variability surrounding a measure's central tendency helps define the reliability of the measure. A "tighter" distribution of variability produces high reliability.

- *Kurtosis* captures the degree to which there is a "peaked" (leptokurtic) or "flat" (platykurtic) distribution of the data, whereas *skew* refers to tendencies of scores to cluster to the higher end of the distribution (negative *skew*) or at the lower end of the distribution (positive *skew*).

Inferential Statistics

- Descriptive statistics describe data; inferential statistics help you reach conclusions that extend beyond the data alone. Inferential statistics include members of a general family of statistical models known as the generalized linear model (GLM). Whereas for the *general linear model* (ANOVA, ANCOVA, regression), the dependent variable follows the *normal distribution*, in the generalized linear model, a flexible generation of ordinary linear regression models allows for the dependent variables to have an error distribution other than normal. The GLM (logistic regression, maximum likelihood, etc.) generalizes linear regression by allowing the linear model to be related to the response variable via a link function, and allowing the magnitude of the variance of each measurement to be a function of its predicted value.

- Some inferential statistical methods may be relatively indeterminate (no one solution) and yet provide insights that permit theorization regarding relationships among variables (e.g., structural equation modeling).

Item Response Theory

- *Item response theory* (IRT) is focused on item-level characteristics rather than on the test-level characteristics that classical test theory typically involves.

- The simplest IRT model is the 1-parameter model, which is algebraically equivalent to the Rasch model. Item-level responses can be analyzed so as to compare the probability of a correct answer against the underlying trait or ability level. This is done using an item characteristic curve. The curve can be studied for various items to examine the discrimination and difficulty level of items.

Probability Theory

The basic foundations of probability theory mirror games of chance. The ratio of outcomes over an infinite number of replays of the game will define the probability of that outcome.

Bayesian Methods

- In 1763, Bayes developed a theorem or law that states that, given a series of mutually exclusive events, the probability of outcome B given an event A is equal to the outcome A given B times the prior probability of outcome B, divided by the prior probability of outcome A. The three elements of any Bayesian model are the prior probability distribution, the likelihood function, and available new data. When all three components are combined, the posterior probability is produced.

- Bayesian models are unique because they allow one to incorporate prior information into a statistical model.

- There have been numerous treatments of the use of Bayesian methods for the identification of noncredible performance and more recent advances in increasing our understanding of latent models. Validity testing has incorporated Bayesian approaches to identify improbable test performances.

Section II: Foundations—Distributions

- Distributions of derived test scores are also known as distribution functions. These distributions can be analyzed and characterized using many mathematical tools.

- The *normal distribution* or "bell curve" distribution represents the classic way in which psychologists expect scores to fall. The *normal distribution* relates to some psychological abilities and attributes, but not all. Many measures in the motor performance and reaction time realms, for example, have positive *skew*, which can make development of useful norms a challenge. A similar challenge is involved in marked peakedness or leptokurtosis. To this end, there may sometimes be a need to transform obtained psychological data for analysis. This will be discussed further later in the chapter.

Central Tendency in Relation to Practice

Central tendency measures are familiar to most; mean, median, and mode should be thoroughly ingrained as constructs for psychologists. Skewed distributions will alter the rank order of the mean, median, and mode. The mean is the first "moment" (i.e., measure of the shape of a collection of points) of a frequency distribution.

Normal Variance

The variance is the average of the squared differences of each observation in a distribution from the mean. The standard deviation (SD) is the square root of the variance. The variance is the second "moment" of a frequency distribution taken about the arithmetic mean. The skewness and *kurtosis* relate to the third and fourth moments.

Normalization and Transformations

- It is possible to take distributions of data points that depart from "true" normality in some way and transform them so as to be "fit" to a normal curve. This may be necessary to solve any one of many problems of distributional shape, and numerous types of transformations may be appropriate depending on the shape of the data (e.g., reciprocals or log transformations for extreme positive *skew*). Every decision to utilize a transformation must be related to an essential measurement concern that can be identified and expressed.

- The creation of normalized standard scores is another common use of transformation, particularly since the operation can be done so as to have virtually any set mean and SD. This is most often done to put all measures of a protocol or battery on the same scale of comparison (see Table 8.1 for list of frequently used score transformations).

- Good performance is expected in unimpaired populations on a number of neuropsychological tests (e.g., judgment of line orientation, naming tasks, etc.), which is what makes them sensitive to brain dysfunction. Such tests, however, will not have a *normal distribution* of scores in the normative sample.

- Some transformation distributions are used on a routine basis in order to change the overall shape of the underlying data that can address this issue of non-normal distribution.

  - Example: percentage distributions render the data into a "rectangular" shape to force artificially even intervals regardless of the underlying values.

TABLE 8.1 Normative Score Transformations

Type of Score	Mean	Standard Deviation
Index or Standard Score	100	15
T score	50	10
Scaled Score	10	3
Z	0	1
Stanine	5	2
Percentile	50	1 SD: 34.13% 2 SD: +13.59% 3 SD: +2.14% 4 SD: +0.13%

- An important attraction of score expression in percentiles is the familiarity and ease in understanding for laypersons and test consumers.

- Percentile scores derived from the natural distribution of raw scores are optimal to minimize misinterpretations of tests with non-normal distributions. A percentile score allows for interpretation of an individual's scores in relation to other scores in the same population and therefore is clear in its presentation of results.

- Clinicians should be aware, however, of the true distribution of scores within the normative sample and should interpret standardized scores (including percentiles) cautiously with this information in mind.

- It is important to consider that transformations may <u>not</u> be appropriate in a variety of circumstances, such as when normative test performance is extremely skewed, and in such cases qualitative analysis of test performance may be the most appropriate interpretative approach.

Section III: Test Construction
Reliability and Validity Considerations

Reliability

- Reliability is fundamentally internal to the test, measurement, or protocol at hand. Reliabilities are a set of operating characteristics that portray the likely outcomes if the techniques of interest are applied once or some multiple of times over some interval.

- Reliability as a measurement construct addresses itself to the consistency of the results under varying test administration conditions. The broadest view of reliability is that it tells to what degree individual differences in test scores can be attributed to technically true differences in the attribute being considered, as contrasted with chance errors.

- All types of reliability can be expressed in terms of a reliability coefficient, varying from 0.0 to 1.0, which is an instance of a correlation coefficient. The classical definition of reliability also can be expressed as the ratio of true variance to total variance.

- Another important concept is the relationship between reliability and sensitivity to change. Perfectly reliable measures will not have sufficient capability to detect change, and reliability versus sensitivity to change is an important trade-off to optimize.

- Reliability can be considered through various types:

  - *Test-retest reliability* is a basic kind of reliability that looks at the stability of scores on repeated administrations of an instrument to the same person. Error variance represents the random fluctuation in performance from one administration to another, although test-retest reliability may also be influenced by the test-retest interval selected or the influence of instruction or *practice effects*.

  - *Alternate forms reliability* is expressed as a reliability coefficient that captures both the stability of the test over time and the consistency of responses to different samples of items tapping the same knowledge or performance. Alternate forms will reduce, but not eliminate the effects of error variance due to *practice effects*. Content sampling is an important construct in alternate form reliability; it answers the question to what extent scores on the alternate forms depend on factors specifically relating to the particular selection of items (i.e., do the items in each pool equivalently sample the content of interest)? Optimizing alternate forms will depend on having been successful in covering the same range of difficulty and span of content between the two tests.

  - *Split-half reliability* involves evaluation of the *internal consistency* of a test by splitting the test in many different ways using only a single administration. Some influences that occur during the taking of the test may vary over the course of the test session. To account for this, odd-even item splitting is utilized. Half scores of the test can be computed for each person, and the resultant correlation will be the reliability of a half-test. The Spearman-Brown formula can be used to calculate the likely effect of lengthening a test to a certain number of items.

  - *Inter-item reliability* or consistency involves the estimation of two sources of error: content sampling (as with the previous two reliabilities) along with the heterogeneity of the domain of knowledge or behavior. Greater homogeneity produces better interterm reliability. The relative homogeneity of a test, however, must match the relative homogeneity of the construct or criterion that the test is trying to measure or predict. The use of the *Kuder-Richardson formula*, also known as the "KR20," results in the reliability coefficient for *internal consistency* of a dichotomously scored test and represents the mean of all half-reliabilities resulting from splitting the test. Unless the content of the test is highly homogeneous, the KR reliability will be lower than the split half-reliability. When a test has the respondent checking a different numeric response for each item (e.g., a Likert-type scale, such as on the Personality Assessment Inventory), *Cronbach's coefficient alpha* serves the inter-item reliability purpose.

  - *Interrater reliability* relates to scorer variance that may systematically affect the outcome of tests when the scoring is not highly standardized or when judgment comes into play. The resulting correlation between separate scorings of the same test materials can be construed as interrater reliability.

Validity

The validity of a test, measurement, or protocol concerns itself with the accuracy with which meaningful and relevant measurements can be made with it. It is aimed at how well a method measures what it was intended to measure, from several perspectives. No procedure can be asserted to have low or high validity without a clear specification of the use to which it is being put. Validity marshals external, independently observable evidence about the behavioral realm a test, measurement, or protocol is assessing. Validity is considered in different ways:

- *Content validity* relates to the degree to which the test, measurement, or protocol covers a representative sample of the knowledge or behavior domain we seek to study. The domain of interest needs to be fully defined at the outset and carefully analyzed to ensure that all the major elements are covered and in correct proportions. The coverage of the content of a domain defines the degree to which the results of the test, measurement, or protocol can be generalized. Content validity should not be confused with *face validity* (i.e., the extent to which the test appears to measure the construct of interest) because it is based on empirical validation. Content validity cannot, however, be expressed as a validity coefficient.

- *Predictive validity* can be expressed as a coefficient and represents the relative success with which the test, measurement, and protocol predicts to a criterion we have defined and set forth in advance.

- *Concurrent validity* is also expressed as a coefficient and represents the degree to which a test, measurement, or protocol measures what it was intended to measure by looking at the performance of a test, measurement, or protocol against a previously validated (concurrent criterion) measure. There are no computational differences between the ways in which predictive validity and concurrent validity are calculated. Concurrent validity can stand in as a substitute for predictive validity.

- *Construct validity* can be thought of as the degree to which a test, measurement, or protocol successfully measures a psychological theoretical construct or trait. The concept is especially useful in situations in which there is no obvious external criterion to benchmark. Construct validity can be tested in several respects:

  - The study of differences between groups that should differ according to the theory for the variable,

  - the study of how test results are influenced by changes in individuals or the environment that should influence or fail to influence the individuals' positions on the continuum,

  - the correlation between different tests that are assumed to measure the same variable (although care needs to be taken that the similarity does not simply arise between similarities in method), and

  - the correlation between single items or different parts of the test, measurement, or protocol. High intercorrelation is desirable if a test is to be regarded as measuring a unitary variable.

Threats to Validity

While slightly different from threats to validity in the context of an experimental design, threats to internal validity in the context of neuropsychological assessment relate to conclusions drawn from the use of a neuropsychological test. Threats to *external validity* relate to limits on generalizability of test results. Both are described in Table 8.2.

TABLE 8.2 Examples of Threats to Internal and External Validity of Clinical Neuropsychological Assessments

Name	Threat Type	Definition
History	Internal	Education level, reading level, age, handedness, gender, and race (can be partially addressed through selection of adequate normative data)
Testing Interval	Internal	Artifact from duration of testing or practice effects.
Order of Test Administration	Internal	Artifact from order of tests administered should be considered given that (1) fatigue over the battery could influence performance and (2) exposure to one test may influence performance on another in the battery
Regression to the Mean	External	By taking a pair of independent measurements from one distribution, samples far from the mean on the first set of scores (due to random variance) will be closer to the mean on the second set. Samples appear to regress because the random variance affecting the samples in the second measurement is independent of the random variance affecting the first. The further from the mean on the first measurement, the stronger the effect.
Multiple Comparisons	External	Within a standard neuropsychological assessment battery are a multitude of scores. As we know, finding one or more scores that fall more than 1 standard deviation below the intraindividual or normative sample mean is not uncommon; based on the assumptions of the *normal distribution*, it will occur 16% of the time. Even a most conservative definition of "score of concern" (such as 2.0 standard deviations below the mean) results in low scores being detected about 4% of the time by chance alone. If we make determinations of impairment based on multiple comparisons of one test score to either other test scores of that individual or to the normative sample, our chance of finding a difference by chance alone that does not reflect a clinically relevant finding is considerable. Correction for multiple comparisons should be considered in deciding whether a test score falling in the low to exceptionally low range represents a clinically interpretable finding.
Situational Variables	External	Medication effects, mood variables, and task engagement (secondary to fluctuating attention, effort, quality of sleep, level of pain, sensory deficits, etc.).

Section IV: Test Evaluation

Multitrait Multimethod Matrix

- The construct validity of a test is often evaluated via convergent and discriminant validity techniques. Convergent validity is demonstrated when two or more approaches to measurement of some trait are positively correlated. Discriminant validity is exemplified by a low correlation coefficient between two similar approaches to measurement of different traits.

- The multitrait multimethod matrix is a composition of correlation coefficients of two or more traits and two or more methods. This matrix contains four types of correlation coefficients: monotrait-monomethod (the correlation between the measure and itself, or the measure's reliability), monotrait-heteromethod (correlation of two different methods of measuring one trait; high value reflects convergent validity), heterotrait-monomethod (the correlation between one method of measurement of two traits; low value reflects discriminant validity), and heterotrait-heteromethod (correlations between two measures of different traits using different methods; low value reflects discriminant validity).

Sensitivity/Specificity and Positive and Negative Predictive Value

- Sensitivity and specificity describe how well the test discriminates between individuals with and without a specified condition. That is, they tell us how good the test is at detecting the presence or absence of a condition that we know exists. To determine the sensitivity and specificity of a test, we must apply the test to a population of individuals in whom the diagnosis is known. Thus, the sensitivity and specificity are generally fixed psychometric properties of the test itself and reveal how good the test of interest is at detecting a known entity, as measured by some gold standard for that condition. For most tests, information regarding sensitivity and specificity in populations of interest is readily available in test manuals. However, caution should be used in applying estimates of sensitivity and specificity to populations that vary from the population on which the sensitivity and specificity were determined. For example, if sensitivity in a particular study is determined with an artificial 50% base rate based on a specific sampling approach, then applying this to a population with a 5% base rate would introduce error; the true sensitivity of test would likely be much lower. If only 5% of the sample has the condition, it will be much harder to detect via use of a test.

- More often, we are interested in knowing whether we are "right" when we make a decision based on a test performance. This refers to the predictive value of the test. Whereas sensitivity and specificity are conditional on the patient having the disease and are not influenced by the *prevalence* of the condition in the population (i.e., the base rate), positive and negative predictive values reflect our diagnostic accuracy in using a specific test in a specific population with a known incidence of a particular condition. That is, positive predictive power tells us what proportion of the time we were correct when we stated that a condition was present based on a test result. Negative predictive power, alternately, tells us what proportion of the time we were correct in stating on the basis of our test that an individual does *not* have a condition.

Likelihood Ratios

Unless a test's sensitivity and specificity are both 100% (which is an unlikely scenario), the *prevalence* of a disease determines how much certainty you can place in your diagnostic conclusions based on a test result. So, how do we really know if a test is any good at making predictions? This question can be answered by calculating likelihood ratios.

- A likelihood ratio of a positive test compares true positives (the likelihood that you were right if you said the condition is present) to false positives (the likelihood that you were wrong if you said the condition is present); a likelihood ratio for a negative test compares false negatives (the likelihood that you were wrong if you said a condition is absent) to true negatives (i.e., the likelihood that you were right if you said the condition is absent).

- A likelihood ratio of 1 indicates that the test result is just as likely in those with and without condition; therefore, the test result does not add much relevant information. Positive likelihood ratio values greater than 1 suggest that a positive test result is indicative of the presence of the condition. The desired negative likelihood ratio is between 0 and 1 (few false negatives as compared to true negatives). As the likelihood ratio moves further away from 1, it indicates that the test provides more useful information in detection of a specific condition.

- An optimal likelihood ratio depends a great deal on the test or measurement characteristics at hand. Measures or criteria with great variability or dispersion will be harder to optimize for this ratio but may be uniquely informative. Likelihood ratios can be compared across tests so that the most useful tests can be chosen to maximize the ability to predict conditions of interest. A benefit of using likelihood ratios over predictive values is that the *prevalence* of the condition does not affect the statistic. However, likelihood ratios can be used in conjunction with probabilities of a condition (i.e., base rates) to calculate a post-test probability of condition detection.

- In practice, what neuropsychologists actually need to know is not the sensitivity and specificity of a test, but rather the probability that a specific individual has a specific condition of interest, given that the test finding was positive. Such information is referred to as a post-test probability and can be calculated using *Bayes' theorem*.

Pre- and Post-Test Probabilities and Incremental Validity

The pre-test probability is the estimated probability that a patient has a condition prior to knowing a test result. In other words, the pre-test probability reflects the base rate of the condition. The post-test probability of a condition is the probability that the patient has the condition given a positive test result; or, in other words, how well the test rules in the condition. Testing, therefore, brings us from a pre-test probability to a post-test probability. The incremental validity of the test is the extent to which the use of the test improves the post-test probability with respect to the pre-test probability, or the positive predictive value of the test (how much of the time am I correct when I identify a condition using the test) minus the base rate of the condition. Alternately, the incremental validity can also be calculated based on negative predictive value, if we are most interested in ruling out a condition, or based on the hit rate, if we are most concerned with the overall accuracy of both our "yes" and "no" decisions. Incremental validity for a test aimed at detecting a very high- or low-frequency condition is generally very hard to achieve. As the base rate approaches 50% of the population, however, it is easier to construct a test that improves on the base rate and therefore demonstrates incremental validity.

Choosing Cut-Offs: Receiver Operating Characteristics (ROC) Curves

- The "costs" of false positive and false negative errors will vary across settings and patients. Thus, there is a need for multiple cut-off scores. The choice of cut-off should be made based on the goal of use for the instrument. For example, detection of suboptimal effort or engagement (i.e., performance invalidity) is integral to appropriate neuropsychological assessment. We want to be very sure in the case of potential suboptimal effort that we are identifying poor task engagement and not an actual level of impairment. We want to minimize false-positive errors (saying an individual's effort is suboptimal when their poor performance instead reflects true impairment). Thus, our goal for performance validity tests is to maximize specificity, recognizing that we do this with some cost to sensitivity to detection of suboptimal effort.

- Alternately, if our goal is to identify all persons showing any degree of impairment in a domain of function, in order to broadly offer some intervention, we would want to choose a cut-off score that maximizes sensitivity (i.e., detecting as many people with the condition as possible), acknowledging the risk of false positives and the sacrifice of specificity. A *receiver operating characteristic (ROC) curve* allows us to visualize the performance of a test by creating a plot of sensitivity (Y axis) and 1-specificity (X axis) based on various cut-off values determining a positive test. The cut-off value chosen should represent the point at which the balance between sensitivity and specificity makes the most sense for a particular condition.

- The area under the ROC curve (AUC) is a statistical measure that reflects the overall accuracy of the test's predictions and can be used to compare the detection accuracy of individual assessment tools.

Standard Error of Measurement (SEM)/ Standard Error of the Estimate (SEE)

- The SEM provides an empirical measure of the error variance around a single true score (i.e., the error of our measurement) based on the theoretical distribution and classical assumptions about errors including equal variances of error distributions.

- The SEM is the SD of the error distribution around the true score and takes into account the SD of the test and the test's reliability coefficient. This calculation is the same for any individual taking the test, regardless of the individual's true or obtained score.

- This index, although theoretically important, is rarely very clinically useful because we generally do not know the true score. We therefore cannot use this information to calculate a confidence interval to aid in data interpretation. The SEE is the SD of true scores if the observed score is held constant. In other words, given the obtained score, a clinician can calculate the range of scores in which the true score is likely to fall and can interpret test performance using a confidence interval. The SEE is often not provided in a test manual but can be calculated based on the SD and reliability of the test. The utility of the SEE in clinical practice is described in the test interpretation section below.

Section V: Test Interpretation

Use of Normative Data

How does a neuropsychologist define an appropriate and psychometrically sound normative set? First, we must ask two questions:

1. Are the test scores normally distributed in the population?

2. Is the *standardization* sample representative of the population to which you wish to compare your patient's performance?

- We need to know when we compare an individual's score to a normative group that the normative sample is representative of a relevant comparison population. A result can appear good or intact when compared with one norm and poor or impaired when compared with another. Thus, utilization of the appropriate reference group when determining whether a score represents true impairment is essential. Due to error inherent in estimating population parameters utilizing modestly sized samples, the smaller the sample, the greater the uncertainty, and the larger the confidence interval of the obtained score, particularly for extreme scores. The larger the sample size, the better, given practical constraints.

Confidence Intervals

Confidence intervals allow for an estimate of the uncertainty of an obtained test score based on both the properties of the test (i.e., reliability as influenced by measurement error) and the properties of the normative sample (i.e., distribution). The estimated true score of the test can be calculated using the obtained score, test mean, and test reliability. As the reliability of the test decreases, the estimated true score is brought closer to the mean, and the confidence band widens. The estimated true score is then the anchor of the confidence band, which is calculated using the desired level of significance based on probability and the SEE. Confidence intervals created using the SEE versus the SEM have smaller bands because of the extra consideration for the test's reliability. This is especially important when reliability is poor because a narrow confidence interval is desirable. Consequently, as the reliability of the test increases, the SEE and SEM (and therefore also the confidence intervals) both decrease. If the test's reliability is very poor, the confidence interval is likely to be very large, and interpretation of the obtained score may yield little useful information.

Low Score Interpretation

- The decision of whether a low score represents an impairment in a specific domain is one central to the role of neuropsychologist. We base this decision on the assumptions of the *central limit theorem* and probability statistics, but whether a low score represents an abnormal difference may be somewhat unclear.

- Binder, Iverson, and Brookes (2009) provide an excellent review of the literature relating to the probability of abnormal neuropsychological test findings in intact individuals with use of various cut-offs for determination of impairment.

- The finding of considerable intraindividual variability has been demonstrated in actual population samples, as well as in statistical simulations (i.e., Monte Carlo and binomial probability methods). It has therefore been recommended that diagnostic inferences be made based on recognizable patterns of test results rather than on psychometric variability alone.

Profile Analysis

- Profile analysis in neuropsychology refers to the practice of plotting standardized scores on a battery of tests in terms of a graph or profile and making inferences about cognitive functioning and probable diagnosis on the basis of the pattern in test performances.

- Both interindividual interpretation (i.e., how this person's profile compares with other people from the presumed diagnostic group) and intraindividual interpretation (examining discrepancies among an individual's scores on different measures) can yield important information. We often want to know how an individual does on a test in terms of some outside reference point (i.e., is their performance "normal"?). However, given large individual differences in baseline cognitive abilities, comparison to the mean performance is inadequate.

- Detection and quantification of individual impairments requires recognition of relative performance across tests and domains within an individual and comparison to what is believed to have been his or her previous level of cognitive functioning.

Statistical Versus Clinical Significance

- Reliable difference informs us of the statistical significance of the difference between two scores (i.e., the likelihood of obtaining some difference between scores by chance at a specified probability level).

- Calculation of the reliable difference involves the difference in obtained score between the tests and the standard errors of the measurement for the two tests.

- The *reliable change index* (RCI) establishes the minimum magnitude of change required for psychometric certainty that two scores actually differ and is discussed further later. Whereas reliable differences refer to the statistical significance of the difference between two scores, an abnormal difference refers to whether the discrepancy between scores is or is not typical and tells us if the magnitude of the discrepancy is rare based on base rates of the observed difference in the population. If it is rare, we can then determine in what way it is clinically meaningful.

- There is a distinction made between *efficacy* and *effectiveness* in intervention trials that parallels the difference between statistically significant and clinically meaningful differences. *Efficacy*, which parallels statistical significance, refers to whether an intervention produces the expected result under ideal circumstances, whereas *effectiveness*, which is similar to clinically meaningful, measures the benefit of an intervention under "real world" conditions.

Reliability of Difference Scores

- The reliability of differences is important for both intra- and interindividual comparison. When working with intraindividual differences, we want to know whether an obtained difference between scores is reliable and that the probability of it arising as a result of measurement error is so small that we are confident in using the score as a means of predicting some phenomenon, such as group membership in a diagnostic category. The reliabilities of the individual tests, therefore, significantly influence the probability that a specific raw score difference is the result of measurement error.

- A reliability coefficient can be used to express the reliability of intraindividual difference scores if the variance of the error distribution of the difference scores and the variance of the distribution of obtained differences are both known. The reliability of the difference score depends partly on the reliability of each of the tests on which the difference scores were based and the extent to which the tests covary.

Repeat Testing: Trend Analysis and Reliable Change

Serial neuropsychological evaluations are now relatively common in a variety of neuropsychological settings, aiding in differential diagnosis and tailored treatment. However, there are multiple sources of change operating in repeated assessments, as well as considerable variability in degree of *practice effects* across tests, even within a cognitive domain. These factors need to be understood for optimal interpretation.

Trend Analysis

Neuropsychological interpretation in serial testing relies on the identification of trends in the analysis of intraindividual change. Interpretations based on change trends are strengthened with multiple complementary findings (i.e., convergent validity). One basic example of trend analysis is the identification of variable engagement within tests or across the testing session. Trend events in this case include implausible increases or decreases in scores, discrepant item responses, or implausible response patterns.

Analysis of Change

- The most straightforward way to statistically evaluate change is to obtain a distribution of observed change scores (the difference from first to second testing) in the normative sample and then convert each individual's change score to a standardized score based on the distribution. Unfortunately, information on test-retest performance in adequate samples is rarely available.

- As neuropsychologists, we want to be sure that changes we see in scores over time are not an artifact of imperfections in our measurements but rather represent true change in cognitive ability. The *reliable change index* (RCI) reflects the probability that the measured change is reliable; that is, that an observed difference between two scores from the same examinee on the same test cannot be attributed to measurement error.

- Calculation of the RCI uses the standard error of the difference (based on the *standard error of measurement* for the test) and computes a *z score* for the difference between the individual's tests based on the normal probability distribution. An RCI falling more than +/– 1.96 reflects a significant difference in the test scores.

- When using test normative sample statistics to calculate RCI, clinicians should not overinterpret a significant RCI value as indisputable evidence that reliable change has occurred. In the context of highly reliable tests, even a very small change score can produce a significant RCI that does not reflect clinically relevant change. Reliable change indexes should also be statistically adjusted for *practice effects* using the mean change score for the reference group.

Discriminant Functions

- Often in the practice of neuropsychology, we want to know whether the profile of obtained test scores from an individual matches what is expected based on membership to a specific diagnostic group (i.e., individuals with Alzheimer's disease). *Discriminant analysis* is the process of utilizing a score profile to determine whether an individual belongs to one group (i.e., a specific diagnosis) or another (i.e., no diagnosis or a different diagnosis).

- *Linear discriminant function* combines information from variables regarding discrimination of the groups with weights for each variable chosen to maximize the F ratio. A specific application of multiple logistic regression yields prediction to one or the other group, denoted 0 or 1, the discriminant function. It is possible to simultaneously predict membership to one of more than two groups utilizing multiple *linear discriminant function*. However, the first discriminant tends to do a better job at discriminating than does any subsequent discriminant and, thus, multiple discriminants are rarely utilized.

- Discriminant function analysis assumes multivariate normality and homogeneity of the variance/covariance matrices and thus, may not always be appropriate. Logistic regression (described in more detail below) makes no assumptions about the distribution of predictors or covariates, has several measures to assess model fit, and allows one to assess the statistical significant of not only the overall model but the individual covariates/predictors in the model.

Use of Regression in Interpretation

- Regression equations are commonly used in neuropsychology as an alternative to normative comparisons. Regression equations can be used to estimate premorbid levels of functioning based on demographic and specific test performances (i.e., predicting a level of test performance based on estimates of baseline abilities), to account for demographic characteristics (i.e., predicting an individual's score on the basis of these characteristics), or to assess change in the neuropsychological functioning of an individual (i.e., predicting a retest score on the basis of their initial test performance). For the latter, the regression approach factors in both *practice effects* and regression to the mean.

- Regression equations are used to generate an expected level of performance for an individual against which an obtained performance can be compared. If an individual has an acquired deficit in functioning, it can be expected that there will be a significant discrepancy between his or her predicted and obtained scores. Consideration must be given, however, to the error inherent in creating the regression equation based on a specific sample, and confidence intervals are, as usual, essential for appropriate interpretation.

- Logistic regression is a type of classification algorithm involving a linear discriminant. Logistic regression allows one to determine the probability that an individual score belongs to one group (e.g., specific diagnosis) or another (e.g., no diagnosis or different diagnosis). Relevant to the practical aspects of neuropsychology, logistic regression can help generate formulas using multiple variables from one test or a battery to help differentiate between groups (i.e., impaired vs. not impaired; adequate vs. inadequate test engagement).

Relevant Definitions

Alpha The first letter of the Greek alphabet; the probability of type I error (i.e., rejecting the null hypothesis when it is true) in making a decision about the tenability of a null hypothesis; a measure of a test's reliability (coefficient alpha) that reflects the internal consistency of the item.

Bayes' theorem Probability/statistics theorem employed in decision analysis to allow the posterior probability of an event to be calculated.

Beta The second letter of the Greek alphabet; the probability of making a type II error (i.e., failing to reject the null hypothesis when it is false) in statistical hypothesis testing.

Central limit theorem If n independent variates have finite variances, then standard expression of their sum will be normally distributed (as n approaches infinity).

Conditional probability The probability of an event or outcome, given that a difference even has occurred. Based on Bayes' theorem.

Cronbach's coefficient alpha The expected correlation of two tests that measure the same construct. The statistic is a function of the number of items in a test, the average covariance between item-pairs, and the variance of the total score.

Discriminant analysis Multivariate statistical technique used to describe differences between two or more groups on a set of measures (descriptive discriminant analysis) or to classify subjects into groups on the basis of a set of measures (predictive discriminant analysis).

Effectiveness The benefit of an intervention under "real world" conditions; analogous to clinically meaningful."

Efficacy Whether an intervention produces the expected result under ideal circumstances; analogous to "statistically significant."

External validity Degree to which results from a particular test or measure can be generalized to situations or related to information beyond the test itself (correlation of measure to another measure of some independent criterion).

General linear model (Not to be confused with multiple linear regression, generalized linear model, or general linear methods). The general linear model or multivariate regression model is a statistical linear model. It may be written as $Y = XB + U$, where Y is a matrix with series of multivariate measurements (each column being a set of measurements on one of the dependent variables), X is a matrix of observations on independent variables that might be a design matrix (each column being a set of observations on one of the independent variables), B is a matrix containing parameters that are usually to be estimated, and U is a matrix containing errors (noise). The errors are usually assumed to be uncorrelated across measurements, and follow a multivariate *normal distribution*. If the errors do not follow a multivariate *normal distribution*, generalized linear models may be used to relax assumptions about Y and U.

Internal consistency Estimate of the reliability of a measure or score based on the average correlation among items within a test. The size of the coefficient depends on both the average correlation among the items *and* the number of items; represented by coefficient alpha.

Item characteristics curves (aka item response function) Shows probability of a correct response as a function of the level of overall performance of the person.

Item response theory Models the response of each test-taker of a given ability to each item on the test; based on the idea that the probability of a correct/keyed response to an item is a mathematical function of person parameters (i.e., the trait or ability) and item parameters (i.e., difficulty or discrimination).

Kappa The 10th letter of the Greek alphabet; a measure of reliability reflecting agreement among raters that is adjusted for the expected level of chance agreement.

Kuder-Richardson formula A formula for estimating the reliability of a dichotomously scored test; influenced by number of items, variance, and item difficulty.

Kurtosis A measure describing the degree to which a distribution of scores is clustered around the mean; if peaked, leptokurtic; if flat, platykurtic.

Linear discriminant function Combines information from variables regarding discrimination of the groups, with weights for each variable chosen to maximize the F ratio. A specific application of multiple logistic regression yields prediction to one or the other group, denoted 0 or 1, the discriminant function. It is possible to simultaneously predict membership to one of more than two groups utilizing multiple linear discriminant function. However, the first discriminant tends to do a better job at discriminating than does any subsequent discriminant and, thus, multiple discriminants are rarely utilized.

Meta-analysis The statistical analysis of results obtained from different independent studies. This technique can be used to create metanorms using data from several independent normative samples.

Normal distribution (aka bell-shaped or Gaussian distribution) A bell-shaped score distribution that is symmetric around the mean. Approximately 68% of the scores fall between −1.0 and +1.0 SDs about the mean, approximately 95% of the scores fall between −2.0 and +2.0 SDs about the mean, and approximately 97.7% of the scores fall between −3.0 and +3.0 SDs.

Person separation index Summary assessment of the ability of a test to discriminate between groups, taking into account measurement error; analogous to reliability statistic.

Power tests Tests in which there is no time restriction or time component.

Practice effects Improvement in performance as a function of having previously taken the test or performed the task.

Prevalence (aka **base rate**) The total number of cases of a particular phenomenon that develop within a given period.

Quantile The expression of a distribution as equal, ordered subgroups. Quantiles can be made by dividing the distribution into any number of equal groups. For example, quartiles create four groups in the distribution.

Receiver operating characteristic (ROC) curve A plot of the probability of detecting a condition against the probability of false alarms; based on signal response theory; used for establishing optimal cut-offs for prediction of binary outcomes.

Regression analysis A method of statistical analysis in which a single outcome variable is related to one or more predictor variables by examining the tendency for scores on the outcome to move in concert with scores on the predictors; usually lines, but curvilinear and nonlinear possibilities exist.

Regression toward the mean The tendency for scores at the extremes of a distribution to migrate toward the mean on repeated assessment due to increased probability closer to the center of the distribution.

Reliable change index (RCI) Used to determine whether changes present on follow-up testing exceed what is considered to result from the methodological aspects associated with repeat assessment; based on test-rest reliability, the standard error of the test, and practice effects; confidence levels are selected based on desired level of precision.

Signal detection theory Ability to detect the presence of a signal from background noise; generates the d' statistic, the distance between the noise distribution and the signal plus noise distribution; has been adapted for use in characterizing response styles in recognition memory testing.

Skew A measure of the asymmetry of a probability distribution; the "tail" of the distribution is in the direction of the skew (i.e., positive or negative).

Standard error of the estimate An estimate of the accuracy of a prediction of test performance; based on the difference between the obtained score and the predicted score, the number of pairs of scores, and the reliability of the test.

Standard error of measurement A measure of the variability of scores obtained on a test relative to the "true scores"; a reliable test has a small standard error of measurement.

Standard error of the mean A measure of the degree to which a sample mean varies from sample to sample around the true mean of the population; the standard deviation of the sampling distribution sample mean; the larger the sample, the smaller the standard error of the mean; standard deviation of the sample divided by the square root of the sample size.

Standardization The process by which data from a group of individuals intended to represent a population of interest are collected and analyzed; can be based on healthy individuals or clinical population. Adequate standardization improves the reliability and validity of test results.

Stratified sample Process of selecting a random sample from specific groups to ensure adequate representation of demographic groups.

Psychometrics, Test Design, and Essential Statistics Questions

NOTE: Questions 3, 28, and 59 on the First Full-Length Practice Examination, Questions 49, 59, and 120 on the Second Full-Length Practice Examination, Questions 11, 75, and 116 on the Third Full-Length Practice Examination, and Questions 6 and 26 on the Fourth Full-Length Practice Examination are from this chapter.

1. The concept of regression to the mean is best expressed by which of the following?
   (a) The apple doesn't fall far from the tree.
   (b) Highly intelligent people have even smarter children.
   (c) People of superior intelligence are likely to have high average children.
   (d) People who are low average are at high risk of having impaired children.

2. You have created a new test that you want to use clinically, but its psychometric properties are unknown. You want to know about the incremental validity of the test, and you have knowledge of the

base rate of the condition that the test was designed to detect. To calculate the incremental validity if you are equally worried about false positives and false negatives, you need to know the test's _____.

(a) overall hit rate

(c) specificity

(b) sensitivity

(d) positive predictive value

3. Which of the following will *not* affect the reliability of an intraindividual difference score (i.e., the reliability of difference in performance between two tests within one individual)?

(a) reliability of test one

(b) correlation between the tests

(c) variance of the distribution of the difference scores

(d) actual difference between the two scores

4. Which of the following is not a well-validated clinical use of regression?

(a) prediction of premorbid ability level

(b) prediction of membership in a clinical group

(c) prediction of performance in one domain based on performances in others

(d) prediction of future test performance based on past test performance

5. Assuming a normal distribution, how many people would score between a 600 and a 900 on a standardized test with a mean of 750 and a standard deviation of 150 (N = 1,000)?

(a) 680

(c) 640

(b) 840

(d) 720

6. When interpreting an obtained test score, one must consider that said score is composed of _____.

(a) true score and random error

(b) true score and both random and nonrandom error

(c) true score only

(d) random error only

7. How does increasing the sample size affect the standard error of the estimate?

(a) A larger sample size produces a larger standard error of the estimate.

(b) A larger sample size produces a smaller standard error of the estimate.

(c) A larger sample size has no effect on the standard error of the estimate.

(d) A larger sample size can produce a larger standard error of the estimate, but only if the sample is larger than 10.

8. Would you conclude impairment in a particular cognitive domain based on one neuropsychological test score falling 1 standard deviation below the mean?

(a) No, finding one or more scores that fall more than one standard deviation below the mean is common, and if using the assumption of the normal distribution of scores, this occurs 16% of the time.

(b) No, finding one or more scores that fall more than one standard deviation below the mean is common, and if using the assumption of the normal distribution of scores, this occurs 4% of the time.

(c) Yes, finding one or more scores falling more than one standard deviation below the mean is uncommon and, and if using the assumption of the normal distribution of scores, this occurs 2% of the time.

(d) Yes, finding one or more scores falling more than one standard deviation below the mean is uncommon and, and if using the assumption of the normal or skewed distribution of scores, this occurs less than 1% of the time.

9. What is the simplest item response theory (IRT) model?

(a) The simplest IRT model is a three-parameter model, which is not algebraically equivalent to the Rasch model.

(b) The simplest IRT model is a two-parameter model, which is not algebraically equivalent to the Rasch model.

(c) The simplest IRT model is a two-parameter model, which is algebraically equivalent to the Rasch model.

(d) The simplest IRT model is a one-parameter model, which is algebraically equivalent to the Rasch model.

10. The Spearman-Brown Formula can be used to _____.

(a) calculate the effect on reliability by lengthening the test

(b) calculate the effect on reliability by removing individual items

(c) assess for the homogeneity of items within the test

(d) assess the interrater reliability of a test

Psychometrics, Test Design, and Essential Statistics Answers

1. **C—People of superior intelligence are likely to have high average children.** *Answers B and D imply regression away from the mean, and answer A indicates no systematic expected change in predictions with repeated measurement. Answer C is the only choice reflective of the idea of regression to the mean.*

   Reference: Nunnally, J. C. & Bernstein, I. H. (1994). *Psychometric theory.* New York, NY: McGraw-Hill.

2. **A—overall hit rate** *Although positive predictive value could be used to calculate incremental validity, it is only useful if we are interested in our test's incremental ability to make a positive diagnosis, not as an indicator for overall diagnostic accuracy. Thus, the overall hit rate is the best choice in this situation because we are interested in both yes and no decisions based on the test (both PPV and NPV).*

   Reference: Spitalnic, S. (2004). Primer in literature interpretation: Test properties 1: Sensitivity, specificity and predictive values. *Hospital Physician, 40,* 27–31.

3. **D—actual difference between the two scores** *The reliability of the tests, the association between them, and the error variance are all included in the formula required to calculate the reliable chance interval. The actual difference between the score is only a point of reference and is compared to the calculated interval.*

Reference: Price, L. D. (2017). *Psychometric methods: Theory into practice* (Methodology in the Social Sciences). New York, NY: Guildford Press.

4. **C—prediction of performance in one domain based on performances in others** *Answers A, B, and D are discussed in the text of the chapter. Answer C is incorrect because performance within each domain is believed to be relatively independent from other domains and there is little basis for prediction of performance in one domain on the basis of others.*

Reference: Lezak, M. D. (2012). *Neuropsychological assessment* (5th ed.). New York, NY: Oxford University Press.

5. **A—680** *500 falls 1 SD below the mean; 900 falls 1 SD above the mean. 68% of a normally distributed sample falls within +/−1 SD from the mean. Thus, in a sample of 1000, 680 (68%) fall +/− 1 SD from the mean.*

Reference: Slick, D. J. (2009). Psychometrics in neuropsychological assessment. In E. Strauss, E. M. S. Sherman, & O. Spreen (Eds.), *A compendium of neuropsychological tests: Administration, norms, and commentary* (3rd ed., pp. 1–55). New York, NY: Oxford University Press.

6. **B—true score and both random and nonrandom error** *As stated in classical test theory, any obtained test score X for an individual consists of a true score and an error component. Some of the error is random while some of the error is systematic (and not random).*

Reference: Gravetter, F., & Wallnau, L. B. (2017). *Statistics for the behavioral sciences* (10th ed.). Boston, MA: Cengage Learning.

7. **B—A larger sample size produces a smaller standard error of the estimate.** *A larger sample size produces a smaller standard error of estimate and increases the likelihood of rejecting the null hypothesis. Recall from the SEM/SEE section, the SEE is the SD of true scores if the observed score is held constant. The SEE helps a clinician calculate the range of scores in which the true score is likely to fall. The larger the sample, the greater the likelihood that one will be able to accurately predict where the true score will fall. Thus, choice B is the only option that correctly answers this question.*

Reference: Gravetter, F., & Wallnau, L. B. (2017). *Statistics for the behavioral sciences* (10th ed.). Boston, MA: Cengage Learning.

8. **A—No, finding one or more scores that fall more than one standard deviation below the mean is common, and if using the assumption of the normal distribution of scores, this occurs 16% of the time.** *As is discussed in the Test Construction section of the chapter (under the reliability and validity subsection), finding one or more scores that fall more than 1 SD below the intraindividual or normative sample mean is not uncommon; based on assumptions of the normal distribution, it will occur 16% of the time. Even a most conservative definition of a low score (such as 2.0 SDs below the mean) results in low scores being detected about 4% of the time by chance alone. Thus, choice A is the correct response to this question.*

Reference: Gravetter, F., & Wallnau, L. B. (2017). *Statistics for the behavioral sciences* (10th ed.). Boston, MA: Cengage Learning.

9. **D—The simplest IRT model is a one-parameter model, which is algebraically equivalent to the Rasch model.** *According to the Rasch model, an individual's response to a binary item (e.g., right/wrong, true/false, agree/disagree) is determined by the individual's trait level and the difficulty of the item. One way of expressing the Rasch model is in terms of the probability that an individual with a particular trait level will correctly answer an item that has a particular difficulty.*

Reference: Price, L. R. (2017). *Psychometric methods: Theory in practice.* New York, NY: Guilford Press.

10. **A—calculate the effect on reliability by lengthening the test** *The Spearman-Brown formula is used to calculate the likely effect of lengthening a test to a certain number of items. The formula predicts the reliability of a new test composed by replicating the current test n times (or, equivalently, creating a test with n parallel forms of the current exam). Thus n = 2 implies doubling the exam length by adding items with the same properties as those in the current exam. Values of n less than one may be used to predict the effect of shortening a test.*

Reference: Gravetter, F., & Wallnau, L. B. (2017). *Statistics for the behavioral sciences* (10th ed.). Boston, MA: Cengage Learning.

Recommended Readings

Anastasi, A., & Urbina, S. (1997). *Psychological testing* (7th ed.). Upper Saddle River, NJ: Prentice-Hall.

Binder, L. M., Iverson, G. L., & Brooks, B. L. (2009). To err is human: "Abnormal" neuropsychological scores and variability are common in healthy adults. *Archives of Clinical Neuropsychology, 24,* 31–46.

De Ayala, R. J. (2009). *The theory and practice of item response theory.* New York, NY: Guildford Press.

Donnell, A. J., Belanger, H. G., & Vanderploeg, R. D. (2011). Implications of psychometric measurement for neuropsychological interpretation, *The Clinical Neuropsychologist, 25,* 1097–1118.

Gravetter, F., & Wallnau, L. B. (2017). *Statistics for the behavioral sciences* (10th ed.). Boston, MA: Cengage Learning.

Millis, S. (2018). What clinicians really need to know about symptom exaggeration, insufficient effort, and malingering: Statistical and measurement matters. In J. E. Morgan & J. J. Sweet (Eds.), *Neuropsychology of malingering casebook* (pp. 21–39). New York, NY: Psychology Press.

Nunnally, J. C., & Bernstein, I. H. (1994). *Psychometric theory.* New York, NY: McGraw-Hill.

Price, L. R. (2017). *Psychometric methods: Theory in practice.* New York, NY: Guilford Press.

Slick, D. J. (2009). Psychometrics in neuropsychological assessment. In E. Strauss, E. M. S. Sherman, & O. Spreen (Eds.), *A compendium of neuropsychological tests: Administration, norms, and commentary* (3rd ed., pp. 1–55). New York, NY: Oxford University Press.

9 Test Administration, Interpretation, and Issues in Assessment

Mike R. Schoenberg, James G. Scott, Eric Rinehardt, and Michelle Mattingly

Introduction

Neuropsychological assessment is a powerful procedure designed to identify the extent and severity of cognitive and behavioral dysfunction. The evaluation is then used to answer a wide range of diagnostic, treatment, and research questions, such as:

- *Differential diagnosis* Differentiates brain dysfunction from non-lesional psychiatric conditions or otherwise reversible causes of cognitive complaints (e.g., depression). This aspect also involves identifying severity and presence of neurocognitive disorders to meet established diagnostic criteria (i.e., dementia, mild cognitive impairment).

- *Describe neuropsychological status* Identifies how a disease or lesion is affecting the cognitive, behavioral, and emotional function of an individual. This also involves identifying the extent and severity of brain dysfunction.

- *Treatment needs* Informs treatment planning, treatment placement, or evaluating for resource utilization needs. This involves tailoring treatment to a particular patient's needs based on results of neuropsychological findings that are integrated with knowledge of neuropathology and known brain mechanisms of recovery and rehabilitation sciences.

- *Treatment effects* Identifies the effects of treatment (often measuring change in neuropsychological function over time with repeated assessments).

- *Screening* Screen for cognitive impairment in persons at risk. Screening may also be used to quickly assess specific cognitive processes that are being treated (e.g., medication and/or rehabilitation interventions).

- *Primary or secondary outcome research measure* Identify basic and central nervous system (CNS) processes and/or the effects of other agents on the CNS.

- *Forensic applications* Assist fact-finding bodies to determine if, or the extent to which, an alleged event resulted in damage to the CNS. Other uses include assisting courts to determine if a defendant is capable of managing his or her affairs independently and/or to evaluate capacity to stand trial.

Although the neuropsychological evaluation can provide unique information in understanding the patient's brain function and behavior, a competent practitioner must have sufficient expertise to obtain, score, and interpret the assessment data to answer specific referral questions. The interpretation of a neuropsychological assessment is one of the last steps in a complex process that requires an in-depth knowledge and appreciation of psychometrics/measurement, research methods/statistics, general psychology, brain–behavior relationships, functional neuroanatomy, and neuropathological etiologies and processes. Thus, interpretation must be integrated with each individual's unique broader health context, including medical history, psychological history, and cultural/societal context to make rational diagnostic and treatment care decisions/recommendations that are guided by the scientific literature. This complex process embodies *evidence-based neuropsychology practice* (Chelune, 2008), defined as providing care that integrates clinical data, research literature, individual patient characteristics, financial realities, and cultural/social norms and values. This chapter endeavors to provide the reader with an overview of an *evidence-based neuropsychology practice* model and its intricacies. Box 9.1 summarizes a series of questions the clinician should be able to answer in the neuropsychological assessment process.

BOX 9.1 Issues in Neuropsychological Assessment and Interpretation

Test selection/normative sample(s)

- Are tests selected sufficient to answer referral question(s)?
- Is normative data adequate for test(s)?
- To what extent is normative data representative of larger population?
- Does normative data include participants similar to the particular patient?
- Is the normative data skewed? Is this individual from a group with a non-normal distribution?
- Are there ceiling/floor effects?
- Were scores in the distribution extrapolated/interpolated?

Comparing test scores across tests

- Are tests scores equally reliable?
- Are sample sizes of normative data for each test similar?
- To what extent are the normative data used to derive test scores comparable? Were tests normed using the same or different samples? If different samples, to what extent are the normative samples similar in terms of demographics? To what extent is the variance in test performances accounted for by demographic factors (e.g., age, education, ethnicity) similar between tests (normative data)?

Identify the likelihood that test score differences are rare and of concern

- What *comparison standard* is being employed? Is the *comparison standard* appropriate to the individual?
- What method or criterion is being used to identify when differences between scores are meaningful (< -1 SD, < -1.5 SD, < -2 SD)? Is the same criterion being used for interpretation of all test scores?
- What is the likelihood one or more low scores on a neuropsychology battery reflect normal variability/ error when compared to other healthy subjects?
- To what extent do the low scores among test(s) reflect a pattern consistent with known neuropathology and are they consistent with the history and behavioral observations?
- Are changes in scores over time due to reliable change or do they reflect normal variability, regression to the mean, and/or measurement error?

Individual patient characteristics

- Does the patient match salient characteristics of the normative samples for each test?
- Does the patient have unique characteristics that require special consideration in assessment planning and test score interpretation (e.g., disability, English as a non-primary language).

Communication of results

- What qualitative classification scheme (e.g., extremely low, very low, below average, average) will be used to communicate results?
- Have the same qualitative classification descriptors been used to communicate all test results?
- How is/are the referral question(s) answered? How are recommendations for care or implications for treatment conveyed?

NOTE: Reproduced (with minor modification) with permission from: Iverson & Brooks. (2011). Improving accuracy for identifying cognitive impairment. In M. R. Schoenberg & J. G. Scott (Eds.), *The little black book of neuropsychology: A syndrome-based approach* (pp. 923–950). New York, NY: Springer.

Introduction to Neuropsychological Assessment and Evidence-Based Neuropsychology Practice

The general organization of an evidence-based neuropsychological evaluation should follow a systematic and organized series of steps guided by the referral question and neuropsychological science. These include:

1. Identification of referral questions and other answerable questions

2. Review of medical records

3. Critical appraisal of the research evidence and its relevance to the particular patient and suspected condition(s)

4. Application of known or suspected neuropathology and brain–behavior relationships to develop an assessment plan

5. Administration of a reliable assessment procedure

6. Interpretation of results

7. Clinical decision-making integrating the evidence with the clinician's expertise, appropriate normative comparisons, and the patient's unique characteristics

8. Communication of these results to the patient and referring party

9. Evaluation of outcomes: Did the evaluation make a difference in the treatment plan or outcome? Quality of care?

Within each step, a series of decisions must be made, each of which affect later steps in the evaluative process and ultimately affect the interpretation of obtained data, the answers to referral questions, and the treatment recommendations. Each of these steps are discussed here.

Practical Neuropsychological Evaluation

A detailed review of all aspects of neuropsychological assessment and interpretation is beyond the scope of this chapter. Here, we provide a brief review of the steps in patient evaluation including the referral, review of medical records, interviewing, and selection of tests. It is essential that the neuropsychologist guide the assessment process to answer referral questions and alert the referring parties if referral questions may not or cannot be answered (or if other services might better answer referral question[s]). Review of medical records should allow for understanding of referral questions, laboratory tests, comorbidities, and medications that may affect the neuropsychological evaluation. The initial clinical interview is critical to understanding the course and history of the problem(s) and associated comorbidities. The interview also allows the clinician to make behavioral observations and obtain critical information not accessible through medical records or test scores. Interview of collateral sources (e.g., family members, caregivers) can also often provide additional insights into the course of symptoms, as well as identify other problems or concerns that may be impacting the patient's function. Here, we turn to a more detailed discussion of the basis for a neuropsychological evaluation and the series of steps involved in the selection and interpretation of tests to answer the referral question.

Test Selection and Neuropsychological Assessment Methods/Process

The overarching assessment process for evidence-based practice is applying neuropsychology expertise with the extant literature to diagnose, treat, and/or identify brain–behavior processes to answer referral questions as efficiently as possible for a particular patient with a unique history and framed by social/

cultural factors. Within this practice framework, one must select from several alternative approaches to neuropsychological assessment. The majority of clinicians use a hypothesis-driven approach termed the *flexible-battery approach*, in which neuropsychological domains are systematically screened, with more detailed assessment when deficits are identified. A flexible battery may also contain core measures specifically used to assess a known (or suspected) neuropathology and/or to answer specific referral question(s). Other assessment methods include the *fixed-battery approach* (e.g., Halstead-Reitan Battery), and the *process* (or Boston) *approach*. The *fixed-battery approach* uses the same set of tests for each patient regardless of the referral question or history. The *process approach* focuses less on the interpretation of tests scores and more on the understanding and interpretation of the behavioral processes that occurred while obtaining that score. Regardless of the assessment method chosen, interpretation is typically based on a *deficit measurement model* and a systematic evaluation of obtained data.

Deficit Measurement in Neuropsychological Evaluation

The neuropsychological evaluation for clinical purposes involves the application of a *deficit measurement model*. Contrasting the scores against a *comparison standard* allows the clinician to determine if reliable improvement or decline has occurred. There are two general *comparison standards*: (1) *normative comparison standards* and (2) *individual comparison standard*.

- **Normative comparison standards** include species specific and population average *comparison standards*:

  - A *species comparison standard* is a capacity shared by all healthy members of the species. For example, all humans have the capacity for language development; lack of language development is abnormal. Such a finding is termed a *pathognomonic sign*.

  - *Population averages* reflect the average performance of a large sample of individuals on a particular skill. When using population normative-based information, a patient's performance is compared to standardization data from a known (often healthy) population. Often, this distribution is assumed to approximate a normal curve (as in the case of intelligence tests), but it can also be skewed, with most individual performances close to either the lowest (positive skew; e.g., failure to maintain set on the Wisconsin Card Sorting Test) or highest score possible (negative skew; e.g., items correct on the Boston Naming Test).

The primary limitation of a population *normative comparison standard* is that it does not provide information sufficient to identify a specific score of concern (SOC) for an individual. For example, is a score concerning if a patient scored at the 14th percentile compared to population *comparison standard* (e.g., age-matched healthy peers) on a verbal memory test? Although below average for a given population (<1 standard deviation [SD] below the mean), this score may be normal for this particular individual depending on their original (premorbid) level of function. The *individual comparison standard* allows the determination of change within an individual, as opposed to referencing a population average expectation. Developing an *individual comparison standard* requires the clinician to establish an estimate of the individual's premorbid level of ability within a reasonable degree of scientific certainty.

- **Individual comparison standards** require the person's level of (neuropsychological) ability(ies) before the onset of known or suspected neurological dysfunction (premorbid functioning) be determined and used to compare current scores against. The *individual comparison standard* may be developed from historical records (e.g., previous cognitive testing, academic records, or vocational indices) or from estimates (often derived from various psychometric methods) and/or behavioral observations. If historical records are available (e.g., prior cognitive test

TABLE 9.1 Considerations in Predicting Premorbid Ability

	If Patient Has A History Of _____			
	Recent acquired dominant hemisphere dysfunction	Recent acquired diffuse brain damage	Remote dominant hemisphere damage	Dyslexia/ learning disorder
Adult	Historical, Demographic, nonverbal	Historical, word reading	Nonverbal, Demographic	Nonverbal, Demographic
Child	Historical, Demographic, nonverbal	Historical, Demographic	Historical, Demographic, nonverbal	Historical, Demographic

NOTE: Historical = using historical records of premorbid ability (previous standardized achievement testing); Demographic = premorbid estimates using demographic variables; nonverbal = methods using current performance on measures minimizing verbal skills; word reading = methods using current performance to read irregularly spelled words.

scores or measures of academic achievement), these can offer the clinician a reliable and valid measure of prior cognitive abilities and can reduce error in determining change in function. Unfortunately, such historical information is rarely available, and premorbid cognitive ability must be estimated. Methods to estimate premorbid cognitive ability can be based on demographic variables (age, education level, occupational history) and/or derived from current performances on cognitive skills and tests less affected by brain dysfunction and/or effects of aging (e.g., reading irregularly pronounced words, vocabulary knowledge, etc.). The best methods to predict premorbid ability:

- Minimize the standard error of estimate
- Are available in rapid time frames (available within hours to days)
- Add no or very little extra time to assessment
- Can be easily obtained/computed

Methods have focused on predicting premorbid IQ scores, but methods to predict attention, processing speed, and memory indexes have been developed as well. Table 9.1 summarizes generally accepted premorbid estimation methods. Once a *comparison standard* has been selected, the next step in interpretation is:

- Evaluate reliability and validity of measures/scores.
- Avoid common interpretation errors (see later in this chapter).
- Answer referral questions, which often (but not always) associates obtained scores to known brain–behavior relationships and neuropathological processes.
- Make evidence-based recommendations for care.

Evaluation of Neuropsychological Data

Neuropsychological assessment includes qualitative and quantitative data, and the clinician must be aware of the types of data obtained and how these data are compared and interpreted. Qualitative data include observations of aberrant behavior during the evaluation, along with clear rule violations (repeatedly interrupting examiner, impulsive errors, forgetting instructions). Other qualitative data are gratuitous responses and incoherent or nonsensical remarks (e.g., flight of ideas, anosognosia, perseveration) that may allude to dysfunction. Quantitative data offer standardized measurements of brain–behavior relationships and typically involve comparison of ordinal (i.e., Likert scale) and interval level data (e.g., T scores). Interpretation errors can result when incorrectly comparing ordinal and interval-level data. The reliability and validity of obtained data must be known for accurate interpretation, which should include appreciation of the psychometrics and normative base of each test (see also Chapter 8, Psychometrics, Test Design, and Essential Statistics).

Reliability and Validity in Test Interpretation

Neuropsychological tests are objective measures designed to reliably and validly sample brain–behavior functions (behaviors). Tests should have published administration procedures, scoring rules, and information about the reliability and validity of derived scores when administered and scored in the standardized manner. Each score is a sample of behavior, reflecting the measurement of a construct and some measurement error. The standard error of measure (SEM) quantifies the error of measurement for a test of a construct. Beyond reliability, tests must be valid measures of brain–behavior constructs and, ideally, have predictive or criterion validity (see also Chapter 8, Psychometrics, Test Design, and Essential Statistics).

Diagnostic Utility of Tests: Sensitivity, Specificity, and Test Accuracy

Table 9.2 provides an example in understanding how neuropsychological interpretation should be guided by knowledge of the effect of base rates on the positive and negative predictive power of each test. Test accuracy is determined by the total true positives and true negatives. Using a test with a high sensitivity rules *out* the diagnosis with a negative test result. The mnemonic *Sn-Nout* can be helpful to remember negative test score (N) on a test with high sensitivity (Sn) rules out a diagnosis. Alternatively, a positive result on a test with a high specificity rules *in* a diagnosis. The mnemonic *Sp-Pin* can help remember a positive test result (P) on a test with high specificity (Sp) rules the diagnosis (condition) in. Please review Table 9.2 for diagnostic statistic terms. The positive predictive value (PPV) and negative predictive value (NPV) provide information about the likelihood the person has the disease when the test score is positive for the condition (PPV and 77.8% in the example) or when it is negative and the condition is absent (NPV and 87.3% in the example). Prevalence rates of the condition affect PPV and NPV but not sensitivity or specificity. As the prevalence rate of the disease decreases (from that found in the published studies), the PPV will also decline. The post-test probability of a positive test is numerically equal to the PPV. The probability of not having the disease when a test result is negative is 1-NPV and termed the post-test probability of a negative test. The pre-test probability is the likelihood of having the disease before performing the test (prevalence rate) and should not be confused with pre-test odds (prevalence/ 1 – prevalence). The likelihood ratio positive (LR+) is the estimate of how much a positive test result will change the odds of having the disease/condition and is based on the ratio of sensitivity and specificity of a test. Likelihood ratio negative (LR-) is the change in odds of not having a disease/condition when a test result is negative. The more the LR deviates from 1, the stronger the likelihood is that the disease is present (LR > 1) or absent (LR < 0.01 indicates the test result is associated with the absence of disease). The

TABLE 9.2 Example of Test Diagnostic Accuracy Values

Diagnostic Test Result	Target Disorder		
	Present	Absent	Totals
Positive	151 (a)	43 (b)	194
Negative	37 (c)	254 (d)	291
Totals	188	297	

post-test odds is the added value of the test over the pretest probability of the condition and may be either positive or negative. The post-test odds-positive (3.51) is the pre-test odds (0.634) multiplied by the likelihood ratio for a positive test (5.54). Post-test odds (pre-test odds × LR) can be converted to the post-test probability [post-test odds/(post-test odds + 1)]. The post-test probability is the probability of the patient having the disease with a positive diagnostic test result. For the example here, without giving the test, the pretest odds of having the disease was 0.63 (or about 4 of every 10 individuals tested). The probability of the disease after a positive test is 0.778 (which is an improvement from 0.388 before the test). As a rule of thumb, a good diagnostic test will increase the post-test odds to above 0.50 in populations in which the prevalence rate (pre-test probability) is low.

- Sensitivity = a/(a + c) [80.3]
- Specificity = d/(b + d) [85.5]
- Positive predictive value = a/(a + b) [77.8]
- Negative predictive value = d/(c + d) [87.3]
- Pre-test probability (prevalence) = (a + c)/(a + b + c + d) [38.8]
- Likelihood ratio for a positive result (LR+) = sensitivity/(1 – specificity) [5.54]
- Likelihood ratio for a negative result (LR–) = (1 – sensitivity)/specificity [0.23]
- Pretest odds = prevalence/(1 – prevalence) [0.634]
- For a positive test result:
  - Post-test odds = pre-tests odds × LR+ [3.51]
  - Post-test probability = post-tests odds/(post-test odds + 1) [0.778 or 77.8%]

Although odds ratios and likelihood ratios are both ratios, these are interpreted differently and used in different clinical contexts. The LR is interpreted as the extent to which a particular test value increases the likelihood of a disease being present (or absent). Odds ratio is interpreted as a measure of effect size and identifies how harmful (or beneficial) a particular exposure is to an individual.

Categorization Versus Interpretation of Scores

Neuropsychologists must establish a criterion (threshold) for determining when a score is low or below expectations. The prior discussion of a *comparison standard* becomes crucial in defining when a score is in the low or exceptionally low range and may be reflective of brain dysfunction. Historically neuropsychologists have employed a wide variety of test score labels for describing similar or equivalent performances. Not surprisingly this has led to confusion, inconsistency, and the potential to negatively impact the communication of neuropsychological results for medical decision-making. Because of this there has been a growing desire to standardize qualitative test score descriptors in neuropsychology. Consequently, a consensus conference was held in 2018 at the American Academy of Clinical Neuropsychology (AACN) Annual Conference and a number of important recommendations were proposed. Although the consensus statement was not published at the time of writing of this chapter, efforts have been made to relay the AACN consensus conference's primary recommendations. Strong recommendations made by the AACN consensus conference can be summarized as follows.

- Scores should not be labeled as "impaired." A person and their abilities can be impaired but a test score can be low for a variety of reasons, only one of which is true cognitive impairment.

- The qualitative labeling, discussion, and interpretation of scores from tests with normal versus non-normal distributions should be approached differently.

- With regard to tests with highly restricted score ranges, test score labels should be based on percentile scores rather than standard scores. The rationale for this recommendation is based upon the fact that percentile ranks are more comparable and meaningful than transformed scores when the distribution is highly skewed. It is also important to stress that the percentiles for non-normally distributed tests are based on actual cumulative counts of individuals who obtained a specific score and thus are not statistical estimations based on standard deviation units around the mean of the reference group.

- If the patient exhibits a specific *pathognomonic sign* or neurobehavioral condition it should be named and/or described in behavioral terms.

Competent neuropsychologists must be aware that a score itself does not verify cognitive "impairment," but rather it is the interpretation of scores (as a measure of brain function constructs) that determines whether or not an impairment is in fact present. Assuming adequate test engagement, a score may reflect an actual brain–behavior relationship *plus* measurement error, along with effects of score bias (normative bias, cultural/educational components not accounted for), error in predicting premorbid ability, fatigue, poor motivation/task engagement, pain, and/or anxiety/depression.

But what is the method for interpreting impairment? There is no universal agreement, but several prevailing thresholds in neuropsychology are used; historical procedures have been based on parametric statistics, whereas others are based on Bayesian statistical modeling.

Statistical Models for Defining Scores of Concern

- *Parametric statistical modeling* to define a SOC is based on extrapolation of the central limit theorem to estimate the performance of an individual relative to a group. In this method, a SOC is defined relative to a normative reference group.

- *Bayesian statistical modeling* is a probability model using a set of corrective variables to improve the accuracy of prediction. Defining SOC using Bayesian statistics, one develops an *individual comparison standard* and uses this individual estimate to identify when a SOC is present.

Establishing Cut-Offs for Scores of Concern

The neuropsychologist may employ different cut-off values (threshold values) for establishing a SOC. Although rarely advisable, some employ a threshold of scores falling 1 SD below the mean (accounting for the bottom 15% of scores in a normal distribution). Using this cut score, index scores of less than 85 or T scores less than 40 are considered to potentially reflect unusually low performance or impairment in the construct being measured. Other commonly used thresholds are -1.5 SD (corresponding to about the lowest 7% of scores) or -2.0 SD (corresponding to bottom 2% of scores) below the mean to identify a score outside of expected performance for an individual. The qualitative test score descriptors recommended by the AACN consensus conference for normally distributed tests were still in development when this book was written and thus have not been included here. However, it is critical to remember that the score labels are only labels and that it is the clinician's interpretation that determines if those scores reflect brain dysfunction.

There are advantages and disadvantages to using various cut-off thresholds to label scores as concerning. Less strict (using a cut-off of -1.0 SD below the mean) thresholds result in increased sensitivity to potential mild dysfunction, but increase the risk of making false-positive errors and incorrectly associating the constellation of scores as brain dysfunction when they are not (e.g., reflect normal variability and measurement error). More conservative standards (i.e., using a cut-off score of -2.0 SD below the mean) result in increased specificity (low scores more likely to actually reflect brain dysfunction) but increase the risk of making false-negative errors (e.g., not identifying mild dysfunction when it is present). It also should be remembered that the frequency of healthy individuals obtaining a low score (or several low scores) in a test battery including 15–30 scores is relatively common. Regardless of which threshold for determining impairment is utilized, it is advantageous to use the same threshold throughout interpretation. This is not just a statistical issue, it is also a clinical one. When the neuropsychologist evaluates and or compares scores, it is ideally done in the context of a known history and hypotheses established before testing. Thus, the test score interpretation should be guided by the literature, qualities of the test instruments employed, and known prototypical patterns for the condition(s) of interest. For example, if the neuropsychologist works in a movement disorders clinic they are probably more likely to interpret below average or low scores on processing speed tests as reflective of disease related impairments. However, similar scores earned by an individual two years post mild TBI are more likely related to other factors besides concussion. Thus, the neuropsychologist's test score labeling approach should stay the same while their interpretive approach should vary depending on the practice setting, assessment goals, and respective base rates with regard to the condition(s) under consideration. In the end objective neuropsychological tests can only do so much and the quality/accuracy of the interpretation is much more dependent on the clinician's skill and acumen.

Know Your Norms (Understand Normative Data)

Interpretation of scores must be guided by knowledge of the strengths and weaknesses of each test's normative sample and representativeness and how the normative sample of a particular test compares to other tests and normative data. The clinician should be aware of the research evidence for the use of various neuropsychological tests in specific patient populations to answer referral questions. It is not uncommon for a neuropsychological evaluation to incorporate a variety of tests assessing different neuropsychological constructs that have normative data derived from different samples. Further, normative data for some tests may be based on age, whereas others provide norms based on age and education or other demographic variables. Thus, within a single neuropsychological evaluation, scores may be derived from age-matched normative data whereas others are based on age and education-normative data whereas still others are based on age, education, ethnic, and gender-normative data (see also Chapter 11, Cultural and Disability Issues in Neuropsychological Assessment). The clinician must be aware that these scores are not directly comparable and have different statistical properties. Additionally, the sample of individuals recruited to provide the normative data may not be representative of a particular individual, leading to gross errors in interpretation. An obvious example of nonrepresentativeness is the use of normative data that does not include anyone of the same age as the patient.

Defining "Rare" Scores: Statistical Significance Versus Cumulative Percentages

The Wechsler Adult Intelligence Scale–4th edition (WAIS-IV; Wechsler, 2008) normative data allow one to better appreciate the difference between statistical differences versus the cumulative prevalence of differences between scores. A statistically significant difference in scores refers to the relative rarity of a difference in scores based on the central limit theorem and the distribution of test scores. Thus, the scores' reliability and standard error of measure will determine the statistical rarity of these obtained scores. Alternatively, prevalence rate refers to the actual occurrence of differences between scores observed for individuals in the normative sample. Having a difference in scores that is statistically rare is still often fairly frequently observed in normative samples. For example, differences of 8–9 points (varies by age group) between WAIS-IV Verbal Comprehension Index (VCI) and Perceptual Reasoning Index (PRI) scores are statistically significant at $p = 0.05$, but this difference between indices was observed in more than 25% of healthy adults in the sample. For a difference in scores to be rare (defined as observed in 5% or less of the sample), the difference between VCI and PRI scores needs to be 22 or more points (Wechsler, 2008). The differences in interpretation of statistical probability on one hand and cumulative percentage on the other highlights the difference between interpreting parametric statistics with assumptions of score frequency and the sequential observation of variability within a population.

Interpreting Single Scores and Patterns of Performance

Another caution in interpreting single low scores as reflective of impairment is family-wise error rate or the increasing likelihood that a positive test finding will occur by chance when multiple tests are administered. If one were to interpret each score falling below the 5th percentile as "impaired," we might expect to make a false positive determination 5% of the time (assuming normal distribution of scores). Although a false-positive rate of 5% may be acceptable for any one test, a neuropsychological evaluation can include 20 to 100+ individual scores, so the family-wise error rate or likelihood of obtaining one score below the 5th percentile is much greater than 5%. Changing the threshold from less than 5% to less than 15% would substantially increase the family-wise error rate and number of scores interpreted as impaired. Figure 9.1 highlights the statistical likelihood of obtaining more low scores with increasing numbers of test scores labeled as concerning. Note that when a test battery includes 36 variables, based on the full Neuropsychological Assessment Battery (NAB; White & Stern, 2003), almost half (48.5%) of the healthy normative sample obtained two or more scores below the 5th percentile, whereas about 15% of the sample had five or more scores below the 5th percentile. This further reinforces the dictum that in most circumstances it is highly inadvisable to use one standard deviation below the mean as a threshold to label scores of concern.

A related issue is the observation that individuals with lower general cognitive ability (IQ) tend to have more low scores, whereas individuals with higher general cognitive ability (IQ) are more likely to have greater variation in scores. Figure 9.2 illustrates the frequency of healthy adults obtaining at least one memory test score below the 5th percentile across two different memory batteries stratified by four qualitative categories of Full-Scale Intelligence Quotient (FSIQ) scores. Among individuals with average FSIQs (90–109), 22–38% of subjects had at least one score below the 5th percentile. The frequency of low scores

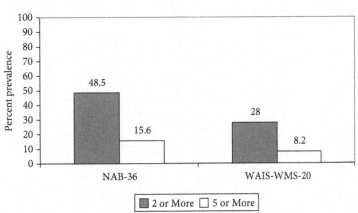

FIGURE 9.1 Base Rates of Low Scores Across Batteries with Different Numbers of Scores Being Interpreted: Cutoff ≤ 5th Percentile

NOTE: Reproduced with permission from Iverson & Brooks. (2011). Improving accuracy for identifying cognitive impairment. In M. R. Schoenberg and J. G. Scott (Eds.) *The little black book of neuropsychology: A syndrome-based approach* (pp. 923–950). New York, NY: Springer.

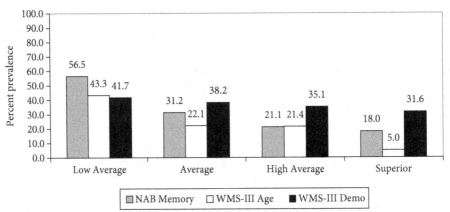

FIGURE 9.2 Percent Healthy Older Adults with Full-Scale IQ (FSIQ) in Four Qualitative IQ Categories with One or More Low Memory Scores Using ≤ 5th Percentile to Identify Memory Impairment

NOTE: Reproduced with permission from: Iverson & Brooks (2011). Improving accuracy for identifying cognitive impairment. In M. R. Schoenberg & J. G. Scott (Eds.) *The little black book of neuropsychology: A syndrome-based approach* (pp. 923–950). New York, NY: Springer. NAB memory module consists of 10 demographically adjusted scores. The WMS-III battery consists of eight scores that may be only age-adjusted or adjusted for age, education level, and ethnicity; Low average = FSIQ 80–89, Average = FSIQ 90–109, High Average = FSIQ 110–119, Superior = FSIQ ≥120.

increased to 41–57% for individuals with FSIQs in the low average range. Figure 9.2 also highlights the impact of using different normative data on interpretation. When using Wechsler Memory Scale (WMS-III) age-based normative data, fewer scores fell below the threshold for being deficient than when WMS-III scores were based on age, education, and ethnicity-matched peers (demo normative data). Clearly, there is intra-individual variation in scores that also varies by level of general cognitive ability.

The occurrence of scores meeting the threshold for concern also varies by the demographic characteristics of the individual. Demographic characteristics' impact on score interpretation can be substantial, particularly for African American samples and patients with less than 7 years of education. Figure 9.3 provides the mean scores of healthy older adults, 50 African American and 50 Caucasian, matched on age, education, and gender on the Repeatable Battery for the Assessment of Neuropsychological Status (RBANS; Randolph, 1998) based on a study by Patton et al. (2003). The effect of ethnicity (which likely reflects quality of education not captured by educational grade/degree obtained; e.g., Manly &

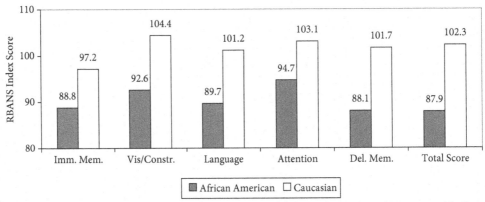

FIGURE 9.3 Comparison of Healthy African Americans to Healthy Caucasians on the Repeatable Battery for the Assessment of Neuropsychological Status (RBANS)

NOTE: Reproduced with permission from: Iverson & Brooks. (2011). Improving accuracy for identifying cognitive impairment. In M. R. Schoenberg & J. G. Scott (Eds.) *The little black book of neuropsychology: A syndrome-based approach* (pp. 923–950). New York, NY: Springer.

Echemendia, 2007) was considerable, ranging from Cohen's $d = 0.52$ (Immediate Memory) to $d = 0.91$ (Total Score).

In interpreting scores, the preceding discussion highlights the importance of clinicians' use of appropriate normative data and the effects that selecting a threshold for a SOC can have on interpretation. Unfortunately, it is frequently necessary for the clinician to utilize neuropsychological measures that are not co-normed and have scores derived from different normative samples.

Interpretation Errors to Avoid

Below are common interpretation errors to avoid:

- ***Do Not Interpret Low Scores Without Context*** Some low scores are bound to occur, and these should not be interpreted as synonymous with brain dysfunction. Determination of impairment requires a *pattern* of scores fitting known brain–behavior relationships that dovetail with the patient's unique history and symptoms. For example, one should *never* interpret an isolated low memory score as evidence of "temporal lobe dysfunction."

- ***Do Not Interpret Education or Ethnicity as Impairment*** Low scores may occur due to differences in cultural, ethnic, and educational backgrounds from the normative group. Low scores are found more commonly among minority ethnic groups in the United States (particularly African Americans) and among individuals with less education (see also Chapter 11, Cultural and Disability Issues in Neuropsychological Assessment).

- ***Overgeneralizing and "if this, then that"*** Do not interpret similar score patterns as reflecting the same type of dysfunction independent of context and neuropathology. For example, although patients with mesial temporal lobe dysfunction typically present with very low to extremely low memory scores, not all patients with low memory scores have mesial temporal lobe dysfunction.

- ***Confirmatory Bias*** Do not exclude contradictory test findings or history when it does not fit with a suspected (or known) disease or condition. Although a patient with depression or somatoform disorders often presents with memory/cognitive complaints not due to neurological disease (e.g., pseudodementia), patients with a history of depression and somatoform disorders may also develop dementia. Thus, one should not dismiss the possibility of dementia in a patient with a known diagnosis of somatoform disorder or depression who presents with memory complaints.

- ***Time as a Moderator*** Clinicians need to be aware of the presenting individual's complaints, course, and severity over time. The temporal presentation of symptoms and medical history likely provides more clues as to the condition or disease than the neuropsychological data themselves. Thus, a clinician should not conclude that a patient presenting with many scores at or below the 15th percentile has a "dementia" if the symptoms have only been present for two weeks.

- ***Absence of Evidence Is Not Evidence of Absence*** Do not interpret the absence of low scores as the absence of neurological (psychiatric) disease. One may not detect dysfunction if a cursory or poorly planned evaluation was completed (e.g., a right homonymous hemianopsia may be unappreciated if not assessed for).

- ***Salient Data Over- or Underinterpretation*** Do not give too much weight to a single dramatic finding (e.g., low score or abnormal neurologic finding) in interpretation as compared to other less eye-catching data (normal laboratory findings) and history (good employment record). Likewise, one or several scores all within a particular domain being low while all other scores are average or better may be discounted as measurement error when these, in fact, relate to neurological impairment if the sampling in that domain was limited. For example, insufficient measurement of processing speed/complex attention in a patient with a history of recent complicated mild traumatic brain injury (TBI).

Special Issues in Interpretation

Pediatric Considerations

A comprehensive review of special issues in pediatric neuropsychological interpretation is beyond the scope of this chapter. However, a summary of major challenges in pediatric neuropsychology interpretation include:

- Test scoring and psychometric data can differ between ages, even for the same test. For example, several test batteries employ different start and stop points for different age groups, resulting in different reliability values for test scores (and sometimes different scores all together).

- Test normative data are often limited for children. For example, normative data for the Boston Naming Test for adolescents aged 14–19 years are very limited.

- Establishing *comparison standards* for children must account for the impact of neuro-developmental factors on the suspected or known neuropathology and how it may alter the clinical presentation.

- Referring questions and suspected progress should be one factor in guiding selection of tests, with some tests being appropriate for wider age bands (2- to 16-year-olds) whereas other tests are designed for narrower age periods (1 to 6-year-olds).

- A child's development trajectory may continue but be altered by acquired neuropathology or in other cases normal development may be stalled or even regress or worsen over time (i.e., delayed consequences). Which pattern occurs (continued, stalled, or regression of function) alludes to etiology and also predicts outcomes. Additionally, the presence of premorbid learning disorders and/or family risk factors can also affect neurodevelopment processes and the recovery/rehabilitative process.

Geriatric Considerations

Geriatric practice must incorporate the effects of aging processes into interpretation and treatment planning and appreciate the changing prevalence patterns for neurodegenerative diseases, sensory changes that occur more often in the elderly, and other medical comorbidities of various age cohorts. The potential impact on neuropsychological function of polypharmacy and increasing sensitivity to medication effects must also be considered. From a psychometric standpoint, normative data for elderly samples may be more restricted, with much smaller cell sizes, particularly for minorities. Furthermore, normative data for older adults can be comprised of individuals with demographic and social characteristics that differ in important ways from a particular patient.

Gender/Cultural/Language Considerations

The impact of demographic (ethnicity, cultural, gender) factors should always be appreciated in neuropsychological evaluation, both in terms of test development and the representativeness of the normative sample to patients with different social/cultural backgrounds. In general, non-native English speakers being assessed in the United States will likely perform differently on tests (e.g., language comprehension limitations, as well as different cultural/educational background) and have inappropriate normative data that extremely limit any interpretation or conclusions that can be drawn. When available, patients should always be assessed in their native language by a clinician speaking this language fluently (preferably a native speaker of that language, see also Chapter 11, Cultural and Disability Issues in Neuropsychological Assessment).

Test Modifications/Testing Special Circumstances

Adaptations and non-standardized administration of standardized tests may be needed in contexts of sensory, motor, or language limitations. In these cases, test modification changes the test and the scores, reducing reliability and therefore associated validity and conclusions that may be drawn from the data obtained. However, these accommodations can be clinically helpful and essential to obtaining meaningful data and thus should not be categorically avoided.

Relevant Definitions

Comparison standard An established benchmark or score against which scores or behaviors are compared to determine if a difference exists. The comparison standard is the value against which all other scores are compared to determine if meaningful differences from this value exist. A comparison standard may be normatively based (determined from an appropriate population) or be an individual comparison standard (determined from the individual's history, demographic characteristics, or obtained from prior cognitive, achievement, behavioral, or other laboratory value). It serves as the basis for the deficit measurement model to determine if there is a meaningful difference between scores.

(Individual) comparison standard Refers to development of a comparison standard specific to a particular individual against which the individual's current scores are compared to determine if meaningful variance in test performance(s) is present. The individual comparison standard differs from a normative comparison standard in that the individual comparison standard takes into account individual variability and allows a comparison standard to be uniquely derived for each person to allow individuals to have premorbid levels of ability that differs from the population average. The individual comparison standard is necessary to make determinations of change for functions or constructs that are normally distributed in the population. The individual comparison standard may be derived from previous neuropsychological, cognitive, or psychological assessment that occurred prior to onset of known or suspected neuropsychological impairment, or it may be estimated from historical data, demographic data, or current performances on measures known to be resistant to effects of brain dysfunction or aging.

(Normative) comparison standard May reflect population average or a species-wide normative standard. Population average refers to the average or median score of an identified sample on a particular test. In neuropsychology/psychology, population average comparison standards are generally most useful in assessing basic cognitive functions that develop throughout childhood (e.g., perception, attention, motor skills, and memory). Species-wide comparison standards are those performance expectations for adults; they display a common course of development and are often fully developed prior to adulthood. Examples include development of receptive and expressive speech, absence of Babinski sign in adults, and symmetric deep tendon reflexes.

Deficit measurement model A central tenet to neuropsychological interpretation in which current performances on measures of neuropsychological, psychological, and behavioral functions are compared against a comparison standard to determine if a change in function has occurred. The discrepancy between the obtained score and the comparison standard provides a basis for asserting that a deficit may be present. This model may also be applied to giftedness when a normative comparison standard is used, such that the discrepancy between the average normative score serves as the reference to evaluate the extent that a score exceeds the population average score.

Evidence-based neuropsychology practice Integrates outcomes research, clinical expertise, the unique aspects of the patient, referral questions, and available costs and resources to the provision of neuropsychology services.

Fixed-battery approach Assessment method in which the selection of tests is fixed, with each patient receiving the same battery of tests that typically assess each basic neuropsychological domain (attention/executive, memory, language, visuoperceptual/constructional) and often screen for psychological disorders.

Flexible-battery approach Assessment method in which the selection of tests to be administered to a patient is guided by test hypothesis developed from a patient's history and/or current performances on tests to answer referral questions about neuropsychological functioning.

Pathognomonic sign A sign whose presence means that a particular disease, condition, or impairment is present beyond any doubt. Examples include aphasia, apraxia, hemispatial inattention, hemiparesis, and agnosia.

Process approach Assessment method in which the interpretation of scores is based more on a careful qualitative and (sometimes) quantitative evaluation of the neuropsychological processes a patient undertook to perform on a test. The assessment method is less guided by the interpretation of test scores and more by the evaluation of the processes by which a patient obtained various test scores.

Test Administration, Interpretation, and Issues in Assessment Questions

NOTE: Questions 41, 62, and 86 on the First Full-Length Practice Examination, Questions 29, 68, and 95 on the Second Full-Length Practice Examination, Questions 15, 40, and 46 on the Third Full-Length Practice Examination, and Questions 62, 66, 91, and 121 on the Fourth Full-Length Practice Examination are from this chapter.

1. Neuropsychological assessment is broadly defined as _____.
   - (a) measuring the impact of psychological impairments on people with neurologic disease.
   - (b) the application of standardized testing techniques to understand and measure underlying brain–behavior relationships
   - (c) non-imaging-based assessment of structural or evolving lesions of the CNS
   - (d) the assessment of the impact of CNS factors on psychological functioning

2. Observation of the plantar (Babinski) reflex in an adult is noted by a neuropsychologist. The comparison standard to determine that this reflex is abnormal is termed the _____.
   - (a) individual comparison standard
   - (b) normative comparison standard
   - (c) species level comparison standard
   - (d) standard individual measurement

3. Negative predictive value (NPV) is defined as the _____.

   (a) true negatives divided by (true negatives plus false negatives)
   (b) percentage of true negatives that can be reliably identified by a test
   (c) absolute number of true negatives out of all cases tested
   (d) absolute number of true positives and true negatives in all cases combined

4. Iverson and Brooks (2011) identified the base rate at which low scores (defined as less than the 5th percentile) occur in the healthy normative population for the Neuropsychological Assessment Battery (NAB), the Extended Halstead Reitan Neuropsychological Battery (E-HRNB), and the Wechsler Adult Intelligence Scale-III/Wechsler Memory Scale-III (WAIS-III/WMS-III). This research identified such low performances occurring on two or more subtests within each battery at what rate?

   (a) rarely (<1% of the time)
   (b) infrequently (5.0% of the time)
   (c) sometimes (15.2–10.4% of the time)
   (d) frequently (48.5–28% of the time)

5. The Wechsler Adult Intelligence Scale–4th Edition (WAIS-IV; Pearson, 2008) has index scores with a mean of 100 and a standard deviation of 15 points. The minimum difference required for statistical significance ($p < .05$) between the Verbal Comprehension Index (VCI) and Perceptual Reasoning Index (PRI) is about _____, whereas the difference between VCI and PRI index scores observed in 5% or less of the normative sample (cumulative percentage) is about _____.

   (a) 8–9 points; 8–9 points
   (b) 8–9 points; 15 points
   (c) 8–9 points; 22 points
   (d) 14–15 points; 8–9 points

6. A 45-year-old accountant is referred for evaluation due to concerns regarding cognitive declines following a slip and fall injury at work. In a detailed test battery he earns multiple scores at the 2nd to 5th percentile, but his scores on various performance validity tests are also below recommended cut-offs. The scores at the 2nd to 5th percentile should be labeled as _____.

   (a) equivocal
   (b) invalid
   (c) impaired
   (d) low

7. Aphasia, agnosia, and apraxia are all examples of _____.

   (a) left hemisphere dysfunction
   (b) pathognomonic signs
   (c) dysconnection syndromes
   (d) diffuse cognitive impairment

8. A neuropsychologist uses a test to help predict which elderly are likely to convert from mild cognitive impairment to dementia within two years. At the two-year follow-up, the neuropsychologist counts how many of the patients who were identified as likely future converters actually did convert to dementia. This statistic is known as the test's _____.

   (a) prior predictive power
   (b) positive predictive power
   (c) negative predictive power
   (d) posterior predictive power

9. A psychologist wants to use a uniform standard for "impairment" across a battery of tests. The psychologist sets the cut-off for impairment at the 10th percentile, with scores falling below that cut-off on any single test being considered indicative of impairment. The battery is then given to 100 consecutively referred clients. Which of the following statements is true?

(a) The percentage of cases identified as having impairment will be larger if the battery includes 30 scores than if it yields 20 scores.

(b) The percentage of cases identified as having impairment will be smaller if the battery includes 30 scores than if it yields 20 scores.

(c) 10% of the cases will be identified as having impairment, regardless of the number of scores in the battery.

(d) 90% of the cases will have at least 1 score in the range of impairment, regardless of the number of scores in the battery.

10. A neuropsychologist is evaluating possible dementia in an 85-year-old African American person who was born and raised in the United States. Which of the following variables is relatively most important in determining whether low scores on a test of psychometric intelligence truly reflect cognitive impairment?

(a) years of completed education, as reflected in available school records

(b) degree to which the patient self-identifies with a particular ethnic subgroup

(c) history of hypertension, diabetes, and heart disease in first-degree relatives

(d) quality of education, as reflected in performance on a word recognition test

Test Administration, Interpretation, and Issues in Assessment Answers

1. **B—the application of standardized testing techniques to understand and measure underlying brain–behavior relationships** *Neuropsychological assessment involves application of standardized assessment testing techniques to the evaluation of current functioning in cognitive, behavioral, and emotional domains and integration of the influences of CNS disease and trauma to understanding performances on neuropsychological tests.*

   Reference: Lezak, M. D., Howieson, D. B., Bigler, E. D., & Tranel, D. (2012). *Neuropsychological assessment* (5th ed.). New York, NY: Oxford University Press.

2. **C—species level comparison standard** *The species comparison standard is a type of normative standard and evaluates an individual's performance relative to a healthy adult member of the species. For example, in humans, bipedal gait, vision, development of language and having intact vision, hearing, smell, taste, and proprioception are species level capacities. .*

   Reference: Lezak, M. D., Howieson, D. B., Bigler, E. D., & Tranel, D. (2012). *Neuropsychological assessment* (5th ed.). New York, NY: Oxford University Press.

3. **A—true negatives divided by (true negatives plus false negatives)** *Negative predictive value is a measure of the accuracy of a negative finding of a test that is affected by the prevalence of the disease/condition in the population. It is defined as the percentage of true negatives divided by true negatives and false negatives.*

   Reference: Irwing, P., Booth, T., & Hughes, D. J. (2018). *The Wiley handbook of psychometric testing.* New York, NY: Wiley.

4. **D—frequently (48.5–28% of the time)** *Performances occurring at the 5th percentile or lower are common in a battery of tests. Their occurrence is demonstrated to be high across a wide variety of neuropsychological batteries and tests and thus, should be expected when using multiple measures.*

Reference: Iverson, G. L., & Brooks, B. L. (2011). Improving accuracy for identifying cognitive impairment. In M. R. Schoenberg and J. G. Scott (Eds.), *The little black book of neuropsychology: A syndrome-based approach* (pp. 923–950). New York, NY: Springer.

5. **C—8–9 points; 22 points** *The statistical difference in WAIS-IV VCI and PRI scores is based on central limit theorem and derives statistical significance based on the mean and standard deviation of standardized scores. The much larger difference in scores needed to be a rare finding, as defined as being observed in 5% or less of the population, is based on Bayesian statistics and observation of normal variation in VCI and PRI scores within the normative sample across different age groups.*

Reference: Wechsler, D. (2008). *Manual for the Wechsler Adult Intelligence Scale* (4th ed.) (WAIS-IV). San Antonio, TX: Pearson Inc.

6. **D—low** *In this case there is reason to suspect that the patient may be engaged in intentional symptom magnification and thus the low scores may not represent his true cognitive abilities. However the question is about test score labeling, not interpretation. According to the AACN consensus conference, scores, no matter how low, should not be labeled as abnormal, deficient, or impaired because this implies an interpretive judgment. It also would not be appropriate to label the scores as indeterminate, equivocal, or invalid although the neuropsychologist may ultimately conclude during the interpretive process that the pattern of test scores is consistent with possible or probable malingering.*

Reference: American Academy of Clinical Neuropsychology, Consensus Conference on Uniform Test Score Labeling of Performance Test Results, San Diego, CA. June 2018.

7. **B—pathognomonic signs** *Aphasia, agnosia, and apraxia, when present, provide clear evidence of underlying brain dysfunction which is commonly referred to as pathognomonic signs.*

Reference: Loring D. W. (2015). *INS dictionary of neuropsychology and clinical neurosciences* (2nd ed.). New York, NY: Oxford University Press.

8. **B—positive predictive power** *This is the proportion of the "positive" test scores that accurately predict the outcome.*

Reference: García-Herranz, S., Díaz-Mardomingo, M. C., & Peraita, H. (2016). Neuropsychological predictors of conversion to probable Alzheimer disease in elderly with mild cognitive impairment. *Journal of Neuropsychology, 10*(2), 239–255.

9. **A—The percentage of cases identified as having impairment will be larger if the battery includes 30 scores than if it yields 20 scores.** *Whenever the number of scores in a battery is increased, the number of cases identified as having impairment will increase, particularly if such a determination is made on the basis of a fixed cut-off for single test scores without consideration of base rates.*

Reference: Binder, L. M., Iverson, G. L., & Brooks, B. L. (2009). To err is human: "Abnormal" neuropsychological scores and variability are common in healthy adults. *Archives of Clinical Neuropsychology, 24*(1), 31–46.

10. **D—quality of education, as reflected in performance on a word recognition test** *Quality of education is a better index of premorbid ability level than absolute level of education.*

Reference: Carvalho, J. O., Tommet, D., Crane, P. K., Thomas, M. L., Claxton, A., Habeck, C., . . . Romero, H. R. (2015). Deconstructing racial differences: The effects of quality of education and cerebrovascular risk factors. *The Journals of Gerontology: Series B: Psychological Sciences and Social Sciences, 70*(4), 545–556.

Recommended Readings

Baron, I. S. (2003). *Neuropsychological evaluation of the child*. New York, NY: Oxford University Press.

Chelune, G. J. (2010). Evidence-based research and practice in clinical neuropsychology. *The Clinical Neuropsychologist, 24*(3), 454–467.Guilmette, T. J., Hagan, L. D., & Giuliano, A. J. (2008). Assigning qualitative descriptions to test scores in neuropsychology: Forensic implications. *The Clinical Neuropsychologist, 22*(1), 122–139.

Heilman, K. M., & Valenstein, E. (2011). *Clinical neuropsychology* (5th ed.). New York, NY: Oxford University Press.

Iverson, G. L., & Brooks, B. L. (2011). Improving accuracy for identifying cognitive impairment. In M. R. Schoenberg & J. G. Scott (Eds.), *The little black book of neuropsychology: A syndrome-based approach* (pp. 923–950). New York, NY: Springer.

Lezak, M., Howieson, D., Bigler, E. D., & Tranel, D. (2012). *Neuropsychological assessment* (5th ed.) New York, NY: Oxford University Press.

Manly, J. J., & Echemendia, R. J. (2007). Race-specific norms: Using the model of hypertension to understand issues of race, culture, and education in neuropsychology. *Archives of Clinical Neuropsychology, 22*(3), 319–325.

Schoenberg, M. R., Osborn, K. E., Mahone, E. M., Feigon, M., Roth, R. M., & Pliskin, N. H. (2018). Physician preferences to communicate neuropsychological results: Comparison of qualitative descriptors and a proposal to reduce communication errors. *Archives of Clinical Neuropsychology, 33*(5), 631–643.

Schoenberg, M. R., & Rum, R. R. (2017). Towards reporting standards for neuropsychological study results: A proposal to minimize communication errors with standardized qualitative descriptors for normalized test scores. *Clinical Neurology and Neurosurgery, 162*, 72–79.

Straus, S. E., Glasziou, P., Richardson, W. S., & Haynes, B. (2019). *Evidence-based medicine: How to practice and teach EBM* (5th ed.). New York, NY: Elsevier.

Strauss, E., Sherman, E. M. S., & Spreen, O. (2006). *A compendium of neuropsychological tests: Administration, norms and commentary* (3rd ed.). New York, NY: Oxford University Press.

Website

The Centre for Evidence Based Medicine (http://www.cebm.net/index.aspx?o=1001) provides many resources and practice tools to assist clinicians' evidence-based practice.

10 Personality Assessment and Self-Report Instruments

Nathaniel W. Nelson, Leslie M. Guidotti Breting, and Jerry J. Sweet

Introduction

A comprehensive neuropsychological evaluation is a multifaceted endeavor that aims to assess the full spectrum of an individual's cognitive, behavioral, and psychological and emotional functioning. Neuropsychologists appreciate that the assessment of psychological and emotional functioning is as, and sometimes even more, essential to the neuropsychological evaluation as the assessment of cognitive function. Related, neuropsychologists administer extended personality inventories, such as the Minnesota Multiphasic Personality Inventory-Adolescent Restructured Form (MMPI-A-RF), Minnesota Multiphasic Personality Inventory Restructured Form (MMPI-2-RF), and the Personality Assessment Inventory with regularity (Martin et al., 2015; Rabin et al., 2016).

The aim of this chapter is to discuss the importance of personality assessment through administration of formal measures of psychological and emotional function. We begin with a general discussion of psychopathology within the context of neuropsychology and the importance of the clinical interview in arriving at a given psychological diagnosis and its most likely etiology. We then provide a brief overview of some of the measures of personality and emotional functioning that clinical neuropsychologists most commonly rely on in pediatric, adult, and geriatric populations. After reading this chapter, the reader will have a basic understanding of how to utilize data via personality inventories and self-report measures in the context of a neuropsychological evaluation. This section focuses only on objective personality measures because surveys have demonstrated that more than 75% of neuropsychologists typically use an objective personality measure, whereas few use projective personality measures (e.g., Brooks, Ploetz, & Kirkwood, 2015; Sweet et al., 2011). Although this chapter discusses specific personality inventories and self-report measures, on the written exam, candidates will most likely not be expected to have memorized extensive details of specific inventories and measures. Still, it would be reasonable to expect questions regarding knowledge of test construction, purpose, strengths, limitations, and fundamentals of test interpretation in diverse clinical samples. Additionally, and perhaps most importantly, one should be able to understand the purpose of using such instruments in diagnostic decision-making and treatment planning.

Assessing Psychopathology Within the Context of Neuropsychology

In this chapter, the term "psychopathology" is used to encompass severe mental disorders (e.g., schizophrenia and psychotic disorders), mood disorders (e.g., bipolar disorder), anxiety disorders, and personality disorders. It is important for clinical neuropsychologists to understand how personality and emotional functioning fits into neuropsychological assessment for differential diagnosis, given that psychiatrists provide a significant number of referrals and that cognitive difficulty may be related to psychopathology. There is also importance in understanding the psychometrics and statistics associated with personality inventories and self-report measures in order to practice as a competent neuropsychologist. Additionally, assessment of personality and affect has a long history in psychology, neurology, and psychiatry, dating back to descriptions such as "frontal lobe syndrome," "catastrophic reactions of patients with missile wounds," and "the epileptic personality."

Assessment of psychopathology is not only important in clinical practice as a neuropsychologist but is also related to the staggering prevalence of mental illness. Prevalence of any form of mental illness among United States adults in 2016 was more than 18% (National Institute of Mental Health; https:// www.nimh.nih.gov). In 2011–2012, one in seven children (14%) aged two to eight years had been diagnosed with a mental, behavioral, or developmental disorder, with highest risk among boys, non-Hispanic white children, and the poor (Centers for Disease Control and Prevention; https://www.cdc. gov/childrensmentalhealth/index.html).

It is essential to recognize that the administration of formal tests of personality and emotional function represents only one aspect of the personality assessment process. Neuropsychologists are discouraged from offering a psychological diagnosis on the basis of personality test results alone. Although results of formal personality and emotional testing certainly provide valuable information regarding the quality and severity of an individual patient's psychological symptoms, test results are rarely if ever regarded as diagnostic in and of themselves. The clinical interview, review of available records pertaining to an individual's medical and psychiatric history, and specific diagnostic criteria are essential in arriving at a formal psychological diagnosis. In preparation for the written examination, we agree with the recommendation of Armstrong et al. (2008, p. 58): "You should most certainly spend time reviewing the current DSM [*Diagnostic and Statistical Manual of Mental Disorders*]." In addition to the basic properties and applications of contemporary psychological tests and measures, candidates are encouraged to familiarize themselves with diagnostic criteria that were revised in the DSM-5 (APA, 2013) in particular.

It is also important to recognize that personality test results are not in and of themselves pathognomonic of any specific brain-based or psychogenic etiologies. Identifying whether psychological disorders are primary in nature, comorbid with a neurological disorder, or causally linked can be a difficult task because many symptoms can appear to be either psychiatric and/or neurological. For instance, early symptoms of multiple sclerosis, frontotemporal dementia, or other neurologic conditions may mimic symptoms of depression; interpretation of personality test results independent of the history and course of a patient's neurologic symptoms and signs might result in an inappropriate diagnosis of Major Depressive Disorder, rather than being recognized as a manifestation of the disease process. As certain non-specific symptoms (e.g., difficulties in attention, learning/memory, expressive language, judgment, impulsivity, mood, and affect) may overlap across such conditions, clinical neuropsychologists must rely on various sources of information (including, but not limited to psychometric test results) to arrive at a well-informed differential diagnosis. Again, personality test results may be invaluable in describing the severity of a given patient's current psychological and emotional symptoms, but it is only when test results are complemented with a thorough history and clinical interview that a neuropsychologist is able to identify the most likely source of a given patient's reported psychological and emotional difficulties.

Within each section of this chapter, some of the most common instruments used in clinical practice will be discussed by age group: pediatric (0–18), adult (18–65), and geriatric (65+). When administering a particular personality inventory or self-report measure, one should examine the original purpose, practical considerations (e.g., reading level, time required), standardization (e.g., population normed on, size of normative sample, specialized subgroup norms), reliability (e.g., test-retest, alternate forms, split half), and validity (e.g., content, criterion, construct) of the measure (see also Chapter 8, Psychometrics, Test Design, and Essential Statistics, for more thorough discussion of these topics).

Extended Personality Tests

Adult/Geriatric

Several extended personality inventories have been developed for use in adult/geriatric populations. The MMPI-2 is among the most widely used and most widely researched personality inventories in adult clinical samples. More recently in 2008, the MMPI-2 was revised and updated to a shorter, 338-item, version titled the MMPI-2 Restructured Form (MMPI-2-RF). Another common personality inventory includes the Personality Assessment Inventory (PAI). These three broadband measures of psychological and emotional functioning will serve as a primary focus below.

The Minnesota Multiphasic Personality Inventory-2nd Edition

Overview and Development

- First developed by Hathaway and McKinley in 1943, the MMPI-2 employs a strategy that treats test items as "unknowns" and incorporates items that optimally differentiate clinical psychiatric groups from healthy community samples, regardless of specific item content. In spite of the great success of the original instrument, researchers and clinicians expressed concern regarding the adequacy of the standardization sample (e.g., sample of convenience from friends and relatives; limited to Caucasians), as well as outdated and sometimes sexist language in test items.

- Published in 1989, the second edition of the MMPI (MMPI-2) was developed using a large normative sample that was more representative of the United States population than the MMPI. Items were reworded in a manner that retained their original meaning but used more acceptable and modern language.

- Raw score responses for the MMPI and MMPI-2 are not normally distributed, and *linear T-score conversions* of the raw scores maintain the same skewed distributions as those of the raw scores. As a result, linear transformations result in T-score (and percentile) values that do not share the same meaning across scales (e.g., T-65 on one scale may have different interpretative value when the same elevation is identified on an alternate scale). Unlike the MMPI, the MMPI-2 clinical scales (excluding 5 and 0) utilize *uniform T-score conversion* to limit skewness and kurtosis differences and to ensure that a given elevation (e.g., T-65) has equivalent interpretive value across scales.

Key Test Properties

- Uses 567 true–false items
- Appropriate for ages 18–84
- Fifth-grade reading level, or higher
- Takes about 60–90 minutes to complete

MMPI-2 Scales and Interpretation

- The full MMPI-2 includes nine validity scales (Cannot Say, VRIN, TRIN, F, Fb, Fp, L, K, S), ten basic Clinical Scales (Hs, D, Hy, Pd, Mf, Pa, Pt, Sc, Ma, Si), nine Restructured Clinical (RC) Scales (RCd, RC1, RC2, RC3, RC4, RC6, RC7, RC8, RC9), fifteen Content Scales, twelve Content Component Scales, and Supplementary Scales that may further elucidate the quality of presenting symptoms. Although interpretations of scale elevations may vary with the context of the evaluation (e.g., inpatient versus outpatient), clinicians typically identify T scores of 65 and greater on the basic Clinical Scales as clinically meaningful and suggestive of symptoms that may be of diagnostic relevance. The MMPI-2 370-item short form may be considered under time constraints, although this version yields only the basic validity and clinical scales.

- Inspection of the *validity scale profile* is usually identified as an initial step in MMPI-2 interpretation. Omission of 30 or more test items on the Cannot Say Scale (CNS) scale suggests that the profile should not be interpreted. The clinician should be mindful of potential random or variable responding to test items (VRIN), disproportionate endorsement of "true" or "false" test items (TRIN), defensive responding or denial of emotional difficulties (L, K, S), and potential exaggeration or embellishment of symptoms (F, Fp, Fb). Certain "post-release" validity scales, such as the Symptom Validity Scale (previously the Fake Bad Scale) and the Response Bias Scale (RBS) are especially useful in identifying exaggeration of somatic and cognitive symptoms.

- When the validity profile is not suggestive of variable responding, or under- or overreporting of symptoms, the next interpretive step entails review of the MMPI-2 clinical scales. Although the basic Clinical Scales may be interpreted individually, there is a long tradition of implementing code types as a strategy for interpreting the basic MMPI-2 Clinical Scales. This approach allows the examiner to identify configurations of scale elevations (e.g., 2- or 3-point) that can then be summarized according to previously established descriptors; individuals demonstrating a given code type may be more similar to samples that have previously demonstrated the code type than other clinical groups.

- The K scale was developed to identify subtle attempts to deny psychopathology or present oneself in an overly favorable light. The K correction was meant to counteract defensive responding and provide a more accurate understanding of an individual's psychological function. However, there is limited empirical support for routine use of the K correction; K correction is typically reserved for code type interpretations, as most code type descriptors were based on K-corrected protocols.

- Interpretation of the basic Clinical Scales considers scale elevations regardless of specific items endorsed. In contrast, content interpretation allows the examiner to understand what emotions and attitudes have been directly communicated. Additional information may be gathered through examination of the Content Scales.

- Significant item overlap exists among the basic Clinical Scales. The RC scales were developed to improve the distinctiveness of psychological constructs by removing an overall emotional complaint or distress factor (Emotional Demoralization; RCd) that is common to each of the basic Clinical Scales. The remaining eight RC scales can be understood as more discrete representations of psychological functioning independent of this general distress factor.

- The MMPI-2 Personality Psychopathology Five (PSY-5) scales assess for signs of personality functioning and trait-related disturbance. Derived from the five-factor model of personality, PSY-5 scales were constructed to assess personality dimensions of Aggressiveness (AGGR), Psychoticism (PSYC), Disconstraint (DISC), Negative Emotionality/Neuroticism (NEGE), and Introversion/Low Positive Emotionality (INTR).

Demographic Considerations

- *Age* Older individuals tend to show slightly higher elevations on clinical scales relevant to somatic complaints, health concerns, and diminished activity and energy. These age-related differences tend to be small (less than five T-score points) and do not warrant age-specific norms for older adults.

- *Gender* Raw score differences have been noted between men and women, which warrants use of gender-specific norms.

- *Ethnicity* Some researchers have documented MMPI-2 scale variations by ethnicity, with African American, Hispanic American, and other minority respondents, endorsing higher and at other times lower symptoms relative to European American respondents. Though MMPI-2 research of culturally diverse samples is warranted, convergent research does not suggest that these variations rise to a level of statistical or clinical significance (see also Chapter 11, Cultural and Disability Issues in Neuropsychological Assessment, for more detailed discussion of this topic).

MMPI-2 and Clinical Neuropsychology

- The MMPI-2 has been studied with various medical and neurological samples to establish psychological effects of medical conditions or related treatments. Medical conditions such as end-stage pulmonary disease, coronary artery disease, and chronic pain have been studied. Several studies have also examined the use of the MMPI-2 among individuals undergoing various medical procedures, such as bariatric surgery, coronary artery bypass graft, and spinal cord stimulator procedures, and have shown benefit in identifying individuals who may be at risk of poor psychological and/or medical outcomes following surgery. A common finding is relatively higher clinical elevations noted on scales related to somatic complaint and physical discomfort (e.g., Hs, Hy, RC1). Reactive emotional difficulties following medical diagnosis and treatment may also be apparent, particularly on scales sensitive to overall emotional distress (RCd), depression (D, RC2), and anxiety (Pt, RC7).

- MMPI-2 profiles may also assist in identification of somatization in various conditions, such as chronic pain, chronic symptoms reported after a concussion, and nonepileptic seizures. Identification of somatization with use of the MMPI-2 may inform appropriate treatment planning (e.g., psychotherapy as an adjunct to medical services).

- Neurological conditions such as multiple sclerosis, seizure disorders, amnestic disorder, stroke, Parkinson disease, and other movement disorders have also been included in MMPI-2 studies. Although a few researchers attempted years ago to establish a "neurocorrection" that essentially parses the extent to which purported brain-based versus psychiatric factors contribute to clinical scale elevations, this practice should be discouraged. Systematic elimination of items corrupts the integrity and interpretative value of the scales as they were originally developed. Neurocorrection tended to underestimate the level of psychopathology that individual patients endorsed and ultimately did not improve diagnostic outcomes.

- Researchers have also attempted to discriminate epileptic seizures from nonepileptic seizures, usually based on the magnitude of somatic complaints (e.g., Hs, Hy). However, classification accuracy was problematic.

- The MMPI-2 is frequently administered in traumatic brain injury (TBI) samples, particularly those who are involved in litigation or other secondary gain contexts related to their injuries. The MMPI-2 has proven useful in identifying premorbid psychological difficulties that are likely to account for or reinforce symptoms following mild TBI (mTBI). A "paradoxical severity effect" has been found in litigants with histories of TBI; litigants with histories of mTBI tend to produce higher validity and clinical scale elevations than those with histories of moderate to severe TBI, particularly on scales related to somatic complaints (e.g., FBS, Hs, Hy, RC1).

- In general, individuals evaluated in litigation or other contexts with higher probability of secondary gain (e.g., workers' compensation) tend to show much higher validity and clinical scale elevations than other clinical groups. Although conventional validity scales, such as F and Fb, may be elevated for some individuals evaluated in neuropsychology contexts, litigants and claimants who undergo neuropsychological evaluations are far more likely to show symptom exaggeration or magnification on scales pertaining to unusual injury complaints (e.g., FBS) and/or cognitive complaints (e.g., RBS).

Minnesota Multiphasic Personality Inventory-2 Restructured Form

Overview and Development

- The MMPI-2-RF, a 2008 revision of the MMPI-2, was developed to maintain the clinical utility of the MMPI-2 with a number of revised and updated psychometrically sound scales.

- The inventory consists of nine validity scales and forty-two substantive scales. Seven of the nine validity scales are revised from the MMPI-2, and one new validity scale (Infrequent Somatic Responses; Fs) was developed to detect endorsement and possible exaggeration of symptoms that are infrequent in medical samples. The forty-two substantive scales consist of the nine previously developed RC scales, three "Higher-Order (H-O) Scales" sensitive to broad areas of psychological dysfunction (Emotional/Internalizing, Thought, and Behavioral/Externalizing Dysfunction), twenty-three "Specific Problems" Scales, two Interest Scales, and revisions of the five MMPI-2 Personality Psychopathology Five (PSY-5) Scales.

Key Test Properties

- Uses 338 true-false items
- Appropriate for ages 18–85
- Requires at least a fifth- to eighth-grade reading level
- Takes about 35–50 minutes to complete

MMPI-2-RF Scales and Interpretation

- MMPI-2-RF interpretation is similar to the MMPI-2; however; the MMPI-2-RF no longer utilizes examination of the 2- or 3-point code types.

- In general, the latest empirical research suggests that RF validity scales operate in a manner that is in keeping with their MMPI-2 counterparts. Like VRIN and TRIN, VRIN-r and TRIN-r have shown utility in identifying non-content-based responding; scales L and K, L-r and K-r show utility in detection of under-reporting of symptoms; Fp-r, F-r, RBS, and FBS-r are effective in the detection of symptom over-report.

- After establishing the validity of the profile, the clinician is able to interpret the substantive scales. The three H-O scales essentially reflect the results of factor analyses of the RC scales, which consisted of:
  - Emotional/Internalizing Dysfunction (EID; with high loadings from RCd RC2, and RC7)
  - Thought Dysfunction (THD; with high loadings from RC6 and RC8)
  - Behavioral/Externalizing Dysfunction (BXD; with high loadings from RC4 and RC9)
- The MMPI-2-RF Specific Problems (SP) scales assess aspects of functioning that were not fully represented by the RC and H-O scales. SP scales are divided by Somatic/Cognitive, Internalizing, Externalizing, Interpersonal, and Interest scales that provide more detailed understanding of an individual's current difficulties and interests. For example, in the context of significant EID and RC1 elevations, the clinician may inspect SP scales to further understand the extent to which difficulties are reflective of cognitive complaints, neurological complaints, or other specific emotional or somatic difficulties. Interpretation of SP scales along with higher-order and restructured clinical scales may also inform specific issues of clinical importance. For example, consideration of EID, RC2, along with the SP suicidality scale (SUI) may assist the determination of whether a given patient with major depression might benefit from inpatient hospitalization related to risk of self-harm.

Demographic Considerations

- *Age* Clinicians should be aware that, as with the MMPI-2, the age range for the normative sample is 18–85, and the proportion of normative participants aged 80 and above is restricted (<1%).
- *Gender* Unlike the MMPI-2, which makes use of gender-based norms, the MMPI-2-RF makes use of non-gender-based norms. However, use of the comparison report function allows for gender-based comparisons.
- *Ethnicity* Ongoing research efforts related to MMPI-2-RF presentations in diverse samples is well warranted. Available studies that have explicitly examined the influence of ethnicity and other cultural variables on MMPI-2-RF validity and substantive scales have not consistently revealed variation of clinical significance but more study is required (see also Chapter 11, Cultural and Disability Issues in Neuropsychological Assessment).

MMPI-2-RF and Clinical Neuropsychology

- The MMPI-2-RF is used by clinical neuropsychologists as often, or even more often, than its predecessor (cf., Martin et al., 2015). A fairly sizable MMPI-2-RF empirical literature relevant to clinical neuropsychology has accumulated in recent years. Much of this research has focused on the validity and classification accuracies of the RF validity scales in litigating versus clinical samples. Results suggest that FBS-r, RBS, and Fs bear particular relevance to symptom exaggeration, cognitive response bias, and potential malingering in forensic neuropsychology applications, relative to other over-reporting validity scales, such as F-r, Fp-r. This is particularly the case among litigants with chronic symptoms attributed to traumatic brain injury. Research has also supported the use of Fs in distinguishing between feigned somatic complaints and somatoform disorders. Other research suggests that F-r and Fp-r may better identify feigned psychological difficulties, such as posttraumatic stress.

- Litigating and simulating TBI samples are more likely to exhibit elevations on RF scales that are sensitive to somatic complaints (e.g., RC1), emotional distress (e.g., RCd, RC2, RC7), and somatic/cognitive problem scales (e.g., HPC, COG) than on scales that are sensitive to psychotic or unusual thought processes.

- Use of the MMPI-2-RF in diverse medical and/or psychiatric samples has also been investigated. Medical samples have included patients with epileptic and non-epileptic seizures, as well as case studies of individuals presenting with neurodegenerative and other disorders of the central nervous system. Use of the MMPI-2-RF as a component of various presurgical protocols has been studied, including bariatric procedures for weight management and spinal cord stimulator implantation for management of chronic back pain. RC1 and somatic specific problem scales (e.g., HPC, MLS, NUC) have shown some utility in distinguishing between patients whose presenting physical symptoms are driven by unresolved psychological and emotional difficulties (somatization).

- Other studies have utilized the RF in samples of patients with psychiatric difficulties, such as depression and other mood disorders, anxiety, posttraumatic stress, bipolar disorder, schizophrenia and psychosis, substance use disorders, and personality and trait disturbance. The RF has also shown utility in the prediction of various clinical outcomes, such as premature termination from therapy and risk of self-harming behavior.

Personality Assessment Inventory

Overview and Development

- Clinical conditions assessed by the personality assessment inventory (PAI; Morey, 2007a) were selected on the basis of (a) their history of importance in current mental disorder nosology and (b) their significance in contemporary diagnostic practice. Indeed, the language used to describe clinical scales resembles the DSM-IV-TR and more recent DSM-5 criteria, although clinicians should be mindful that, as with the MMPI-2, the PAI is not in isolation able to render an accurate diagnosis.

- Items comprise twenty-two non-overlapping scales: four validity scales (ICN, INF, NIM, PIM), eleven clinical scales (SOM, ANX, ARD, DEP, MAN, PAR, SCZ, BOR, ANT, ALC, DRG), five treatment scales (AGG, SUI, STR, NON, RXR), and two interpersonal scales (DOM, WRM). Ten of the clinical scales include subscales that provide further understanding of specific difficulties that underlie full-scale elevations. Cut scores may vary without evaluation context (e.g., inpatient or outpatient), but validity and clinical scale elevations at or above a T score of 70 relative to the community sample usually heralds an area of clinical significance.

Key Test Properties

- Uses 344 items with four anchors available for each item ("false," "slightly true," "mainly true," "very true")

- Appropriate for ages 18–89

- Requires a fourth-grade reading level or higher

- Takes about 45–75 minutes to complete

PAI Scales and Interpretation

- The first step in profile interpretation entails the identification of how many of the 344 items were not answered. Omission of seventeen or more items suggests that the profile should not be interpreted.

- The four validity scales should be inspected before determining that the clinical profile is acceptable for interpretation. These scales are sensitive to carelessness or confusion in responding (Inconsistency; ICN), idiosyncratic response style that is atypical of normative and clinical samples (Infrequency; INF), symptom exaggeration (Negative Impression Management; NIM), and denial of minor faults or defensive responding (Positive Impression Management; PIM). Other supplemental validity indicators, such as the malingering index (MAL) and defensiveness index (DEF), may further inform the validity of the clinical profile.

- The eleven clinical scales are sensitive to somatic complaints, anxiety and related disorders, depression, mania, paranoia and psychotic symptoms, borderline and antisocial tendencies, and alcohol and drug problems. Clinical subscales may also be interpreted to provide a better understanding of the specific aspects of a given constellation of symptoms that may underlie clinical scale elevations. For example, the anxiety (ANX) scale includes Cognitive (ANX-C), Affective (ANX-A), and Physiological (ANX-P) subscales that further inform the precise quality of anxiety that likely accounts for the full-scale elevation.

- Treatment scales exemplify areas that may be of particular importance with regard to clinical care and prognosis (e.g., suicidal ideation, nonsupport). Interpersonal scales (Dominance, Warmth) assess one's approach and tendencies to interpersonal relationships.

Demographic Considerations

- *Age* Age exhibits some degree of influence on PAI scores, particularly at the extremes of the normative sample. Individuals 30 years of age or younger show mean scores on select clinical scales that are 5–7 T-score points above the mean for the normative sample. Individuals 60 and older tend to show T scores that are below the normative sample on most clinical scales.

- *Gender* There is no evidence that men and women exhibit variations in scale means that are meaningfully different from standard error of measurement.

- *Ethnicity* Differences in PAI scores related to race and ethnicity appear to be small.

- *Education* Education appears to have the most significant effect across scales, with individuals with 4–11 years of education showing 4–5 T-score points higher on most scales and subscales than individuals with higher levels of education.

PAI and Clinical Neuropsychology

- Similar to the MMPI-2 and MMPI-2-RF, researchers have examined the utility of the PAI in assessing psychopathology in medical and neurologic samples. Psychometric characteristics of the PAI has been shown to be satisfactory in diverse medical and psychiatric samples. Some researchers have found the PAI to be useful in discriminating epileptic and nonepileptic seizure samples, substance abuse samples, and general psychiatric outpatient samples in the context of clinical neuropsychological assessment.

- Much of the relevant PAI literature in clinical neuropsychology has examined validity and clinical scale differences among compensation-seeking claimants and non-compensation-seeking samples. Claimants and those who show signs of cognitive response bias tend to display significantly greater elevations on validity scales associated with symptom exaggeration (NIM) than non-claimants and those who show sufficient effort on cognitive testing. NIM has also shown some utility in the detection of feigned pain symptoms. NIM and PAI clinical scales, most notably those that associated with physical complaints (SOM) and emotional distress (ANX, DEP), tend to be significantly higher in claimants relative to non-claimants. There is some evidence that the PAI validity scales may be less effective in detecting symptom exaggeration relative to the MMPI-2 and MMPI-2-RF.

Pediatric

Assessing personality traits in children and adolescents is somewhat controversial because, by definition, a personality disorder must be long-standing. However, there are several objective measures specifically aimed at the pediatric population and psychopathology/personality, including the MMPI-Adolescent-Restructured Format (MMPI-A-RF), MMPI-Adolescent (MMPI-A), the PAI-Adolescent (PAI-A), the Personality Inventory for Children-2nd Edition (PIC-2), and the Personality Inventory for Youth (PIY). The most commonly used pediatric personality inventories are discussed here. It is important to note that the pediatric measures have been developed more recently than the adult measures and therefore have a less developed research literature.

Minnesota Multiphasic Personality Inventory-Adolescent-Restructured Form

Overview and Development

- The MMPI-A-RF is a 2016 revision of the MMPI-A. The MMPI-A-RF mirrors the structure of the MMPI-2-RF.

- There are seven validity scales, ten clinical scales, and fifteen content scales.

- The normative data is from the same standardization sample as the MMPI-A. No new normative data was collected.

Key Test Properties

- Uses 241 true-false items

- Appropriate for ages 14–18

- 4.9 reading level or higher is recommended

- Takes about 30–45 minutes to complete via paper and pencil, which is about 15 minutes quicker than the MMPI-A

MMPI-A-RF Scales and Interpretation

The MMPI-A-RF has forty-eight empirically validated scales, which includes six validity scales as well as cannot say, three higher-order scales, nine RC scales, and thirty other scales examining specific somatic/cognitive complaints, internalizing, externalizing, interpersonal, interest, and temperament-oriented perspectives (PSY-5).

Demographic Considerations

- *Age* The MMPI-A-RF was developed for use with a limited age range and should be used with caution in children younger than 14 and may be developmentally inappropriate for children under 12.
- *Gender* There are separate norms based on gender.

MMPI-A-RF and Clinical Neuropsychology

Given how recently this measure was developed, there is limited empirical research. In fact, there are only four published journal articles and one book chapter, but there have been over twenty poster presentations related to the MMPI-A-RF.

Minnesota Multiphasic Personality Inventory-Adolescent

Overview and Development

- The MMPI-A is an extension and revision of the MMPI-2, discussed earlier. The MMPI-A has seven validity scales, ten clinical scales, and fifteen content scales.
- The standardization sample was 1,620 adolescents (805 boys and 815 girls) who lived in eight different states (CA, MN, NY, NC, OH, PA, VA, WA).
- It is the most widely used objective personality measure with adolescents.

Key Test Properties

- Uses 478 true-false items
- Appropriate for ages 14–18
- Sixth-grade reading level or higher is recommended
- Takes about 45–60 minutes to complete

MMPI-A Scales and Interpretation

- The MMPI-A is composed of many of the original MMPI items, some new items developed for MMPI-2, and a number of new items that specifically address adolescent issues and behaviors, such as attitudes about school and parents, peer group influence, and eating problems.
- The MMPI-A uses slightly different T-score cut-offs than the MMPI-2. The MMPI-2 uses a T-score cut-off of 65, whereas the MMPI-A uses a range of 60–65 to indicate that the score is approaching a level of clinical concern or attention. The MMPI-2 and MMPI-A norms were developed using the same target distribution to assure the percentile equivalence across the two forms. If an adolescent is tested with the MMPI-A and later tested with the MMPI-2, the T scores can be meaningfully compared.
- The MMPI-A 350-item short form may be considered under time constraints, although this version of the MMPI-A yields only the basic validity and clinical scales.
- Some of the changes from the MMPI-2 to the MMPI-A included three of the Content Scales developed using primarily new adolescent-specific items (School Problems, Low Aspirations, and Alienation). The Family Problems Scale (A-fam) was improved with the addition of adolescent-specific content. A new scale, Conduct Problems (A-con), was substituted for the MMPI-2 Antisocial Practices (ASP) Scale on the MMPI-A.

- The most significant changes from the MMPI-2 to the MMPI-A were on the F, Mf, and Si scales.

Demographic Considerations

- *Age* The MMPI-A was developed for use with a limited age range and should be used with caution in children younger than 14 and may be developmentally inappropriate for children under 12.
- *Gender* There are separate norms based on gender.

MMPI-A and Clinical Neuropsychology

- Adolescents who are 18 years old may be given the MMPI-2 or the MMPI-A because normative and clinical samples for both instruments include 18-year-olds. The clinician should make a case-by-case judgment regarding which assessment to use with 18-year-old patients. A suggested guideline is to use the MMPI-A instrument with 18-year-olds who are still in high school and the MMPI-2 instrument with 18-year-olds who are in college, working, or living an otherwise independent adult lifestyle. Some studies have found the MMPI-2 to overpathologize 18-year-olds compared to the MMPI-A and a self-report symptom checklist.
- The MMPI-A has been well studied in juvenile delinquent as well as in other clinical populations including, anxiety disorders, ADHD, depression, eating disorders, psychiatric inpatients, suicidal adolescents, and substance abusing adolescents.

Personality Assessment Inventory-Adolescent (PAI-A)

Overview and Development

- The PAI-A (Morey, 2007b) was designed to complement its parent instrument, the PAI, which was described in detail earlier. Development of the PIA-A started in 1999, with the goal being to retain the structure of the PAI and as many of the items as possible; a limited number of items were reworded to be more applicable and meaningful to adolescents.
- The PAI-A is slightly shorter in length than the PAI and consists of 264 items. The structure of the PAI-A, like the PAI, contains twenty-two non-overlapping scales: four validity scales, eleven clinical scales, five treatment scales, and two interpersonal scales.

Key Test Properties

- Uses 264 items rated as "false," "slightly true," "mainly true," "very true"
- Appropriate for ages 12–18
- Fourth-grade reading level recommended
- Takes about 45 minutes to complete

PAI-A Scales and Interpretation

- The interpretation and information about the scales described earlier for the PAI are generally also applicable to the PAI-A, so will not be reiterated here. One difference is that omission of 14 or more items (17 on the PAI) suggests that the profile should not be interpreted.

- An advantage of the PAI-A is in assessing borderline personality features, which most other instruments used with adolescents do not include.

Demographic Considerations

- *Gender* There is no evidence that boys and girls exhibit variations in scale means that are meaningfully different from the standard error of measurement.
- *Ethnicity* Differences in PAI scores related to race and ethnicity appear to be small.

PAI-A and Clinical Neuropsychology

The PAI was developed for use among individuals aged 12–18; however, adolescents aged 18 year may be administered either the PAI-A or PAI. Clinical judgment should be used to determine which version to administer.

Personality Inventory for Children-Second Edition (PIC-2)

Overview and Development

- The PIC-2 is a parent rating scale of children's behavior, which was revised from the original PIC that was developed in 1977. The PIC-2 is used to evaluate the emotional, behavioral, cognitive, and interpersonal adjustment of children and adolescents.
- Normative data were based on ratings from 2,306 parents of children in grades K–12 with additional data collected from 1,551 parents of children referred for educational or clinical intervention.

Key Test Properties

- Uses 275 true-false items; the brief form has 96 items.
- Appropriate for ages 5–19
- Takes about 40 minutes to complete; brief version is about 15 minutes

PIC-2 Scales and Interpretation

The structure of the PIC-2 contains three validity scales, nine adjustment scales, and twenty-one adjustment subscales. The nine adjustment scales include cognitive impairment, family dysfunction, psychological discomfort, impulsivity/distractibility, reality distortion, social withdrawal, delinquency, somatic concern, and social skills deficits.

Demographic Considerations

T scores are normed by child's gender.

PIC-2 and Clinical Neuropsychology

- Developed from theoretical constructs, then validated using populations with specific maladaptive functioning.
- Based on empirical research, primary factors of personality based on behavioral observations, and areas of interest believed to be useful for practicing clinicians.

Personality Inventory for Youth (PIY)

Overview and Development

The PIY is a self-report measure to be used in conjunction with the PIC-2, which is completed by a parent. The PIY is an adolescent self-report inventory that assesses emotional and behavioral adjustment, family interaction, and school and academic functioning.

Key Test Properties

- Uses 270 true-false items
- Appropriate for ages 9–19
- Third-grade reading level required
- Takes about 30–60 minutes to complete

PIY Scales and Interpretation

- Four validity scales, nine non-overlapping clinical scales, and twenty-four non-overlapping subscales. The nine non-overlapping clinical scales mirror those on the PIC-2 and include nine adjustment scales, which consist of cognitive impairment, family dysfunction, psychological discomfort, impulsivity/distractibility, reality distortion, social withdrawal, delinquency, somatic concern, and social skills deficits.
- The abbreviated format includes only the first 80 items and is often used as a classroom screening measure.

Demographic Considerations

T scores are normed by child's gender.

PIY and Clinical Neuropsychology

Young children have been found to have a tendency to under-report problematic behaviors or difficult emotions, when compared to parent report on the PIC-2 in terms of identification of behavior problems and emotional states. In older children and adolescents there tends to be a greater correlation between child and parent ratings.

Self-Report Screening Measures of Emotional Function

Self-report measures are used to determine attitudes, behaviors, feelings, or thoughts. There are three major approaches to developing self-report measures: theory-guided, factor analysis, and criterion-key. Questionnaires typically use one of three formats: a Likert scale, true–false, or multiple choice. Hundreds of self-report measures have been developed to assess different symptomatology. It is outside the realm of this chapter to discuss each self-report measure individually; a few of the most common are highlighted here.

Pros

- Brief and straightforward
- Easy to administer
- Examine many symptoms quickly

Cons

- Majority are face-valid without embedded validity indicators:
  - The lack of validity indicators makes it difficult to detect over- or under-reporting of symptoms.

- Not diagnostic
- Often unreliable due to overlapping symptoms with other disorders.
- Often not psychometrically robust, with a limited number of items, lack of validity studies, and limited normative data.

Adult/Geriatric

Beck Depression Inventory-2nd Edition (BDI-II)

Overview and Development

- The BDI-II is a 21-item self-report measure that specifically assesses depressive symptoms in adults and adolescents aged 13–86 years. Items are rated on a 4-point scale ranging from 0 to 3, and symptoms are meant to be endorsed within the last two weeks. The measure was developed to correspond with depressive disorders criteria outlined by the DSM-IV. Administration time is approximately 5–10 minutes, although individuals with severe depression or obsessive tendencies may take longer to complete the measure.

- Factor analyses have disclosed a two-factor solution consisting of Somatic-Affective (e.g., fatigue, loss of energy, changes in sleep/appetite) and Cognitive (e.g., pessimism, guilt, suicidal thoughts) dimensions.

- Total raw scores determine overall descriptors of depressive symptoms severity. Scores ranging from 0 to 13 are suggestive of "minimal" symptoms, 14 to 19 are "mild," 20 to 28 are "moderate," and 29 to 63 are suggestive of "severe" depressive symptoms.

- In addition to establishing overall symptom severity on the basis of respondents' endorsement of symptoms across the inventory, review of individual item contents may inform important clinical issues related to depression. For example, the BDI-II includes critical items related to suicidal ideation that may be of particular clinical concern and that may inform clinical decision-making (e.g., whether symptoms might warrant inpatient hospitalization to prevent self-harm).

Demographic Considerations

- *Age* There is no consistent evidence of a significant relationship between age and BDI-II symptom endorsement. Some researchers have reported minimal relationships in outpatients, college students, adolescents, and geriatric inpatients. Other studies have found that BDI-II scores are more likely to increase with age in both adolescent and adult samples.

- *Gender* There is no consistent evidence of a significant gender effect on BDI-II symptom endorsement. Some researchers have reported no significant gender differences, whereas several other studies have found that females tend to endorse higher depressive symptoms than males.

- *Education* BDI-II symptoms tend to be inversely correlated with education.

- *Ethnicity and Socioeconomic Status (SES)* Researchers have not generally found BDI-II scores to be differentially associated with ethnicity, although some have identified a modest negative relationship between SES and BDI-II symptom endorsement.

BDI-II and Clinical Neuropsychology

Although age has not in itself been identified as directly related to BDI-II symptom endorsement, some clinicians use the Geriatric Depression Scale (GDS) as an alternative among individuals with age-related cognitive decline.

Beck Anxiety Inventory (BAI)

Overview and Development

- The BAI is a 21-item self-report measure that assesses symptoms of anxiety in adults and adolescents aged 17–80 years. Although the test developers acknowledge the frequent co-occurrence of depression and anxiety, the BAI was constructed to assess anxious symptoms that overlap minimally with depression. Items are rated on a 4-point scale ranging from 0 to 3, and symptoms are meant to be endorsed within the last week. Administration time is approximately 5–10 minutes, although individuals with severe depression or obsessive tendencies may take longer to complete the measure.

- Total raw scores determine overall descriptors of anxiety. Scores ranging from 0 to 7 are suggestive of "minimal" symptoms, 8 to 15 are "mild," 16 to 25 are "moderate," and 26 to 63 are suggestive of "severe" symptoms of anxiety.

Demographic Considerations

- *Age* The 1993 BAI manual describes a significant negative correlation between anxious symptoms and age.

- *Gender* The 1993 BAI manual describes a significant gender effect, with women endorsing significantly higher anxious symptoms than men.

BAI and Clinical Neuropsychology

Many of the BAI items reflect physical manifestations of anxiety. This suggests that the instrument may be of lower utility among aging individuals with physical complaints that reflect a normal aspect of the aging process.

Depression Anxiety Stress Scale (DASS)

Overview and Development

- The DASS (Lovibond & Lovibond, 1995) is a 42-item self-report measure that was designed to measure the negative emotional states of depression, anxiety, and stress related to the dimensional conceptualization of psychological disorder. The measure is within the public domain, so permission is not needed to use it. The DASS questionnaires and scoring key may be downloaded from the DASS website and copied without restriction (http://www2.psy.unsw.edu.au/dass/). The measure is designed for those 17 years of age and older, but has also been used down to age 14. Alternatives to the DASS for younger children include the Children's Depression Inventory (CDI) for depression, and the State Trait Anxiety Inventory for Children (STAIC) or the Revised Children's Manifest Anxiety Scale (RCMAS) for anxiety.

- Items are rated on a 4-point severity/frequency scale to the extent to which an examinee has experienced each state over the past week.
- Total raw scores are then given cutoff descriptors of normal, mild, moderate, severe, or extremely severe for depression, anxiety, and stress.

Demographic Considerations

- *Age* There is no consistent evidence of a significant relationship between age and DASS symptom endorsement.

Geriatric Depression Scale (GDS)

Overview and Development

- The GDS is a 30-item self-report measure that was developed to specifically assess depressive symptoms. Although the measure can be used with individuals aged 17 years and older, the measure was developed to specifically identify depressive symptoms in the elderly.
- Items are dichotomous ("yes" or "no") and request the examinee to endorse whether given statements accurately describe his or her feelings at the time of administration.
- Total raw scores determine overall descriptors of depressive symptoms severity. Scores ranging from 0 to 9 are described as "normal," 10 to 19 are "mild," and 20 to 30 suggest "severe" symptoms. A 15-item version of the GDS is also available and includes descriptors for "normal" (0–4), "mild" (5–8), "moderate" (8–11), and "severe" (12–15) depressive symptoms. Administration time is approximately 5–10 minutes for the 30-item version and 5–7 minutes for the 15-item version.

Demographic Considerations

- *Age* There is no consistent evidence of a significant relationship between age and GDS symptom endorsement.
- *Gender* There is some indication that men may be at risk of false-negative results compared with women, suggesting that different cut scores may be needed by gender.

GDS and Clinical Neuropsychology

- The content of the GDS items does not include somatic symptoms that may be a normal aspect of the aging process. This is one reason why the GDS may be more appropriate for use relative to other self-report measures (e.g., BDI-II) in elderly samples.
- The yes–no format is also thought to be less cognitively demanding relative to measures that include multiple item response anchors. The GDS should not be administered among aging adults with evidence of moderate cognitive impairments (as defined by Mini Mental State Examination score of 20 or less).

Trauma Symptom Inventory—2 (TSI-2)

Overview and Development

- The TSI-2 (Briere, 2011) is a substantially revised version of the Trauma Symptom Inventory, a widely used self-report instrument that is intended to assess acute and chronic symptoms of posttraumatic stress, as well as other related areas of psychological, behavioral, and emotional dysfunction. The measure consists of 136 items that reflect symptoms related to such traumatic events as physical violence, sexual assault, combat-related trauma, motor vehicle accidents, and natural disasters. Items are endorsed according to 4-point anchors ("0" being "never"; "3" being "often") and contribute to two validity scales (Response Level, RL; Atypical Response, ATR), four factors (Self-disturbance, SELF; Posttraumatic Stress, TRAUMA; Externalization, EXT; and Somatization, SOMA), and twelve clinical scales (Anxious Arousal, AA; Depression, D; Anger, ANG; Intrusive Experiences, IE; Defensive Avoidance, DA; Dissociation, DIS; Somatic Preoccupations, SOM; Sexual Disturbance, SXD; Suicidality, SUI; Insecure Attachment, IA; Impaired Self-Reference, ISR; Tension Reduction Behavior, TRB).

- The measure is appropriate for use among individuals aged 18–90 and at a reading level of fifth grade and beyond. Administration time is approximately 20 minutes.

- A 126-item alternate version that does not contain any sexual symptom items is also available, the TSI-2-A.

TSI-2 Scales and Interpretation

- T scores for each of the validity and clinical scales have a mean of 50 and a standard deviation of 10, T scores of 65 or higher are regarded as being of clinical significance or diagnostic relevance.

Demographic Considerations

- *Age* Younger respondents tend to exhibit subtly higher scale elevations than do older respondents.

- *Gender* Test results are normed by gender.

Pediatric

Behavior Assessment System for Children, Third Edition (BASC-3)

Overview and Development

- The BASC-3 (Reynolds and Kamphaus, 2015), is a comprehensive set of rating scales and forms developed to understand the behaviors and emotions of children and adolescents that includes: the Teacher Rating Scales (TRS), Parent Rating Scales (PRS), Self-Report of Personality (SRP), Student Observation System (SOS), and Structured Developmental History (SDH).

- The measure yields three validity scales, many subscales (depending on the version self-report or parent/teacher only) to reflect specific aspects of externalizing problems, internalizing problems, behavioral symptoms index, and adaptive skills. The measure also includes clinical probability indices and a functional impairment index.

- Teachers or other qualified observers can complete forms at three age levels—preschool (ages 2 to 5), child (ages 6 to 11), and adolescent (ages 12 to 21) by rating specific behaviors on a four-point scale of frequency, ranging from "Never" to "Almost Always." The TRS contains 105–165 items.

- The BASC-3 provides specific behavioral intervention recommendations in a detailed guide.

Key Test Properties

- Appropriate for ages 2–25
- Teacher Rating Scales measure adaptive and problem behaviors in the preschool or school setting in ~10–20 minutes.
- Parent Rating Scales measure both adaptive and problem behaviors in the community and home setting in ~10–20 minutes.
- Self-Report of Personality Gain insight into a child's or young adult's thoughts and feelings in 30 minutes.
- There are three sets of norms to choose from, which include: (1) Same Sex Normative Tables (male, female); (2) Combined Gender Normative Tables (male+ female); (3) ADHD and General Clinical Norm Group, which are all presented by age level.

Demographic Considerations

- *Age* T scores and percentile ranks are normed by age.
- *Gender* Test results are normed by gender.

BASC-3 and Clinical Neuropsychology

- The BASC-3 includes a behavioral intervention guide, which utilizes Tier two and three interventions. Tier two interventions for targeted risk and initial problem development is different from tier three interventions where individualized treatments address specific, chronic, and debilitating problems. The BASC-3 can be especially helpful when formulating recommendations for use within an IEP.
- The multimethod, multidimensional approach of the BASC-3 has allowed this instrument to be studied extensively with individuals diagnosed with ADHD.

Behavior Rating Inventory of Executive Function, Second Edition (BRIEF2)

Overview, Development, and Interpretation

- The BRIEF2 is a 2015 revision of the BRIEF (Gioia, Isquith, Guy, & Kenworthy, 2000), which is a parent- and teacher-rating scale that was developed to examine behavior and executive functioning in a pediatric population. The BRIEF2 was designed to be used as an adjunctive external validation of neuropsychological assessment findings on executive functioning measures. There is also the BRIEF-A, which is a similar version for use with adults; however, this chapter will only focus on the version for children.
- The measure yields three validity scales, seven to nine subscales to reflect specific aspects of executive functioning within three broad components, the Behavioral Regulation Index, Emotion Regulation Index, and the Cognitive Regulation Index. Specifically, the BRIEF2 assesses inhibition, self-monitoring, shifting, emotional control, initiation, task completion, working memory, planning, organization, and organization of materials. The new infrequency validity scale helps identify unusual responding.
- Other versions of the BRIEF2 exist for preschool-aged children (BRIEF-P) and (as a self-report version) for adolescents (BRIEF-SR).

Key Test Properties

- Uses 86 items rated on a 3-point scale using "never," "sometimes," and "often"

- Appropriate for ages 5–18

- Takes about 5–10 minutes to complete

Demographic Considerations

- *Age* T scores are normed by age.

- *Gender* T scores are normed by child's gender. However, the gender of the parent completing the rating form has not been shown to result in significantly different ratings.

- *Education* A low, negative correlation has been demonstrated between parental education and BRIEF2 rating.

- *Ethnicity and SES* Children from low-SES families tend to be rated as having more executive difficulties.

BRIEF2 and Clinical Neuropsychology

- The BRIEF2 is often used to assist in the diagnosis of ADHD as some theories of ADHD propose that a central problem is with executive functioning.

- The BRIEF2 has been studied with many other pediatric populations including children with ADHD, Autism spectrum disorder, a specific learning disorder, anxiety, TBI, epilepsy, neurofibromatosis type 1, cancer, and diabetes

- Interrater agreement between parent and teacher ratings is moderate, as is the agreement between parent and adolescent self-ratings.

Child Behavior Checklist (CBCL)

Overview, Development, and Interpretation

- The CBCL is among the most widely used instruments to assess behavioral problems and personality in children. The CBCL is a parent rating scale that was developed for ages 1.5–18 years. There is also a Teacher's Report Form (TRF), Youth Self-Report (YSR), and a semistructured interview.

- The YSR is for adolescents ages 11–18, contains 119 items, and requires a fifth-grade reading level.

- There are two versions of the rating forms: the preschool checklist (CBCL/1½–5) is intended for use with children aged 18 months to 5 years and the school-aged version (CBCL/6-18) is for children aged 6–18 years.

- The scores result in empirically based syndrome scales and DSM-oriented scales. The instrument assesses internalizing (i.e., anxious, depressive, and overcontrolled) and externalizing (i.e., aggressive, hyperactive, noncompliant, and undercontrolled) behaviors.

- The CBCL has factorially derived scales that examine social withdrawal, somatic complaints, anxiety and depression, destructive behavior, social problems, thought problems, attention problems, aggressive behavior, and delinquent behaviors.

Key Test Properties

- Uses 99 items (preschool) and 118 (school-aged) rated on a 3-point scale of "very true or often true," "somewhat or sometimes true," or "not true."
- Takes about 10–15 minutes to complete the CBCL; about 10 for the TRF; about 60 for the semistructured interview.

CBCL Scales

- The 1.5- to 5-year-old form examines aggressiveness, depressive symptoms, destructive symptoms, sleep problems, social withdrawn, and somatic problems.
- The 6- to 18-year-old form examines the Total score, Externalizing (Aggressive, Delinquent), Internalizing (Anxious/Depressed, Somatic Complaints, Withdrawn), and Social Competence (Activities, Social, School) scales.
- The TRF examines the Total score, Externalizing (Aggressive, Delinquent), Internalizing (Anxious/Depressed, Somatic Complaints, Withdrawn), and Adaptive Functioning (Behaving Appropriately, Happy, Learning, School Performance, Working Hard) scales.

Demographic Considerations

- *Age* T scores are normed by age.
- *Gender* T scores are normed by gender.

CBCL and Clinical Neuropsychology

- The CBCL is able to significantly differentiate clinically referred from nonreferred children.
- Items were factor analyzed to empirically identify the forms of psychopathology that occur in children. The items are presented in alphabetical order to reduce the bias that might occur as a result of informants' preconceived notions regarding the presence or absence of a particular disorder.

Conners' Rating Scales-Revised (CRS-R)

Overview, Development, and Interpretation

- The CRS-R utilizes cross-informant assessment to examine behavior problems in children and adolescents, with a focus on externalizing behaviors and symptoms of ADHD.
- There are several versions, including parent, teacher, and self-report forms, as well as long and short versions.

Key Test Properties

- Appropriate for ages 3–17 for parent and teacher versions
- Appropriate for ages 12–17 for self-report version
- All versions use a 4-point rating scale ("not true at all," "just a little true," "pretty much true," or "very much true").
- Takes about 30 minutes to complete the long parent version; about 15 minutes to complete the long teacher version.

Demographic Considerations

- *Age* T scores are normed by age.
- *Gender* T scores are normed by gender.

CRS-R and Clinical Neuropsychology

- The CRS-R Parent Form, long version, examines fourteen factors: oppositional, cognitive problems/inattention, hyperactivity, anxious-shy, perfectionism, social problems, psychosomatic, Global Index (Restless-Impulsive, Emotional Lability), ADHD Index, and DSM-IV Symptoms subscale (DSM-IV Inattentive, DSM-IV Hyperactive-Impulsive).

- The CRS-R Teacher Form, long version, examines thirteen factors: oppositional, cognitive problems/inattention, hyperactivity, anxious-shy, perfectionism, social problems, Global Index (Restless-Impulsive, Emotional Lability), ADHD Index, and DSM-IV Symptoms subscale (DSM-IV Inattentive, DSM-IV Hyperactive-Impulsive).

- Reliability between parents has been found to be moderate to high, as well as between teachers. However, reliability between parent and teacher has been found to be low, with parents indicating more deviancy than teachers.

- A weakness of the CRS-R is that all questions are negatively worded.

Relevant Definitions

Clinical scale profile Result of personality testing that depicts the magnitude and quality of psychological/emotional difficulties across various symptom-specific scales. The profile may reveal the full range of symptom severity, from relatively subtle and not diagnostically relevant, to severe and potentially over-reported. The profile may reveal such symptoms as depression, anxiety, somatic complaints, paranoia, and psychotic processes, and, when used in conjunction with the clinical interview, assist in the differential diagnosis process. For measures such as the MMPI-2, MMPI-2-RF, and PAI, the clinical scale profile may be interpreted only if the validity scale profile suggests a forthright approach to testing (i.e., absence of variable responding, or under- or over-reporting of symptoms).

Code type interpretation An interpretative strategy that allows the examiner to identify configurations of scale elevations (e.g., 2- or 3-point) that can then be summarized according to previously established descriptors; individuals demonstrating a given code type may be more similar to samples who have previously demonstrated the code type than other clinical groups.

Face validity A simplistic form of validity that allows examiners to easily determine if a measure assesses a construct of interest (e.g., depression). Face-valid test items are usually what comprise tests developed with the logical keying approach, often at the expense of discriminative validity.

Linear T-score conversion A method of conversion that entails the direct transformation of raw scores into T-score equivalents. Raw score distributions on the MMPI, for example, are non-normally distributed, and linear T-score equivalents retain the same skewed distributions as the raw score distributions from which they are derived. As a result, linear T scores at a given level of elevation (e.g., T-65) may not share the same meaning or interpretative value across scales.

Uniform T-score conversion A method of converting raw scores into T scores that ensures that skewness and kurtosis are similar across scales. Unlike linear T scores, which may not share the same meaning at a given elevation (e.g., T-65), uniform T scores can be regarded as having equivalent percentiles and retain similar interpretive meaning across scales.

Validity scale profile Result of personality testing that informs test-taking attitude and credibility of self-reported symptoms. Validity scales may reveal inconsistent response consistency (e.g., MMPI-2 VRIN, TRIN), underreporting of symptoms (e.g., MMPI-2 L, K), or overreporting of symptoms (e.g., F-family; FBS). Evidence of inconsistent responding or underreporting or overreporting of symptoms suggests that the clinical scale profile is unlikely to represent an accurate reflection of psychological and emotional function.

Personality Assessment and Self-Report Instruments Questions

NOTE: Questions 8, 35, and 55 on the First Full-Length Practice Examination, Questions 51, 77, and 109 on the Second Full-Length Practice Examination, Questions 61 and 96 on the Third Full-Length Practice Examination, and Questions 39 and 80 on the Fourth Full-Length Practice Examination are from this chapter.

1. In clinical psychology and neuropsychology, formal diagnosis of a psychological disorder is _____.
   - (a) accomplished through the administration of personality inventories and other measures sensitive to psychopathology
   - (b) a process that entails the integration of information obtained through the clinical interview and results of personality test findings
   - (c) rarely feasible, given the premium that is placed on the assessment of cognitive function
   - (d) feasible only to the extent that subsequent therapeutic services may be reimbursed

2. The benefits of personality testing relative to brief self-report measures of emotional function are that extended personality tests _____.
   - (a) are pathognomonic of specific DSM-5 diagnoses and help with differential diagnosis
   - (b) can be tailored to the individual patient's condition and symptoms; and used to plan treatment
   - (c) provide a more detailed and elaborate assessment of the quality, validity, and magnitude of self-reported symptoms
   - (d) provide more detail regarding symptom longitudinal course, validity, and duration

3. When compared to the MMPI-2, the PAI _____.
   - (a) takes longer to administer in its entirety
   - (b) has a more extensive research literature attesting to its utility
   - (c) includes norms that are less likely to be impacted by age and gender
   - (d) includes language that is directly relevant to modern diagnostic systems, such as the DSM-5

4. Limitations of most self-report measures of emotional function include _____.
   - (a) low convergent validity with other measures and often discrepant findings from the clinical interview
   - (b) greater reliance on face validity and limited ability to detect response bias

(c) the frequent use of a Likert scale approach, which can be confusing to patients with cognitive impairment

(d) limited incremental validity above/beyond extended personality measures

5. In keeping with the general advice regarding how one uses the results of personality testing, when diagnosing somatization a prudent clinician would _____.

(a) consider elevations of relevant scales in the context of history and medical findings

(b) base the diagnosis primarily on elevations of relevant validity and clinical scales

(c) not include the results of personality testing, which have been shown to have less relevance to the diagnosis

(d) disregard personality test findings when discrepant from interview and history information

6. The MMPI-2-RF is distinct from the MMPI-2 in that the former includes _____.

(a) an updated normative comparison group based on United States Census information

(b) a more expansive and culturally-appropriate set of test items

(c) "higher-order" scales that examine internalizing, externalizing, and thought dysfunction

(d) polytomous, as opposed to dichotomous, response options, similar to the PAI

7. Which of the following would represent an invalid profile on the PAI-A?

(a) NIM T = 75 and DEP T = 80

(b) ICN T = 80 and PIM T = 72

(c) INF T = 68 and SCZ T = 64

(d) NIM T = 70, PIM T = 30, and ANX T = 60

8. If on self-report measures of emotional functioning a patient receives scores of BDI-II = 0, BAI = 0 and PHQ-9 = 0, then one should carefully examine the PAI for _____.

(a) elevated ICN indicating inconsistent responding

(b) elevated NIM indicating negative impression management

(c) elevations on DEP and ANX clinical scales indicating possible depression and anxiety

(d) elevated PIM indicating positive impression management

9. Which measure would be most appropriate to use to evaluate current emotional functioning in a 32-year-old woman who is reporting a significant traumatic event followed by nightmares, avoidance, and re-experiencing of the event?

(a) BDI-2

(b) STAI

(c) TSI-2

(d) MMPI-A-RF

190

10. When evaluating adjustment issues in a 13-year-old adolescent with acquired neurological injury by means of standardized rating scales that include self-report by the adolescent and a corollary parent report version, it is relatively more common to find that the adolescent will _____.

    (a) report fewer problematic behaviors and emotions than the parent

    (b) report more problematic behaviors and emotions than the parent

    (c) generate a profile of concerns that closely mirrors that of the parent

    (d) generate a profile of concerns that is opposite that of the parent

Personality Assessment and Self-Report Instruments Answers

1. **B—a process that entails the integration of information obtained through the clinical interview and results of personality test findings** *Neuropsychologists recognize the importance of exploring the individual patient's history and background information, review of records, and formal DSM-5 diagnostic criteria in addition to personality test results to establish formal psychological diagnoses.*

   Reference: Lamberty, G. J., & Nelson, N. W. (2012). Case formulation in clinical neuropsychology. In *Specialty competencies in clinical neuropsychology* (pp. 44–59). New York, NY: Oxford University Press.

2. **C—provide a more detailed and elaborate assessment of the quality, validity, and magnitude of self-reported symptoms** *The MMPI-2, MMPI-2-RF, and PAI are examples of extended personality inventories that include well-researched validity and clinical scales that establish symptom plausibility, quality, and severity in a way that face valid self-report measures do not. They also provide more detailed and elaborate assessment of the quality and magnitude of self-reported symptoms.*

   References:
   (a) Graham, J. R. (2006). *MMPI-2: Assessing personality and psychopathology* (4th ed.). New York, NY: Oxford University Press.
   (b) Graham, J. R. (2012). *MMPI-2: Assessing personality and psychopathology* (5th ed.). New York, NY: Oxford University Press.
   (c) Morey, L. C. (2007). *Personality Assessment Inventory professional manual* (2nd ed.). Lutz, FL: Psychological Assessment Resources.
   (d) Tellegen, A., & BenPorath, Y. S. (2008). *MMPI-2-RF (Minnesota Multiphasic Personality Inventory-2-Restructured Form) technical manual.* Minneapolis, MN: University of Minnesota Press.

3. **D—includes language that is directly relevant to modern diagnostic systems, such as the DSM-5** *Clinical conditions assessed by the PAI were selected on the basis of (a) their history of importance in current mental disorder nosology and (b) their significance in contemporary diagnostic practice. Indeed, the language used to describe clinical scales resembles what is included within the DSM-IV-TR criteria, although clinicians should be mindful that, like the MMPI-2, the PAI is not in itself a diagnostic measure.*

   Reference: Morey, L. C. (2007). *Personality Assessment Inventory (PAI) professional manual* (2nd ed.). Lutz, FL: Psychological Assessment Resources.

4. **B—greater reliance on face validity and limited ability to detect response bias** *The BDI-II, BAI, GDS, and other self-report measures of emotional function typically include face-valid test items and do not include validity scales that examine response validity issues. Items may also be common to various psychological conditions and lack diagnostic specificity.*

Reference: Strauss, E., Sherman, E. M. S., & Spreen, O. (2006). *A compendium of neuropsychological tests: Administration, norms, and commentary* (3rd ed.). New York, NY: Oxford University Press.

5. **A—consider elevations of relevant scales in the context of history and medical findings** *The clinical interview, review of available records pertaining to an individual's medical and psychiatric history, and specific diagnostic criteria are essential in arriving at a formal psychological diagnosis.*

Reference: Boone, K. B. (2017). *Neuropsychological evaluation of somatoform and other functional somatic conditions: Assessment primer.* New York, NY: Routledge.

6. **C—"higher-order" scales that examine internalizing, externalizing, and thought dysfunction.** *Factor analyses have demonstrated personal variations in the endorsement of affect, thought, and behavior. The broadband H-O scales can be likened to the Wechsler indices, in that they provide a broad overview of functioning across these common domains, and can be understood further through closer inspection of "narrower-band subdomains" contained on other scales.*

Reference: Ben-Porath, Y. S., & Tellegen, A. (2008). *Minnesota multiphasic personality inventory -2 restructured form (MMPI-2-RF) manual for administration, scoring, and interpretation.* Minneapolis, MN: Pearson.

7. **B—ICN T = 80 and PIM T = 72** *Inconsistency (ICN) is the degree to which respondents answer similar questions in the same way and Positive Impression (PIM) is the degree to which respondents describe themselves in a positive or overly positive light. Each of the validity scales has a separate T score to indicate an invalid profile. To be considered invalid the scales have the following interpretations to invalidate the profile: ICN T ≥ 73, INF T ≥ 75, NIM T ≥ 92, PIM T ≥ 68.*

Reference: Morey, L. C. (2007b). *Personality Assessment Inventory-Adolescent (PAI-A) professional manual.* Lutz, FL: Psychological Assessment Resources.

8. **D—elevated PIM indicating positive impression management** *Positive Impression (PIM) is the degree to which respondents describe themselves in a positive or overly positive light. Given that the face-valid self-report measures in this case suggest no complaints but do not contain validity scales it is important to consider the PAI scores.*

Reference: Strauss, E. Sherman, E. M. S., & Spreen, O. (2006). *A compendium of neuropsychological tests: Administration, norms, and commentary* (2nd ed.). New York, NY: Oxford University Press.

9. **C—TSI-2** *The TSI-2 is a widely used test of trauma-related symptoms and behaviors, which includes two validity scales and 12 clinical scales.*

Reference: Briere, J. (2011). *Trauma symptom inventory—2: Professional manual.* Odessa, FL: Psychological Assessment Resources.

10. **A—report fewer problematic behaviors and emotions than the parent** *In clinical settings, adolescents tend to report their problems as less severe than their parents perceive them. This discrepancy can be magnified after acquired adolescent brain injury because of a lack of deficit awareness due to the injury.*

Reference: Wilson, K. R., Donders, J., & Nguyen, L. (2011). Self and parent ratings of executive functioning after adolescent traumatic brain injury. *Rehabilitation Psychology, 56,* 100–106.

Recommended Readings

Archer, R. P., Handel, R. W., Ben-Porath, Y. S., & Tellegen, A. (2016). *Minnesota Multiphasic Personality Inventory-Adolescent-Restructured Form (MMPI-A-RF): Manual for administration, scoring, interpretation, and technical manual.* Minneapolis, MN: University of Minnesota Press.

Armstrong, K., Beebe, D. W., Hilsabeck, R., & Kirkwood, M. (2008). *A step-by-step guide to ABPP/ABCN certification in clinical neuropsychology: How to become board certified without sacrificing your sanity.* Oxford Workshop Series: American Academy of Clinical Neuropsychology. New York, NY: Oxford University Press.

Baron, I.S. (2018). *Neuropsychological evaluation of the child: Domains, methods, case studies* (2nd ed.). New York, NY: Oxford University Press.

Boone, K.B. (2017). *Neuropsychological evaluation of somatoform and other functional somatic conditions: Assessment primer.* New York, NY: Routledge.

Brooks, B. L., Ploetz, D. M., & Kirkwood, M. K. (2015). A survey of neuropsychologists' use of validity tests with children and adolescents. *Child Neuropsychology, 22*(8), 1001–1020.

Hoelzle, J. B., Nelson, N. W., & Arbisi, P. A. (2012). MMPI-2 and MMPI-2-Restructured form validity scales: Complementary approaches to evaluate response validity. *Psychological Injury & Law,* 174–191.

Kessler, R. C., Chiu, W. T., Demler, O., & Walters, E. E. (2005). Prevalence, severity, and comorbidity of twelve-month DSM-IV disorders in the National Comorbidity Survey Replication (NCS-R). *Archives of General Psychiatry, 62*(6), 617–627.

Rabin, L. A., Paolillo, E., & Barr, W. B. (2016). Stability in test-usage practices of clinical neuropsychologists in the United States and Canada over a 10-year period: A follow-up survey of INS and NAN members. *Archives of Clinical Neuropsychology, 31,* 206–230.

Strauss, E. Sherman, E. M. S., & Spreen, O. (2006). *A compendium of neuropsychological tests: Administration, norms, and commentary* (2nd ed.). New York, NY: Oxford University Press.

Sweet, J., Giuffre Meyer, D., Nelson, N., & Moberg, P. (2011). The TCN/AACN "Salary Survey": Professional practices, beliefs, and incomes of U.S. neuropsychologists. *The Clinical Neuropsychologist, 25,* 12–61.

Weiner, I. B., & Greene, R. L. (2008). *Handbook of personality assessment.* Hoboken, NJ: John Wiley & Sons.

Testing Instrument References

Achenbach, T. M. (1991). *Manual for child behavior checklist 4-18 and 1991 profile.* Burlington: University of Vermont Psychiatry Department.

Archer, R. P., Handel, R. W., Ben-Porath, Y. S., & Tellegen, A. (2016). *Minnesota Multiphasic Personality Inventory-Adolescent-Restructured Form (MMPI-A-RF): Manual for Administration, Scoring, Interpretation, and Technical Manual.* Minneapolis, MN: University of Minnesota Press.

Beck, A. T., & Steer, R. A. (1993). *Beck anxiety inventory manual.* San Antonio, TX: The Psychological Corporation.

Beck, A. T., Steer, R. A., & Brown, G. K. (1996). *Beck depression inventory* (2nd ed.). San Antonio, TX: The Psychological Corporation.

Ben-Porath, Y. S. (2012). *Interpreting the MMPI-2-RF.* Minneapolis, MN: University of Minnesota Press.

Briere, J. (2011). *Trauma symptom inventory—2: Professional manual.* Odessa, FL: Psychological Assessment Resources.

Conners, C. K. (1997). *Conners' rating scales-revised: Technical manual.* North Tonawanda, NY: Multi-Health Systems.

Gioia, G. A., Isquith, P. K., Guy, S. C., & Kenworthy, L. (2015). *Behavior rating inventory of executive function* (2nd ed.). Lutz, FL: Psychological Assessment Resources.

Lachar, D., & Gruber, C. P. (1995). *Personality Inventory for Youth (PIY) manual: Technical guide.* Los Angeles, CA: Western Psychological Services.

Lovibond, S. H., & Lovibond, P. F. (1995). *Manual for the Depression Anxiety Stress Scales* (2nd ed.). Sydney, AU: Psychology Foundation.

Morey, L. C. (2007a). *Personality Assessment Inventory (PAI) professional manual* (2nd ed.). Lutz, FL: Psychological Assessment Resources.

Morey, L. C. (2007b). *Personality Assessment Inventory-Adolescent (PAI-A) professional manual.* Lutz, FL: Psychological Assessment Resources.

Reynolds, C. R., & Kamphaus, R. W. (2015). *Behavior assessment system for children* (3rd ed.). Circle Pines, MN: American Guidance Service.

Wirt, R. D., Lachar, D., Seat, P. D., & Broen, W. E., Jr. (2001). *Personality inventory for children* (2nd ed.). Los Angeles, CA: Western Psychological Services.

11   Cultural and Disability Issues in Neuropsychological Assessment

Daryl Fujii, Tedd Judd, Donna Morere, and Desiree Byrd

Introduction

Culture and language can impact all aspects of the neuropsychological assessment. Its impact can be distilled into three components: (1) collecting accurate data, (2) providing a context for interpreting data, and (3) generating useful recommendations.

For accurate data collection, *culture*, language, and disability can impact rapport and communication between the examinee and neuropsychologist (NP), willingness of the examinee to disclose information or participate in the evaluation, the presentation of emotional disorders, appropriate test selection, and test administration. Thus it is essential that NPs attain cultural knowledge and develop skills in working with culturally diverse examinees (CDEs) prior to commencing the assessment. NPs should be cognizant that interviewing and psychological testing is a Western, able-bodied technology associated with the values, assumptions of knowledge, and behavioral expectations of Western *culture*, which are not universally shared. When testing a CDE or one with a motor or sensory disability, NPs should be aware of American Education and Research Association (AERA), American Psychological Association (APA), and the National Council on Measurement in Education (NCME) (2014) standards for fairness in testing, appreciate potential disadvantages for a CDE, and adapt tests or test administration to maximize fairness and accuracy in testing. AERA identifies four issues:

1. Test takers (TTs) must be comfortable with the testing situation. This standard entails TTs' comfort with the testing process and rapport with the examiner.

2. Tests must be free of *measurement bias*es that include equivalencies in *content* and *construct validity*, and what is considered a correct response.

3. Accessibility, or the ability to process and respond to test items, must be equivalent across cultures.

4. Tests should be valid for the purpose of the construct being measured. This standard entails that fairness for all of the conditions must be met.

In addition, the TT must have had an opportunity to learn the content and skills targeted by the tests. NPs should also consider that for many CDEs, assessment of functionality and adaptive behavior are essential, as tests may be less valid for predicting behaviors.

Test scores cannot be interpreted in isolation. Characteristics of the TT are crucial for determining meaning. For example, reading at grade level has different meanings for a native English speaking 10-year-old versus a native Farsi-speaking child of the same age who immigrated a year ago. The same principles also apply to behavior. For example, the complaint "feeling tired" may have different diagnostic implications for a 45-year-old Chinese female who is experiencing a major depressive disorder after losing her oldest son in an accident versus a 45-year-old white male with multiple sclerosis. In this regard, it is imperative that NPs are aware of a CDE's life experiences, values, learning opportunities, norms for behavior, and idioms of distress so that data can be interpreted within a proper context. Important moderating factors include language skills, education, and level of *acculturation*.

Finally, neuropsychological assessments should generate recommendations and interventions that are useful to the CDE. Again, it is crucial that the NP possesses a good appreciation of the CDE's life context and functionality, which also entails knowledge of a CDE's social roles and expectations, conception of disease and treatment, and resources.

This chapter describes cultural and linguistic considerations in conducting a culturally-informed neuropsychological assessment with CDEs and examinees with disabilities. First, ethical issues are discussed concerning NPs' obligations for providing services to CDEs and also includes the broader role of NPs as advocates. Next, preparatory steps for a neuropsychological evaluation are described that entail acquiring a cultural knowledge base and making accommodations for addressing AERA expectations for fairness in testing and collecting accurate data. Recommendations for data interpretation and report writing are then described. The chapter closes with specific recommendations for working with individuals with disabilities.

Ethical Issues

Overview: Non-Discrimination

Federal law and professional ethics mandate that NPs may not discriminate in their services on the basis of disability, race, color, or national origin, which includes language, spoken or signed. NPs are required to provide meaningful access to all programs, services, and information they offer to Limited English Proficient (LEP) persons. Interpreter services are to be free of charge to the examinee. Those services are to be offered in equal quality. This overarching mandate has ethical implications not only for access to services, but also for professional competency, use of interpreters, test selection, and interventions. It remains an unfulfilled challenge to our profession to develop the research and training that allows us to fulfill this obligation.

Access to Services

NPs have both individual and institutional obligations to provide equitable access to services. As such, NPs, when involved in institutional policy and governance, are obliged to advocate for workplace diversity and evidence-based accountability for changes that facilitate equitable access and service, such as budgeting for interpreters, cultural consultation, community referrals, testing materials, extra clinical time, continuing education, disability accommodations equipment, etc.

Professional Competence

Ethics require that NPs only provide services for which they are competent (APA Ethics 2.01(a)). Providing non-discriminatory, culturally competent access presents potentially conflicting ethical and legal mandates. How can an NP who is not culturally competent serve a CDE without discrimination? NPs are obliged individually and collectively as a science and profession to continually improve their cultural competence, and to find an optimal balance of ethical concerns for each individual case. An essential aspect of providing competent services entails learning about the neuropsychologically relevant aspects of an examinee's language and *culture* in advance of, during, and after the evaluation. Specifics of this preparatory work are described in the sections on Culture and Acculturation, Education and Literacy, Language Knowledge, Bilingualism, and Disabilities. Resources for obtaining this material are available through Internet medical and/or mental health population profiles and language profiles, for example, through Ethnomed.org, Omniglot.org, Ethnologue.org, and everyculture.com, as well as the social sciences, medical, psychology, and neuropsychology literature. Other options may include referral to a linguistically/culturally competent NP, collaboration or consultation with a linguistically/culturally-competent allied health professional, and/or culturally competent work with an interpreter.

Interpreter Use

NPs are responsible for the ethics and cultural competence of those who work under them, such as psychometrists, students, clerical staff, and interpreters (APA Ethics 2.05). It is greatly preferable to use trained, professional interpreters who abide by their professional code of ethics. When interpreters are not professionals, NPs need to train and guide them in interpreter ethics, including competence, accuracy, confidentiality, and impartiality. Interpreters need to establish good relationships with both (all) parties so as to inspire trust, but not ally too strongly with any party so as to show no partiality. NPs must respect this balance; for this reason, interpreters are limited in sharing cultural knowledge, impressions, opinions, and knowledge of the examinee. Impartiality also means that interpreters avoid dual relationships, such as family members, friends, attorneys, etc. Some dual roles, such as healthcare provider, may be compatible.

Test Selection

The NP is responsible for selecting tests that reliably measure the variable of interest in a population representative of the TT (APA Ethics 9.02; AERA, APA, NCME). This usually means that the test is in the TT's best language. Testing may also be appropriate in the TT's less-good language if the purpose is to measure their competence in that language, but such testing may only be diagnostically useful with respect to specific language-learning functions. Many neuropsychological tests are now available in multiple languages. A collective challenge to professional neuropsychology is facilitating access to such tests and information about them. The technology for test translation, adaptation, renorming, and revalidation has been well worked out for tests that are based upon their semantic content (inventories, fund of knowledge, etc.). Many neuropsychological tests, however, are not based upon their semantic content. It is the NP's responsibility, therefore, to use their knowledge of cognitive processes along with the International Test Commission's guidelines on test translation and adaptation to select tests and responsibly interpret the results. Having the interpreter perform on-the-spot translations or interpretations of test instructions and especially of test content is a substandard and generally obsolete practice. NPs should also have competence in incorporating disability accommodations into testing (see the "Disabilities" section of this chapter).

Interventions and Recommendations

Cultural competence is also called for in providing interventions and recommendations (APA Ethics 9.06, 9.10). Where pertinent, the NP should provide guidance regarding the best language(s) for oral and written communication, healthcare, and education. NPs should know or discover linguistically and culturally competent community referral sources, for example, psychotherapists, educational resources, and legal services. They should likewise be familiar with pertinent assistive technologies, disability support groups, communities, and state services appropriate to individuals with disabilities. NPs are also in a good position to provide recommendations for medical and other treatments and education that are congruent with the CDE's beliefs, health understanding, *culture*, and resources. Interventions and recommendations should be in the best interests of the patient, including cultural and linguistic adaptations chosen to increase the likelihood of success of the interventions and recommendations.

Culture

Psychological assessment was developed within the context of Western *culture*, including its values, expectations, and experiences, to measure Western defined constructs. The more similar a CDE's *culture* is to Western *culture*, or the more acculturated the CDE is to Western *culture*, the more valid Western testing and assessment is for that individual. Typically absent in these findings, however, are specifics of how *culture* and language can influence different performances on Western tests.

This section identifies specific pertinent cultural components, the contextual implications of each cultural component for understanding a CDE, and their potential impact on the assessment process. As education, literacy, and language have ubiquitous impacts on the assessment process, these topics will be discussed in subsequent sections. Cultural categories include: (a) macro-societal structures; (b) values, beliefs, and social structures; (c) medical conditions and beliefs about illness; (d) communication style; and (e) concept of intelligence. These descriptions will be followed by ways to assess for *acculturation*, context of immigration, and application to different ethnic groups.

Learning about an evaluee's cultural context is merely a starting point for understanding their individuality through (a) conceptualizing their behaviors, cognitive functioning, and cultural influences; (b) developing hypotheses for clinical conceptualization; and (c) guiding the interview for obtaining more specific information with the purpose of (d) refining the NP's conceptualization of the CDE.

Macro-Societal Structures

Macro-societal structures, the physical, historical, and economic contexts in which a people have lived in over centuries, strongly influence a people's specific characteristics, including cognition and brain functioning. Geography and climate largely determine economies and many features of *culture*. Historical events such as natural disasters, wars, and colonization, and the philosophy and stability of government can impact a population's worldview, external cultural influences, languages spoken, and economic development. A country's natural resources, geographic location, sociopolitical history, and economy influences the people's standard of living; access to learning tools such as books, computers, and the Internet; and the quality of the educational system. A related issue is that low socioeconomic status is associated with increased exposure to stress and trauma and smaller frontal and hippocampal structures.

Values, Beliefs, and Social Structures

Religious beliefs and political systems have important implications for values, attitudes, and worldview. Social structures and belief systems have strong influences on cognition and what are considered appropriate behaviors and in which contexts. Social norms such as expectations for family relationships, interactions with strangers of different status, or collectivist versus individualistic allegiance, have strong implications for understanding a CDE's behaviors, which would include interactions with the NP. Thus, awareness of these cultural characteristics can help the NP develop rapport, guide optimal approaches for communication, appreciate a CDE's experience of the testing situation, and generate useful recommendations that are consistent with cultural values and the CDE's social environment. These skills are ideally developed through guided practice and experience.

Medical Conditions and Beliefs About Illness

Knowledge of the psychiatric and neuroepidemiology of the population, as well as their traditional beliefs about illness, spiritual/social medical interventions, and idioms of distress, can provide important contextual information for diagnosis, case formulation, and making useful recommendations for treatment. For example, illnesses such as cerebral malaria, cisticercosis, or organophosphate pesticide poisoning, are only common in specific countries. Many Muslim cultures frame what we regard as mental disorders as spiritual or family disorders, while other cultures, such as Somalis, do not have concepts such as depression. In addition, there are many culturally specific intervention practices that CDEs may be either considering or using such as Chinese medicine, Latin/x curanderos, and Christian faith healers. Neuropsychologists should be aware that treatments differ in empirical support and efficacy. Knowledge of traditional treatments can assist the neuropsychologist to probe CDEs on what has been tried before and appreciate barriers to seeking or accepting recommendations for Western treatments, increase the neuropsychologist's awareness of culturally consistent efficacious treatments, and cue strategies to convince CDEs to try Western interventions if appropriate.

Communication Style

Communication involves not only language content, but also pragmatic characteristics or communication styles that often differ across cultures. Such differences may include: (a) expectations re: in which situations talking is acceptable, (b) what is considered appropriate to disclose to strangers, (c) the pace of speech and duration of pauses to indicate one has finished speaking and it is the listener's turn to respond, (d) the meaning of and comfort with silence, (e) directness of communication, (f) preference for linear thinking, and (g) norms for emotional expressiveness which can be a perceived as either a sign of honesty or lack of emotional modulation. Many collectivist cultures rely on indirect statements and nonverbals to avoid conflicts, thus the listener must be attuned to not only what is said, but what is not said to appreciate the speaker's intent. Cultures which rely on storytelling or other non-linear communication styles may not respond well to direct, sequential interviewing style that is typically used by NPs.

Incongruence in communication style between the NP and CDE can easily result in miscommunication and misinterpretation of behaviors, but may have other implications as well. In communication mismatches the other speaker may be seen as rude or socially inappropriate. For example, many cultures consider it respectful to avoid eye contact, to show little affect, and to volunteer little information toward an authority figure such as an NP. The NP may misinterpret this as resistance or depression. If the NP gives very direct feedback to CDE and their family that uses indirect communication, s/he may be seen as rude, insensitive, and/or not trustworthy. These perceptions can harm rapport and reduce test cooperation. Consequently, the CDE may misunderstand test instructions and expectations and they may distrust the findings and not adhere to recommended interventions. In essence, the NP's naiveté regarding a CDE's communication style can result in inaccurate data and ineffective treatment.

Concept of Intelligence

Many leading theorists have purported that intelligence is intimately tied to one's physical and social environment. The implication is that what is considered intelligent behavior will differ across cultures insofar as differences exist in the social problems associated with their environments. In this regard, standards of intelligence for a CDE may differ from Western notions of intelligence that emphasize reasoning, problem solving, understanding complex abstract ideas, and quick learning. For example, many traditional African cultures equate intelligence with skills in facilitating and maintaining harmonious group relationships and with being slow and thoughtful rather than quick and possibly impulsive. Interestingly, high performances on tests evaluating these skills are negatively correlated with scores on Western intelligence tests. Cultural differences in the conceptualization of intelligence have several important ramifications for testing such as nonequivalence in the construct of intelligence (*measurement bias*), what would be considered a correct response (accessibility), and interpretation of performances (validity). A special consideration for neuropsychological testing is the Western notion that intelligence is equated with quick responding, which is the premise for scoring on timed tests. The implication is that a CDE's score on intelligence tests may not be predictive of functional behaviors, hence diagnoses.

Perhaps the most important clinical application of the concept of intelligence in neuropsychology concerns intellectual disability. This diagnosis has enormous implications for education and adult competencies. The two principle diagnostic criteria—intelligence test performance and adaptive behavior—are both highly variable culturally and across processes of *acculturation*. Useful and accurate diagnosis and interventions require flexible clinical thinking, sensitivity to cultural expectations and trajectories, and sensitivity to diverse conceptualizations of intellectual disability.

Acculturation

Understanding a CDE's *acculturation* to Western *culture* is critical to be able to estimate the impact of a CDE's *culture* on the assessment process. The degree to which one has adopted mainstream *culture* can be estimated by collecting a thorough history from the CDE and, to some extent, through *acculturation* scales. Age at immigration, amount of education in the United States, proficiency in English, and cultural identification are most strongly associated with *acculturation*. *Acculturation* and English-language acquisition are often more rapid in children and young adults than in older adults, and generational differences and conflicts are common.

There is a selection bias regarding who emigrates from a given country that varies enormously by country of origin and by historical epoch. For documented immigration, the applicant must meet eligibility criteria for the different immigration categories, which include family reunification, employment, political affiliation, and selection by lottery. For undocumented immigration, the person must be highly motivated and have access to resources to travel to and enter the United States. Understanding the context of immigration can help the NP appreciate how the CDE fits within his/her *culture* of origin, prevent stereotyping, and provide insight into possible mental health issues associated with the stressors of immigration. At the same time, the NP must realize that inquiring about documentation status can be threatening to some and may damage rapport. *Acculturation* status varies widely according to individual histories for CDEs whose communities have been in the United States for many generations, such as Native Americans, African Americans, Puerto Ricans, American Samoans, Native Hawaiians, Amish, etc.

Communication styles also vary by *culture*; for example, indirect communication is common for many Asian cultures. Nonlinear narration is common for traditional Native Americans. Many Native Americans, Asians, and Latinos are reticent to disclose about self or family, and this may further vary with the ethnicity of the clinician and purpose of the encounter. Historical conflicts between the NP's and examinee's cultures or country of origin can impact rapport and disclosure.

NPs should be aware of specificities within ethnicities. For example, the 2010 United States census lists nineteen specific and three group categories for country origins of Hispanics, and twenty-four categories for Asians, while persons from Kenya, Nigeria, Jamaica, and Haiti among others are included under African Americans. There are over 350 languages spoken in the United States, with about nine languages with over one million speakers each, and over 60 million in the United States speak a language other than English at home. Even when a country of origin is accurately identified, there may be much cultural and linguistic diversity within that country to be specified. For example, India has 780 languages and a multitude of cultures. In addition, there are 567 federal recognized Native American tribes with 33% of the population living in native areas. On a micro-level, most persons are *multicultural*, thus NPs need to be aware of the different characteristics and experiences, and intersectionalities that influence a CDE's behavior and cognition.

Education

The impact of education and literacy on cognition is immense, with both processes significantly moderating performances on neuropsychological testing. Education (a) develops skills in using writing, drawing, and memorization; (b) instills a value for learning; and (c) exposes students to test taking situations. On a cognitive level, education (a) exposes students to information outside of the immediate environment and language not used in everyday conversation, (b) teaches reading, (c) develops *taxonomic classification*, (d) improves *semantic processing*, and (e) helps to develop *formal operational thinking*.

By contrast, persons with a limited amount of or no formal education develop a different skill set and ways of thinking based on learning from and about their environment and exposure to media. The relationship between education and performance on neuropsychological testing is not linear. For example, individuals with zero years of education perform profoundly worse than individuals with three years, while smaller differences exist between those with three and six years of education, and six and nine years.

In addition to years of education, quality of education has been found to impact performance on neuropsychological testing. Resources such as availability of books, computers, or the Internet, as well as qualifications of teachers vary between and within countries. For example, a CDE with "6 years" of education may have received 4 hours/day, 7 months/year instruction not in their native language in a rural classroom with a roof but no walls, benches but no desks, a teacher with 11 years of education, and few books to share among the 70 students. Given the significant impact education has for developing cognitive skills, it is important that NPs be familiar with the details surrounding the CDE's educational experiences. The number of years of education received in the United States versus other countries is pertinent, as well as the resources the school has for teaching foreign students, particular for the CDE's country of origin.

Quality of education within the United States is also pertinent to neuropsychological evaluation and test expectations. For example, many older African Americans were educated in segregated schools in the South that were grossly underfunded and had excessively high student:teacher ratios. Helpful tools for deciphering education quality for English-speaking CDEs educated in the United States are single-word reading tests that have been validated against objective markers of education quality and offer grade-equivalent scores that can be used to anchor test interpretation when education quality level is significantly below achieved grade level.

Providing equitable educational neuropsychology services to immigrant children can be challenging, beginning with service access. Parents may be unaware of services or reluctant to ask for them. They may not view difficulties as disabilities. Schools may assume that difficulties are due to English as a Second Language status rather than disability and may wait for a few years for the child to learn English before flagging a problem. NPs need to be particularly skilled at history-taking, with an approach that is multilingual, dynamic, and longitudinal.

Literacy

The process of reading exposes individuals to visual symbols that are distinct from the world they represent. This experience fosters the development of decontextualized communication, which is the ability to discuss and inquire about things that are not present. In this manner, reading is a foundation for abstract and *formal operational thinking*. Additionally, reading facilitates *semantic processing*, develops *taxonomic classification*, is a limitless source for acquiring information that is outside of one's immediate environment, and can also act as an external storage to facilitate memory. An important implication of literacy is its impact on problem solving. Individuals who are literate use more abstract strategies while those who are illiterate employ more visual, procedural, and pragmatic, sensory-based strategies.

Literacy rates vary across countries and writing systems. Lack of education opportunities due to poverty, the need to work, and/or governmental failure results in social illiteracy. Personal illiteracy is due to a reading disorder or other neurological condition and occurs despite educational opportunities. If a CDE is illiterate or semi-literate, it is important for NPs to determine the reason.

Language Issues

Language is fundamental to neuropsychological assessment. Therefore, the NP should seek a thorough understanding of the TT's language history, education, and use, even when the TT's best language is English (or other language of evaluation). This understanding includes features of the TT's language(s), and understanding of the TT's language history.

Language Knowledge

The great diversity in the cognitive, phonetic, grammatical, pragmatic, and written features of the world's languages has major importance for understanding a TT's brain processes, learning, and communication potential. The NP can learn fundamental linguistic and cognitive features of non-English language(s) online (e.g., Omniglot.org, Ethnologue.com) and through various texts. Interpreters may offer insight about specific features, but most are not trained linguists and should not be relied upon as the only source of information. Some languages have special features, such as tones, clicks, or unusual grammar.

Many major languages have two writing systems, such as Chinese, Japanese, Korean, Punjabi, and Hindi-Urdu; many languages have no effective writing system; it is important to understand these in order to understand what system(s) the TT uses. The nature of the writing system has tremendous impact on literacy abilities and reading disorders. Transparent orthographies are relatively easy to learn and read (e.g., most romance languages, most recently literate languages, the Japanese and Korean phonetic systems), sometimes without formal schooling. Other systems take many years to master (e.g., Arabic, Hindi-Urdu, Chinese, the Japanese and Korean ideographic systems).

CDE's Language History and Use

Individual histories of language learning and use impact how language abilities will be affected by brain disorders, how language abilities may recover, and treatment strategies. The TT's language history is most usually learned through interview with the TT and/or family members. This includes which languages they learned at what ages; which languages were involved in their formal education; their levels and components of literacy in each; current usage, competencies, and preferences; and language use goals, especially for education and employment. While this may sound intimidating, with experience and skill these components can usually be determined within a few minutes. Thorough guidance is available from interviews such as in the Bilingual Aphasia Test. Language questionnaires can contribute to the evaluation but are not yet a substitute for a thorough interview.

Bilingualism

Although more than half of the world's population is bilingual, bilingual norms for neuropsychological tests are rare. NPs therefore need understanding of the complex nature of bilingualism and multilingualism in order to apply clinical judgment to the interpretation of evaluation results. Bilinguals may have variable competencies and preferences across languages, such as being literate in one but not another, preferring one language for emotions and another for work and academics, etc. Bilingualism confers both cognitive advantages and disadvantages especially in details of language use and certain executive functions, and potentially in cognitive reserve.

Knowledge of the processes of becoming bilingual is critical in evaluating language functions in bilinguals, but it is especially critical if a second language is still being acquired, and especially in pediatrics and education. For example, it may take a child only a year to develop Basic Interpersonal Communication Skills (BICS) in their host and educational language, but up to 6 years to develop Cognitive and Academic

Language Proficiency Skills (CALPS). So children may communicate fluently on the playground within a year, but may struggle academically for many years, but not for reasons of cognitive impairment. They may pass through a period of not being fully proficient (for age) in either language. In such contexts NPs should be prepared to evaluate types of language exposure and use, methods and intensity of instruction, and educational goals. Knowledge of specific language features such as the nature of writing systems is particularly important when these are at issue in education.

Choosing Language(s) of Evaluation

The choice of language(s) of an evaluation depends upon the purposes of the evaluation. For diagnosis it is generally best to evaluate someone with tests in their best language, normed and validated for diagnosis on a population representative of the TT. This is best carried out by professionals who speak that language and are knowledgeable about testing. NPs therefore need skills in locating and collaborating with such professionals and in obtaining and interpreting such tests. For academic placement or various other competencies it is typically best to evaluate in the language in which that academic placement or competence is to be carried out, regardless of what is the person's best language. For example, if the language of the workplace is Spanish then workplace competence should be tested in Spanish; if the language of instruction is English then academic placement testing may be best in English. For complete evaluation of the TT's cognitive and linguistic status evaluation should be in all of their languages, although this often is not pragmatic or necessary. In educational settings, it is particularly important to be clear about language choice and the purposes of evaluation, such as whether the evaluation is to determine cognitive abilities, language dominance, language abilities, and/or academic achievement.

Language issues are most pertinent for first-generation CDE immigrants, with more variability for the second generation. About 35% of Hispanic Americans and 60% of Asian Americans are immigrants. Native American language issues vary greatly by tribe. Those who are better in their native language than English are mostly among the elderly and the Navajo. Native peoples from Latin America who speak their native language better than Spanish or Portuguese are common, for example, there are more Maya than Navajo in the United States. Native American English and African American English have dialectical variations from mainstream United States English. Language is also highly salient for deaf individuals, as there is variability in use of American Sign Language (ASL) and its variants versus speechreading which can significantly impact best approaches for an evaluation.

Interpreter Use

When professionals who are clinically competent in the TT's language are not available, then NPs need to evaluate through interpreters. Interpreters deal with spoken language, and translators deal with written language. Interpreter use is a basic skill for all health professionals who have patient contact requiring practiced skill in the pragmatics of such communication, in the manners of speaking that will interpret well, and in clarification of ambiguity and miscommunication. Closely related skills are establishing cross-cultural rapport and obtaining accurate information from those with distinct perspectives. Such evaluations depend more heavily upon interviews, observations, history, and cultural and linguistic knowledge and competence rather than testing.

In general, the sight-translation of tests and application of non-representative norms is an obsolete practice that is inaccurate and often unethical. However, there are circumstances and tests for which such practices may give qualitative information and a behavioral sample that can legitimately contribute to clinical and forensic decision-making. Most professional interpreters are not trained in testing and need extra preparation by the NP.

Assessment

Preparatory work should assist the NP in developing: (1) expectations for cognition, English proficiency/language(s) spoken, and behavior for persons from the examinee's *culture*, (2) an appreciation of salient cultural experiences that shape these characteristics, (3) working hypotheses of how specifics of the CDE's *culture* interfaces with mainstream *culture*, and (4) working hypotheses of how suspected neurological disorders would present in the CDE and impact functioning within the CDE's environment. This conceptualization will then guide the NP's approach to assessment, specifically to meet AERA standards to maximize rapport, facilitate acquisition of interview data, select appropriate tests, and review individual items for *content validity*. Assessment plans need to be prioritized and flexible to deal with uncertainties and time constraints.

It is highly recommended that NPs use cultural consultants such as colleagues, other professionals, or interpreters (see Interpreter Use and Language sections regarding constraints on using interpreters as a cultural consultants). Cultural consultants may be identified through community cultural organizations and special interest groups within professional organizations. Ultimately and ideally, the culturally competent NP may serve as a cultural broker for the CDE and family, assisting them in understanding and dealing with disability concepts, pertinent institutions, and sectors of society.

Data Interpretation

In addition to the aforementioned cultural facets, NPs should be aware of the literature on (a) pertinent neurological disorders, (b) the CDE's group level performance on neuropsychological tests, and (c) pertinent neuropsychological literature regarding potential issues such as bilingualism, illiteracy, poverty, *acculturation*, and impact of *culture* on Performance Validity Tests (PVTs).

Data interpretation entails several steps. Ideally, tests should be scored with norms based upon samples that are similar in *culture* and demographics to the CDE. Such cultural norms are available for African American and Latin/x examinees, but vary considerably for CDEs of other cultures. That being said, neuropsychologists should evaluate educational experiences, *acculturation*, and languages carefully to choose the norms and interpolations most appropriate to the individual and the evaluation questions. For example, standard age- and education-corrected United States norms would likely be appropriate for a third-generation English-only-speaking Korean American attending college.

If specific cultural norms are unavailable, NPs could utilize the "most appropriate" norms from ethnic groups with similar cultures, educational levels and educational quality, and economies. For example, there are limited neuropsychological norms for Argentines that are available in English. Spain and Mexico are two predominantly Spanish-speaking countries with cultures similar to Argentina's that have norms that can be found in the neuropsychological literature. Norms from Mexico may be more appropriate than those from Spain, as Argentina is more similar to Mexico in terms of gross domestic product per capita and educational attainment.

A third option is to use the individual comparison method, where an estimate of premorbid functioning "on Western tests" (e.g., IQ score) is used as a benchmark to interpret test data with Western norms. This entails adjusting norms using the premorbid estimate as the mean (e.g., setting mean as -1 SD of each score). The determination of premorbid functioning on Western tests for a CDE can be challenging. One approach entails a multistep process whereby the NP first estimates the functional level of the *culture* on Western tests based on the literature, academic test scores for the country (e.g., Programme for International Student Assessment), or country's economy, and then adjusts this score based upon the functioning of the CDE within his/her *culture* (e.g., CDE's level of education versus country's mean, occupation, etc.). For example, a composite of educational test scores, economy, and education resources would suggest the average American Samoan person with a high school education would score about a standard deviation below Western norms on neuropsychological tests. Based upon this benchmark, an instructor at the community college with a master's degree may be estimated to score in the average range. Although imperfect, as cultures differ in their experiences and skills that can differentially impact performances on specific tests, this method can provide a ballpark figure of general functioning on Western tests. It should not be used as the sole indicator for interpreting test scores. When scoring test data, NPs may consider using both standard and adjusted norms to see how the CDE performs in relation to similar others from their *culture/language/country* of origin and also in comparison to the United States general population.

The guiding principle in case formulation for CDEs is determining how the data "makes sense" given the CDEs' education, skills, language, life experiences, and impact of neurological disorder on functioning. An important consideration and moderating factor is the accuracy of the data. Data accuracy for specific components or tests and in general can be determined by assessing for potential threats to AERA fairness in testing categories and the NP's ability to address these issues. When a CDE is vastly different from available normative populations a functional assessment that does not include norm-referenced cognitive testing, may be most relevant. Examples of functional assessments include charting behavioral changes over time (e.g., Informant Questionnaire on Cognitive Decline in the Elderly-IQCODE) or estimating cognition based upon real-world functioning (e.g., Clinical Dementia Rating-CDR). PVTs can be helpful in determining if data interpretation based on mainstream norms may be valid. If PVT performance falls in abnormal ranges then the burden is upon the NP to determine, if possible, reasons for such performances and how those reasons impact other tests. This may require debriefing of their understanding of the task and of the nature of the evaluation, their perception of the materials, and other possible factors. Malingering cannot be presumed.

Report Writing

The general principle when writing up a neuropsychological report about a CDE is to make the implicit explicit. However, the length and level of detail a NP chooses to include in his/her write up will vary across setting, purpose, and individual style. The following are aspects of the evaluation process a NP should include for a comprehensive description of the process: (a) a cultural contextual description of the CDE (e.g., birthplace, educational history, age at immigration, languages spoken, etc.); (b) identified impact of *culture* on the assessment process; (c) accommodations made by the NP, such as language(s) the evaluation was administered in, rationale, use of interpreters, and interpreter's name and qualifications; (d) rationale for test and norm selection; and (e) potential weaknesses in data gathering (e.g., suboptimal rapport or interpreter, test naiveté). The formulation should include supportive and conflicting data, caveats for one's diagnostic conclusions, and confidence in the findings. Finally, recommendations should be culturally adapted by: (a) identifying and making suggestions for utilizing cultural strengths, resources, and community; (b) being appropriate for the CDE's social and physical environment; and (c) addressing the CDE and/or family's concerns.

Disabilities

Disability has only recently been considered an aspect of diversity. Skilled clinicians who would consider cultural competence when accepting a referral may assess persons with disabilities (PWDs) without realizing that they lack the knowledge and skills needed to work with those individuals. While training in neuropsychology rarely includes instruction in working with PWDs, current testing standards recognize that PWDs require special consideration (AERA, APA, & NCME, 2014), and the APA website offers Guidelines for Assessment of and Intervention with Persons with Disabilities (APA, 2011), which emphasize the need for clinicians to be aware of their own attitudes toward and beliefs about disabilities and PWDs. This discussion will focus on the practical aspects of evaluating individuals with physical and sensory disabilities.

Presumptions and Attitudes

The clinician must avoid making assumptions about the disability or its likely effects on the TT. Clinicians may assume that TTs who are deaf or blind experience total sensory loss, leading to the belief that auditory (deaf TT) or visual (blind TT) distractions will not be an issue. In reality, most deaf and blind individuals have some residual hearing or vision, and often the auditory and visual noise that is perceived is more distracting to the TT than it is to the typical TT. A clinician may assume that a blind TT requires Braille, and so a referral may be dismissed as the clinician has no Braille materials. However, many blind individuals can see stimuli or read print if the items are enlarged or the print is an appropriate font. Similarly, a clinician may assume that a deaf TT will require ASL or be able to speechread (commonly called lipreading). Alternatively, a clinician may assume that a TT with a motor impairment such as cerebral palsy (CP) may be able to speak and plan to focus on speech-based tasks; however, CP may affect speech production. Thus, the TT may use sign language or an alternative communication device, which may require additional test modifications. The appropriate mode of communication can only be determined by asking the right questions prior to determining whether the clinician is competent to provide an accurate and ethical evaluation.

Deaf individuals range from those who communicate solely via ASL and identify with Deaf Culture to those who function primarily orally, use speechreading and residual hearing via hearing aids or cochlear implants, and are integrated into the hearing world, to various communication approaches on a continuum between the two. Simply providing an interpreter is not an adequate accommodation, as deafness has widespread effects on a range of skills, knowledge, and life experiences. Culturally Deaf individuals may have difficulty understanding instructions even when interpreted into ASL, and may respond in ways that are readily misinterpreted by the naïve clinician, resulting in misdiagnosis. The considerations above concerning language and *culture* also apply to the Culturally Deaf whose language, ASL, has a unique, visual vocabulary and linguistic structure distinct from spoken languages. Direct translation of stimuli and instructions into ASL may alter the complexity of the task or provide either too much or inadequate information for the TT. Clinicians may be tempted to test deaf individuals who have oral skills using spoken language; however, despite their oral skills, if their primary mode of communication involves signing, this is comparable to testing a primary Spanish speaker in English because they have "adequate" English skills. Such approaches routinely result in misdiagnosis and can cause the TT considerable harm.

Pre-Information

Prior to scheduling an assessment of a PWD, the clinician should ensure that they know the relevant information related to the person's disability. While each disability involves specific sets of information, they share a number of questions in common. It is always important to determine the nature, etiology, onset, duration, and severity of the disability. A person with a recent onset will have different needs than one with a congenital or early onset. The former may be in the process of grieving their loss and still lack the skills to manage their environment, making it more difficult to obtain valid data. The latter may function well given appropriate test modifications and accommodations or may have secondary developmental impacts. The severity of the disability will affect the types of accommodations and modifications required. Information about adaptive strategies the person uses and the degree to which they find them beneficial will inform the clinician as to the types of testing accommodations that may be required or most effective.

Accommodations

The need for test accommodations and modifications will depend on the nature and extent of the impairment. While a person with paralysis of a limb might require the omission or substitution of tasks requiring responses involving that limb, those with limited strength or early onset pain or fatigue may simply require additional breaks, added time, or the use of keyboards or adaptive equipment. Some tasks which typically require a motor response may be administered orally or the examiner may perform the task under the direction of the TT for tasks measuring cognitive process (e.g., card sorting). The modifications and accommodations that are effective during testing can inform the recommendations. For example, if a TT with motor limitations is able to respond to writing tasks by using a keyboard and it is demonstrated that their ability to write is otherwise limited, laptop use could be recommended for writing tasks.

Some accommodations involve making the test environment and materials physically accessible. Wheelchair users may require larger rooms, while visually limited TTs may require specific lighting arrangements. These types of accommodations will be less likely to affect test validity than modifications to the tests themselves. Again, the key is to inquire adequately prior to the assessment so that the clinician has a plan to address any needed accommodations or modifications and is able to obtain access to materials, engage in research and consultation, and schedule the appointments accordingly. Blind TTs may vary from total blindness to adequate vision restricted to a small area. Braille, tactile tasks, and the omission of visually based measures may better address the needs of the former, but be inappropriate for the latter, who would be better served by carefully selected visual tasks which allow for enlarged stimuli and the additional time needed to view the items.

Tests

Few tests are designed to accommodate the needs of PWD. While "motor free" and "nonverbal" measures are now available, the heterogeneity of each type of disability makes the development of measures that can address a broad group (e.g., deaf TT) impractical. While such measures may be appropriate, clinicians may overlook issues such as the use of stimuli (e.g., musical instruments for a deaf TT), which may be outside of the life experience of the individual. Thus, the selection of appropriate tests requires knowledge and understanding not only of the disability involved, but also of the test content. While the manual may provide information about the test's use with PWD, this does not guarantee that such issues will be avoided. Often, the clinician must use an available measure with accommodations or modifications and address the limitations in the test interpretation. This will require understanding of the task demands involved in each instrument and knowledge of subtle, often secondary, effects of the disability. For example, deafness may not only affect language and communication development but also limit literacy and academic achievement, family and peer relationships, and world knowledge and experiences. The clinician's task is to ensure that the data obtained reflect the individual's skills and abilities rather than the effects of their disability, and interpretation of the data must be informed by an understanding of the effects of the TT's disabilities on life experience as well as test performance. Many effects of disabilities on assessments are subtle and require the clinician to be aware of the broad range of impacts on test taking that can result from disabilities. For example, deaf TTs cannot look at stimuli while simultaneously receiving task instructions, placing them at a disadvantage to TTs who are able to do so. Similarly, a TT with a visual or motor impairment may not be able to quickly scan response arrays, again placing them at a disadvantage.

Interpretation and Report

Modifications or accommodations used should be described in the report. The use of modifications and accommodations may be necessary in order to obtain valid and useful data; however, breaking standardization affects the validity of the normative data for the TT. Even so, the availability of specialized norms for PWD does not imply validity of the instrument for the individual. Research on the effects of test modifications on validity has been mixed. Even a specific type of modification (e.g., allowing pointing responses) may inflate scores for some tasks but not others. Common modifications for deaf or blind TT (e.g., Braille/large print or signing) may differentially make individual test items either easier or harder for the TT compared to the standard administration. Omission of subtests or sections of tests may result in construct underrepresentation and cause deficits to be overlooked. The clinician should consider carefully whether the targeted construct has been evaluated accurately by the modified task. The issue of test validity is further complicated by the fact that many PWD require multiple test modifications. Thus, the clinician is cautioned to modify standard administration only when the disability limits access to the test, resulting in *construct-irrelevant variance*, and must take care to ensure that the modifications themselves do not result in added variance. When modifications are used, the clinician must report potential limitations and interpret the data with caution.

Summary of Knowledge and Skills

The assessment of PWD requires the development of knowledge-based competence. The clinician must collect comprehensive information about the disability as it is experienced by the individual prior to the appointment to inform their test selection and assessment process. They must know the content and task demands of measures to be used so that issues that may arise can be addressed, either through accommodations and modifications or interpretation of the data. They must have knowledge of both the primary and secondary effects of the individual's disability on social and emotional functioning, relationships, academic and vocational performance, and other life experiences in addition to its effects on performance on neuropsychological tests or other measures. This knowledge must be used to provide a comprehensive, integrated report that reflects the individual in context and provides realistic, appropriate recommendations. Perhaps most critically, they must approach the individual with a disability with respect; otherwise they are likely to be met with suspicion and resistance to the assessment process.

Relevant Definitions

Acculturation The socialization process by which a foreign-born individual adopts the values, customs, norms, attitudes, and behaviors of the dominant host culture. An important consideration of acculturation for neuropsychological evaluation as it relates to fairness in testing is the similarity of a CDE's culture and experiences to mainstream culture.

Construct-irrelevant variance This represents variance in test performance involving factors that are irrelevant to the interpreted construct (e.g., not what the test was intended to measure), which can inflate or decrease scores and decrease the construct validity of the test for the individual.

Content validity A test has content validity if test items adequately and representatively sample the content area it was intended to measure. A test item is unfair if a test taker is overly familiar or unfamiliar with a test item due to differing experiences.

Construct validity Construct validity is the degree to which a test measures what it claims, or purports, to be measuring. A test is unfair if a construct, for example intelligence behavior, differs across cultures.

Culture Belief systems and value orientations that influence customs, norms, practices, and social institutions, including psychological processes (language, care-taking practices, media, educational systems) and organizations (media, educational systems). Culture has been described as the embodiment of a worldview through learned and transmitted beliefs, values, and practices, including religious and spiritual traditions. It also encompasses a way of living informed by the historical, economic, ecological, and political forces on a group.

Formal operational thinking The last stage in Piaget's model of cognitive development whereby a child is able to think about and manipulate information beyond his/her personal experience. At this stage, the child is able to think abstractly, performing operations such as thinking about the ideas of others, applying a principle across situations, and pondering "what-if" scenarios with potential outcomes.

Intersectionality The confluence of cultural, historical, political sociobiological, economic, institutional, and social contexts that shape an individual and with which they identify.

Measurement bias A test is biased if it systematically favors a particular result, thereby overstating or understating the true value of the measure. Biases can result from a CDE's difficulty understanding instructions, familiarity with tasks, experiences with content, differences in the construct being measured, or what is considered a correct response.

Multicultural Refers to the coexistence of diverse cultures that reflect varying reference group identities. Multicultural can refer to the coexistence of cultures within an individual, family, group, or organization.

Semantic processing Semantic processing entails encoding the meaning of a word and relating it to other words with similar meanings. This placement of the word into an existing mental context allows for a deeper processing and stronger memory traces.

Taxonomic classification A classification system based upon a hierarchy of attributes from broad to specific. This is the preferred and highest scoring classification system of objects and concepts for WAIS Similarities responses.

Cultural and Disability Issues in Neuropsychological Assessment Questions

NOTE: Questions 20 and 33 on the First Full-Length Practice Examination, Question 6 on the Second Full-Length Practice Examination, Question 118 on the Third Full-Length Practice Examination, and Question 30 on the Fourth Full-Length Practice Examination are from this chapter.

1. American Samoans have been found to miss the animal naming items on the Montreal Cognitive Assessment significantly more than Westerners. Poor performances appear to stem from unfamiliarity with these animals. This is an example of bias in ____.

   (a) accessibility
   (b) content validity
   (c) construct validity
   (d) reliability

2. In the Tagalog translation of the Montreal Cognitive Assessment, NPs are allowed to repeat instructions for the similarities section if the examinee needs clarification. This administrative

adaptation was based upon a pilot study of elderly, cognitively intact Filipinos who often required repetition of instructions for this section to understand the task. This adaptation best exemplifies which American Education and Research Association (AERA) principle?

(a) accessibility

(c) content validity

(b) construct validity

(d) comfort with the testing situation

3. Non-discrimination in neuropsychological services with respect to language spoken by the evaluee is _____.

(a) an aspirational option of the new APA Multicultural Guidelines

(b) a requirement of federal law and the Civil Rights Act of 1964

(c) not required as it places undue burden of competence on the clinician

(d) now possible due to a proliferation of culturally validated tests and norms

4. Regarding responsibility for learning about the evaluee's languages and cultures, it is the _____.

(a) evaluee's responsibility to inform the neuropsychologist about any way in which the evaluee's cultures or languages diverge from mainstream culture and English language

(b) interpreter's responsibility as a cultural broker to educate the neuropsychologist about the evaluee's languages and cultures

(c) neuropsychologist's responsibility to inquire of the evaluee about any way in which the evaluee's cultures or languages diverge from mainstream culture and English language

(d) neuropsychologist's responsibility to acquire knowledge about the evaluee's languages and cultures and to determine the evaluee's language and cultural history while minimally burdening the evaluee

5. When evaluating bilingual children for possible language disorder or learning disability, they should be evaluated in _____.

(a) their best spoken and written language

(b) the language of instruction at school

(c) both their home and their school languages

(d) the language for which the best tests are available

6. Education facilitates cognitive development by _____.

(a) helping the individual survive in their immediate environment

(b) socializing with peers and facilitating outdoor exercise

(c) providing students with good nutrition to enhance brain development

(d) exposing students to information outside their immediate environment

7. Reading develops decontextualized communication by _____.

(a) acting as an external storage for memorizing information from the environment

(b) facilitating a discussion of things that are in the person's immediate environment

(c) exposing the person to visual symbols that are distinct from the world they represent

(d) exposing the person to allegorical stories that teach life lessons

8. On average, Native Americans prefer visual/holistic processing and perceive intelligent responding as resulting from a slow and thoughtful reasoning process versus rapid problem solving. Would a timed test such as WAIS-IV Block Design be a valid measure of nonverbal reasoning for Native Americans? Why or why not?

    (a) No, Native Americans would be disadvantaged for valuing a slower response style.

    (b) No, unfamiliarity with test materials would invalidate the test results.

    (c) Yes, because it is emphasizes visual processing which is a strength.

    (d) Yes, it's a nonverbal test, which would make it a cultural fair measure.

9. A native Jamaican adolescent earns a score that is 1–3 points below the standard thresholds on two commonly administered stand-alone PVTs, though no behavioral evidence of suboptimal effort was detected. The best course of action is to _____.

    (a) adhere to the manuals' published cut points for this age group, render the evaluation invalid and explain your conclusion in the report

    (b) examine the results of embedded measures and administer additional stand-alone measures to assess for consistency

    (c) review the literature on the psychometric properties of these PVTs in ethnic minorities and interpret the result in light of this research

    (d) given the unknown validity for these tests in people from other cultures, ignore the finding and omit it from the final report

10. An elderly Caucasian man from a small rural Appalachian town reports the completion of 12 years of education, but the results of a reading recognition test place his reading ability at the 6th grade level. When deciding the appropriate education level to set normative data interpretation at, you should _____.

    (a) use the achieved level value of 12th grade, to reflect data accuracy and respect the examinee's academic experience

    (b) use the 6th grade value, which better reflects the quality of this examinee's education and then contextualize the Appalachian school experience

    (c) decide to forego the use of normative data that adjusts for education and use the age-corrected tables available in the test manuals

    (d) generate and report standard scores that adjust for 6th and 12th grades and decide which scores best address the referral question

Cultural and Disability Issues in Neuropsychological Assessment Answers

1. **B—content validity** *Content validity entails equivalencies in test items across cultures whereby there are no advantages or disadvantages across cultures in attaining a correct response. In this example, American Samoans are less familiar with the animals as they have less opportunities for exposure to the test items stemming from the remoteness of the islands, absence of zoos, and less access to books or the Internet.*

Reference: American Education Research Association. American Psychological Association, and the National Council on Measurement in Education. (2014). *Standards for educational and psychological testing* (2nd ed.). Washington DC: American Education Research Association.

2. **A—accessibility** *This administrative adaptation allows for the Filipino examinee to process what is required from the test item so they can respond appropriately. The content of the items has not changed, nor the task itself, thus repetition of instruction does not impact construct or content validity. Although repetition may increase comfort with the testing process, the main purpose was to allow for fairness in responding to the test items.*

Reference: American Education Research Association. American Psychological Association, and the National Council on Measurement in Education. (2014). *Standards for educational and psychological testing* (2nd ed.). Washington DC: American Education Research Association.

3. **B—a requirement of federal law and the Civil Rights Act of 1964** *Language use is covered under non-discrimination based on national origin in APA ethics and the Civil Rights Act of 1964 (Judd, et al., 2009). Psychology has been slow to respond to these mandates with respect to needed training and research, and so this remains a mandate requiring continuous professional improvement.*

Reference: Judd, T., Capetillo, D., Carrión-Baralt, J., Mármol, L. M., San Miguel-Montes, L., Navarrete, M., . . . Silver, C. H., (2009). Professional considerations for improving the neuropsychological evaluation of Hispanics. Hispanic Neuropsychological Society/National Academy of Neuropsychology. *Archives of Clinical Neuropsychology, 24*, 127–135.

4. **D—neuropsychologist's responsibility to acquire knowledge about the evaluee's languages and cultures and to determine the evaluee's language and cultural history while minimally burdening the evaluee** *Professional competence requirements oblige neuropsychologists to have the knowledge and skills to serve their examinees adequately. This includes adequate knowledge about their examinee's language and cultural background and skills in working with that background. Non-discrimination requirements oblige neuropsychologists to eliminate any unnecessary barriers to care, such as having to be articulate about their own cultures and languages and educating the neuropsychologist about that. Neuropsychologists may choose to fulfill this obligation, in part, by hiring interpreters for the additional job of cultural broker, but in doing so they need to determine that the interpreter has that competence and make that an explicit part of their professional agreement.*

Reference: American Psychological Association. (2017). *Ethical principles of psychologists and code of conduct.* (2.01a, 3.01)

5. **C—both their home and their school languages** *When a person is bilingual both languages are important to their cognition. Evaluation in their home language will reflect their development and may reveal a disorder in their development and deficiencies of language skills. Evaluation in their home language may also be needed to reveal the full extent of their fund of knowledge and cognitive abilities. Evaluation in their school language will reflect current learning struggles, levels of language functioning, and instructional needs.*

Reference: Judd, T., Capetillo, D., Carrión-Baralt, J., Mármol, L. M., San Miguel-Montes, L., Navarrete, M., . . . Silver, C. H. (2009). Professional considerations for improving the neuropsychological evaluation of Hispanics. Hispanic Neuropsychological Society/National Academy of Neuropsychology. *Archives of Clinical Neuropsychology, 24*, 127–135.

6. **D—exposing students to information outside their immediate environment** *Education broadens the individual's awareness and knowledge beyond immediate experience including new vocabularies not used in everyday conversation.*

   Reference: Ardila, A., Bertolucci, P., Braga, L., Castro-Caldas, A., Judd, T., Kosmidis, M., . . . Rosselli, M. (2010). Illiteracy: The neuropsychology of cognition without reading. *Archives of Clinical Neuropsychology, 25,* 689–712.

7. **C—exposing the person to visual symbols that are distinct from the world it represents** *Decontextualized communication is the ability to discuss things that are not present. Reading is the process of using symbols to represent objects, which facilitates abstract thinking.*

   Reference: Ardila, A., Bertolucci, P., Braga, L., Castro-Caldas, A., Judd, T., Kosmidis, M., . . . Rosselli, M. (2010). Illiteracy: The neuropsychology of cognition without reading. *Archives of Clinical Neuropsychology, 25,* 689–712.

8. **A—No, Native Americans would be disadvantaged for valuing a slower response style** . *Although Native Americans prefer visual holistic processing, and WAIS–IV Block Design is visuospatial task, their preference for slow and thoughtful processing would place them at a disadvantage due to time limits for responding and bonus points for completing items quickly. Visuospatial tests are not found to be culturally fair and there are no known tests that are fair for all cultures. Tests of executive functioning are often novel and unfamiliar to most.*

   Reference: Prescott, S. (1991). *The American Indian: Yesterday, today, and tomorrow: A handbook for educators.* Sacramento, CA: California State Department of Education.

9. **C—review the literature on the psychometric properties of these PVTs in ethnic minorities and interpret the result in light of this research** *The available literature, though mixed, suggests that cut points of some PVTs are not generalizable to examinees from cultures outside of those represented in the normative sample, particularly those born outside of the United States.*

   Reference: Salazar, X., Lu, P., Wen, J., & Boone, K. (2007). The use of effort tests in ethnic minorities and non-English-speaking and English as a second language populations. In K. Boone (Ed.), *Assessment of feigned cognitive impairment: A neuropsychological perspective* (pp. 405–427). New York, NY: Guilford Press.

10. **D—generate and report standard scores that adjust for 6th and 12th grades and decide which scores best address the referral question** *The choice of demographic corrections depends upon the specific referral question and whether it is more appropriate to interpret performance in light of the examinee's unique characteristics or in reference to the larger population.*

    Reference: Testa, S. M., Winicki, J. M., Pearlson, G. D., Gordon, B., & Schretlen, D. J. (2009). Accounting for estimated IQ in neuropsychological test performance with regression-based techniques. *Journal of the International Neuropsychological Society, 15,* 1012–1022.

Recommended Readings

American Psychological Association. (2017). *Multicultural guidelines: An ecological approach to context, identity and Intersectionality.* Washington, DC: American Psychiatric Publishing.

Fujii, D. (2017). *Conducting a culturally informed neuropsychological assessment.* Washington, DC: American Psychological Association.

Fujii, D. E. (2018). Developing a cultural context for conducting a neuropsychological evaluation with a culturally diverse client: the ECLECTIC framework. *The Clinical Neuropsychologist, 32*(8), 1356–1392.

Hill-Briggs, F., Dial, J., Morere, D., & Joyce, A. (2007). Neuropsychological assessment of persons with physical disability, visual impairment or blindness, and hearing impairment or deafness. *Archives of Clinical Neuropsychology, 22*, 389–404.

Judd, T., Capetillo, D., Carrión-Baralt, J., Mármol, L. M., San Miguel-Montes, L., Navarrete, M., . . . Silver, C. H. (2009). Professional considerations for improving the neuropsychological evaluation of Hispanics. Hispanic Neuropsychological Society/National Academy of Neuropsychology. *Archives of Clinical Neuropsychology, 24*, 127–135.

Julayanont, P., & Ruthirago, D. (2018). The illiterate brain and the neuropsychological assessment: from the past knowledge to the future new instruments. *Applied Neuropsychology: Adult, 25*(2), 174–187.

12 Symptom and Performance Validity Testing

Glenn J. Larrabee and Michael W. Kirkwood

Introduction

Neuropsychological assessment is dependent upon the accuracy of information provided by the examinee during a clinical interview, as well as upon the accuracy of symptom endorsement on behavioral rating scales and omnibus personality tests such as the MMPI-2-RF. Additionally, the major portion of the neuropsychological evaluation, the measurement of cognitive and sensorimotor abilities, requires an actively engaged participant so that the examiner can rely upon the accuracy of the examinee's performances in reaching conclusions about an examinee's neuropsychological status. The results from the most reliable and valid test procedures can be completely invalid for an examinee who intentionally underperforms on the various measures of ability, and who feigns or exaggerates on measures of emotional status, pain, or personality. Consequently, each neuropsychological evaluation must evaluate both performance and symptom validity.

Performance validity tests or measures (*PVTs*) allow determination of whether examinees are demonstrating their actual level of ability, while *symptom validity tests* or measures (*SVTs*) allow determination of whether examinees are presenting an accurate report of their actual subjective experience. This terminology was preceded by less precise descriptions that were inconsistently used by neuropsychologists including "response bias," as well as the use of "symptom validity" to refer to both *PVTs* and *SVTs*. Last, the term "effort tests" was commonly employed, which was misleading, since successful completion of *PVTs* requires very little effort in order to produce a valid performance and intentional underperformance can actually require a great deal of mental effort.

History of PVTs and SVTs

Formal examination of performance validity in neuropsychological evaluation dates to the work of Rey with the Dot Counting Test in 1941, and the 15-item Test in 1964. In the early 1960s, Spreen and Benton conducted what is known as a simulation research designed to compare Benton Visual Retention Test performance of normal persons feigning impairment with that of clinical patients who had bona fide clinical disorders. Rey's research characterized the first "free-standing" or stand-alone measures of performance validity (i.e., *PVTs* that were designed solely for the purpose of detecting invalid performance). By contrast, the Spreen and Benton research was the first to demonstrate that actual clinical tests of specific neuropsychological abilities, in this case, visual memory, could also yield information about performance validity. Consequently, these clinical tests could do "double duty;" in other words, they measured a primary ability such as memory, but also contained "embedded" measures of performance validity. The intended purpose of these measures of performance validity was to identify invalid performance that differed from the level and patterns of performance that characterized persons with bona fide cognitive impairment. In this early work, Spreen and Benton discovered that variability in clinical patient performance precluded routine clinical application of the patterns of simulated impairment they had derived for the Visual Retention Test.

Subsequent developments in the 1970s included the use of two-alternative forced choice testing by Pankratz and colleagues, to evaluate the validity of an examinee's claim of deafness. With two-alternative forced choice testing, a person with zero ability should perform at chance; as a result, significantly worse-than-chance performance (based on the normal approximation to the binomial) could be assumed to represent intentional selection of the incorrect items. This can be determined statistically using the normal approximation to the binomial. With two alternatives, the probability of a correct response, p, is .5 and equal to the probability of an incorrect response, q. In a four-alternative task, p equals .25 and q equals .75. In the normal approximation to the binomial for a two-alternative task, the mean equals the number of trials, n, multiplied by p. With 100 trials, this becomes (100)(.5) = 50. The standard deviation of the normal approximation to the binomial is ($\sqrt{\ }$) of npq or in this case, ($\sqrt{\ }$)(100)(.5)(.5) = 5. If an examinee obtains 40 correct out of 100, this can be transformed to a z score by the equation 40-50/5 or –2.00. Thus, the probability of getting 40 correct out of 100 by simply guessing is .02, the value under the normal curve corresponding to a z score of –2.00. Obtaining such a rare score, by chance (guessing) is .02; it can be assumed that factors other than chance were operative.

Pankratz has referred to significantly below-chance performance as the "smoking gun of intent." His work influenced subsequent applications of this technique for evaluation of feigned memory impairment such as the Portland Digit Recognition Test of Binder in 1990, the Test of Memory Malingering developed by Tombaugh in 1996, and the Word Memory Test developed by Green and colleagues in 1999.

A landmark paper by Heaton and colleagues in 1978 demonstrated two things:

(1) Experienced clinicians could not reliably discriminate tests scores produced by non-injured persons simulating impairment from test scores indicating actual neuropsychological impairment due to severe brain injury on performances from the Halstead-Reitan Battery, with correct classification ranging between 50% to 69%; and (2) atypical patterns of performance that actually did separate the two groups could be derived statistically; i.e., discriminant function analysis correctly classified 100% based on their Halstead-Reitan and WAIS performance, and 94% correct on the basis of their MMPI profiles. This paper showed that persons simulating impairment performed atypically compared to the bona fide brain injury group, doing more poorly on measures such as the Seashore Rhythm Test and Finger Tapping. Nearly 20 years later (1996), Mittenberg and colleagues replicated the Heaton group's findings with new samples of non-injured simulators, and persons who had sustained traumatic brain injury (TBI) with bona fide impairment.

Symptom validity testing also dates to the 1940s, with the original publication of the MMPI. Hathaway and McKinley included three validity scales: "Cannot Say" (representing unanswered items), L, and F. Research has demonstrated the utility of the F scale in detecting exaggeration of severe psychopathology, demonstrating one of the key features of detection of invalid symptom report: over-endorsement of rarely endorsed symptoms. Subsequent research with the MMPI-2 and MMPI-2-RF has also incorporated scales capturing unusual response patterns associated with personal injury litigation, such as the Symptom Validity Scale (FBS), and scales associated with failure of PVTs such as the Response Bias Scale (RBS). Whereas the F and Fp scales are useful for detection of exaggerated symptoms suggestive of psychosis as might occur in criminal legal settings, the FBS and RBS are more suited for detection of exaggerated injury or physical illness in civil legal settings. Further discussion of these issues is provided in Chapter 10: Personality Assessment and Self-Report Instruments.

Presently, research on *PVTs* and *SVTs* is continuing the logarithmic growth that began since the 1990s. This research is a major part of applied clinical research in neuropsychology. The major neuropsychology practice journals almost always have at least one paper per issue devoted to *PVT* and *SVT* research.

Multiple position papers and practice guidelines (e.g., National Academy of Neuropsychology, American Academy of Clinical Neuropsychology) have established the importance of validity testing in every case, both clinical and forensic. Recent practice surveys have clearly demonstrated that *PVT* and *SVT* use is commonplace among both adult and pediatric practitioners.

The research base supporting *PVT* and *SVT* use is one of the most extensive in all of psychology. Over the past several decades, more than 1,000 scientific articles, 20 comprehensive reviews, a dozen meta-analytic studies, and a dozen textbooks have appeared in the literature. The bulk of this work has been focused on adults, though increasing attention in recent years has been devoted to pediatric populations as well. In adults, multiple *PVTs* and *SVTs* have now been validated. Above certain ages, children have also been found capable of passing a number of stand-alone *PVTs* using cutoffs established with adults. For example, children as young as five or six consistently pass the TOMM, and children with at least a third-grade reading level can pass the WMT and Medical Symptom Validity Test (MSVT).

Across both adult and child populations, free-standing *PVTs* are heavily weighted toward procedures that appear to measure memory, such as the TOMM, PDRT, WMT, MSVT, Victoria Symptom Validity Test, ACS Word Choice Test, Rey Word Test, Rey-15-item test, and Memory Validity Profile. Some free-standing *PVTs* also appear to measure processing speed, such as the Dot Counting Test and the b Test. Again, these procedures are sufficiently easy that most patients with bona fide neurologic, psychiatric, or developmental disorders can perform validly.

Numerous embedded or derived measures of performance validity are also available. Since these procedures are derived from actual clinical measures of neuropsychological abilities such as tests of memory or sensorimotor function, great care needs to be taken to ensure that performances are truly atypical for a bona fide disorder, and at the same time, characteristic of invalid performance. For example, an embedded *PVT* for the Category Test was derived by identifying those items rarely missed by persons with moderate to severe TBI, but more commonly missed by non-injured persons instructed to believably feign impairment. For the Continuous Visual Memory Test, the *PVT* was derived by finding those items answered correctly by persons with moderate and severe TBI but failed by persons in litigation for claimed mild disorders, who had no other medical or neuroradiologic abnormalities and who also performed significantly worse-than-chance on the PDRT (i.e., met criteria for definitely invalid performance). The *PVT* developed for one version of the Rey Auditory Verbal Learning Test, a widely used measure of verbal learning and memory, was based on multiple invalid patterns of performance, such as failing to recognize words that were consistently provided over the five learning trials for this test procedure.

Poor performance on recognition relative to recall on text recall, paired associate learning, and verbal list learning tests is a common feature of embedded/derived *PVTs*, as is abnormally poor performance on measures of simple motor function such as the Finger Tapping Test, particularly when such failure occurs in the context of relatively normal performance on more demanding measures of motor function such as the Grooved Pegboard Test. In summary, successfully developed measures of embedded/derived performance validity are atypical in either pattern or level of performance in comparison to the performance on these measures by patients with bona fide neuropsychological disorder.

As of 2018, *SVTs* have not been validated in pediatric populations referred for neuropsychological assessments specifically. In adults, *SVTs* are available for omnibus personality tests such as the MMPI-2-RF, and the Personality Assessment Inventory (PAI). The PAI, however, only allows evaluation for exaggerated psychopathology, and does not contain *SVT* scales sensitive to exaggeration of injury or illness, unlike the MMPI-2-RF. Scores that are atypical for patients presenting valid pain complaints have been identified for pain scales including the Modified Somatic Perception Questionnaire (MSPQ) and the Pain Disability Index (PDI). In both cases, examinees exaggerating pain effects and disability endorse more symptoms than are typical of chronic pain patients. Free-standing *SVTs* also exist, including the

Structured Interview of Reported Symptoms-2nd edition (SIRS-2), which is useful in criminal forensic settings for detection of feigned psychosis, and the Structured Inventory of Malingered Symptomatology (SIMS), with a broader set of symptoms considered in comparison to the SIRS-2; the SIMS evaluates symptom report across five scales: Psychosis, Low Intelligence, Neurological Impairment, Affective Disorders, and Amnestic Disorders. It is noteworthy that the original cutting scores on the SIMS were based on comparisons of normal subjects instructed to feign versus normal subjects asked to respond accurately, absent the presence of patients with bona fide clinical problems. The SIMS was found in subsequent post publication investigations involving clinical patients to have an elevated false positive rate; consequently, more conservative cutoffs are necessary than those published in the test manual.

Importance of Performance Validity Testing

Failure to take into account performance validity in the individual case can lead to misdiagnosis of the presence and severity of impairment. It is generally accepted that in the presence of failed *PVTs* and *SVTs*, poor performances are more likely secondary to invalid performance, whereas normal-range performances may themselves be underestimates of true level of ability.

In clinical research, failure to take into account performance validity can distort relationships with external criteria. Thus, grade point average did not show the expected relationship with IQ until subjects failing a *PVT* were excluded. Olfactory identification did not show the expected linear association with severity of TBI until those examinees failing *PVTs* were excluded. The median memory test correlation with hippocampal volume in Mild Cognitive Impairment was .49 for those passing *PVTs* but -.11 for those failing *PVTs*. Memory test performance did not differ between examinees with and without CT scan abnormalities until those subjects failing *PVTs* were excluded. Memory complaints only correlated with memory test performance in those examinees who failed *PVTs*. Neuropsychological test performance was only associated with the presence or absence of brain injury in those persons who passed *PVTs*.

Numerous studies in adults have demonstrated that *PVT* failure is associated with significantly worse performance on a wide variety of neuropsychological tests. As performance on *PVTs* diminishes, examinee scores on neuropsychological tests decline dramatically as well. *PVT* failure in adults accounts for approximately 50% of the variance on ability-based tests, far more than that explained by educational level, age, neurological condition, and neuroimaging results. Only a few studies have investigated the relationship between *PVT* performance and ability-based tests in children. Available work suggests that similar relationships exist, at least in pediatric samples with relatively high rates of noncredible effort such as youth with persistent symptoms after mild head injury or those being evaluated for Social Security Disability benefits.

In adults, the base rate of *PVT* and *SVT* failure is high in settings with external incentive. One survey of 11 studies with over 1,000 cases showed a failure rate of 40% in civil settings. A consecutive series of criminal defendants showed that 54% met diagnostic criteria for either probable or definite malingering. Base rates appear equally high regardless of external incentive including personal injury litigation, disability applications, or the criminal court. At a base rate of 40%, Chafetz and Underhill estimated Social Security Disability costs of $20 billion for malingered mental disorders, and $14 billion for malingered musculoskeletal disorder (commonly associated with chronic pain).

In mixed studies with clinical pediatric populations, noncredible presentations do not occur frequently, but they have been found consistently, with at least a small percentage of children (~3–5%) presenting noncredibly across most case series. Children and adolescents being seen clinically for persistent symptoms of concussion display higher rates of noncredible effort overall, typically 15% or more. By comparison, 8% of adults in general medical/psychiatric clinical settings are estimated to feign or exaggerate symptomatology, with higher rates seen when clear external incentive is apparent as mentioned. The only base rate work conducted to date examining a child population with a clear external incentive is in the context of Social Security Disability evaluations; rates of *PVT* failure here are similar to those seen in adults (40+%), though the noncredible presentation is thought to typically be driven by the caregivers in what is considered "malingering by proxy."

Diagnosis of Malingering

Malingering is defined as the fabrication and/or exaggeration of deficits in pursuit of an external incentive, such as potential monetary reward in personal injury litigation or avoidance or mitigation of punishment in a criminal setting. Failure on *PVTs* and *SVTs* alone does not support a diagnosis of malingering. Rather, this failure must occur in the context of an identifiable external incentive. Diagnostic criteria have been published for *malingered neurocognitive dysfunction (MND)* by Slick and colleagues, with the criteria being considered relevant for both adults and children (see Table 12.1). To date, *MND* research has focused almost exclusively on adults. Bianchini, Greve, and colleagues also modified the *MND* criteria for *malingered pain-related disability (MPRD)*.

TABLE 12.1 Malingering Criteria from Slick, Sherman, and Iverson (1999)

A. Presence of substantial external incentive	
B. Evidence from neuropsychological testing	
1. Definite negative response bias	
2. Probable response bias	
3. Discrepancy between test data and known patterns of brain functioning	
4. Discrepancy between test data and observed behavior	
5. Discrepancy between test data and reliable collateral reports	
6. Discrepancy between test data and documented background history	
C. Evidence from self-report	
1. Self-reported history is discrepant with documented history	
2. Self-reported symptoms are discrepant with known patterns of brain functioning	
3. Self-reported symptoms are discrepant with behavioral observations	
4. Self-reported symptoms are discrepant with information obtained from collateral informants	
5. Evidence from exaggerated or fabricated psychological dysfunction	
D. Behaviors meeting necessary criteria from Groups B and C are not fully accounted for by psychiatric, neurological, or developmental factors	
Definite	Meets Criterion A **AND** Criterion B1 and Criterion D
Probable	Meets Criterion A **AND** two or more B Criteria (excluding B1); or meets one B Criterion (excluding B1) **AND** one of more C Criteria. Meets Criterion D
Possible	Meets Criterion A **AND** one or more C Criteria **but NOT** Criterion D; or meets all criteria for Definite or Probable **but DO NOT** meet Criterion D

Both *MND* and *MPRD* start with a gate-keeper criterion of the presence of an external incentive. Note that in the case of pain, the incentive may be obtaining narcotic analgesics. Both *MND* and *MPRD* approach the diagnosis of malingering in a probabilistic manner, relying on both *PVTs* and *SVTs*, as well as on atypical findings on physical examination for *MPRD*, and presence of "compelling inconsistencies" regarding pain symptom disability (e.g., moving in dramatically impaired fashion when in the doctor's office undergoing examination, but without apparent problems when engaged in activities of daily living while unaware of being observed). Additionally, both *MND* and *MPRD* require that *PVT* abnormalities cannot be attributed to neurologic (e.g., Alzheimer's disease), psychiatric (e.g., schizophrenia), or developmental (e.g., intellectual disability) abnormalities. These latter rule-out criteria are important to ensure that *PVT* failure does not represent a "false positive"; that is, a failure due to bona fide inability to perform the task due to severe neurologic, psychiatric, or developmental disability. In this vein, various disorders have been identified as showing elevated risk for *PVT* failure as a result of true inability to perform the task, with one investigation showing an elevated false positive rate in persons requiring 24-hour supervision. *PVT* failure also frequently occurs in patients with Alzheimer-type dementia.

If *PVT* and *SVT* failure occur in the context of external incentive, and such failure cannot be attributed to neurologic, psychiatric, or developmental factors, then determination can be made as to whether the results are consistent with definite, probable or possible *MND* or *MPRD*. A diagnosis of definite *MND* or definite *MPRD* is made when there is evidence of significantly worse-than-chance performance on a two-alternative forced choice *PVT*, or in the case of *MPRD*, when there is evidence of a compelling inconsistency. Probable *MND* or *MPRD* is diagnosed when there is evidence of failure of two or more *PVTs*, or failure of one *PVT* and one *SVT*. If there is failure of only one *PVT*, or multiple *SVT* failures with no accompanying *PVT* failure, a diagnosis of possible *MND* is made; however, a diagnosis of probable *MPRD* can be made based upon multiple *SVTs* and/or *PVT* or *SVT* failure in combination with abnormal physical examination results.

The consensus paper of AACN endorses the use of *PVTs* and *SVTs*, recommending use of *PVTs* throughout the examination so that the clinician can continuously monitor the validity of the examination results. This consensus committee also endorsed the ability of the clinician to reach a conclusion of malingering, following careful assessment and consideration of the context of the examination.

Research Designs, Empirical, and Statistical Issues

There are two basic research designs for creating *PVTs* and *SVTs* in neuropsychological practice: the *simulation design* and the "known groups" or criterion groups design. Both designs involve a comparison group with bona fide neurologic disorder and measurable neuropsychological deficits; often this is a group of patients with moderate and/or severe TBI. Such a comparison group is critical, since the basic goal of *PVT* and *SVT* research is to identify patterns that are invalid for actual, acquired impairment; consequently, use of clinical groups (preferably without external incentive) is essential to control for *false positive error* (i.e., identifying a valid impairment as an indication of invalid performance). The simulation group uses a group of non-injured persons instructed to intentionally underperform to some extent but not so much that it would be obvious. The performance of the simulating group on the *PVT* or *SVT* being investigated is then compared for the simulators vs. the actual clinical patients. The strength of this type of design is that the researcher is certain who is feigning because the persons in the *simulation design* have been instructed to feign. An oft-cited weakness is the concern over generalizability; specifically, are the simulators actually performing as would non-injured or minimally injured persons seeking real-world incentives?

The criterion groups or "known groups" design uses the same type of clinical comparison group as would be utilized for a *simulation design*. The group with invalid performance, though, is a group seeking external incentive, usually through civil litigation or disability claim, who also show evidence of invalid performance by failing two or more *PVTs* or *SVTs*, or one *PVT* at worse-than-chance level. On occasion, known-group investigations will form these invalid performance groups through use of the diagnostic criteria for *MND* or *MPRD*. The performance of the known invalid group and the valid clinical group is contrasted on the *PVT* being investigated as a predictor of invalid performance. The strength of the known groups design is that it employs an invalid performance group that has "real-world" external incentives. The weakness is that the generalizability of the results is only as good as the classification accuracy of persons comprising the group characterized as demonstrating invalid clinical presentation. With both the simulation and known groups designs, one needs to ensure valid presentation in the clinical case comparison group.

Larrabee and colleagues observed how the results from simulators and known groups have provided statistical support for both the *MND* and *MPRD* criteria. First, several studies showed similar levels of performance for simulators and for litigants who performed significantly worse-than-chance on two-alternative forced choice testing, establishing that worse-than-chance performance was intentional since these litigants performed similarly to persons intentionally underperforming (because they had been instructed to do so). These authors then demonstrated the similarity of performance of litigants failing two or more *PVTs* to that of litigants who performed significantly worse-than-chance, showing that multiple *PVT* failure was intentional, because it matched below-chance performance. Last, the finding that *PVT* failure and malingering increased linearly in association with degree of external incentive (no incentive vs. Louisiana workman's compensation vs. Federal workman's compensation), supported the role of external incentive in the *MND* criteria.

Chapter 8: Psychometrics, Test Design, and Essential Statistics reviews diagnostic statistics in detail so this will not be recapitulated here. We will instead focus on important major diagnostic issues in research on *PVTs* and *SVTs*. *PVTs* and *SVTs*, as noted previously, are designed to discriminate between valid and invalid clinical presentation. Traditionally, the focus has been on keeping the false alarm rate (mis-identifying a valid impairment as invalid performance) at a minimum for two reasons: (1) it is better to make an error of omission than commission due to the negative consequences for the individual examinee, and (2) false positives play a significant role in "ruling in" the conclusion of invalid presentation. Diagnostically, the specificity (Sp) of a test is the percent of the persons without the condition of interest correctly identified as not having the conditions (the converse of the false positive rate). Specificity then becomes important for ruling in a condition of interest (think of the mnemonic SpIN). On the other hand, sensitivity (Sn) is the percentage of the persons who actually have the condition of interest identified correctly as having the condition, and is important for ruling out the condition of interest (think of the mnemonic SnOUT). The diagnostic probability (Positive Predictive Probability, PPP) for the presence of malingering when the examinee actually has the condition of interest (produces a positive score) is defined by the ratio of true positives/(true positives + false positives) in association with that positive score. The diagnostic probability (Negative Predictive Power, NPP), for the absence of a diagnosis of malingering when the examinee actually does not have the condition of interest, is defined by the ratio of true negatives/(true negatives + false negatives) in association with that negative score.

The base rate of the condition of interest impacts these computations. Often, when a PVT or SVT is developed the sample sizes for the credible and non-credible performance groups are generally equal. By contrast, a new application of the PVT or SVT may occur in a setting with either higher or lower base rate of invalid examination results. Consider a PVT with an Sn of .60 and an Sp of .90. If you have 100 cases and a high base rate of .90, 90 cases are non-credible. Your True Positive values for cases detected by your PVT becomes 54 (.60)(90). Your False Positive value for mis-identified cases is 9 (.10)(90). Your PPP is then 54/54 + 9 = .857. In a new sample, with a low base rate of non-credible performance of .10, the calculations for the PPP now start with 10 credible cases (.10)(100). The True Positive value for your test becomes (.60)(10) = 6. Your false positive value then becomes (.10)(90) = 9. Your new PPP becomes 6/6 + 9 = .40. These computations show how using a test with a predetermined Sn and Sp can yield vastly different PPP in high and low base rate conditions. Moreover, in this particular PVT example, with Sn of .60 and Sp of .90 and a high base rate of .90, use of the base rate alone identifies more invalid cases than application of the PVT; in other words, simply identifying all cases as non-credible correctly identifies 90 out of 100, for a PPP of .90, compared to the computed PPP of .857.

A convention has developed in neuropsychological research to keep the false positive rate for an individual PVT at 10% or less; in other words, 90% or more of patients with a bona fide clinical disorder will be correctly identified by the PVT in question as validly performing. Because of this convention, individual PVTs typically have high Specificity (Sp; low false positive rate), but lower Sensitivity (Sn; higher false negative rate). The first meta-analysis of PVTs in 2001 reported an average sensitivity of .56 (false negative rate of .44) and specificity of .95 (false positive rate of .05). A subsequent meta-analysis in 2011 reported a mean sensitivity of .69 (false negative rate of .31) and mean specificity of .90 (false positive rate of .10).

The diagnostic probability of a particular condition of interest is dependent upon the ratio of true positives/(true positives + false positives); (also see previous discussion of PPP). Another way to represent this is with the positive likelihood ratio (LR+), obtained by dividing the true positives by the false positives associated with a specific PVT score. The LR+, when multiplied by the base rate odds of invalid performance, yields the odds of an invalid performance, which can then be transformed back to a probability by the formula of odds/odds + 1. Obviously, the smaller the false positive rate, the larger the LR+ (to a degree). Another way to consider the meaning of the LR+ is that it reflects how much more likely the performance is to represent the performance of someone with the condition of interest (invalid performance) compared to the performance of someone without the condition of interest.

If we return to the meta analyses described earlier, the LR+ for the 2001 study (Sn = .56, Sp=.95) is .56/.05 = 11.2, and the LR+ for the 2011 study (Sn = .69, Sp = .10) is .69/.10 or 6.9. These values can be compared to the Heaton et al. data on the Halstead Reitan Average Impairment Rating contrasting brain injured versus normal subjects (Sn = .771, Sp = .854), for an LR+ of .771/.146 = 5.28. Importantly, this shows that with properly developed PVTs, the discrimination of invalid impairment from valid impairment is actually superior to the discrimination of valid impairment from normal performance.

The above data are pertinent to individual PVTs and SVTs, but in actual clinical practice, multiple PVTs and SVTs are employed in both clinical and forensic cases (more so with forensic than with non-forensic clinical evaluation). A recent general survey of neuropsychologists practicing with adults showed an average of 4.8 free-standing and embedded/derived PVTs in clinical cases, and 6.3 in forensic cases. For forensic neuropsychology experts, another survey reported an average of 5.93 PVTs per clinical case, and 8.02 per forensic case. These surveys showed that multiple validity measures are also used in conducting research on PVTs and SVTs, either relying upon failure of two or more PVTs, or attaining the Slick probable MND criteria (which also require multiple sources of evidence). Finally, the proliferation of PVTs and SVTs reflected in the past 10 years of journal publications raises questions regarding the impact of multiple PVTs and SVTs on diagnostic accuracy.

Some have utilized Monte Carlo simulation to investigate false positive failure rates for PVTs using per-test specificity rates of .90, for statistically simulated data, reporting failure rates that exceed the expected per test failure rate of .10. Whereas Monte Carlo simulation appears to accurately match expected pass/fail rates compared to standard normative data on tests such as the subtests comprising the WAIS-IV, the same is not true for simulated PVT vs. actual PVT performances; rather, the Monte Carlo simulations appear to overestimate false positive rates compared to actual *PVT* patient performances. It has been argued that this is the consequence of skewed distributions for actual *PVTs* whereas the Monte Carlo simulations rely upon normally distributed data. Skew is evident, for example, in the TOMM manual containing clinical data, with several patients including those with stroke causing aphasia or TBI (including severe TBI) performing perfectly or near-perfectly on the TOMM. For patients with aphasia, the average percent correct on TOMM trial 2 was 98.7%, in patients with TBI, with one day to over three months of coma, producing an average TOMM trial 2 of 98.3%. Again, these numbers are the product of the focus on *PVT* development to minimize false positive rates for individual measures of performance and symptom validity.

Presently, it is unusual to see elevated false positive rates when using a cutoff of impairment on two or more *PVTs* and/or *SVTs* to define invalid clinical presentation. To further minimize diagnostic error, there has been an ongoing focus on specifying the clinical conditions likely to result in *false positive errors*. As noted earlier, this includes severe neurologic, psychiatric and developmental disorders that often result in a need for 24-hour supervised living.

It has also been suggested that a false positive analysis be conducted for the individual case, including determining whether the examinee has a condition likely to result in *PVT* or *SVT* failure (e.g., Alzheimer's disease, schizophrenia). Also, since *PVTs* mimic actual neurobehavioral domains of ability, the neuropsychological data should be scrutinized for evidence that the examinee has sufficient native ability to perform the *PVT*. Someone who performs normally on the AVLT should not be failing the Word Memory Test. Someone who produces a normal performance on Trail Making B should not be failing the b Test. Someone who performs normally on the Grooved Pegboard should not be producing extremely poor scores on Finger Tapping. Last, the examinee with multiple *PVT* failures should not be able to drive independently to the examiner's office, if the *PVT* failures reflect bona fide rather than invalid impairment.

Relevant Definitions

False positive error (in relation to performance validity) Refers to failure on a PVT due to ability-based problems rather than non-credible performance. Very young age, Alzheimer-type dementia, and impairment severe enough to warrant 24-hour supervision are all associated with elevated false positive rates on *PVTs*. Conventionally, cut-scores for PVTs are chosen conservatively such that the false positive rate for an individual PVT is 10% or less.

Known groups design Along with the simulation design, one of two basic research designs for creating PVTs and SVTs. Also known as the "criterion groups" design. Consists of two groups: (1) a group of individuals with high risk for invalid performance (e.g., individuals seeking compensation) who also show clear evidence of invalid performance by failing two or more PVTs or SVTs or one PVT at worse-than-chance level and (2) a group of individuals with bona fide neurologic disorder and measurable neuropsychological deficits (e.g., patients with moderate to severe TBI). The strength of the design is that it employs individuals with "real-world" external incentives. The weakness is that the generalizability of the results is only as good as the classification accuracy of the groups.

Malingered neurocognitive dysfunction (MND) Diagnostic criteria for malingering proposed by Slick and colleagues. The diagnosis is probabilistic, allowing for determination of definite, probable, and possible malingering. The diagnosis of MND first requires the presence of an external incentive. Data from both PVTs and SVTs are then aggregated. In order for a diagnosis to be made, PVT/SVT abnormalities cannot be attributed to neurologic (e.g., Alzheimer's disease), psychiatric (e.g., schizophrenia) or developmental (e.g., intellectual disability) problems.

Malingered pain-related disability (MPRD) Diagnostic criteria for pain malingering proposed by Bianchini, Greve, and colleagues, who based the criteria on MND. Similar to MND, the diagnosis is probabilistic, allowing for determinations of definite, probable, and possible malingering of pain-related disability. It also requires the presence of an external incentive. Data from both PVTs and SVTs are aggregated, as are atypical findings on physical examination and the presence of "compelling inconsistencies" regarding pain symptom disability. In order for a diagnosis to be made, abnormalities cannot be attributed to neurologic (e.g., Alzheimer's disease), psychiatric (e.g., schizophrenia), or developmental (e.g., intellectual disability) problems.

Performance validity test (PVT) Performance-based measures that allow for determination of whether examinees are providing an accurate measure of their actual level of ability. There are two general types: stand-alone and embedded. Stand-alone or free-standing PVTs are designed solely for the purpose of detecting invalid performance. Embedded measures are derived from clinical tests of specific neuropsychological abilities capturing clinically atypical performance that also yield information about performance validity.

Symptom Validity Test (SVT) Self- and other-report measures that allow for determination of whether examinees and others (e.g., caregivers) are presenting an accurate report of actual symptom experience during questionnaire responding.

Simulation Design Along with the *known groups design*, one of two basic research designs for creating PVTs and SVTs. Consists of two groups: (1) a group of non-injured persons instructed to intentionally underperform on PVTs and (2) a group of individuals with bona fide neurologic disorder and measurable neuropsychological deficits (e.g., patients with moderate to severe TBI). The strength of the design is that the researcher is certain who is feigning. The primary weakness relates to generalizability (i.e., are the simulators actually performing as would non-injured or minimally injured persons seeking real-world incentives?).

Symptom and Performance Validity Testing Questions

NOTE: Question 76 on the First Full-Length Practice Examination, Question 11 on the Second Full-Length Practice Examination, Question 2 on the Third Full-Length Practice Examination, and Questions 57 and 92 on the Fourth Full-Length Practice Examination are from this chapter.

1. A 42-year-old woman sustained a mild TBI in a motor vehicle crash 9 months ago. She is reporting persistent symptoms including increased difficulties with focus and memory. She is planning on hiring an attorney. During your evaluation, she failed multiple PVTs. On the MMPI-2 RF, which of the following scales is most likely to be elevated?

   (a) F-r

   (b) Fp

   (c) Fp-r

   (d) FBS-r

2. You are seeing a 9-year-old for a neuropsychological evaluation. Which of the following has the most empirical support to detect intentional feigning?

   (a) stand-alone PVTs

   (b) embedded PVTs

   (c) parent-reported SVTs

   (d) self-reported SVTs

3. Diagnoses of both malingered neurocognitive dysfunction (MND) and malingered pain-related disability (MPRD) are best described as:

(a) continuous

(b) dimensional

(c) probabilistic

(d) quantitative

4. The rate of noncredible presentations in adult civil litigants presenting for neuropsychological evaluation is about ____.

(a) 5%

(b) 10%

(c) 20%

(d) 40%

5. With properly developed PVTs, the discrimination of invalid impairment from valid impairment has been found to be ____ the discrimination of valid impairment from normal performance.

(a) superior to

(b) worse than

(c) equivalent to

(d) unrelated to

6. The primary reason Monte Carlo simulations are misleading when used to investigate false positive failure rates for PVTs is because the distribution for PVT scores is ____.

(a) multivariate

(b) kurtotic

(c) skewed

(d) truncated

7. Complaints in the context of which of the following conditions has been found to be associated with the highest rates of PVT failure in school-aged pediatric populations?

(a) mild TBI

(b) moderate to severe TBI

(c) fetal alcohol syndrome

(d) perinatal stroke

8. In which of the following clinics is the Personality Assessment Inventory (PAI) likely to be most useful as an SVT?

(a) neurology

(b) psychiatric

(c) rehabilitation

(d) general medical

9. The diagnostic probability of malingering when the examinee is actually malingering is defined by the ratio of ____.

(a) true positive/(true positives + false positives)

(b) true negative/(true negatives + false negatives)

(c) false positive/(true positives + false positives)

(d) false negative/(true negatives + false negatives)

10. In the setting in which you practice, the base rate of noncredible effort is relatively low, happening about 10% of the time. Assuming the sensitivity of a PVT is .50 and the specificity is .90 across settings, the positive predictive probability in your setting will be ____ a setting with a base rate of noncredible effort of 50%.

(a) lower than

(b) higher than

(c) equivalent to

(d) indeterminate in

Symptom and Performance Validity Testing Answers

1. **D—FBS-r** *FBS-r (and RBS) is sensitive to exaggerated symptoms of injury or illness. Civil litigants have been shown to have higher risk for elevated FBS (and RBS). The other scales are sensitive to exaggerated psychopathology rather than exaggerated injury-related complaints.*

   Reference: Wygant, D. B., Sellbom, M., Gervais, R. O., Ben-Porath, Y. S., Stafford, K. P., Freeman, D. B., & Heilbronner, R. L. (2010). Further validation of the MMPI-2 and MMPI-2-RF Response Bias Scale: Findings from disability and criminal forensic settings, *Psychological Assessment, 22*, 745–756.

2. **A—stand-alone PVTs** *Dozens of studies have now demonstrated that school-aged children can pass at least some stand-alone PVTs using cut-off scores developed originally for adults. Embedded PVTs and SVTs are not nearly as strongly supported at this point in pediatric populations for detecting feigned or exaggerated cognitive problems.*

   References:
   (a) DeRight, J., & Carone, D. A. (2015). Assessment of effort in children: A systematic review. *Child Neuropsychology, 21*, 1–24.
   (b) Kirkwood, M. W. (Ed.). (2015). *Validity testing in child and adolescent assessment: Evaluating exaggeration, feigning, and noncredible effort.* New York, NY: Guilford Press.

3. **C—probabilistic** *Because it is not often possible to determine whether or not a patient is malingering with absolute certainty, the proposed criteria for MND and MPRD were designed to include formal specification of probabilistic levels of diagnostic certainty (i.e., possible, probable, and definite malingering).*

   References:
   (a) Bianchini K. J., Greve, K. W., & Glynn, G. (2005). On the diagnosis of malingered pain-related disability: Lessons from cognitive malingering research. *Spine, 5*, 404–417.
   (b) Slick, D. J., Sherman, E. M., & Iverson, G. L. (1999). Diagnostic criteria for malingered neurocognitive dysfunction: Proposed standards for clinical practice and research. *Clinical Neuropsychologist, 13*, 545–561.

4. **D—40%** *Larrabee et al. review results of several investigations of base rate of invalid performance in both civil and criminal settings falling in the range of 40% +/− 10. Base rates appear equally high regardless of external incentive including personal injury litigation, disability applications, or the criminal court.*

   Reference: Larrabee, G. J., Millis, S. R., & Meyers, J. E. (2009). 40 plus or minus 10, a new magical number: Reply to Russell. *The Clinical Neuropsychologist, 23*, 841–849.

5. **A—superior** *With properly developed PVTs, the discrimination of invalid impairment from valid impairment is superior to the discrimination of valid impairment from normal performance.*

   Reference: Larrabee, G. J. (2015). Performance and symptom validity: A perspective from the adult literature. In M. W. Kirkwood (Ed.), *Validity testing in child and adolescent assessment* (pp. 62–76). New York, NY: Guilford Press.

6. **C—skewed** *Monte Carlo simulations rely upon normally distributed data so simulations reasonably match expected classification rates when using tests with normally distributed data. In contrast, Monte Carlo simulations appear to overestimate false positive rates compared to those seen in actual patient performances on PVTs. This is because the distributions for PVTs are skewed, with performances at the ceiling and in a restricted range (i.e., most people perform perfectly or near perfectly).*

   Reference: Larrabee, G. J. (2014). False-positive rates associated with the use of multiple performance and symptom validity tests. *Archives of Clinical Neuropsychology, 29*, 364–373.

7. **A—mild TBI** *The base rates of noncredible performance in children and adolescents undergoing neuropsychological evaluation have been found to be relatively elevated in those with persistent problems after mild TBI, even in clinical settings (15–20% or higher). Rates of PVT failure in school-aged children with moderate to severe brain injury and FAS are relatively low (5%).*

References:
(a) Araujo, G. C., Antonini, T. N., Monahan, K., Gelfius, C., Klamar, K., Potts, M., . . . Bodin, D. (2014). The relationship between suboptimal effort and post-concussion symptoms in children and adolescents with mild traumatic brain injury. *The Clinical Neuropsychologist, 28*, 786–801.
(b) Carone, D. A. (2008). Children with moderate/severe brain damage/dysfunction outperform adults with mild-to-no brain damage on the Medical Symptom Validity Test. *Brain Injury, 22*, 960–971.
(c) Gidley Larson, J. C., Flaro, L., Peterson, R. L., Connery, A. C., Baker, D. A., & Kirkwood, M. W. (2015). The Medical Symptom Validity Test measures effort not ability in children: A comparison between mild TBI and fetal alcohol spectrum disorder samples. *Archives of Clinical Neuropsychology, 30*, 192–199.

8. **B—psychiatric** *The PAI allows for evaluation of exaggerated psychopathology so would be most useful in a psychiatrically focused clinic; it does not contain SVT scales sensitive to exaggeration of injury or illness like the MMPI-2-RF does, so it would be less useful for a neurological, rehabilitation, or general medical setting where feigned/exaggerated psychopathology is less common than feigned/exaggerated illness- or injury-related complaints.*

Reference: Morey, L. C. (2007). *Personality Assessment Inventory Professional Manual*. Odessa, FL: Psychological Assessment Resources.

9. **A—true positive/(true positives + false positives)** *The diagnostic probability of a particular condition of interest is dependent upon the ratio of True Positives/(True Positives + False Positives). Another way to represent this is with the positive likelihood ratio (LR+), obtained by dividing the True Positive by the False Positives associated with a specific PVT score.*

Reference: Larrabee, G. J. (2015). Performance and symptom validity: A perspective from the adult literature. In M. W. Kirkwood (Ed.). *Validity testing in child and adolescent assessment* (pp. 62–76). New York, NY: Guilford Press.

10. **A—lower than** *Sensitivity and specificity are not affected by base rates. In contrast, both positive predictive probability (PPP) and negative predictive power (NPP) are influenced by the base rate of the condition of interest. The less frequent a condition occurs, the lower the PPP will be, assuming sensitivity and specificity remain the same.*

Reference: Larrabee, G. J. (2015). Performance and symptom validity: A perspective from the adult literature. In M.W. Kirkwood (Ed.). *Validity testing in child and adolescent assessment* (pp. 62–76). New York, NY: Guilford Press.

Recommended Readings

Bush, S. S., Ruff, R. M., Troster, A. I., Barth, J. T., Koffler, S. P., Pliskin, N. H., . . . Silver, C. H. (2005). Symptom validity assessment: Practice issues and medical necessity. NAN policy and planning committee. *Archives of Clinical Neuropsychology, 20*, 419–426.

DeRight, J., & Carone, D. A. (2015). Assessment of effort in children: A systematic review. *Child Neuropsychology, 21*, 1–24.

Heilbronner, R. L., Sweet, J. J., Morgan, J. E., Larrabee, G. J., Millis, S. R., & Conference Participants. (2009). American Academy of Clinical Neuropsychology consensus conference statement on the neuropsychological assessment of effort, response bias, and malingering. *The Clinical Neuropsychologist, 23*, 1093–1129.

Kirkwood, M. W. (Ed.). (2015). *Validity testing in child and adolescent assessment: Evaluating exaggeration, feigning, and noncredible effort*. New York, NY: Guilford Press.

Larrabee, G. J. (2012). Performance validity and symptom validity in neuropsychological assessment. *Journal of the International Neuropsychological Society, 18*, 625–631.

Larrabee, G. J. (2014). False-positive rates associated with the use of multiple performance and symptom validity tests. *Archives of Clinical Neuropsychology, 29*, 364–373.

Martin, P. K., Schroeder, R. W., & Odland, A. P. (2015). Neuropsychologists' validity testing beliefs and practices: A survey of North-American professionals. *The Clinical Neuropsychologist, 29*, 741–776.

Schroeder, R. W., Martin, P. K., & Odland, A. P. (2016). Expert beliefs and practices regarding neuropsychological validity testing. *The Clinical Neuropsychologist, 30*, 515–535.

Section III Disorders and Conditions: Neurodevelopmental

13   Intellectual Disability

Jennifer L. Huffman

Definition

As part of a multimethod approach, the identification of intellectual disability (ID), formerly known as mental retardation, involves several aspects:

- Intellectual functioning is typically measured with individually administered intelligence tests, with an intelligence quotient (IQ) score of approximately two standard deviations below the population mean (65–75) needed to diagnose ID.

- Individuals with ID also need to show deficits in *adaptive functioning* relative to expectations for chronological age and sociocultural background in conceptual, social, and practical domains across multiple environments, such as home, school, work, and community.

- The onset of symptoms occurs during the developmental period, specifically during childhood or adolescence.

- Severity of ID is defined on the basis of *adaptive functioning* (not IQ scores) because *adaptive functioning* determines the level of supports required, and IQ measures are less valid in the tail end of the IQ range.

Neuropathology

The majority of cases of ID result from changes in early brain development, which can be influenced to some extent by environmental factors. Research is growing regarding neuropathology for specific etiologies of ID.

- Changes in early brain development can result in reduced cerebral volume or severe diffuse pathology.

- In some cases, microcephaly with differential volume reduction in certain regions of the brain is evident (e.g., fetal alcohol syndrome).

- In other cases (e.g., autism), enlarged head circumference is accompanied by mild ventricular enlargements and/or enlargement of some brain structures.

- These changes are believed to be related to a disruption of neuronal proliferation, apoptosis, migration, synaptogenesis, and/or dendritic pruning.

Epidemiology

The overall prevalence of ID globally is estimated to be less than 1%. The bell curve model that predicts 2.5% would have an IQ score of 70 or less does not take into account delayed diagnosis (especially for cases of *mild ID*) and the association between life expectancy and severity of ID. The ratio of males to females is 1.5:1, in large part due to the number of X-linked syndromes that cause ID (e.g., fragile X syndrome).

Causes of ID can be *genetic* (e.g., Down syndrome, fragile X syndrome, Williams syndrome, Tay-Sachs disease, maple syrup urine disease, Prader-Willi syndrome, Angelman syndrome, Klinefelter syndrome, tuberous sclerosis) or *acquired* (e.g., prematurity/low birth weight, exposure to alcohol and other drugs, environmental toxins, traumatic brain injury, infections, iodine deficiency, stroke, epilepsy, meningitis, whooping cough, anoxia). The remaining cases are idiopathic or of unknown cause.

Down syndrome is the most prevalent form of ID with a known genetic etiology. Fragile X syndrome is the most common familial or inherited form of ID with a known genetic etiology (see Chapter 18, Chromosomal and Genetic Syndromes, for more detail). The leading worldwide preventable cause of ID is iodine deficiency causing thyroid hormone deficiency during pregnancy. Another common environmental and preventable cause of ID is fetal alcohol syndrome.

Current guidelines recommend chromosome microarray as a first-line test for children with ID of an unknown cause, which replaces the standard karyotype and fluorescent in situ hybridization (FISH) tests. Other important tests include fragile X testing, testing for inborn errors of metabolism, and brain MRI in certain children. Establishing an etiologic diagnosis confers certain benefits, such as: clarifying etiology, understanding prognosis or expected clinical course, discussing genetic recurrence risks, identifying potential complications, and providing condition specific family support.

Morbidity depends on the severity of ID, as well as comorbid diagnoses.

- Approximately 85% of individuals with ID are classified in the mild range. Individuals with *mild ID* show delays in language but are usually fluent speakers in adolescence. They may acquire academic skills up to the sixth-grade level. They are immature in social interactions, with more concrete language and problem-solving skills compared to same-age peers. They may function appropriately with personal care but need some support with complex daily living skills relative to peers. Competitive employment is often attained in jobs that do not emphasize conceptual skills. They often require support for making healthcare/legal decisions and raising a family.

- Approximately 10% are classified as *moderate ID*. They normally attain functional language by adolescence, acquire academic skills up to the second-grade level, and require moderate levels of supervision. They demonstrate a capacity for establishing meaningful relationships with family and friends but have difficulty accurately perceiving social cues, with limited social judgment and decision-making skills. With extensive teaching, they can care for basic personal needs and participate in household tasks (reminders may be needed). Independent employment in jobs requiring limited conceptual and communication skills is possible, with considerable support needed to manage certain aspects, such as social expectations, scheduling, and financial management. Development of recreational skills requires additional supports and learning over an extended period of time. Maladaptive behavior (present in a significant minority) can cause social problems.

- About 3–4% show *severe ID* and display limited language (e.g., single words or phrases and use of gestural communication), demonstrate poor academic-related skills (e.g., may demonstrate familiarity with the alphabet and simple counting), and require extensive supervision. They depend on family members and familiar others for pleasure and help. They cannot make responsible decisions regarding well-being of self or others. Work and recreation skills require ongoing supervision and support. Maladaptive behavior (present in a significant minority) can include self-injury.

- The remaining 1–2% exhibit *profound ID* and may learn single words, acquire no academic skills, and require pervasive supervision and support for all activities. Conceptual skills generally involve using physical objects in a goal-directed manner. They may understand simple instructions or gestures and express themselves primarily through nonverbal, non-symbolic communication. They enjoy relationships with well-known family members or familiar others. They might be able to participate in some activities of daily living. Simple actions with objects form the basis of vocational activities. Comorbid physical and sensory impairments may prevent functional use of objects and participation in many social, home, recreational, and vocational activities. Maladaptive behavior is present in a significant minority.

Persons with limited intellectual development learn more slowly than persons with typical intellectual development, making it difficult for them to acquire new information and learn skills important for independent living. The majority of individuals with ID reside with family members, although others reside in group homes or live semi-independently with some supervision. Individuals with *mild ID* often work successfully in supported employment settings, with some success being reported for the other three types of ID as well.

Research suggests that persons with different forms of ID differ behaviorally (e.g., boys with fragile X syndrome and Down syndrome). Furthermore, behavioral differences can be found depending on the type of transmission. For example, Angelman syndrome results from a deletion on chromosome 15 contributed by the mother, whereas Prader-Willi syndrome results from a deletion on the same chromosome contributed by the father or by receiving two chromosome 15's contributed by the mother (maternal uniparental disomy). Angelman syndrome involves ID, sleep disturbance, seizures, jerky movements, frequent laughter or smiling, and usually a happy demeanor. In contrast, Prader-Willi syndrome involves low muscle tone, short stature, incomplete sexual development, ID, compulsive behaviors, and chronic feelings of hunger that lead to excessive eating. Moreover, individuals with Prader-Willi syndrome caused by the deletion show greater maladaptive behaviors and cognitive impairment than individuals with Prader-Willi syndrome caused by uniparental disomy. Certain personality characteristics associated with particular syndromes might affect morbidity. For example, an outgoing nature might predict increased vulnerability to being taken advantage of by others, and mood disturbance could impact the ability to live or work with others.

Individuals with ID have a shorter life expectancy (in the 60s) than individuals without ID (in the 70s). Although life expectancy has improved overall in recent years, a good deal of variability is apparent depending on the cause and severity of the ID. For example, the life expectancy for individuals with Tay-Sachs disease is 4 or 5 years, and the life expectancy for individuals with Down syndrome is 60 years.

Determinants of Severity

By definition, an ID diagnosis requires a combination of an individually administered intelligence test and a formal measure of *adaptive functioning*. Deficits in intellectual functions such as reasoning, problem solving, planning, abstract thinking, judgment, academic skills, and learning from experience need to be confirmed by both clinical assessment and individualized, standardized intelligence testing. Current diagnostic guidelines emphasize the importance of assessing *adaptive functioning* and relying on this information to specify the severity of ID. Deficits in adaptive skills limit functioning in one or more activities of daily living, such as competence in language, memory, academic skills, practical knowledge, judgment in novel situations, social communication skills, social judgment, friendships, personal care, job responsibilities, financial management, self-management of behavior, recreation, and work.

Scales administered early in development were not designed as measures of intelligence, and research suggests they are most predictive of subsequent identification of ID for children who score lowest in the developmental quotient range. Commonly used measures of developmental functioning include the Bayley Scales of Infant Development and the Mullen Scales of Early Learning. Frequently used measures of intellectual functioning include the Wechsler series intelligence tests, the Differential Abilities Scales, the Kaufman series intelligence tests, the Stanford-Binet Intelligence Scales, and the Leiter International Performance Scales. Interpretation of scores on these measures needs to take into account the standard error of measurement for a given test because scores falling at the border could reasonably be categorized as ID depending on *adaptive functioning* level. See Chapter 8, Psychometrics, Test Design, and Essential Statistics, and Chapter 9, Test Administration, Interpretation, and Issues in Assessment, regarding psychometric issues in general and confidence intervals in particular.

Commonly used measures of *adaptive functioning* include the Vineland Scales of Adaptive Behavior, Adaptive Behavior Assessment System (ABAS), and Scales of Independent Behavior (SIB). These measures are questionnaires or interviews administered to family members, caregivers, or teachers who know the individual well. Commonly evaluated adaptive skills include conceptual skills (e.g., competence in memory, language, basic academic skills, problem-solving, judgment in novel situations), social skills (e.g., awareness of the thoughts and feelings of others, empathy, interpersonal communication skills, peer relationships, social judgment), and practical skills (e.g., personal care, job responsibilities, financial management, recreation, self-management of behavior). Adaptive measures also may include ratings of fine and gross motor functioning. It is critical to include multiple measures of *adaptive functioning* from multiple sources, and interpret scores from standardized measures and information gathered from interviews with clinical judgment given the potential for bias and the importance of these measures in determining severity of ID.

Presentation, Disease Course, and Recovery

The first indicators of ID often include failure to meet developmental milestones and/or physical characteristics associated with certain conditions that cause ID (e.g., facial features in Down syndrome, growth deficiency and/or craniofacial abnormalities in fetal alcohol syndrome). Individuals with ID often exhibit simple, concrete play. Behavioral outbursts and temper tantrums early on are common. In less affected individuals, indications may not be apparent until they enter school and fail to meet educational expectations for their age, particularly on tasks requiring abstract reasoning, retention, and generalization of information. Individuals with ID often exhibit motor and language developmental delays, have a hard time remembering information, struggle to understand social rules, have difficulty understanding the consequences of their actions, and have difficulty solving problems. Their skill development tends to level out in early adolescence, with growing gaps between them and normally developing peers once expectations for abstract thinking and problem-solving increase.

In the United States, early intervention services are provided by each state from birth to 3 years of age. Individuals with ID are eligible to receive special education services under federal law from ages 3 to 21. In Canada, similar services are provided but vary by province.

- Mainstreaming for children with *mild ID* is the preferred option by many parents and educators and has the advantage of exposing individuals with ID to children with normally developing social and emotional skills. However, individualized attention may be more limited in a mainstream setting.

- Children with more severe disability are often placed in self-contained classrooms or attend schools for students with special needs in order to receive appropriate support for their multiple needs.
- Children with ID require special accommodations and modifications to their curriculum for optimal learning such as:
  - having tasks broken down into small component steps to be learned in sequence.
  - hands-on, concrete approaches and visual materials when being taught.
  - immediate feedback regarding performance.
- As children reach junior high school, emphasis typically shifts from acquiring academic skills to acquiring functional skills, such as learning how to count money, management of personal hygiene, learning social communication/norms, and low-skill job preparation.
- In some states, students with a diagnosed ID are eligible to receive support services through the educational system for longer than federal law requirements. However, after age 21, individuals with ID are typically serviced through the state departments of developmental disabilities.

Because it is most often not possible to normalize the core cognitive deficits in ID, interventions focus on prevention and improving quality of life. Prevention efforts for reducing the incidence of ID include:

- Education regarding proper nutrition and eliminating alcohol and drug use during pregnancy
- Childhood helmet utilization
- Childhood vaccinations
- Screening of medical and genetic conditions that are known to cause ID if not treated early (e.g., phenylketonuria, hypothyroidism)

Agencies around the world provide assistance for individuals with ID through the development of individual service plans. Such plans are developed following an assessment of individual needs and competencies to optimize the functioning and life satisfaction of the individual with ID. Interventions are recommended to improve social and independent living skills and create a match between the environment and abilities of the individuals being assessed. *Applied behavior analysis* (ABA) is an evidence-based intervention program used to treat problem behaviors in ID. Individuals with ID are often placed in supported employment situations with a goal of helping them reach the least restrictive level of supervision and support. Medical intervention and medication treatment are used to address comorbid conditions.

Recovery is not expected in individuals with ID. Stable performance on IQ and *adaptive functioning* measures is expected over time, with some exceptions. Depending on the underlying etiology of ID, certain individuals are at increased risk for problems as they age. For example, evidence suggests that individuals with Down syndrome and fragile X syndrome show declining IQ scores into adulthood. Additionally, individuals with Down syndrome are prone to developing Alzheimer disease and tend to die within 8 years of this diagnosis. Associated illnesses, such as heart disease or diabetes, are common in certain conditions (e.g., Williams syndrome, Down syndrome) and require special treatment considerations to prevent premature death.

Expectations for Neuropsychological Assessment Results

Historically, ID has been thought to affect cognition in a global way, with general slowing in development. However, recent evidence suggests that specific cognitive and behavioral profiles occur across various ID conditions.

- *Intelligence/Achievement* Performance on intelligence tests usually measures at 70 or below, although it is sometimes as high as 75. Declining scores are expected for certain causes of ID (e.g., Down syndrome, fragile X syndrome). In certain conditions, relative differences in verbal and nonverbal abilities are expected such as in autism (verbal worse than nonverbal) or Williams syndrome (verbal better than nonverbal). Performance on measures of academic achievement vary, with some individuals with ID performing quite well on rote measures such as word recognition, spelling, and solving simple mathematics problems. These individuals often perform much more poorly on higher level academic tasks such as reading comprehension, written production, mathematics reasoning, and other similar tasks that involve increased inferential reasoning and problem-solving.

- *Attention* Problems with attention are common in individuals with ID. Research suggests that the prevalence of attention problems varies according to the etiology of the ID. In other words, some individuals with ID exhibit worse attention deficits than would be predicted by intellectual level alone. Proper diagnosis and treatment of attention disorders is important in treating individuals with ID because these comorbid problems often go untreated.

- *Processing Speed* Slowed processing speed and extra time needed to process cognitive information is a common problem for individuals with ID.

- *Language* Language functioning varies by severity and cause of ID, as well as by environmental influences. For example, individuals with Williams syndrome often show relative strengths in language tasks compared to their visuospatial skills. One-word receptive language skills are often a relative strength in individuals with ID who have received extensive language support through early intervention or an enriched home environment.

- *Visuospatial* Visuospatial problems are often found in individuals with ID and vary by etiology. For example, spatial cognition is below mental age expectations for individuals with Williams syndrome yet is often a relative strength for individuals with autism or Down syndrome.

- *Memory* Evidence of different profiles of memory difficulties for different causes of ID are emerging from the literature, including differences in verbal and spatial immediate memory and short-term memory among groups that do not fully correspond to general differences in cognitive functioning. In general, individuals with ID exhibit weaknesses with long-term memory.

- *Executive Functions* Executive functions are generally impaired in individuals with ID, and a growing body of research is attempting to explore the specific executive functioning differences for individuals with ID. For example, some individuals with ID have good working memory skills yet poor pragmatic judgment and trouble-shooting abilities. Some have shown deficits with sequential processing or inhibitory control. Others show specific problems with updating working memory. Yet others display behavioral problems associated with attention disorders such as inattention, hyperactivity, impulsivity, and transition problems.

- *Sensorimotor Functions* Significant delays in the development of all sensorimotor skills is expected in individuals with ID.

- *Emotion and Personality* Individuals with ID often exhibit problems with impulse control, frustration tolerance, behavioral regulation, mood, and low self-esteem that vary with diagnosis type and age. For example, children with fetal alcohol syndrome often exhibit increasing behavioral problems during puberty. Specific syndromes have certain associated personality characteristics, such as the outgoing nature and associated fears and anxieties in children with Williams syndrome. Additionally, young children with Prader-Willi syndrome are described as friendly and affectionate but the onset of hyperphagia is associated with increased temper tantrums, stubbornness, impulsivity, food stealing, and compulsive behaviors.

- *Symptom and Performance Validity* Assessment of test engagement is important in individuals with ID, although research suggests that a cautious approach is needed when using common measures of performance validity. Considered in isolation, performance validity tests (PVTs) might result in misclassification of individuals with ID as providing noncredible effort, given the possibility of false-positive errors. At the same time, well-motivated individuals with IQs in the mild ID range rarely fail PVTs that have been demonstrated to have high specificity. In choosing PVTs for an individual with ID, consideration needs to be given to the specific task demands of the test, as well as the individual's areas of cognitive deficit, reading level, behavioral problems, neurological disease, and age. For individuals with ID, more stringent cutoff scores (to maintain at least 90% specificity) might be needed on some PVTs and alternate administration might be required (e.g., a combined oral-computer administration with the examiner operating the mouse, trackpad, or keys). When possible, consider the use of PVTs specifically designed for individuals with ID. Sensitivity and specificity for determining poor validity is maximized by failure on two or three PVTs using appropriate adjusted cutoffs. Keep in mind that below-chance performance is still indicative of malingering, and research suggests that approximately 10% to 13% of low-IQ individuals seeking disability benefits obtain significantly below-chance performance. Carefully considering developmental history and utilizing multiple PVTs, qualitative analysis of response errors, and observations of behavioral inconsistencies are crucial when evaluating the validity of results for individuals with ID.

Considerations when Treating Patients with ID

- *Driving* Research indicates that individuals with *mild ID* are capable of learning the skills necessary to drive, particularly if their driving is limited to short distances and familiar routes. However, few programs provide needed assistance with obtaining a license.

- *Work* As noted, individuals with *mild ID* are often successful in supported work settings.

- *School and Vocational Training* Individuals with ID qualify for educational programming from age 3 to 21 under United States federal law; additional services before and after these ages may be provided, but the duration varies by state. Individual service plans are developed based on needs and competencies with a goal of utilizing competencies while addressing needs to optimize functioning. Individuals with *mild ID* are often successful in vocational training programs with supervision and support.

- *Capacity* Assessment of the decision-making capacity for individuals with *mild ID* requires careful consideration of the specific capacity in question, along with relevant laws.

- *Psychological and Emotional Issues* Individuals with ID are about four or five times more likely to be diagnosed with a psychiatric disorder than normally developing peers. Thus, assessment and treatment for comorbid psychiatric disorders is important.

- *Severe Psychiatric Complications* Individuals with severe psychiatric complications are at increased risk for behavioral problems and need for extensive supervision. Psychiatric treatment and specialized group home placement are often required.

- *Medications* Medication management is recommended to treat comorbid problems with ID, including problems with attention, underlying seizures, diabetes, heart disease, and mood disorders. Supervision to ensure proper administration of medications is often needed.

- *Risk Factor Modification* Primary prevention of ID includes improving the nutritional status of women of child-bearing age (e.g., folic acid and iodine supplementation), immunizations prior to pregnancy, avoiding exposure to harmful chemicals during pregnancy (e.g., alcohol, nicotine, or illicit drugs), education regarding increased risk of complications in pregnancy with advancing maternal age, detection and care for high-risk pregnancies, maternal screening and treatment (e.g., syphilis, Rh incompatibility), provision of high-quality neonatal intensive care services, reduction of environmental pollutants (e.g., lead), immunization of children, and genetic counseling. Advances in prenatal screening and diagnosis also offer preventative options but carry ethical implications. Secondary prevention includes neonatal screening and appropriate medical treatment (e.g., phenylketonuria, galactosemia, hypothyroidism) and intensive early intervention services for children at risk for developing ID. Tertiary prevention includes appropriate education, training, and support for families and caregivers.

- *Interpersonal Relationships* Individuals with ID are often capable of establishing interpersonal relationships with peers of a similar mental age. As they age, keeping up with rapid-paced conversation becomes increasingly difficult, given slowed processing speed and communication limitations. Many individuals with ID form intimate relationships, although they are also generally at risk for being exploited, including sexually.

- *Practical Issues* Care needs to be taken as individuals with ID transition from pediatricians to adult-oriented healthcare providers, who may be ill-prepared to treat their associated medical and mental health conditions. Because individuals with ID often live with their aging parents, parents should be advised to set up caregiving arrangements in the event of their incapacity. Such a transition should be made prior to the event of their incapacity to prevent an adult child with ID from coping with a major transition and the incapacity of their parents at the same time.

- *Rehabilitation Considerations* An individualized approach should be taken when developing a treatment program for individuals with ID because many individual differences influence appropriate programming. Providers need to fully understand the patient's premorbid level of functioning by conducting a careful review of available records. Providers also need to pay special attention to any behavioral needs that can be addressed through a formal behavioral modification system in addition to necessary rehabilitation services.

- *Cultural Issues* Caution is needed when testing individuals from minority groups, given controversy with possible test bias. Sensitivity to cultural and language issues and use of a multimethod approach is recommended.

Relevant Definitions

Adaptive functioning Abilities in the areas of communication, self-care, home living, social skills, community use, self-direction, health and safety, functional academics, leisure, and work.

Applied behavior analysis (ABA) A highly structured behavioral treatment with empirical support for treating problem behaviors in individuals with ID.

Mild ID Approximately 85% of individuals with ID score in the mild range. Such individuals show delays in language but are usually fluent speakers in adolescence. They may acquire academic skills up to the sixth-grade level. They often require intermittent supervision and guidance.

Moderate ID Approximately 10% of individuals with ID score in the moderate range. Such individuals normally attain functional language by adolescence, acquire academic skills up to the second-grade level, and require moderate levels of supervision.

Profound ID Approximately 1–2% of individuals with ID score in the profound range. Such individuals may learn single words, acquire no academic skills, and require extensive supervision. They are dependent on others for physical care.

Severe ID Approximately 3–4% of individuals with ID score in the severe range. Such individuals display limited language, may demonstrate familiarity with the alphabet and simple counting, and require extensive supervision.

Intellectual Disability Questions

NOTE: Questions 19, 78, and 112 on the First Full-Length Practice Examination, Questions 22 and 56 on the Second Full-Length Practice Examination, Questions 25, 94, and 109 on the Third Full-Length Practice Examination, and Questions 31, 71, 88, and 122 on the Fourth Full-Length Practice Examination are from this chapter.

1. Susan mentioned that her adopted child is short in stature and has ID. It is possible that she could have a diagnosis of this most common known environmental cause of ID in the United States.
   - (a) prematurity
   - (b) anoxia at birth
   - (c) lead toxicity
   - (d) fetal alcohol syndrome

2. A child's mother expresses frustration that a comprehensive chromosome microarray test did not identify a genetic cause for her son's diagnosis of ID. You explain that the child could still have a genetic disorder not detected by the test to explain the ID diagnosis because there are _____ known genetic causes of ID.
   - (a) more than 1,000
   - (b) 500
   - (c) 100
   - (d) 10

3. Sally is 10 years of age and earned a score of 30 on measures of intelligence and adaptive functioning. She has little understanding of written language. She speaks in single words or phrases, such as requesting food or drink. She understands simple commands. She is learning the alphabet and can

count to 3. She requires support for carrying out activities of daily living, and her parents provide her with constant supervision. Sally's level of ID is best classified as _____.

(a) mild

(c) severe

(b) moderate

(d) profound

4. Maple syrup urine disease is an example of what classification of disorders associated with ID?

(a) disorders of brain formation

(c) chromosomal disorders

(b) inborn errors of metabolism

(d) environmental influences

5. The United States and Canada mandate newborn screening for which two preventable causes of ID?

(a) phenylketonuria (PKU) and congenital hypothyroidism

(b) maple syrup urine disease and Down syndrome

(c) PKU and fetal alcohol syndrome

(d) galactosemia and fragile X syndrome

6. The leading preventable cause of ID globally is _____.

(a) prematurity

(c) lead toxicity

(b) iodine deficiency

(d) fetal alcohol syndrome

7. Current guidelines recommend _____ as a first-line test for children with ID.

(a) chromosome microarray

(c) blood lead levels

(b) magnetic resonance imaging of the brain

(d) fluorescent in situ hybridization (FISH)

8. Kim is 35-years-old and earned a total standard score of 75 on an individually administered intelligence test, a score that was consistent with previous measures of intellectual functioning as a child. Kim lives at home with her parents. She makes small purchases but cannot manage her checking account. Her parents now administer her diabetes medication to her because medication noncompliance has led to several hospitalizations. She rides the bus to her job at a local cafeteria where she receives close supervision in clearing tables and washing dishes. She reads at a 4th grade level. Her parents remind her to take showers. She seemed to have a strong and supportive network of friends with learning problems. She is most likely to have _____.

(a) borderline intellectual functioning

(c) mild ID

(b) severe learning disability

(d) adaptive living skill disorder

9. Joe is nonverbal but demonstrates an understanding of the word "no" and his mother shaking her head by crying out. He smiles broadly in response to calling his name or playing his favorite music. He is incontinent and needs to use a wheelchair. Fine motor impairments prevent functional use of objects, and Joe takes most of his nutrition from nightly tube feedings. He enjoys watching movies and children playing in the park. Joe requires constant supervision from his parents. Which severity level of ID best describes Joe's functioning?

(a) mild ID

(c) severe ID

(b) moderate ID

(d) profound ID

10. A child with mild ID presents to an inpatient psychiatric unit for increased symptoms of depression and aggressive behavior. He is short for his age and seems "floppy" in tone. He is overweight, and his parents reported that they had to put locks on all the cupboards and refrigerator at home given his insatiable appetite. He is quite stubborn and engages in repetitive behaviors including asking constant questions and skin picking. He has been gaining weight steadily over the past few years, and his pediatrician sent him to a nutritionist for a consultation. Based on the description, which genetic cause of ID should be suspected?

(a) Down syndrome

(b) Prader-Willi syndrome

(c) Angelman syndrome

(d) fragile X syndrome

Intellectual Disability Answers

1. **D—fetal alcohol syndrome** *Fetal alcohol syndrome is the most common known environmental and preventable cause of ID in the United States.*

   Reference: Mattson, S. N., & Vaurio, L. (2010). Fetal alcohol spectrum disorders. In K. O. Yeates, M. D. Ris, H. G. Taylor, & B. F. Pennington (Eds.), *Pediatric neuropsychology: Research, theory, and practice* (2nd ed., pp. 447–470). New York, NY: Guilford Press.

2. **A—more than 1,000** *The number of known genetic causes of ID is growing exponentially with advances in genetic testing. The incidence of idiopathic or unknown causes of ID is decreasing as a result.*

   Reference: King, B. H., Toth, K. E., Hodapp, R. M., & Dykens, E. M. (2009). Intellectual disability. In B. J. Sadock, V. A. Sadock, & P. Ruiz (Eds.), *Comprehensive textbook of psychiatry* (9th ed., pp. 3444–3474). Philadelphia, PA: Lippincott, Williams, & Wilkins.

3. **C—severe** *Sally's performance on standardized testing, activities of daily living, and need for supervision fit best in the severe category.*

   Reference: American Psychiatric Association. (2013). *Diagnostic and statistical manual of mental disorders* (5th ed.). Arlington, VA: American Psychiatric Publishing.

4. **B—inborn errors of metabolism** *Maple syrup urine disease is a rare genetic disorder characterized by deficiency of particular enzymes to metabolize certain protein amino acids properly. The condition gets its name from the characteristic sweet odor of affected infants' urine, which resembles maple syrup.*

   Reference: Levy, P. A. (2009). Inborn errors of metabolism: Part 2: Specific disorders. *Pediatrics in Review, 30,* e20–e28.

5. **A—phenylketonuria (PKU) and congenital hypothyroidism** *All states and provinces/territories screen for PKU and congenital hypothyroidism.*

   Reference: Therrell, B. L., Padilla, C. D., Loeber, J. G., Kneisser, I., Saadallah, A., Borrajo, G. J. C., & Adams, J. (2015). Current status of newborn screening worldwide: 2015. *Seminars in Perinatology, 39,* 171–187.

6. **B—iodine deficiency** *Iodine deficiency disorders are one of the biggest worldwide public health problems. Iodine deficiency during pregnancy results in impaired synthesis of thyroid hormones by the mother and fetus, often resulting in ID.*

   Reference: Zimmerman, M. B., Jooste, P. L, & Pandav, C. S. (2008). Iodine-deficiency disorders. *The Lancet, 372,* 1251–1262.

7. **A—chromosome microarray** *Recently published guidelines by the American Academy of Pediatrics lists chromosome microarray as a first-line test for ID, replacing the standard karyotype and fluorescent in situ hybridization (FISH) tests for the child with ID of unknown etiology.*

Reference: Moeschler, J. B., Shevell, M., & Committee on Genetics. (2014). Comprehensive evaluation of the child with intellectual disability or global developmental delays. *Pediatrics, 134*(3), e903–e918.

8. **C—mild ID** *Kim's IQ score falls within the mild ID range when considering the margin of error (± 5), and descriptors of Kim's adaptive functioning and need for supervision suggests a level of functioning in the mild ID range.*

Reference: American Psychiatric Association. (2013). *Diagnostic and statistical manual of mental disorders* (5th ed.). Arlington, VA: American Psychiatric Publishing.

9. **D—profound ID** *Descriptions of Joe's behavior indicate extremely low cognitive functioning and need for constant supervision, with maximum assistance needed to carry out basic activities of daily living.*

Reference: American Psychiatric Association. (2013). *Diagnostic and statistical manual of mental disorders* (5th ed.). Arlington, VA: American Psychiatric Publishing.

10. **B—Prader-Willi syndrome** *Overeating and obesity are defining features of Prader-Willi syndrome, likely resulting from a disruption in the functioning of the hypothalamus of affected individuals.*

Reference: King, B. H., Toth, K. E., Hodapp, R. M., & Dykens, E. M. (2009). Intellectual disability. In B. J. Sadock, V. A. Sadock, & P. Ruiz (Eds.), *Comprehensive textbook of psychiatry* (9th ed., pp. 3444–3474). Philadelphia, PA: Lippincott, Williams, & Wilkins.

Recommended Readings

American Psychiatric Association. (2013). *Diagnostic and statistical manual of mental disorders* (5th ed.). Arlington, VA: American Psychiatric Publishing.

Chafetz, M. (2018). Disability. In J. E. Morgan & J. H. Ricker (Eds.), *Textbook of clinical neuropsychology* (2nd ed., pp. 980–999). New York, NY: Routledge.

Harris, J. C. (2010). *Intellectual disability: A guide for families and professionals.* New York, NY: Oxford University Press.

King, B. H., Toth, K. E., Hodapp, R. M., & Dykens, E. M. (2009). Intellectual disability. In B. J. Sadock, V. A. Sadock, & P. Ruiz (Eds.), *Comprehensive textbook of psychiatry* (9th ed., pp. 3444–3474). Philadelphia, PA: Lippincott Williams & Wilkins.

McGrath, L. M., & Peterson, R. L. (2009). Intellectual disabilities. In B. F. Pennington (Ed.), *Diagnosing learning disorders* (2nd ed., pp. 181–226). New York, NY: The Guilford Press.

Mervis, C. B., & John, A. E. (2010). Intellectual disability syndromes. In K. O. Yeates, M. D. Ris, H. G. Taylor, & B. F. Pennington (Eds.), *Pediatric neuropsychology: Research, theory, and practice* (2nd ed., pp. 447–470). New York, NY: The Guilford Press.

14   Autism Spectrum Disorder

Deborah Fein and Eva Troyb

Definition

Autism spectrum disorder (ASD) is a spectrum of autism phenotypes characterized by deficits in communication and socialization, as well as by the presence of *restricted and repetitive behaviors (RRBs)*. In the fourth edition of the Diagnostic and Statistical Manual of Mental Disorders (DSM-IV), the autism spectrum included autistic disorder (AD); pervasive developmental disorder, not otherwise specified (PDD-NOS); Asperger's disorder; childhood disintegrative disorder; and Rett's disorder. However, in DSM-5, the disorders have been collapsed into a single diagnostic category of "autism spectrum disorder." This was done because the American Psychiatric Committee responsible for the DSM-5 revision concluded that while ASD vs. non-ASD is a reliable distinction, distinctions among the subtypes are not.

Deficits in Communication and Socialization

A diagnosis of ASD requires that individuals present with a persistent deficit in social communication and social interaction across multiple contexts, defined as *all of the following* in DSM-5 (Table 14.1):

1. Impaired social-emotional reciprocity, ranging, for example, from abnormal social approach and failure of normal back-and-forth conversation; to reduced sharing of interests, emotions, or affect; to failure to initiate or respond to social interaction.

2. Deficits in nonverbal communicative behaviors used for social interaction, ranging, for example, from poorly integrated verbal and nonverbal communication; to abnormalities in eye contact and body language or deficits in understanding and use of gestures; to a total lack of facial expressions and nonverbal communication.

3. Deficits in developing, maintaining, and understanding relationships, ranging, for example, from difficulties adjusting behavior to suit various social contexts; to difficulties in sharing imaginative play or in making friends; to absence of interest in peers.

Presence of Restricted and Repetitive Behaviors (RRBs) and Interests

A core feature of ASDs is *restricted and repetitive* patterns of behaviors or interests, defined as *at least two of the following* in DSM-5:

1. Stereotyped or repetitive motor movements, use of objects, or speech

2. Insistence on sameness, inflexible adherence to routines, or ritualized patterns of verbal or nonverbal behavior

3. Highly restricted, fixated interests that are abnormal in intensity or focus

4. Hyper- or hypo-reactivity to sensory input or unusual interest in sensory aspects of the environment

TABLE 14.1 Diagnostic and Statistical Manual of Mental Disorders (DSM-5) Diagnostic Criteria

Impairment in social communication and social interaction (all three must be present)	• Impaired social-emotional reciprocity • Impaired nonverbal communication • Failure to develop or maintain appropriate peer relationships
Restricted, repetitive patterns of behavior and interest (at least two must be present)	• Repetitive behaviors or speech • Insistence on sameness • Unusual preoccupations or interests • Sensory interests

NOTE: The DSM-5 requires both social/communicative impairments and RRBs. In the DSM-5, children with social communication deficits but no or only one repetitive behavior or interest may qualify for a diagnosis of Social (Pragmatic) Communication Disorder, which is a subcategory of Communication Disorder. The practical and research consequences of this change in diagnosis remain to be seen.

In addition, DSM-5 provides a severity dimension, along which symptoms should be rated, from Level 1 (requiring support) to Level 2 (requiring substantial support) to Level 3 (requiring very substantial support). Language disorder and intellectual disability (ID) are separately coded as ancillary features.

Asperger's Disorder

Note: Asperger's disorder is no longer a separate diagnosis in DSM-5 but is discussed here for historical background. Many individuals and families still identify as having Asperger's disorder.

Asperger's disorder was defined in DSM-IV by the presence of impaired social ability and RRBs *in the absence of a language delay or significant impairment in adaptive functioning.* Children and adolescents with Asperger's disorder were said to be interested in interacting with others, but these interactions were thought to be often odd or awkward. Controversy remains regarding the distinction between autistic disorder and Asperger's, including whether differences exist in genetic risk factors, family history, pathophysiology, treatment, and outcome of these conditions.

Rett's Disorder

Note: Rett's disorder is no longer a separate diagnosis in DSM-5 but is discussed here for historical background.

Rett's disorder is a rare (affects 1 in 10,000–15,000) genetic disorder that occurs primarily in females. It is associated with the *MeCP2* gene and is characterized by early typical development until the age of 6 to 18 months, followed by significant deterioration of motor and social skills. Rett's disorder is marked by a loss of purposeful hand movements, which are replaced by repetitive hand mannerisms, the most common of which is described as "hand-wringing" or "hand-washing." The disorder is also accompanied by progressive cerebral atrophy. After a period of regression, there is usually a plateau lasting months to years, followed by slow growth of skills. Outcome for these children is generally poor, with nonambulatory status and severe cognitive deficits expected.

Neuropathology

Autism is a neurodevelopmental syndrome highly determined by genetics that affects complex brain functions. Investigations into the neuroanatomy of autism implicate numerous structures and systems throughout the brain. The pathological effects are varied and have an unclear anatomical basis. There is no single region of abnormality that is consistent across individuals with autism, and brain structure and function often present in different ways across individuals and throughout development. Neuroanatomical investigations are complicated by the heterogeneity of clinical presentation, high rates of psychological and medical comorbidity, and early-life onset and presentation in a still developing brain. Current theories posit that dysfunction originates on both a biological level (e.g., genes, proteins, molecules) and across the hierarchy of levels of integration (e.g., subcellular assemblies to cells, tissues, brain regions, neural systems, and large brain units). It is thought that feedback from the environment shapes the phenotypic expression of autism's core symptomatology. High concordance rates in monozygotic twins and low concordance rates in dizygotic twins suggest that ASDs are complex genetic disorders with multiple loci contributing to a global phenotype.

Despite heterogeneity, a number of anatomical findings have been demonstrated consistently across studies. The most replicated biological finding is that brain size (i.e., weight, volume, and/or head circumference) is often larger than average in younger subjects. This shows a distinctive developmental course: brain size is normal or slightly small at birth, followed by a growth spurt between six and 24 months that results in larger than average brains, followed by a slowed growth that returns the brain size to average by later childhood. The corpus callosum is typically undersized and not enlarged proportionally to overall enlargement of the brain. There is involvement in the cerebellum, limbic system, basal ganglia, thalamus, and white matter, although this involvement varies markedly across age group and studies. Perfusion within the brain is lower, although the distribution of this perfusion has varied in measures across studies. Metabolic and diffusion tensor imaging measures suggest a reduction in fiber integrity and the density of metabolites, and recent studies suggest that some of these differences can be detected as young as 6 months of age. Research into the neurochemical basis of autism has demonstrated that monoamines may have an influence on systems that are commonly impaired in autism including mood, arousal, and attention. Hyperserotonemia (an increase in the serotonin levels in blood platelets) in blood was the earliest biological finding in autism and is generally replicated. The glutamate and gamma aminobutyric acid (GABA) systems show decreased activation and abnormalities in receptors across individuals with ASDs. In the last several years, researchers have focused on connections among brain networks as likely to be fruitful. For example, although not confirmed across multiple studies, some findings have suggested overconnected close brain areas and underconnected long-distance areas. Others have suggested atypical connections among the default mode network, social cognition network, and reward network. Some research centers are attempting to follow the growth of connections from the first year of life, for children likely to be at risk for autism (e.g., baby siblings of affected children, premature infants).

A growing body of empirical evidence supports a number of neuropsychological theories of ASDs, none of which is mutually exclusive. Individuals with ASDs are thought to have impairment of the higher level cognitive skills that underlie goal-oriented behavior in executive functioning, contributing to multiple aspects of executive functions, especially impairments in working memory, inhibition, flexibility, and self-monitoring. Individuals with autism are thought to have "weak central coherence," which contributes to difficulties in the integration of information from the environment into a meaningful whole. In particular, these individuals process featural and local elements of stimuli at the expense of global meaning. They have strengths in understanding and acquiring rote skills rather than those that require abstract thinking, inferences, or complex problem solving. Social motivation theories suggest that individuals with ASDs have a decreased level of motivation to orient to social stimuli, which derails emergence of normal developmental pathways of social and communication skills. Social cognitive theories focus on impairments in the capacity to represent and reason about the thoughts, intentions, beliefs, desires, feelings, memories, and knowledge of others (poor "*theory of mind*"). In addition, individuals with poor *theory of mind* may fail to understand that the points of view or knowledge of others may differ from their own. They will, therefore, be able to predict specific concrete actions of others from their experience but will not be able to modify these predictions based on the others' nonverbal communication cues or the social context.

Risk Factors

The heritability of autism, based on twin studies, is high. It is currently thought that genetic polymorphisms acting together, influenced by environmental contributions, are related to a complex etiology. There is some convergence of risk gene research on genes controlling synaptic functioning. Research currently suggests that heredity and early fetal development may play a causal role in autism, possibly in interaction with environmental risk factors. Other factors that may confer some risk for autism are being a younger sibling of an affected child, prematurity, advanced paternal age, and obstetric complications.

Epidemiology

Estimates of prevalence depend on the methods used and have generally increased over the last 30 years. Estimates across different countries and different ascertainment methods range from one in 38, to one in 200. Using 2014 data, the CDC reported an overall prevalence of one in 68, with prevalence in boys of one in 42 and in girls of one in 189. There is ongoing debate about the reality of the apparent increase in prevalence. One study in England that cast some doubt on the increase found similar prevalence across the adult lifespan, rather than increased prevalence in younger adults. Fombonne (2009) concludes: "There is evidence that the broadening of the concept, the expansion of diagnostic criteria, the development of services, and improved awareness of the condition have played a major role in explaining this increase, although it cannot be ruled out that other factors might have also contributed to that trend."

ASDs occur more commonly in males than females, with the most commonly accepted gender ratio of 4:1 male to female.

- The sex ratio appears to vary based on IQ, with females with ASDs tending to have lower verbal and nonverbal IQs. The male-to-female ratio approaches 2:1 in those with ASD and moderate to severe ID.

- Current evidence and research suggests that, on the whole, individuals with ASDs have reduced life expectancy. Elevated death rates have been linked to several specific causes, including seizures and accidents such as suffocation and drowning. Excess mortality is more significantly increased among individuals with ASDs with severe ID.

Comorbidity

Autism spectrum disorder is commonly comorbid with a number of psychological and emotional conditions. These comorbid conditions include: ID (comorbidity estimates vary from 40–70%), anxiety disorders (22–84% of cases, with high rates of specific phobia), depression (4–58%), tic disorders (6%), and seizure disorders (11–39%). Seizure disorders are more common in cases with comorbid ID. As many as 55% of individuals with ASD also commonly demonstrate symptoms of ADHD. The relationship between ASD and ADHD is still unclear and under active investigation. Some findings indicate that children with both diagnoses have more severe social impairments than children with ASD alone, that children with ASD plus ADHD combined subtype are more likely to have more deficits in social and adaptive functioning than children with ASD plus ADHD-inattentive subtype, and that ASD and ADHD may share genetic vulnerability.

Determinants of Severity

A diagnostic evaluation, involving both direct behavioral observation and parent interview, is helpful in determining the severity of an autism spectrum disorder. If the child is in an early intervention or school program, teacher informants can also be very helpful. The Autism Diagnostic Interview-Revised (ADI-R) is a parent interview that gathers information about early development and core deficits involved in ASDs. The ADI-R is useful in evaluating repetitive behaviors, stereotyped interests, and rigid preferences that may not be directly observable during an evaluation. It is more valid for children over the age of 2. The Autism Diagnostic Observation Schedule (ADOS) and ADOS-2 and ADOS-Toddler are interactive tools that involve direct observation of a behavioral sample through a series of reciprocal play and social routines. The ADOS allows a clinician to directly observe the presence and severity of ASD symptomatology, and there are different modules for children with different levels of language. The Modified Checklist for Autism in Toddlers (M-CHAT) and M-CHAT-Revised are autism-specific screening tools that identify children at elevated risk for autism. The American Academy of Pediatrics advises broad developmental screening at multiple ages, and autism specific screening at 18 and 24 months. The Childhood Autism Rating Scale (CARS) is a behavior rating scale that helps to identify children with an ASD and differentiate them from developmentally disabled children who do not have an ASD. The clinician rates a child on 15 items that are each representative of a characteristic, ability, or behavior common to children with autism and/or developmental disability more generally. Scores for each item are assigned based on severity and indicate how noticeably the child's behavior deviates from the behavior expected of a typically developing child of the same developmental level. The severity of an ASD is noted by elevated scores in each core domain for all of these measures; higher scores indicate more severe impairment in social and communicative abilities and elevated amounts and intensity of repetitive behaviors and stereotyped interests. Severity of cognitive delay and language delay are other very important measures of severity of impairment.

Presentation, Disease Course, and Outcome

Clear stages of progression of ASD are only evident in Rett's disorder. The behavioral presentation of the remaining phenotypes of ASD varies considerably across individuals, as well as across development.

- *First Year of Life*
  - Autism spectrum disorder can be reliably diagnosed as early as 18–24 months; however, some signs of ASD may be evident in children as young as 6 months of age.
  - Between 6 and 12 months of age, children who later receive an ASD diagnosis may exhibit the following behaviors:
    - Delayed vocal sound production
    - Decreased frequency of simple babbling
    - Reduced frequency of pointing or failure of pointing to develop
    - Atypical eye contact or gaze avoidance
    - Lack of social smiling
    - Failure to respond to name
    - Emotional flatness
    - Atypical disengagement of visual attention
    - Diminished interest in social interaction and adult language
    - Unusual and repetitive hand and finger mannerisms
  - Several biologic markers for ASD may also be present during this period and may include accelerated head growth, macrocephaly, and enlarged brain volume (including cerebral white and gray matter). Recent studies suggest that hyper-growth of the cortical surface can be seen in the second half of the first year.

- *Second Year of Life*
  - During the second year of life (12–24 months), symptoms described above become more evident. Additional symptoms that are generally noted during the second year include:
  - Delayed speech:
    - Delayed comprehension of phrases
    - Limited use of complex babble, single words, and phrases
    - Unusual prosody
    - Delayed and immediate echolalia
  - Limited use of nonverbal communication:
    - Reduced frequency of pointing and use of other gestures
    - Limited range of facial expressions
    - Facial expressions less commonly directed at others
    - Less integration of gaze with vocalization
  - Lack of interest in peers
  - Limited imitation of others
  - Low rates of joint attention (pointing, showing, following gaze and point)
  - Restricted range of functional and imaginative play
  - Greater frequency and duration of repetitive hand and finger mannerisms and preoccupation with parts of objects
- *Regressive Onset* Between 20% and 47% of children with ASDs appear to exhibit few symptoms of ASDs until they experience a marked loss of language and/or socialization skills around the age of 15–24 months of age. Whether any developmental abnormalities are present before the onset of the regression remains unclear. Some longitudinal studies do suggest subtle delays or abnormalities before the frank regression, and some suggest a plateau rather than regression in some children. The relationship between vaccines and regressive onset of ASDs has received much attention in the media; however, a causal relationship is not empirically supported in multiple high-quality studies.
- *Third, Fourth, and Fifth Years* Symptoms of ASDs during the third, fourth, and fifth years of life appear similar. In many, communicative ability improves with time. Often, as it improves, language begins to contain other abnormalities, including *echolalia*, unusual prosody, and limited ability to engage in reciprocal conversation. Nonverbal communication continues to be impaired and includes limited use of gesture and joint attention, unusual eye contact, and limited range and use of facial expression. Functional and imaginative play continues to be restricted in range and/or frequency. The frequency of restricted interests and repetitive behaviors often increases during this period. In children with phrase speech and full sentences, they tend to repeat immediately what they have heard or repeat favorite phrases; conversation is one-sided rather than reciprocal.
- *Middle Childhood* With time and intervention, children may gain daily living skills during middle childhood and become more capable of acquiescing to the demands of their environments. Some children with ASDs become more aware of societal rules and more interested in fulfilling the wishes of others, resulting in a decrease of public displays of repetitive behaviors. However, abnormalities in verbal and nonverbal communication and socialization

skills generally remain. However, there is strong evidence that a small minority (perhaps 5–20%) of individuals with ASD can lose symptoms of autism and function within the normal limits of social relationships; most of these individuals got intensive early intervention.

- *Adolescence* Symptoms during this period may be particularly challenging to treat. As many as 11–39% of individuals with ASDs experience seizures that most commonly begin in infancy or adolescence; seizures are often associated with significant intellectual impairment. Some adolescents with ASDs may also present with behavioral difficulties including resistance to change, *self-injurious behaviors*, compulsive behaviors, tantrums, and aggressive behaviors, which can be severe. In addition, daily living skills often continue to be impaired in adolescence. However, increased communicative and social skills may allow adolescents with ASDs to become more interested in participating in therapeutic interventions to help alleviate difficult behaviors and other remaining deficits. Aggression and irritability often worsen with the beginning of puberty and abate somewhat toward the end of adolescence, but some adolescents remain aggressive and irritable.

- *Adulthood* Little is known about ASD symptomatology during adulthood. Recent reports indicate that 50% of adults have poor outcomes (i.e., require high level of residential assistance, have few friends, and have supported or no employment). Although most adults with ASDs continue to require support from others, many are employed for at least several hours each week.

Rett's Disorder

Rett's disorder is associated with the X-linked gene *MECP2*; it typically progresses through four stages:

- *First Stage* Marked by head growth deceleration, reduced interest in play, atypical hand mannerisms, deterioration in communicative abilities, and unusual eye contact. This often follows a period of 6 to 18 months of apparently normal development.

- *Second Stage* Marked by the presence of classic symptoms of autism, frequent and unusual motor stereotypies, loss of cognitive and language skills, and deteriorating motor abilities.

- *Third Stage* Symptoms of ASD typically diminish, and cognitive gains are made. However, motor skills continue to decline, and seizure onset is common. Daily living skills are poor, impacted by intellectual impairment and motor disability.

- *Fourth Stage* Motor abilities continue to deteriorate during the fourth stage of RD, and the majority of children with RD become wheelchair dependent during this time.

Rule-Outs

Numerous medical conditions present with similar symptomatology as in ASD including, but not limited to, Landau-Kleffner syndrome, fragile X syndrome, Heller's syndrome, and Klinefelter's syndrome. Appropriate medical and genetic tests can help identify the presence of these disorders, in addition to the autism phenotype. ASD is a behavioral syndrome, and often occurs in association with more established medical, especially genetic and metabolic, disorders.

Expectations for Neuropsychological Assessment Results

- *Intelligence/Achievement* Individuals with ASDs exhibit cognitive profiles with a high degree of variability between domains and subtests. There is no standard profile of intelligence for an individual with an ASD. As noted above, 40–70% of cases score within the ID range (IQ < 70). Individuals with ASD tend to demonstrate most difficulty on tasks that require language, abstract reasoning, flexible thinking, inferential reasoning, and sequencing. Strongest performance is often seen on tasks that require visuospatial processing, rote memory skills, and attention to detail. Many studies show that individuals with ASD overall tend to score higher on measures of nonverbal as compared to verbal reasoning, with significant variability observed among subtests. However, this pattern has not been consistently found among high-functioning individuals with ASD. As such, IQ should not inform diagnostic definitions.

- *Attention/Concentration* As noted above, many individuals with ASD exhibit attentional deficits, but significant variability has been reported across different forms of attention. Individuals with ASD appear to have particular difficulty disengaging and shifting attention. In contrast, sustained attention is relatively spared, especially with materials of interest to them. Individuals with ASDs may also have heightened attention to personally salient stimuli.

- *Processing Speed* Processing speed is likely to be impaired if measured with a verbally loaded task. In spatial, nonverbal tasks, processing speed may be unimpaired. When processing speed is unimpaired on testing, it is still often found to be slowed in natural settings where distractions place burdens on attention.

- *Language* There are many components to language, each of which may be differentially affected across individuals with ASDs. Often, children with ASD exhibit language delays as toddlers and preschoolers. Many of these children begin speaking with time and appropriate intervention; however, approximately 20–30% remain nonverbal. Verbal individuals with ASDs generally show relative strengths in phonology and articulation, basic grammar, and single-word receptive and expressive vocabulary. Grammar is important to assess because a subgroup of children may have grammatical difficulties similar to those with specific language impairment. Semantics, higher-level output (e.g., conversation, constructing narratives), prosody, comprehension of formulated speech, and pragmatic use of language are areas of particular difficulty.

- *Visuospatial Abilities* A subset of individuals with ASDs have enhanced visual-perceptual processing abilities. These individuals with ASD excel on visuospatial tasks that require identifying, matching, and copying visual stimuli. However, studies suggest that individuals with ASD tend to focus on details of visual stimuli and have difficulty integrating the details in context. Many individuals with ASD display deficits in face processing, and some in face recognition ability. Typically, individuals with ASDs attend significantly less to the eyes when viewing a face, which can contribute to social skill difficulties.

- *Memory* The memory skills of individuals with ASDs vary widely, but memory impairments are well established in this population. Nondeclarative memory (e.g., facts, procedures, perceptions, routines, associations) generally appears to be appropriate for mental age. Some individuals with ASDs may also have strong memory capacity for topics of interest. Declarative memory tends to be impaired mildly in high-functioning individuals, and more extensively in low-functioning individuals. Across most individuals with ASD, memory for social and emotional information tends to be selectively impaired. Free and cued recall of lists of unrelated items appears appropriate for mental age. Paired associate learning is also generally intact. Among high-functioning individuals, recognition memory is generally unimpaired (with the exception of memory for social information), but moderately impaired among low-functioning individuals. Some studies also suggest that individuals with ASD tend to be less efficient when learning contextually organized material.

- *Executive Functions* Executive functioning deficits are common in individuals with ASD. High-functioning individuals with ASD sometimes perform normally on standardized tests of executive functioning in a structured, laboratory environment. However, parent and teacher reports of executive functioning skills on standardized questionnaires (e.g., BRIEF) often reveal more difficulty in daily life. Problems with planning, inhibition, working memory, monitoring performance, cognitive and behavioral flexibility and shifting attention, and initiation are often seen in individuals with ASD. According to the "executive dysfunction" theory, deficits in this domain underlie ASD symptomatology, including social communication deficits, rigidity, stereotyped behaviors, adherence to routines, and restricted interests in ASD. It is worth noting that impairment in this domain is less consistently observed when measured during the preschool period.

- *Sensorimotor Functions* Impairment in fine motor skills, gross motor skills, balance, coordination, and motor planning have been observed among individuals with ASDs. Delayed or abnormal motor development has been noted across numerous studies. Assessing motor skills without requiring imitation is important due to deficits in imitation skills. Individuals with ASDs also often have sensory impairments (over- and/or undersensitivity) that can impact subsequent cognition and behavior patterns. A tendency to experience overstimulation can predispose an individual to engage in a limited range of behaviors in a limited range of environments. Others have difficulty distinguishing relevant stimuli from the extraneous, which can lead to both hyper- and hyposensitivity in any of the sensory domains. Auditory oversensitivity and visual self-stimulation are the most common.

- *Social Behavior* Social impairment is a core deficit in ASD, yet social functioning is difficult to effectively assess. In observational measures, one would expect an individual with ASD to have a poor quality of reciprocal social interaction, characterized by a degree of impairment in any of the following: eye contact; social referencing and engagement with others; integration of verbal and nonverbal social overtures; imitation; and giving, sharing, and showing behaviors. Social overtures may be unusual in quality and restricted to the personal demands or interests of the individual, with variable attempts to involve others in that interest. Social overtures may entirely lack integration into context or be socially inappropriate, diminished, or nonexistent. Individuals with ASD often have difficulty with theory of mind or the ability to understand the states of mind in other people. Individuals with ASD may also struggle to perceive and/or respond appropriately to the emotional displays of others.

- *Academic Skills* Academic skills that require rote memorization tend to be stronger than skills that require abstract thinking and inference making. High-functioning students with ASD often present with age-appropriate decoding, spelling, and math calculation skills. Difficulties are most commonly observed in reading comprehension, solving math word problems, and written expression.

- *Performance and Symptom Validity* Pragmatic language deficits may prevent an individual from understanding the nature of the testing situation and may exaggerate his or her difficulties with staying on task, paying attention to the examiner, and answering questions in a relevant manner. Individuals who have difficulty disengaging their attention may perseverate on topics or tasks of interest. Individuals with ASDs may have difficulty with stimuli presented at a fast rate, which could lead to hyperarousal and performance deficits; ample time to complete tasks should be provided. Some individuals may lack the social motivation to please the examiner or experience social anxiety, which could impact performance. They may need assistance to say "I don't know." Lack of social motivation should be addressed by providing nonsocial reinforcers for good effort (e.g., edibles, points to earn a break or small tangible rewards).

- *Adaptive Behavior/Skills* Individuals with ASD show a highly variable profile on measures of adaptive functioning in the areas of communication, daily living, socialization, and motor skills. The most pronounced deficits are typically in the socialization and communication domains. Individuals with ASDs may show a varying degree of deficit in both daily living skills and motor ability. Adaptive skills of children with ASD are often lower than their IQs would predict.

Considerations when Treating Patients with ASDs

Role of Early Intervention

Studies comparing the gains made by children with ASDs of various ages after receiving intervention have demonstrated that the younger the child begins to receive treatment, the better the outcome. Intervention appears to have the greatest likelihood for success if begun prior to age 5 years, with some research suggesting that the optimal age for initiating treatment falls between 2 and 3 years. Two recent studies, however, suggest that starting behavioral treatment before the second birthday can result in even better functioning, although this requires a diagnosis well before the second birthday, which is often not feasible.

Behavioral Management and Skills

Intensive applied behavioral analysis (ABA; 15–25 hours per week) has been shown to be effective in treating children with ASD. Task analysis and contingent reinforcement can aid in guiding preferred behaviors and help teach skills in a stepwise fashion. Sustained attention in individuals with ASD improves when strong incentives are used. For very low-functioning children, an assessment of their memory abilities is informative in teaching the child basic skills; often, procedural or rote memory is relatively intact. Restricted, repetitive, stereotypical, and ritualistic behaviors are commonly elevated among individuals with ASD. Younger and often lower-functioning individuals with ASD may demonstrate a great deal of repetitive behavior in the clinical setting due to its unfamiliarity and testing demands. Younger and lower-functioning individuals often show high rates of motor stereotypies, whereas older and higher-functioning individuals show more cognitive symptoms such as resistance to change and preoccupying interests.

Intelligence and Adaptive Skills

Knowledge of an individual's cognitive profile is useful to a clinician making recommendations for treatment planning. These recommendations should utilize a child's cognitive strengths and provide intervention and accommodations for areas of weakness. Individuals with ASDs typically have difficulty with top-down processing, leading to difficulties in seeing the "big picture." Treatment approaches need to incorporate explicit task instructions and expectations for skills that typically developing individuals may naturally acquire. As noted above, IQ often exceeds measures of adaptive functioning ability, and this is particularly true among high-functioning individuals with ASD. Results on adaptive functioning measures are useful in planning intervention, which should include a focus on developing functional skills, generalization across skills and settings, and independence. In adolescence and adulthood, consideration should be given to educational and vocational placement and career planning. Individuals with lower IQs are more likely to have poorer outcomes in later life in terms of adaptive functioning skills and independence, and they should receive intensive intervention services to bring cognitive functioning to as high a level as the individual can achieve.

Language

Early language skills are a strong predictor of outcome, making early language intervention an integral element of an early education plan. For children who are not verbal, intervention should primarily focus on advancing functional communication. To accomplish this goal, alternative forms of communication may be considered (e.g., *picture exchange communication system*, sign language, augmentative and alternative communication device). For children who are verbal, speech and language therapy should focus on semantic and grammatical skill acquisition, as well as social use of language. Communication goals should be targeted throughout the day in both structured educational settings, as well as during naturalistic day-to-day tasks and activities. Specific targets of therapy can include but are not limited to increasing semantic knowledge and knowledge of words, increasing grammatical understanding, and encouraging social use of language. Children with ASDs are typically impaired in their active conversational skills, such as turn- and perspective-taking, exploring the interests of others that are different from their own, and appropriately initiating and maintaining a conversation. They have difficulties with maintaining eye contact, respecting personal space, and using idioms and figures of speech. Programs should be designed to target an individual's deficits both in semantic and pragmatic language ability.

Executive Function

Executive function impairment can be targeted with provision of supports and environmental changes. Daily routines and reinforcements are used to teach students strategies to compensate for executive functioning deficits. When appropriate, a visual schedule of the day's activities can be developed to keep a child appropriately on task. Cognitive behavioral principals have also been used to develop programs to advance cognitive and behavioral flexibility in children and adolescents with ASD (e.g., "Unstuck and On Target" curriculum). Fluency and processing speed impairments can be addressed with extended time for tasks and activities, and shifting difficulties can be counteracted with clear, time-dependent instructions, warnings for transitions, and barriers set to prevent perseveration.

Attention/Imitation

Few interventions specifically target attention. Despite this, environmental supports such as removing distracters, simplifying complex tasks, using high-interest materials, and providing frequent breaks can help to improve attention. Deficits in sustained attention can be remediated using strong and immediate reinforcers for nonpreferred activities. Typically, social reinforcers will not be as effective in this population, and, instead, one could incorporate the interests of the individual into the material or behavioral targets being taught, as well as providing extrinsic reinforcers (e.g., food, breaks, money, points). Children with ASDs commonly present with imitation impairments, which can impede learning. Programs should focus as early as possible on the development of imitation skills. Programs can target simple vocal and motor imitation and progress to complex verbalizations and actions.

Social Cognition

Interventions involving explicit teaching of social skills should be applied and adapted to the needs of the individual. Younger children and lower functioning individuals with ASDs should be taught basic skills such as eye contact, imitation, requesting, and simple reciprocal interactions. As a child matures, more interactive play skills can be taught, and more complex understanding of social interactions can be fostered in older individuals. High-functioning children with ASDs often have social anxiety; interventions for these individuals should include relieving anxiety through cognitive-behavioral therapy, which increases skills and confidence. In some cases, medication is also used to reduce anxiety. Children with ASDs often lack social motivation, and interventions should be targeted toward teaching them the inherent rewards associated with social interaction.

Sensory and Motor Function/Impairment

Sensory impairments, ranging from sensory-seeking and self-stimulatory behaviors to extreme aversion toward certain sensory input, can significantly impact an individual's functioning. Occupational therapy can target sensorimotor impairment by teaching specific motor skills and helping caregivers and teachers to modulate the environment to reduce unpleasant stimuli, whereas behavior therapy can help desensitize the individual to aversive stimuli and teach relaxation and cognitive strategies. If motor difficulties are suspected, assessment by a neurologist, a physical therapist, or an occupational therapist is required. In addition, hearing should be tested before diagnosis and considered during treatment.

Repetitive Behavior

If repetitive or other interfering behaviors are present, a functional assessment of the behavior is needed. This involves taking data on antecedents and consequences of the behavior with the goal of identifying the function of the behavior or the factor(s) that may be maintaining or reinforcing the behavior. Common functions of such behavior include escape from demands, positive or negative attention from adults or peers, access to preferred objects or activities, and intrinsic reinforcement (inherently pleasurable activities). A functional behavior assessment allows the clinician to understand the function and context of the behavior and determine how to alter the environment so that inappropriate behaviors are no longer being rewarded. Instead, the individual should be able to access the reward by engaging in appropriate behaviors. Intrinsically reinforcing behaviors are, obviously, the most difficult to treat, since the reinforcement is not under the therapist's control. Repetitive behaviors should be actively reduced, when possible, to prevent an individual from focusing his or her attention inward and neglecting the physical and social environments. Some behaviors are especially resistant to extinction; the caregiver should be enlisted to ensure that these behaviors are not reinforced and that they are extinguished as early as possible. Individuals with low IQs and adaptive abilities are most likely to engage in repetitive self-injury and violent behaviors toward objects or others, which should be targeted aggressively by intervention specialists.

Psychological and Emotional Issues

Autism spectrum disorder commonly co-occurs with a number of psychological and emotional conditions that can complicate assessment and treatment (see the section "Comorbidity" earlier in the chapter). Comorbid conditions should be given consideration and appropriate treatment alongside an intervention specifically targeting ASD symptomatology. Medical conditions, such as seizures, should be treated with standard medical care. Psychiatric comorbidities can be treated with cognitive-behavioral therapy if the child is high functioning enough and motivated to participate. Behavioral therapy and relaxation training can help with anxiety in lower-functioning children. Medication may be used as well (see below).

Medications and Diet

Medication alone does not alleviate the core symptoms of ASD. However, medications are often used to treat co-occurring psychiatric conditions, and emotional and behavioral difficulties experienced by individuals with ASD. In fact, as many as 70% of children with ASDs who are older than 8 years have received some form of psychoactive medication treatment. Two atypical antipsychotics (aripiprazole and risperidone) have been approved by the United States Food and Drug Administration to treat irritability in children and adolescents with ASD. Both medications have received some empirical support to reduce hyperactivity and stereotypy. Methylphenidate has consistently been shown to reduce ADHD symptoms in children with ASD. Atomoxetine, clonidine, and guanfacine have also received some empirical support in treating ADHD symptoms in this population. Some studies have supported the use of buspirone in the treatment of repetitive behaviors in children with ASD, but more studies are needed. GABA-ergic, glutamatergic medications, and oxytocin are currently being explored as potential treatments for core features of ASDs; however, further investigation is necessary. Selective serotonin reuptake inhibitors (SSRIs) have been studied as a possible treatment for repetitive behaviors. In adults with ASDs, SSRIs have shown some improvement in *RRBs*, but no benefit has been found in the pediatric population. With regard to diet, nutrition is certainly known to impact cognition and behavior; however, there is no empirical support for the use of any special diet to manage ASD symptomatology (e.g., gluten-free, casein-free). Experimental treatments are on the horizon, including transcranial magnetic stimulation, intranasal oxytocin, and manipulating the gut biome.

Relevant Definitions

Echolalia The repetition of sounds, words, phrases, or several sentences. Immediate echolalia refers to the repetition of vocalization immediately after hearing it, whereas delayed echolalia refers to the repetition of vocalizations heard previously. Echolalia is observed in typical development between the ages of 12 and 30 months but generally fades with vocabulary growth. In ASDs, the frequency of echolalia persists past 30 months and is often used to initiate conversation or to respond.

Idiosyncratic speech The use of words in an inappropriate way to form meaningful but unusual phrases.

Picture exchange communication system An augmentative communication system used to aid children who have difficulties with spoken language. These systems most commonly employ the use of small pictures, which represent objects, actions, or words, that a child can select and present to communicate with others and that adults can arrange as well to communicate with the child.

Restricted and repetitive behaviors (RRBs) Include repetitive stereotypic motor behaviors (e.g., hand flapping), ritualistic behaviors (e.g., lining up objects), and insistence of sameness behaviors (e.g., resistance to change in daily schedule), as well as interests that are unusual in their focus or in the degree of intensity. These behaviors are often noticed during the second year of life, and the frequency and severity of these behaviors often increase during the first 5 years of life.

Self-injurious behaviors Behaviors that inflict injury on the individual. A wide range of such behaviors is observed among individuals with ASDs, including banging the head on walls, tables, or floors, as well as hitting, scratching, or biting oneself. The frequency of self-injurious behaviors also varies considerably, with some individuals with ASD engaging in such behaviors countless times each day, whereas others engage in these behaviors several times each year. Self-injurious behaviors are more commonly observed in individuals with moderate to profound levels of ID.

Theory of Mind The understanding that other people have mental states (beliefs, knowledge, emotions, perspectives, etc.) that are different from one's own and that can help one to predict and understand their behavior.

Autism Spectrum Disorder Questions

NOTE: Questions 13, 30, and 66 on the First Full-Length Practice Examination, Questions 3, 30, 65, and 96 on the Second Full-Length Practice Examination, Questions 6, 36, 56, 68, and 87 on the Third Full-Length

Practice Examination, and Questions 5, 50, and 83 on the Fourth Full-Length Practice Examination are from this chapter.

1. Which of the following interventions for young children with ASD has been demonstrated empirically to lead to significant improvement in skills and cognitive functioning?

    (a) applied behavior analysis

    (b) interpersonal therapy

    (c) cognitive therapy

    (d) selective norepinephrine reuptake inhibitors (SNRIs) and SSRIs

2. The best estimate of the male-to-female sex ratio in cases diagnosed with high-functioning ASD is ____.

    (a) ten males for every female

    (c) two females for every male

    (b) one male for every female

    (d) four males for every female

3. Children with ASD display deficits in face processing and atypical attentional strategies when attending to faces. They typically pay significantly reduced attention to which facial feature?

    (a) cheeks

    (c) mouth

    (b) nose

    (d) eyes

4. In individuals with ASDs, which type of memory is most likely unimpaired?

    (a) episodic memory

    (c) memory for person-related information

    (b) procedural memory

    (d) memory for emotion-related information

5. Which is most characteristic of nonverbal communication in children with ASDs?

    (a) preference toward verbal communication and presence of echolalia

    (b) communicating emotions through facial expressions

    (c) poor integration of gaze with vocalization

    (d) nonverbally commenting rather than requesting

6. Approximately what percentage of high-functioning adults with ASD have poor outcomes (i.e., require high level of residential assistance, have few reciprocal social relationships, and have supported or no employment)?

    (a) 10–15%

    (c) 50–60%

    (b) 30–35%

    (d) 80–90%

7. Executive functioning deficits in high functioning individuals with ASD are most likely to be apparent ____.

    (a) across measures beginning in the preschool period

    (b) on direct testing in clinical settings

    (c) on behavior rating scales completed by caregivers

    (d) after the preschool period when measured using computerized assessments

8. Twin studies show some shared environment influence on the ASD phenotype; they also show _____.

   (a) about equal concordance in monozygotic and dizygotic twin pairs

   (b) similar concordance rates in dizygotic twin pairs and full biological siblings

   (c) strong genetic association with schizophrenia in one or both parents

   (d) high concordance in monozygotic twins and low concordance in dizygotic twins

9. Which of the following is most consistently associated with the onset of ASD during the first two years of life?

   (a) delayed language acquisition   (c) stranger anxiety

   (b) restricted interests   (d) stereotypies

10. Which of the following genetic syndromes present with symptoms commonly associated with autism spectrum disorders?

    (a) Turner's syndrome   (c) Angelman syndrome

    (b) fragile X syndrome   (d) Williams syndrome

Autism Spectrum Disorder Answers

1. **A—applied behavior analysis**   *15–25 hours per week of intensive behavioral intervention has the greatest effect on the developmental trajectory of individuals with an ASD, particularly their adaptive skills and IQ.*

   Reference: Howard, J. S, Stanislaw, H., Green, G. Sparkman, C. R., & Cohen, H. G. (2014). Comparison of behavior analytic and eclectic early interventions for young children with autism after three years. *Research in Developmental Disabilities, 35*(12), 3326–3344.

2. **D—four males for every female**   *A review of epidemiological studies conducted by Fombonne (2009) revealed that the median male-to-female ratio of ASD is 4.2:1.*

   Reference: Fombonne, E. (2009). Epidemiology of pervasive developmental disorders. *Pediatric Research, 65*(6), 591–598.

3. **D—eyes**   *Eye-tracking studies have shown that children with autism pay significantly less attention to the eyes than do typically developing children. This difference is first observed in early infancy.*

   Reference: Jones, W., & Klin, A. (2013). Attention to eyes is present but in decline in 2–6 month-old infants later diagnosed with autism. *Nature, 504*(7480), 427–431.

4. **B—procedural memory**   *Studies of high- and low-functioning individuals with ASD reveal impaired episodic memory and diminished recall of person- and emotion-related information. Nondeclarative memory has repeatedly been found to be appropriate for mental age.*

   Reference: Boucher, J., Mayes, A., & Bigham, S. (2012). Memory in autistic spectrum disorder. *Psychological Bulletin, 138*(3), 458–496.

5. **C—poor integration of gaze with vocalization**   *Children with ASD often demonstrate deficits in nonverbal communication, including poorly integrated verbal and nonverbal communication, abnormalities in eye contact, limited gesture use, restricted range of facial expressions, and difficulty understanding the nonverbal communication of others.*

   Reference: Chiang, C., Soong, W., Lin, T., & Rogers, S. J. (2008). Nonverbal communication skills in young children with autism. *Journal of Autism and Developmental Disorders, 38*, 1898–1906.

6. **C—50–60%** *Studies examining adult outcomes of individuals diagnosed with ASD in childhood suggest that around 50% of participants were rated as having "poor" or "very poor" outcome. Similar rates are found among adults who had broadly average nonverbal reasoning skills in childhood. Approximately 20% were rated as having "good" or "very good" outcomes (e.g., living independently or with minimal supports, employed in skilled work with minimal supports, have reciprocal social relationships).*

Reference: Howlin, P., Moss, P., Savage, S., & Rutter, M. (2013). Social outcomes in midlife to later adulthood among individuals diagnosed with autism and average nonverbal IQ as children. *Journal of the American Academy of Child & Adolescent Psychiatry, 52,* 572–581.

7. **C—on behavior rating scales completed by caregivers** *Executive functioning deficits in high functioning children with ASD are most commonly observed when situational demands require the use of multiple abilities at once. As a result, parent report of these abilities in everyday settings are most likely to reveal deficits. Studies using computerized assessments appear to be less likely to display deficits than when tasks are administered by humans. Additionally, multiple studies examining these abilities in the preschool period have found age-appropriate skills.*

Reference: Kenworthy, L., Yerys, B. E., Anthony, L. G., & Wallace, G. L. (2008). Understanding executive control in autism spectrum disorders in the lab and in the real world. *Neuropsychology Review, 18,* 320–338.

8. **D—high concordance in monozygotic twins and low concordance in dizygotic twins** *Suggests that ASD has multiple and complex but significant genetic contributions.*

Reference: Hallmayer, J., Cleveland, S., Torres, A., Phillips, J., Cohen, B., Torigoe, T., . . . Lotspeich, L. (2011). Genetic heritability and shared environmental factors among twin pairs with autism. *Archives of General Psychiatry, 68*(11), 1095–1102.

9. **A—delayed language acquisition** *Delayed language acquisition is one of the earliest indicators of an ASD during early childhood.*

Reference: Mitchell, S., Cardy, J. O., & Zwaigenbaum, L. (2011). Differentiating autism spectrum disorder from other developmental delays in the first two years of life. *Developmental Disabilities Research Reviews, 17*(2), 130–140.

10. **B—fragile X syndrome** *ASDs are frequently comorbid with fragile X syndrome. The prevalence of ASD in fragile X syndrome has been estimated at as high as 50%, with some studies suggesting that as many as 90% of individuals with fragile X syndrome present with some ASD symptomatology.*

Reference: Abbeduto, L., McDuffle, A., & Thurman, A. J. (2014). The fragile X syndrome-autism comorbidity: What do we really know? *Frontiers in Genetics, 5*(355), 1–10.

Recommended Readings

Ecker, C., Bookheimer, S. Y., & Murphy, D. G. (2015). Neuroimaging in autism spectrum disorder: Brain structure and function across the lifespan. *The Lancet. Neurology, 14*(11), 1121–1134.

Fein, D. A. (Ed.). (2011). *The neuropsychology of autism.* New York, NY: Oxford University Press.

Hollander, E., Hangerman, R., & Fein, D. (2018). *Autism spectrum disorders.* Washington, DC: American Psychiatric Association Publishing,

Jones, E. J., Gliga, T., Bedford, R., Charman, T., & Johnson, M. H. (2014). Developmental pathways to autism: A review of prospective studies of infant risk. *Neuroscience and Biobehavioral Reviews, 39,* 1–33.

Moss, J., & Howlin, P. (2009). Autism spectrum disorders in genetic syndromes: Implications for diagnosis, intervention and understanding the wider autism spectrum disorder population. *Journal of Intellectual Disability Research, 53*(10), 852–873.

Sacrey, L. A., Bennett, J. A., & Zwaigenbaum, L. (2015). Early infant development and intervention for autism spectrum disorder. *Journal of Child Neurology, 30*(14), 1921–1929.

15   Learning Disabilities

E. Mark Mahone, Robert L. Mapou, and Emily C. Maxwell

Introduction

Learning disabilities are neurobiologically based, developmental disorders that affect the brain's ability to receive, process, store, and respond to information. They typically arise in childhood, persist into adulthood, and are associated with unexpected academic underachievement. The underachievement is considered "unexpected" when it is not explained by low intelligence, sensory impairments, emotional disturbances, or lack of opportunities to learn. Learning disabilities occur along a continuum, with variability in severity and characteristic features, rather than as discrete, dichotomous entities. Learning disabilities also occur across the full spectrum of intellectual functioning.

Learning disabilities are also associated with a variety of risks. For example, the majority of students with learning disabilities will be suspended from school at least once. The presence of a learning disability also confers a greater risk for school dropout, especially among low-income students, and a well-documented connection exists between school dropout and incarceration.

This chapter focuses on three learning disabilities that have been broken into several subtypes:

- *Reading disabilities* (word recognition/dyslexia, reading fluency, comprehension)
- *Mathematics disabilities* (computation, problem solving)
- *Written expression disabilities* (handwriting, spelling, composition)

Of note, some neuropsychologists have supported the notion of a nonverbal learning disability (NLD), which involves deficits in nonverbal reasoning, visuospatial skills, mathematical skills, fine motor skills, and social/interpersonal skills. However, several critical reviews have concluded that there is insufficient empirical and clinical support for such a disorder, and so NLD is not presently recognized as an official diagnosis in the medical, psychological, or educational fields. Nevertheless, neuropsychologists should be mindful that some patients and families (particularly those with diagnoses in which NLD features are commonly discussed in their communities (e.g., Turner syndrome, 22q11.2 deletion, and congenital hydrocephalus) find the cognitive profile associated with NLD useful in understanding their difficulties. The prevailing (narrower) definition of learning disability places the emphasis on problems that cause academic dysfunction.

Definitions

The most recent legal definition of learning disability was included in the Individuals with Disabilities Education Improvement Act of 2004. It states:

> Specific learning disability means a disorder in one or more of the basic psychological processes involved in understanding or in using language, spoken or written, that may manifest itself in an imperfect ability to listen, think, speak, read, write, spell, or do mathematical calculations. The term includes such conditions as perceptual handicaps, brain injury, minimal brain dysfunction, dyslexia, and developmental aphasia. The

term does not include children who have learning problems that are primarily the result of visual, hearing, or motor handicaps; of intellectual disability; of emotional disturbance; or of environmental, cultural, or economic disadvantage.

Despite advances in our knowledge of learning disabilities, this definition has remained essentially unchanged since it was first written in 1969. In 1985, the Rehabilitation Services Administration incorporated a different definition of learning disability, specific to adults, into disability law:

A specific learning disability is a disorder in one or more of the central nervous system processes involved in perceiving, understanding, and/or using concepts through verbal (spoken or written) language or nonverbal means. This disorder manifests itself with a deficit in one or more of the following areas: attention, reasoning, processing, memory, communication, reading, writing, spelling, calculation, coordination, social competence, and emotional maturity.

DSM-5 Definition of Specific Learning Disorder

The diagnostic criteria in the American Psychiatric Association's Diagnostic and Statistical Manual of Mental Disorders-Fifth Edition (DSM-5) for Specific Learning Disorder reflect a hybrid model of identification. Note that the DSM nomenclature uses the term "Disorder," while other educational and legal definitions use the term "Disability." Both definitions are highly similar and overlapping. The DSM-5 definition additionally reflects the recognition that individuals may "grow into" their learning deficits and may not fully manifest problems until a later age.

- Diagnosis is made using a synthesis of the individual's history (developmental, medical, family, education), psychoeducational reports of test scores and observations, and response to intervention. A Specific Learning Disorder is now defined as:

  - Difficulty learning and using academic skills, as indicated by the presence of at least one of the following symptoms that have persisted for at least 6 months, despite the provision of interventions that target those difficulties.

    o Inaccurate or slow and effortful word reading (e.g., reads single words aloud incorrectly or slowly and hesitantly, frequently guesses words, has difficulty sounding out words)

    o Difficulty understanding the meaning of what is read (e.g., may read text accurately but not understand the sequence, relationships, inferences, or deeper meanings of what is read)

    o Difficulty with spelling (e.g., may add, omit, or substitute vowels or consonants)

    o Difficulty with written expression (e.g., makes multiple grammatical or punctuation errors within sentences, employs poor paragraph organization; written expression of ideas lacks clarity)

    o Difficulty mastering number sense, number facts, or calculation (e.g., has poor understanding of numbers, their magnitude, and relationships; counts on fingers to add single-digit numbers instead of recalling the math fact as peers do; gets lost in the midst of arithmetic computation and may switch procedures)

    o Difficulty with mathematical reasoning (e.g., has severe difficulty applying mathematical concepts, facts, or procedures to solve quantitative problems)

- The affected academic skills are substantially and quantifiably below those expected for the individual's chronological age, and cause significant interference with academic or occupational performance, or with activities of daily living, as confirmed by individually administered standardized achievement measures and comprehensive clinical assessment. For individuals age 17 years and older, a documented history of impairing learning difficulties may be substituted for the standardized assessment.

- The learning difficulties begin during the school-age years but may not become fully manifested until the demands for those affected academic skills exceed the individual's limited capacities (e.g., as in timed tests, reading or writing lengthy complex reports for a tight deadline, excessively heavy academic loads).

- The learning difficulties are not better accounted for by intellectual disabilities (see also Chapter 13, Intellectual Disability), uncorrected visual or auditory acuity, other mental or neurological disorders, psychosocial adversity, lack of proficiency in the language of academic instruction, or inadequate educational instruction.

Epidemiology

Approximately 15–20% of the United States population (i.e., more than one in six Americans) has a learning disability. Approximately 13–14% of students in the United States (more than 8 million children) are identified as having a federally defined handicapping condition and receive special education services in school. Half of those identified for special education are classified as having a Specific Learning Disability. The number of affected individuals varies depending on the assessment methods and the threshold used to define the "deficit" in academic achievement. Many research studies have utilized the classification of either less than the 25th percentile (low achieving) or less than the 10th percentile (extremely low achieving) as cutoff points for defining a learning disability. Not surprisingly, research findings involving outcomes, comorbidities, and biological correlates all differ depending on the definition (and threshold) used.

- Difficulties with basic reading and language skills make up the most common learning disabilities. Approximately 85% of those students having a primary learning disability have a learning disability in reading and language processing.

- Males are about 1.5 times as likely as females to have reading disabilities.

- Learning disabilities often run in families, with heritability for reading ranging from approximately 0.3 to 0.9, and for math ranging from 0.5 to 0.8.

Presentation, Disorder Course, and Recovery

- For most individuals with learning disabilities, the core functional deficits can first be observed in childhood, usually in the preschool or early elementary school years.

- A learning disability typically represents a persistent functional deficit, rather than a developmental lag. These disabilities frequently persist over time, despite intervention efforts, and typically do not spontaneously remit or normalize with time or age.

  - For some, the manifestations and impact may not become evident until later in childhood, in the teenage years, or even in the adult years (although this is rarer).

- In those diagnosed for the first time as adults, the disorders may be milder, although some adults have found ways to compensate despite having significant learning disabilities (e.g., avoidance of tasks that emphasize deficits, self-selection of career path, informal accommodations throughout schooling).

- Among individuals with early-onset learning disabilities who have received intervention by early elementary school, deficits in word-reading accuracy and/or mathematics calculation can improve; however, weaknesses in phonological processing, automaticity of word recognition, and reading fluency tend to persist.

- Anxiety can amplify academic difficulties among individuals with learning disabilities. Rich connections between the limbic and frontal systems interact, such that anxiety can serve to flood frontal brain systems with excessive dopamine, pushing the system to the impairing side of the inverted U-shaped curve.

Diagnosis of Learning Disabilities

Aptitude-Achievement Discrepancy Model

- Some states and school districts still identify children with learning disabilities based on a discrepancy between measured intelligence and a specific academic skill.

- In particular, individuals diagnosed using a discrepancy method do not differ functionally or behaviorally from individuals diagnosed using a low-achievement method alone.

Low-Achievement Model

- Models based primarily on low achievement have been shown to have substantial validity and are frequently used in research.

- Because youth who perform below average on achievement tests (and do not have intellectual disability) can be differentiated on external variables, low achievement is considered a viable definition for learning disability.

Intraindividual Differences Model

- This model takes into account individual profiles of strengths and weaknesses in cognitive functioning and information processing. Students are identified as having learning disabilities when their profiles are markedly uneven.

- The validity of this model has been challenged.
  - Cognitive profiles derived from neuropsychological assessment do not translate readily into individualized instruction.
  - It assumes that a "flat" profile is inconsistent with a learning disability.
  - Variability ("test scatter") is the rule rather than the exception and, alone, cannot be used to diagnose a learning disability.

Response to Intervention (RTI) Model

- The premise of RTI is that students should receive adequate instruction with appropriate monitoring before being considered to have a learning disability.

- In the RTI model, the response of all students to standard and adequate instruction is evaluated from the start of school.
  - Those who do not acquire a specific academic skill undergo selective assessment of that skill (often within the context of curriculum-based measurement).
  - Assessment can include limited neuropsychological testing of the abilities important for that academic skill (e.g., phonological awareness for reading). Following assessment, a new instructional plan is developed and implemented, its impact is assessed, and the instructional plan is further modified as needed.
- A potential problem of the RTI model is that little consensus exists regarding how to define "inadequate response to appropriate instruction," and how to ensure adequate fidelity for implementation of each of the three "tiers" of intervention. There also is no research support for an RTI approach in adults.

Section 1: Reading Disabilities

Definition

The scientific literature has shifted to definitions that reflect more specific types of reading problems. Three subtypes are reflected in the descriptors for reading disabilities included in diagnostic criteria in the DSM-5: word decoding (dyslexia), reading fluency, and reading comprehension. The most common reading disability, and the only one for which there is an evidence-based definition, is dyslexia. Dyslexia is a specific learning disability that is neurobiological in origin. It is characterized by difficulties with accurate and/or fluent word recognition and by poor spelling and decoding abilities. These difficulties typically result from a deficit in the phonological component of language that is often unexpected in relation to other cognitive abilities and the provision of effective classroom instruction. Secondary consequences may include problems in reading comprehension and reduced reading experience that can impede growth of vocabulary and background knowledge.

DSM-5 Descriptive Feature Specifiers for Impairment in Reading

The following descriptive specifiers highlight the domains of academic difficulties and the subskills that are affected at the time of assessment:

- Word reading accuracy
- Reading rate or fluency
- Reading comprehension

Neuropathology

- There are currently at least thirteen candidate genes that have been linked to dyslexia. Of these, four genes were initially identified in speech/language disorders. Research in molecular genetics has also demonstrated that neuronal migration, neurite outgrowth and guidance, and ciliary biology are involved in the development of dyslexia.
- Children at genetic risk for the development of dyslexia display differences (as early as a few days to 6 months of age) in brain response and orienting to speech sounds.

- Postmortem studies of individuals with developmental dyslexia in the 1970s and 1980s revealed consistent (unexpected) symmetry of the planum temporale, polymicrogyria of the left planum temporale, and cortical dysplasias in the left hemisphere.

- Some researchers have implicated a region in the left occipitotemporal cortex, including the middle part of the left fusiform gyrus, devoted to rapid processing of words, and referred to as the *visual word form area.*

- Recent neuroimaging studies have generally suggested alterations in structure (gray and white matter volumes) of several regions primarily in the left cerebral hemisphere regions and right cerebellum in children and adults with dyslexia, as well as alterations in functional activation in association with various reading tasks. Differences between typically developing individuals and those with dyslexia have also been found with respect to white matter microstructure predominantly in the left hemisphere.

- During tasks requiring phonological analysis, underactivation is seen in Wernicke's area, angular gyrus, and striate cortex, with concurrent overactivation in the inferior frontal gyrus—sometimes referred to as the *neural signature of dyslexia* (although, to be clear, functional neuroimaging is not used clinically to diagnosis a learning disability).

Epidemiology

Reading disabilities are estimated to occur in 10–15% of school-aged children and adolescents; however, estimates differ depending on the methods used for defining impairment. It is also true that some children who meet research definitions for a learning disability may not meet state or district definition for the federally handicapping educational disability (and vice versa). Reading disabilities are slightly more common in males. Socioeconomic status has been found to account for approximately 10% of the variance in reading outcomes.

- According to the 2017 United States National Assessment of Educational Progress (NAEP), 32% of fourth-graders and 24% of eighth-graders performed at the "below basic" level in reading.

Co-Occurring Conditions with Dyslexia

- Approximately 55% of children with dyslexia have oral language deficits, and about 50% of children with language difficulties (i.e., DSM-5 Language Disorder and Speech Sound Disorder) exhibit deficient reading.

- Deficits in language skills are also common in adults with dyslexia.

- Incidence of mathematics disabilities in those with dyslexia is as high as approximately 55%.

- Approximately 25–40% of children with dyslexia have ADHD, and approximately 25–40% of children with ADHD have dyslexia. The two disorders co-occur more often than would be expected by chance.

- Deficits in processing speed have been reported in both dyslexia and ADHD and are independent of specific deficits in phonological awareness and language skills, perhaps a cognitive reflection of the genetic overlap.

Presentation and Disorder Course

Skills Considered Fundamental for Acquisition of Reading

- *Phonological Awareness* The individual's ability to understand that words are comprised of specific speech sounds (phonemes). Phonological skills involve the ability to parse out the component sounds of words and to put them back together. Most individuals with dyslexia have deficient phonological awareness and have difficulty converting graphemes (written units of sound) into phonemes.

- *Decoding* The individual converts letters into sounds and combines them to form a recognizable word. The ability to convert letters to sounds is based on knowledge of the alphabet and phonological awareness.

- *Sight Reading* The individual retrieves or recognizes words from sight that are already known. As this skill develops, the recognition becomes faster and more automatic, and the number of sight words grows.

- *Prediction* The reader applies context, linguistic and background knowledge, and memory to text to anticipate or guess the meaning of unknown words. This is a top-down (executive) skill, facilitated by knowledge of word-letter associations.

Automaticity, Rapid Naming, and Reading

- Rapid automatized naming (RAN) has been shown to be strongly predictive of reading, independent of phonological awareness.

  - Failure to automatize skills necessary for rapid serial naming is considered a core difficulty among children with reading disabilities.

  - The most widely used measures of RAN require the individual to quickly and accurately name sets of overlearned visual stimuli (e.g., letters, simple objects, digits, and colors). For adults, however, measures of object naming are likely to be most sensitive, because naming of letters, digits, and colors is far more automatic.

The Double-Deficit Model of Reading Disabilities

- The model argues for the presence of two "single-deficit" subtypes of reading disabilities with more limited reading deficits and one "*double-deficit*" subtype with more pervasive and severe deficits.

- Rapid naming speed (single-deficit) and phonological awareness (single-deficit) variables contribute uniquely to different aspects of reading according to this model.

  - The implications of processing speed as a core deficit are also considered.

- There is some limited support for this model in adults.

Reading Fluency

- Development of reading fluency is critical for becoming a competent reader.

- Reading fluency depends on skills that include phonological awareness, phonics, automaticity of sound-symbol relationship retrieval, decoding, recognition of sight words, vocabulary, and processing speed.

- Individuals with dyslexia typically have problems with fluent reading of text; however, poor reading fluency is also observed in individuals who do not have basic word recognition difficulties (e.g., children with ADHD commonly have poor reading fluency even in the absence of dyslexia).

- For some, fluency may normalize, especially if the problem is addressed by third grade, but for others, reading and understanding text remains difficult throughout school and into adulthood.

- Deficits in reading comprehension tend to improve among individuals who have had direct instruction in methods to develop vocabulary, reading fluency, and strategy use.

- The primary problem for adults is slow, inefficient reading, even when decoding and single-word reading are adequate. This can be due to associated problems with spoken language and working memory.

Reading Comprehension

- Functional deficits related to reading comprehension tend to fit into three categories:

  - Basic word recognition skills and reading fluency

  - Broad oral language skills (including expressive and receptive vocabulary, as well as oral language comprehension)

  - Attention and executive functions (including sustained attention, working memory, cognitive inhibition, planning, organized memory search, estimation)

- The "simple view" of reading emphasizes the necessity of both decoding and language comprehension skills for proficient reading comprehension.

- Reading comprehension is dependent on orthographic (visual word form) and morphologic (word meaning) processing, in addition to phonologic processing.

- Deficits in attention and executive functioning in children and adults with reading disorders can prevent smooth coordination of the component skills needed for effective reading comprehension.

  - Children with specific reading comprehension disorders (i.e., those with poor comprehension despite intact word recognition skills) often have deficits in the planning elements of executive function.

  - Adults can have more difficulty with interpreting what they have read than with literal or fact-based understanding.

- In a meta-analysis, adults with reading comprehension deficits showed effect sizes that supported deficits in decoding, word reading, language, and working memory similar to deficits in children.

Late-Emerging Reading Disabilities

- Learners can struggle with fluency and comprehension in the absence of basic word recognition/decoding problems.

- Approximately 40% of all students with reading disabilities have *late-emerging reading disabilities*; that is, deficits are not evident until at least third grade.

  - This pattern is sometimes known as the "fourth-grade slump," can be associated with the transition from "learning to read" to "reading to learn," and may also be related to reduced vocabulary development in students of low socioeconomic status backgrounds.

  - *Late-emerging reading disabilities* are often associated with coexisting conditions, especially ADHD.

- Children who received early intervention and showed improvement may start to struggle again with the increased demands and volume of middle and high school reading and when they are expected to work more independently.

Expectations for Neuropsychological Assessment Results

Although some researchers have concluded that only brief assessment is necessary for any learning disability diagnosis prior to starting treatment, others have suggested that comprehensive assessment is valuable to understand the full range of functional strengths and weaknesses. Comprehensive evaluations can be even more important for adults, for whom there can be a variety of reasons for learning problems. Comprehensive assessment can help:

- Diagnose co-occurring conditions
- Determine if an intellectual disability better accounts for underachievement
- Determine if another disorder, such as ADHD, better accounts for underachievement
- Determine if emotional factors explain or exacerbate underachievement
- Provide additional targets and recommendations for intervention (e.g., language therapy for deficits in spoken language; occupational therapy to improve motor skills, handwriting, and keyboarding; psychotherapy to address emotional issues)

Regarding reading disabilities, Box 15.1 includes the skills most likely to be affected. By focusing on the expected areas of difficulty, assessment can be streamlined.

BOX 15.1 Areas of Functional Weakness in Reading Disabilities

- Phonological awareness
- Listening comprehension/immediate memory (single word, discourse)
- General knowledge and vocabulary
- Auditory verbal span
- Executive function (planning, estimation) as related to reading comprehension
- Processing speed
- Word retrieval (confrontation naming, rapid automatized visual naming, timed word generation/word fluency)
- Phonological and orthographic skills (decoding, single word reading, encoding when reading, spelling)
- Fluency (non-contextual—single words; contextual—text)
- Timed versus extended time reading comprehension (for adolescents and adults)

NOTE: Adapted from Mapou, 2009, and used with permission of Oxford University Press

---

Considerations when Treating Patients with Reading Disabilities

The National Reading Panel reviewed the scientific literature on reading instruction and specifically recommended phonological awareness, phonics, sight word acquisition, vocabulary, and comprehension of text as essential domains for instruction in normal reading development for all students. They also concluded:

- Oral reading enhances reading fluency better than silent reading practice.
- Instruction in vocabulary should be taught directly, as well as augmented via computer interface.

- Comprehension is developed by a combination of direct instructional methods to develop vocabulary, reading fluency, and strategy use.

Overall, reading interventions have been found to be most effective in one-to-one or small group settings. Structured literacy approaches involve explicit, systematic, and cumulative instruction of word identification and decoding, and are recommended for individuals with dyslexia.

- Repeated reading has been the most effective intervention for improving reading fluency. Additionally, reading fluency has been improved by reading with audiobooks, using an easier level of text, setting a performance criterion, giving performance feedback, and modeling (teacher or by more proficient peer).

- Interventions for reading comprehension include explicit instruction of strategies (e.g., how to make inferences, identify themes, summarize) use of non-written media (e.g., listening to a text, visual presentation) while teaching these strategies, and structured questioning during reading.

- Intrinsic motivation tends to increase voluntary reading, which in turn increases reading comprehension. This finding has been found particularly true when children express wanting to read in order to experience involvement (e.g., getting lost in a story, experiencing imagination). An increase in voluntary reading has not been demonstrated for extrinsic motivation (e.g., competition). Therefore, in order to increase voluntary reading, instructors may wish to encourage reading activities through high-interest material.

- Some emerging research has demonstrated that training in morphological awareness (i.e., understanding how words can be broken down into smaller units of meaning, such as roots, prefixes, and suffixes) can be useful as a compensatory strategy in adults with dyslexia.

Controversial and/or Unproven Treatments for Reading Disabilities

While there are many evidence-based treatments for learning disabilities in reading, there are also numerous programs that claim to improve reading abilities but have no research to support their effectiveness. The following are two examples of such programs that are not evidence-based.

- *Vision Therapy and Associated Treatments* A joint report from the American Academy of Pediatrics and the American Academy of Ophthalmology concluded:

    Scientific evidence does not support the claims that visual training, muscle exercises, ocular pursuit-and-tracking exercises, behavioral/perceptual vision therapy, "training" glasses, prisms, and colored (Irlen) lenses and filters are effective direct or indirect treatments for learning disabilities. There is no valid evidence that children who participate in vision therapy are more responsive to educational instruction than children who do not.

- *Fast ForWord* This program is a set of computer-based interventions designed to improve oral language and literacy skills in children with language learning weaknesses. The program is based on the principle that language-based learning disabilities are due to a rapid auditory temporal processing deficit that compromises the development of phonological representations. A meta-analysis of treatment studies indicated that there was no significant effect of Fast ForWord as a treatment for children's oral language or reading difficulties.

Section 2: Mathematics Disabilities

Definition

DSM-5 Descriptive Feature Specifiers for Impairment in Mathematics

The following descriptive specifiers highlight the domains of academic difficulties and their subskills that are impaired at the time of assessment:

- Number sense
- Memorization of arithmetic facts
- Accurate or fluent calculations
- Accurate math reasoning

Other Subtypes of Mathematics Disabilities

- The *semantic memory subtype* Characterized by deficient, inaccurate, or inconsistent arithmetic fact retrieval.
- The *procedural errors subtype* Characterized by the use of developmentally immature procedures or errors in the execution of procedures.
- The *visuospatial subtype* Characterized by misalignment of numbers or place value errors in decimals. This subtype characterization is based largely on adult lesion data and has not been validated in studies of children.

Neuropathology

- Studies have indicated that several brain regions within the posterior parietal cortex are involved in math processing, especially the intraparietal sulcus, the supramarginal gyrus, and the angular gyrus.
- Across a variety of anatomic and functional imaging studies, there is a developmental trend in numerical processing in typically developing individuals such that young children who are just learning math skills have greater activation in prefrontal regions, whereas older adolescents and adults demonstrate decreased dependence on working memory and attentional resources mediated by prefrontal regions.

Epidemiology

Emerging data suggest that mathematics disabilities are nearly as prevalent as reading disabilities and should receive similar attention.

- Recent studies suggest that up to 20% of individuals have some form of math learning disability.
- According to the 2017 NAEP, 20% of fourth-graders and 30% of eighth-graders performed at the "below basic" level in mathematics achievement.

Co-Occurring Conditions with Mathematics Disabilities

Reading and mathematics disabilities frequently co-occur.

- Skills in automaticity, processing speed, and working memory needed to read single words are necessary for automatizing math fact retrieval.

- Phonological awareness has been proposed to be associated with mathematics computation in elementary school children.

- Both working memory and phonological awareness contribute shared variance among disorders of reading, math, and attention.

- In adults, deficits in semantic knowledge, attention, visuospatial skills, and executive functioning affect mathematics performance.

- Math difficulties in children have also been associated with math-specific anxiety, as well as anxiety more generally. Anxiety must also be considered for adults in whom math skills have normalized.

Genetic and Neurodevelopmental Disorders Associated with Mathematics Disabilities

See also Chapter 18, Chromosomal and Genetic Syndromes, and Chapter 20, Congenital and Acquired Hydrocephalus.

- Turner syndrome
- Fragile X syndrome (girls)
- Congenital hydrocephalus
- Neurofibromatosis type I
- Spina bifida
- Congenital hypothyroidism
- 22q deletion syndrome
- Williams syndrome
- Preterm birth/very low birth weight

Presentation and Disorder Course

Skills Involved in Mathematics Acquisition

- *Domain-specific skills* Several skills that are often collectively referred to as *numerosity* (i.e., understanding and recognizing the concept of quantity) have been demonstrated to be important for mathematical achievement. These include the ability to decipher whether an Arabic number is greater or less than another (symbolic comparison), the ability to determine which of two arrays contains more or less objects (non-symbolic comparison), and the ability to accurately place a given Arabic numeral on a number line (number line estimation). Furthermore, an individual's ability to count forward and backward (i.e., procedural counting), as well as the ability to articulate a specific quantity after counting (i.e., conceptual counting) are also vital in the early development of math skills.

- *Domain-general skills* Many of the same fundamental cognitive processes underlying reading development are also critical for the development of math abilities. Cognitive skills often involved in mathematical achievement include language, phonological awareness, visuospatial skills, nonverbal reasoning, working memory (spatial and verbal), processing speed, attention, and executive functions (especially planning and estimation).

- An important difference between math and reading is that math achievement is cumulative throughout and beyond the elementary school years.

Expectations for Neuropsychological Assessment Results

Box 15.2 includes the neuropsychological skills most likely to be impaired in mathematics disabilities.

BOX 15.2 Areas of Functional Weakness in Mathematics Disabilities

- Attention
- Executive functions: Planning, organization, and problem solving
- Processing speed
- Working memory
- Visuospatial skills
- Semantic knowledge
- Fluency for simple math facts (speed of retrieval)

NOTE: Adapted from Mapou, 2009, and used with permission of Oxford University Press

Considerations when Treating Patients with Mathematics Disabilities

- Math concepts should be taught in an explicit, step-by-step manner. Math instruction should be supplemented with concrete examples, demonstration, modeling, and verbal descriptions. These concepts should always be linked to previously learned skills.

- When students have co-occurring difficulties in math calculation and word problem solving, focused instruction on math problem solving has been demonstrated to translate into improving calculations as well, but not vice versa.

Section 3: Written Expression Disabilities

Definition

A variety of terms have been used to characterize problems with written expression, including developmental output failure, *dysgraphia*, writing disorder, writing problems, disorder of written expression, problems in written expression, writing difficulties, and writing disabilities. There is a paucity of research conducted on those with written expression disabilities in comparison to reading disabilities. However, it should be noted that many students struggle with writing and fall below grade expectations. These students have been referred to as the "silent majority," given their lack of a diagnosis and intervention.

As a result, much of the literature addresses writing difficulties as opposed to a group of individuals diagnosed with a learning disability in written expression.

DSM-5 Descriptive Feature Specifiers for Impairment in Written Expression

The following descriptive specifiers highlight the domains of academic difficulties and their subskills that are impaired at the time of assessment:

- Spelling accuracy
- Grammar and punctuation accuracy
- Clarity or organization of written expression

Neuropathology

Research on the neural basis of written expression difficulties in children remains limited. However, recent imaging studies have begun to explore the structural and functional difficulties in children with dysgraphia. As with all types of learning disabilities, the neuroimaging correlates of the condition vary with the age of the individual, the presence (or absence) of co-occurring disorders, and the imaging methods used. Given the overlap between disorders of written expression and other conditions (e.g., dyslexia, ADHD), the interpretation of imaging findings is even more challenging.

- Children with dysgraphia have been found to have alterations in white matter microstructure in several brain regions, predominantly within the left hemisphere.

Epidemiology

- Incidence rates of written expression disabilities vary from 7% (using a regression formula) to 15% (using a low-achievement method).
- Boys are two to three more times more likely to have written expression disability than girls.
- Approximately 75% of individuals with dyslexia also have written expression disabilities.
- According to the 2011 NAEP, 20% of eighth-graders and 21% of twelfth-graders performed at the "below basic" level in writing.

Co-Occurring Conditions with Written Expression Disabilities

Most children with learning disabilities in reading or math have significant problems in at least one area of written expression. Among children with a written expression learning disability, up to 75% also exhibit a reading learning disability.

Presentation and Disorder Course

- *Dysgraphia* Has been defined as including deficits in legible automatic letter writing, orthographic coding (i.e., storing written words and processing letters in them), and finger sequencing (i.e., emphasizing the motor deficits involved in writing).
- Cognitive phenotypes observed among children with poor written expression include those with only handwriting problems (dysgraphia), those with only reading and spelling problems (dyslexia), and those with oral language and written language problems.

- Students with dyslexia tend to have problems with automatic letter writing and naming that contribute to weaknesses in inhibition and verbal fluency and may explain spelling problems.

- Several components of language are involved in translation of mental information into written format.

  - *Transcription* involves the subword level (handwriting) and word level (spelling) of written language.

  - *Syntax* is a level of language that provides structure for organizing words.

- *Processing speed* Also plays an important contributing role in written expression disorders. Writing fluency alone may be a better predictor of overall writing success in school than performance on writing samples alone.

- *Working memory* Is important in written expression because it allows the individual to engage in multiple cognitive tasks at the same time (e.g., retrieval of information from memory, maintenance of multiple ideas; see also Chapter 5, Domains of Neuropsychological Function and Related Neurobehavioral Disorders).

- *Executive functioning* Several additional components of executive functions have been found to be particularly important in written expression tasks, given their involvement in the three primary stages of writing: (1) planning, (2) translating ideas into words, and (3) revising.

- Many individuals with ADHD can be vulnerable to difficulties with written expression, even in the absence of reading disabilities, because of executive function difficulties. These difficulties often manifest in mid to late elementary school years and beyond.

  - Among college students, behaviors associated with ADHD have also been shown to be associated with written expression difficulties.

- In early elementary school, difficulties on measures of orthographic choice (i.e., selecting the appropriate written word versus a pseudo-homophone, for example, rain versus rane), working memory, inhibition, visual memory, and planning have been predictive of poor written expression skills in grades three and four.

- Additionally, children who are at-risk for developing written expression difficulties have been found to exhibit lower performance on spelling, writing mechanics, quality, length, and syntax as early as the first grade.

- Factors found to be associated with writing disabilities in adults include slow writing speed, poor handwriting, spelling errors, weak vocabulary, and low verbosity. Men with dyslexia may be more affected in writing skills than women with dyslexia.

Expectations for Neuropsychological Assessment Results

Box 15.3 includes the neuropsychological skills most likely to be affected in individuals with written expression disabilities.

> **BOX 15.3** Areas of Functional Weakness in Written Expression Disabilities
>
> - Motor speed and dexterity
> - Handwriting quality (including copying from both desktop and blackboard)
> - Attention and executive functioning (particularly working memory)
> - Phonological and orthographic skills (encoding, spelling dictation)
> - Language abilities
> - Oral sentence formulation
> - Verbal organization (oral, written)
> - Fluency for writing words and sentences
> - Essay writing
>
> **NOTE:** Adapted from Mapou, 2009, and used with permission of Oxford University Press

Considerations when Treating Patients with Written Expression Disabilities

- Systematic and explicit instruction on transcription skills has been demonstrated to improve writing fluency and quality.

- Supporting the development of oral language skills can also improve written expression.

- Research has demonstrated the utility of self-regulated strategy development (SRSD) instruction, which teaches self-regulation strategies (e.g., goal setting, self-monitoring) to improve the writing process.

Considerations when Evaluating and Treating Individuals with Learning Disabilities

Shift in Emphasis

As seen in Figure 15.1, when moving from childhood to adolescence to adulthood, the emphasis on how one treats the learning disability changes. For the early years of school, identification and prevention of the learning disability is most important. For children identified later, evidence-based intervention is crucial. However, for adolescents and adults, in whom early intervention may have provided the maximum benefit or in whom intervention may have less impact on a well-established and poorly treated learning disability, accommodations become very important.

Accommodations

The most common accommodation is extended time on tests, typically from 25% to 100% of the standard amount of time, used to mitigate the impact of a learning disability on speed when reading, writing, or doing math. This becomes increasingly important, as tests become more complex in late elementary and middle school. Other common accommodations include the use of a computer for tests that require writing, extra breaks during lengthy tests, note-taking supports (permission to record lectures, access to PowerPoint presentations ahead of class, in-class note-taker), and course substitutions.

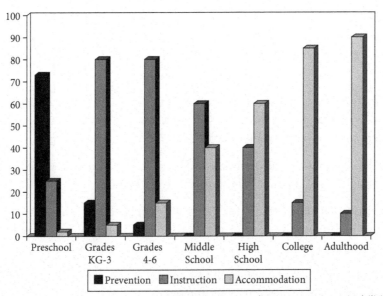

FIGURE 15.1 Prevention, Intervention, and Accommodation: Approaches to Learning Disabilities Over the Lifespan

NOTE: Morris, R. (2009, February) Discussant for the invited International Neuropsychological Society Symposium, "Cognitive/neuro-psychological assessment is critical to learning disabilities—Or is it?" Reprinted with Permission.

Documentation Guidelines for High-Stakes Testing

Documentation guidelines have been published to guide neuropsychological assessment of adolescents and adults in secondary and postsecondary education. Originally developed by the Association on Higher Education and Disability and subsequently modified and revised by Educational Testing Service, testing agencies, such as the College Board, Law School Admission Council, Association of American Medical Colleges, the National Board of Medical Examiners, and state bar examiners, as well as universities, have adopted these guidelines. Because requirements differ, guidelines should be consulted before completing an assessment. Also, because of guidance for documentation issued by the Association on Higher Education and Disability, requirements for updated neuropsychological evaluations for secondary and postsecondary education students may be eased. In addition, evaluators must be familiar with recent updates to laws following implementation of the 2008 Amendments to the 1990 Americans with Disabilities Act and with documentation guidelines for high-stakes testing issued in 2015 by the Department of Justice Civil Rights Division, Disability Rights Section. Finally, because some high school, college, and post-secondary education students may try to "get an edge" through accommodations to which they are not truly entitled, evaluators should (1) be conservative when making a learning disability diagnosis and (2) always include measures of performance and symptom validity that are now part of standard neuropsychological practice.

Relevant Definitions

Double-deficit model A model of reading disabilities that hypothesizes two "single-deficit" subtypes of reading disabilities (phonological awareness or rapid automatized naming) with more limited reading impairments and one "double-deficit" subtype with more pervasive and severe impairments.

Dysgraphia Impairment in legible automatic letter writing, orthographic coding (i.e., storing written words and processing letters in them), and finger sequencing.

Late-emerging reading disabilities A pattern observed in approximately 40% of all students with reading disabilities in which problems are not observed until at least third grade and are often associated with the transition from "learning to read" to "reading to learn." This pattern is sometimes referred to as the "fourth-grade slump."

Neural signature of dyslexia A pattern observed in functional magnetic resonance imaging (fMRI) studies of reading in which underactivation is seen in Wernicke's area, the angular gyrus, and striate cortex, and concurrent overactivation is observed in the inferior frontal gyrus.

Numerosity The understanding and recognizing of the concept of quantity, which can include symbolic comparison, non-symbolic comparison, and number line estimation.

Response to intervention (RTI) A model for defining learning disabilities based on the premise that students should receive adequate instruction with appropriate monitoring before being considered to have a learning disability.

Visual word form area A region in the left occipitotemporal cortex, including the middle part of the left fusiform gyrus, devoted to rapid processing of written words.

Learning Disabilities Questions

NOTE: Questions 32, 57, 74, and 84 on the First Full-Length Practice Examination, Questions 37, 60, and 113 on the Second Full-Length Practice Examination, Questions 50, 79, and 115 on the Third Full-Length Practice Examination, and Questions 21, 67, and 107 on the Fourth Full-Length Practice Examination are from this chapter.

1. You are evaluating an employed adult who believes that he has a learning disability. Obtaining a detailed history from this adult _____.

   (a) is crucial for establishing the developmental onset of these disorders, in combination with information on current functioning

   (b) is desirable, although a definitive diagnosis may be made on the basis of current functioning

   (c) should include childhood academic records and a parent interview if possible combined with information on current functioning

   (d) is not helpful without looking at records and obtaining a current evaluation of the adult's skills

2. When evaluating for a learning disability a child who has not shown progress with standard instruction, which model has the best research support for diagnosis?

   (a) aptitude-achievement discrepancy

   (b) intra-individual differences

   (c) response to intervention

   (d) low-achievement model

3. Although some researchers and clinicians believe there is usefulness in diagnosing _____, there is disagreement over whether it exists as a separate learning disability.

   (a) nonverbal learning disability

   (b) written language disability

   (c) reading disability

   (d) mathematics disability

4. A college student with a history of a written language disorder and accommodations for that is asking for use of a computer on writing tests. You would like to do a streamlined evaluation to document his need for accommodation. What skills will be most important to assess?

    (a) visuospatial skills, organizational abilities, and spoken language comprehension

    (b) handwriting speed, visuospatial skills, and visual learning and memory

    (c) spelling, handwriting quality and speed, and vocabulary

    (d) visuospatial skills, spoken language skills, and attention

5. The double-deficit model of reading posits that deficits in _____ are associated with persistent and severe reading disabilities.

    (a) pseudoword decoding and reading of real words

    (b) rapid automatized naming and phonological awareness

    (c) phonological awareness and verbal working memory

    (d) single word reading and reading comprehension

6. You have evaluated an 11-year-old girl and diagnosed a specific learning disability with impairment in written expression. An evidence-based recommendation would be school instruction and support in _____.

    (a) transcription skills and visuospatial skills

    (b) transcription skills and listening comprehension

    (c) transcription skills and self-regulation strategies

    (d) listening comprehension and self-regulation strategies

7. The brain region most consistently found to be involved in math processing is the _____.

    (a) cingulate gyrus

    (c) inferior temporal sulcus

    (b) intraparietal sulcus

    (d) postcentral sulcus

8. The visual word form area is a region in the brain that has been associated with rapid processing of written words. This region can be found in the _____.

    (a) left frontotemporal cortex

    (c) right occipitotemporal cortex

    (b) right frontotemporal cortex

    (d) left occipitotemporal cortex

9. Late-emerging reading disabilities refer to difficulties in reading not observed until at least _____.

    (a) third grade

    (c) ninth grade

    (b) sixth grade

    (d) adulthood

10. You have determined that a child has dyslexia and want to recommend evidence-based intervention. What else in addition to phonological awareness should be the initial focus of intervention?

    (a) reading comprehension

    (c) fluent reading of sentences

    (b) word reading

    (d) spelling

Learning Disabilities Answers

1. **C—should include childhood academic records and a parent interview if possible combined with information on current functioning** *A learning disability is a developmental disorder. It does not appear in adult life without evidence of earlier problems. The history can be the most important part of the assessment. However, memory is fallible, and some adults may be motivated to distort their history so that they can get accommodations. Therefore, a better option is to review academic records and to interview a parent, rather than relying only on self-report. It is also necessary to show the expected academic and neuropsychological profile at the time of assessment. Adults who have no history of early learning problems but are reporting difficulty with reading, writing, or math most likely have another cause for their problems.*

   References:
   (a) American Psychiatric Association (2013). *Diagnostic and statistical manual for mental disorders* (5th ed.; DSM-5). Washington, DC: American Psychiatric Press.
   (b) Mapou, R. L. (2009). *Adult learning disabilities and ADHD: Research informed assessment.* New York, NY: Oxford University Press.

2. **D—low-achievement model** *Of these four models, the low-achievement model has the best validity, especially when standard instruction has not been effective.*

   References:
   (a) Fletcher, J. M. (2009). Dyslexia: The evolution of a scientific concept. *Journal of the International Neuropsychological Society, 15,* 501–508.
   (b) Fletcher, J. M., Lyon, G. R., Fuchs, L. S., & Barnes, M. A. (2018). *Learning disabilities: From identification to intervention* (2nd ed.). New York, NY: Guilford Press.

3. **A—nonverbal learning disability** *There is far less empirical support for nonverbal learning disability as a separate learning disability. The educational impact is less specific, and there is overlap between the features of nonverbal learning disability and ADHD.*

   References:
   (a) Fletcher, J. M., Lyon, G. R., Fuchs, L. S., & Barnes, M. A. (2018). *Learning disabilities: From identification to intervention* (2nd ed.). New York, NY: Guilford Press.
   (b) Pennington, B. F., McGrath, L. M., & Peterson, R. L. (2019). *Diagnosing learning disorders: From science to practice* (3rd ed.). New York, NY: Guilford Press.
   (c) Spreen, O. (2011). Nonverbal learning disabilities: A critical review. *Child Neuropsychology, 17,* 418–443.

4. **C—spelling, handwriting quality and speed, and vocabulary** *Research on college students with dyslexia has shown that these four skills are highly predictive of writing problems. Although individuals with poor visuospatial skills, organizational skills, and attention can have difficulty with writing, these are less important components of an assessment.*

   References:
   (a) Connelly, V., Campbell, S., MacLean, M., & Barnes, J. (2006). Contribution of lower order skills to the written composition of college students. *Developmental Neuropsychology, 29,* 175–196.
   (b) Gregg, N., Coleman, C., Davis, M., & Chalk, J. C. (2007). Timed essay writing: Implications for high-stakes tests. *Journal of Learning Disabilities, 40,* 306–318.

5. **B—rapid automatized naming and phonological awareness** *The presence of deficits in both phonological awareness (single deficit) and rapid automatized naming (single-deficit) contribute to the double-deficit condition, which is associated with persistent reading disability.*

   Reference: Wolf, M., O'Rourke, A. G., Gidney, C., Lovett, M., Cirino, P., & Morris, R. (2002). The second deficit: An investigation of the independence of phonological and naming-speed deficits in developmental dyslexia. *Reading and Writing, 15,* 43–72.

6. **C—transcription skills and self-regulation strategies** *Transcription training and self-regulated strategy development (SRSD) have been found to result in higher-quality story writing than control conditions.*

   Reference: Limpo, T., & Alves, R. A. (2017). Tailoring multicomponent writing interventions: Effects of coupling self-regulation and transcription training. *Journal of Learning Disabilities, 51*(4), 381–398.

7. **B—intraparietal sulcus** *While several brain regions have been demonstrated to be involved in mathematics and number processing, the intraparietal sulcus has been repeatedly found to be activated in brain imaging studies.*

   References:
   (a) Bugden, S., Price, G. R., McLean, D. A., & Ansari, D. (2012). The role of the left intraparietal sulcus in the relationship between symbolic number processing and children's arithmetic competence. *Developmental Cognitive Neuroscience, 2*(4), 448–457.
   (b) Butterworth, B., & Walsh, V. (2011). Neural basis of mathematical cognition. *Current Biology, 21*(16), R618–R621.
   (c) Kaufmann, L., Wood, G., Rubinsten, O., & Henik, A. (2011). Meta-analyses of developmental fMRI studies investigating typical and atypical trajectories of number processing and calculation. *Developmental Neuropsychology, 36*(6), 763–787.

8. **D—left occipitotemporal cortex** *The visual word form area is located in the left occipitotemporal cortex and has been implicated in word recognition.*

   Reference: Raschle, N. M., Chang, M., & Gaab, N. (2011). Structural brain alterations associated with dyslexia predate reading onset. *Neuroimage, 57*(3), 742–749.

9. **A—third grade** *Also known as the "fourth-grade slump," late-emerging reading disabilities refers to the transition from "learning to read" to "reading to learn." These difficulties are not seen until at least third grade.*

   Reference: Etmanskie, J. M., Partanen, M., & Siegel, L. S. (2016). A longitudinal examination of the persistence of late emerging reading disabilities. *Journal of Learning Disabilities, 49*(1), 21–35.

10. **B—word reading** *Dyslexia at its core is a disorder of phonological awareness and word reading. Once these skills are built, intervention can progress to work on fluency when reading sentences and reading comprehension.*

    Reference: Fletcher, J. M., Lyon, G. R., Fuchs, L. S., & Barnes, M. A. (2018). *Learning disabilities: From identification to intervention* (2nd ed.). New York, NY: Guilford Press.

Recommended Readings

Barnes, M. A., Martinez-Lincoln, A., & Raghubar, K. P. (2017). Mathematical learning disabilities: What does the science tell us about assessment and diagnosis? *Perspectives on Language and Literacy, 43*, 10–19.

Coker, D. L., Jr., & Kim, Y. S. G. (2017). Critical issues in the understanding of young elementary school students at risk for problems in written expression: Introduction to the special issue. *Journal of Learning Disabilities, 51*, 315–319. [Refer to articles within the special issue]

Fletcher, J. M., Lyon, G. R., Fuchs, L. S., & Barnes, M. A. (2018). *Learning disabilities: From identification to intervention* (2nd ed.). New York, NY: Guilford Press.

Mapou, R. L. (2009). *Adult learning disabilities and ADHD: Research-informed assessment.* New York, NY: Oxford University Press.

Pennington, B. F. (2009). *Diagnosing learning disorders: A neuropsychological framework* (2nd ed.). New York, NY: Guilford Press. [Especially chapters 6, 12, 14, and 15]

Peterson, R. L., & Pennington, B. F. (2015). Developmental dyslexia. *Annual Review of Clinical Psychology, 11,* 283–307.

Swanson, H. L., Harris, K. R., & Graham, S. (Eds.). (2013). *Handbook of learning disabilities* (2nd ed.). New York, NY: Guilford Press.

Wolf, L. E., Schreiber, H., & Wasserstein, J. (Eds.). (2008). *Adult learning disorders: Contemporary issues.* New York, NY: Psychology Press.

16 Attention-Deficit/Hyperactivity Disorder

John W. Kirk and Richard Boada

Definition

Attention-deficit/hyperactivity disorder (ADHD) is a neurodevelopmental disorder that begins during childhood and frequently persists into adulthood. The clinical phenotype consists of short attention span, overactivity, and impulsivity. Historically, the relative importance of each of these behavioral symptoms has waxed and waned in the formulation of the disorder, mirroring an evolving conceptualization of the core deficit.

History

The disorder presently termed ADHD was viewed initially as one of motor overactivity that brought individuals into conflict with environmental expectations and also prevented on-task behavior. Subsequently, emphasis shifted to the central role of attentional impairment in the disorder, resulting in two diagnostic categories: attention deficit disorder (ADD) with hyperactivity and ADD without hyperactivity. Accumulating research eventually called into question the role of inattention as the primary or core deficit, which led to the collapse of these two diagnoses into a single construct: attention-deficit/hyperactivity disorder.

The Diagnostic and Statistical Manual of Mental Disorders—Fifth Edition (DSM-5, 2013) has kept the overarching ADHD diagnosis and continued to divide it into three subtypes: ADHD-Predominately Hyperactive/Impulsive Presentation (ADHD-H), in which hyperactive/impulsive symptoms predominate; ADHD-Predominately Inattentive Presentation, in which inattention symptoms predominate (ADHD-I); and ADHD-Combined Presentation, in which both sets of symptoms are prominent (ADHD-C).

Epidemiology

- ADHD is the most common behavioral disorder of childhood, affecting approximately 10% of United States children ages 4 to 17 years. Prevalence rates have risen from 7% in 1998–2000 to 10% in 2011–2013. The increase in prevalence is thought to be secondary to several factors including clinicians more accurately diagnosing the disorder in recent years and broader diagnostic criteria.

- Worldwide estimates of ADHD are lower at around 5%, likely secondary to varying diagnostic methods, practice guidelines, and access to specialized healthcare services.

- Boys are diagnosed with ADHD about twice as often as girls (prevalence rates of 12% vs. 6%, respectively), with this being especially true at younger ages and in clinically referred samples.

This difference is often attributed to differential manifestations of ADHD symptoms by gender (e.g., less disruptive symptoms in females, later age of onset) and lower rates of the ADHD-H subtype compared to the ADHD-I subtype in girls.

- Incidence rates increase with age, with estimates of ADHD among 10- to 17-year-olds being almost twice as high as rates of ADHD in children 5 to 9 years of age.

- Recent studies suggest that prevalence rates of ADHD do not differ significantly between non-Latin/x whites and African American children. Rates for Latin/x children seem to be lower.

- The prevalence of ADHD varies by subtype. In children aged 8 to 15 in the United States, approximately twice as many are diagnosed with ADHD-I as with the ADHD-C or ADHD-H. Interpretation of this statistic, however, is confounded by the fact that there is less than optimal stability of subtype classifications over time.

- ADHD diagnosis is associated with various socioeconomic factors. Diagnosis is more common in children of families whose incomes are closer to the poverty level, in single-parent households, and in those having Medicaid as opposed to private insurance or no insurance.

Diagnosis of ADHD

Diagnostic Criteria Changes with DSM-5

The DSM-5 has addressed some of the issues in ADHD diagnostic criteria that were problematic in the DSM-IV. Some of the improvements are:

- ADHD is characterized as a *neurodevelopmental disorder*, which more appropriately recognizes its onset and chronic developmental course.

- Increasing the age by which impairing symptoms must be present from 7 to 12, reflecting research finding little difference in symptom expression and outcome between children diagnosed by these different ages.

- Presence of autism spectrum disorder is no longer exclusionary.

- Symptoms of inattention and/or hyperactivity/impulsivity are required to be merely "present" rather than cause "impairment." There is still the stipulation that symptoms interfere with functioning or development. "Functional impairment" is rated more wholistically and separately, with modifiers of mild, moderate, or severe.

- Examples were added to each symptom item to improve clarity and relevance across the lifespan.

- Downward adjustment of the cut point for diagnosis in adolescents 17 years and older and in adults was made, to improve validity and reliability at older ages. Older adolescents and adults must have at least five of nine symptoms (down from six of nine symptoms for individuals < 17 years of age) in each symptom category (inattention or hyperactivity/impulsivity).

Limitations of Diagnostic Criteria and Their Application

While the ADHD diagnostic criteria underwent the changes outlined in the previous section, and these changes likely make these diagnostic criteria among the most rigorous and empirically derived available for diagnostic purposes, there are still some important limitations to consider.

First, there continues to be lower stability than is optimal for ADHD subtypes at the individual level over time, especially with individuals diagnosed as having ADHD-C at a young age reverting to ADHD-I as they get older. Although the latter could be influenced by lower sensitivity of hyperactive-impulsive

(HI) items in older individuals, studies have also shown that declining HI symptoms with increasing age are likely to be a part of the natural history of the disorder.

Second, there is continued debate in the literature regarding the validity of the ADHD-H subtype (i.e., without ever having inattentive symptoms). If internal and external validity or ADHD-H is in question, then reliability of symptoms may also fluctuate.

Third, clinical decision-making processes differ across providers, with some clinicians relying on rating scales completed by others, while others interview raters in depth regarding the presence and severity of symptoms. Differences in clinical practice, especially across providers of different disciplines (pediatricians, psychologists, psychiatrists), likely introduce additional variability in diagnostic accuracy and reliability.

Fourth, the longitudinal stability of a diagnosis is also affected by the imposition of a cutoff (whether it be five or six symptoms), when the underlying symptom dimension is continuous. Factors such as changing contextual demands, fluctuation in interests and motivation, and reduced inter-rater reliability, can all affect the ratings on symptom questionnaires, or the description of severity on interview, at a given point in time.

Fifth, the ADHD criteria and cutoffs are applied equally across gender, while the literature indicates that there are significant gender differences in the manifestation and symptom severity of ADHD. While this may be due to differing neurobiological mechanisms of the disorder across males and females, or interaction with other cognitive factors, researchers have also questioned whether item bias or method variance may contribute to the clinical prevalence disparity.

And last, the items in the DSM-5 still do not reflect some of the more recent conceptualizations of the disorder including theories that propose that executive functioning deficits (e.g., response inhibition, self-regulation, and motivation) are primary.

Continuous Symptom Dimensions Versus Categorical Subtypes

It is important to note that although symptoms of inattention, hyperactivity, and impulsivity are what clinicians use to diagnose ADHD, the clinical symptoms are just one end of a continuum of skill or ability in each of these domains. Researchers find it more beneficial to study traits or abilities continuously, as it increases the variance that can be used in analyses (rather than dichotomizing the dimension). This use of a symptom dimension approach, rather than a case/control approach, has allowed researchers to add important information to our understanding of ADHD and its underlying constructs.

The main findings from these dimensional approach studies are:

- DSM criteria for ADHD identify individuals who demonstrate significant functional impairment in social, academic, occupational, and overall global and adaptive functioning.

- These deficits occur even when IQ, demographic factors, and concurrent psychopathology are controlled.

- The validity of ADHD-H beyond the preschool years remains unclear. The latter is less heritable than other ADHD subtypes and is associated with less academic and cognitive impairment.

- There is support for the concurrent, predictive, and discriminant validity of the inattentive and hyperactive-impulsive symptom dimensions, arguing for their inclusion in future diagnostic systems.

- The influence of the symptom dimension approach is already seen in the DSM-5, as the latter no longer uses a "subtype" classification scheme; instead, it has clinicians choose the predominant "presentation" (Inattentive, Hyperactive/Impulsive, or Combined).

- Studies that have identified participants by clinical subtype (ADHD-C and ADHD-I) have found that they are associated with similar academic, neuropsychological, and adaptive impairments.

- ADHD-C and ADHD-I share etiological influences and respond to the same pharmacological and psychosocial interventions.

Sluggish Cognitive Tempo and ADHD-I

Recent research in ADHD has led to a hypothesis that the inattentive dimension of ADHD-I may be associated with a different set of inattentive behaviors than those associated with ADHD-C. This set of inattentive behaviors is known as *sluggish cognitive tempo* (SCT) and is characterized by difficulty sustaining attention, daydreaming, lethargy, mental confusion or "mental fogginess," low motivation/initiation, physical underactivity, slowed movement, and decreased responsiveness. Children identified as having SCT are often described as spacey, having slowed information processing, easily confused, having erratic retrieval of information from memory, and being socially reticent and uninvolved. They are rarely aggressive and are less likely to have comorbid oppositional defiant disorder (ODD) or conduct disorder (CD). Sluggish cognitive tempo symptoms are correlated with the inattentive items found in ADHD-C, such that children with the latter also display higher levels of SCT than do children without ADHD. Recent factor analytic studies have consistently shown that many symptoms of SCT covary with the inattentive ADHD symptoms; however, there is consistent evidence that there are unique components of SCT (lethargy, underactivity, and slowness) which appear to be distinct from the inattention associated with ADHD. Although SCT is related to anxiety and depression (especially in older children and adolescents), the unique characteristics of SCT seems to be separable from anxiety and depression among factor analytic studies. Sleep difficulties may be a contributing factor in children with SCT, as they are rated to have greater parent-reported difficulty waking in the morning. There may be less efficacy with traditional stimulant medication in treating children with SCT, as these medications target hyperactive/impulsive symptoms better than the core features of SCT. Additional research is needed to clarify the validity of SCT symptoms and their relationship to external correlates, as well as potential biomarkers for this subtype.

Neuropathology

Pathophysiology

- ADHD has long been associated with abnormalities in frontal brain regions. Structural and functional imaging evidence indicates underactivation in frontocortical and frontosubcortical networks that persists into adulthood despite a relative symptomatic improvement in adults with the disorder.

- Structural brain differences found in children with ADHD include reduced total brain volume, delayed cortical maturation in frontal and temporal regions, and abnormalities in the corpus callosum; prefrontal, temporal, and parietal cortex; and basal ganglia (especially the caudate nucleus). Basal ganglia abnormalities are the most consistent finding across samples and methods.

- Functional imaging studies using single photon emission computed tomography (SPECT) and positron emission tomography (PET) techniques have also revealed differences in the frontal lobe and basal ganglia regions in ADHD. Functional magnetic resonance imaging (fMRI) studies have shown decreased activation in dorsolateral prefrontal cortex and dorsal anterior cingulate cortex on tasks requiring inhibitory control.

- These various structural abnormalities are thought to lead to deficits in a distributed neural network that includes frontal cortex and its striatal-thalamic-cerebellar connections. The links between specific frontal regions to subcortical structures are thought to influence modality-specific mechanisms that modulate the interaction with the environment. The wide array of neural systems affected in ADHD underscores the fact that the disorder has a more complex set of cognitive, motor, and behavioral/emotional symptoms at the endophenotypic level than is represented by the DSM-based symptom lists.

Genetics

- ADHD is familial and significantly heritable: 30–35% of first-degree relatives of children with ADHD also have the disorder, for a *relative risk* of 6 to 8 times that of the general population.

- Twin studies show that there is a heritability of 70–80% in both children and adults, with little or no evidence that environmental risk factors shared by siblings significantly impact etiology. The two main symptom dimensions of ADHD are also significantly heritable, with genetic influences accounting for upward of 75% of the variance in most cases. Most of the rest of the phenotypic variance in ADHD is accounted for by nonshared environmental influences and measurement error.

- Molecular genetic studies of ADHD have used candidate gene approaches, as well as linkage and association analyses, to identify possible genes affecting the disorder. The candidate gene approach has mostly targeted genes that affect the *dopamine* pathway (e.g., the *dopamine transporter gene DAT1*), due to the mechanism of action of psychostimulant medication. Association studies, testing *polymorphisms* in functional genes affecting both *dopamine* and serotonin pathways, have yielded some positive results.

- Genome-wide linkage and association analyses have identified linkage regions with small effect sizes on chromosomes 5, 6, 10, 12, and 16. Multiple genes have been found to be linked with ADHD, but their cumulative effect only accounts for a small percentage of the genetic variance in the disorder.

- Most of the genetic variance in ADHD symptomatology remains unexplained, highlighting the complex relationship between genetic and brain factors and a heterogeneous phenotype.

Risk Factors

Various additional environmental risk factors have been identified as being associated with ADHD symptoms. These include prematurity, birth complications, maternal smoking, lead exposure/toxicity, and moderate to severe traumatic brain injury.

Determinants of Severity

- ADHD symptoms vary in their severity, which is not surprising given that, in a multifactorial, polygenic disorder, accumulation of risks along the liability spectrum will be associated with a more severe phenotypic presentation.

- Gender differences in phenotypic severity have also been documented, with girls showing a milder clinical manifestation of the disorder.

- Various studies have found that comorbidity is often a marker for a more severe manifestation of the disorder. Thus, children with ADHD who also have a comorbid condition often have a more severe presentation than do those children with ADHD alone. For example, in comparison to children with ADHD or dyslexia alone, children with dyslexia plus ADHD exhibit a more extensive and severe profile of neuropsychological weaknesses and have a stronger genetic loading for both dyslexia and ADHD.

- There is a significant interaction between dyslexia and ADHD in terms of functional impairment. Children with both dyslexia and ADHD are at significantly higher risk of being retained in school, as well as of having legal difficulties and academic, social, and occupational impairment, compared with controls or children with either condition in isolation.

- Comorbidity with ODD and CD is associated with more severely impaired psychosocial outcomes, including a higher risk of legal difficulties and antisocial behavior.

Presentation, Developmental Course, and Recovery

- Children with ADHD represent a highly heterogeneous group. Although the two latent traits of inattention and hyperactivity/impulsivity are highly correlated, they differ in profile and impairment.

- Parents of young children with ADHD often complain of excessive gross motor activity, difficulty delaying gratification, short attention span, distractibility, and difficulty completing routine daily tasks (e.g., dressing, mealtime, and bedtime routines). Some young children with ADHD have motor difficulties and, as such, are described as being clumsy, getting injured more often, and having poor fine motor dexterity and coordination.

- During the school years, parents often report that their child with ADHD has difficulty sitting still for reading time, walks around or talks inappropriately in the classroom, impulsively starts tasks, daydreams, needs instructions repeated, and leaves tasks unfinished. Social difficulties are often identified as well, with fewer friendships and more conflicts reported. At times, children with ADHD are seen as a source of "entertainment" in the classroom, although this frequently leads to trouble with teachers.

- In higher elementary school grades, lack of or inconsistent academic progress is a key complaint. Children often do well for the first few weeks of the school year, but then grades worsen. Parents frequently report that their child does not like to sit and read, finds school tasks boring, has reduced written output (e.g., can't put thoughts down on paper), is disorganized with materials, loses belongings, forgets to turn in homework (e.g., multiple missing assignments), and has difficulties organizing and multitasking during more complex tasks.

- Children with ADHD often negotiate peer interactions impulsively, do not fully appreciate social nuances and expectations, do not plan or take into consideration the potential consequences of their actions, and get into arguments with caregivers. They continue to be restless and fidgety.

- Children with ADHD have lower academic achievement than their non-ADHD peers. They achieve lower grades and have weaker study skills (e.g., taking notes in class, preparing for tests, completing long-term projects, using reference materials). They are more likely to receive special education services.

- By early adolescence, signs of excessive gross motor activity are less common, and hyperactivity symptoms tend to be confined to fidgetiness or an inner feeling of jitteriness or restlessness.

- In adulthood, restlessness may lead to difficulty participating in sedentary activities and avoiding pastimes or occupations that provide limited opportunity for spontaneous movement.

- Persons with ADHD have difficulty identifying causal relationships in social situations and generating effective solutions to social problems. These social cognition deficits, in combination with frequently occurring executive functioning difficulties and aggression, increase the likelihood of peer rejection and association with deviant peers. Affiliation with the latter can contribute to further negative outcomes, such as delinquency and substance use.

- Children with ADHD have more conflicts with parents, and the latter report more stress, poorer coping, and less perceived competence in parenting. Marital difficulties and higher divorce rates are common.

- Young adults with ADHD engage in riskier activities, including having sex at earlier ages and with more partners. They are less likely to use contraception and thus become pregnant and contract sexually transmitted diseases more often than do young adults without ADHD. Young adults with ADHD have less stable romantic relationships and eventually also divorce at higher rates.

- Adults with ADHD have lower academic achievement, have lower high school and college graduation rates, and are less capable in terms of organization and time management skills. All of these contribute to poorer employment outcomes. When employed, they are less likely to work in a professional job setting. They experience more changes in employment and are at higher risk of being terminated from their jobs due to tardiness or absenteeism. As adults, these risks and associated problems result in significant reductions in earning and an increase in the use of social assistance. Adults with ADHD are more prone to accidents while driving, as well as to infractions. Overall, they tend to attain lower socioeconomic status than their peers.

Comorbidity of ADHD

- ADHD without a comorbid disorder (i.e., ADHD alone) is the exception rather than the rule. Since ADHD is a behaviorally defined disorder, many of the symptoms are also seen in other medical, psychiatric, and behavioral disorders.

- Significant ADHD symptoms have been associated with the following medical conditions (note: this is not an inclusive list): thyroid dysfunction, bipolar disorder, autism spectrum disorder, Klinefelter syndrome and its variants, neurofibromatosis and other genetic conditions, moderate to severe brain injury, stroke, epilepsy, sleep disorders, and lead toxicity.

- ADHD co-occurs significantly with a variety of psychiatric and other developmental conditions including obsessive-compulsive disorder, Tourette syndrome, developmental coordination disorder, developmental dyspraxia, dyslexia, speech-sound disorder, language disorder, ODD, CD, depression, and anxiety.

- Although increased comorbidity can be due to factors such as selection biases (e.g., clinical ascertainment), symptom overlap, and *assortative mating*, in other instances the comorbidity is due to shared etiological influences or cognitive deficits. For example, the locus on chromosome 6p has been found to be pleiotropic (i.e., affecting more than one phenotype) for both inattentive symptoms and dyslexia.

- Recent studies have investigated the shared and unique cognitive factors that predict reading, math, and attention skills. Following a multiple deficit framework of neurodevelopmental disorders, processing speed accounted for the overlap between reading and attention as well as the overlap between math and attention, while verbal comprehension mediated the relationship between reading and math.

- Discrete executive functions were associated with outcomes: working memory predicted math, while cognitive inhibition predicted attention ratings. This model did not vary significantly across younger and older participants. While 80–90% of the variance in reading and math was accounted for by these cognitive predictors, only 28% of the variance in attention was explained.

- Meta-analyses of studies of children, adolescents, and adults indicate that hyperactivity-impulsivity symptoms are more strongly associated with symptoms of externalizing disorders (ODD, CD), whereas inattention symptoms are more strongly associated with withdrawal and depressive symptoms across the age spectrum. Studies of substance-use disorders have yielded inconsistent results; some studies have reported that substance use or abuse was independently associated with both symptom dimensions, whereas others have found an association mainly with hyperactive-impulsive symptoms.

Assessment Methods

- Clinical interview and behavioral rating scales (e.g., Child Behavior Checklist, Conners Comprehensive Behavior Rating Scales, ADHD Rating Scale) are most often used to diagnose ADHD. Teacher and parent versions are often administered to ensure that symptoms are present across at least two settings.

- There has been significant debate as to the clinical utility of a neuropsychological evaluation for the diagnosis of ADHD. Sensitivity, specificity, and positive and negative predictive power of specific neuropsychological tests (e.g., continuous performance tests [CPTs], executive functioning measures, etc.) have been insufficient to propose using them as sole determinants of an ADHD diagnosis.

- Complexity in the diagnostic process arises because clinically significant symptoms of inattention, hyperactivity, and impulsivity are not confined to ADHD; they occur in many other developmental, psychiatric, and neurological conditions. Additionally, children with ADHD often have comorbid learning and psychiatric disorders that require appropriate evaluation in their own right, so that a comprehensive treatment plan can be devised.

- Individuals may be motivated to feign or exaggerate ADHD symptoms in order to gain medication or accommodations on high-stakes examinations or to enhance their performance in school or at work.

Expectations for Neuropsychological Assessment Results

- *Intelligence* Full Scale IQ in community samples of children and adolescents with ADHD is approximately half a standard deviation below the normative mean. Differences are found in verbal and nonverbal reasoning, processing speed, and working memory.

- *Attention/Concentration* By definition, attention is impaired in children with ADHD, as measured by parent and teacher rating scales. Continuous performance tests often show higher rates of omission and commission errors, slower response time, and increased response time variability. Continuous performance tests are more sensitive at younger ages, but, even then, not all children with ADHD will be impaired on them.

- *Language* Basic semantic and syntactic skills are often a relative strength in children with ADHD, unless they have comorbid dyslexia or language impairment. However, even for children with ADHD alone, tasks that require increased working memory capacity (e.g., sentence repetition, processing lengthy verbal instructions) will show weaker performance. In addition, children with ADHD will often write less than their peers on written tasks, and their organization and coherence will be less mature than expected.

- *Visuospatial Abilities* Children with ADHD typically have visual perceptual and visuospatial skills in the average range. Performance may fluctuate depending on task demands (e.g., timed tasks, increased number of details requiring organization). If the child has comorbid fine motor difficulties, copying tasks will likely be affected.

- *Memory* Children with ADHD do not typically demonstrate abnormal forgetting. On verbal list-learning tests, they often show deficits in how consistently and reliably they encode novel information. Spontaneous retrieval of learned information can also be hindered by their attentional disorder, especially if they present with a comorbid learning disability. Recognition of information is usually within normal limits. Performance on story recall-type tasks can be hindered by relative weakness in coherence and organization.

- *Executive Functions* Deficits in response inhibition, execution, and vigilance have been noted in stop-signal tasks, with children with ADHD having slower stop-signal reaction times (e.g., increased time to stop a prepotent response). Individuals with ADHD-I and ADHD-C likely perform differentially. Set-shifting and task-switching measures (e.g., Wisconsin Card Sorting Test, Trails—Part B) have shown small to moderate effect sizes when comparing children with and without ADHD. Interference control tasks, such as the Stroop Test, have shown mixed results, with small to large effect sizes reported. The variable findings of executive function deficits in ADHD, and the fact that differences between children with ADHD and those with other clinical conditions are usually not as large, has led some researchers to suggest that this is not a primary deficit in ADHD.

- *Sensorimotor Functions* A subgroup of children with ADHD demonstrate motor impairment, with deficient performance on tasks that measure fine motor dexterity, motor planning, praxis, and visual–motor precision. Poor handwriting can be a function of these motor deficits, but also due to a hasty approach.

- *Emotion and Personality* Evidence from studies looking at state regulation (arousal, activation, and reward motivation) show decreased performance in children and adolescents with ADHD. Children with ADHD are also at greater risk of manifesting various externalizing and internalizing disorders, including ODD, CD, anxiety, and depression.

- *Performance and Symptom Validity Testing* Some patients may feign or exaggerate symptoms in order to obtain medication or academic accommodations; therefore, performance validity testing (PVTs) and symptom validity testing (SVTs) are essential in evaluating for an overly negative response bias on behavioral rating forms, as well as overly poor performance on measures of cognitive functioning (e.g., attention and memory). The base rate for suspected symptom exaggeration or feigning of ADHD in college students ranges from at least 15% to nearly 50%. While there are limited data on base rates of PVT or SVT failure in children with ADHD, a number of case studies highlight symptom exaggeration and noncredible performance in this patient population.

Considerations when Treating Patients with ADHD

The multimodal treatment study of children with ADHD (MTA Cooperative Group, 1999, 2004) is the largest, best-controlled study to date assessing the efficacy of medication and behavioral therapy. This study enrolled 579 children with ADHD, ages 7 to 9 years and randomized them to one of four treatment conditions: medication alone (i.e., psychostimulant medication), behavioral intervention alone (i.e., intensive behavioral therapy with parent training, school intervention, and summer treatment in a camp setting), a combination of the medication and behavioral interventions, and community control (i.e., no treatment beyond that typically provided in the community).

Children were treated for 14 months, with follow-up at 10 months after the conclusion of active treatment. Results at 14 months found a sizable reduction in symptoms, with those in the medication alone and combined group showing the greatest improvement. Behavioral therapy and community control groups showed less improvement than the medication alone or combined group, but did not significantly differ from each other. The behavioral intervention did improve outcome in some nonsymptom areas (e.g., improved social skills and reduction of disruptive behavior at school), but, even then, the effect was larger in the group of children receiving the combined medication and behavior therapy.

At 24 months follow-up, the medication and combined groups continued to show persistence of improvement, but with decreased effects over time. Over time, the combined treatment of medication and behavioral therapy appeared to be superior to the medication alone, possibly addressing the contribution of comorbidities among these children (i.e., especially anxiety).

The Preschool ADHD Treatment Study (PATS) was a large multi-site, double-blind, crossover, placebo-controlled clinical trial which studied the effect of methylphenidate in preschoolers with ADHD ranging in age of three to 5.5 years. The results indicated that the medication led to improvements in symptoms, but with the effect size smaller than those noted in the MTA trials. Most of the children receiving medication maintained symptom improvement at 10-month follow-up, but side effects were more common (i.e., slowed growth rate). Based on the results from the PATS research, the American Academy of Pediatrics has recommended behavioral therapy as a first line of treatment in children within this preschool age range.

Medication

Recent reviews of the effects of medication treatment of ADHD indicate that various medications have the potential to significantly reduce symptoms and high-risk behaviors, as well as improve quality of life.

- Psychostimulant medications, including various forms of methylphenidate and salts of amphetamine (e.g., Ritalin, Adderall, and Concerta) are the first-line psychopharmacological treatment for ADHD. These drugs have the largest effects and the greatest frequency of response, with approximately 70–90% of patients benefiting from them. Response rate is improved by switching from one stimulant (or form of delivery) to another if initial response is inadequate and by careful titration and management.

- Serious adverse effects (mainly hypertension) are rare, although mild unwanted effects such as insomnia and anorexia are reasonably common.

- Comorbid disorders can elevate the risk for adverse effects, emphasizing the need for careful differential diagnosis and monitoring.

- Atomoxetine (Strattera) is a noradrenergic reuptake inhibitor that may reduce tics. It is often effective in children with ADHD who have comorbid anxiety, but in general these nonstimulant medications have been found to have smaller effect sizes (0.57) as compared to the stimulant medications (0.95 to 0.99) and therefore are not considered a first-line treatment of ADHD.

- Guanfacine (Tenex, Intuniv) and clonidine are alpha 2a adrenergic receptor agonists, often used as second-line medications for ADHD.

- Modafinil (Provigil) has shown efficacy in the treatment of ADHD in two double-blind, placebo-controlled trials, but the United States Food and Drug Administration (FDA) declined to approve it for clinical use for ADHD in children.

- When treating patients with psychiatric comorbid conditions, the rule of thumb is to treat the most serious disorder first. For example, the recommendation would be to treat an active mood disorder first, then assess the need to treat secondary ADHD symptoms.

Behavior and Cognitive Behavior Therapy

Psychopharmacological treatments for ADHD are effective in reducing core symptoms but do not address co-occurring social skills deficits or poor parent–child and peer–peer relationships. Considerable evidence exists for the effectiveness of behavioral treatments in reducing core symptoms of ADHD and improving co-occurring impairments.

- *Behavioral Parent Training (BPT)* Is a first-line behavioral treatment often administered adjunctively with medication. It is based on foundations of social learning theory that focus on teaching the child more socially acceptable behavior by training the primary caregivers in contingency management strategies. Techniques target cues, consequences, and reward systems and emphasize consistent discipline. It reduces ADHD symptoms, improves parenting skills and parents' sense of competence, and decreases family stress.

- *Behavioral classroom interventions* Have been widely employed with children diagnosed with ADHD. Direct classroom contingency management strategies frequently use a token economy or point system to reward positive or on-task behavior. These rewards may be implemented individually or for the entire classroom or school.

- *Academic interventions* Often involve changes in the level of the curriculum used, as well as modification to how instructions are delivered. Teachers may shorten the length of a task, increase opportunities for students to make choices, allow children to respond orally rather than in written format, and utilize hands-on approaches to maintain engagement.

- *Peer-related interventions*, such as social skills groups, address the difficulties that children with ADHD have in initiating and maintaining appropriate peer relationships. They are most beneficial when combined with behavior management techniques.

Alternative Treatments

Electroencephalographic (EEG) biofeedback, also known as neurofeedback, attempts to treat ADHD by training the individual to increase the ratio of high-frequency beta-EEG activity to low-frequency theta-EEG activity. Recent reviews suggest that EEG biofeedback may be effective in treating inattentive symptoms, but caution that it should not be used as the sole treatment modality. Recent studies looking at computerized cognitive training programs, such as Cogmed, have shown initial improvements in visual and verbal working memory skills; however, these studies have a number of limitations including a lack of investigation into the potential long-term academic benefit of these programs. In order for neurofeedback and computerized training programs to be considered evidence-based treatments for ADHD, further study will be required, which will need to include additional high-quality randomized controlled trials and an emphasis on measuring generalizability to real-world outcomes. Dietary interventions have also been investigated with these interventions divided into two general types: supplements (e.g., free fatty acids) and dietary exclusions (e.g., avoiding artificial additives). Meta-analytic studies have concluded that dietary treatments have potentially positive health benefits, but have minimal therapeutic benefit in treating ADHD symptoms, particularly beyond stimulant medications alone. Dietary interventions may be indicated in children with known food intolerances.

Considerations when Treating Select Populations with ADHD

Pediatric Considerations

The child's age at the time that behavioral or cognitive-behavioral interventions are delivered is likely to influence outcome. Younger children typically are more responsive to direct behavioral management strategies and parent training programs. The effectiveness of the latter will depend on factors such as parental education, investment of time, and cultural parenting styles. Treatment with adolescents, who are asserting their independence, will often benefit from programs that focus on improving parent–child interactions and communication. Monitoring of growth and medication compliance is even more important as children enter middle and high school.

Adult Considerations

Some people believe that children outgrow symptoms of ADHD and that it does not need to be treated in adulthood; counseling may be needed to negate this misconception. Although the primary symptoms of ADHD typically begin in early childhood, symptoms persist into adulthood for as many as 85% of individuals. Pharmacological treatment often continues to be useful in adulthood, in addition to other interventions focusing on marital counseling, job coaching, and parenting. Care should be taken in young adults to detect feigning of symptoms for the purpose of acquiring medications or accommodations for high-stakes examinations. Due to the higher risk for psychiatric disorders, including anxiety, mood, personality, and substance abuse disorders, careful assessment of comorbid conditions is important in developing a comprehensive and effective treatment plan.

Relevant Definitions

Assortative mating A nonrandom mating pattern in which individuals with similar genotypes and/ or phenotypes mate with one another more frequently than would be expected under a random mating pattern. If a person with one disorder marries a spouse with another disorder, this will increase the probability that their children could manifest symptoms of both disorders. This is a potential explanation for increased rates of comorbidity between two disorders in the population.

Dopamine A monoamine neurotransmitter in the catecholamine family produced in several areas of the brain, including the substantia nigra and the ventral tegmental area. Dopamine receptors (D_1–D_5) are sensitive to dopamine release into the synaptic cleft. Genetic studies of ADHD have implicated genes that are involved in the dopamine pathway (e.g., *DAT1*).

Heritability The extent to which variability in a measured trait (either cognitive, behavioral, or physical) can be explained by genetic factors. This measure is often derived from twin studies, in which the difference in genetic similarity between monozygotic and dizygotic twins can be used to compute an estimate of heritability. The latter can be computed for an extreme score or for the entire distribution of scores.

Pleiotropy The situation in which one gene influences multiple phenotypic traits. A gene locus on chromosome 6p affects both inattentive symptoms and dyslexia.

Polymorphism Often referred to as a single nucleotide polymorphism (SNP), it refers to variation at the level of a base pair (A, T, C, or G) in the DNA sequence. Single nucleotide polymorphisms can occur in coding or noncoding regions of the genome. Single nucleotide polymorphisms are used in genome-wide association studies (GWAS) to attempt to identify genes that are associated with a trait, disorder, or disease.

Relative risk Relative risk is a ratio of the probability of the event occurring in the exposed group versus a nonexposed group. As used in this chapter, it refers to the ratio of the probability of a family member of an ADHD proband also having ADHD compared to the probability of a family member of a control proband having ADHD.

Attention-Deficit/Hyperactivity Disorder Questions

NOTE: Questions 46, 90, and 115 on the First Full-Length Practice Examination, Questions 8, 54, 74, and 100 on the Second Full-Length Practice Examination, Questions 16, 76, 95, and 123 on the Third Full-Length Practice Examination, and Questions 35, 69, 98, and 120 on the Fourth Full-Length Practice Examination are from this chapter.

1. The base rate of ADHD among children in the United States is approximately _____ within community-based samples.
   (a) 2–3%
   (b) 5%
   (c) 10%
   (d) 25%

2. You are working with a 7-year-old boy with ADHD in the context of poor reading and writing skills. How likely is this child to have comorbid developmental dyslexia?
   (a) 10–25%
   (b) 25–40%
   (c) 35–50%
   (d) 60–75%

3. When comparing children with ADHD to their typically developing peers, which of the following structural brain imaging findings has been reported?
   (a) abnormalities in the supplementary sensorimotor area
   (b) abnormalities in the thalamic nuclei
   (c) abnormal symmetry of the planum temporale
   (d) abnormal cortical maturation within the frontal and temporal lobes

4. When evaluating for ADHD among adults, it is important to rule out competing psychiatric diagnoses that may have a similar presentation. Which one of the following disorders is most likely to be confused with ADHD?
   (a) bipolar disorder
   (b) delusional disorder
   (c) factitious disorder
   (d) schizophrenia

5. Which of the following statements is true regarding adults with ADHD and psychosocial functioning?

    (a) Adults with ADHD are at lower risk for driving difficulties, traffic citations, crashes, or license suspensions.

    (b) Academic outcome in those diagnosed with ADHD in adulthood is better than the academic outcome of adults who were diagnosed with ADHD as children.

    (c) The risk for psychiatric disorders in adults with ADHD is not greater than that of the general population.

    (d) Adults with ADHD (without comorbid learning disabilities) do not significantly benefit from extended time on standardized exams.

6. Abnormalities in which brain structure have been most consistently associated with ADHD?

    (a) cerebellar vermis   (c) basal ganglia

    (b) substantia nigra   (d) frontal lobe

7. Which of the following statements is true regarding the diagnosis of ADHD according to the DSM-5?

    (a) Symptoms must be present prior to 12 years of age.

    (b) Adults use the same diagnostic criteria as children.

    (c) Symptoms must be described as "impairing."

    (d) An autism spectrum disorder is exclusionary.

8. You are evaluating a 28-year-old male who has a history of unstable employment, substance abuse, and depression. He believes that he has ADHD. From an assessment and treatment perspective, what would you consider to be most important?

    (a) This adult likely has engaged in substance abuse and suffered from depression secondary to undiagnosed/treated ADHD, and therefore the ADHD is thought to be the primary diagnosis with a strong recommendation for a trial of stimulant medication.

    (b) This adult needs to be treated for his depression and substance abuse before a diagnosis of ADHD should be considered.

    (c) Adults with substance abuse are less likely to abuse stimulant medications and therefore a trial of stimulant medication could be indicated.

    (d) This adult likely has ADHD and a comorbid learning disability as the primary diagnosis and therefore intensive reading remediation treatment is warranted.

9. Which of the following statements is true regarding the prevalence and incidence of childhood ADHD?

    (a) Younger girls are more likely than boys to be diagnosed with ADHD.

    (b) Incidence and prevalence rates of ADHD decrease with age.

    (c) Boys are diagnosed with ADHD twice as often as girls.

    (d) ADHD is specific to certain geographic, cultural, and socioeconomic status groups.

10. Based on recent cognitive studies, which of the following cognitive endophenotypes is most likely to account for the comorbidity between ADHD and dyslexia?

    (a) working memory   (c) response inhibition

    (b) processing speed   (d) phoneme awareness

Attention-Deficit/Hyperactivity Disorder Answers

1. **C—10%** *ADHD is now recognized as the most common behavioral disorder of childhood, affecting nearly 10% of children ages 4–17 years within the United States alone, which is an increase from the estimated rates published by the DSM-IV TR (3–7%).*

   Reference: Pastor, P., Reuben, C., Duran, C., & Hawkins, L. (2015). Association between diagnosed ADHD and selected characteristics among children aged 4–17 years: United States, 2011–2013. *NCHS Data Brief, 201,* 1–8.

2. **B—25–40%** *ADHD is comorbid with a variety of neurodevelopmental disorders, including dyslexia, language impairment, and autism spectrum disorder. Specifically, the comorbidity of ADHD and dyslexia ranges between 25% and 40%.*

   Reference: Boada, R., Willcutt, E. G., & Pennington, B. F. (2012). Understanding the comorbidity between dyslexia and attention-deficit/hyperactivity disorder. *Topics in Language Disorders, 32,* 264–284.

3. **D—abnormal cortical maturation within the frontal and temporal lobes** *A number of structural brain imaging findings have been reported in ADHD, with abnormal cortical maturation in frontal and temporal lobes being one of them. Planum temporale differences have been reported in dyslexia. Specific thalamic nuclei or supplementary sensorimotor area differences have not been reported.*

   Reference: Nakao, T., Radua, J, Rubia, K., & Mataix-Cols, D. (2011). Gray matter volume abnormalities in ADHD: Voxel-based meta-analysis exploring the effects of age and stimulant medication. *American Journal of Psychiatry, 168,* 1154–1163.

4. **A—bipolar disorder** *Symptoms of ADHD are often seen in many other psychiatric conditions among adults such as bipolar disorder, alcohol and substance abuse, depression, and anxiety; it is important to investigate the presence of these psychiatric disorders when making a diagnosis of ADHD among adults.*

   Reference: Halmoy, A., Fasmer, O. B., & Gillber, C. (2009). Occupational outcome in adult ADHD: Impact of symptom profile, comorbid psychiatric problems, and treatment. *Journal of Attention Disorders, 13,* 175–187.

5. **D—Adults with ADHD (without comorbid learning disabilities) do not significantly benefit from extended time on standardized exams.** *Extended time on reading comprehension tests has been found to improve performance of adults with LD, but resulted in far less improvement for those with ADHD alone. One possible explanation for this is that adolescents and adults with ADHD tend to rush through tests as a result of impulsivity, so having difficulty completing the test on time is not as much of an issue.*

   Reference: Miller, L. A., Lewandowski, L. J., & Antshel, K. M. (2015). Effects of extended time for college students with and without ADHD. *Journal of Attention Disorders, 19,* 678–686.

6. **C—basal ganglia** *A meta-analysis of structural brain imaging studies has shown that the most consistent finding in ADHD are abnormalities in the basal ganglia and, in particular, the caudate nucleus.*

   Reference: Nakao, T., Radua, J, Rubia, K., & Mataix-Cols, D. (2011). Gray matter volume abnormalities in ADHD: Voxel-based meta-analysis exploring the effects of age and stimulant medication. *American Journal of Psychiatry, 168,* 1154–1163.

7. **A—Symptoms must be present prior to 12 years of age.** *With the DSM-5, the age of onset was raised from 7 years to 12 years, with a separate criteria for adolescents and adults ages 17 years and older.*

   Reference: American Psychiatric Association (2013). *Diagnostic and statistical manual for mental disorders* (5th ed.). Washington, DC: American Psychiatric Publishing.

8. **B—This adult needs to be treated for his depression and substance abuse before a diagnosis of ADHD should be considered.** *When treating patients with psychiatric comorbid conditions, the rule of thumb is to treating the most serious disorder first. For example, treating an active mood disorder and/or significant substance abuse first then assessing the need to treat secondary ADHD symptoms. There would be significant concerns in recommending stimulant medication in an individual with history of substance abuse, especially if this individual has not been effectively treated for this behavior.*

   Reference: Faraone, S. V., Asheron, P., Banaschewski, T., Biederman, J., Buitelaar, J. K., Ramos-Quiroga, J. A., . . . Franke, B. (2015). Attention-deficit/hyperactivity disorder. *Nature Reviews: Disease Primers, 1,* 1–23.

9. **C—Boys are diagnosed with ADHD twice as often as girls.** *All of these statements are false with the exception of A. Boys are about twice as likely as girls to be diagnosed with ADHD.*

   Reference: Pritchard, A. E., Nigro, C. A., Jacobson, L. A., & Mahone, E. M. (2012). The role of neuropsychological assessment in the functional outcomes of children with ADHD. *Neuropsychology Review, 22,* 54–68.

10. **B—processing speed** *Cognitive studies investigating the etiology of the comorbidity between ADHD and dyslexia have found that processing speed is the cognitive endophenotype that best accounts for the phenotypic covariance among the two disorders.*

    Reference: Willcutt, E. G., Betjemann, R. S., McGrath, L. M., Chhabildas, N. A., Olson, R. K., & DeFries, J. C., (2010). Etiology and neuropsychology of comorbidity between RD and ADHD: The case for multiple-deficit models. *Cortex, 46*(10), 1345–1361.

Recommended Readings

Barkley, R. A. (2014). *Attention-deficit hyperactivity disorder: A handbook for diagnosis and treatment* (4th ed.). New York, NY: Guilford Press.

Faraone, S. V., Asheron, P., Banaschewski, T., Biederman, J., Buitelaar, J. K., Ramos-Quiroga, J. A., . . . Franke, B. (2015). Attention-deficit/hyperactivity disorder. *Nature Reviews: Disease Primers, 1,* 1–23.

Fletcher, J. M. (2014). The effects of childhood ADHD on adult labor market outcomes. *Health Economics, 23,* 159–181.

Mahone, E. M., & Denckla, M. B. (2017). Attention-deficit/hyperactivity disorder: A historical neuropsychological perspective. *Journal of the International Neuropsychological Society, 23,* 916–929.

Mapou, R. L. (2009). *Adult learning disabilities and ADHD.* New York, NY: Oxford University Press.

MTA Cooperative Group (1999). A 14 month randomized clinical trial of treatment strategies for attention-deficit/hyperactivity disorder: The MTA Cooperative Group multimodal treatment stud of children with ADHD. *Archives of General Psychiatry, 56,* 1073–1086.

MTA Cooperative Group (2004). National Institute of Mental Health multimodal treatment study of ADHD follow-up: 24-month outcomes of treatment strategies for attention-deficit/hyperactivity disorder. *Pediatrics, 113,* 754–761.

Peterson, R. L., Boada, R., McGrath, L. M., Willcutt, E. G., Olson, R. K., Pennington, B. F. (2017). Cognitive prediction of reading, math, and attention: Shared and unique influences. *Journal of Learning Disabilities, 50,* 408–421.

Pritchard, A. E., Nigro, C. A., Jacobson, L. A., & Mahone, E. M. (2012). The role of neuropsychological assessment in the functional outcomes of children with ADHD. *Neuropsychology Review, 22,* 54–68.

Willcutt, E. G., Nigg, J. T., Pennington, B. F., Solanto, M. V., Rohde, L. A., Tannock, R., . . . Lahey, B. B. (2012). Validity of DSM–IV attention deficit/hyperactivity disorder symptom dimensions and subtypes. *Journal of Abnormal Psychology, 121,* 991–1010.

Section III Disorders and Conditions: Medical

17   Prematurity

Amy K. Connery and Jennifer C. G. Larson

Definition

Prematurity is defined as a birth that occurs before 37 weeks *gestational age* and refers specifically to *gestational age* and immaturity of body systems. Birth weight is often used as a proxy for *gestational age* due to the high correlation between the two and the difficulty of precisely determining *gestational age*. Table 17.1 describes the generally agreed upon terms for defining prematurity and low birth weight.

TABLE 17.1 Terms for Defining Prematurity and Low Birth Weight

Category	Gestational Age	Birth Weight
Late preterm birth	<37 weeks	
Low birth weight		<2,500 g (5lbs., 8 oz.)
Very preterm	<33 weeks	
Very low birth weight		<1,500 g (3 lbs., 5 oz.)
Extremely preterm	<29 weeks	
Extremely low birth weight		<1,000 g (2 lbs., 3 oz.)
Micropremature	<26 weeks	<750 g (1 lb., 10 oz)

Neuropathology

Prematurity confers increased risk for neurological complications that can lead to structural neuroanatomical changes and increased rates of morbidity and mortality. Additionally, early neurologic injury as a result of prematurity can compromise brain function and disrupt future brain development. Preterm infants are at risk for certain neurological complications, with the most common being *periventricular hemorrhagic infarction (PVHI)* and *periventricular leukomalacia (PVL)*. An evolving sequence of events beginning with reductions in cerebral oxygen and blood flow (hypoxia-ischemia) can result in *intraventricular hemorrhage (IVH)* and then *PVHI*. See Table 17.2. Problems with cerebrovascular autoregulation, inflammatory response, and impaired cerebral blood flow can result in PVL. Premature infants are also vulnerable to post-hemorrhagic hydrocephalus, focalized neuronal injury, and cerebral ischemic lesions, all less common than PVHI and PVL. *Hypoxic-ischemic encephalopathy* (HIE) can also be seen in preterm infants after a sentinel hypoxic-ischemic event with a corresponding clinical presentation (e.g., poor Apgar scores, cord blood metabolic acidosis, need for resuscitation). HIE is a clinical diagnosis with varying diagnostic criteria across studies and sites. PVL can be also considered a type of HIE lesion when observed on neuroimaging (see also Chapter 28, Hypoxic and Ischemic Brian Injury).

TABLE 17.2 Intraventricular Hemorrhage Grade and Associated Neurological Sequelae

Grade I	Bleeding is confined to the germinal matrix
Grade II	Bleeding into the ventricles, but without ventricular dilation
Grade III	Bleeding resulting in ventricular dilation
Grade IV	Large hemorrhage with associated PVHI in the parenchyma

Risk Factors for Premature Birth

- Maternal history of previous preterm birth
- Short spacing between pregnancies
- Multiple birth pregnancy
- Maternal age:
  - Younger than 16 years
  - Older than 35 years
- Maternal health problems:
  - Diabetes
  - Obesity
  - High blood pressure
  - Kidney or heart disease
  - Infections during pregnancy
  - Stress
- Abnormalities of the uterus or cervix
- Maternal alcohol, drug, or cigarette use
- Low socioeconomic status
- Lack of prenatal care
- African American ethnicity

Epidemiology

- According to vital statistics, the number of live births in the United States in 2016 was estimated at approximately 4 million. Of these approximately:
  - 10% were preterm (i.e., <37 weeks gestation)
    - Of these, 7% were late preterm and 3% were <33 weeks gestation
  - 8% were low birth weight (<2,500 g; 5 lbs., 8 oz.)
  - 1% were very low birth weight (<1,500 g; 3 lbs., 5 oz.)
- Multiple births (twin and triplet/+) account for the vast majority of preterm and low/very low birth weight births. In 2016, an estimated 33/1,000 of live births were twins and 10/1,000 births were triplet/+. The rate of triplet/+ births has been declining since the peak in 1998.

- Of these births, approximately one of two twins and nine of ten triplet/+ babies were born low birth weight and/or preterm.

• In 2017, the infant mortality rate in the United States was six per 1,000 births, with premature birth being the second leading cause of death in infants under 1 year of age and accounting for approximately one third of all infant deaths.

• Despite advanced technologies and practices, the United States has one of the highest rates of preterm births in the world among high-income countries.

• The rate of preterm births in the United States steadily increased from 1981 until 2006. From 2007 to 2014, the overall preterm birth rate declined primarily for late preterm births and not in other categories. The decline is believed to be related to a lower incidence of births to younger mothers. The rate of preterm birth did not decline for African American and Hispanic women during this time. The preterm birth rate has been increasing since 2015 primarily for late preterm births. The causes for this are not yet well understood.

• Non-Hispanic African American women have higher rates of preterm infants, low and very low birth weight infants, and infant mortality. The rate of preterm birth is approximately 50% higher for African American women than for all other women. Even when controlling for known risk factors for preterm birth, the risk for African American women persists.

• In high-income countries:

  - Approximately a third of babies born at <25 weeks gestation survive (although there is wide variability across studies), with 7–15% developing cerebral palsy (CP), and 2–5% developing moderate to severe hearing loss and/or blindness. 30–70% have moderate to severe cognitive impairment (i.e., mental developmental index (MDI <70), 14–25% of which is profound impairment (i.e., MDI < 50) at 18 to 22 months corrected age. Across all studies lower *gestational age* was associated with poorer outcome.

  - Over 80% of babies born at 25–27 weeks gestation survive, with approximately 4–10% developing CP and 1–6% developing moderate to severe hearing loss and/or blindness. Up to 20% have moderate to severe cognitive impairment at 3-year follow-up, and up to 50% have learning and behavioral problems at school age.

  - Approximately 96% of babies born 28–31 weeks gestation survive. Those with very low birth weight are at increased risk for disabilities. Cognitive deficits without major motor problems are common.

  - Approximately 98% of babies born 32–33 weeks gestation survive. These infants are at lower risk for developing complications associated with preterm birth than other preterm babies, but remain at increased risk compared with term babies for developing learning and behavioral problems.

  - Greater than 99% of babies born 34 to 36 weeks gestation survive. However, they are four times more likely than their full-term peers to die within the first year of life. They are at higher risk (almost twice the rate compared to typically developing peers) for developmental delay at 3.5 to 4 years of age, and are at higher risk for developing learning and/or behavioral difficulties.

• The current threshold of biological viability is considered to be 23 weeks *gestational age* in high-income countries and approximately 34 weeks in low- and lower middle-income countries. The threshold has been lowered over the years as neonatal medical advances have been made.

- Premature birth is the leading cause of death in children under 5 worldwide with over 95% of the low birth weight infants worldwide born in low- and middle-income countries. There are significant inequalities in survival rates between high- and low- and middle-income countries, as well. More than 90% of children born extremely preterm in low-income countries do not survive compared to a mortality rate of less than 10% in this group in high-income countries.

Determinants of Severity

A definitive relationship exists between the degree of prematurity, birth weight, and functional outcome. In fact, for the preterm infant, each week of increasing *gestational age* and every additional gram of birth weight leads to decreased risk for long-term impairment. Additionally, it is important to consider the relationship between weight relative to *gestational age* (e.g., *small for gestational age [SGA]* and *intrauterine growth restriction [IUGR]*). However, consideration of the severity of prematurity and birth weight alone do not sufficiently account for and do not fully predict functional outcome. In fact, recent studies have demonstrated that other medical complications associated with prematurity may be better predictors than gestational age alone. Other factors include:

- The severity of medical and neurological complications, with the presence of grades III and IV IVH (see Table 17.2) conferring the greatest risk.
- Use of prenatal and postnatal steroids to hasten infant lung development and *germinal matrix* maturation.
- Care center factors, including birth in a hospital with a neonatal intensive care unit (NICU) and/or transfer to a NICU in the first 24 hours of life, availability of a neonatologist, and integrated NICU care.
- Familial and environmental factors, including socioeconomic status, maternal educational level and mental health, quality of responsive care, and environmental stimulation.
- Male preterm infants are at a greater risk for poor outcome than females, although the specific reasons for this increased vulnerability are not yet understood.
- Length of NICU stay and NICU growth velocity.
- Some studies have found reduced gray and white matter volumes, as well as larger ventricle size in premature infants even when controlling for medical risk factors and birth weight. This knowledge may be useful in predicting cognitive, motor, and neurosensory impairments.
- While outcome prediction models for premature infants have been proposed, results are variable across studies indicating how complex and multifaceted the determinants of severity are in this population.

Presentation, Disease Course, and Recovery

Acute Hospitalization

Recovery Course

- Recovery course during the acute period is often variable and dependent on the degree of prematurity and birth weight, as well as on the presence and severity of medical complications.

- The first hours of life are critical, with approximately 50% of all IVH occurring in the first 6 to 8 hours of life and 95% occurring within the first 4 to 5 days. Transfer to a NICU with an on-staff neonatologist during this period positively affects outcome.

Assessment Methods

- Different neuroradiological techniques can be useful in detecting various neurological complications.
  - Serial cranial ultrasound is the most commonly used imaging technique and is performed routinely in the context of prematurity to detect neurological events and abnormalities. Ultrasound is useful for detection of IVH and severe white matter abnormalities, but is not sensitive to mild to moderate white matter abnormalities.
  - Brain magnetic resonance imaging (MRI) can be done in an MRI-compatible incubator and has been deemed safe for the preterm infant. Magnetic resonance imaging can be useful in monitoring brain development and detecting a wide variety of neurologic abnormalities and injury, including PVL.
  - Computed tomography (CT) scans are utilized in the care of preterm infants; however, the value of the information gained through a CT scan may not outweigh the risk of the high dose of radiation delivered to the preterm infant.
  - Continuous video electroencephalogram (EEG) is used to monitor for seizures.
- Several non-imaging tools can also be useful in the detection of neurological complications:
  - In children younger than 5 months corrected age, General Movement Assessment (GMA) combined with neonatal MRI is 95% accurate in predicting CP. GMA is a non-invasive method designed to qualitatively assess spontaneous movements in children born preterm through approximately 20 weeks post-term corrected age.
  - In children older than 5 months corrected age, Hammersmith Infant Neurological Examination (HINE) combined with neonatal MRI is more than 90% accurate in predicting CP.

Treatment

- Aggressive intervention for babies born at the threshold of viability is a complex ethical decision generally made in consultation with both parents and medical providers. Multiple factors must be considered, including the risk of severe long-term neurodevelopmental sequelae and reduced quality of life.
- Some NICUs immediately perform coagulant studies on admission to assess risk for a hemorrhagic or thrombotic event. If concerns arise, prophylactic treatment is initiated. Neuroprotective agents, such as magnesium sulfate, as well as agents to assist with neuroregeneration and repair are under investigation.
- Premature babies are often treated with synthetic *surfactant* to assist in keeping air sacs in the lungs open during respiration.
- Hypothermia and hyperbaric chambers are used as neuroprotective therapies in an effort to decrease the incidence of HIE.
- Inhaled nitric oxide has been used in an effort to reduce the incidence of *bronchopulmonary dysplasia (BPD)*, although its use has been controversial in improving short- and long-term outcomes.

- Postnatal steroid (e.g., glucocorticoid dexamethasone) treatment has been used to prevent and treat respiratory complications in preterm infants. Although improved pulmonary compliance has been observed, the use of postnatal steroids is somewhat controversial. Early reports suggested that postnatal steroid use was associated with chronic hypoxia, reduced cerebral volumes, neurodevelopmental delay, and other adverse effects within the central nervous system. However, these findings are inconsistent across the literature. Despite the reported adverse effects, a study found that factors other than postnatal steroid use (i.e., length of NICU stay and gender) contributed to functional outcome.

Inpatient Hospitalization

Recovery Course

Possible complications in preterm infants include hypoxic/ischemic neurological events, chronic lung disease, *apnea of prematurity, necrotizing enterocolitis (NEC), retinopathy of prematurity*, septicemia, *patent ductus arteriosus*, respiratory distress syndrome, pulmonary hypertension, and *bronchopulmonary dysplasia (BPD)*. Major morbidities for premature infants include:

- Grade III or IV IVH, occurring in approximately 10–25% of babies born <28 weeks, 10–20% of babies born 28–32 weeks, and <10% of babies born 33–36 weeks.
- Approximately 40% of babies born <28 weeks, 20% born 28–30 weeks, 10% born 30–32 weeks, and <5% born <32–36 weeks have major morbidities at the time of discharge from the NICU including Grade III or IV IVH, as well as NEC stage II/III, pulmonary hypertension, seizures, HIE, and/or BPD.

Assessment Methods

- Advanced, integrated monitoring of brain function is critical during the inpatient hospitalization phase.
- Continuous monitoring of the neonate's basic physiology is also important during the inpatient stay to prevent secondary neurologic injury. This includes monitoring of the maintenance of body temperature, blood oxygenation and pressure, and cardiac function.

Treatment

- Intensive, integrated NICU care, such as the *Newborn Individualized Developmental Care and Assessment Program (NIDCAP)*, are models of medical management used in various NICUs. These programs attempt to replicate the intrauterine environment to the extent possible. Some studies have shown improved long-term outcome in infants treated in these types of care models, including improved growth velocity and infant self-regulatory functioning, as well as reduced family stress.
- The nutritional and dietary needs of the infant may be critical because poor postnatal growth has been associated with decreased motor and cognitive functioning.

Outpatient Rehabilitation

Recovery Course

- The long-term course of recovery is likely predicted by complex and multifactorial considerations, many of which have been listed previously.
- Long-term consequences of prematurity have been documented in children born late preterm (34–36 weeks) and in those children without significant medical or neurological complications associated with birth.

Assessment Methods

- The Neonatal Behavioral Assessment Scale, the Bayley Scales of Infant and Toddler Development-III, and the Mullen Scales of Early Learning are common assessment measures used after NICU discharge. These measures are primarily used for monitoring and intervention planning and not as predictors of long-term future success or functioning.
- Certain types of white matter injury (e.g., PVL) are not consistently detected by ultrasound, the most commonly used imaging technique in the NICU. As a result, some neurologic injury may not be diagnosed. Therefore, follow-up neuroimaging may be helpful in understanding the full extent of the neurologic sequelae.
- Follow-up with a neurologist is recommended if CP is suspected (see also Chapter 19, Cerebral Palsy).

Treatment

- Early intervention services and ongoing intervention from speech/language pathologists, occupational and physical therapists, and psychologists are often recommended.
- Along with early intervention, an enriching and stimulating home environment has been found to improve cognitive outcome in young children. Therefore, intervention programs that focus on familial support and education are important.
- Cognitive rehabilitation strategies can be useful in addressing attentional and information processing problems.
- Academic support, depending on the specific needs of the school-aged child, is important.
- Early intervention and repeated assessment, including neuroimaging, of the developing child is important in continuing to monitor development and support the planning and modification of intervention services.

Expectations for Neuropsychological Assessment Results

Due to advances in the medical management of prematurity, functional outcomes vary substantially depending on the birth cohort year. As a result, caution should be used in extrapolating study results from one birth cohort to another. Although medical advances have improved the mortality rate over generations of preterm infants, the rate of neurodevelopmental disability has been relatively stable, with perhaps a recent trend toward improved functional outcome, particularly in the late and very preterm babies. Despite considerable heterogeneity in neuropsychological outcome in this population, patterns in neuropsychological test performance are commonly seen.

- *Intelligence/Achievement* Full-Scale IQ (FSIQ) scores may be lower, although significant variability in index scores is often noted, rendering the FSIQ a less useful construct in this population. In group studies, those with a history of prematurity often score in the average range for FSIQ, but below their full-term peers. In preterm infants, mean IQ tends to be higher with increasing *gestational age.* Increased rates of intellectual disability are found in the smallest and most premature infants. Notably, even children born preterm with average general intelligence scores are more vulnerable to subtle or more significant neuropsychological deficits that can affect overall functioning in the school and social environments. Higher rates of learning disabilities, grade retention, and special education are apparent in this population. Learning problems are seen most commonly in math computation and application skills and in written output. These children often remain behind academically because their rate of progress is slower than that of their peers.

- *Attention/Concentration* Attention problems are commonly noted, with increased rates of diagnosed ADHD. Specific problems with selective attention, sustained attention, shifting attention, and impulsivity have been identified.

- *Processing Speed* Slowed speed of processing is a common problem. The frequency of white matter pathology in preterm infants is thought to explain the common deficits in speed of processing in this population.

- *Language* Generally, crystallized verbal abilities, such as semantic knowledge and expressive/receptive vocabulary, are spared. However, difficulties in more fluid verbal skills, such as verbal comprehension, fluency, and pragmatics can be seen. Naming difficulties have also been reported. Language skills often progress and improve over time; however, higher order language problems frequently persist.

- *Visuospatial* Visuospatial skills appear to be particularly vulnerable in those with a history of prematurity. Problems are frequently seen even in children without associated motor or visual deficits. The proximity of the vulnerable periventricular region to the optic radiations, as well as dorsal stream dysfunction involved in the integration of visual information, are hypothesized to be the source of this dysfunction.

- *Memory* Slower rates of information acquisition for both verbal and visual information and deficits in information retrieval and delayed recall are commonly seen. Spatial memory deficits have been found in children born micropremature (<26 weeks). Marked reductions in hippocampal volumes are hypothesized to underlie the memory deficits frequently observed in those with a history of prematurity.

- *Executive Functions* Problems with working memory, planning, set-shifting, inhibition, vigilance, and organization can be seen in this population. This is likely due to the increased rates of abnormalities in frontal and subcortical functional systems resulting from premature birth and its complications, as well as overall reduced processing speed.

- *Sensorimotor Functions* Motor and sensory (e.g., vision and hearing) deficits are relatively common in this population. Although CP is less common, more subtle deficits in fine and gross motor dexterity and coordination are frequently observed. Specifically, problems in motor persistence, dexterity and coordination, speed, visuomotor integration, and motor quality (overflow) are commonly seen even in preterm children with normal cognition.

- ***Emotion and Personality*** Both internalizing and externalizing behaviors have been reported in this population. Those with a history of prematurity are more likely to exhibit behavioral problems than their term-born peers, with concerns for hyperactivity and poor social skills commonly reported. Increased rates of anxiety are also common, as are reduced adaptive skills. Recent research suggests increased prevalence of autism spectrum disorders in extremely preterm and very low birth weight children. Lower general cognitive ability and the presence of motor, visual, hearing, or other chronic health problems are predictive of deficits in independent, adaptive functioning.

- ***Performance and Symptom Validity*** Objective measures of performance or symptom validity have not yet been studied in this population. However, because of the ubiquitous effects of suboptimal test engagement on neuropsychological test performance, PVTs are recommended clinically in school-aged children.

Considerations when Treating Select Populations with Prematurity

Pediatric Considerations

Advances in the medical management of prematurity have led to better short- and long-term outcomes for infants born today in the United States than in past decades. After 2000, survival rates have continued to increase, and there appears to be a trend toward lower morbidity. Of course, longitudinal data on adult functional outcomes for preterm infants born in the last decade are not yet available.

Testing Considerations

Age corrections for prematurity are generally made until 24 months of age; however, some practitioners believe that the age correction should be used for a more extended period. There is little empirical support for designating the appropriate length of time for which age corrections should be made.

Geriatric Considerations

Because there have been many advances in the medical management of premature babies over the past decades, including the emergence of NICUs in the 1970s and introduction of *surfactant* in the 1980s, patients born during or before this time may have considerably different outcomes related to a history of prematurity than a child born today. Older patients are more likely to have had more medical complications and worse long-term outcome related to premature birth. Early neurologic insult can continue to impact functioning into adulthood. Some individuals with a history of prematurity, particularly in earlier born cohorts, struggle with chronic health problems related to motor, visual, and hearing impairments, as well as with respiratory problems due to pulmonary injury.

Acknowledgments

We would like to thank Ida Sue Baron, Ph.D., ABPP-CN, and Megan N. Scott, Ph.D. for reviewing a previous version of this chapter.

Relevant Definitions

Apnea of prematurity (AOP) Refers to unexplained cessation of breathing and is associated with bradycardia, cyanosis, pallor, and/or hypotonia. AOP tends to be caused by an immature respiratory control system and is associated with decreased arterial oxygen saturation. It typically does not persist beyond 40 weeks postconceptual age. Research on AOP and functional outcome is variable, with some research indicating poorer cognitive and academic outcomes and other research reporting no differences in outcome. Apnea of prematurity is treated both inpatient and outpatient using a variety of techniques including medication, continuous positive airway pressure (CPAP), and mechanical ventilation.

Bronchopulmonary dysplasia (BPD) Also known as chronic lung disease. Refers to long-term respiratory problems. Bronchopulmonary dysplasia is caused by lung damage that occurs as a result of requiring mechanical ventilator support (i.e., breathing machine) or receiving high levels of oxygen for long periods shortly after birth. Although the use of a ventilator or high oxygen levels may be necessary to facilitate breathing and survival in a neonate, these interventions may damage the fragile lung tissue through inflammation and irritation. Treatment of BPD often includes continued use of a mechanical ventilator and supplemental oxygen in which pressure and oxygen levels are decreased over time. Bronchopulmonary dysplasia is most common in premature infants. Given that extra calories are needed due to effortful breathing, infants with BPD are typically fed using nasogastric tubes. Both oxygen treatment and tube feedings may continue for several months and may cause long-term lung damage. Diffuse neurocognitive impairments are associated with severe BPD.

Germinal matrix This highly cellular and highly vascularized region of the brain is found below the lining of the lateral ventricle. It is from this region that cells migrate during development, most commonly between 22 and 30 weeks gestation. The germinal matrix diminishes gradually and has mostly disappeared by 36 weeks gestation. Because of its location in a vascular watershed zone, the germinal matrix is the most common location of IVH in preterm infants.

Gestational age Refers to the age of an embryo or fetus and is typically calculated from the first day of the last menstrual period.

Hypoxic-ischemic encephalopathy (HIE) A term commonly used to describe encephalopathy caused by a reduction in cerebral oxygenation and blood flow. In the preterm infant, HIE is often recognized as the result of a sentinel hypoxic-ischemic event. However, due to the multiple other neurological risk factors in the preterm infant, the specific cause or contribution of each risk factor to HIE is often uncertain.

Intrauterine growth restriction (IUGR) Refers to poor growth of a fetus during pregnancy. Specifically, IUGR is said to occur when the developing fetus's weight falls below the tenth percentile compared to other babies of equal *gestational age*. Intrauterine growth restriction can be caused by many factors, but most commonly it is associated with a fetus not receiving enough oxygen and nutrition from the placenta during pregnancy. Research indicates that IUGR, independent of prematurity and neonatal complications, results in lower IQ and specific neuropsychological impairments (e.g., inattention, executive functioning, visuomotor organization, and higher order verbal skills). Additionally, IUGR is associated with abnormal development of frontal brain regions.

Intraventricular hemorrhage (IVH) Refers to increased vascular pressure and consequent vessel rupture and hemorrhage. Earlier onset of IVH is associated with more severe grade. There is an increasing incidence of higher grade IVH for the most preterm infants. Severity of grade is associated with increased rate of mortality and neurological sequelae (see Table 17.2). However, even in infants with the lowest grades of IVH, increased incidence of learning disability is apparent.

Newborn Individualized Developmental Care and Assessment Program (NIDCAP) An example of an integrated care model found in NICUs. These care models can include limiting bright lights, noise, and exposure to other noxious stimuli; "kangaroo care" or skin-to-skin contact with the baby; and creation of a comfortable, soothing environment for family members to partner in the neonate's care.

Necrotizing enterocolitis The death of intestinal tissue that occurs when the lining of the intestinal wall dies and tissue falls off. Necrotizing enterocolitis most often occurs in preterm or sick infants, and the cause is currently unknown. Prognosis for infants with necrotizing enterocolitis is poor, with death occurring in approximately 25% of cases.

Neonatal respiratory distress syndrome (RDS) A condition characterized by difficulty breathing that occurs almost exclusively in premature infants whose lungs are not yet fully developed. Respiratory distress syndrome is primarily caused by the lack of *surfactant* in the infant's lungs. Most cases of RDS are seen in infants born before 28 weeks *gestational age*. Mortality rates associated with RDS have decreased considerably since the introduction and use of artificial *surfactant* and prenatal glucocorticoids that help to speed lung development.

Neonatal septicemia Also known as sepsis. Refers to a severe infection in the blood that spreads throughout the body. In premature infants, sepsis is believed to be caused by pregnancy complications that increase the likelihood of infection (e.g., premature rupture of the membranes, difficult delivery, infection in uterus or placenta, fever in mother) but can also be contracted in the NICU due to the neonate's vulnerability to infection.

Patent ductus arteriosus (PDA) A heart condition in which the ductus arteriosus of the heart does not close, resulting in abnormal blood flow between the aorta and the pulmonary arteries, which are connected to the heart. Patent ductus arteriosus can be associated with other morbidities common to preterm infants (e.g., IVH, BPD, NEC, feeding intolerance, etc.). Patent ductus arteriosus occurs more commonly in preterm infants (approximately 8/1,000 premature births) and in those infants with RDS.

Periventricular hemorrhagic infarction (PVHI) A venous infarction that is most frequently a complication of a large IVH. This infarction obstructs the terminal veins, causing periventricular ischemia and then hemorrhagic venous infarction. This results in asymmetric necrosis of the periventricular white matter.

Periventricular leukomalacia (PVL) Results from ischemic injury to the white matter surrounding the lateral ventricles. Focal necrotic lesions occur in the border end zones of the medial cerebral artery (MCA), posterior cerebral artery (PCA), and anterior cerebral artery (ACA). Abnormalities in cortical neuronal organization may occur due to injury of subplate neurons (i.e., the first neurons generated in the cortex that facilitate neuronal connectivity and functional maturation). Periventricular leukomalacia increases the risk for CP, specifically spastic diplegia. More extensive PVL can include involvement of the upper extremities as well.

Retinopathy of prematurity (ROP) Occurs when blood vessels in the retina of the eye develop abnormally. Premature birth can disrupt eye development and may cause the blood vessels to stop growing or to grow abnormally. Also the use of excessive oxygen after birth can result in oxygen toxicity and lead to abnormal growth of the blood vessels. Those babies who are the smallest and most premature are at greatest risk for developing ROP. Most infants who develop ROP have stage 1 or 2 and recover with minimal to no long-term visual problems. Stages 3+ may result in significant vision problems or blindness. In a small number of preterm babies, ROP worsens over time, sometimes very rapidly, and can lead to significant vision problems, including blindness. Early intervention is critical in the treatment of ROP.

Small for gestational age (SGA) When a developing baby's weight falls below the tenth percentile compared to other babies of equal *gestational age*. Babies born SGA may be proportionally small (small all over) or they may be of normal size, but have decreased body weight. In some cases, SGA may be the result of IUGR, but it may also result from maternal factors (e.g., high blood pressure, anemia), uterus or placental factors (e.g., placental previa or abruption, infection), or fetal development factors (e.g., multiples, chromosomal abnormality).

Surfactant A naturally occurring substance that helps the lungs to inflate and prevents the alveoli (air sacs) from collapsing. Surfactant is produced by fetuses between 24 and 28 weeks *gestational age*. By approximately 35 weeks *gestational age*, there is enough surfactant to prevent the alveoli from collapsing. If there is a high risk that a baby will be born prematurely, the mother is given prenatal corticosteroids (i.e., glucocorticoids) to hasten lung development and surfactant production in the fetus. This helps reduce the need of surfactant replacement therapy in the newborn. If, however, there was not time for a course of prenatal corticosteroids or the infant is born with low blood oxygen levels and respiratory distress, postnatal delivery of artificial surfactant is required. Both treatments attempt to ameliorate or prevent RDS and increase the likelihood of survival.

Prematurity Questions

NOTE: Questions 54, 87, 102, and 108 on the First Full-Length Practice Examination, Questions 67, 88, and 106 on the Second Full-Length Practice Examination, Questions 23, 41, and 59 on the Third Full-Length Practice Examination, and Questions 53, 77, and 111 on the Fourth Full-Length Practice Examination are from this chapter.

1. Due to location of injury, a patient with a history of periventricular leukomalacia may present with abnormalities in function of the _____.
   - (a) vestibulospinal tract
   - (b) corticospinal tract
   - (c) tectospinal tract
   - (d) reticulospinal tract

2. A 70-year-old patient with a history of preterm birth and current neurocognitive concerns presents for neuropsychological assessment with complaints of subtle motor abnormalities, respiratory problems, deficits in visuospatial skills, and problems in working memory and organization. Which of the following might be considered?
   - (a) Symptoms are consistent with the development of dementia with Lewy bodies.
   - (b) Symptoms are consistent with her birth history.
   - (c) Symptoms are consistent with her birth history or the development of a subcortical dementia.
   - (d) Symptoms are consistent with the development of a subcortical dementia.

3. Which of the following factors presents an increased risk for preterm birth?
   - (a) multiple birth pregnancy, intensive maternal exercise, in vitro fertilization, and maternal age
   - (b) alcohol or drug use, high blood pressure, selective serotonin reuptake inhibitor (SSRI) use, and cervix abnormalities
   - (c) caffeine consumption, excessive maternal weight gain, maternal age, and diabetes
   - (d) multiple-birth pregnancy, maternal infection, low socioeconomic status, and maternal age

4. Visuospatial skills appear particularly vulnerable in patients with a history of prematurity due to _____.

   (a) vulnerability of cranial nerves II, III, and VI to hypoxic injury

   (b) the use of prenatal corticosteroids to hasten lung development

   (c) the proximity of the vulnerable periventricular region to the optic radiations

   (d) abnormal development of blood vessels in the retina (i.e., retinopathy of prematurity)

5. During an intake interview with the parents of a 7-year-old, they report that their child was diagnosed with a grade III IVH as the result of preterm birth. A grade III IVH is associated with which of the following neurological sequelae?

   (a) bleeding resulting in ventricular dilation

   (b) bleeding confined to the germinal matrix

   (c) large hemorrhage with associated PVHI in the parenchyma

   (d) bleeding into the ventricles, but without ventricular dilation

6. Early _____ is the most commonly used imaging technique to detect neurological insult in the preterm infant; however, _____ is better at detecting more subtle white matter damage, particularly PVL, and at predicting final diagnoses of neurological sequelae in preterm infants.

   (a) magnetic resonance imaging; ultrasound

   (b) ultrasound; computed tomography

   (c) computed tomography; magnetic resonance imaging

   (d) ultrasound; magnetic resonance imaging

7. You have just administered the Bayley Scales of Infant and Toddler Development to a 14-month-old child with a history of preterm birth. You have identified significant motor, language, and cognitive delays. Which of the following are you most likely to recommend?

   (a) referral to a neurologist and to community-based resources for children with intellectual disabilities

   (b) referral to a neonatologist and to early intervention services

   (c) serial cranial ultrasound and referral to a neurologist

   (d) early intervention services and family support and education

8. Identical twins are born at 28 weeks gestational age. In the first 24 hours after birth, an IVH is identified in one twin. By day five, the other twin has not experienced any significant complications. Which of the following is true about the twins?

   (a) The IVH is more likely to be severe in the first twin. It is most likely that IVH will not occur in the second twin.

   (b) The IVH in the first twin is likely to be mild. The second twin should be monitored closely as the IVH is more likely to be severe if it occurs later.

   (c) Because they are identical twins, it is likely the second twin will have an IVH and so should be monitored closely.

   (d) Because ultrasound is not sensitive to IVH detection, it is highly likely that that second twin had an IVH that was not identified.

9. The germinal matrix is more vulnerable in the preterm infant than the full-term infant because ____.

   (a) it is not yet developed in the preterm infant and is fully developed in term infants

   (b) it is located in a vascular watershed zone and has largely disappeared by 36 weeks gestation

   (c) full-term infants have better developed respiratory systems and so are not vulnerable to injury in watershed zones, such as the germinal matrix

   (d) its vascular structure is different in preterm babies and so more susceptible to injury

10. In reviewing the birth records of a patient born at 30 weeks gestation, including ultrasound reports, there is no mention of neurological injury. What is your conclusion?

   (a) No neurological injury occurred, but the child is still at risk due to the preterm birth.

   (b) The child may have sustained an IVH as ultrasound is not sensitive to IVH detection.

   (c) No neurological injury occurred and therefore any deficits are unlikely to be related to preterm birth.

   (d) As certain types of white matter injury are not detected by ultrasound, you cannot rule out that an injury was sustained.

Prematurity Answers

1. **B—corticospinal tract** *The corticospinal tracts are proximal to the periventricular area.*

   Reference: Rutherford, M. A., Supramaniam, V., Ederies, A., Chew, A., Bassi, L., Groppo, M., . . . Ramenghi, L. A. (2010). Magnetic resonance imaging of white matter diseases of prematurity. *Neuroradiology, 52*(6), 505–521.

2. **C—Symptoms are consistent with her birth history or the development of a subcortical dementia.** *Taking a thorough history will reveal if symptoms are long-standing and potentially related to the patient's birth history, which could still be relevant at this age. Certainly, the patient's age should be considered and the likelihood that she received less advanced medical care and may have greater neurocognitive effects of prematurity than had she been born today. If symptoms have arisen recently, concerns for the onset of a more recent neurological condition, such as subcortical dementia, could be considered. Symptoms of prematurity can mimic those of the subcortical dementias due to injury location.*

   Reference: Baron, I. S., & Rey-Casserly, C. (2010). Extremely preterm birth outcome: A review of four decades of cognitive research. *Neuropsychology Review, 20*, 430–452.

3. **D—multiple-birth pregnancy, maternal infections, low socioeconomic status, and maternal age** *Low to moderate caffeine consumption, maternal exercise, maternal weight gain, and use of SSRIs have not been shown to increase the risk for preterm delivery.*

   Reference: Taylor, H. G. (2008). Low birth weight. In J. E. Morgan & J. H. Ricker (Eds.), *Textbook of clinical neuropsychology*. New York, NY: Taylor and Francis Group.

4. **C—the proximity of the vulnerable periventricular region to the optic radiations** *Visuospatial skills appear impacted even in those patients without a history of motor or visual deficits (e.g., ROP).*

   Reference: Bassi, L., Ricci, D., Volzone, A., Allsop, J. M., Srinivasan, L., Pai, A. . . . Counsell, S. J. (2008). Probabilistic diffusion tractography of the optic radiations and visual function in preterm infants at term equivalent age. *Brain, 131*, 573–582.

5. **A—bleeding resulting in ventricular dilation** *Grade I IVH refers to bleeding that is confined to the germinal matrix, grade II IVH refers to bleeding into the ventricles without ventricular dilation, and grade IV IVH refers to a large hemorrhage with associated PVHI in the parenchyma.*

Reference: Inder, T., Perlman, J., & Volpe, J. (2017). Preterm intraventricular hemorrhage/posthemorrhagic hydrocephalus. In J. Volpe, T. Inder, B. Darras, L. S. De Vries, A. Plessis, J. Neil, & J. Perlman (Eds.), *Volpe's neurology of the newborn* (6th ed., pp. 637–698). Philadelphia, PA: Elsevier.

6. **D—ultrasound; magnetic resonance imaging** *There are many neuroimaging techniques used to detect neurological complications in preterm infants. Ultrasound is the most commonly used. Although early ultrasound is helpful in the detection of IVH and more severe white matter damage, it is limited in its ability to detect more subtle forms of white matter damage. In contrast, MRI is more sensitive in detecting more subtle forms of white matter damage in preterm infants. Additionally, in preterm infants, white matter damage found at approximately 3 weeks after birth using MRI was highly predictive of term MRI findings. Although MRI has been deemed safe for use in this population and there are MRI-compatible incubators, routine use of MRI in preterm infants may be difficult due to medical complications common to this population.*

Reference: Glass, H. C., Costarino, A. T., Stayer, S. A., Brett, C. M., Cladis, F., & Davis, P. J. (2015). Outcomes for extremely premature infants. *Anesthesia and Analgesia, 120*(6), 1337–1351.

7. **D—early intervention services and family support and education** *Both of these factors have been found to improve outcome in young children. While infant-toddler assessment tools have improved predictive validity for lower functioning children, they are not IQ tests and so intellectual disability should not be diagnosed. Referral to a neurologist can be useful when motor delays are present and if CP is suspected.*

Reference: Jarjour, I. T. (2015). Neurodevelopmental outcome after extreme prematurity: A review of literature. *Pediatric Neurology, 52*(2), 143–152.

8. **A—The IVH is more likely to be severe in the first twin. It is most likely that IVH will not occur in the second twin.** *Earlier occurring IVH is associated with increased severity. 90% of all IVH occur in the first four days of life, so it is probable that the second twin will not have an IVH.*

Reference: Inder, T., Perlman, J., & Volpe, J. (2017). Preterm intraventricular hemorrhage/posthemorrhagic hydrocephalus. In J. Volpe, T. Inder, B. Darras, L. S. De Vries, A. Plessis, J. Neil, & J. Perlman (Eds.), *Volpe's neurology of the newborn* (6th ed., pp. 637–698). Philadelphia, PA: Elsevier.

9. **B—it is located in a vascular watershed zone and has largely disappeared by 36 weeks gestation** *Germinal matrix IVH is the most common type of neonatal hemorrhage and is vulnerable to hypoxic ischemic injury. However, by 36 weeks gestational age the germinal matrix has largely disappeared reducing risk for hemorrhage in this area.*

Reference: Inder, T., Perlman, J., & Volpe, J. (2017). Preterm intraventricular hemorrhage/posthemorrhagic hydrocephalus. In J. Volpe, T. Inder, B. Darras, L. S. De Vries, A. Plessis, J. Neil, & J. Perlman (Eds.), *Volpe's neurology of the newborn* (6th ed., pp. 637–698). Philadelphia, PA: Elsevier.

10. **D—As certain types of white matter injury are not detected by ultrasound, you cannot rule out that an injury was sustained.** *Ultrasound is sensitive to IVH and so IVH can likely be ruled out. However, ultrasound is not sensitive to certain types of white matter injury and therefore, if ultrasound was the only imaging modality, neurological injury cannot be ruled out definitively.*

Reference: Kinney, H. C. & Volpe, J. J. (2017). Encephalopathy of prematurity: Neuropathology. In J. Volpe, T. Inder, B. Darras, L. S. De Vries, A. Plessis, J. Neil, & J. Perlman (Eds.), *Volpe's neurology of the newborn* (6th ed., pp. 389–404). Philadelphia, PA: Elsevier.

Recommended Readings

Anderson, P. J. (2014). Neuropsychological outcomes of children born very preterm. *Seminars in Fetal and Neonatal Medicine, 19,* 90–96.

Baron, I. S., Litman, F. R., Ahronovich, M. D., & Baker, R. (2012). Late preterm birth: A review of medical and neuropsychological childhood outcomes. *Neuropsychology Review, 22,* 438–450.

Baron, I. S., & Rey-Casserly, C. (2010). Extremely preterm birth outcome: A review of four decades of cognitive research. *Neuropsychology Review, 20,* 430–452.

Stoll, B. J., Hansen, N. I., Bell, E. F., Walsh, M. C., Carlo, W. A., Shankaran, S., . . . Eunice Kennedy Shriver National Institute of Child Health and Human Development Neonatal Research (2015). Trends in care practices, morbidity, and mortality of extremely preterm neonates, 1993–2012. *Journal of the American Medical Association, 314,* 1039–1051.

Spittle, A., Orton, J., Anderson, P. J., Boyd, R., & Doyle, L. W. (2015). Early developmental intervention programmes provided post hospital discharge to prevent motor and cognitive impairment in preterm infants. *Cochrane Database of Systematic Reviews,* (11), CD005495.

Volpe, J., Inder, T., Darras, B., De Vries, L. S., Plessis, A., Neil, J., & Perlman, J. (2017). *Volpe's neurology of the newborn* (6th ed.). Philadelphia, PA: Elsevier.

MEDICAL

18 Chromosomal and Genetic Syndromes

Jennifer Janusz

Introduction

A number of genetic disorders can impact cognitive, behavioral, and emotional functioning. This chapter reviews twelve different chromosomal and genetic disorders, describing the neurocognitive and behavioral presentation of each. The following disorders are covered in this chapter: neurofibromatosis type 1, tuberous sclerosis complex, Sturge-Weber syndrome, Williams syndrome, 22q11.2 deletion syndrome, adrenoleukodystrophy, Klinefelter syndrome, fragile X syndrome, Turner syndrome, phenylketonuria, Prader-Willi syndrome, and Angelman syndrome. The American Board of Clinical Neuropsychology (ABCN) exam will most likely not require that you memorize all of the physical symptoms of each of these conditions, but you will be expected to know/understand the central features of each and characteristics that distinguish one from another. Furthermore, please note that due to the large number of conditions covered, the section "Expectations for Neuropsychological Assessment Results" is in a summarized format for each disorder rather than in a bullet format as in other chapters.

Section 1: Neurofibromatosis Type 1

Definition

Three disorders comprise the neurofibromatoses: neurofibromatosis type 1 (NF1), neurofibromatosis type 2 (NF2), and schwannomatosis. All have the development of nerve sheath tumors in common. Neurofibromatosis type 1 is characterized by skin and bone abnormalities resulting from tumors growing along the nerves. Neurofibromatosis type 2 is characterized by bilateral acoustic *schwannomas* on the eighth cranial nerve, *meningiomas*, and *ependymomas*. Schwannomatosis is associated with *schwannomas* and chronic pain. Neurofibromatosis type 1 will be highlighted in this section because it is the most common of the three disorders and also associated with neuropsychological deficits.

Neurofibromatosis type 1 is a neurocutaneous autosomally dominant genetic disorder, with symptoms affecting the central nervous system (CNS) and the skin. Diagnostic criteria for NF1 have been developed by the National Institutes of Health (NIH); the presence of two of the following clinical criteria are considered positive for NF1:

- Six or more café-au-lait macules more than 5 mm in diameter in prepubertal individuals and more than 15 mm in diameter in postpubertal individual
- Two or more *neurofibromas* or one *plexiform neurofibroma*
- Freckling in the axilla or groin
- Optic *glioma*
- Two or more Lisch nodules (iris *hamartomas*)

- A distinctive bony lesion (such as sphenoid dysplasia or pseudoarthrosis)
- A first-degree relative with NF1

Neuropathology

- *Brain Tumors* Brain tumors are seen in 15% of people with NF1, with the majority present by age 6 years. Most are benign optic *gliomas* and do not require treatment. While optic *gliomas* themselves are not thought to have cognitive impact, treatment with radiation can effect neurocognitive functioning.
- *T2 Hyperintensities (T2Hs)* Focal areas of hyperintensity are seen on T2-weighted magnetic resonance images (MRIs) in 60–70% of children with NF1. Some literature refers to these as "unidentified bright objects" or UBOs. They frequently occur in the basal ganglia, cerebellum, thalamus, brainstem, and subcortical white matter. They are not consistently associated with the presence or degree of cognitive impairment.
- *Macrocephaly/Megalencephaly* Seen in 30–50% of people with NF1.

Morbidity and Mortality

- 30–65% diagnosed with learning disability (LD); diagnoses include disorders of reading, math, and written expression.
- 30–50% diagnosed with ADHD; occurs equally in boys and girls.
- Average lifespan is 50–60 years; mortality typically due to vascular dysplasia or malignancy; individuals with milder symptoms have average life expectancy.

Presentation, Disease Course, and Recovery

Clinical features tend to present at different ages, which complicates diagnosis because younger children may not yet exhibit all characteristics, thus not meeting clinical criteria for NF1 until later in childhood. Most symptoms worsen over time, and there are certain periods in life when symptoms increase. Specifically, *neurofibromas* increase in number during puberty (in males and females) and during pregnancy. The one exception to this are T2H, which resolve by early adulthood. Clinical features vary considerably, with some individuals having milder characteristics that do not impact daily living and others having severe, debilitating symptoms.

Individuals do not recover from NF1. Cognitive deficits can be identified early and continue through life. Children with NF1 can present with delays in development. Preschool-aged children present with a similar neurocognitive profile to school-aged children. In adults, deficits continue to be present in these same domains. Indeed, growth curve analyses suggest that, over time, the profile of neurocognitive skills does not change; in other words, areas of deficit do not improve, but skills that are intact remain so. However, children may show increasing difficulties in school as academic demands change and become more challenging.

Expectations for Neuropsychological Assessment Results

"Leftward shift" of IQ is seen, with Full-Scale IQ (FSIQ) averaging from 89 to 98. Intellectual disability (ID) is diagnosed in 4–8% of individuals with NF1. Approximately 75% of children with NF1 are estimated to have academic difficulties, although not all meet traditional, discrepancy-based criteria for LD. Deficits in attention and executive functioning (EF) skills are commonly seen. Visuospatial weaknesses were one of the first cognitive deficits to be identified, although more recent research has not replicated earlier findings of verbal IQ greater than nonverbal IQ discrepancies. Furthermore, more recent research has documented language deficits as well, specifically in word-list generation, naming, reading comprehension, and written expression. Deficits are seen in manual dexterity, coordination, and balance; however, no deficits in motor speed are seen once processing speed is controlled for. In contrast, verbal and visual memory skills are intact.

Internalizing disorders (anxiety, depression) are more common than externalizing disorders, although poor impulse control can be associated with ADHD. Children with NF1 are at greater risk for social difficulties and often present as socially awkward. However, individuals with NF1 are not at greater risk for severe psychiatric problems.

Section 2: Tuberous Sclerosis Complex

Definition

Tuberous sclerosis complex (TSC) is a variably expressed, autosomally dominant neurocutaneous disorder affecting multiple organ systems including the skin, heart, kidney, lungs, and brain. Clinical diagnostic criteria are complex and involve major and minor criteria; the major criteria are listed as the first eleven physical characteristics in Table 18.1 under "Defining Characteristics." Tuberous sclerosis complex arises from one of two genes: *TSC1* or *TSC2*. Although some research suggests that clinical presentation of *TSC1* may be milder, there is considerable overlap of the two phenotypes and prediction of neurological/cognitive status should not be made based on genetic mutation alone.

Neuropathology

- *Cortical Tubers* This feature gave rise to the name "tuberous sclerosis" to describe the potato-like appearance of these lesions. Cortical tubers are characterized by a proliferation of glial and neuronal cells and loss of the six-layered structure of the cortex. They are variable in size and number and are often the focus for epileptiform discharges.

- *Subependymal Nodules* These are *hamartomas* that form in the walls of the ventricles. Although these are usually asymptomatic, some will evolve into subependymal giant-cell astrocytomas, particularly in familial cases of TSC and in those presenting before age 20.

- *Subependymal Giant-Cell Astrocytomas (SEGA)* A slow-growing tumor that is the most common brain tumor in TSC. It is primarily seen in children/adolescent and rarely develops after 20 years of age. It occurs in 5–20% of children/adolescents. Tumors at the foramen of Monro can block the flow of cerebrospinal fluid, leading to increased intracranial pressure.

Epidemiology

- 80–90% of individuals with TSC are diagnosed with epilepsy. Seizures typically begin in infancy, with focal seizures preceding, coexisting with, or evolving into infantile spasms. Various other seizure types are seen in TSC, and they are often intractable.

- 45% diagnosed with ID; children with TSC who have ID are at greater risk for behavioral and psychiatric disorders.

TABLE 18.1 Summary of Disorders

Disorder	Incidence	Gene Location	Key Physical/Medical Characteristics	Cognitive/Behavioral Characteristics
Neurofi-bromatosis Type 1	1 in 3,500	Chromosome 17	Café au lait macules Inguinal/axillary freckling Neurofibromas Plexiform neurofibromas Lisch nodules Optic glioma T2 hyperintensities	Learning Disabilities Attention-deficit / hyperactivity disorder (ADHD)
Tuberous Sclerosis Complex	1 in 6,000	TSC1 gene (chromosome 9q34) TSC2 gene (chromosome 16p13.3)	Cortical tubers Facial angiofibromas/ Hypomelanotic macules Shagreen patch Subependymal nodules Subependymal giant-cell astrocytoma (SEGA) Cardiac rhabdomyoma Lymphangiomyomatosis Renal angiomyolipoma Epilepsy	Intellectual Disability Autism
Sturge-Weber Syndrome	1 in 5,000	Somatic mosaic mutation in GNAQ gene on chromosome 9q21	Port wine stain Vascular malformation of eye Vascular malformation of brain Seizures Migraines Stroke-like episodes	Intellectual Disability Varying deficits related to medical complications
Williams Syndrome	1 in 7,500 to 1 in 20,000	Deletion of 20–28 genes from chromosome band 7.11.23q	Connective tissue abnormalities Cardiovascular disease; supravalvar aortic stenosis Ocular/visual abnormalities; hyperopia, strabismus Ear/auditory abnormalities: chronic otitis media, hypersensitivity to sound Kidney/urinary tract abnormalities Facial dysmorphology • "Elfin" appearance • Broad brow • Flat nasal bridge • Short upturned nose • Wide mouth with full lips • Starburst iris pattern • Irregular dentition	Intellectual Disability Better verbal than nonverbal skills Hypersociability Anxiety/Phobias

(continued)

TABLE 18.1 Continued

Disorder	Incidence	Gene Location	Key Physical/Medical Characteristics	Cognitive/Behavioral Characteristics
22q11.2 Deletion Syndrome	1 in 2,000 to 5,000	Deletion at chromosome 22q11.2	Cardiac defects • Tetralogy of Fallot • Interrupted aortic arch • Ventricular septal defect • Vascular ring • Truncus arteriosus Hypocalcemia Mild conductive hearing loss Palatal defects • Submucosal cleft palate Velopharyngeal dysfunction Facial dysmorphology • Long face • Long, pear-shaped nose • Small ears with overfolded helices • Vertically narrow eyes	Borderline IQ Better verbal than nonverbal skills Anxiety Schizophrenia
Adrenoleuko-dystrophy	1 in 17,000	Defect in *ABCD 1* gene on Xq28	Nervous system Adrenocortical insufficiency	Nonverbal deficits EF deficits Psychiatric symptoms in adults
Klinefelter Syndrome (47,XXY)	1 in 600–800	Additional X chromosome	Tall stature Hypogonadism Fertility problems Hypotonia Hypertelorism Clinodactyly Hyperextensible joints Flat feet	Language deficits Dyslexia ADHD Anxiety/Depression
Fragile X syndrome	1 in 4,000 males 1 in 8,000 females	Repetition of CGG trinucleotide sequence at Xq27.3	Prominent ears Hyperextensive joints Flat feet Soft skin Macroorchidism Long face Epilepsy	Autism ADHD Intellectual Disability
Turner Syndrome	1 in 2,500	Absence/ abnormality of second X chromosome	Short stature Low posterior hairline Webbed neck Downward slanting palpebral fissures Epicanthal folds Broad chest Poor nail growth Cardiovascular malformations Congenital heart disease Kidney malformations Hearing loss Strabismus	ADHD Math disability Nonverbal deficits Deficits in social cognition Depression in adults

(continued)

TABLE 18.1 Continued

Disorder	Incidence	Gene Location	Key Physical/Medical Characteristics	Cognitive/Behavioral Characteristics
			Hypothyroidism Infertility due to absent or minimal ovarian tissue resulting in diminished estrogen	
Phenyl-ketonuria	Ethnic variation; 1 in 10,000 in North America	Mutation in phenylalanine hydroxylase (PAH) gene	Elevated phenylalanine in blood Low levels of tyrosine	*Untreated:* Significant neurological dysfunction *Treated:* Relationship between Phe levels and cognition ADHD Math deficits Reduced processing speed
Prader-Willi Syndrome	1 in 15,000	Lack of paternally expressed genes in region of q11-q13 on chromosome 15	Neonatal hypotonia Hypogonadism Hyperphagia Obesity Facial dysmorphology • Almond shaped eyes • Narrow temple and nasal bridge • Downturned mouth with thin upper lip Short stature Small hands and feet Hypopigmentation	Intellectual Disability Autism Behavioral problems related to hyperphagia
Angelman Syndrome	1 in 12,000 to 1 in 15,000	Lack of maternally expressed genes in region of q11-q13 on chromosome 15	Ataxic gait Epilepsy Microcephaly Facial dysmorphology • Prominent chin • Deep set eyes • Wide mouth with protruding tongue	Severe Intellectual Disability Severe speech delays Happy disposition with easily provoked laughter

- 40–50% diagnosed with an autism spectrum disorder (ASD) and there is an increased risk of ASD in individuals with ID.

- 25–50% diagnosed with ADHD; higher prevalence in children with seizures.

- Life expectancy is variable and depends on severity of symptoms; those with mild symptoms have normal life expectancy, whereas those with life-threatening symptoms including brain tumors, kidney lesions, and lung lesions may have shortened life expectancy.

Presentation, Disease Course, and Recovery

Cortical tubers and cardiac rhabdomyomas can be seen prenatally on ultrasound, and some individuals may present in infancy with seizures. Global delays and ASDs are usually identified in the preschool years; ADHD is typically diagnosed in school-aged children. Psychological disorders, including anxiety and depression, are typically diagnosed in adolescence and adulthood.

Disease course is variable. Those with profound intellectual impairment often show little cognitive progression past the sensorimotor stage. Infants with early developmental delays tend to remain delayed compared to peers over time. Even children who do not exhibit early delays fall behind peers during the school years (i.e., delayed consequences). However, TSC is not associated with intellectual or behavioral regression.

There is no cure for TSC. The most common treatment is the use of antiepileptic drugs for seizures, which can affect both cognition and behavior. Everolimus, an mTOR inhibitor, is also used to treat both SEGA and epilepsy. Individuals with TSC are not typically good candidates for epilepsy surgery because they generally have multiple seizure foci.

Expectations for Neuropsychological Assessment Results

A bimodal distribution of IQ is seen, with a substantial minority of individuals (30%) with IQ in the range of profound ID and a relatively larger proportion (70%) with near-normal to 130 IQ. Some research indicates a downshift of mean IQ to 93. However, high rates of LD are seen in children with normal IQ. Deficits in attention and EF skills, including working memory, organization, and planning, are seen in those with average IQ. No studies have investigated visuospatial and language skills, although survey data suggest only 30% have normal language development, with deficits in expressive vocabulary, abstract language, and grammar. Deficits are seen in memory recall, while recognition is spared.

More than 50% of children with TSC exhibit behavioral problems including aggressive outbursts, temper tantrums, and self-injury. Intellectual disability is a risk factor, but behavioral problems are seen in children with normal intelligence as well. Anxiety and depression can develop in adolescence and adulthood. Severe psychiatric problems are not common, although temporal lobe epilepsy and psychosis can be seen.

The comprehensive term "tuberous sclerosis-associated neuropsychiatric disorders" (TAND) is now used to describe the constellation of intellectual, behavioral, and psychosocial difficulties associated with TSC. A TAND checklist has been validated for use in screening symptoms.

Section 3: Sturge-Weber Syndrome
Definition

Sturge-Weber syndrome (SWS) is a neurocutaneous disorder with the defining characteristic of a facial capillary malformation or port-wine birthmark (PWB). Other major characteristics include vascular malformation of the brain (leptomeningeal angioma) and glaucoma. The PWB typically affects the face in the region of the ophthalmic division of the trigeminal nerve. Leptomeningeal angiomas are usually seen on the same side as the PWB, typically affecting the occipital and parietal lobes; bilateral brain involvement is less common. Sturge-Weber syndrome is caused by a somatic mosaic mutation in the *GNAQ* gene located on chromosome 9q21.

Neuropathology

- *Leptomeningeal Angioma* This is a capillary-venous vascular malformation of the brain. A PWB increases the risk of brain involvement by 10–20%, and the risk increases with the size and extent of the birthmark.

- *Cerebral Atrophy and Cortical Calcification* These are most commonly lateralized and seen in the occipital and parietal regions. Over time, calcification appears to "spread" into frontal areas; however, it is likely that this just becomes easier to capture on imaging over time rather than truly "spreading."

Epidemiology

- 75% of individuals with unilateral brain involvement and 95% of individuals with bilateral brain involvement have seizures. Seizures typically occur on the side of the body contralateral to the PWB.
- Headaches and migraines are common. In adults, these can have a more significant impact on quality of life than seizures.
- Stroke-like episodes can be associated with seizures and/or migraines and typically present with weakness and/or sensory disturbance on the side contralateral to brain involvement. Motor weakness can persist or become permanent following prolonged/clustered seizures or a stroke-like episode.
- Risk of central nervous system manifestations is greatest when the PWB involves the upper division of the trigeminal nerve
- 30–60% of individuals have glaucoma
- Eighteen-fold increased prevalence of growth hormone deficiency is seen.
- 50–60% are diagnosed with ID; risk factors include cerebral atrophy, cortical calcification, leptomeningeal angioma, and seizures that have early onset and are poorly controlled.

Presentation, Disease Course, and Recovery

Neurological deficits evolve over time as the result of stroke-like episodes and seizures. Toddlers and young children are especially vulnerable to stroke-like episodes precipitated by falls. Individuals with SWS are to avoid recreational activities associated with increased head injury risk. Most adults have some focal neurological deficit, usually some degree of hemiparesis.

Although seizures typically begin in childhood, they can present in adults who had been otherwise neurologically normal. Seizures occur in the first year for most individuals with unilateral brain involvement. These are usually focal motor seizures, but complex partial seizures are common as well. Status epilepticus, usually associated with a stroke-like episode, can also be seen. Seizures tend to stabilize in older childhood, but can again worsen in adolescence. Severe headaches and migraines worsen with age, but can be seen in younger children as well. If not properly treated in younger children, migraines can trigger seizures and stroke-like episodes.

Later seizure onset (after 9–12 months of age), good seizure control, and unilateral brain involvement have all been associated with better neurological outcome. However, individuals with SWS are at risk for neurological deterioration, which is thought to be secondary to venous occlusions and associated hypoxia and worsened by seizures. Prognosis is worse when there is an onset of seizures and/or stroke-like episodes before six months of age. Although neurological deterioration is seen more commonly in infants and young children, new neurological deficits can present in adults. Early-onset dementia has also been reported in individuals with SWS in their 50s and 60s. Individuals with more mild or well-controlled symptoms have average life expectancy, whereas the lives of those with more severe symptoms are shortened.

There is no cure for SWS. Antiepileptic drugs (AEDs) are used to control seizures, with some research suggesting better cognitive functioning in children treated prophylactically compared to those treated after their first seizure. Surgery, including surgical lobectomy, hemispherectomy, and callosotomy, has also been used in individuals with intractable seizures. Because microvascular thrombosis is thought to contribute to neurological decline, low-dose aspirin is commonly recommended. Stimulant medications are also used to treat children with attentional deficits.

Expectations for Neuropsychological Assessment Results

Few large studies of cognitive and behavioral functioning of individuals with SWS have been completed. Only one study has investigated specific neuropsychological domains through a case series of four individuals (Zabel et al., 2010). Understanding neuropsychological functioning in SWS is further complicated by the variable course and outcome of the disease, which are related to frequency/severity of seizures, stroke-like episodes, and recovery from such events. Indeed, neuropsychological presentation may fluctuate even on an individual basis. Although there is not a "typical" SWS neuropsychological profile, the case series just referenced identified several risk factors for worse cognitive outcome, including more frequent seizures, seizures onset in infancy, more extensive/diffuse cortical involvement, and a history of stroke-like episodes.

Among individuals with SWS, 60% have IQ scores in the range of ID, although IQ scores can range from extremely low to above average. Although no studies have specifically examined academic performance, "learning problems" are frequently reported. Attention problems are also common. Processing speed is slow, and sensorimotor function varies, with deficits often seen following stroke-like episodes. In the case series (Zabel et al., 2010), mild to moderate impairments in language comprehension, word-list generation, and verbal memory were seen in children with left hemisphere involvement. Deficits are also seen in visual-perceptual skills.

Lower IQ and frequent seizures increase risk for psychological and behavioral problems. Disruptive behavior disorder is the most common psychiatric diagnosis in children, and noncompliance and oppositional behaviors have been reported. Mood problems, particularly anxiety symptoms, are seen in children. Physical characteristics may contribute to emotional adjustment because emotional distress has been related to the size of PWB in children over 10. Depression is frequently seen in adults who are cognitively intact. Substance-related disorders and mood disorders are the most common psychiatric conditions diagnosed in adults. Aggression and self-injurious behaviors can be seen in children and adults with intellectual impairment. Social problems are common.

Section 4: Williams Syndrome

Definition

Williams syndrome (WS) is characterized by mild to moderate cognitive deficits with an uneven neuropsychological profile, connective tissue abnormalities, cardiovascular disease, and characteristic facial dysmorphology, including elf-like features. Williams syndrome is caused by a deletion of 26 to 28 genes on chromosome 7. This is typically a spontaneous genetic mutation.

Neuropathology

- *Reduction of Cerebral Volume with Preservation of Cerebellar Volume* In general, gray matter volume is preserved, with reduction in cerebral white matter volume.

- *Narrowing of the Corpus Callosum* This is primarily seen in the splenium and isthmus.

- *Abnormal Cell Density in the Primary Visual Cortex* Studies have linked this to decreased activation in visual cortices during face processing tasks.

- *Reduced Sulcal Depth in the Intraparietal/Occipitoparietal Sulcus* Studies have linked this to abnormal dorsal stream function, resulting in visuospatial deficits.

- *Abnormal Neural Pathways* In functional imaging studies, increased amygdala activation was seen in response to threatening scenes, whereas reduced amygdala activation was seen in response to threatening faces. This was thought to relate to the hypersocial and anxious traits seen in WS. Also, dorsal stream hypoactivation has been observed during visual processing tasks.

Epidemiology

- 70% experience failure to thrive as infants.

- 50–75% develop cardiovascular disease, typically supravalvar aortic stenosis.

- 50% are diagnosed with strabismus, cataracts, and visual acuity problems.

- 85–95% have hypersensitivity to sound.

- Majority have IQ in the range of ID, with uneven skills. Individuals with larger gene deletions are at greater risk for more severe intellectual disabilities.

- 50–65% are diagnosed with ADHD.

- Cardiovascular disease accounts for most cases of shortened lifespan.

Presentation, Disease Course, and Recovery

Motor delays and hypotonia are typically seen in infancy. Typical language developmental sequences are not seen. For example, children with WS typically start using single words before they start pointing, they typically look at an adult's face rather than where the adult is pointing, receptive and expressive vocabularies are comparable, and grammatical errors continue into adolescence. Emergence of first words is delayed by an average of 2 years; however, once they begin speaking, their vocabulary development and ability to combine words continues at a rate consistent with typically developing peers. Despite their atypical language development, individuals with WS are described as "talkers" and clearly use language for social purposes.

By age 30, the majority of adults have sensorineural hearing loss, which can begin in some individuals as early as late childhood. The majority of adults also have diabetes or prediabetes. Premature gray hair and wrinkling of the skin can also be seen. Individuals with WS typically have a hoarse voice related to connective tissue abnormalities.

Individuals with WS often have an enhanced affinity for music. They show an earlier interest in music, spend more time listening to music, and have a greater emotional response to music. Rhythm and timbre are often particular strengths in individuals with WS.

There is no cure for WS. Given their interest in music, musical activities and music therapy have been found to be effective in lowering anxiety and maladaptive behaviors.

Expectations for Neuropsychological Assessment Results

Average FSIQ is 55, with ranges from 40 to 90; few studies document IQs greater than 70. Verbal IQ tends to exceed nonverbal IQ, and, after initial delays, language skills are better than nonverbal skills. Impaired visuospatial functioning is a hallmark of WS, including deficits in visual-constructional tasks, perceptual grouping, orientation discrimination, mental imagery, and spatial relationships. In contrast, object and face recognition are often intact. Individuals with WS tend to take a local/featural rather than a global/configurational approach when completing constructional tasks and processing faces, suggesting that the dorsal visual stream is dysfunctional while the ventral visual stream remains intact. Consistent with verbal/nonverbal differences, auditory rote memory is a relative strength, whereas visual rote memory is deficient. Short- and long-term visuospatial memory is also impaired, with greater deficits on spatial memory tasks than object memory tasks. Reading is relatively better than math, with adults with WS attaining a fifth-grade reading level; however, reading decoding is often better than comprehension. Rates of ADHD are higher than the general population. Fine and gross motor deficits are seen.

Anxiety and persistent fears are common, with the number of individuals meeting criteria for generalized anxiety disorder increasing in adulthood. From 54–96% have specific phobias. "Hypersociability" is seen, and individuals with WS are described as overly friendly, willing to approach others, and having a strong emotional/empathic response. Increased interest in others, with an intent focus on faces, and preference for social over nonsocial stimuli can be seen in infancy. Despite this, individuals with WS tend to lack social judgment and "social intelligence," resulting in difficulty forming friendships and social isolation. Children with WS also exhibit *conversational stereotypies*. Individuals with WS tend to do well in open-ended, less constrained social situations in which they can take the initiative. However, they struggle more in constrained social context where they must adapt to the situation.

Section 5: 22q11.2 Deletion Syndrome

Definition

22q11.2 deletion syndrome (22q11DS), also called DiGeorge syndrome, Shprintzen syndrome, or velocardio-facial syndrome, is characterized by multiple congenital anomalies including cardiac malformations, hypocalcemia, mild conductive hearing loss, and palatal defects. Approximately 90% of cases are de novo *mutations*, whereas 10% are inherited from a parent in an autosomally dominant pattern.

Neuropathology

- *Decrease in Total Brain Volume* Brain volume is decreased by about 10%; white matter is more reduced than gray matter. Frontal lobe volume is more preserved, whereas parietal lobe volume is reduced. There is a general anterior to posterior pattern of progressive volume reduction.
- *Reduced Cerebellar Volume* Observed with associated decrease in the size of the vermis and pons.
- *Hippocampal Reduction* Can be commensurate or disproportionate to overall volumetric decrease.
- *Disorganized Axonal Tracts* In parietoparietal, frontofrontal, and frontotemporal connections.
- *Cortical Thinning* In parieto-occipital and orbitofrontal regions.

Epidemiology

- 75–80% have a congenital heart defect.
- 69% have palatal abnormalities resulting in speech and feeding difficulties.
- 30–40% are diagnosed with ADHD.
- 30–40% are diagnosed with anxiety disorders, especially specific phobias and separation anxiety.
- 10–30% are diagnosed with ASD.

- 82–100% have learning difficulties.
- 20–30% are diagnosed with mood disorder, including major depression and bipolar disorder.
- 25–35% are diagnosed with psychotic disorder.
- Congenital heart defects account for most cases of mortality.

Presentation, Disease Course, and Recovery

During infancy, much focus is on cardiac and palatal malformations, and developmental delays can be erroneously attributed to health problems. Delays are seen in both motor and speech/language development even in children with IQs greater than 70. Expressive language is more often delayed than receptive language, and many children with 22q11DS are nonverbal until 3 years of age. Although language improves over time, higher order language and language pragmatics remain impaired.

Although individuals with 22q11DS have relatively stronger verbal than nonverbal skills, controversy remains whether this represents a nonverbal learning disorder (NLD). This is mainly due to the finding that many studies document only a 4- to 5-point discrepancy between verbal and performance indices. However, individuals with 22q11DS exhibit many other characteristics traditionally associated with NLD, including strong rote memory skills, good reading decoding in contrast to poor math skills, impaired attention and EF skills, and mood/psychiatric disorders.

One of the greatest concerns in 22q11DS is the increased risk for psychosis and schizophrenia. The average age of onset of psychosis is in the late teens to early 20s. However, subthreshold psychotic symptoms are present in 30–50% of adolescents with 22q11DS. Research has suggested that subthreshold symptoms (including hallucinations and delusions), anxiety (especially obsessive-compulsive disorder), symptoms of depression, and relatively lower verbal IQ scores are the best predictors of the onset of psychotic disorders in adolescence. Adults with 22q11DS and schizophrenia perform more poorly on neuropsychological measures associated with prefrontal systems, including spatial working memory, strategy formation, verbal reasoning, visual recognition, and attention, compared to those without schizophrenia.

Stimulant medications are often effective for attention problems; however, individuals with 22q11DS tend to respond less well to antipsychotic medications.

Expectations for Neuropsychological Assessment Results

IQ scores range from mild ID to average range, with mean IQ scores in the borderline range. Language skills are generally better than nonverbal skills, although children with 22q11DS typically perform worse on language testing than would be expected given verbal IQ scores, with weaknesses in expressive and pragmatic skills. Deficits in nonverbal skills, including visuospatial, visual-perceptual, and visual-motor skills are common, and visuospatial and spatial attention deficits have been linked to difficulties with math and numerical processing. Math difficulties are commonly seen in manipulation of quantities, execution of calculation strategies, and word problem solving. However, verbally based math skills, such as number reading and retrieval of math facts, are intact. Reading, spelling, and phonological processing are areas of relative strength, although typically behind peers, and reading comprehension lags behind reading decoding. Consistent with verbal/nonverbal differences, verbal memory is better than visual memory. However, individuals tend to do better on rote verbal learning task (lists) as opposed to more complex verbal memory tasks (stories). Deficits are also seen in facial memory. Deficits are seen across visual, spatial, and auditory attention tasks; more attention problems are seen as tasks increase in load and complexity. Executive functioning is an area of concern, with difficulties seen in cognitive flexibility, nonverbal problem solving, and nonverbal working memory. Children tend to be rigid, perseverative, and inflexible in their problem-solving approach. Problems with response inhibition and impulsivity are also seen. Deficits in temporal processing are reported, and studies using Wechsler scales to assess overall cognitive ability show deficits on the Processing Speed Index, as well. Deficits in gross motor skills are more marked than fine motor deficits.

Anxiety, including specific fears and separation anxiety, is common. Obsessive-compulsive disorder is also frequently seen, although children tend to show more "obsessive" features and fewer compulsive behaviors. Extremes in behavior can be seen and are considered "person and situation dependent," many of the behaviors are not uncommon for children with developmental delay. Problems with social functioning are common, and individuals with 22q11DS are described as having bland affect with minimal facial expression. Social skills deficits may be partially related to communication difficulties, especially in younger children, as well as to deficits in visuospatial and EF skills.

The risk of developing schizophrenia is twenty-five times that of the general population. Individuals are also at greater risk for mood disorders. Although reports generally find greater prevalence of ASD than in the general population, there is some controversy surrounding this because some believe that social deficits are secondary to language and cognitive delays.

Section 6: Adrenoleukodystrophy

Definition

Adrenoleukodystrophy (ALD) is an X-linked, recessive disorder affecting CNS myelin and adrenal cortex caused by a defect in the gene *ABCD1*. This results in abnormal breakdown of very-long-chain fatty acids (VLCFA), which then accumulate in plasma, brain, and adrenal cortex. Adrenoleukodystrophy is neurodegenerative in nature, with death occurring within 2 to 5 years after clinical onset.

Because this is an X-linked disorder, males show greater deficits. Heterozygous females may demonstrate mild to moderate myeloneuropathy, typically after the age of 40; cerebral and adrenal involvement is rare. There are four main phenotypes of ALD in males: cerebral inflammatory, adrenomyeloneuropathy (AMN), Addison-only, and asymptomatic. The cerebral inflammatory phenotype is further divided into childhood cerebral (CCALD), adolescent (AdolCALD), and adult (ACALD); CCALD is considered the "classic" form and is the most common, representing 31–35% of cases. Please see Table 18.2 for specifics regarding each.

Neuropathology

- *Inflammatory Brain Demyelination* A posterior pattern is seen in 80%, with demyelination starting at the splenium of the corpus callosum and spreading out into the parieto-occipital white matter. Arcuate fibers are spared.

- *Noninflammatory Distal Axonopathy* This involves long tracts of the spinal cord and is associated with the AMN phenotype.

Epidemiology

- 90% have adrenal insufficiency.

- 56% of adults have psychiatric symptoms.

- 100% of males with cerebral inflammatory ALD (this includes CCALD, AdoCALD, and ACALD), will have neurologic deterioration; death occurs within several years of cerebral involvement.

- Death in males with AMN occurs after several decades.

TABLE 18.2 Adrenoleukodystrophy Phenotypes

Phenotype	Description
Childhood Cerebral (CCALD)	Onset age 3–10 years. Characterized by progressive behavioral, cognitive, and neurological decline, with total disability within 3 years.
Adolescent Cerebral ALD (AdolCALD)	Onset age 11–21 years. Similar to CCALD but slower progression.
Adult Cerebral ALD (ACALD)	Onset age 21–35. Dementia, behavioral disturbance; sometimes focal deficits. Progression parallels CCALD.
AMN-No Cerebral disease	Onset 28 years + 9. Involves mainly spinal cord and peripheral nerve involvement. Progression of symptoms is slow.
AMN-Cerebral Disease	Onset 28 years + 9. Involves mainly spinal cord and peripheral nerve involvement, as well as behavioral and cognitive symptoms. Progress of symptoms is rapid.
Addison-only	Onset before 7.5 years. Primary adrenal insufficiency without neurologic involvement.
Asymptomatic	Common < 4 years; very rare > 40 years. Gene abnormality without adrenal or neurologic deficit.

NOTE: Adapted from Engelen et al. (2012). X-linked adrenoleukodystrophy (X-ALD): Clinical presentation and guidelines for diagnosis, follow-up, and management. *Orphanet Journal of Rare Diseases, 7*(51), 1–14.

Presentation, Disease Course, and Recovery

For children with CCALD, development is typically normal prior to onset. CCALD has onset between the ages of 3 and 8, first presenting with ADHD-like symptoms. This is then followed by intellectual, behavioral, and neurological deterioration, including withdrawal, aggression, poor memory, poor school performance, impaired auditory discrimination, visual disturbances (including blindness), poorly articulated speech, spatial disorientation, disturbances of gait and coordination, progressive ataxia, and seizures. A minimally responsive state is seen within 2 years of disease onset, followed by death.

In adolescent cerebral adrenoleukodystrophy (AdolCALD), initial progression of symptoms is usually slower than in CCALD, and may first present with adrenal insufficiency, neurological dysfunction, or psychiatric symptoms. Death is seen within 1 to 2 years of symptom onset. For adult cerebral adrenoleukodystrophy (ACALD), early cognitive decline can be subtle, and is not always immediately noticed by others. This is followed by psychiatric symptoms mimicking schizophrenia or psychosis, which at times results in misdiagnosis and delay of diagnosis of ACALD. Motor impairments, including abnormalities of gait and upper motor neuron involvement, are typically seen after development of psychiatric symptoms. Death is seen within 3 to 4 years of symptom onset.

Medical therapies have focused on adrenal hormone replacement therapy for those with primary adrenocortical insufficiency. A low-fat diet with lipid supplement with Lorenzo's oil (LO) normalizes plasma VLCFA but does not seem to significantly alter the progression of the disease, particularly in individuals who were symptomatic when therapy started and had cerebral inflammatory phenotypes. For asymptomatic boys, the use of LO may reduce (but not eliminate) their risk for developing CCALD.

Currently, *hematopoietic stem cell transplant* (HSTC) is the only effective long-term treatment if done at an early stage of cerebral disease. After HSTC, improvement can be seen in nonverbal IQ, whereas verbal IQ remains stable. Children also often show few functional impairments or behavioral difficulties after treatment. Predictors of good outcome following HSTC include few or no neurologic deficits (i.e., early disease), nonverbal IQ greater than 80, and less significant findings on MRI. Studies suggest a 68% 5-year survival rate for those receiving stem cells from a related donor, and a 54% survival rate for those receiving stem cells from an unrelated donor.

Expectations for Neuropsychological Assessment Results

Studies have investigated the neuropsychological functioning of asymptomatic boys and found no deficits in intellectual ability, adaptive skills, academic skills, language skills, memory, or EF. Although visuoperceptual and visual-motor skills were within normal limits, there was an inverse correlation with age possibly suggestive of decline as children matured.

Both children and adults with ALD present with a cognitive pattern typically seen in other demyelinating diseases such as multiple sclerosis. Attention problems are one of the first clinical symptoms to emerge in children, whereas psychiatric symptoms are among the first in adults. Greater deficits are seen in nonverbal IQ tasks as opposed to verbal IQ tasks, with difficulties on visuospatial, visual-perceptual, and visual-motor tasks. Deterioration in nonverbal IQ occurs over time, related to progressing cerebral lesions in parietal and occipital regions. Although language skills are relatively stronger, weaknesses are seen in word-list generation and naming. Consistent with verbal/nonverbal differences, auditory short-term sequential memory is better than visual short-term sequential memory. Deficits in memory, particularly visual, are seen in adults with AMN. EF deficits are common in both children and adults. Worsening motor and sensory functioning are seen with disease progression. Increased behavioral problems are also seen as the disease progresses.

Section 7: Klinefelter Syndrome (47,XXY)

Definition

Klinefelter syndrome (KS; 47,XXY) is the most common sex chromosome *aneuploidy* seen in males, resulting from the presence of an extra X chromosome. It is associated with characteristic physical features including tall stature, *hypogonadism*, and fertility problems. The specific genes have not been identified. Current estimates indicate that 10% of individuals are diagnosed prenatally, with another 25% diagnosed during childhood and the remaining 65% not diagnosed until puberty. However, with the development and increased use of noninvasive prenatal screening (NIPT), which tests fetal DNA extracted from the mother's blood for certain chromosomal disorders, the rate of prenatal diagnosis will likely be higher in the future.

Neuropathology

- *Reduced Overall Brain Volume* This includes reduced volume of limbic areas, reduced volume of caudate nucleus and cerebellum, and enlarged lateral ventricles.
- *Differences in Temporal Lobe Characteristics* Reduced overall temporal lobe gray matter volume (with greater reduction on left then right) and reduced temporal lobe asymmetry are

seen. Relative preservation of the temporal lobe is seen in individuals treated with testosterone during development.

- **_Increased Rates of Anomalous Cerebral Dominance_** Dichotic listening tasks report decreased right-ear advantage for verbal material. Studies using functional MRI (fMRI) report that language is less lateralized in men with KS, primarily due to increased activity in the right hemisphere as opposed to reduced activity in the left hemisphere. This was most prominent in the superior temporal gyrus (STG) and the supramarginal gyrus region, which is close to the posterior STG and part of Wernicke's area.

Epidemiology

- 35–65% are diagnosed with ADHD.
- 5–10% are diagnosed with ASD.
- 50–75% are diagnosed with LD, predominantly dyslexia.
- Increased mortality risk with a median loss of 2.1 years.

Presentation, Disease Course, and Recovery

Characteristics of KS may be subtle or absent in early childhood. Many children present with motor and/or speech delay. Language milestones are typically delayed, and early speech/language deficits are seen in sentence building, speech production, intonation, and word finding. Tall stature can be seen in childhood, but becomes more apparent in adolescence. Adults with KS are approximately 3 inches taller than would be predicted given family history.

Physical development tends to be normal until puberty when testosterone deficiency results in slow or incomplete pubertal development. This may involve absent or diminished growth of facial, chest, and pubic hair. *Microorchidism* is seen in almost all, and *gynecomastia* is seen in 25–30%. The rates of breast cancer are higher in this population (9 in 1,000) than in males without KS. Testosterone replacement therapy (TRT) is started in adolescence to support physical pubertal changes, muscular development, bone density, physical endurance, and sexual functioning. With advanced reproductive techniques, a subset of males can father children. Some studies have shown improvement in word-list generation and motor skills following TRT. Other medical problems that emerge in adolescence and adulthood include osteoporosis, autoimmune diseases, thyroid problems, intention tremor, and type II diabetes.

Expectations for Neuropsychological Assessment Results

IQ is generally in the average range, although 5–10 points lower than sibling/population cohorts. An overall pattern of better nonverbal than verbal skills is seen, with deficits in specific language skills (verbal comprehension, verbal conceptual abilities, higher level language processing, verbal expression, and grammatical construction) and verbal executive tasks. Language-based learning disabilities (dyslexia) are common, posited to be related to underlying language difficulties. Individuals also have difficulty with verbally presented math problems and written computations. However, language deficits are more common in children than adults, and longitudinal and adult outcome studies report less of a discrepancy between nonverbal and verbal IQ scores than in childhood. Although verbal and nonverbal immediate and delayed memory are intact, performance on visual memory tasks tends to be enhanced. There is a high rate of ADHD diagnosis, with more reports of symptoms of inattention than hyperactivity; this is most common in children under 10. Processing speed is slow. Deficits are also seen in strength, agility, hand/finger dexterity, hand speed, and running speed.

Individuals with KS have elevated rates of anxiety and depression, including social anxiety and social withdrawal, as well as more behavioral difficulties, including emotional lability, irritability, and perseverative questioning. Individuals with KS are described as shy, emotionally sensitive, and socially immature; as such, peer and social difficulties are common. Language deficits (including problems with language pragmatics) and learning disorders may be contributing factors, as are social cognitive deficits consists with ASD. There is a higher rate of ASD and psychotic symptoms in this population.

Section 8: Fragile X Syndrome

Definition

Fragile X syndrome (FXS) results from a repetition in the CGG trinucleotide sequence at Xq27.3. In typical individuals, there are up to 44 repeats. Individuals with 45–54 repeats are in the "gray zone" (they do not have expression of the disease but the repeats may expand with future generations). Premutation carriers have 55–200 repeats, and more than 200 repeats is considered a full mutation. The mutation causes a deficit or absence of the FMR1 protein (FMRP), which causes the physical, cognitive, and behavioral features. Males are more significantly affected than females. As females have two X chromosomes, with the FXS mutation on only one of those, the other one can normally produce FMRP, thus lessening the mutation's impact on development. Fragile X syndrome is the leading cause of inherited ID and the most common single gene disorder associated with autism.

Neuropathology

- Most imaging studies have been conducted with females and higher functioning adults, which may limit generalizability of findings.

- *Enlarged hippocampus, caudate nucleus, thalamus, and amygdala* Caudate nucleus is, on average, over 20% larger than controls and correlates with increased severity of autistic behavior and stereotypic tendencies.

- *Reduction in size of cerebellar vermis.*

- *Dysmorphia of cerebellar vermis and caudate nucleus* Is predictive of poorer cognitive testing and lower IQ scores.

Epidemiology

- 10–20% are diagnosed with epilepsy, more predominantly in males. Epilepsy in FXS has its own characteristic electroencephalogram (EEG) abnormalities, including rhythmic theta waves with decreased and slower alpha waves, overall slowing of general background activity, and abnormal bursts of electrical activity in the centrotemporal region (pattern closely resembles benign rolandic epilepsy). Seizures often resolve after childhood or adolescence.

- 40% of premutation males and 10% of premutation females develop fragile X-associated tremor/ataxia syndrome (FXTAS), characterized by progressive gait ataxia, intention tremor, parkinsonism, peripheral neuropathy, short-term memory loss, and executive dysfunction.

- 25–47% of males are diagnosed with autism. Autism is associated with poorer developmental outcomes and more behavior problems.
- 70–90% of males and 30–50% of females are diagnosed with ADHD; this usually reflects symptoms of hyperactivity, impulsivity, inattention, and hyperarousal.
- 80% of males and 30% of females are diagnosed with ID; most males diagnosed with moderate to severe ID; females are more often diagnosed with mild ID.
- Lifespan is normal.

Presentation, Disease Course, and Recovery

Most males manifest ID, whereas females exhibit less severe cognitive and behavioral/social problems. Male and female premutation carriers usually have normal IQ, but ADHD, anxiety, shyness, and social difficulties can be seen. Some studies indicate that premutation carriers are also at risk for EF deficits.

Developmental delays are usually the first signs of FXS. However, as other physical features may be subtle or not emerge until adolescence, FXS is usually diagnosed later than other developmental disabilities, with a mean diagnosis at 8 years.

The development of large testicles occurs during puberty. An increase in size is seen until they are 2–4 times normal size at about 15 years of age, when they stabilize. Fertility is normal, although cognitive deficits typically interfere with reproduction. There is no cure for FXS, although clinical trials are underway investigating the efficacy of drugs targeting metabotropic glutamate receptors and GABA receptors to address behavioral difficulties.

Expectations for Neuropsychological Assessment Results

Mean IQ for FXS males is in the mid 40s, whereas scores for FXS females range from mild ID to the average range. IQ scores tend to decline in males over time, reflecting a lack of expected progress rather than a regression in skills. In females without ID, increased risk of math disability can be identified as early as kindergarten. This has been related to problems understanding mathematical principles and number facts (despite adequate retrieval of rote learned information), as well as poor spatial reasoning and working memory. In contrast, reading is a relative strength. Deficits are seen in visuospatial, visual-constructional, and visual-motor skills, whereas visuoperceptual skills are relatively intact. "Cluttering" has been used to describe the speech of individuals with FXS. This is characterized by incomplete sentences, short bursts of two- to three-word phrases, *echolalia, palilalia,* perseveration, poor articulation, and stuttering. Memory is better for more structured, cohesive information (stories) than for more abstract information. Deficits in working memory and cognitive flexibility have been described in all individuals with FXS; studies with boys document further deficits in inhibition and planning. In general, executive deficits are greater than would be expected given IQ. Attention problems are seen, although generally consistent with overall cognitive ability. Processing speed is also consistent with cognitive level. Hypotonia is common in infants and children, with balance problems continuing in adulthood. Problems are also seen with fine motor and oral motor skills.

Poor eye contact and gaze aversion are common and frequently the presenting symptoms in males. Diagnosis of ASD typically reflects poor social and communicative abilities. Individuals with FXS tend to be rigid and have difficulty with transitions, and social anxiety and abnormal social behaviors are common. Many individuals with FXS demonstrate "approach-withdrawal" behavior, in that they want to interact but instead withdraw. They also exhibit hyperarousal in response to unusual sensitivity to auditory, visual, and tactile stimuli. Self-injurious behaviors are seen more commonly in males. Other behavior problems are frequently related to ADHD symptoms.

Section 9: Turner Syndrome

Definition

Turner syndrome (TS) results from a missing or abnormal second X chromosome. As such, it occurs only in females. Approximately 50% of individuals with TS have chromosome constitution of 45,X, whereas the other 50% have chromosomal or structural abnormalities of the second X chromosome. Girls with TS have characteristic physical features, including short stature and a webbed neck. Cardiovascular malformations, congenital heart disease, and kidney malformations are common.

Neuropathology

- *Decreased volumes of parietal and occipital cortices* Have been associated with deficits in visuospatial processing.
- *Abnormal structure and function of amygdala, insula, anterior cingulate, ventromedial prefrontal cortex, and orbitofrontal cortex* Are surmised to relate to social/affective deficits.
- *Dysfunctional frontoparietal circuitry* Is associated with deficits in visuospatial working memory.
- *Agenesis or anatomical differences of the corpus callosum.*

Epidemiology

- 17–45% have cardiovascular malformations, with higher prevalence in those with 45, X as opposed to *mosaic karyotype*.
- Almost all have short stature. In the absence of growth hormone treatment, average height is 4 feet, 7 inches.
- Many develop osteoporosis and are infertile due to inadequate estrogen production secondary to minimal or absent ovarian tissue.
- 30% have thyroid disorder, usually hypothyroidism.
- 25% are diagnosed with ADHD.
- 45–55% diagnosed with math disability.
- There is a reduced life expectancy of up to 13 years compared to the general population. Cardiovascular malformations are the most common cause of death.

Presentation, Disease Course, and Recovery

Developmental motor delays can be seen early. Individuals with 45,X are usually diagnosed earlier than those with mosaicism. Median age of diagnosis is 6 years, although 22% are diagnosed after the age of 12, typically when the girl fails to begin puberty.

Although 20–30% of girls undergo puberty spontaneously, this is usually in girls with mosaicism. Estrogen/progesterone replacement therapy is typically required for breast/pubertal development and bone density. Studies have found that treatment with estrogen and androgen can result in improvements in processing speed, motor skills, and math. Growth hormone therapy is typically initiated in childhood.

Expectations for Neuropsychological Assessment Results

Given spatial, math, and social skills deficits, many girls with TS display traditional features of NLD. However, there is considerable variability in the neurocognitive profile, so this diagnosis cannot be applied broadly to all girls.

Mean IQ scores range from 92 to 102, with significantly stronger verbal than nonverbal IQ (although this discrepancy becomes less apparent over time). Nonverbal deficits are a hallmark of TS, and nonverbal IQ may be the most sensitive measure of cognitive deficits in TS. Deficits are seen across visuospatial, visual-perceptual, and visual-motor skills. Greater problems are seen on tasks of "how things go together" and spatial location/orientation than on object identification. Greater deficits are seen in visual than verbal memory. Although reading is a strength, with some girls demonstrating hyperlexia, math disabilities are common. Early math skills are average, but deficits in automaticity of math skills and timed calculations, as well as procedural errors during problem solving, are often seen by mid- to late-elementary school. Deficits in planning, cognitive flexibility, and spatial working memory are common. Studies have suggested that deficits in spatial working memory and slow processing/response speed may be the primary deficits underlying more general nonverbal and EF difficulties and math problems. This is unlike in girls with FXS, in whom math problems have been linked to visuospatial deficits. Despite relatively intact verbal skills, deficits are seen in retrieval and rapid naming. Girls also have difficulty with language concepts related to spatial and temporal relationships, and executive skills of sequencing, working memory, and planning also interfere with narrative story-telling. Difficulties are also seen on certain verbal executive tasks, such as word list generation. Early motor deficits are common and continue through childhood; tasks that require both motor and spatial skills are significantly impaired. There is a risk for hearing loss, especially prematurely in middle age.

Some studies show few emotional/behavioral problems, whereas others suggest increased risk for anxiety, depression, and low self-esteem. Social difficulties are often related to impairments in social and emotional processing. Girls with TS are described as socially immature, lacking connectedness with peers, and having poor social competence. They have difficulty accurately and/or efficiently reading social and nonverbal cues and struggle to maintain appropriate eye gaze or interpersonal boundaries. Pragmatic language deficits are also seen, and social cognitive and "theory of mind" deficits have been identified. Problems forming and maintaining relationships continue into adulthood. Body image issues are reported, even after treatment with growth hormone. Women with TS report less interest in sexual relationships and less sexual activity related to lower levels of sex hormones. Although there is not a higher incidence of severe psychiatric problems, adult women with TS are more likely to exhibit depressive symptoms. They also frequently struggle with issues related to infertility.

Section 10: Phenylketonuria

Definition

Phenylketonuria (PKU) results from a mutation in the phenylalanine hydroxylase (PAH) gene, which normally inhibits the metabolism of phenylalanine (Phe) into tyrosine (Tyr). In untreated individuals, this dysfunction results in an accumulation of Phe in the blood and other tissues and low levels of Tyr. Standard treatment requires a Phe-restricted diet; adherence to the diet can mitigate many cognitive and neurological difficulties. Phenylketonuria is usually identified through newborn screening blood tests. Approximately 1 in 50 people are carriers; it is an autosomal recessive disorder. Prevalence rates vary by population; PKU is more common in North America and Europe and less common in Asia and Africa.

Phenylketonuria is classified based on Phe level at diagnosis: classical PKU (blood Phe >1,200 mmol/L), moderate PKU (blood Phe 900–1,200 mmol/L), mild PKU (blood Phe 600–900 mmol/L), and non-PKU (blood Phe 120–599 mmol/L). More than half of individuals with PKU have one of the milder phenotypes.

Neuropathology

Untreated PKU

- *Hypomyelination and gliosis* Is seen in systems that myelinate postnatally.
- *Progressive white matter degeneration* Is seen less frequently and mostly in adults.
- *Delay or arrest in development of cerebral cortex* Is seen.
- *Diffuse cortical atrophy and reduced dendritic arborization* Is seen.

Treated PKU

- *White Matter Abnormalities* Abnormal myelination occurs. T2 hyperintensities are seen, most commonly in the occipital-parietal regions but may extend to frontal and parietal lobes in more severe cases.
- *Volume loss* Is seen in cerebrum, corpus callosum, hippocampus, and pons.

Epidemiology

- 75% of untreated individuals have significant neurological dysfunction.
- 5% of untreated adults have a progressive neurological disorder, usually supranuclear motor disturbance.
- 13–46% of treated individuals are diagnosed with ADHD; typically the inattentive subtype.
- Those treated can have a normal lifespan.

Presentation, Disease Course, and Recovery

The course for children untreated or late-treated for PKU is considerably different from those treated early. Untreated infants appear physically normal, but may present with nonspecific symptoms such as hypotonia, irritability, and feeding difficulties. Untreated babies typically have a musty odor due to excretion of phenylacetic acid. At 4 to 6 months, infants gradually develop progressive psychomotor retardation and may develop seizures. Cognitive deterioration occurs over the next 3 to 4 years. Significant behavior problems are seen, including obsessive-compulsive rituals, self-injurious behavior, and extreme tactile sensitivity. The IQ of untreated individuals is usually below 50 and remains stable into and throughout adulthood.

Many children who are initially "missed" on newborn screen are eventually diagnosed in early childhood when they start exhibiting significant developmental delays. Starting treatment at this age usually results in much better cognitive and neurologic outcomes. However, eventual developmental outcome is variable, and most have IQs in the mild to moderate ID range. Even when IQ is average, late-treated individuals almost always exhibit learning problems.

Individuals who are treated early do much better cognitively and neurologically. However, they can exhibit more subtle neuropsychological deficits, as described here.

Although there is no cure for PKU, early treatment with a low-Phe diet can be effective. Phe levels and age at initiation of treatment are highly related to degree of cognitive deterioration. Furthermore, white matter abnormalities noted on imaging are reversible with treatment. Research is clear that a low-Phe diet should continue through childhood and adolescence. There has been some controversy regarding whether treatment can be discontinued in adulthood. However, recent research suggests that individuals should remain on a low-Phe diet throughout their lives. Sapropterin dihydrochloride has been found effective in lowering blood Phe levels and can be prescribed to supplement a low-Phe diet. Stimulant medication has been used to treat attention problems with benefit.

Expectations for Neuropsychological Assessment Results

This section refers to individuals with early treated PKU. IQ tends to be in the average range, although lower than sibling controls. IQ and blood Phe levels are highly correlated, even in those receiving early treatment. Reading and spelling are intact, whereas math is deficient, surmised to be related to visuospatial/perceptual weaknesses, EF/working memory deficits, parietal myelin abnormalities, and/or frontal transmitter abnormalities. Academic scores are related to length of dietary treatment, with better scores seen for those treated longer. Studies regarding language skills are not consistent, although there is a relationship between Phe levels and language skills, with declines on language measures seen in children who discontinue the diet after age 6. Visuoperceptual and visuospatial deficits are common, although may be partially related to EF deficits. Executive functioning deficits can be identified in preschool-aged children. The most common deficits are seen in working memory and prepotent response inhibition, although some studies also identify problem with word list generation, initiation of problem solving, concept formation, and reasoning. Although memory is intact, EF deficits impact strategies used. A direct correlation between Phe level and EF has not been consistently identified; however, when groups are divided into high-Phe and low-Phe, the high-Phe group consistently performs more poorly. Deficits are seen in selective and sustained attention and related to Phe levels. Reduced processing speed is a major component of PKU phenotype and is the primary deficit in adults; this has been correlated with structural white matter abnormalities but not Phe level. Gross motor deficits are rare in those treated early, but fine motor deficits are seen and related to Phe level.

Individuals with PKU are at risk for emotional and behavioral problems, including hyperactivity, impulsivity, and limited task persistence. In children, diet discontinuation, lower IQ, and higher Phe levels are associated with more behavior problems. Individuals with PKU have poor social competence and are at risk for social isolation. Depression is common, especially among women. Anxiety disorders, including phobias and panic attacks, are also common. Agoraphobia has been related to higher Phe levels.

Section 11: Prader-Willi Syndrome

Definition

Prader-Willi syndrome (PWS) results from the lack of paternally expressed genes in the q11-q13 region of chromosome 15 (called the PWS critical region or PWSCR). Hyperphagia (excessive eating) is a hallmark of PWS. This disorder is also characterized by neonatal hypotonia, *hypogonadism*, obesity, and mild to moderate intellectual disability.

Neuropathology

- *Structural neuroanatomical abnormalities* Include morphological changes in pituitary gland, reduction in number of cells in paraventricular nucleus of hypothalamus, ventriculomegaly, decreased tissue volume in parieto-occipital lobe, Sylvian fissure polymicrogyria, and incomplete insular closure.

- *Connectivity abnormalities* Are seen diffusely in studies looking at trace value and fractional anisotropy (FA). Higher trace value is seen in the left frontal white matter and left dorsomedial thalamus; FA is significantly reduced in posterior limb of internal capsule, right frontal white matter, and splenium of the corpus callosum.

- *Abnormalities in brain regions related to eating* Functional imaging has documented differences in the amygdala and orbital frontal cortex, including delayed response to glucose ingestion in areas related to satiety (hypothalamus, insula, ventromedial prefrontal cortex, and nucleus accumbens).

Epidemiology

- Majority have an IQ in the range of mild to moderate ID.

- Approximately 25% are diagnosed with ASD; there is an increased risk of psychiatric disorders.

- Hypotonia is present at birth and continues throughout life.

- *Hypogonadism* is present at birth in males and females. Females may have phenotypic puberty (breast and body hair development) but abnormal menstrual cycles and early menopause. Males are generally infertile and do not progress past mid-puberty.

- Respiratory issues including restrictive lung disease, obstructive sleep apnea (usually neuromuscular in origin), and decreased oxygen saturation occur.

- Gastrointestinal complications are common, as well as viscous saliva and decreased saliva production resulting in swallowing difficulties and decreased or absent ability to vomit.

- Obesity (secondary to hyperphagia) is common, with related complications of type II diabetes and cardiovascular problems.

- Short stature is noted, with average height of around five feet.

- Diminished lifespan is seen; mortality is most often related to respiratory failure. Secondary causes include choking (related to binge eating with salivary and swallowing problems) and gastric necrosis and rupture. It has been suggested that individuals with PWS have less sensitivity to pain, which may delay seeking medical attention in cases of gastric rupture.

Presentation, Disease Course, and Recovery

Prader-Willi syndrome has two clinical phases: the neonatal phase and the hyperphagic phase. The first phase starts at birth and can last 1 to 3 years. Hypotonia and hyporeflexia are typically seen. Feeding difficulties, including poor suck, lethargy, and little interest in feeding, result in decreased weight gain and failure to thrive. Developmental motor and language milestones are delayed; problems with language processing continue into adulthood.

The hyperphagic phase often begins between 2 and 6 years of age. At first, after early feeding problems, interest in food becomes more normal. However, it then becomes excessive, with constant requests for food or active foraging. During this time, food-related problem behaviors such as covert eating and stealing food often start, as do a variety of other behavioral problems. Although hyperphagia was originally thought due to constant hunger, a current alternative hypothesis is that it is more related to lack of satiety after eating.

There is no cure for PWS. Early diagnosis and intervention are important for behavioral and dietary problems. Standard medical interventions, including growth hormone treatments, are used for medical complications. Dietary recommendations are consistent with other overweight individuals, including a reduction in caloric intake and exercise. Individuals with PWS typically have lower metabolic rates, so are often restricted to even fewer calories. Complete food restriction (including locked kitchens) is commonly recommended, as is heightened supervision in the community. Behavioral interventions have been successful in training individuals with PWS to discriminate between prohibited and permitted foods. Psychotropic medications have been used for behavioral issues, including selective serotonin reuptake inhibitors (SSRIs) for compulsive and self-injurious behavior and antipsychotic medications for aggression and disruptive behaviors.

Expectations for Neuropsychological Assessment Results

IQ scores tend to fall in the mild to moderate range of ID, with a mean IQ of 62 to 73 and a range from 39 to 96. Adaptive functioning is typically worse than IQ, even for higher functioning individuals. Performance IQ tends to be higher than verbal IQ, and nonverbal skills are a relative strength. Individuals with PWS do better on visuospatial and simultaneous processing tasks than verbal and sequential processing tasks. Visual processing is also better than auditory processing. Individuals with PWS also do well on visual recognition tasks, as well as on tasks involving perceptual closure and attention to detail, such as jigsaw puzzles. In contrast, speech deficits are typically above what would be expected given cognitive level, including poor speech-sound development and reduced oral motor skills. Language deficits are typically attributed to cognitive impairment and include deficits in vocabulary, grammar, morphology, narrative abilities, and pragmatic skills. More academic difficulties are seen than would be expected by IQ. Little research has been done regarding attention; one study found half the sample met ADHD criteria, whereas another study found a quarter of their sample demonstrated symptoms of ADHD. In both studies, hyperactivity and impulsivity were the most common symptoms. Findings have been mixed regarding EF and memory performance. Hypotonia and motor problems are seen throughout life.

Behavioral problems related to food/eating behaviors, including a preoccupation with food, are seen. However, compulsive behaviors not related to food are also common, including ordering/arranging, concerns with symmetry/exactness, and a need to tell, ask, or know. Ritualistic behaviors (insistence on routines, hoarding, repetitive actions) and self-injurious behaviors (particularly skin picking) are common. Other common behavior problems include temper tantrums, rigidity, lack of inhibition, impulsiveness, and low frustration tolerance. Compulsive and other behavior problems emerge in the first two years and increase during childhood. Although behavior problems can be seen in young adults, they diminish in older adults. Individuals with PWS have difficulty interpreting social information, and there is an overlap in symptoms seen in PWS and ASD, including repetitive and compulsive behaviors, maladaptive behaviors, and social deficits. There is a greater risk for psychiatric disorders, including bipolar with psychotic features, nonpsychotic mood disorders, and anxiety.

Section 12: Angelman Syndrome

Definition

Angelman syndrome (AS) results from the lack of maternally expressed genes in the q11-q13 region of chromosome 15. Characteristics of AS include severe ID, ataxic gait, epilepsy, severe speech/language delays, repetitive/stereotyped behaviors, and sensory-seeking behaviors. Individuals with AS tend to have a happy disposition with easily provoked and inappropriate laughter.

Neuropathology

- *Generally Normal Brain Structures* Cerebral atrophy and ventricular dilation seen in a minority.
- *Characteristic EEG Pattern* Three patterns are seen in childhood in those with and without seizures:
  1. Persistent symmetrical high-voltage slow-wave activity (4–6 cycles/second) not associated with drowsiness,
  2. Very large amplitude slow activity (2–3 cycles/second) occurring in runs and more prominent in frontal regions, and
  3. Spike and sharp waves mixed with large amplitude 3–4 cycles/second seen posteriorly and provoked by eye closure.
- In individuals over 10 years of age, the background rhythm is slower than normal and there may be focal spikes and intermittent or continuous triphasic delta activity over frontal regions. There is no correlation between EEG findings and paroxysms of laughter.

Epidemiology

- 80–90% are diagnosed with epilepsy. Seizure types include tonic-clonic, atypical absence, complex partial, myoclonic, atonic, and tonic.
- 100% have movement or balance disorder with ataxia of gait and/or tremulous limb movement.
- 100% have severe developmental delay, particularly in speech and language
- Sleep disorders are common, especially frequent night waking, early awakening, decreased need for sleep, and abnormal sleep–wake cycles.
- Lifespan is normal.

Presentation, Disease Course, and Recovery

Developmental delay is first noted around 6 months, and children are slow to progress thereafter; most individuals plateau in development between 24 and 30 months of age.

Seizure onset is typically between 1 and 5 years of age, and it may be difficult to distinguish seizures from hyperkinetic limb movements. Seizures are difficult to control and typically require multiple AEDs. It seems as though seizures may diminish during late childhood and adolescence but then return in adulthood, typically presenting as atypical absence or myoclonic seizures.

Hyperkinetic movements of the trunk and limbs may present in infancy. Voluntary movements are often irregular, varying from slight jerking to uncoordinated movements that prevent walking, reaching for objects, and the like. About 10% fail to achieve walking. Motor stereotypies, including hand flapping and waving, are commonly seen. Stereotypies involving the mouth, including chewing inedible objects, are also frequent.

Through adolescence and into adulthood, facial characteristics become more pronounced. Mobility tends to decrease due to limb hypertonicity and development of thoracic scoliosis, as well as a reluctance to walk. As a result, many individuals become obese.

There is no cure for AS. Multiple AEDs are usually required for seizure control. Medications typically are not used for hypermotoric or hyperactive behavior, although some benefit from stimulant medications. Speech therapy focused on nonverbal methods of communication, including use of gestures, sign language, and assisted communicative devices is essential.

Expectations for Neuropsychological Assessment Results

Few studies have examined IQ or academics, as testing is difficult due to attention problems, hyperactivity, and lack of speech and motor control. Language is significantly impaired, and speech tends to be absent or consists of a few single words. Although receptive language is better than expressive, it is still far below age expectation. Attention span is typically short and can interfere with social interactions and ability to learn communication techniques. Hyperactivity and impulsivity are common. Movement disorders compromise motor development, and milestones are delayed. Muscle tone is abnormal, with truncal hypotonia and hypertonicity of the limbs.

"Behavioral uniqueness" is listed as a main clinical characteristic of AS. This includes frequent laughter/smiling, happy demeanor, easily excitable personality (often with hand flapping), and hypermotoric behavior. The characteristic frequent and easily provoked laughter can be seen as early as infancy. Individuals with AS tend to present with a happy disposition and smile frequently. Relative strengths are noted in social skills; they have a sociable disposition and are often more social than would be expected given their overall cognitive ability. Eye contact is good, and they are typically curious about and seek out others for interaction. However, those with more profound cognitive deficits and severe seizure disorders demonstrate more irritability and temper tantrums. Some individuals with AS have a fascination with water and reflective surfaces. The prevalence of ASD is disputed because ASD can be incorrectly diagnosed given repetitive motor behaviors.

Relevant Definitions

Aneuploidy An abnormal number of chromosomes.

Conversational stereotypies Repetitive use of certain overlearned phrases during conversation.

De novo mutation A genetic mutation that is present for the first time in a family member and not passed down by either parent.

Echolalia Repetitions of another's verbalizations.

Ependymoma Tumor arising from the ependyma (the membrane lining the ventricular system).

Glioma Tumor arising from glial cells in the brain or spine.

Gynecomastia Male breast enlargement.

Hamartoma Benign, focal malformation of tissue that has developed in a disorganized manner.

Hematopoietic stem cell transplant Treatment where stem cells are collected from bone marrow or peripheral blood from a donor (autologous transplant) or the patient (allogeneic) and infused intravenously to produce new blood cells and enhance immune function.

Hypogonadism Diminished function of testes and ovaries resulting in reduced sex hormones and cell production.

Hypomyelination Abnormal formation of myelin in the brain or spinal cord resulting in reduced myelin.

Karyotype Number and appearance of chromosomes.

Macroorchidism Abnormally large testicles.

Meningioma Tumor arising from the meninges, the membranes enveloping the CNS.

Microorchidism Abnormally small testicles.

Mosaic karyotype Cells with two different karyotypes present in the same individual.

Neurofibroma Benign nerve sheath tumor that forms on the peripheral nervous system

Non-epileptic myoclonus Jerking of the limbs lasting seconds to several hours, usually starting in the hands and spreading to the upper and lower extremities, face, and entire body.

Palilalia Repetition of one's own word or phrase.

Plexiform neurofibroma Large, non-encapsulated tumor that diffusely involves long nerve segments and has an increased risk of malignant transformation.

Schwannoma Benign nerve sheath tumor composed of Schwann cells. Schwann cells produce the myelin sheath covering peripheral nerves.

Chromosomal and Genetic Syndromes Questions

NOTE: Questions 10, 39, 49, and 96 on the First Full-Length Practice Examination, Questions 15, 80, 97, and 110 on the Second Full-Length Practice Examination, Questions 20, 52, and 110 on the Third Full-Length Practice Examination, and Questions 48, 60, 75, and 105 on the Fourth Full-Length Practice Examination are from this chapter.

1. Despite having different cognitive, behavioral, and neurological phenotypes, which of the following two disorders are caused by an absence or lack of expression at the same region of chromosome 15?

    (a) neurofibromatosis and tuberous sclerosis

    (b) Klinefelter syndrome and fragile X syndrome

    (c) Prader-Willi syndrome and Angelman syndrome

    (d) Turner syndrome and Williams syndrome

2. A child presents to your clinic for evaluation of developmental delays. In reading the history, you note that he has a history of seizures and migraines. Upon meeting the child, he has a large facial capillary malformation. This child is most likely to have which disorder?

   (a) tuberous sclerosis

   (b) neurofibromatosis type 1

   (c) neurofibromatosis type 2

   (d) Sturge-Weber syndrome

3. Individuals with tuberous sclerosis are at increased risk for seizures due primarily to ____.

   (a) cortical tubers

   (b) T2 hyperintensities

   (c) hamartomas

   (d) subependymal giant-cell astrocytomas

4. One of the first clinical symptoms of adrenoleukodystrophy is ____.

   (a) a decline in verbal skills

   (b) symptoms consistent with ADHD

   (c) motor impairment

   (d) severe psychiatric symptoms

5. Individuals with early-treated PKU tend to show ____.

   (a) no cognitive deficits

   (b) significant cognitive impairments

   (c) deficits in visuospatial and math skills

   (d) deficits in language and reading skills

6. A 32-year-old male presents for evaluation. Upon meeting him, you note his tall stature and, during the interview, you learn that he and his wife have been having fertility problems. His neuropsychological evaluation reveals language-based difficulties and dyslexia. He is most likely to have which of the following?

   (a) Klinefelter syndrome

   (b) fragile X syndrome

   (c) 22q11.2 deletion syndrome

   (d) adrenoleukodystrophy

7. A 45-year-old man presents to your office for evaluation due to concerns with attention that are interfering at work. During the interview, you learn that he struggled in school. You note that he has many small bumps up and down his arms, as well as several on his face. When you ask him about this, he states that many of his family member's on his father's side also have these bumps. He is most likely to have which disorder?

   (a) tuberous sclerosis

   (b) Klinefelter syndrome

   (c) neurofibromatosis type 1

   (d) Prader-Willi syndrome

8. While individuals with this disorder may present with failure to thrive and feeding difficulties in infancy, later in childhood they develop food-related problem behaviors, including covert eating and stealing food, and obesity.

   (a) Turner syndrome

   (b) Prader-Willi syndrome

   (c) Angelman syndrome

   (d) Williams syndrome

9. Treatment with a specialized diet can help to preserve cognitive functioning in individuals with this disorder.

   (a) adrenoleukodystrophy

   (b) fragile X syndrome

   (c) tuberous sclerosis

   (d) phenylketonuria

10. Which disorder cannot be seen in females?

    (a) Klinefelter syndrome   (c) Turner syndrome

    (b) fragile X syndrome   (d) Angelman syndrome

Chromosomal and Genetic Syndromes Answers

1. **C—Prader-Willi syndrome and Angelman syndrome**   *Both result from absence or lack of expression of chromosome 15q11-13.*

   Reference: Buiting, K. (2010). Prader-Willi syndrome and Angelman syndrome. *American Journal of Medical Genetics Part C (Seminars in Medical Genetics), 154C,* 365–375.

2. **D—Sturge-Weber syndrome**   *A facial capillary malformation is a defining characteristic of Sturge-Weber syndrome and is not seen in the other syndromes.*

   Reference: Zabel, T. A., Reesman, J., Wodka, E. L., Gray, R., Suskauer, S. J., Turin, E., . . . Comi, A. M. (2010). Neuropsychological features and risk factors in children with Sturge-Weber syndrome: Four case reports. *The Clinical Neuropsychologist, 24*(5), 841–859.

3. **A—cortical tubers**   *While subependymal giant-cell astrocytomas are frequently seen in tuberous sclerosis, cortical tubers are the primary cause of seizures. T2 hyperintensities are commonly seen in neurofibromatosis type 1, not tuberous sclerosis, and they do not cause seizures.*

   Reference: Byars, A. W. (2010). Tuberous sclerosis complex. In K. O. Yeates, M. D. Ris, H. G. Taylor, & B. F. Pennington (Eds.), *Pediatric neuropsychology: Research, theory, and practice* (2nd ed.). New York, NY: Guilford Press.

4. **B—symptoms consistent with ADHD**   *Following an initial period of normal development, ADHD-like symptoms are the first to present between 3 and 8 years of age. This period is then followed by progressive behavioral, cognitive, and neurological decline. Psychiatric symptoms are seen in adult onset.*

   Reference: Cox, C. S., Dubey, P., Raymond, R. V., Mahmood, A., Moser, A. B., & Moser, H. W. (2006). Cognitive evaluation of neurologically asymptomatic boys with X-linked adrenoleukodystrophy. *Archives of Neurology, 63,* 69–73.

5. **C—deficits in visuospatial and math skills**   *Children with treated PKU tend to have IQ scores in the average range. Language and reading skills are better than visuospatial and math skills. Deficits in visuospatial skills may be partially related to executive functioning problems.*

   Reference: Antshel, K. M. (2010). ADHD, learning, and academic performance in phenylketonuria. *Molecular Genetics and Metabolism, 99,* S52–S58.

6. **A—Klinefelter syndrome**   *Fertility problems are associated with Klinefelter syndrome but not the other disorders listed. Visuospatial deficits, rather than language deficits, are associated with adrenoleukodystrophy and 22q11.2 deletion syndrome. Fragile X syndrome is associated with more broad-based cognitive deficits.*

   Reference: Temple, C. (2010). Klinefelter syndrome. In R. D. Nass & Y. Frank (Eds.), *Cognitive and behavioral abnormalities of pediatric diseases* (pp. 188–201). New York, NY: Oxford University Press.

7. **C—neurofibromatosis type 1** *Individuals with NF1 have neurofibromas, which look like small bumps on the skin. NF1 is inherited in an autosomal dominant fashion, so it typically is seen in multiple family members. Those with NF1 are also at increased risk for learning and attentional problems.*

> **Reference:** Rosser, T. (2018). Neurocutaneous disorders. *Continuum, 24*(1, Child Neurology), 96–129.

8. **B—Prader-Willi syndrome** *Individuals with Prader-Willi syndrome demonstrate early feeding problems but then develop problematic food-related behaviors that can lead to obesity.*

> **Reference:** Buiting, K. (2010). Prader-Willi syndrome and Angelman syndrome. *American Journal of Medical Genetics Part C (Seminars in Medical Genetics), 154C*, 365–375.

9. **D—phenylketonuria** *Cognitive functioning can be preserved when a low-Phe diet is initiated soon after birth. Adrenoleukodystrophy can be treated with hematopoietic stem cell transplant. There are no specific treatments for fragile X syndrome or tuberous sclerosis.*

> **Reference:** Romani, C., Palermo, L, MacDonald, A., Limback, E., Hall, S. K., & Geberhiwot, T. (2017). Impact of phenylalanine levels on cognitive outcome in adults with phenylketonuria: Effects across tasks and developmental stages. *Neuropsychology, 31*, 242–254.

10. **A—Klinefelter syndrome** *Klinefelter syndrome is only seen in males, as it is the presence of an extra X in a male (XXY). Turner syndrome cannot be seen in males, as it is the presence of only one X chromosome. Fragile X syndrome is seen in both males and females, but males are more significantly affected. Angelman syndrome is seen in both males and females and both are equally affected.*

> **Reference:** Wilson, R., Bennett, E., Howell, S. E., & Tartaglia, N. (2011). Sex chromosome aneuploidies. In A. S. Davis (Ed.), *Handbook of pediatric neuropsychology* (pp. 805–820). New York, NY: Springer.

Recommended Readings

Camp, K. M, Parisi, M. A. Acosta, P. B., Berry, G. T., Blau, N., Bodamer, O. A., . . . Young, J. M. (2014). Phenylketonuria scientific review conference: State of the science and future research needs. *Molecular Genetics & Metabolism, 112*, 87–122.

Cassidy, S. B., Dykens, E., & Williams, C. A. (2000). Prader-Willi and Angelman syndromes: Sister imprinted disorders. *American Journal of Medical Genetics (Seminars in Medical Genetics), 97*, 136–146.

Davis, A. S. (Ed.). (2011). *Handbook of pediatric neuropsychology.* New York, NY: Springer Publishing Company.

Hall, D. A., & Berry-Kravis, E. (2018). Fragile X syndrome and fragile-X associated tremor ataxia syndrome. *Handbook of Clinical Neurology, 147*, 377–391.

Hutaff-Lee, C., Cordeiro, L., & Tartaglia, N. (2013). Cognitive and medical features of chromosomal aneuploidy. *Handbook of Clinical Neurology, 111*, 273–279.

Mauger, C., Lancelot, C., Roy, A., Coutant, R., Cantisano, N., & Le Gall, D. (2018). Executive functions in children and adolescents with Turner syndrome: A systematic review and meta-analysis. *Neuropsychology Review, 28*(2), 188–215.

Moberg, P. J., Richman, M. J., Roalf, D. R., Morse, C. L., Graefe, A. C., Brennan, L., . . . Gur, R. E. (2018). Neurocognitive functioning in patients with 22q11.2 deletion syndrome: A meta-analytic review. *Behavior Genetics, 48*(4), 259–270.

Moser, H. W., Mahmood, A., & Raymond, G. V. (2007). X-linked adrenoleukodystrophy. *Nature Clinical Practice Neurology, 3*, 140–151.

Nass, R. D., & Frank, Y. (2010). *Cognitive and behavioral abnormalities of pediatric diseases.* New York, NY: Oxford University Press.

Reily, J., Lai, P., Bernicot, J., & Bellugi, U. (2010). Williams syndrome. In R. D. Nass & Y. Frank (Eds.), *Cognitive and behavioral abnormalities of pediatric diseases* (pp. 267–283). New York, NY: Oxford University Press.

Rosser, T. (2018). Neurocutaneous disorders. *Continuum, 24*(1, Child Neurology), 96–129.

MEDICAL

Tara V. Spevack

Definition

Cerebral palsy (CP) has been recognized as a neurodevelopmental motor condition involving compromised posture, balance, muscle control, and movement since the mid-nineteenth century yet remains a challenge to define. In part the difficulty reflects that CP, rather than representing a unitary construct, encompasses a collection of motor disorders with a wide range of etiologies, functional manifestations, and comorbidities. Moreover, the conceptualization of CP continues to evolve based on advances in understanding the mechanisms and sequelae of early damage to the developing brain. The most widely used definition of CP was published in 2007 and represents the consensus of an international committee (see Rosenbaum et al., 2007). It reads:

> Cerebral palsy (CP) describes a group of permanent disorders of the development of movement and posture, causing activity limitation, that are attributed to non-progressive disturbances that occurred in the developing fetal or infant brain. The motor disorders of cerebral palsy are often accompanied by disturbances of sensation, perception, cognition, communication, and behaviour, by epilepsy, and by secondary musculoskeletal problems.

It is worth noting that the definition does not distinguish between CP in which the presumed etiology is prenatal or perinatal in origin ("congenital") and CP in which the presumed etiology is postnatal in origin ("acquired"), terminology that was more common alongside earlier definitions of the condition but fraught with methodological and conceptual difficulties. The paper includes an annotated explanation of each term used in the definition which serves as a useful framework for understanding CP. Key concepts are summarized in Table 19.1.

Two limitations of the consensus definition are important to recognize. (1) It indicates that the causal insult occurs early in brain development but does not specify an upper age limit. Most CP registries include individuals with onset before 2 years of age whereas others use a cut-off of 3 years. Less frequently, allowances have been made for a later endpoint. Regardless, there is agreement that the damage occurs before the affected motor functions have fully developed thereby altering the developmental trajectory. (2) The definition does not establish a lower threshold of severity. Manifestations can range from subclinical abnormalities to severe mobility and activity limitations.

Neuropathology

CP is a clinical diagnosis predicated on findings of brain-based abnormalities upon formal neurodevelopmental examination (or, more realistically, serial examinations) together with either observation or a history of activity limitations. Neuroimaging studies (typically MRI) as part of the diagnostic evaluation are standard practice and reveal brain abnormalities in 80–90% of children with CP. Of those cases, white matter damage is the most frequent finding, followed by cortical or subcortical lesions

TABLE 19.1 Key Concepts Related to the Formal Definition of Cerebral Palsy

Terminology	Annotation
a group	CP is an umbrella term.
	There is heterogeneity in the etiology, type, and severity of motor problems.
permanent	CP is not transient (although it can be outgrown); it is a chronic condition.
	Clinical evolution as a person ages is to be expected.
disorders	CP disrupts the typical orderly processes of child development.
development	Due to its early age of onset, CP impacts the subsequent acquisition of motor skills.
movement and posture	Abnormal motor control is the hallmark feature of CP and is reflected in problems with movement and posture.
activity limitation	This is updated terminology that replaces the term "disability" while emphasizing that individuals with CP have some difficulty in executing certain motor-dependent tasks.
attributed to	This phrasing acknowledges that further progress in understanding the causal mechanisms of CP is needed.
non-progressive	Although the brain insult that causes CP is static, it can be associated with changing or additional manifestations over time (e.g., improvements in response to brain maturation and intervention; worsening due to activity limitation and aging).
fetal or infant brain	CP arises from an inciting event that occurs early in brain development.
	Motor disorders originating in the spinal cord, peripheral nerves, or muscles preclude a diagnosis of CP.
accompanied by	Comorbid developmental problems with sensation, perception, cognition, communication, and behavior are common.
secondary musculoskeletal problems	Typical musculoskeletal problems include muscle contractures, spinal deformity, and hip displacement.

(particularly involving the basal ganglia), brain malformations, and postnatal injuries (including focal infarction). Importantly, neuroimaging has disproven the historical belief that birth asphyxia is the major cause of CP. In fact, birth asphyxia accounts for the minority (10% to 20%) of cases. Regardless of the etiology, CP originates in either or both of the two semi-independent motor systems of the brain (i.e., *pyramidal* and *extrapyramidal*) thereby resulting in distinctive patterns of physical impairments that are used to classify subtypes of the disorder (Table 19.2).

Pyramidal System

Simply put, the pyramidal system connects regions of the cortex involved with motor control to muscle via the corticospinal tract. It is responsible for initiating and carrying signals that enable voluntary skilled movements.

- Damage to the *pyramidal system* results in spastic CP, which represents the majority (70–85%) of cases. Spastic CP:
  - is characterized by abnormally high muscle tone;

TABLE 19.2 Classification of Cerebral Palsy According to Motor System

Pathogenesis	% of CP Population	CP Subtype	Most Frequent MRI Finding/ Neuropathology	Typical Time of Injury
Pyramidal Motor System	70–85	**Spastic hemiplegic**	Unilateral middle cerebral artery stroke	Prenatal
		Spastic diplegic	White matter damage of prematurity	Prenatal
		Spastic quadriplegic	Anoxia or other generalized insult/bilateral gray matter injury	Prenatal in 50% of cases
Extrapyramidal Motor System	15–30	**Dyskinetic**	Hypoxic-ischemic injury often with basal ganglia involvement	Perinatal
		Ataxic-hypotonic	Cerebellar malformation	Prenatal

- occurs more frequently in children born preterm than full-term; and

- is most often associated with underlying *periventricular leukomalacia (PVL), intraventricular hemorrhage (IVH)*, or both.

• *Topographical subtypes* (i.e., phenotypes) of spastic CP are delineated based on which limbs are affected.

  ▪ *Spastic hemiplegic CP* involves the arm and leg on one side of the body, typically with greater involvement of the arm than the leg. It is the most common subtype of spastic CP in children born full-term and usually results from loss of blood flow along the middle cerebral artery in one hemisphere (i.e., perinatal stroke). The left hemisphere is affected in two thirds of these cases. Nearly all children with hemiplegic CP learn to walk; more than half have normal intellectual functioning.

  ▪ *Spastic diplegic CP* primarily involves the lower extremities, although the upper extremities often are affected to a lesser degree such that hand movements can be clumsy. It is the most common form of CP in children born preterm. White matter damage, especially PVL, is the predominant underlying neuropathology. In children born at term, no risk factors may be apparent, or the cause may reflect multiple etiologies. The severity of the motor disability is positively, but not perfectly, correlated with the severity of the cognitive impairment.

  ▪ *Spastic quadriplegic CP* involves all four extremities and the trunk and neck (i.e., full body). Insult to the brain occurs prenatally in approximately 50% of cases, perinatally in 30% of cases, and postnatally in 20% of cases. Spastic quadriplegia is typically caused by a generalized event such as anoxia. It is the most severe subtype of CP and is frequently accompanied by epilepsy and impaired intellectual functioning.

  ▪ In recent years, new terminology for characterizing the topography of pyramidal CP has emerged mainly in Europe. Specifically, the terms "diplegia" and "quadriplegia" have been replaced because they are imprecise (e.g., diplegia sometimes is used to refer to individuals with lower extremity involvement only, whereas at other times it is used to refer to individuals with arm involvement of lesser severity than leg involvement). Instead, CP is classified based on whether limbs on one side versus both sides of the body are affected;

"unilateral CP" replaces the term "hemiplegic CP" and "bilateral CP" replaces the terms "diplegic CP" and "quadriplegic CP."

Extrapyramidal System

The *extrapyramidal motor system* is comprised of the cerebellum, basal ganglia, and brainstem. It functions to "fine tune" the movements of the *pyramidal system* by making adjustments to posture and coordination.

- Damage to the *extrapyramidal system* results in non-spastic CP, which represents the minority (15–30%) of cases. This form of CP:
  - typically involves all extremities, upper more than lower; and
  - often is associated with normal intellectual functioning.
- The subtypes of extrapyramidal CP are delineated based on the kind of abnormal motor movements that occur.
  - *Dyskinetic CP* is characterized by variations in muscle tone and involuntary *athetoid* or *dystonic* movements that often are caused by an underlying hypoxic-ischemic injury typically in full-term infants. The abnormal movements can make it difficult to sit comfortably and coordinate the muscles necessary for walking and speaking.
  - *Ataxic CP* applies when the predominant abnormality reflects cerebellar dysfunction and is characterized by a lack of coordination during voluntary gross and fine motor movements. Typical manifestations are poor balance, unsteadiness, a wide-based gait, and shakiness or tremors during activities involving manual dexterity.

Mixed Cerebral Palsy

Mixed CP accounts for approximately 20% of cases. It is characterized by abnormalities that reflect involvement of both the *pyramidal* and *extrapyramidal motor systems.* In practice, many individuals with CP exhibit mixed motor signs but are classified according to the predominant motor impairment.

Risk Factors

The risk factors associated with CP are diverse, can have complex interactions, and are rarely pathognomonic. Preterm birth is the most important risk factor for CP followed by low birth weight. The majority of children ultimately diagnosed with CP are first identified as high-risk newborns and their development is closely monitored, ideally allowing for early intervention. A second group of newborns has no identified risk factors and tends to be diagnosed only after developmental motor delays or abnormalities become apparent.

- *Prenatal*
  - Maternal risk factors
    - intellectual disabilities
    - infection or toxic exposure during pregnancy
    - certain diseases during pregnancy (e.g., epilepsy, thyroid disorder, high blood pressure)
  - Fetal risk factors
    - multiple birth gestation
    - death in-utero of a co-twin
    - male sex of the fetus
    - *intrauterine growth restriction*

- ○ developmental brain malformations
- ○ thrombophilic disorders

- *Perinatal*
  - *Prematurity* is the foremost risk factor for CP. The lower the gestational age of a baby, the greater the risk. It is important to emphasize, however, that a little more than half of children with CP are born at or near term. In other words, full-term infants account for the majority of CP cases. That contradiction can be explained by the fact that there are more full-term than preterm live births.
  - Low *birth weight* represents the second most important risk factor for CP. The lower the *birth weight*, the greater the risk. Lending support to the notion that CP etiology is multifactorial, many children with low *birth weight* do not develop CP, and many children who develop CP have a normal *birth weight*.
  - Anoxic damage to the brain during a difficult labor or delivery, although once considered the major risk factor for CP, is present in only a minority (10–14%) of cases. Even when birth asphyxia occurs, prenatal factors may have contributed to the fetal distress.
  - Other perinatal risk factors include a low *Apgar* score at 5 minutes, abnormal muscle tone (particularly *hypotonia*) in a newborn, and perinatal stroke.

- *Postnatal*
  - The major postnatal risk factors for CP are infections (e.g., meningitis, encephalitis) and brain injury.
  - In the case of children with onset of motor problems consistent with CP due to a brain insult that occurred after the age of 3 years, convention holds that a diagnosis of CP is not technically correct. Instead, the diagnosis should reflect the underlying cause (e.g., traumatic brain injury, stroke).

- *Socioeconomic Status (SES) and Race*
  - Preterm birth, low birth weight, and postnatal acquired brain trauma are documented risk factors for CP. An association between SES and each of those factors also has been documented (i.e., lower SES confers a greater risk; higher SES has a protective effect). In contrast, a direct link between SES and increased risk for CP has not been well established. That is, when controlling for known perinatal risk factors, an association between SES and CP risk has been demonstrated in some studies but not others.
  - There is a higher prevalence of CP among black children than white children in the United States. Whether that finding can be explained by disparities in SES (i.e., lower overall SES in the black population than white population) is an ongoing subject of investigation.

Epidemiology

Prevalence/Incidence

With a prevalence of 2–2.5 out of every 1,000 live births in developed countries, CP is the leading cause of physical disability in childhood. As noted previously, prematurity is a major risk factor for CP, with risk increasing steadily as gestational age decreases. *Intrauterine growth restriction* and low *birth weight* are also major risk factors, with a similar inverse relationship. Advances in obstetric and neonatal care have reduced not only the incidence of infant mortality but also the incidence of CP in babies born prematurely. Despite those improvements, the overall prevalence of CP has remained relatively constant due to an unchanged incidence of CP in full-term infants, an increasing number of multiple births due to more frequent use of in vitro fertilization, improved survival rates in preterm and other medically fragile infants, and improved life expectancy for individuals with CP.

Physical Morbidity

Physical morbidity in the form of abnormal muscle tone or movement is a defining feature of CP and can adversely impact functional mobility and the ability to perform activities of daily living. The more severe the primary motor disturbance, the greater the likelihood that a child will experience accompanying medical problems and functionally significant disabilities. Common neurological and physical comorbidities of CP are listed below.

- Approximately 33% of children with CP are unable to walk, 17% require assistance to walk, and 50–60% walk unaided.

- Musculoskeletal complications are a frequent concern. For example, *spasticity* can cause constant extension in limbs and result in contractures, hip dislocation, and scoliosis.

- Up to 75% of children and 70% of adults with CP experience chronic pain, often associated with musculoskeletal problems. Chronic pain is a major contributor to quality of life concerns in this population.

- The incidence of epilepsy is much higher (28–50%) than in the general population.

- Oral-motor impairments can negatively impact chewing, swallowing, and control of saliva. In severe cases respiratory complications may develop due to aspiration associated with oral-motor dysfunction or gastroesophageal reflux. A feeding tube is sometimes necessary due to failure to thrive and undernutrition. Oral-motor impairments also can cause problems with speech articulation and volume resulting in a need for augmentative and alternative communication.

- Visual and ocular-motor impairments of varying severity occur in 28% of children with CP, with approximately 10% experiencing blindness. The incidence of hearing impairments is 10–12%.

- Bladder control problems, including urinary incontinence, have been reported in approximately 25% of the CP population.

- Positioning issues and discomfort can disrupt sleep. Sleep disorders occur in 20–25% of individuals with CP. Fatigue, not only from sleep problems but also the extra energy expended to complete daily activities, is a common complaint.

- Skin complications, such as pressure sores secondary to reduced mobility, warrant careful monitoring.

Cognitive Morbidity

Cognitive impairments and learning disabilities occur more frequently in children with CP than in typically developing peers.

- Studies of intellectual functioning in children with CP indicate IQ lower than 70 in 30–50% and IQ lower than 50 in approximately a third of this population. When less significant but functionally important cognitive problems are included the estimates are higher.

- The prevalence of cognitive morbidities varies across subtypes, increasing when motor impairments are severe and when epilepsy is present. Thus, quadriplegia is more highly associated with intellectual disabilities than any other form of CP. The degree of motor involvement, however, is not a reliable indicator of the degree of cognitive impairment since individuals with severe CP can have normal intellectual functioning and individuals with mild CP can experience severe cognitive disabilities. CP, then, is heterogeneous not only with respect to motor, but also cognitive, manifestations.

Social-Emotional Morbidity

Cerebral palsy is associated with an increased prevalence of social difficulties, depression, and low self-esteem. Behavior problems also occur more frequently in children with CP (25% based on parent report) than in the general population.

Mortality

- The life expectancy of people with CP has increased in part due to medical advances. Also, a shift in attitudes toward individuals with disabilities has improved societal inclusion as well as access to health and social services.

- The major risk factors for a shortened lifespan are medical fragility (especially when associated with respiratory diseases or feeding problems/dependence on a feeding tube) and severe motor problems that cause immobility. The leading cause of death in individuals with severe CP is chronic respiratory infection.

- Although children with the most severe motor impairments are less likely to survive into adulthood compared with the general population, survival rates continue to improve and most children with CP now survive into adulthood.

- Life expectancy of individuals with mild CP is approximately that of individuals in the general population.

Determinants of Severity

In a broad sense, the severity of impairment correlates with the severity of the causal factors. Yet interindividual differences in the level and pattern of impairments are the norm. It is becoming increasingly apparent that CP is the result of a complex and variable multifactorial causal pathway. Genetic and epigenetic factors can influence the predisposition to one or more of the causes of CP, the response to the underlying brain insult, and resiliency. With respect to environmental determinants, early interventions can help prevent or minimize the associated medical and developmental complications of CP and improve longer-term functioning.

Classifying CP based on the degree of functional impairment is important for purposes of monitoring development, guiding treatment planning and determining response to intervention. In a clinic setting, CP often is as characterized as mild (i.e., minimal functional limitations), moderate (i.e., some assistance is required to accomplish ambulation and daily activities), or severe (i.e., nonambulatory and extensive assistance is required to accomplish daily activities). This method offers an easily understood and meaningful language for discussing problems, particularly with parents and other caregivers. Its major drawback is the absence of quantitative rating criteria and poor sensitivity to functional changes.

Published in the late 1990s, the *Gross Motor Function Classification System (GMFCS)* has become the most widely used standardized measure of CP severity in children by researchers, epidemiologists, and healthcare and rehabilitation providers. The instrument is reliable and valid and provides a quick five-level ordinal rating based on functional mobility and activity limitation; a higher number indicates a higher degree of severity and higher level of required assistance. Specifically, Level I describes children who can walk and climb stairs independently and without limitation; other gross motor skills such as running and jumping may reflect problems with speed, balance, or coordination. Level V describes children with severe limitations in voluntary control of movement and impaired mobility even with assistance. They are transported in a wheelchair in all settings. More recently, analogous and complementary measures of fine motor skills (Manual Ability Classification System) and communication (Communication Function Classification System) have been developed making it possible to gain a more comprehensive understanding of an individual's functioning.

Presentation, Disease Course, and Recovery

Gestation/Newborn (1–28 days)

Because CP is diagnosed based on clinically observable motor manifestations of underlying brain pathology, the disorder cannot be identified in utero. Unless the outward motor signs are severe, CP typically is not apparent during the newborn period either. Concerns tend to be based on the presence of prenatal or perinatal factors that place a baby at high risk for CP.

Infancy (1–12 months)

With the exception of severe cases, accurate detection of CP during infancy is difficult. Not only is normal development characterized by flux (i.e., changing motor patterns and marked increases in voluntary motor skills) but early motor abnormalities can be transient. Signs of possible CP that warrant vigilance include persisting infantile reflex patterns and delays in achieving developmental motor milestones. Of note, precocious acquisition of certain motor skills can also be a harbinger of CP. For example, standing well before the age of 12 months can reflect hypertonia (stiffness and rigidity) in the legs, and a strong hand preference in the first 12 to 18 months can indicate weakness in the other hand. Adding to the complexity of the diagnostic process, the absence of motor abnormalities in an infant does not preclude CP. Approximately 50% of children ultimately diagnosed with CP have a seemingly unremarkable pre- and perinatal history.

Toddler Stage (1–3 years)

Persisting or emerging motor delays are common during the toddler years. Most children do not manifest full motor signs of CP until 2 years of age or beyond, and a definitive diagnosis usually is made in the second or third year of life. Thereafter, motor signs of the disorder can change as brain development and physical growth continue (e.g., *hypotonia* often evolves into *spasticity*). Serial examinations provide important prognostic information by tracking the age at which pivotal milestones are achieved (e.g., sitting independently by the age of 2 years is predictive of eventual ambulation).

Childhood (3–18 years)

In cases of mild CP, a definitive diagnosis may not be made until 4 or 5 years of age. Conversely, approximately half of all children with the diagnosis "outgrow" the disorder (i.e., no longer exhibit motor signs of CP) by the age of 7 years, particularly those with mild, monoparetic (weakness in only one extremity), diplegic, or *extrapyramidal* subtypes. Those same children, however, experience a higher rate of other neurological problems (e.g., seizures, intellectual disabilities) than typically developing peers.

Adulthood

Despite the fact that CP is not progressive, per se, its motor manifestations can worsen. Prolonged stress on the body and limitations in mobility and physical activity can result in secondary complications during adulthood such as a premature deterioration of functional skills. Cerebral palsy also carries an increased risk of diseases of aging such as osteoporosis and arthritis.

Expectations for Neuropsychological Assessment Results

Studies of neuropsychological functioning in individuals with CP are scarce but have recently begun to increase. Several methodological challenges add to the complexity of the research process and difficulty achieving optimal sample sizes.

- The cognitive sequelae of CP may not be immediately apparent since children may "grow into" deficits. Conversely, any detectable early problems may change with time.

- Most available instruments require verbal and visual-motor responses that are not always possible for patients with CP-associated speech, vision, ocular-motor or fine motor impairments. The practice in some studies of classifying participants who are "untestable" as having an intellectual disability results in flawed data.

- To avoid confounding an inability to respond or a slow rate of responding with low cognitive functioning or specific neuropsychological impairments, tests can sometimes be adapted to improve accessibility. Strategies include incorporating assistive technology into test administration; allowing alternate response modalities such as finger pointing, eye gaze, or a communication device; removing or extending time limits; and prorating scores based on partial test completion. Although modified test protocols provide important clinical information, the trade-off is compromised standardization. To address those limitations, efforts to develop accessible technology-assisted neuropsychological instruments are ongoing.

Beyond the expected motor abnormalities, CP is not associated with a prototypical neuropsychological profile although better language-based than visually-based functioning is the norm. When present, diffuse white matter and subcortical involvement tend to be associated with weaknesses in attention, processing speed, and executive functioning; however, preliminary research suggests that when cognition is assessed independent of motor functioning using assistive technology, problems with executive functioning are no longer apparent. Summaries of neuropsychological functioning in this population such as those that follow are fraught with intricacies and exceptions that require further study.

- *Intelligence/Achievement* Individuals with CP demonstrate a full spectrum of abilities from severe impairment to giftedness, but estimates suggest that general cognitive functioning is affected to some degree in 75% of the CP population. Approximately 50% of individuals with CP have intellectual functioning in the borderline to impaired range. The severity of impairment is positively, but not perfectly, correlated with the degree of motor impairment such that intellectual disabilities occur more frequently with quadriplegic CP than any of the other subtypes. With respect to academic achievement, 25–30% of individuals with CP have specific learning disabilities.

- *Attention/Concentration* Attention is negatively affected by periventricular white matter and subcortical damage. Another adverse influence on attention is epilepsy, which occurs at higher than average rates in the CP population.

- *Processing Speed* Measuring processing speed independent of response speed is particularly important, albeit challenging, in this population. There is some evidence of slowed information processing even when the potential confound of motor speed is removed. Further investigation is needed.

- *Speech and Language* Compromised oral-motor control can preclude speech or cause dysarthria and reduced speech intelligibility. For some, a technology-assisted communication system can improve self-expression and social engagement. Apart from the motor aspects of speech, language skills span the ability spectrum but are near normal or normal in many individuals with mild to moderate CP. Evidence of hemisphere-specific language deficits has been mixed. There is mounting research to suggest that in the presence of damage to either hemisphere, novel brain organization will occur when possible to allow for preserved language even at the expense of visually-based functions. Bilateral insults place greater constraints on the capacity for sparing of language.

- *Visuospatial* The most robust finding in neuropsychological studies of CP is of visuoperceptual and visuospatial impairments beyond what can be accounted for by problems with visual acuity, ocular-motor control, or eye-hand coordination.

- *Memory* The previously mentioned attention problems, as well as primary visual (and less frequently, auditory) impairments, can contribute to memory difficulties. Particular problems with executive aspects of learning and memory have been documented.

- *Executive Functions* Cerebral palsy is associated with an increased risk of problems with executive functions and life skills. Although some research has demonstrated that such impairments cannot be explained by motor impairments alone, other investigations have called those findings into question.

- *Sensorimotor Functions* By definition, individuals with CP experience motor abnormalities. In addition, visual/ocular-motor impairments are present in 28% of patients (with some higher estimates). Hearing impairments occur in 10–12% of patients. Sound sensitivity and disturbances in the sensory perception of touch, pain, and proprioception also have been documented at higher rates than in the general population. Understanding the potential impact of sensorimotor impairments on test accessibility and resulting scores is essential for accurately interpreting assessment results and providing useful clinical recommendations.

- *Emotion and Personality* Cerebral palsy, depending on its severity, can limit the ability of a young child to communicate, interact with others, play, and explore the environment, all of which are important for behavioral adjustment, social-emotional and psychological development, and general well-being. In addition, when impairments in self-care necessitate assistance from caretakers, opportunities to exercise control over the environment, make choices, and gain independence are reduced. In fact, children with CP are at increased risk of behavior problems and social difficulties (including rejection and bullying by peers, being perceived as having a lower social status, fewer reciprocated friendships) and associated loneliness, low self-esteem, and depression. Stress in the family system also can occur due to the added demands on caregivers. As adults, individuals with CP are at higher risk for social-emotional adjustment problems, isolation, and low community participation. Cerebral palsy is not associated with a particular personality type.

- *Performance and Symptom Validity* Cerebral palsy-related fatigue and pain are common and can interfere with alertness, test engagement, and task persistence. Furthermore, motor and speech impairments can make it necessary for patients to invest painstaking effort to complete each item of each test. Conversely, when testing is restricted to a forced-choice format to circumvent the need for oral language and fine motor responses, boredom can play a major role. Frustration tolerance and motivation therefore represent critical influences on performance. Multiple, brief test sessions may be necessary to optimize participation.

Considerations when Treating Patients with Cerebral Palsy

- *School* Most children with CP benefit from an individualized education program to facilitate appropriate access to physical, academic, and social aspects of the school environment.

  - Modifications and accommodations may be necessary due to fatigue and discomfort, as well as problems with functional mobility, sitting posture and balance when at a desk, and completion of daily living activities.

  - A mechanism for completing missed work is helpful if attendance is regularly interrupted by medical and therapy appointments.

  - In addition to special education to address any cognitive and learning problems, some children need communication devices and other forms of assistive technology to be incorporated into the classroom.

  - Because children with CP can experience difficulty keeping up with peers, and stigmatization and rejection due to motor disabilities and medical issues such as drooling and incontinence, strategies to facilitate social acceptance and inclusion are of paramount importance.

- *Psychological and Emotional Issues* Early interventions that are continually updated based on progress can improve functioning and longer-term outcome. A family-centered approach to treatment is considered best practice. Therefore, parents should be considered active participants in goal-setting and assessing progress, and therapies should occur in a child's real-world home and school environments whenever possible. Parents often benefit from support and education related to the stresses of having a child with disabilities. Family-centered care also focuses on facilitating positive parent–child interactions, social connectedness, school and community participation, and healthy emotional adjustment.

- *Medications* Medications for CP tend to be more effective at reducing *spasticity* than addressing muscle weakness, incoordination, or movement abnormalities. The most commonly used anti-*spasticity* medications are listed in Table 19.3.

- *Risk Factor Modification* One focus of risk factor modification is the reduction or elimination of preventable and treatable causes of CP including maternal health problems, inadequate prenatal care, premature birth, complications of *prematurity*, newborn infections, and traumatic brain injury in young children. Promising medical advances are being made in the areas of neuroprotection of the fetus, neonatal intensive care, and earlier detection of CP. Taken together, these innovations are reducing the prevalence and severity of CP, particularly in developed countries. A second focus involves early intervention for children who already have CP to optimize development, adaptive functioning, and outcome while preventing secondary complications of the disorder.

TABLE 19.3 Medication Management of Spasticity

Medication	Class	Mechanism	Result
Generic Name: *baclofen* **Common Name:** Lioresal	Muscle relaxant	**Brain** Inhibits descending excitatory motor pathways that activate reflexes at the spinal level	* Reduced spasticity, hyperreflexia, and painful muscle spasms and increased muscle flexibility; allows an improved response to therapy
Generic Name: *botulinum toxin type A* **Common Name:** BOTOX®	Neuromuscular blocker	**Muscle** Injected into select muscles, especially in the extremities, to cause focal muscle paralysis and reduce muscle contractions	Reduced spasticity, improved range of motion or mobility; used to help the patient fit into a brace, splint or serial cast, improve positioning, and allow other treatments (especially occupational and physical therapies) to work better
Generic Name: *diazepam* **Common Name:** Valium	Benzodiazepine	**Brain** Relaxes muscles by enhancing the effect of the inhibitory neurotransmitter gamma-aminobutyric acid (GABA)	** Reduced spasticity, hyperreflexia, and painful muscle spasms; improved sleep; reduced anxiety

NOTE: *Oral dose is limited by central nervous system side effects (e.g., drowsiness); higher doses are tolerated via intrathecal delivery of the drug through a surgically implanted pump. **Side effects (including sedation, increased drooling, ataxia, and cognitive dullness) limit its use.

- *Interpersonal Relationships* Children with CP are more likely than typically developing children to experience peer rejection, social isolation, and victimization. Social skills training, particularly when integrated into the everyday school environment, can improve relationships. Involvement in carefully selected extracurricular activities, preferably with a child's input, can provide important opportunities to develop friendships and a sense of belonging and self-efficacy. Adults with CP, particularly those with lower cognitive functioning or higher levels of motor disability, are more likely to experience isolation and less likely to live with a domestic partner or marry, making ongoing involvement with community agencies that provide social opportunities especially important.

- *Rehabilitation Considerations* Rehabilitation for individuals with CP is designed to minimize impairment, prevent secondary disabilities, maximize independence, and improve quality of life. Physical, occupational, and speech/language therapies to optimize gross and fine motor functioning, mobility, daily living skills, swallowing, feeding, and communication are the keystones of treatment and are most effective when started at a young age and continued on an as-needed and flexible basis into adulthood. Without those therapies deterioration in physical functioning and mobility can occur. Specialized equipment, mechanical aids, and assistive technology including communication devices are used to maintain or increase the level of independent functioning and facilitate participation at home and school, and in the community. Rehabilitation also involves implementation of classroom and workplace modifications and supports. Recreational therapies such as therapeutic horsemanship and adaptive sports not only improve gross motor functioning and endurance, but also foster increased social participation, self-esteem, and physical and emotional well-being. Because the motor manifestations of CP change with time, as do the needs of patients as they age, treatment plans must be updated frequently so that they remain developmentally and clinically appropriate. Since few medical professionals have experience caring for adults with CP, the transition from adolescence to young adulthood can be complicated by difficulty locating providers of routine medical care, let alone management and treatment of CP-associated problems. Moreover, there have been more concerted efforts to promote community accessibility and integration for children than for adults. The result can be a disruption to continuity of care and unmet medical, vocational, therapy, and social-emotional needs.

Relevant Definitions

Apgar score Named after its developer, Virginia Apgar, MD, the Apgar score is a quick exam performed 1 minute and 5 minutes after birth. The 1-minute score indicates how well the baby has tolerated the birthing process. The 5-minute score indicates how well the baby is doing outside of the womb. To make the key features of the rating system easy to remember, the name Apgar has been turned into an acronym: *A*ppearance (skin color), *p*ulse (heart rate), *g*rimace response (reflex irritability in response to stimulation), *a*ctivity (muscle tone), and *r*espiration (breathing effort). Apgar scores range from 0 to 10. Higher scores are better (7, 8, and 9 are normal; a perfect score of 10 rarely occurs even in healthy babies). A very low Apgar score at 5 minutes, especially when it is less than 3, is associated with an increased risk of CP, particularly in newborns with a normal birth weight; however, an Apgar score in isolation cannot predict outcome. Most babies with low Apgar scores do not exhibit any lasting sequelae. Conversely, many children with CP have a history of normal Apgar scores.

Athetosis Slow and writhing involuntary movements that can affect any part of the body and typically are repetitive, sinuous, and rhythmic. Athetoid CP typically involves the extremities, mouth, and tongue.

Birth weight Extremely low birth weight (i.e., <1,000 g or 2 lbs., 3 oz.) is a risk factor for CP. Very low birth weight (i.e., <1,500 g or 3 lbs., 5 oz.) also is a risk factor but not to the same degree. In other words, the lower the abnormal birth weight, the greater the risk.

Dystonia Involuntary sustained or intermittent muscle contractions that cause repetitive and often twisting movements, as well as awkward, irregular postures. Dystonia can be triggered or worsened by, and interfere with, voluntary actions.

Extrapyramidal system One of the two semi-independent motor systems of the brain. It is comprised of the cerebellum, basal ganglia, and brainstem and serves to make adjustments to posture and coordinated motor movements. Extrapyramidal CP is characterized by abnormal involuntary movements, especially athetosis or dystonia.

Hypotonia Low muscle tone. A child with hypotonia is "floppy" or "loose" with poor head control.

Intrauterine growth restriction A condition characterized by poor growth of a baby during gestation as reflected by weights less than the 10th percentile for gestational age.

Intraventricular hemorrhage (IVH) Bleeding inside the ventricular system of the brain. When severe, the bleeding can spread to the surrounding brain tissue. Intraventricular hemorrhage frequently occurs in the context of prematurity, especially at gestational ages of 30 weeks or less (when the intra- and periventricular region is particularly sensitive to insult). Intraventricular hemorrhage is rarely present at birth and usually occurs in the first few days of life.

Periventricular leukomalacia (PVL) Cerebral white matter necrosis around the ventricles that interrupts the throughput of motor tracts. Periventricular leukomalacia results from interrupted blood flow and oxygen to the area, particularly in preterm babies of less than 32 weeks. In fact, PVL is sometimes referred to as "white matter damage of prematurity."

Prematurity When a baby is born more than 3 weeks before the "due date" (i.e., at a gestational age of less than 37 weeks). The more severe the prematurity (particularly below gestational ages of 30–31 weeks), the greater the risk of CP.

Pyramidal system One of the two semi-independent motor systems of the brain. It includes motor cortex, spinal motor neurons, and the corticospinal tract that connects the two and is responsible for initiating and carrying signals for voluntary muscle contractions that enable skilled movements. Damage to the pyramidal system is associated with spastic CP.

Spasticity Abnormally increased muscle tone or muscle stiffness that can interfere with functional movement and daily activities. When severe, spasticity is characterized by uncontrollable muscle spasms. Spasticity can be accompanied by discomfort or pain.

Cerebral Palsy Questions

NOTE: *Questions 7, 31, 72, 89, and 121 on the First Full-Length Practice Examination, Questions 4, 26, 52, 94, and 123 on the Second Full-Length Practice Examination, Questions 4, 44, 64, and 102 on the Third Full-Length Practice Examination, and Questions 93, 94, and 95 on the Fourth Full-Length Practice Examination are from this chapter.*

1. Cerebral palsy is the most common cause of childhood ____.
   - (a) ambidexterity
   - (b) cognitive impairment
   - (c) motor stereotypies
   - (d) physical disability

2. A risk factor for cerebral palsy is ____.
   - (a) female sex of the fetus
   - (b) maternal infection
   - (c) a first pregnancy
   - (d) cesarean delivery

3. Cerebral palsy most often results from a brain insult during which developmental stage?
   - (a) prenatal
   - (b) neonatal
   - (c) infancy
   - (d) toddlerhood

4. Typical neuroimaging findings in patients with cerebral palsy include ____.
   - (a) ventricular dilatation or aqueductal stenosis
   - (b) arteriovenous malformation or Chiari II malformation
   - (c) middle cerebral artery stroke or subdural hemorrhage
   - (d) intraventricular hemorrhage or periventricular leukomalacia

5. Spasticity refers to ____.
   - (a) motor incoordination
   - (b) involuntary muscle contractions
   - (c) increased muscle tone
   - (d) impaired voluntary motor control

6. Pyramidal cerebral palsy implies damage to brain pathways originating in the ____.
   (a) cortical gray matter
   (b) basal ganglia
   (c) thalamus
   (d) corona radiata

7. Which of the following is true of spastic quadriplegia?
   (a) the underlying brain insult typically occurs during delivery
   (b) neuroimaging tends to reveal diffuse underlying neuropathology
   (c) cognitive impairments are less likely than in ataxic cerebral palsy
   (d) problems with trunk, but not head, control persist into adulthood

8. A patient with dyskinetic cerebral palsy is most likely to present with involvement of which brain region?
   (a) cortical gray matter
   (b) thalamus
   (c) basal ganglia
   (d) corona radiata

9. A definitive diagnosis of cerebral palsy is usually made between the ages of 2 to 3 years rather than at birth because ____.
   (a) head ultrasonography is contraindicated in medically fragile newborns
   (b) abnormal reflex patterns and muscle tone in a newborn can resolve
   (c) it is advisable to wait until the cerebral palsy subtype can be accurately identified
   (d) if seizures develop in infancy a diagnosis of cerebral palsy would not apply

10. Most children with cerebral palsy ____.
    (a) can walk without assistance
    (b) require assistance to walk
    (c) learn to walk after 3 years of age
    (d) do not learn to walk

11. Evidence-based treatments of cerebral palsy–related spasticity include ____.
    (a) anti-inflammatory corticosteroid medication
    (b) hyperbaric oxygen therapy
    (c) botulinum toxin injections
    (d) ventriculoperitoneal shunt implantation

12. Which statement about cerebral palsy is true?
    (a) preterm birth is the major risk factor
    (b) preterm infants account for the majority of cases
    (c) neuroimaging is normal in 25–30% of cases
    (d) it is permanent and cannot be outgrown

13. One reason the diagnostic process for cerebral palsy (CP) can result in a false positive error is ____.
    (a) an infant with a normal neurological exam can show signs of CP at follow-up
    (b) there can be a latency between a perinatal brain insult and its manifestations
    (c) an infant can present with an unremarkable birth history and no risk factors
    (d) neurological and motor abnormalities in an infant can be transient

14. A 5-year-old boy has been referred for a neuropsychological assessment. He was born at 29 weeks gestation and spent 2 months in a neonatal intensive care unit due to feeding problems which subsequently resolved. His fine motor, language, and social development have been on track. He uses a walker and receives physical therapy at school but participates in a regular kindergarten classroom and is doing well. What subtype of cerebral palsy is most likely?

(a) dyskinetic

(c) ataxic

(b) spastic diplegic

(d) mixed

15. In the case described in Question 14, what is an MRI most likely to show?

(a) hypoxic-ischemic injury

(c) periventricular leukomalacia

(b) focal internal capsule lesion

(d) perinatal middle cerebral artery stroke

Cerebral Palsy Answers

1. **D—physical disability**   *CP is considered a cause of physical disability whereas cognitive problems are considered a common comorbidity.*

References:
(a) Glader, L., & Tilton, A. (2009). Cerebral palsy. In W. B. Carey, A. C. Crocker, E. R. Elias, H. M. Feldman, & W. L. Coleman (Eds.), *Developmental-behavioral pediatrics* (4th ed., pp. 653–662). Philadelphia, PA: Elsevier.
(b) Oskoui, M., Shevell, M. I., & Swaiman, K. F. (2017). Cerebral palsy. In K. F. Swaiman, S. Ashwal, D. M., Ferriero, N. F. Schor, R. S. Finkel, A. L. Gropman, . . . M. Shevell (Eds.), *Swaiman's pediatric neurology: Principles and practice* (6th ed., pp. 734–740). Philadelphi, PA: Elsevier.

2. **B—maternal infection**   *Male sex of the fetus is a risk factor; first pregnancies and cesarean deliveries are not considered risk factors.*

References:
(a) Karlsson, P., Sarah McIntyre, S., & Msall, M. E. (2014). Cerebral palsy in an era of neuroprotection and evidence based interventions: Risk factors, therapeutic management, and prognoses for long term functioning and participation. In H. Yates (Ed.), *Handbook on cerebral palsy: Risk factors, therapeutic management and long-term prognosis* (pp.1–24). New York, NY: Nova Science Publishers.
(b) Platt, M. J., Panteliadis, C. P., & Häusler, M. (2018). Aetiological factors. In C. P. Panteliadis (Ed.), *Cerebral palsy: A multidisciplinary approach* (3rd ed., pp. 49–58). Cham, Switzerland: Springer International.

3. **A—prenatal**   *Perinatal and postnatal causes are less common.*

References:
(a) Badawi, N., & Keogh, J. M. (2012). Causal pathways in cerebral palsy. *Journal of Paediatrics and Child Health, 49*, 5–8.
(b) Singer, H. S., Mink, J. W., Gilbert, D. L., & Jankovic, J. (2016). Cerebral palsy. In H. S. Singer, J. W. Mink, D. L. Gilbert, & J. Jankovic, *Movement disorders in childhood* (2nd ed., pp. 453–475). San Diego: Academic Press.

4. **D—intraventricular hemorrhage or periventricular leukomalacia**   *Perinatal stroke and brain malformations are less frequent findings.*

Reference: Marret, S., Vanhulle, C., & Laquerrier, A. (2013). Pathophysiology of cerebral palsy. In M. J. Aminoff, F. Boller, & D. F. Swaab (Series Eds.) & O. Dulac, M. Lassonde, & H. B. Sarnat (Eds.), *Handbook of clinical neurology: Pediatric neurology* (Vol 3, Part 1, pp. 169–176). Amsterdam, NL: Elsevier B.V.

5. **C—increased muscle tone**   *Stiffness and tightness are also descriptors.*

Reference: Singer, H. S., Mink, J. W., Gilbert, D. L., & Jankovic, J. (2016). Cerebral palsy. In H. S. Singer, J. W. Mink, D. L. Gilbert, & J. Jankovic, *Movement disorders in childhood* (2nd ed., pp. 453–475). San Diego: Academic Press.

6. **A—cortical gray matter**   *Pyramidal CP involves brain pathways originating in cortical, not subcortical, regions.*

   Reference: Oskoui, M., Shevell, M. I., & Swaiman, K. F. (2017). Cerebral palsy. In K. F. Swaiman, S. Ashwal, D. M., Ferriero, N. F. Schor, R. S. Finkel, A. L. Gropman, . . . M. Shevell (Eds.), *Swaiman's pediatric neurology: Principles and practice* (6th ed., pp. 734–740). Philadelphia, PA: Elsevier.

7. **B—neuroimaging tends to reveal diffuse underlying neuropathology.**   *Spastic quadriplegia is often associated with generalized insults such as anoxia.*

   Reference: Marret, S., Vanhulle, C., & Laquerrier, A. (2013). Pathophysiology of cerebral palsy. In M. J. Aminoff, F. Boller, & D. F. Swaab (Series Eds.), & O. Dulac, M. Lassonde & H. B. Sarnat (Eds.), *Handbook of clinical neurology: Pediatric neurology* (Vol 3, Part 1, pp. 169–176). Amsterdam, NL: Elsevier.

8. **C—basal ganglia**   *Damage to the basal ganglia associated with a hypoxic-ischemic event is a typical finding.*

   Reference: Singer, H. S., Mink, J. W., Gilbert, D. L., & Jankovic, J. (2016). Cerebral palsy. In H. S. Singer, J. W. Mink, D. L. Gilbert, & J. Jankovic, *Movement disorders in childhood* (2nd ed., pp. 453–475). San Diego: Academic Press.

9. **B—abnormal reflex patterns and muscle tone in a newborn can resolve**   *Conversely, motor manifestations of CP (unless very severe) are not always apparent during the newborn period.*

   Reference: Novak, I. (2014). Evidence-based diagnosis, health care, and rehabilitation for children with cerebral palsy. *Journal of Child Neurology, 29*(8), 1141–1156.

10. **A—can walk without assistance**   *A minority require assistance to walk.*

    Reference: Novak, I. (2014). Evidence-based diagnosis, health care, and rehabilitation for children with cerebral palsy. *Journal of Child Neurology, 29*(8), 1141–1156.

11. **C—botulinum toxin injections**   *Hyperbaric oxygen therapy lacks research support. Corticosteroids and shunts are not typical treatments.*

    Reference: Spevack, T. V. (2012). Cerebral palsy. In C. A. Noggle, R. S. Dean, & A. M. Horton Jr. (Eds.), *The encyclopedia of neuropsychological disorders* (pp. 174–178). New York, NY: Springer.

12. **A—preterm birth is the major risk factor**   *Although prematurity is a major risk factor, full-term infants account for the majority of CP cases.*

    Reference: Novak, I., Morgan, C., Adde, L, Blackman, J., Boyd, R. N., Brunstrom-Hernandez, J., . . . Badawi, N. (2017). Early, accurate diagnosis and early intervention in cerebral palsy: Advances in diagnosis and treatment. *JAMA Pediatrics, 171*(9), 897–907.

13. **D—neurological and motor abnormalities in an infant can be transient**   *The other choices would result in false negative errors.*

    Reference: Singer, H. S., Mink, J. W., Gilbert, D. L., & Jankovic, J. (2016). Cerebral palsy. In H. S. Singer, J. W. Mink, D. L. Gilbert, & J. Jankovic, *Movement disorders in childhood* (2nd ed., pp. 453–475). San Diego: Academic Press.

14. **B—spastic diplegic**   *Features of this child's presentation that are consistent with spastic diplegia are his history of premature birth and his primary problem with walking (suggesting bilateral lower extremity involvement).*

    Reference: Glader, L., & Tilton, A. (2009). Cerebral palsy. In W. B. Carey, A. C. Crocker, E. R. Elias, H. M. Feldman, & W. L. Coleman (Eds.), *Developmental-behavioral pediatrics* (4th ed., pp. 653–662). Philadelphia, PA: Elsevier.

15. **C—periventricular leukomalacia** *Spastic diplegia is often associated with diffuse white matter injury.*

> **Reference:** Marret, S., Vanhulle, C., & Laquerrier, A. (2013). Pathophysiology of cerebral palsy. In M. J. Aminoff, F. Boller, & D. F. Swaab (Series Eds.), & O. Dulac, M. Lassonde, & H. B. Sarnat (Eds.), *Handbook of clinical neurology: Pediatric neurology* (Vol 3, Part 1, pp. 169–176). Amsterdam, NL: Elsevier.

Recommended Readings

Graham, H. K., Rosenbaum, P., Paneth, M., Dan, B., Lin, J. P., Damiano, D. L., . . . Lieber, R. L. (2016). Cerebral palsy. *Nature Reviews Disease Primers, 2*, 1–24.

Novak, I., Morgan, C., Fahey, M., Finch-Edmondson, M., Galea, C., Hines, A., . . . Badawi, N. (2020). State of the evidence traffic lights 2019: Systematic review of interventions for preventing and treating children with cerebral palsy. *Pediatric Neurology and Neuroscience Reports, 20*(Article No. 3).

Oskoui, M., Shevell, M. I., & Swaiman, K. F. (2017). Cerebral palsy. In K. F. Swaiman, S. Ashwal, D. M., Ferriero, N. F. Schor, R. S. Finkel, A. L. Gropman, . . . M. Shevell (Eds.), *Swaiman's pediatric neurology: Principles and practice* (6th ed., pp. 734–740). Philadelphia, PA: Elsevier.

Rosenbaum, P., Paneth, N., Leviton, A., Goldstein, M., Bax, M., Damiano, D., . . . Jacobsson, B. (2007). A report: The definition and classification of cerebral palsy April 2006. *Developmental medicine and child neurology* [Suppl. 2007, January 31]. 109, 8–14.

Singer, H. S., Mink, J. W., Gilbert, D. L., & Jankovic, J. (2016). Cerebral palsy. In H. S. Singer, J. W. Mink, D. L. Gilbert, & J. Jankovic, *Movement disorders in childhood* (2nd ed., pp. 453–475). San Diego: Academic Press.

Stadskleiv, K., Jahnsen, R., Andersen, G. L., & von Tetzchner, S. (2018). Neuropsychological profiles of children with cerebral palsy. *Developmental Neurorehabilitation, 21*(2), 108–120.

20 Congenital and Acquired Hydrocephalus

Jack M. Fletcher

Definition

Hydrocephalus is the accumulation of cerebrospinal fluid (CSF) in or around the ventricles, which usually results in ventricular expansion and pressure on other parts of the brain. Hydrocephalus is usually secondary to another condition that interferes with the flow of CSF and can be congenital or acquired. Normal pressure hydrocephalus (NPH) can occur idiopathically in adults or secondary to atrophy, strokes, and other conditions.

When hydrocephalus occurs acutely in children or adults, the accumulation of CSF often results in impairment of gait, atypical eye movements, headaches, vomiting, and cognitive difficulties. Treatment is required to prevent additional injury to the brain and death. As a chronic condition, hydrocephalus must be monitored on a long-term basis and can be associated with cognitive and motor difficulties in children and adults.

Neuropathology

The most common cause of hydrocephalus is an obstruction that blocks the normal flow of CSF in the brain. Ventricular dilation can also result from inadequate absorption or overproduction of CSF or loss of brain tissue because of atrophy. When ventricular dilation occurs, animal and human studies show that there is stretching and enlargement of the periventricular white matter fibers. This process unleashes a host of complications, including reductions in blood flow because of impairment to blood vessels serving the white matter. Multiple neurochemical changes also affect glucose and oxygen utilization. Because one purpose of CSF flow in the brain is to remove potentially toxic metabolic byproducts, these toxins accumulate in the brain and may induce further injury. In infants and young children, these changes impede brain development and can cause neuronal death affecting development of gray matter. Demyelination and disruption of the development of the cerebral white matter can result as well, primarily from ventricular expansion and stretching of axons.

At a neuropathological level, the general effects of hydrocephalus can be understood as a subcortical disconnection syndrome because of injury to the long periventricular pathways (e.g., corpus callosum, projection pathways) that support communication across different brain regions. However, hydrocephalus is not strictly an injury to the white matter nor is it an isolated condition. Rather, hydrocephalus is usually secondary to another disease process and rarely occurs as the only entity affecting outcomes.

Classification and Causes

The mechanical effects of hydrocephalus are likely universal, and different classifications may have more to do with the age of origin, site of the disruption, and whether there is increased and sustained intracranial pressure (ICP). There are multiple, overlapping classifications of hydrocephalus (see Table 20.1).

TABLE 20.1 Classification and Causes

Congenital versus Acquired	In **congenital** (or "early" hydrocephalus, see below), the origin is typically very early in development, whereas **acquired** forms of hydrocephalus may occur across the lifespan as a consequence of a disorder such as a tumor, infection, traumatic brain injury, or dementia.
Common Types of Congenital Hydrocephalus (Four types; see descriptions next page)	• **Spina bifida myelomeningocele** • **Aqueductal stenosis** • **Dandy-Walker syndrome** • **Prematurity intraventricular hemorrhage**
Internal versus External	**Internal hydrocephalus** usually refers to obstructive hydrocephalus involving the foramen of Monro or a narrowing of the aqueduct of Sylvius (aqueductal stenosis). These are classic forms of congenital hydrocephalus that result in accumulation of CSF, increased intracranial pressure, ventricular expansion, and compression of the brain. **External hydrocephalus** involves the subarachnoid spaces and is most often used to describe individuals with disorders of CSF absorption (e.g., meningitis), but is also used to describe other forms of hydrocephalus external to the ventricles that do not necessarily involve increased intracranial pressure.
Communicating (versus Noncommunicating; also called ex vacuo, arrested, or compensated hydrocephalus**)**	**Communicating hydrocephalus** is not an obstructive process, but refers to abnormalities of CSF absorption. In adults, communicating hydrocephalus occurs after injuries affecting the subarachnoid space around the ventricles that are involved in absorption of CSF. Intracranial pressure is not always increased in these cases involving ventricular enlargement with accumulated CSF. An example is the development of enlarged ventricles in people with dementia and other conditions that are associated with loss of brain tissue.
Noncommunicating	**Noncommunicating** is the obstructive form of hydrocephalus associated with congenital disorders, but can be associated with other disorders (e.g., cysts) that obstruct the outflow of CSF into the subarachnoid space. These forms of hydrocephalus are often classified according to the location of the obstruction.
Normal Pressure Hydrocephalus (NPH)	The most common type of hydrocephalus with adult onset is **NPH**, representing the accumulation of CSF in the ventricles with ventriculomegaly. NPH may be associated with increased intracranial pressure that is sporadic and fluctuating. In some cases, NPH has no obvious cause, but it may also be due to another insult to the brain, such as a tumor, hemorrhage, or traumatic brain injury. Except for idiopathic NPH, which is not well understood, the disorder producing the hydrocephalus is the key to understanding outcomes and hydrocephalus is a secondary complication. Risk factors for idiopathic NPH include hypertension, vascular disease, and diabetes.

Common Types of Hydrocephalus

There are four types of congenital ("early") hydrocephalus, three of which are disorders of embryogenesis (spina bifida, aqueductal stenosis, and Dandy-Walker syndrome [DWS]). The fourth is acquired and associated with prematurity and intraventricular hemorrhage (IVH). All are typically obstructive, internal, and noncommunicating. In addition, NPH most commonly occurs in older adults. It is a communicating form of nonobstructive hydrocephalus due to impaired reabsorption of CSF, but obstruction can be a factor in secondary forms of the disorder.

Spina Bifida Myelomeningocele

Spina bifida ("split spine") is a typically nonlethal neural tube defect that occurs in the first 30 days of gestation. It is the most common form of spina bifida and the most common cause of congenital hydrocephalus, accounting for about 70% of all childhood cases. In spina bifida, the portion of the neural tube that eventually forms the vertebral column fails to fuse during early embryogenesis. The degree of closure leads to different kinds of spinal lesions apparent at birth, including *myelomeningocele*, which, is an "open" neural tube defect because central nervous system (CNS) tissue is exposed. Closed spinal defects ("dysraphisms") include *meningocele, lipomas* (fatty tumors), and defects of the vertebrae, such as *diastomyelia*, that split the cord. *Spina bifida occulta* is a common form of spinal abnormality with no protruding spinal sac that is usually not overtly apparent at birth (i.e., "hidden"); it is often identified because a person experiences back pain, with the abnormality identified only on radiological examination. The relation of *spina bifida occulta* to other forms of spina bifida is unclear and, like other closed forms of spina bifida, is rarely associated with hydrocephalus or other brain abnormalities.

In spina bifida *myelomeningocele*, the spinal cord protrudes through the meninges. The brain is rarely normal, and hydrocephalus develops in about 90% of infants because of the Chiari II malformation of the hindbrain, which causes obstruction at the fourth ventricle. The Chiari II malformation is virtually ubiquitous in association with *myelomeningocele*, involving a small posterior fossa in which the cerebellum is herniated and downwardly extends through the foramen of Monro. The cerebellum itself is abnormal, with additional crowding effects on the medulla (kinking) and tectum (beaking). The corpus callosum is also usually abnormal because of failure of the rostrum or splenium to develop (hypogenesis) in about half of people with spina bifida *myelomeningocele*, with most also showing thinning of the corpus callosum (hypoplasia) secondary to hydrocephalus. In addition to the direct effects of these brain malformations on cognitive and motor functions, hydrocephalus, per se, and its treatment, further injures the brain. There may be additional long-term effects of the underlying defect in neural migration that impair brain function that are not well understood.

Quantitative assessments of the shunted *myelomeningocele* brain show overall reductions in gray and white matter volumes, with increased CSF. The reductions in thickness and volume are most apparent posteriorly, with the brain thicker and showing little volume loss in the frontal regions. The basal ganglia are usually visibly normal, but assessments of integrity using diffusion tensor imaging show abnormalities of the caudate and palladium, as well as of long projection fibers and the corpus callosum. Gyrification is reduced frontally and enhanced posteriorly, coinciding with areas of enlarged and reduced thickness. The hippocampus is reduced in volume and integrity, but the amygdala is often normal. There is little evidence that the quantitative changes in the frontal regions are compensatory. More generally, quantitative studies, as well as qualitative reading of magnetic resonance imaging (MRI) scans show significant amounts of variability. Spina bifida *myelomeningocele* is an interesting example of the capacity of the brain to reorganize and support cognitive functions in the face of an ongoing injury that begins prenatally.

Aqueductal Stenosis

Hydrocephalus develops in aqueductal stenosis because of a congenital narrowing of the aqueduct of Sylvius and usually without a spinal defect, although people with closed neural tube defects may develop hydrocephalus because of aqueductal stenosis despite no Chiari II malformation. In the absence of a spinal defect, hydrocephalus is the primary problem affecting brain development, and the brain often appears otherwise normal. In particular, the cerebellum is generally normal, although some downward extension of the cerebellum may be present because of pressure effects from hydrocephalus. In addition, partial callosal hypogenesis is apparent in about 20% of cases. The origins of aqueductal stenosis are not well understood, but the co-occurrence with spina bifida and callosal hypogenesis suggests that it is a form of a neural tube defect. Children with only aqueductal stenosis and hydrocephalus may have better outcomes in cognitive and motor functions than those with aqueductal stenosis and additional callosal and cerebellar abnormalities.

Dandy-Walker Syndrome (DWS)

About 70–80% of children with DWS develop hydrocephalus because of a cystic fourth ventricle with partial to complete agenesis of the cerebellar vermis. In contrast to the small posterior fossa in spina bifida *myelomeningocele*, the posterior fossa is enlarged with expansion of the fourth ventricle. Although the ventricular dilation is characterized as hydrocephalus, it is a cystic malformation often requires shunting around the blockage created by the cyst. Partial agenesis of the corpus callosum may be common. In addition to the classic presentation of DWS, there are also variants in which only some of the features are apparent, but with malformation of the vermis. Because of its rarity, we know relatively little about outcomes in DWS.

Prematurity Intraventricular Hemorrhage (IVH)

Children with prematurity IVH develop hydrocephalus because of a hemorrhage involving the germinal matrix shortly after birth. Intraventricular hemorrhage is a consequence of perinatal asphyxia, usually in low-birth-weight infants, occurring as part of a complex sequence of events involving problems with cerebral blow flow and perfusion. The germinal matrix bleeds into the ventricles, obstructing the flow of CSF. The IVH is typically graded according to severity as I (germinal matrix hemorrhage not bleeding into the ventricles), II (germinal matrix hemorrhage with bleeding into the ventricles), III (bleeding with ventricular enlargement), and IV (bleeding into the tissue around the ventricles with ventricular enlargement). By definition, only grades III and IV are associated with hydrocephalus. Infants are monitored and may change categories depending on the progression of the IVH. Unlike spina bifida *myelomeningocele* and aqueductal stenosis, hydrocephalus is more often arrested and nonprogressive. Despite progress in treatment, IVH remains a significant problem associated with prematurity, especially in extremely low birth weight infants.

Epidemiology

For all forms of congenital hydrocephalus, mortality rates are about 0.7 deaths per 100,000 person years over a 20-year period (1979–1998). The rate has declined because of advances in treatment. The death rate is highest for infants. The causes of various hydrocephalus disorders are listed in Table 20.2.

TABLE 20.2 Causes of Congenital and Acquired Hydrocephalus

Neural tube defects	In spina bifida myelomeningocele, hydrocephalus results from the obstruction caused by the Chiari II malformation of the hindbrain
Aqueductal stenosis	Hydrocephalus is caused by congenital narrowing of the aqueduct of Sylvius
Dandy-Walker syndrome	Cystic fourth ventricle with partial to complete agenesis of the cerebellar vermis
Prematurity-IVH	Hydrocephalus is caused by bleeding into the ventricles from a germinal matrix hemorrhage in very-low-birth-weight infants
Normal pressure hydrocephalus	In older adults, idiopathic hydrocephalus occurs as a communicating disorder with impaired reabsorption of CSF; may be secondary to obstructive process

Neural Tube Defects (Spina Bifida, Anencephaly, Encephalocele)

The worldwide incidence of neural tube defects is about 1–10 per 1,000 births and roughly equal for spina bifida and anencephaly "without brain." In contrast, encephalocele, in which the brain protrudes from the skull, is much rarer, as are hydranencephaly (missing hemispheres) and lissencephaly (bending of head to spine). These defects are apparent at birth, but risk can also be detected through prenatal blood tests and directly assessed with ultrasonography. Because of antenatal diagnosis, the birth prevalence (about 1 per 10,000) of anencephaly in North America is much lower than spina bifida (about 3.5 per 10,000). Anencephaly is lethal, representing a failure of the neural tube to close at the cephalad end, so that there is little development of the cortex. The rarer neural tube defects range in severity and may not always be lethal. Although neural tube defects have a multifactorial genetic etiology, effects of individual genes are small and environmental factors (poverty, maternal diet, environmental toxins) account for some of the worldwide variability in incidence. In North America, prevalence rates of neural tube defects were declining because of increased emphasis on folate acid supplementation for women in childbearing years and through dietary fortification of bread and other product, but rates have stabilized since these efforts at folate supplementation. There is sufficient influence of hereditable factors (genetics) and noncompliance with dietary recommendations that spina bifida will likely maintain its status as the most common severely disabling CNS birth defect compatible with life. Interpretation of incidence is complicated by the possible increase in elective terminations due to advances in prenatal diagnosis. *Myelomeningocele* accounts for about 70% of all forms of congenital hydrocephalus. Neural tube defects occur slightly more frequently in girls and, in North America, are more common in Latin/x and Caucasian than African and Asian ethnicities. Before the advent of shunting in the 1970s, spina bifida with hydrocephalus was often fatal, primarily because of complications associated with the Chiari II malformation. Now people with spina bifida commonly live into adulthood, with the Spina Bifida Association estimating that 70,000 people with spina bifida live in the United States. Known fatalities typically occur early in development and often because of the Chiari malformation and its effects on brainstem functioning. Nonetheless, the spontaneous death rate of spina bifida with hydrocephalus in older children and adults remains relatively high, presumably because of documented and undocumented problems with the shunt used for treatment.

Aqueductal Stenosis

Occurs in about 5–10 per 100,000 live births and accounts for about 5–15% of cases with congenital hydrocephalus. These figures often include X-linked hydrocephalus, a genetic disorder affecting males and associated with hydrocephalus and intellectual disabilities. Although usually detected in infancy because of problems with head size and control and gaze, aqueductal stenosis is also detected because of radiological studies in people complaining of headaches and unexpected vomiting. Prenatal ultrasonography may identify hydrocephalus.

Dandy-Walker Syndrome

Occurs in about in 3–5 per 100,000 live births and accounts for 5–10% of all cases with congenital hydrocephalus. It can be detected in prenatal diagnosis, but is usually identified in the first year of life because of head size, poor control, and gaze problems. Dandy-Walker is often fatal (about half of cases), but the prognosis has improved with advances in early diagnosis and treatment.

Prematurity IVH

Intraventricular hemorrhage is generally determined by grade and not by overall incidence. It occurs with the highest incidence and severity at the lowest levels of gestational age and birthweight. For example,

37% of premature infants born below 23 weeks gestation sustain Grades III–IV IVH, but these rates dramatically decline by 28 weeks gestation, which usually reflects higher birth weights. There are multiple causes, with half occurring in the first 6 hours after birth and another third after the first day because of different causes, but all involving a germinal matrix bleed. IVH, especially at the more severe grades, is associated with long-term problems at school. The incidence has been declining because of advances with treatment.

Normal Pressure Hydrocephalus (NPH)

Normal pressure hydrocephalus has an incidence of at least 5 to 6 per 100,000 people and is most common in people over 65, in whom the overall prevalence rate is estimated at 0.5%. The incidence increases with age. These figures are regarded as minimal estimates because it is often not identified. In patients with dementia, where it would be considered idiopathic because there is no direct CNS pathology causing increased intracranial pressure, NPH has been estimated as occurring in 2–6% of all affected patients. It is usually diagnosed by radiological study in people presenting with headaches, urinary incontinence, gait abnormalities, and mental decline. It can be confused with Parkinson's disease and different forms of dementia. When it is not identified, it can be very incapacitating; identification is important because many of the difficulties associated with NPH are reversible with correct treatment for ventricular expansion and accumulated CSF, usually shunting.

Determinants of Severity

Hydrocephalus can be understood as a complex cascade of events resulting from the impedance of CSF flow and accumulation. Animal and human studies show that the process is somewhat mechanical and predictable according to fluid and pressure dynamics and is related to the degree of CSF accumulation, increased ICP, and ventricular expansion. Although severity of hydrocephalus is one determinant of outcomes, the other factors relate to the underlying disorder and associated malformations. In children with spina bifida (again, largely *myelomeningocele*), outcomes vary in part because of the severity of the Chiari II malformation and the direct effects on cerebellar functions involving motor control and precision, rhythmicity, and timing. In addition, people with spina bifida who have other features of the Chiari II malformation, such as tectal beaking, or who have hypogenesis of the corpus callosum, tend to have poorer outcomes. Another factor specific to spina bifida is the level of the spinal lesion, which can range from the lower thoracic to sacral levels (spinal lesions of the upper thoracic and cervical levels are usually fatal). In all forms of spina bifida, there are bowel and bladder problems, and difficulties with ambulation are predictable based on the level of the spinal lesion. Higher-level spinal defects are often associated with paraplegia of the lower limbs and an inability to ambulate, as well as with more severe brain malformations. Because of the obvious orthopedic and urinary problems, spina bifida is often viewed publicly as an orthopedic disorder, which is how it is often classified in public schools despite the fact that the brain is often impaired. The direct effects from the injury to the brain on upper extremity coordination (especially writing) and different cognitive skills are often misinterpreted as problems with motivation and behavior.

In other forms of congenital hydrocephalus, the determinants of severity are directly related to hydrocephalus and the underlying disorder. Aqueductal stenosis is often a relatively pure form of early hydrocephalus and may present with no other brain malformations. The primary determinant of severity is hydrocephalus and its treatment, although some with aqueductal stenosis present with abnormalities of the cerebellum and corpus callosum that are associated with more severe outcomes. In DWS, the severity of the cystic malformation and the degree of vermis hypogenesis directly influence outcomes, with particular difficulties with gait and upper extremity control. In prematurity IVH, the complications of prematurity (birth weight, lung disease) clearly influence outcomes independently of hydrocephalus (recognizing that the occurrence of hydrocephalus is a manifestation of severity of prematurity). Unlike congenital forms of hydrocephalus, in which the skull can expand to accommodate ventricular expansion, the brain has no place to go in NPH. If idiopathic, severity is a direct product of the increase in ICP and compression of the ventricles on other parts of the brain. In all other forms of hydrocephalus secondary to hemorrhage, infection, trauma, and atrophy in adults and children, severity is determined primarily by the disorder itself, with hydrocephalus adding to severity.

Presentation Course and Treatment

Presentation: Acute Course

In the acute phase, most forms of hydrocephalus associated with CSF accumulation can cause severe brain damage and death if not treated. Headaches, urinary incontinence, and mental decline can be associated with all acute presentations of hydrocephalus in older children and adults. In infants, detection of neural tube defects is possible through alpha-fetal protein tests of the blood because of the open spinal lesion, although these are risk indicators with relatively high false-positive rates. Prenatal (and postnatal) ultrasonography can potentially detect all forms of early hydrocephalus, but false-negative errors are possible. Radiological studies are essential for people suspected of NPH. Spina bifida is usually identified at birth because of the spinal lesion; if the lesion is a *myelomeningocele*, it triggers immediate concern for the Chiari II malformation and hydrocephalus. Aqueductal stenosis and DWS are often identified in infancy because of the expansion in head circumference and abnormalities of head control and gaze; for DWS, gait abnormalities are common. Intraventricular hemorrhage is identified and monitored based on routine ultrasonography.

Presentation: Chronic Course

Hydrocephalus is also a chronic disorder after treatment. The long-term effects are variable and depend on the cause of the disorder but can be identified early in development. In spina bifida *myelomeningocele*, problems with attention and motor control can be identified in infants and clearly persist into adulthood. The specific manifestations depend on the stage of development of the person, but are relatively consistent from early childhood if the hydrocephalus is stable over time. People with hydrocephalus require a lifetime of monitoring, especially if treated with shunts.

Treatment

The most common treatment for hydrocephalus is implantation of a shunt that diverts the flow of CSF around the site of blockage. The most common shunt placement is in a right posterior ventricle with a valve that drains fluid into the peritoneal cavity. However, any ventricle is a candidate for shunting, and it is not unusual to see a patient with left or bilateral shunts. Other surgical approaches to CSF diversion include *endoscopic third ventriculostomy (ETV)*, in which the floor of the third ventricle is perforated to drain CSF into an open CSF space, usually the subcistern. Because this procedure avoids a shunt, its use is increasing in all forms of congenital hydrocephalus. It is most frequently used with aqueductal stenosis and in developing countries without shunt technology. For problems with CSF absorption, medications that absorb excessive fluid may be used. In prematurity, treatments for lung problems are used to prevent IVH. As rates of shunting decline, there is relatively little data on children treated with prenatal surgery, ETVs, and other alternatives to shunting.

Shunts often fail and need to be revised, which may involve replacing the shunt, lengthening the tube, or other procedures. Failure can occur because of blockage. In addition, shunt sites sometimes become infected. Although shunt technology has evolved, many neurosurgeons view shunt treatment as undesirable because of the risk for failure and infection and the multiple operations required. Many neurosurgical centers no longer immediately implant a shunt when the spine is repaired at birth, monitoring the progression of hydrocephalus over time. Newer forms of treatment involve prenatal surgery to correct the spinal defect. In one large clinical trial, such surgery reduced the risk of a Chiari II malformation, reduced shunting, and resulted in better motor (but not cognitive) outcomes at 3 years of age, with these effects persisting in a follow-up at 6 to 10 years. Studies of lifetime shunt revisions and infections with childhood outcomes have not shown strong relations, with a meta-analysis observing a relationship of lifetime shunt revisions and IQ of about 3 points.

Shunts do alleviate pressure on the brain and in animal studies are associated with partial restoration of brain function. In adults with NPH, treatment is essential and may restore motor and mental functions. Shunt diversion is often necessary, but the issues with monitoring and revisions apparent with children are also apparent with older adults.

Expectations for Neuropsychological Assessment Results

Generalizations about neuropsychological performance should be made cautiously because of the variability of the different disorders associated with hydrocephalus. In completing neuropsychological assessments, it is important to understand the cause of hydrocephalus and to evaluate the host of factors influencing outcome in order to provide a good formulation of each case. Most data on outcomes in congenital hydrocephalus are from studies of shunted spina bifida. In most studies with spina bifida, the cause of hydrocephalus is the Chiari II malformation associated with *myelomeningocele*. In the few cases with no Chiari and either arrested or shunted hydrocephalus, there is aqueductal stenosis. The difference in outcomes between these two disorders, when shunted, is largely a matter of degree, with aqueductal stenosis showing higher levels of performance. The largest differences are on tests of fine motor skills, where children with spina bifida have more significant difficulties because of the Chiari malformation. More generally, intellectual disabilities occur infrequently. Attention problems are common, and children with early hydrocephalus often meet criteria for ADHD, predominantly inattentive presentation. However, it is not obviously the same disorder as in developmental forms of ADHD. Children with developmental forms of ADHD most commonly have difficulties with self-regulation, reflecting problems with "top-down" control associated with frontostriatal function and other aspects of an anterior attention system (see also Chapter 16, Attention-Deficit/Hyperactivity Disorder). In contrast, children with congenital hydrocephalus have difficulties with orienting and disengaging, but stronger regulation when oriented and engaged, which may be consistent with a disorder of the posterior attention system. Children and adults with any form of hydrocephalus often appear under-aroused and lethargic.

The problems seen with cognitive functions in congenital hydrocephalus are commonly interpreted as examples of executive function deficits. However, this generalization does not always match well with the strengths of children with congenital hydrocephalus or the underlying neuropathology. On average, children with congenital hydrocephalus will do poorly on executive function measures, but the reasons are not as simple as frontal lobe dysfunction. Rourke interpreted the neuropsychological performance of children with congenital hydrocephalus as a nonverbal learning disability characterized by strengths in verbal skills involving phonology, vocabulary, and grammar, auditory attention, auditory and verbal memory, word decoding, and spelling. In contrast, weaknesses in motor, tactile, spatial, concept forma-tion, and problem-solving skills; verbal comprehension, prosodics, and reading comprehension; and in math, writing, and social skills are apparent. Although many of these patterns are apparent in congen-ital hydrocephalus, certain aspects do not fit well, especially the presence of both verbal and nonverbal memory and attention difficulties and the hypersociality characteristic of many with spina bifida and aqueductal stenosis. Neuropsychological evaluations are facilitated by interviews and rating scales that address the consequences of the disorder in everyday function, especially addressing adaptive beha-vior, executive functions, and behavioral adjustment. On adaptive behavior assessments, characteristic patterns show strengths in social/communication domains, severe problems with motor functions, and weaknesses in daily living skills, often because of the orthopedic and bladder complications associated with spina bifida. General problems with multiple domains of executive function emerge on rating scales like the BRIEF, which are highly correlated with ratings on inattention scales. Behavior rating scales are also sensitive to internalizing problems that emerge as children move into adolescence and adulthood.

Inattention, dysexecutive, and white matter hypotheses do not address the complexity of outcomes associated with congenital hydrocephalus. Dennis, Landry, Barnes, and Fletcher (2006) proposed that there are prototypic patterns that are most clearly apparent for spina bifida and early hydrocephalus and that outcomes are variable. Core deficits involve timing, attention, and motor functions, which persist throughout development. The deficits that manifest themselves are general problems in assembling, constructing, and integrating information that cut across domains. In contrast, prototypical strengths involving associative learning of rote verbal material, facial recognition, vocabulary and grammar, and word decoding and spelling emerge. The pattern is not terribly different from what Rourke (1995) identified except for the greater emphasis on the pervasiveness of attention and motor problems, the lack of domain-specificity, and identification of factors that reduce strengths in associative processing. For example, the prototypical patterns identified by Rourke and Dennis are not apparent in the child with spina bifida and hydrocephalus who is lower in socioeconomic status (SES), Latin/x (although SES is the critical variable), has additional complications of hydrocephalus, a very severe Chiari malformation, other neurological problems (e.g., seizures), callosal hypogenesis, and/or an upper level spinal defect.

In DWS, a prototypical pattern is not apparent except for the severe difficulties with upper motor co-ordination apparent because of the cerebellar hypoplasia. Intellectual disabilities are more common than in spina bifida or aqueductal stenosis. In prematurity IVH, there is a clear progression according to level of IVH, with children at grades I and II performing higher than children with grades III and IV. Children with grade IV IVH and shunted hydrocephalus show no particular pattern of strengths and weaknesses, with clearly poorer outcomes than children with IVH who are not shunted.

Neuropsychological performance of adults with idiopathic NPH tends to show a variable and diffuse pattern of performance that often improves with shunting. Neuropsychological deficits are especially apparent on motor-based tasks, but extend to most areas assessed, including attention, memory, spatial skills, and concept formation. Improvement after shunting is more likely in patients who have not shown severe gait difficulties or evidence of dementia or stroke. In patients with secondary NPH, the primary disorder is obviously a major determinant of neuropsychological outcomes.

In the summary here, the basis is the prototypical child (and adult) with congenital hydrocephalus. This is the most common type of referral for both child and adult neuropsychologists, especially given the number of adults who have survived congenital hydrocephalus. The prototype assumes a child or adult who has not grown up in poverty, has not experienced significant complications of hydrocephalus and its treatment, and, in spina bifida, has a spinal lesion below the thoracic level.

- *Intelligence* On Wechsler-type tests, higher verbal than visuospatial performance may be present; poor scores on tests with a timed motor component is common. Performance is more comparable on verbal and nonverbal tasks that are not timed and have no motor component.

- *Achievement* Word reading and spelling are better developed than reading comprehension, writing, and math, with the last domain sometimes profoundly impaired.

- *Attention/Concentration* On paper and pencil assessments of focused attention, significant impairment is present because of the motor component. On sustained attention tasks with minimal motor requirements, initial levels of task performance are well below normative expectations, but there is relatively stable performance over time. Major problems orienting and disengaging attentional focus.

- *Processing Speed* Extremely deficient, especially if a paper-and-pencil timed task is employed.

- *Speech and Language* Preservation of vocabulary, grammar, and expressive language; weaknesses in language comprehension, prosodics, and pragmatics.

- *Visuospatial* Categorical perception intact, but complex configurational skills impaired.

- *Memory* Often intact for rote, associative material (e.g., digit recall and faces); verbal and nonverbal learning and retrieval are usually impaired.

- *Executive Functions* Impaired on most tests of executive functions, although often with a pattern of initial difficulties and subsequent improvement over trials (e.g., Wisconsin Card Sorting, Tower of Hanoi). Difficulties often reflect attention and motor problems.

- *Sensorimotor Functions* Upper extremity motor deficits on simple and complex tasks, especially if cerebellar involvement; simple tactile sensation intact, but complex tactile impaired. Procedural learning intact.

- *Emotion and Personality* High interest in people, with interpersonal skills often being a strength; can be hypersocial, overly talkative, and intrusive. In adolescence and adulthood, depressive feelings may emerge because of social isolation and difficulties related to the disability.

- *Performance and Symptom Validity* Interested in pleasing examiner and tend to treat assessments as a social opportunity. May be under aroused and lethargic, which is not usually a motivational deficit.

Considerations when Treating Patients with Congenital Hydrocephalus

- *Level of Supervision* Level of independence is of concern for children and adults. They often do not have opportunities to develop optimal level of independence because of caregiver's overcompensation.

- *Driving* Often unable to drive without modifications for physical disabilities; attentional and processing speed need to be considered.

- *Employment* Many adults are independent and able to work, but rates of unemployment and underemployment are high.

- *School/Vocational Training* Academic problems with math, reading comprehension, and writing are often not identified or treated. Schools often fail to recognize that the basis for learning difficulties is the brain and not motivation or personality. Accommodations are needed in high school and college, especially for writing and mathematics. Transition plans involving academics, vocational, and social domains are essential for children with congenital hydrocephalus as they move into adulthood.

- *Capacity* Highly variable, but general intellectual disability is infrequent, and caregiver relations are very important in developing independence.

- *Emotional and Psychological Issues* Hypersociality can be an issue that responds to intervention. Issues with disability identification, social relations, and isolation often emerge in adolescents and adults. Family issues can emerge in a minority of patients, often revolving around academic and attention problems. Difficulties with acceptance of personal appearance and disability, social development (fewer friends, some isolation), and reduced influence on familial interactions are more apparent, especially in girls with spina bifida *myelomeningocele*. Development parallels typical adolescence despite these risk factors, with evidence of resilience. Family-based interventions are sometimes needed.

- *Psychiatric Complications* Infrequent as a primary problem, but common as a secondary problem, especially as children move into adolescence.

- *Medications* Although inattention is a common problem, response to stimulants generally is less positive than in developmental disorders. Commonly overmedicated when stimulants are used.

- *Interpersonal Relationships* Often very social, especially when young. Social issues can involve hypersociality and isolation, with fewer friends. Sometimes have difficulty sustaining relationships, especially in adolescence.

- *Functional Issues* Level of independence needs constant attention throughout development, especially in relation to parental expectations and tendencies toward reduced levels of physical activity and obesity.

- *Rehabilitation Considerations* Optimal rehabilitation interventions depend on a variety of factors including age and functional status. PT, OT, and speech-language therapy are routinely provided to support mobility and communication. Assistive devices (e.g., orthotics, braces, and wheelchairs) are often used.

Considerations when Treating Select Populations with Hydrocephalus

Pediatric Considerations

Children have variable outcomes and needs. A careful neuropsychological assessment should be conducted, especially in relation to academic skills and attention problems. Family issues often emerge for children with congenital hydrocephalus, especially in terms of the relation between parenting and level of independence. Parents need help in structuring environments and expectations to promote independence, especially because of motoric deficits that may prevent exploration in the young child and excessive parental responsiveness in older children. Tendencies to be protective are common, and many parents benefit from education about the nature of the disorder, parenting, and related areas. Close collaboration with other disciplines involved in care of this chronic disability, including neurosurgery, orthopedics, urology, and physical and occupational therapy, is vital. Interventions usually parallel those for children with developmental disorders of behavior, academic skills, and attention. For attention problems, response to stimulants is less positive than in developmental disorders, and other interventions need to take into account neuropsychological strengths and weaknesses. Public perception is often focused on orthopedic components, and schools often classify children as orthopedically impaired in terms of special needs. Hydrocephalus, per se, is not well understood as a factor in learning and development.

Transition

Many children with congenital hydrocephalus have trouble with major developmental transitions: childhood to adolescence and adolescence to adulthood. In the former, overall emotional adjustment may decline because of social isolation, the degree of disability, increased leaning difficulties in school, and sexual maturity. The child may seem to change from happy and outgoing to increasingly withdrawn. In moving into adulthood, many with congenital hydrocephalus experience difficulties adjusting to advanced academic placements and a vocation. Considerable support may be needed to help the adult achieve sufficient independence to live without assistance, form sustaining relations, and deal with the cumulative effects of long-term neuropsychological deficits. In adults, collaborations with vocational services and training are essential.

Geriatric Considerations

Older patients may have grown up with congenital hydrocephalus, and there is little information on this age group. Normal pressure hydrocephalus is a separate disorder that emerges idiopathically in people with hypertension, diabetes, and cardiovascular disease and as a secondary factor in people with dementia and stroke. Normal pressure hydrocephalus is often not identified and is frequently mistaken for dementia or Parkinson's disease. It is important to identify NPH, especially when it is idiopathic, because major sequelae may be reversible with shunting.

Acknowledgments

This research was supported by Eunice Kennedy Shriver National Institute of Child Health and Human Development Grant P01 HD35946 "Spina Bifida: Cognitive and Neurobiological Variability," Jack M. Fletcher and Maureen Dennis, Principal Investigators. The opinions expressed in this paper are not necessarily the opinions of the NICHD.

Relevant Definitions

Diastomyelia Rare spinal dysraphisms represented by congenital cleft or cavity in the spinal cord that gives the appearance of a split (tethered) or duplicated spinal cord.

Endoscopic third ventriculostomy An alternative to shunt implantation in which the floor of the third ventricle is perforated to permit the flow of CSF into an open CSF space (usually the subcistern). Only patients with specific characteristics are candidates for this procedure, which is more typically used with aqueductal stenosis and in developing countries where shunt technology is not widely available.

Hydrocephalus ex vacuo Expansion of the ventricles with no increase in ICP; also called arrested or compensated hydrocephalus.

Meningocele A rare spinal dysraphism in which the meninges protrude through the spinal cord, causing a bulge in the skin. There is a sac with CSF, but usually no CNS tissue. The brain of children with meningocele is often normal, although some develop hydrocephalus because of aqueductal stenosis. Problems with lower limb control and urinary problems occur below the level of the spinal lesion.

Myelomeningocele The most common form of spina dysraphism in which there is protrusion of the meninges through an incompletely formed spinal cord with a sac containing CSF and CNS material. A myelomeningocele is usually associated with the Chiari II malformation and is the primary cause of hydrocephalus in children.

Spina bifida occulta A common condition in otherwise healthy people in which the outer part of the spinal vertebrae are not completely closed. This form of spina bifida is often not identified except through radiological study and, in many cases, represents a normal variation that is asymptomatic.

Spinal lipoma A fatty tumor with fibrous material interlaced with the spinal cord. People with lipomas typically have normal brains, but orthopedic and urinary difficulties occur below the mass.

Congenital and Acquired Hydrocephalus Questions

NOTE: Questions 63, 79, 106, and 119 on the First Full-Length Practice Examination, Questions 17, 78, and 104 on the Second Full-Length Practice Examination, Questions 47, 73, and 120 on the Third Full-Length Practice Examination, and Questions 11, 45, and 101 on the Fourth Full-Length Practice Examination are from this chapter.

1. Spina bifida is a neural tube defect _____.
   (a) that is usually associated with hydrocephalus because of a stenosis of the aqueduct of Sylvius
   (b) in which hydrocephalus occurs largely in association with a myelomeningocele
   (c) that is increasing in prevalence in North America because of environmental toxins
   (d) that affects word reading skills more frequently than computational math skills

2. Shunt treatment for children with early hydrocephalus is _____.
   (a) always required because of the pressure it puts on parenchymal tissue
   (b) required in most cases because of severity of aqueductal stenosis
   (c) not required because over time the flow of CSF typically stabilizes
   (d) essential in children with elevated ICP and progressive ventricular expansion

3. Aqueductal stenosis is _____.
   (a) a brain malformation characterized by congenital narrowing of the aqueduct of Sylvius
   (b) typically a form of communicating hydrocephalus
   (c) usually identified at birth because of the enlarged head
   (d) not identified until the person develops symptoms like headaches and vomiting

4. The incidence of neural tube defects has been _____.
   (a) stable over the past several decades since the advent of shunting
   (b) declining due to folate acid supplementation and dietary fortification
   (c) traditionally much higher in boys than in girls
   (d) increasing for spina bifida and decreasing for anencephaly

5. Acute hydrocephalus ____.

   (a) needs to be monitored because it will normalize as fluid dynamics stabilize

   (b) primarily affects motor function and gait, not cognition

   (c) has primary effects on neuropsychological tests of higher cortical functions

   (d) requires monitoring and may require intervention, usually through a new shunt or shunt revision

6. Social skills in children and adults with congenital hydrocephalus ____.

   (a) are a problem because of introversion

   (b) can be a relative strength

   (c) are usually severely impaired

   (d) are like those seen in children with ADHD

7. Hydrocephalus develops in infants born prematurely ____.

   (a) because of secondary effects of cerebral palsy

   (b) due to another disorder that causes hydrocephalus

   (c) as a consequence of an intraventricular hemorrhage

   (d) because of extremely low birth weight

8. Prenatal surgery for myelomeningocele ____.

   (a) improves motor and cognitive functions

   (b) is dangerous and ineffective

   (c) improves motor but not cognitive functions

   (d) improves cognitive but not motor functions

9. In children and adults with spina bifida, neuropsychological assessments are most useful for ____.

   (a) determining the type of neural tube defect that caused hydrocephalus

   (b) evaluating shunt status

   (c) inferring brain dysfunction

   (d) determining strengths and weaknesses for treatment planning

10. Communicating hydrocephalus is ____.

   (a) always obstructive

   (b) usually due to abnormalities of CSF absorption

   (c) associated with increased intracranial pressure

   (d) different from hydrocephalus ex vacuo

11. It is important to identify, monitor, and treat normal pressure hydrocephalus ____.

   (a) because treatment that reduces elevated ICP may restore cognitive and motor functions

   (b) to ensure that the patient does not have dementia

   (c) to ensure that a hemorrhagic stroke does not lead to more bleeding

   (d) because Medicare requires treatment

12. Intraventricular hemorrhage in low birth weight infants ____.

    (a) is decreasing because of interventions that prevent germinal matrix hemorrhage

    (b) is increasing because more extremely low birth weight infants are born each year

    (c) is reliably associated with hydrocephalus

    (d) requires shunting

13. Neuropsychological assessment is important in normal pressure hydrocephalus to determine ____.

    (a) the type of dementia affecting the patient

    (b) the presence of increased ICP

    (c) the presence of cognitive difficulties and restoration after intervention

    (d) whether the effect on the brain is focal or diffuse

14. Dandy-Walker syndrome is ____.

    (a) a form of communicating hydrocephalus

    (b) a fourth ventricle cyst often with agenesis of the vermis

    (c) similar to the Chiari II malformation in myelomeningocele

    (d) a common form of congenital hydrocephalus

15. Hydrocephalus ____.

    (a) predominantly affects the white matter in the right hemisphere

    (b) affects white matter and gray matter of the brain

    (c) only affects the gray matter of the brain

    (d) predominantly affects the gray matter in the left hemisphere

Congenital and Acquired Hydrocephalus Answers

1. **B—in which hydrocephalus occurs largely in association with a myelomeningocele** *Myelomeningocele usually presents with the Chiari II malformation that obstructs the flow of CSF.*

   Reference: Barkovich, A. J., & Raybaud, C. (2018). *Pediatric neuroimaging* (6th ed.). Philadelphia, PA: Lippincott Williams and Wilkins.

2. **D—essential in children with elevated ICP and progressive ventricular expansion** *Progressive hydrocephalus can be fatal.*

   Reference: Swaiman, K. F., Ashwal, S., Ferriero, D. M., Schor, N. F., Finkel, R. S., Gropman, A. L., . . . Shevell, M. I. (2017). *Swaiman's pediatric neurology: Principles and practices* (6th ed.). New York, NY: Elsevier.

3. **A—a brain malformation characterized by congenital narrowing of the aqueduct of Sylvius** *Since the CSF cannot flow freely from the aqueduct into and out of the fourth ventricle, this would be a non-communicating form of hydrocephalus.*

   Reference: Swaiman, K. F., Ashwal, S., Ferriero, D. M., Schor, N. F., Finkel, R. S., Gropman, A. L., . . . Shevell, M. I. (2017). *Swaiman's pediatric neurology: Principles and practices* (6th ed.). New York, NY: Elsevier.

4. **B—declining due to folate acid supplementation and dietary fortification** *Rates of all NTDs have declined by about 30% since the advent of folate supplementation.*

Reference: Au, K. S., Ashley-Koch, A., & Northrup, H. (2010). Epidemiologic and genetic aspects of spina bifida and other neural tube defects. *Developmental Disabilities Research Reviews, 16,* 6–25.

5. **D—requires monitoring and may require intervention, usually through a new shunt or shunt revision** *Progressive hydrocephalus can be fatal and cause additional injury to the brain if it persists and is not treated.*

Reference: Swaiman, K. F., Ashwal, S., Ferriero, D. M., Schor, N. F., Finkel, R. S., Gropman, A. L., . . . Shevell, M. I. (2017). *Swaiman's pediatric neurology: Principles and practices* (6th ed.). New York, NY: Elsevier.

6. **B—can be a relative strength** *People with early hydrocephalus, especially spina bifida, are often amiable and extraverted. Some children are hypersocial to the point of being overly friendly and not safe.*

Reference: Fletcher, J. M., & Dennis, M. (2010). Spina bifida and hydrocephalus: Modeling variability in outcome domains. In K. O. Yeates, M. D. Ris, H. G. Taylor, & B. F. Pennington (Eds.) *Pediatric neuropsychology: Research, theory, and practice* (2nd ed., pp. 3–25). Hillsdale, NJ: Erlbaum.

7. **C—as a consequence of an intraventricular hemorrhage** *The germinal matrix hemorrhage is so severe that it obstructs the flow of CSF.*

Reference: Swaiman, K. F., Ashwal, S., Ferriero, D. M., Schor, N. F., Finkel, R. S., Gropman, A. L., . . . Shevell, M. I. (2017). *Swaiman's pediatric neurology: Principles and practices* (6th ed.). New York, NY: Elsevier.

8. **C—improves motor but not cognitive functions** *The management of myelomeningocele (MOMS) clinical trial found that children were more likely to walk independently and had higher overall motor and sensorimotor functions than children treated postnatally. There were no differences in cognitive functions.*

Reference: Adzick, N. S., Thom, E. A., Spong, C. Y., Brock, J. W., 3rd, Burrows, P. K., Johnson, M. P. . . . MOMS Investigators (2011). A randomized trial of prenatal versus postnatal repair of myelomeningocele. *New England Journal of Medicine, 364,* 993–1004.

9. **D—determining strengths and weaknesses for treatment planning** *Because of the variability in outcomes, children and adults with spina bifida need neuropsychological evaluations to identify patterns of cognitive, adaptive, and behavioral strengths and weaknesses in order to plan an intervention program addressing their individual needs.*

Reference: Fletcher, J. M., & Dennis, M. (2010). Spina bifida and hydrocephalus: Modeling variability in outcome domains. In K. O. Yeates, M. D. Ris, H. G. Taylor, & B. F. Pennington (Eds.) *Pediatric neuropsychology: Research, theory, and practice* (2nd ed., pp. 3–25). Hillsdale, NJ: Erlbaum.

10. **B—usually involves abnormalities of CSF absorption** *Communicating hydrocephalus, also known as hydrocephalus ex vacuo, is not an obstructive process and may not involve increased ICP. The ventricles are enlarged because CSF is not adequately reabsorbed.*

Reference: Swaiman, K. F., Ashwal, S., Ferriero, D. M., Schor, N. F., Finkel, R. S., Gropman, A. L., . . . Shevell, M. I. (2017). *Swaiman's pediatric neurology: Principles and practices* (6th ed.). New York, NY: Elsevier.

11. **A—because treatment that reduces elevated ICP may restore cognitive and motor functions** *NPH should be identified and treated because increased ICP and ventricular dilation leads to motor and cognitive difficulties that may be reversible with treatment.*

Reference: Sinforiano, E., Pacchetti, C., Picascia, M., Pozzi, N. G., Todisco, M., & Vitali, P. (2018). Clinical and cognitive features of idiopathic normal pressure hydrocephalus. In B. Gürer (Ed.), *Hydrocephalus—Water on the brain* (pp. 43–74). IntertechOpen.

12. **A—is decreasing because of interventions that prevent germinal matrix hemorrhage** *Successful interventions in the Neonatal Intensive Care Unit have reduced the incidence and severity of IVH.*

    Reference: Swaiman, K. F., Ashwal, S., Ferriero, D. M., Schor, N. F., Finkel, R. S., Gropman, A. L., . . . Shevell, M. I. (2017). *Swaiman's pediatric neurology: Principles and practices* (6th ed.). New York, NY: Elsevier.

13. **C—the presence of cognitive difficulties and restoration after intervention** *Neuropsychological evaluation can assist in identifying the extent of cognitive impairment associated with NPH and the degree of restoration after intervention.*

    Reference: Sinforiano, E., Pacchetti, C., Picascia, M., Pozzi, N. G., Todisco, M., & Vitali, P. (2018). Clinical and cognitive features of idiopathic normal pressure hydrocephalus. In B. Gürer (Ed.), *Hydrocephalus—Water on the brain* (pp. 43–74). IntertechOpen.

14. **B—a fourth ventricle cyst often with agenesis of the vermis** *Although there are variants of Dandy-Walker syndrome, the classic form is with a fourth ventricle cyst and partial to complete agenesis of the cerebellar vermis.*

    Reference: Barkovich, A. J., & Raybaud, C. (2018). *Pediatric neuroimaging* (6th ed.). Philadelphia, PA: Lippincott Williams and Wilkins.

15. **B—affects white matter and gray matter of the brain.** *At a neuropathological level, the general effects of hydrocephalus can be understood as a subcortical disconnection syndrome because of injury to the long periventricular pathways (e.g., corpus callosum, projection pathways); however, hydrocephalus is not strictly an injury to the white matter, as it has widespread effects on the brain including on gray matter as well.*

    Reference: Del Bigio, M. (2010). Neuropathology and structural changes in hydrocephalus. *Developmental Disabilities Research Reviews, 16,* 16–23.

Recommended Readings

Barkovich, A. J. & Raybaud, C. (2018). *Pediatric neuroimaging* (6th ed.). Philadelphia, PA: Lippincott Williams and Wilkins.

Copp, A. J., Adzick, A. S., Chitty, L. S., Fletcher, J. M., Holmbeck, G. N., & Shaw, G. M. (2015). Spina bifida. *Nature Disease Primers, 1,* 1–18.

Fletcher J. M., & Dennis, M. (2010). Spina bifida and hydrocephalus: Modeling variability in outcome domains. In K. O. Yeates, M. D. Ris, H. G. Taylor, & B. F. Pennington (Eds.), *Pediatric neuropsychology: Research, theory, and practice* (2nd ed., pp. 3–25). Hillsdale, NJ: Erlbaum.

Sinforiano, E., Pacchetti, C., Picascia, M., Pozzi, N. G., Todisco, M., & Vitali, P. (2018). Clinical and cognitive features of idiopathic normal pressure hydrocephalus. In B. Gürer (Ed.), *Hydrocephalus—Water on the brain* (pp. 43–74). IntertechOpen.

Swaiman, K. F., Ashwal, S., Ferriero, D. M., Schor, N. F., Finkel, R. S., Gropman, A. L., . . . Shevell, M. I. (2017). *Swaiman's pediatric neurology: Principles and practices* (6th ed.). New York, NY: Elsevier.

21   Toxic Exposure in Utero

Doug Bodin and Christine Clancy

Section 1: Drugs of Abuse—Alcohol

Definition

Alcohol (ethanol) is a teratogen that passes through the placental barrier and affects the developing fetus throughout gestation. Intrauterine alcohol exposure results in a heterogeneous pattern of neurological, cognitive, behavioral, and physical symptoms that have been defined differently across a variety of classification systems. Fetal alcohol spectrum disorder (FASD) is an umbrella term, not a diagnostic term, that describes the craniofacial, cardiovascular, skeletal, and neurological deficits that can occur when alcohol is consumed during pregnancy. Per the Institute of Medicine (IOM), the medical disorders that collectively comprise FASD include fetal alcohol syndrome (FAS) and partial FAS (pFAS), alcohol-related birth defects (ARBD), and alcohol-related neurodevelopmental disorder (ARND) (see Tables 21.1 and 21.2). The most recent edition of the *Diagnostic and Statistical Manual of Mental Disorders* (DSM-5; American Psychiatric Association, 2013) now includes the diagnosis, Neurobehavioral Disorder Associated with Prenatal Alcohol Exposure (ND-PAE). Many children with histories of prenatal alcohol exposure do not meet the diagnostic criteria of FAS. These children lack the characteristic facial features of FAS and have variously been labeled as having pFAS or ARND. Fetal alcohol spectrum disorders are the leading cause of preventable intellectual disability (ID), birth defects (i.e., heart, kidney, and bone problems and other malformations; difficulty seeing and hearing; and reduced immune function) and developmental disorders in the Western hemisphere and result in a substantial burden of cost. Consensus at this time is that no level of alcohol consumption during pregnancy is considered safe.

Neuropathology

Prenatal alcohol exposure leads to alterations in size and structure across brain regions. During the first and second trimester, prenatal alcohol consumption interferes with the migration, proliferation, and organization of brain cells, resulting in varying craniofacial and brain malformations. During the third trimester, consumption is associated with damage to the cerebellum, hippocampus, and prefrontal cortex. Neurochemical effects of alcohol may include:

- Increased turnover of norepinephrine and dopamine
- Decreased transmission in acetylcholine systems
- Increased transmission in gamma-aminobutyric acid (GABA) systems
- Increased production of beta-endorphin in the hypothalamus

Structural Neuroimaging Studies

Neuroimaging techniques continue to change and improve, which has resulted in inconsistencies within the literature with respect to structural and functional research findings. However, mounting evidence

TABLE 21.1 Institute of Medicine Diagnostic Classifications for Fetal Alcohol Spectrum Disorder (FASD)

Fetal Alcohol Syndrome (FAS)
FAS with confirmed maternal alcohol exposure
A. Confirmed maternal alcohol exposure
B. Evidence of a characteristic pattern of facial anomalies that includes features such as short palpebral fissures and abnormalities in the premaxillary zone (e.g., flat upper lip, flattened philtrum, and flat midface)
C. Evidence of growth retardation
D. Evidence of central nervous system (CNS) abnormalities such as structural brain abnormalities or neurologic hard or soft signs
FAS without confirmed maternal alcohol exposure
B, C, and D as above
Partial FAS with confirmed maternal alcohol exposure
A. Confirmed maternal alcohol exposure
B. Evidence of some components of the pattern of characteristic facial anomalies, as well as either C or D or E
C. Evidence of growth retardation
D. Evidence of CNS abnormalities such as structural brain abnormalities or neurologic hard or soft signs
E. Evidence of a pattern of behavior or cognitive abnormalities that are inconsistent with developmental level and cannot be explained by familial background or environment alone (e.g., learning difficulties, poor impulse control)

across various studies reveals that white matter may be disproportionately impacted in FASD. Additional structural brain abnormalities associated with FASD include, but are not limited to, the following:

- Microcephaly
- Migrational anomalies (e.g., heterotopias)
- Disproportionate reductions in gray and white matter volumes, particularly in frontal, parietal, and temporal lobes
- White matter hypoplasia > gray matter hypoplasia.

Diagnosis of FAS

As a consequence of the heterogeneity of clinical presentation, a variety of medical classification systems have been developed. Although some variability exists across classifications, the following four criteria must be met for a medical FAS diagnosis (See Table 21.1):

1. *Growth Deficiency* Defined as below average height and/or weight. Babies with FAS are often small for gestational age and may continue to show growth deficiency as adolescents and adults.

2. *Craniofacial Features* Specific pattern of facial anomalies that include short palpebral fissures (eye width decreases with increased prenatal alcohol exposure), a flat midface, a short upturned nose, a smooth or long philtrum (the ridges running between the nose and the lip), and a thin vermilion (the upper lip thins with increased prenatal alcohol exposure). See Figure 21.1.

TABLE 21.2 Institute of Medicine Diagnostic Classifications for Alcohol-Related Effects

Alcohol-Related Effects	
Clinical conditions in which there is a history of maternal alcohol exposure, and where clinical or animal research has linked maternal alcohol ingestion to an observed outcome. There are two categories which may co-occur. If both diagnoses are present, then both diagnoses should be rendered	

Alcohol-Related Birth Defects (ARBD)	
Congenital anomalies, including malformations and dysplasias	
Cardiac	
Atrial septal defects	Aberrant great vessels
Ventricular septal defects	Tetralogy of Fallot
Skeletal	
Hypoplastic nails	Clinodactyly
Shortened fifth digits	Pectus excavatum and carinatum
Radioulnar synostosis	Klippel-Feil syndrome
Flexion contractures	Hemivertebrae
Camptodactyly	Scoliosis
Renal	
Aplastic, dysplastic, hypoplastic kidneys	Ureteral duplications
Horseshoe kidneys	Hydronephrosis
Ocular	
Strabismus	Refractive problems secondary to small globes
Retinal vascular anomalies	
Auditory	
Conductive hearing loss	Neurosensory hearing loss
Other	
Virtually every malformation has been described in some patient with FAS. The etiologic specificity of most of these anomalies to alcohol teratogenesis remains uncertain.	

Alcohol-Related Neurodevelopmental Disorder (ARND)	
Presence of A or B or both	
A. Evidence of central nervous system (CNS) abnormalities such as structural brain abnormalities or neurologic hard or soft signs	
B. Evidence of a pattern of behavior or cognitive abnormalities that are inconsistent with developmental level and cannot be explained by familial background or environment alone (e.g., learning difficulties, poor impulse control)	

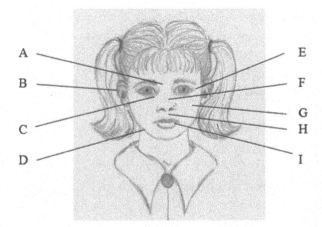

FIGURE 21.1 Facial Dysmorphology Characteristic of Fetal Alcohol Syndrome

Associated Features: A—low nasal bridge; B—minor ear anomalies; C—epicanthal folds; D—small jaw. **Discriminating Features:** E—short palpebral fissures; F—short nose; G—flat mid-face; H—indistinct philtrum; I—thin upper lip.

3. *Central Nervous System Dysfunction* Central nervous system (CNS) damage can be assessed structurally, neurologically, and functionally:

- *Structural abnormalities*: Includes microcephaly of two or more standard deviations (SD) below the mean, callosal agenesis, or cerebellar hypoplasia.

- *Hard neurologic signs*: May include seizure disorders or another diagnosable disability. Soft neurological signs, which require more clinical judgment, may be also apparent, including fine or gross motor problems and hearing loss.

- *Functional abnormalities*: Includes general cognitive deficits, deficits in memory, executive functions, attentional deficits, and learning disabilities.

4. *Prenatal Alcohol Exposure* Confirmed or unknown prenatal alcohol exposure. Women often have difficulty accurately recalling the frequency or amount of alcohol consumption during pregnancy. At present, no biochemical marker can reliably confirm maternal alcohol consumption in pregnancy; however, studies are investigating the utility of fatty acid ethyl esters in meconium as markers for prenatal exposure.

DSM-5 Diagnostic Criteria for Neurodevelopmental Disorder Associated with Prenatal Alcohol Exposure (ND-PAE)

The DSM-5 diagnostic criteria of ND-PAE is listed as a diagnosis under Other Specified Neurodevelopmental Disorder. To meet criteria for a psychiatric diagnosis of ND-PAE, an individual must have been exposed to alcohol at some point during gestation, and that the exposure was more than "minimal," although that determination is left up to clinical judgment. In addition, an individual must also display impaired neurocognitive functioning, self-regulation, and adaptive functioning.

Epidemiology

The incidence rates of FAS vary widely across countries due to different screening measures and underidentification or misdiagnosis. Recent data estimate the global prevalence of FAS to be 10%. The general incidence of FAS is more than two times higher in the United States (1–3 per 1,000) compared to Europe and other countries (0.8 per 1,000). The rate of FASD in the United States is as high as 9.1 per 1,000 live births. In European studies, the major factor associated with FAS is low socioeconomic status (SES) rather than racial background, whereas in the United States, race and SES are often confounded. In the United States, FAS is associated with higher maternal age and lower education level, diverse racial, educational, and economic backgrounds, untreated or undertreated mental health issues, social isolation, and a history of abuse. African American or Native American populations, which are typically characterized by lower SES, have incidence rates approximately 10 times higher (2.29 per 1,000) than those of middle and upper SES and Caucasian backgrounds (0.26 per 1,000). The rate of FASDs is reported as being as high as 9.1 per 1,000 live births in the United States, comparable with or higher than rates for other developmental disabilities such as Down syndrome or spina bifida.

Determinants of Severity

- *Quantity (Dose) Consumed* Although alcohol is a known teratogen, there is no clear consensus as to what level of exposure is considered toxic; however, the diagnostic criteria developed at the University of Washington (Astley, 2004) state the following:
  - *High risk*: A blood alcohol concentration (BAC) greater than 100 mg/dL delivered at least weekly in *early* pregnancy (roughly equivalent to a 55 kg/121 pound woman drinking 6 to 8 beers in one sitting)
  - *Some risk*: The confirmed use of alcohol during pregnancy with use less than high risk or unknown usage patterns
  - *Unknown risk*: The unknown use of alcohol during pregnancy
  - *No risk*: The confirmed absence of prenatal alcohol exposure, which rules out a diagnosis of FAS.
- *Pattern of Exposure* Chronic consumption (four to five drinks daily) and binge drinking, which equates to five or more standard drinks (e.g., 12 oz. of beer; 5 oz. table wine; 1.5 oz. of spirts) in one sitting or more than nine drinks per week, are associated with FAS. Lesser quantities consumed during pregnancy are associated with ARBD and ARND.
- *Timing of Exposure* First trimester drinking increases the likelihood of FASD 12x; drinking during the first and second trimester increases the likelihood of FASD 61x, and drinking in all three trimesters increases the likelihood of FASD 65x.
- *Additional Risk Factors*
  - Polydrug use (e.g., licit or illicit drugs) and their synergistic interactions
  - Higher maternal age
  - Maternal mental health issues
  - Lower education level
  - Reduced access to prenatal and postnatal care and services
  - Inadequate nutrition
  - An environment that includes stress, abuse, and/or neglect

Presentation, Disease Course, and Recovery

Children with FAS have CNS damage that leads to lifelong neurocognitive and behavioral problems. Adolescents and adults with FAS face:

- School failure/greater likelihood to drop out of high school
- Inability to secure and hold employment
- Mental health issues
- Delinquency; involvement with the law

Expectations for Neuropsychological Assessment Results

- *Intelligence/Achievement* Great variability in intellectual performance: IQ scores range from 20 to 120, with an average between 65 and 72. Children with more dysmorphic features tend to have lower IQ scores. Approximately 25% of people with FAS and 10% of people with ARND have IQ scores of 70 or below. Even if a child with FASD does not have an ID, the child often has learning problems that interfere with sound judgment and can cause behavioral problems that significantly impact his or her life. Some studies report greater impairment in verbal than nonverbal abilities, but findings are not consistent. Learning difficulties, lower overall school performance, disrupted school attendance, lower performance in reading and spelling, and deficits in mathematical skills have been reported.

- *Attention/Concentration* A large proportion of children (60–95%) with FASDs qualify for a diagnosis of ADHD; the disorder is 3–9 times higher in children with FASD than in the general population. Pervasive deficits in visual sustained attention have been found. Deficits in auditory visual attention are task dependent and occur when intertarget intervals are long.

- *Processing Speed* Deficits in reaction time and cognitive efficiency have been found when tasks are more challenging and require complex cognition and the use of working memory.

- *Speech and Language* Secondary to craniofacial abnormalities, some studies have reported problems with oral-motor function and speech production. Deficits in confrontation naming have been reported, as well as expressive and receptive language disorders. Problems with comprehension of higher level language, such as metaphors, sarcasm, and idioms, as well as deficits in pragmatic language and social discourse, have been documented.

- *Visuospatial* Deficits in local versus global analysis of hierarchical visual stimuli have been documented. Deficits in visuospatial construction (e.g., copying task) have been reported, although reduced performance is thought to be associated with motor deficits.

- *Memory* Verbal learning and memory deficits have been documented in children exposed to alcohol secondary to dysfunction in hippocampal dendrites; retention is intact when an implicit strategy is used. Deficits in memorizing verbal and nonverbal information result from difficulties with the acquisition of the information rather than the ability to remember the information over time. Studies examining visual memory are inconsistent in their findings. Some show impaired spatial recall, others show sparing of spatial retention and object recall.

- *Executive Functions (EF)* Deficits have been documented across many EF domains, including verbal and nonverbal fluency, response inhibition, planning and organization, cognitive flexibility, and concept formation.

- *Sensorimotor Functions* Delayed motor development and fine motor deficits associated with reduced cerebellar size have been reported including tremors, weak grasp, and poor eye-hand coordination. Balance is particularly affected secondary to cerebellar involvement, but performance varies across task demands. Sensory integration problems, tactile defensiveness, and reduced or undersensitivity to stimulation have been reported.

- *Emotion and Personality* Children exposed prenatally to alcohol are often classified as restless, impulsive, inattentive, disruptive, aggressive, or delinquent. Some children display socially disinhibited behavior, such as boundary issues, social intrusiveness, and lack of awareness of social dangers. Elevated levels of both internalizing and externalizing behavior disorders have been documented. Lack of social judgment, deficits in moral development, and failure to learn and generalize from experience contribute to problems with socialization. In later childhood and young adulthood, they are more likely to engage in antisocial behaviors and juvenile delinquency. There is significantly more sleep disturbance, shortened sleep duration and an increased rate of night awakenings, which interfere with school performance, learning, memory, academic performance, mood and behavior. Deficits in adaptive behavior exist across communication, socialization, and daily living skills domains.

Considerations when Treating Patients with FASDs

The Importance of Early Diagnosis

Only a fraction of those exposed to alcohol in utero currently receive a diagnosis because of limited expertise and the need for comprehensive multidisciplinary diagnostic evaluation. Early diagnosis is essential because early interventions and resources may:

- Mitigate the development of secondary disabilities in childhood and adulthood (e.g., disrupted school experience/school failure, unemployment, mental health problems, trouble with the law, alcohol and drug problems)

- Allow appropriate intervention, counseling, and treatment to the mother to prevent the birth of additional affected children

- Prompt caregivers, physicians, and other professionals to seek diagnosis and support for siblings who may also be affected

Comorbid Diagnoses

Fetal alcohol spectrum disorders are associated with increased rates of ADHD, conduct disorder (CD), oppositional defiant disorder (ODD), and obsessive-compulsive disorder (OCD).

Protective Factors

- *Early diagnosis* is a universal protective indicator for all secondary disabilities. In one study, only 11% of individuals with FASD were diagnosed by age 6. Every effort must be made to attain early diagnoses for children with FASD.

- *Services* from governmental developmental disabilities programs. These services are needed by most individuals with FASD, yet most do not qualify.

- *Living in a stable home* with nurturing parents.

- *Protection from violence*, specifically from witnessing or being victimized by violence.

Section 2: Drugs of Abuse—Cocaine

Definition

Cocaine is a crystalline alkaloid derived from leaves of the coca plant. In utero exposure occurs primarily through maternal use of crack cocaine.

Neuropathology

In utero exposure to cocaine affects the CNS via its effects on the monoamine system, especially dopamine. Exposure early in gestation affects neural proliferation and migration, whereas exposure during later gestational stages may affect neuronal maturation and synaptogenesis. In utero exposure to cocaine may lead to abnormalities in the frontocingulate cortex, including the anterior cingulate gyrus.

Epidemiology

In the United States, prenatal exposure to cocaine occurs in 30,000–160,000 infants annually. Approximately 0.5–3% of pregnant women worldwide are estimated to use cocaine. Infants prenatally exposed to cocaine are often born with small head circumference and low birth weight.

Determinants of Severity

Studies have found a dose-response relationship between amount of in utero exposure and later neurobehavioral problems.

Presentation, Disease Course, and Recovery

Infants exposed to cocaine in utero often display many neurobehavioral characteristics during the neonatal period including poor sleep cycles, abnormal startle response, abnormal brainstem evoked potentials, and other evidence of immature neurological functioning. Toddler/preschoolers who were exposed prenatally often show impulsivity and emotional lability in response to frustration.

Expectations for Neuropsychological Assessment Results

- *Intelligence/Achievement* Studies have documented lower overall IQ in children exposed to cocaine in utero. Deficits in academic achievement may be more related to environmental variables, such as parent education and SES.
- *Attention/Concentration* Deficits in sustained and selected attention are the most consistently documented neuropsychological deficits.
- *Processing Speed* Slower reaction times have been documented on continuous performance tasks, although this may be a function of poor attention regulation.
- *Language* Language delay has been documented, with expressive language being most affected
- *Visuospatial* Deficits in visual perceptual organization are common.
- *Memory* Primary deficits in working memory are consistently documented.
- *Executive Functions* Perseveration, disinhibition, and poor task orientation have been found.
- *Emotion and Personality* Children exposed to cocaine prenatally are often impulsive and display poor emotional control. Emotional/behavioral problems are more likely to be seen in frustrating or novel contexts.

Considerations when Treating or Evaluating Patients with Cocaine Exposure

Research on the neurobehavioral/neuropsychological outcomes of children exposed to cocaine in utero is made difficult by several confounding variables including maternal use of multiple substances during pregnancy, low SES, lack of prenatal care, and poor pre- and postnatal nutrition. Although many studies have documented deficits in emotional and behavioral regulation in children exposed to cocaine prenatally, the literature on specific treatments for these children is sparse.

Section 3: Drugs of Abuse—Marijuana (Cannabis)

Definition

Marijuana is the most commonly used illicit drug. Marijuana is derived from the Cannabis plant and is used for its psychoactive and medicinal properties (e.g., it is used medically for the stimulation of hunger, pain relief, and reduction of nausea and vomiting). Cannabis preparations are largely derived from the female plant of Cannabis sativa, and consist of approximately 60 plant-derived cannabinoid compounds (phytocannabinoids), with Δ9-tetrahydrocannabinol (THC) being the predominant psychoactive constituent. The cannabinoid receptor type 1 (CB1) is the primary target in the brain for THC, and the rewarding property of cannabis has been associated with the mesocorticolimbic dopamine system. Delta-9 (Δ9) THC, the main psychoactive compound, produces changes in mood, perception, motor coordination, short-term and working memory, and concentration.

THC readily crosses the placenta during gestation. THC is secreted in maternal milk during lactation at estimates of up to eightfold higher concentrations in breast milk than in maternal plasma concentrations.

Neuropathology

The endocannabinoid system exists from the earliest stage of pregnancy, in the preimplantation embryo and uterus, placenta, and in the developing fetal brain, presenting multiple points of vulnerability throughout gestation. Prenatal cannabis exposure (PCE) has been found to be associated with fetal growth restriction in mid and late pregnancy, and also with lower birthweight. Continued PCE affects dopamine signaling within and beyond the mesolimbic system.

Infants exposed to cannabis in utero have not been found to be at increased risk of birth defects, but an increased risk of stillbirth among women who used marijuana in pregnancy has been demonstrated. Altered sleep patterns have been found, with cannabis-exposed infants displaying increased irritability, excitability and arousal 24–72 hours after birth. Heavy marijuana exposure is reported to cause delay in infant visual maturation and visual attentiveness. The most consistent and visible consequences of regular heavy marijuana consumption is significantly heightened tremors, exaggerated startle and visual responses, and poor habituation to novel stimuli, which is thought to reflect nervous system immaturity and/ or drug withdrawal. Other motor differences observed among the infants of heavy marijuana users include an exaggerated Moro reflex, increased occurrence of athetoid movements, and disinhibition in a number of motor tests, which are behaviors similar to those observed in infants undergoing narcotic withdrawal.

Epidemiology

Three longitudinal studies of PCE have been conducted (Canada, United States, Europe):

- After alcohol and tobacco, it is the next most used drug during pregnancy.

- The Substance Abuse and Mental Health Services Administration estimates that 7% of pregnant women aged 18–25 used illicit drugs in the month prior to being surveyed. Marijuana was the most prevalent substance abused, ranging from 2–6% usage as determined by interview or self-report.

- Marijuana use in pregnancy is expected to rise with increased legalization of the drug throughout the Canada and the United States and with increased use in alternative forms, such as vaping, lotions, and edibles.

- Women with severe nausea and vomiting in pregnancy are more likely to report usage.

- Heavy marijuana use has been associated with increased alcohol consumption, as well as tobacco and other illicit drugs during pregnancy.

- Using marijuana six or more times per week on average during pregnancy has been associated with a significant reduction in length of gestation (by 1.1 weeks) after statistically adjusting for nicotine, alcohol, parity, mother's prepregnancy weight, and the child's sex.

- Boys exhibit greater vulnerability when tested for performance in attention, learning, and memory after PCE.

Determinants of Severity

The effects of prenatal marijuana exposure are difficult to parse out from other environmental risk factors such as polydrug use, low SES, maternal mental health, exposure to violence, and limited access to medical and social services.

Expectations for Neuropsychological Assessment Results

- *Intelligence/Achievement* Prenatal marijuana exposure does not appear to affect overall IQ, but it has been associated with underachievement in reading and spelling. Lower scores occur in reading, math and spelling, most notably in those exposed to heavy marijuana use in the first trimester when home environment, race/ethnicity, socioeconomic status, and other prenatal substance use were controlled.

- *Attention/Concentration* Studies have shown problems with attention and concentration; however, prenatal alcohol exposure was often a confounding factor. One study showed that of children exposed prenatally, the first- and third-trimester exposures predicted increased hyperactivity, inattention, and impulsivity in later childhood and adolescence.

- *Executive Functions* Deficits evident in top-down processing, including working memory, focused attention, behavioral inhibition, self-regulation and monitoring, and cognitive flexibility.

- *Visuospatial* A neuroimaging study has shown altered neural functioning during visuospatial working memory processing after controlling for other prenatal and current drug use.

One study showed prenatal exposure predicted visual memory, analysis, and integration deficiencies. Problems with abstract and visual reasoning, and visual-perceptual functioning have also been documented.

- *Sensorimotor Functions* Prenatal exposure to marijuana is associated with decreased rates of visual habituation and increased tremors in 4-day-old infants. By 1 year of age, however, no adverse behavioral effects of prenatal marijuana exposure were noted.

- *Emotion and Personality* One study showed that offspring of heavy marijuana users were significantly more likely to report delinquent behavior in middle adolescence, after controlling for maternal substance use, household income, home environment, maternal IQ, and child's race. PCE is a contributory factor for increased vulnerability to neuropsychiatric disorders (e.g., schizophrenia). There is an increased rated of mood (i.e., depressive symptoms) and behavior dysregulation (impulsivity and hyperactivity) and delinquent behavior in children with PCE

Section 4: Environmental Toxicants–Mercury

Definition

Mercury (Hg) is a natural element that exists in the environment in metallic, inorganic, and organic forms. The most common compound, methylmercury, is formed in water and soil by microscopic organisms. Mercury is widely used in industry, agriculture, and healthcare. Common sources of mercury include fungicides and pesticides (most contain methylmercury), cosmetics, dental fillings, commercial thermometers, and high-efficiency compact fluorescent bulbs (CFL). Coal-fired power plants, which release mercury into the air when coal is burned, are the largest man-made source of mercury. Airborne mercury makes its way into water sources and bioaccumulates in fish. Eating fish contaminated with methylmercury is the primary human exposure. The highest concentrations occur in predatory species (e.g., shark, tuna, and swordfish) and shellfish.

Neuropathology

Mercury in its many forms can be ingested, inhaled, or absorbed through the skin. Neurologic, gastrointestinal, and renal systems are the most commonly affected organ systems in mercury exposure. When handled, elemental mercury (e.g., silvery liquid found in barometers) is absorbed very slowly through the skin; mercury vapor is absorbed about 50 times faster through the lungs. Methylmercury, an organic mercury compound, binds to proteins and compounds and gains access to brain tissues by active transport into the endothelial cells in the blood-brain barrier. Methylmercury destroys neurons and causes cerebral atrophy in both hemispheres. Dimethylmercury is the deadliest of the mercury compounds. It easily permeates the skin, gets into the bloodstream, and is deposited in the brain, kidneys, and other organs, resulting in acute mercury poisoning. Symptoms begin with paresthesia, deterioration in fine motor coordination, and restriction of the visual fields, and then progresses to severe ataxia, dementia, and death.

Pre- and Postnatal Exposure to Mercury

Pregnant women with a diet high in fish and shellfish are at greatest risk of methylmercury exposure. Because it is lipophilic (fat soluble), methylmercury crosses the placental barrier and the blood-brain barrier and is poorly excreted by the fetus, allowing accumulation in the CNS. Neuropathology in fetal cases is more widespread than in children or adults and can result in atrophy and hypoplasia of the cerebral cortex and corpus callosum, abnormal cytoarchitecture, and dysmyelination of the pyramidal tract.

Mercury's harmful effects to the fetus include brain damage, intellectual disability, poor motor coordination, blindness, seizures, and inability to speak. Infants and children may also be exposed postnatally to mercury through breast milk.

Epidemiology

- Blood level is measured in micrograms of mercury per deciliter of blood (µg/L). The United States Environmental Protection Agency (EPA)'s *reference dose (RfD)* for methylmercury is 0.1 µg/kg body weight/day (equivalent to a 5.8 µg/L blood mercury level). Mercury levels in women of childbearing age dropped 34% from a survey conducted in 1999 to 2000 to follow-up surveys conducted from 2001 to 2010. Additionally, the percentage of women of childbearing age with blood mercury levels above the level of concern decreased 65% between the 1999–2000 survey and the follow-up surveys from 2001–2010.

- More than 300,000 newborns each year are estimated to be at increased risk of learning disabilities associated with in utero exposure to methylmercury.

Common Exposures to Mercury

Three widely publicized topics of concern to the general population are fish consumption (especially in children and pregnant women), vaccines, and dental amalgams.

Consumption of Fish and Shellfish

The allowable intake of methylmercury according to the EPA is 0.1 µg of mercury per kilogram per day. The United States Food and Drug Administration (FDA) recommends that pregnant women, breastfeeding mothers, and young children avoid eating fish with a high mercury content (>1 ppm), such as shark, swordfish, tilefish, and king mackerel and fresh, frozen, and canned albacore tuna (mercury content between 0.5 ppm and 1.5 ppm). Recent studies, however, have not shown any deleterious associations between intellectual functioning and behavior and the consumption of recommended serving sizes of various types of fish during pregnancy. In fact, several studies have demonstrated a protective association for fish consumption (.2 servings/week), particularly with respect to ADHD-related impulsivity and hyperactivity.

Vaccines

Thimerosal (~50% methylmercury) was used as a preservative in pertussis, diphtheria, tetanus, and influenza vaccines. In 2000, the United States Public Health Service ordered the removal of thimerosal from all vaccines. No good empirical evidence has linked vaccines containing thimerosal with autism spectrum disorders or other neurodevelopmental problems.

Dental Amalgams

The Public Health Service concluded that dental amalgams do not pose a serious health risk of mercury poisoning so are not a likely source of in utero exposure.

Determinants of Severity

- A linear dose-response relationship exists.
- Fetuses have greatest risk because of their inability to excrete mercury.

Presentation, Disease Course, and Recovery

All forms of mercury are toxic to the fetus, but methylmercury most readily passes through the placenta. Offspring of women exposed to significant mercury have progressive cortical degenerative disease, cerebral palsy, ID, severe sensory deficits, microcephaly, and limb malformations (now coined Congenital Minamata disease). Neuropathology indicates the occipital cortex and cerebellum are most affected.

Expectations for Neuropsychological Assessment Results

- *Seychelles Prospective Cohort Study* Methylmercury levels were unrelated to any neurodevelopmental parameters; however, activity level in boys decreased as maternal hair methylmercury concentrations increased.
- *Faroe Islands Prospective Study* Higher cord blood methylmercury levels were associated with deficits in motor skills, attention, language, visuospatial skills, and memory.
- *New Zealand Study* Higher prenatal exposure (>6 ppm in maternal hair samples) were significantly associated with expressive language and visuospatial deficits and lower overall intelligence scores.

Section 5: Environmental Toxicants— Polychlorinated Biphenyls (PCBs)

Definition

Polychlorinated biphenyls are part of a family of man-made organic chemicals known as chlorinated hydrocarbons. Prior to 1979, PCBs were commonly used in transformers, adhesives and tapes, plastic and rubber products, oil-based paint, electrical devices and appliances, and carbonless copy paper. The primary human exposure occurs through the food chain, via highly contaminated fish and sea mammals.

Neuropathology

The principal route of prenatal exposure is maternal consumption of seafood before and during pregnancy. The PCBs are noted to be endocrine disruptors. Polychlorinated biphenyl exposures have been associated with changes in thyroid hormone levels in infants and decreased size of the splenium of the corpus callosum.

Epidemiology

Large scale studies conducted in Oswego, New York, Michigan, the Netherlands, and Germany show similar impact of PCBs on neurodevelopment.

Determinants of Severity

- Dose-dependent associations exist between PCB level and neurobehavioral impairment.
- The neurotoxic effects of PCBs on dopamine activity are potentiated by methylmercury.

Presentation, Disease Course, and Recovery

Asian studies showed that exposure in utero was associated with low birth weight and delays in sensorimotor and cognitive abilities.

Expectations for Neuropsychological Assessment Results

Limited studies suggest that the general profile of neurocognitive performance after in utero exposure to PCBs shows reduced verbal abilities and deficits in executive functions.

Section 6: Environmental Toxicants—Inorganic Lead (Pb)

Definition

Inorganic lead (Pb) is a common environmental metal that is a known neurotoxin. Sources of exposure in humans include drinking water from lead pipes, as well as imported candies, toys, cosmetics, and pottery. In the United States, lead was banned in paint and gasoline in the 1970s; however, pregnant mothers, infants, and children can still be exposed to lead via paint chips and/or paint dust during renovations. Currently, in utero exposure to lead is most likely to occur from maternal occupational exposure.

Neuropathology

Inorganic lead can mimic calcium and thus pass through the blood-brain barrier. Once in the CNS, lead interferes with neurulation, migration, synaptogenesis, and neurotransmission. In the fetus, lead crosses the placenta and accumulates in fetal organs. Animal studies have suggested that lead may specifically affect the dopamine system. Imaging studies in children exposed to lead have been equivocal. Magnetic resonance imaging studies have documented decreased cerebral volume in the frontal gray matter, anterior cingulate, and prefrontal cortex. Magnetic resonance spectography (MRS) studies have documented decrease in the N-acetylaspartate-to-creatine ratio, which is a possible indicator of neuronal loss.

Epidemiology

Approximately 250,000 United States children aged 1 to 5 years have blood lead levels that are above the action level recommended by the CDC. Incidence rates have declined sharply in recent years but remain high in low-income areas, minority children, and children living in older homes. Unborn children and young children are at greatest risk for poor health and neurobehavioral outcomes from lead exposure.

Determinants of Severity

- Blood lead level is measured in micrograms of lead per deciliter of blood (µg/dL). The United States Centers for Disease Control and Prevention (CDC) determines the current "action level" or level at which public health actions are recommended. The CDC recommends case management for children with blood levels of 5 µg/dL or higher.

- There appears to be a dose-response relationship between blood lead level and neuropsychological outcomes, although recent research has documented mild neuropsychological deficits even at low lead levels.
  - <30 μg/dL = low lead level
  - >80 μg/dL can result in lead encephalopathy
  - >44 μg/dL = pharmacological intervention

Presentation, Disease Course, and Recovery

Signs of acute elevated lead levels include headache, irritability, abdominal pain, vomiting, weight loss, attention problems, hyperactivity, learning problems, and slowed speech development.

Expectations for Neuropsychological Assessment Results

Declines in IQ and academic achievement have been documented even at low blood lead levels. The most common neuropsychological domain affected by lead exposure is executive functions. Deficits in visuospatial skills are also commonly found. Children exposed pre- or postnatally to elevated lead levels are often restless, impulsive, inattentive, and aggressive. Elevated levels of both internalizing and externalizing behavior disorders have been documented, including increased rates of ADHD and ODD. In later childhood and young adulthood, individuals with a history of elevated blood lead levels are more likely to engage in juvenile delinquency and antisocial behaviors. These difficulties are seen more commonly in males than females.

Considerations when Treating and Evaluating Select Populations with Pb

Age Considerations

Children absorb approximately 50% of ingested lead, whereas adults only absorb 10–15%. More severe neurocognitive and neurobehavioral effects are seen when lead exposure occurs in utero and during infancy, as opposed to during later childhood and adulthood.

Chelation Treatment

Children with blood lead levels of greater than 44 μg/dL are often treated with *chelation therapy*. Chelation treatment uses dimercaptosuccinic acid to trap lead in the body and remove the lead through urine. This treatment is effective in reducing blood lead levels but is likely not effective in reversing cognitive or behavioral deficits.

Methodological Considerations

Use of biomarkers of exposure, such as lead levels in blood, hair, teeth, and breast milk, are relied on as measures of lead exposure. Exposure to lead is not a random event. Numerous confounding variables exist, including lowered parental IQ, worse SES, maternal drug use, and poorer caregiving quality.

Section 7: Other Toxic Substances with Neuropsychological Relevance

Nicotine/Tobacco

- Nicotine exposure in-utero can lead to reduced fetal oxygen supply, fetal undernourishment, and vasoconstrictor effects on the placenta and umbilical cord
- Equivocal findings regarding neuropsychological effects
- Externalizing behavior disorders are common, particularly ADHD

Amphetamines

- Motor deficits during infancy
- Deficits in executive functions during childhood
- Poor emotional regulation

Opiates

- In utero exposure to opioids, predominately heroin, can lead to decreases in neural plasticity and increased cell death. There is also an increased risk for lower birth weight.
- Motor deficits during infancy with later deficits in executive functions and ADHD symptoms during childhood.

Pesticides

- Organophosphate pesticides (OPs) disrupt the enzyme that regulates acetylcholine.
- Prenatal exposure to OPs has been linked to various neuropsychological and behavioral deficits in childhood.

Air Pollution

- Animal models suggest that particulate matter in air pollutants can cross the blood-brain barrier and affect the developing brain.
- Studies have documented slightly lower IQ scores, as well as academic and behavioral deficits, in children exposed prenatally to high levels of air pollution.

Prescription Medications

- Exposure to antiepileptic medications during the first trimester can lead to major anatomical birth defects whereas exposure during the third trimester has been linked to cognitive and behavioral deficits. Valproic acid and polytherapy appear to have the most significant risk. Exposure to Valproic acid has been linked to verbal deficits, as well as increased risk for ADHD and autism spectrum disorder (ASD).
- In utero exposure to the blood thinner warfarin (Coumadin) has been linked to developmental delays and Dandy-Walker malformation.
- In utero exposure to the acne medication isotretinoin (Accutane) has been linked to an increased risk for birth defects and ID.
- In utero exposure to selective serotonin reuptake inhibitors (SSRIs) can lead to *neonatal abstinence syndrome* (NAS), but the long-term effects, if any, are unknown.

Relevant Definitions

Acrodynia ("painful extremities") is a rare disease that primarily affects young children exposed to mercury. It is often misdiagnosed in children as measles, other viral exanthems, or Kawasaki disease. Symptoms include irritability, photophobia, pink discoloration and edema of the hands and feet, hair loss, irritability, anorexia, insomnia, poor muscle tone, profuse sweating, and polyneuritis.

Blood-brain barrier A semi-permeable membrane made up of endothelial cells that separates circulating blood from brain tissue. The blood-brain barrier allows passage of oxygen, certain gases, and nutrients from the circulating blood to brain tissue but blocks passage of most harmful toxins. Some toxins, such as lead and alcohol, pass through the blood-brain barrier. Importantly, the blood-brain barrier is not fully developed until approximately 6 months gestation.

Chelation therapy The use of a chemical substance that removes excess or toxic metals (e.g., lead, iron, copper, calcium, mercury) before they can cause damage to the body.

Neonatal abstinence syndrome (NAS) A nonspecific group of symptoms that can be displayed by some newborns whose mothers used illicit or prescription drugs during pregnancy. Symptoms are variable but may include excessive crying, irritability, hyperactive reflexes, seizures, and increased muscle tone.

Reference dose (RfD) An exposure without recognized adverse effects.

Toxic Exposure in Utero Questions

1. The highest exposure risk to mercury is _____.
   (a) accidentally ingesting a drop of liquid mercury from a broken thermometer
   (b) dropping a compact fluorescent bulb
   (c) eating canned tuna every day for one week
   (d) spilling dimethylmercury on your latex gloves while conducting an experiment

2. How is an absolute level of maternal alcohol consumption over the course of a pregnancy determined in a child who has a diagnosis of fetal alcohol syndrome?
   (a) via the use of biomarkers
   (b) testing maternal blood alcohol levels during each trimester of pregnancy
   (c) through maternal self-report
   (d) there is no reliable way to determine maternal alcohol consumption

3. The neurotoxicity of PCBs is potentiated by _____.
   (a) lead
   (b) mercury
   (c) arsenic
   (d) copper

4. You are the clinical neuropsychologist consultant on a study evaluating the potential effects of in utero cocaine exposure on various neurotransmitters in the fetal brain. Which of the following neurotransmitters would you predict to be most affected by cocaine exposure?

   (a) dopamine

   (b) serotonin

   (c) norepinephrine

   (d) glutamate

5. A neuropsychologist is asked to evaluate the neuropsychological functioning of an 8-year-old boy with a documented blood lead level of 35 μg/dL. Which of the following sources of data will be essential in assisting the neuropsychologist in ruling out alternative explanations for any neuropsychological problems in this child?

   (a) cognitive testing

   (b) clinical interview with parents

   (c) teacher interview

   (d) school record review

6. Which of the following is the leading cause of preventable intellectual disability?

   (a) cocaine use during pregnancy

   (b) Down syndrome

   (c) Fetal Alcohol Spectrum Disorder

   (d) lead exposure during pregnancy

7. Alcohol exposure during the first and second trimesters interferes with which of the following processes in brain development?

   (a) neuronal migration and proliferation

   (b) programmed cell death

   (c) cerebellar formation

   (d) basal ganglia formation

8. You are a clinical neuropsychologist consulting on a study examining the potential cognitive effects of in utero exposure to marijuana. Which of the following factors would be most important to consider when evaluating study outcomes?

   (a) gender

   (b) use of other substances

   (c) geographic region

   (d) type of marijuana used

9. You are evaluating a child who was exposed to cocaine in utero. Given what is known about the common neuropsychological effects of cocaine exposure, which of the following cognitive domains should be most important when designing your test battery?

   (a) sensorimotor functions

   (b) delayed memory

   (c) language

   (d) attention

10. In utero exposure to tobacco has been consistently linked to the development of which of the following?

   (a) depression

   (b) anxiety

   (c) ADHD

   (d) autism

Toxic Exposure in Utero Answers

NOTE: Questions 42 and 70 on the First Full-Length Practice Examination, Questions 69, 118, and 121 on the Second Full-Length Practice Examination, Questions 38, 71, and 105 on the Third Full-Length Practice Examination, and Questions 29, 64, and 114 on the Fourth Full-Length Practice Examination are from this chapter.

1. **D—spilling dimethylmercury on your latex gloves while conducting an experiment** *Elemental (metallic) mercury is poorly ingested by the gastrointestinal tract and 99.9% is excreted through feces; a 150 g can of albacore tuna has approximately 0.030 mg of methylmercury that will be absorbed into the body; but, if only ingested for a short period of time, it will also be excreted from the body; compact fluorescent bulbs release mercury vapors into the air that are toxic and require particular clean-up, as per the EPA; dimethylmercury is extremely toxic and only a tiny drop on latex gloves has been shown to cause death.*

   Reference: US Environmental Protection Agency. (2018, December 31). *Mercury in your environment.* http://www.epa.gov/hg/effects.htm

2. **D—there is no reliable way to determine maternal alcohol consumption** *Taking maternal blood or cord blood samples throughout pregnancy is ineffective; samples drawn at delivery may show current blood alcohol levels, but they will not show the absolute amount over the course of the pregnancy. Maternal self-report is often erroneous and can be confounded by the use of other drugs that impact accurate recollection. At this time, various biomarkers are being studied, but none has proven to be reliable.*

   Reference: Glass, L., & Mattson, S. N. (2016). Fetal alcohol spectrum disorders: Academic and psychosocial outcomes. In C. A. Riccio & J. R. Sullivan (Eds.), *Pediatric neurotoxicology: Academic and psychosocial outcomes* (pp. 13–50). Cham, Switzerland: Springer International.

3. **B—mercury** *Methylmercury has been shown to potentiate the neurotoxic effects of polychlorinated biphenyls on dopamine activity.*

   Reference: Dietrich, K. N. (2010). Environmental toxicants. In K. O. Yeates, M. D. Ris, H. G. Taylor, & B. F. Pennington (Eds.), *Pediatric neuropsychology: Research, theory, and practice* (pp. 211–264). New York, NY: Guilford Press.

4. **A—dopamine** *In utero exposure to many toxic substances, namely lead and cocaine, appears to affect the developing CNS via its actions on the monoamine system, namely dopamine.*

   Reference: Gilbert, S. G., Miller, E., Martin, J., & Abulafia, L. (2010). Scientific and policy statements on environmental agents associated with neurodevelopmental disorders. *Journal of Intellectual and Developmental Disability, 35,* 121–128.

5. **B—clinical interview with parents** *When evaluating children exposed to high blood lead levels, numerous confounding variables exist, including lowered parental IQ, worse SES, maternal drug use, and poorer caregiving quality. These variables can best be gathered via a thorough clinical interview with family.*

   Reference: Dietrich, K. N. (2010). Environmental toxicants. In K. O. Yeates, M. D. Ris, H. G. Taylor, & B. F. Pennington (Eds.), *Pediatric neuropsychology: Research, theory, and practice* (pp. 211–264). New York, NY: Guilford Press.

6. **C—Fetal Alcohol Spectrum Disorder** *Fetal alcohol spectrum disorder is the leading cause of preventable intellectual disability in the United States. Cocaine and lead exposure can affect IQ but not typically to the level of intellectual disability. Down syndrome is not preventable.*

   Reference: Janke, K., & Jacola, L. (2018). Intellectual disability syndromes. In J. Donders & S. Hunter (Eds.), *Neuropsychological conditions across the lifespan* (pp. 61–78). New York, NY: Cambridge University Press.

7. **A—neuronal migration and proliferation** *Prenatal alcohol consumption during the first and second trimester interferes with neuronal migration and proliferation, whereas prenatal alcohol consumption in the third trimester leads to structural damage to the cerebellum, hippocampus, and prefrontal cortex*

   Reference: Glass, L., & Mattson, S. N. (2016). Fetal alcohol spectrum disorders: Academic and psychosocial outcomes. In C. A. Riccio, & J. R. Sullivan (Eds.), *Pediatric neurotoxicology: Academic and psychosocial outcomes* (pp. 13–50). Cham, Switzerland: Springer International.

8. **B—use of other substances** *The relation between prenatal exposure to marijuana and neuropsychological outcomes is confounded by factors such as polysubstance use and low SES.*

   Reference: Parris, L. (2016). Opiates and marijuana use during pregnancy: Neurodevelopmental outcomes. In C. A. Riccio, & J. R. Sullivan (Eds.), *Pediatric neurotoxicology: Academic and psychosocial outcomes* (pp. 77–89). Cham, Switzerland: Springer International Publishing.

9. **D—attention** *Prenatal exposure to cocaine affects several neuropsychological functions but tends to have a specific effect on sustained and selective attention.*

   Reference: Singer, L. T., Min, M. O., Lang, A., & Minnes, S. (2016). In utero exposure to nicotine, cocaine, and amphetamines. In C. A. Riccio, & J. R. Sullivan (Eds.), *Pediatric neurotoxicology: Academic and psychosocial outcomes* (pp. 51–76). Cham, Switzerland: Springer International Publishing.

10. **C—ADHD** *In-utero exposure to tobacco has been consistently linked to the development of ADHD.*

   Reference: Singer, L. T., Min, M. O., Lang, A., & Minnes, S. (2016). In utero exposure to nicotine, cocaine, and amphetamines. In C. A. Riccio, & J. R. Sullivan (Eds.), *Pediatric neurotoxicology: Academic and psychosocial outcomes* (pp. 51–76). Cham, Switzerland: Springer International.

Recommended Readings

Dietrich, K. N. (2010). Environmental toxicants. In K. O. Yeates, M. D. Ris, H. G. Taylor, & B. F. Pennington (Eds.), *Pediatric neuropsychology: Research, theory, and practice* (pp. 211–264). New York, NY: Guilford Press.

Mattson, S. N., & Vaurio, L. (2010). Fetal alcohol spectrum disorders. In K. O. Yeates, M. D. Ris, H. G. Taylor, & B. F. Pennington (Eds.), *Pediatric neuropsychology: Research, theory, and practice* (pp. 265–293). New York, NY: Guilford Press.

Riccio, C. A., & Sullivan, J. R. (Eds.) (2016). *Pediatric neurotoxicology: Academic and psychosocial outcomes*. Cham, Switzerland: Springer International.

Michael Westerveld

Definition

According to the International League Against Epilepsy (ILAE), the accepted definition of a seizure is "a transient occurrence of signs and/or symptoms due to abnormal excessive or synchronous neuronal activity in the brain." The clinical manifestation, which includes behaviors exhibited during a seizure (also referred to as "ictal semiology") varies considerably depending on the underlying cause of the seizure and the manner in which the seizure spreads or engages networks in the brain. Seizures are classified based on the observed behavior during the event, with the behavioral features at the onset being key to classification. The classification terminology for seizure types was most recently updated in 2017, with the goal of providing a more practical, operational definition that would facilitate communication among clinicians, patients, and researchers. The new system emphasizes clinical features while minimizing confounds with diagnostic inferences and epilepsy syndromes. Changes to the terminology were carefully considered and several more commonly used terms are no longer a part of the new terminology. The main features for classification are determination of whether the onset is focal, generalized, or undetermined. Focal seizures, as defined by the ILAE, have onset originating in networks limited within one cerebral hemisphere and may be discretely localized within the hemisphere, more widely distributed within the hemisphere, or originate in subcortical structures. As with the previous update, the degree of impairment in consciousness or awareness is considered in seizure classification, but the terms "simple" and "complex" are replaced by "aware" and "impaired awareness." A summary of the updated classification system can be seen in Figure 22.1.

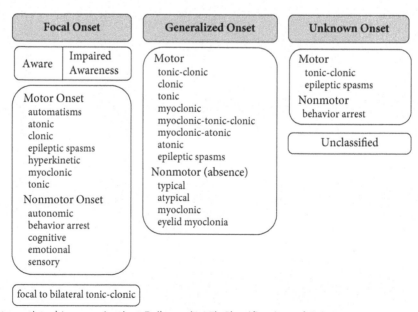

FIGURE 22.1 International League Against Epilepsy (ILAE) Classification of Seizures

NOTE: Reproduced with permission from *Epilepsia*, a journal of the International League against Epilepsy

Seizures are discrete events and, in most cases, a symptom of an underlying pathological condition or process affecting brain function. Some conditions that cause seizures are acquired (e.g., trauma or injury to the brain, neoplasm, autoimmune disorders), whereas others are congenital (e.g., cortical dysplasia) or genetic. Not all conditions that cause seizures lead to epilepsy, and many can be adequately treated or resolved without development of recurrent seizures (e.g., high fever in children, substance use and/ or withdrawal). A single seizure may be treated by addressing the underlying cause (if known), such as correcting a transient metabolic problem. However, a diagnosis of epilepsy, or recurrent seizures, implies that there is an underlying condition that is not related to transient factors and is an intrinsic property of the brain where there is an enduring predisposition to generate epileptic seizures. A diagnosis of epilepsy is made when there have been at least two unprovoked seizures, at least 24 hours apart, or after a single unprovoked seizure when the risk for another is known to be high (>60%) based on other medical factors (e.g., positive imaging findings), or an epilepsy syndrome has been diagnosed (e.g., childhood absence epilepsy).

Classification of recurrent seizures into epileptic syndromes presents a unique challenge given the heterogeneity of seizure types and causes. Ongoing review of classification systems is needed given research advances that fundamentally alter understanding of pathological mechanisms and management of seizure disorders. The classification system adopted in 2017 provides a simplified framework that considers etiology at all stages of classification, considers comorbidities, and eliminates confusing or ambiguous terminology. The working model for classification of epilepsies is shown in Figure 22.2. Eliminated terminology includes replacement of the term "benign" with "self-limiting" or "pharmacoresponsive," where appropriate. While there are no "ILAE approved" epilepsy syndromes, Table 22.1 provides a summary of commonly encountered syndromes by age of typical presentation.

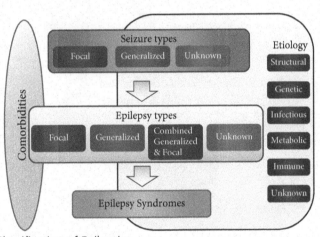

FIGURE 22.2 Model for Classification of Epilepsies

NOTE: Reproduced with permission from *Epilepsia*, a journal of the International League against Epilepsy

Neuropathology

There are numerous underlying causes of seizures and epilepsy, and epileptic seizures should be considered a symptomatic expression of some type of underlying neuronal dysfunction. The precipitating factor may be genetic, structural, metabolic, autoimmune mediated, or related to transient factors, and epilepsy syndromes may have more than one contributing etiology. However, the common mechanism involves a fundamental disruption of the balance between inhibitory and excitatory neuronal activity and the development of recurrent excitatory networks. This disruption can be caused by acquired or congenital/

TABLE 22.1 Classification of Epileptic and Electroclinical Syndromes Arranged by Age of Onset

Neonatal Period	• Neonatal seizures • Familial neonatal epilepsy • Ohtahara syndrome • Early myoclonic encephalopathy	
Infancy	• Febrile seizures • Self-limited infantile epilepsy • Self-limited familial infantile epilepsy • West syndrome • Dravet syndrome • Myoclonic epilepsy of infancy • Myoclonic encephalopathy in non-progressive disorders • Epilepsy of infancy with migrating focal seizures	
Childhood	• Febrile seizures, Febrile seizures plus • Early onset childhood occipital epilepsy • Epilepsy with myoclonic atonic seizures (formerly "astatic" seizures) • Childhood absence epilepsy (CAE) • Self-limited epilepsy with centrotemporal spikes (BECTS) • Late-onset childhood occipital epilepsy • Autosomal dominant nocturnal frontal lobe epilepsy (ADNFLE) • Epilepsy with myoclonic absences • Lennox-Gastaut syndrome • Epileptic encephalopathy with continuous spike and wave during sleep (CSWS; also referred to as Electrical Status Epilepticus during Slow Sleep (ESES) • Landau-Kleffner syndrome	
Adolescence/Adult	• Juvenile absence epilepsy • Juvenile myoclonic epilepsy (JME) • Epilepsy with generalized tonic-clonic seizures alone • Autosomal dominant epilepsy with auditory features (ADEAF) • Other familial temporal lobe epilepsies	
Variable at Age of Onset	• Familial focal epilepsy with variable foci • New onset refractory status epilepticus (NORSE) • Febrile illness related epilepsy syndrome (FIRES) • Progressive myoclonus epilepsies • Reflex epilepsy	
Distinctive Constellations/ Surgical Syndromes	• Mesial temporal lobe epilepsy with hippocampal sclerosis • Rasmussen syndrome • Gelastic seizures with hypothalamic hamartoma • Hemiconvulsive-hemiplegic epilepsy	
Nonsyndromic Epilepsies	**Epilepsy attributed to structural metabolic causes**	• Malformations of cortical development • Neurocutaneous syndromes (tuberous sclerosis complex, Sturge-Weber) • Tumor, infection, trauma, vascular, antenatal/ perinatal insults, etc.
	Epilepsies of unknown cause	

genetic conditions affecting the brain and, in many cases, may be difficult to identify or be unknown (e.g., so-called idiopathic or cryptogenic epilepsy). A comprehensive review of all types of neuropathology associated with epilepsy is beyond the scope of this chapter. Some of the more common known pathological substrates are reviewed briefly.

MEDICAL

Epilepsy is a lifespan disease, can occur at any time, and may persist throughout the lifespan in some syndromes. However, common types of underlying neuropathology differ in children and adults. The temporal lobe, in particular the hippocampus, is the most common site of pathology in adults and adolescents with seizures that include alteration of awareness, accounting for as many as two thirds of cases. In surgical series that report on pathology, the most common pathology in adults is hippocampal sclerosis (HS), with estimates generally around 65–75% of surgical cases. Hippocampal sclerosis is a histopathologically defined pattern of cell loss along with astrogliosis in the hippocampal formation. While common among patients with temporal lobe epilepsy, HS may also be seen to varying degrees in other conditions (e.g., dementia, hypoxic injury). The ILAE classification scheme for HS identifies three subtypes, with the most common (Type 1) found in 60–80% of surgical cases and involving prominent cell loss in all hippocampal subfields. Types 2 and 3 are less common, and have cell loss more limited to the CA1 and CA4 subfields, respectively. In addition, the remaining neurons may become part of an "epileptogenic network" that is marked by synaptic reorganization and may be associated with "dual pathology" or cell loss in the hippocampus along with the presence of other abnormalities, such as focal cortical dysplasia. Hippocampal sclerosis is frequently detected by neuroimaging, characterized by the appearance of atrophy, with increased signal intensity on T2 weighted magnetic resonance imaging (MRI) and fluid-attenuated (FLAIR) sequences.

New onset epilepsy in a previously healthy adult is uncommon, and often associated with primary CNS neoplasm, neurovascular event, trauma, infection, or autoimmune disorders. In particular, the role of autoimmune disorders in previously unclassified or unknown etiologies is increasingly recognized. Autoimmune epilepsies may be associated with primarily temporal lobe pathology with secondary involvement of other cortical areas ("limbic encephalitis"), or encephalopathies with diffuse brain involvement. Autoimmune mediated epilepsy may be associated with paraneoplastic syndromes, or infectious etiology. Autoimmune antibodies associated with NMDA receptors, GABA, AMPA, and voltage gated potassium channel receptors have been linked to epilepsy.

TABLE 22.2 Classification of Malformations of Cortical Development

MCD caused by abnormal neuronal and glial proliferation or apoptosis	Decreased proliferation/increased apoptosis (microcephalies)	
	Increased proliferation/decreased apoptosis with normal cell types (megalencephalies)	
	Abnormal proliferation (abnormal cell types)	• Non-neoplastic (e.g., hamartomas of tuberous sclerosis, focal cortical dysplasia, hemimegencephaly) • Neoplastic (e.g., dysembryoplastic neuroepithelial tumor, or DNET, ganglioglioma)
MCD caused by abnormal neuronal migration	• Lissencephaly and subcortical band heterotopias • Cobblestone brain malformation with congenital muscular dystrophy • Heterotopia (subependymal heterotopias, subcortical [other than band] heterotopias)	
MCD caused by abnormal cortical organization (including late neuronal migration)	• Polymicrogyria and schizencephaly • Cortical dysplasia without balloon cells • Microdysgenesis	
MCD not otherwise classified	• Malformations due to inborn errors of metabolism • Other unclassified malformations (e.g., sublobar dysplasia)	

NOTE: MCD, Malformations of Cortical Development; from Barkovich et al., 2001, updated 2012 and Desikan, 2016.

Underlying pathology in pediatric epilepsy syndromes is age dependent, much more variable, and more often unknown than in comparable adult samples. Neonatal seizures are frequently associated with hypoxic ischemic encephalopathy, which comprises 35–45% of cases. Other common causes in neonatal epilepsy include infarction/hemorrhage, genetic or syndromic epilepsy, and brain malformations. Causes for childhood onset epilepsy are also quite variable, and include increasingly recognized contributions of genetic variants, and autoimmune epilepsies. The developmental differences in underlying pathology can also be seen in surgical case series. As noted, adult surgical series report up to 75% of cases have hippocampal sclerosis as the primary pathology. However, in children, malformations of cortical development (MCD; see Table 22.2) and low-grade brain tumors comprise the majority of pathological substrates.

Malformations of cortical development are a frequent cause of epilepsy and can be present anywhere in the cerebral cortex. These malformations vary considerably in their origin and presentation and can be macro- or microscopic. The MCD classification is based on genetic and embryologic principles and on pathologic, histologic, and imaging criteria. Although the malformations themselves may be associated with regional or localized alterations in metabolic activity that generate seizures, MCD may also be a marker of more widespread alteration in the metabolic balances that predispose to epileptogenesis.

Genetic causes of, or contributors to, epilepsy are increasingly recognized, and may potentially lead to more effective treatments. Genes associated with epilepsy can be grouped into monogenic (e.g., genes that cause epilepsies or syndromes with epilepsy as the core symptom), neurodevelopment-related genes (e.g., genes associated with gross brain developmental malformations and epilepsy), epilepsy-related genes (e.g., genes associated with gross physical or other systemic abnormalities that may be accompanied by epilepsy) and potential epilepsy-associated genes that may represent a susceptibility factor but require further investigation. Many epilepsy genes may have multiple phenotypic expressions, such as the SCN1A gene associated with Dravet syndrome that is also associated with febrile seizure syndromes (familial febrile seizures; generalized epilepsy with febrile seizures +, or GEFS+). Similarly, many epilepsy syndromes are associated with multiple genetic variants.

Epidemiology

Epilepsy is considered one of the most common acute neurological conditions affecting children and adults. According to the World Health Organization, approximately 50 million people worldwide have epilepsy. Regional estimates of incidence and prevalence vary considerably, but the majority (up to 80%) of cases occur in developing regions. This may be related to higher rates of epilepsy-related conditions (e.g., malaria, neurocysticercosis, birth-related injuries) as well as lack of access to preventive care or treatment. In the United States, the incidence (number of new cases per year) is estimated to be approximately 50 per 100,000 individuals, and the prevalence is estimated at 5–10 per 1,000, or more than 3 million cases. Onset is most common among children less than 5 years of age and in adults over 65 years. While the majority of seizures with alteration of consciousness or awareness occur before age 15, the number of new onset cases is growing fastest in the elderly population.

Mortality

Many of the known causes of epilepsy include neurological disease such as neurovascular disease or neoplasms, and, as a result, there is increased mortality. In general, there is a slight increase in mortality for epilepsy without a known cause, but a more significant increase for symptomatic epilepsy. However, even in epilepsy without a known cause, risk of mortality is increased for both children and adults. Causes of increased mortality in epilepsy in the absence of other mortality risk factors have been widely studied and include SUDEP (sudden unexplained death in epilepsy), unintentional injury (e.g., falls, drowning), suicide, and complications associated with status epilepticus. The risks appear balanced between males and females with epilepsy, but are substantially higher for younger age groups compared with elderly, when other mortality risk factors rise. Overall, the standard mortality ratio (SMR) in epilepsy ranges from 1.2 to 9.3 depending on the region and methods used. However, it is clear that there is ample evidence of increased mortality in epilepsy.

Determinants of Severity

Given that epilepsy refers to a broad range of disorders with varying pathological substrates, localizations within the brain, and electroclinical features, it is difficult to list determinants of severity for each. It becomes even more challenging to list determinants of cognitive comorbidities associated with epilepsy, given the diverse underlying causes. However, generally speaking, severity increases with seizure recurrence and frequency. Known risk factors for seizure recurrence include prolonged febrile convulsions that may induce neurological injury, neoplasm, disorders of neuroblast migration such as cortical dysplasia and heterotopias, traumatic brain injury, and genetic factors.

Cognitive impairments related to seizure severity are multidetermined. Specific cognitive deficits are often associated with focal neuropathological substrates producing localized seizures in brain regions associated with specific functions (e.g., memory disturbance in temporal lobe epilepsy). Generalized cognitive deficits (e.g., attention problems, decreased psychomotor speed) may be associated with seizures themselves or be associated with other factors, such as treatment of seizures with antiepileptic medications.

Seizure frequency is the most significant factor in determining severity of cognitive impairment. Other variables associated with severity of cognitive impairment include the type of epilepsy risk factor (e.g., tumor, central nervous system [CNS] infection, trauma), younger age of seizure onset, and the number of antiepileptic drugs (AEDs). Genetic epilepsies are more likely to be associated with epileptic encephalopathy and other developmental disorders such as autism and intellectual disability.

Presentation, Disease Course, and Recovery

The natural history of epilepsy is highly dependent on the syndrome and pathology, with each syndrome having a unique course, treatment, and prognosis. Comprehensive review of the course of all epilepsy syndromes is beyond the scope of the chapter and, instead, the discussion is focused on the more commonly encountered epilepsy syndromes of temporal lobe epilepsy with hippocampal sclerosis and childhood absence epilepsy.

Temporal Lobe Epilepsy (TLE)

Temporal lobe epilepsy with hippocampal sclerosis (HS) is associated with a history of febrile seizures as an infant or toddler. Febrile seizures that are prolonged, or in cases when there are recurrent episodes of febrile seizures, present a greater risk for later development of TLE. Other factors associated with increased risk for HS include a history of perinatal complications, hypoxic-ischemic injury, CNS infections, and limbic encephalitis. Although some children may develop epilepsy shortly after febrile seizures, a latent period during which there are no seizures and development is normal is not uncommon. Temporal lobe epilepsy is typically treated with one or more anticonvulsant medications, which have varying mechanisms of action. However, one of the reasons that surgical series in epilepsy are dominated by temporal lobectomy reports is that TLE with HS can be very difficult to treat, and as many as one third of patients with TLE develop medically intractable seizures.

The behaviors associated with TLE can vary, but a few behaviors occur relatively frequently. For example, warning signs or auras are common among individuals with TLE associated with HS. Auras vary but often involve GI symptoms (e.g., rising epigastric sensation or "butterflies" in the stomach) or psychic phenomena (e.g., déjà vu). Seizure onset in TLE is associated with an alteration of awareness and gradual alteration of awareness, but not necessarily with loss of consciousness. During a seizure, behavior may be disorganized and include repetitive movements of the hands, tongue, mouth, or lips. Repetitive movements of the hand are typically ipsilateral to the side of seizure onset (e.g., left TLE associated with left-hand repetitive movement), whereas the opposite hand is typically in a forced tonic posture. Some patients may continue to speak during a temporal lobe seizure, depending on the laterality of the seizure focus. Speech patterns during or immediately following a seizure in TLE are significant for lateralization; absence of speech is not necessarily lateralizing, but the ability to continue speaking clearly is associated with non–language dominant temporal lobe onset in the overwhelming majority of cases. Postictal speech patterns are also typically lateralizing, with aphasic or dysnomic speech typically following dominant TLE seizures. Postictal confusion and/or fatigue is common, and the duration can vary from a few minutes to a few hours. Secondary generalization to a tonic-clonic seizure occurs up to 50% of the time in TLE.

Temporal lobe epilepsy that is resistant to medications can be treated by other means, including surgery to remove the epileptogenic temporal lobe and mesial temporal structures. Common surgical interventions (standard temporal lobectomy, modified anterior temporal lobectomy, selective amygdalahippocampectomy) are effective in the majority of well selected cases. However, these procedures also convey some risk of cognitive morbidity (e.g., decreased efficiency in learning and memory, word-finding deficits, visual field defects). However, newer treatment approaches may mitigate some of this risk. Particularly with respect to memory and, in the case of dominant temporal lobectomy, also to aspects of language (e.g., naming). A relatively newer application of thermal laser ablation applied to mesial temporal lobe structures has shown promise both with respect to seizure control and reduced cognitive morbidity, although additional research is needed to replicate early findings. The minimally invasive nature of the laser ablation procedure is an advantage that may appeal to patients who are reluctant to undergo more extensive surgery.

Application of the responsive neurostimulation system ("Neuropace") to temporal lobe epilepsy also holds promise, particularly for patients with bilateral temporal lobe seizure onset for whom resection is not an option. In this technology, subdural electrodes are implanted in the brain over the epileptic zone. The device is programmed to constantly monitor neural activity and triggers stimulation of the implanted electrodes when abnormal activity concerning for seizures is detected. An advantage of this technology is that it can also collect and analyze data that can be used to enhance performance of the system. Early trials in patients with TLE have shown significant seizure reduction.

Childhood Absence Epilepsy (CAE)

Childhood absence epilepsy is a primary generalized epilepsy in that it involves widespread neural networks at seizure onset. Childhood absence accounts for approximately 15% of childhood seizures, making it among the most common epilepsy syndromes of childhood. Childhood absence epilepsy is a self-limiting epilepsy syndrome in that seizures typically do not persist past adolescence. CAE inheritance is polygenic, with genes for γ-aminobutyric acid (GABA) receptors, calcium channels, and nonion channel genes such as *SLC2A1* all implicated in contributing to the disorder. Imaging findings are typically negative, and there are no other pathological findings or other risk factors that have been described. Age of onset is typically between 3 and 8 years, with the peak occurring around 6 years. Children with CAE are typically otherwise neurologically normal, although there is a high incidence of comorbid learning and/or attention disturbance. Other than familial history, there are no associated risk factors.

The electroencephalogram (EEG) is characterized by 3 Hz spike-wave discharges that begin suddenly and typically last five to 10 seconds, but can be as brief as 3 seconds or last longer than 20 seconds. Children with untreated CAE may have very frequent seizures (e.g., in some cases, up to 100 or more) on a daily basis.

Behaviors that characterize typical absence seizures are fairly nondescript. During a seizure, a sudden behavior arrest with alteration in awareness is apparent, often described as "staring." There may be some associated minor motor automatisms, such as eyelid fluttering or lip movements, but these are not always present, and, when they do occur, they can be subtle. Seizures end as suddenly as they begin, and individuals are often unaware of the seizure. They will typically resume the activity that they were engaged in prior to the seizure but may be briefly disoriented and need prompting to resume activity or repetition of instructions. It is commonly believed that if a child is redirected during a staring spell that it is not an absence seizure. However, the seizures are usually very brief and, by the time the child is redirected, the seizure is likely to be over, giving the appearance that they were "daydreaming" instead of having an absence seizure.

Medical management in CAE can be variably effective. Common medications used to treat CAE include ethosuximide, lamotrigine, and valproic acid. Although a large-scale randomized clinical trial found that ethosuximide (Zarontin) provided the best seizure relief with the least significant side effects related to cognitive function, treatment failure with the first line medication can show a short-term failure rate as high as 47%. Recent studies have suggested that genetic profiling and computer modeling of affected ion channels may lead to novel treatment approaches with improved efficacy.

Childhood absence epilepsy is often considered a benign, age-limited epilepsy syndrome, with most children having seizure remission during adolescence. However, seizures can persist into adolescence and adulthood and, in approximately 15% of cases, can develop into juvenile myoclonic epilepsy.

Other Epilepsy Syndromes

Other less common but well-known epilepsy syndromes with distinctive features include Landau-Kleffner syndrome, Lennox-Gastaut syndrome, and Rasmussen syndrome.

- *Landau-Kleffner syndrome (LKS)* is associated with a progressive encephalopathy (sometimes referred to as acquired epileptic encephalopathy) that particularly affects language. The typical course is normal language development prior to onset, which is usually between the ages of three and seven years. A progressive aphasia begins with development of receptive language impairment and verbal auditory agnosia, followed by gradual development of expressive language deficits. In many cases, there are also more general impairments in cognitive function, including regression of overall intellectual ability and deficits in attention. In some cases, there is also regression in sociability and development of autistic behaviors, although some attribute these behaviors to frustration associated with loss of language. There is no known cause for LKS, although approximately 20% of cases with genetic testing are associated with variations in a glutamate receptor gene (GRIN2A). Additionally, there are clinical reports of response to immunotherapy, suggesting a possible role for autoimmune antibody in the development of the disorder. The clinical picture in LKS is dominated by the language and cognitive deficits that characterize the disorder; clinical seizure types (e.g., behaviors observed during seizures) actually may vary, and some children do not have clinically evident seizures despite an abnormal EEG. Electrophysiological findings in LKS implicate the language-dominant perisylvian region but can be bilateral and also include frontal lobe pathology. Typically, the course does not typically include spontaneous recovery of language, and treatment of the seizures and EEG abnormalities do not provide relief of cognitive impairments. There have been some reports of improvement following surgery involving multiple subpial transections in Wernicke's area, but results are inconsistent, and there is no consensus regarding patients that may benefit from more aggressive treatment. As noted above, some patients have shown response to immunotherapy although this has not been widely studied. More conventional approaches that include speech and language interventions are critical, including development of compensatory skills (e.g., sign language).

- **Lennox-Gastaut syndrome** Lennox-Gastaut (LGS) is often referred to as an encephalopathic generalized epilepsy syndrome due to the progressive and severe cognitive impairments that are typically observed. Like many epilepsy syndromes that were previously thought to be "idiopathic," genetic causes are suspected. Several associated genetic findings have been associated with LGS, although the specifics are not well understood.

  Clinically, individuals with Lennox-Gastaut may present with multiple different seizure types, including atypical absence seizures, tonic seizures, and atonic seizures. Risk factors for Lennox-Gastaut include a history of infantile spasms, as well as other known causes including MCD, neurocutaneous disorders (e.g., tuberous sclerosis [TS] complex), CNS infection (meningitis, encephalitis), and hypoxic-ischemic injury. Thus, the disorder is not defined by a single underlying pathology or clinical seizure type, but instead is characterized by the EEG pattern, which may consist of bursts of fast activity, especially during slow wave sleep. The background EEG is usually dominated by slow activity but can be disorganized and may exhibit a hypsarrhythmia pattern (i.e., disorganized background with high-amplitude, irregular spike-and-wave activity). More important than the EEG is the cognitive and behavior presentation, which typically includes severe global cognitive impairments. Although cognitive impairments associated with risk factors may be present at the onset, cognitive abilities typically regress.

- **Rasmussen syndrome** is characterized by a progressive unilateral encephalopathy and medically refractory seizures. Although presentation can vary, the most commonly reported presentation is in children between 3 and 14 years. In nearly all of the children presenting with the disorder, premorbid cognitive and behavior development is normal. Once seizures begin, a progressive course generally results in loss of cognitive skills related to the side of seizure onset (e.g., language decline in dominant hemisphere; visuospatial decline in nondominant hemisphere). Ultimately, there is nearly complete loss of function in the affected hemisphere, including hemiparesis. Rasmussen syndrome is widely considered to have an autoimmune basis, although specific markers have not been identified. Some patients respond well to immunotherapy. However, aggressive surgical intervention (modified functional hemispherectomy) is often considered the best course. Early surgical intervention may provide the best opportunity for reorganization of function, particularly in children with language-dominant hemisphere disease.

Expectations for Neuropsychological Assessment Results

No clearly identified profile or pattern of cognitive function exists among persons with epilepsy. Neuropsychological presentation is highly dependent on multiple disease factors, including age of onset, existence of a clearly identified syndrome or underlying pathology, localization of pathology, disease course, and iatrogenic factors such as treatment with anticonvulsant medications.

- **Intelligence/Achievement** Many forms of epilepsy are associated with global cognitive impairments, of which one manifestation is low intelligence. However, many persons with epilepsy have normal overall intelligence even when more specific cognitive deficits exist. For both children and adults, IQ serves generally as a proxy for outcome, disease severity, and extent of underlying pathology. Persons with less severe epilepsy and those with more focal seizure onset are more likely to have normal IQ.

One of the most important risk factors for low IQ is age of seizure onset, with earlier onset associated with lower overall IQ. This association appears to be independent of other factors thought to be related to cognitive decline, such as seizure frequency or location of seizure onset. In fact, localization of seizure onset may not have the expected influence on IQ; for example, verbal–nonverbal intellectual skill discrepancies have not been found to be a lateralizing sign in focal epilepsy syndromes.

Whether seizures and epilepsy are a cause of low IQ is questioned. Progressive deterioration is seen in a subset of individuals who have recurrent seizures, but the majority do not show progressive decline. Risk factors for decline include seizure severity and treatment with multiple medications (which may also be a result of seizure severity). Secondary factors such as comorbid learning disabilities may also lead to low IQ in adults with childhood onset epilepsy.

Many epilepsy syndromes have a significant effect on intellectual development. In particular, epilepsies associated with several types of MCD, such as subcortical band heterotopias, are also associated with severe cognitive impairments and low IQ. Syndromic epilepsies, such as encephalopathic generalized epilepsy (including Lennox-Gastaut and LKS), are also associated with extremely low IQ. However, epilepsy is not necessarily always the causally related risk factor; children with intellectual deficiency due to other causes also have a higher frequency of seizures. For example, there is a high comorbidity of epilepsy in children with autism and intellectual disability.

- *Attention/Concentration* Approximately 30–50% of persons with epilepsy have difficulties with attention regardless of seizure type/syndrome. Predominantly inattentive types of attention-deficit/hyperactivity disorder (ADHD) are more common than hyperactive or combined types, and boys and girls with epilepsy appear to be equally affected. Combined inattentive-hyperactive ADHD may be related to severity of epilepsy. The combined subtype is associated with earlier age of onset and a higher degree of intractability, and it results in lower quality of life.

Although attention problems are present in many types of epilepsy, absence seizures tend to be more highly associated with attention problems and, in some cases, may be mistaken for an attention disorder due to the characteristic behaviors. Attention problems in absence seizures are associated with impaired function in an attention network comprising anterior insula-frontal operculum and medial frontal cortex.

The mechanism of attention problems in other seizure syndromes can vary depending on the nature of the seizures and underlying pathology. For example, nocturnal seizures are believed to affect attention and cognitive function by altering sleep patterns. Attention problems in localization-related partial epilepsy are observed in relation to interictal discharges (e.g., so-called transient cognitive impairment). Attention abnormalities associated with epilepsy appear to differ from those in children with ADHD alone. More difficulties with sustained attention are observed in children with epilepsy, compared with more complex and divided attention problems in children with ADHD who do not have epilepsy.

Treatment with some antiepileptic medications may produce attention difficulties as a side effect, but, in most cases, attention problems are not accounted for by medication effects alone. Problems with attention often precede development of seizures, suggesting that there may be antecedent neurobiological insult or developmental abnormality. This raises the question of how to effectively treat attention problems in children with epilepsy. There is a historical reluctance to treat attention problems with stimulants in persons with epilepsy. However, the data to address this question are surprisingly sparse, with variable results. While there is mounting evidence that stimulant treatment for ADHD symptoms is not associated with increased risk of seizures or seizure-related hospitalizations in children with epilepsy, there are also reports that show some children do experience increased seizures. Children with active seizures at the time stimulant treatment is initiated may be more likely to experience increased seizure activity with stimulants compared with children whose seizures are well controlled. In general, there is a small risk of increased seizures in individual patients. However, it is also important to acknowledge the limited data and methodological problems. Seizures are naturally variable in frequency, and attributing increased seizures to stimulant medication in a small number of patients over a brief time frame with inadequate baseline frequency is tenuous. It seems that the majority of the limited evidence suggests that stimulant treatment can be effective, but careful assessment of patient characteristics may identify some children at increased risk for seizure exacerbation. However, given the extensive literature on the adverse effects of ADHD symptoms on academic, intellectual, behavioral, and psychosocial outcomes, the benefits may outweigh the risk when the additive effects on these outcomes in epilepsy are also considered.

Newer nonstimulant treatments for ADHD symptoms have not been well studied in terms of efficacy or safety in epilepsy populations. There is some evidence that children taking atomoxetine are not at increased risk of having seizures; however, there is little information on efficacy in managing ADHD symptoms in the context of epilepsy. Similarly, there are no studies to evaluate efficacy of alpha-2 agonists (guanfacine, clonidine) on ADHD symptoms in persons with epilepsy. Pharmacologically, there are no reported interactions between the alpha-2 agonists and antiepileptic medications but since a potential side effect of these medications is sedation, caution is advised when using them in conjunction with sedating antiepileptic medications.

Differences in underlying pathology for comorbid ADHD symptoms in persons with epilepsy may account for the phenotypic and differential treatment response. Increased gray matter volume, specifically in sensorimotor, supplementary motor, and prefrontal regions, has been identified in children with comorbid ADHD and epilepsy. Decreased brainstem volumes have also been identified, implicating both frontal-cortical and subcortical systems regulating attention in epilepsy-associated attention problems.

- *Processing Speed* Processing speed deficits may have a structural or neuroanatomical basis or be related to side effects of AEDs used to treat epilepsy. Decreased white matter volume and frontal lobe epilepsy have been found to be associated with processing speed deficits. Other factors associated with slower processing speed include frequency of interictal epileptiform discharges and number of seizures.

  Processing speed deficits are among the commonly cited side effects of anticonvulsant medications. Antiepileptic drugs tend to reduce hyperexcitability and neuronal transmission by increasing inhibitory action (e.g., GABA-ergic inhibition) or reducing availability and function of excitatory neurotransmitters (e.g., glutamate). As one would expect with decreased excitatory potential, one of the effects is often reduced processing speed, independent of the impact of epilepsy, per se, and has been demonstrated in healthy volunteers as well as persons with epilepsy.

- *Language* Language deficits are commonly reported in children with various forms of epilepsy. Depending on the age of onset, impaired verbal skill development is not necessarily limited to epilepsy affecting the dominant hemisphere. Onset of seizures during critical language development can disrupt important networks involved in language even when the seizures arise from the right hemisphere and particularly when seizures involve bilateral networks.

Many of the epilepsy syndromes that have early onset (neonatal period, infancy; see Table 22.1.) are associated with failure to develop normal language.

More subtle language deficits may also be associated with localization-related epilepsy, particularly frontal and temporal lobe epilepsy involving the dominant hemisphere. Adults with TLE frequently demonstrate deficits in word finding and semantic knowledge, a finding that is as robust in TLE as verbal memory deficits. Confrontation naming and word-finding deficits in TLE indicate a network that involves both hippocampal and extrahippocampal structures in language deficits associated with TLE. Variations in anatomical volume and connectivity and changes in functional activation patterns that include mesial and lateral temporal lobe, and insula are noted in TLE and may be implicated in TLE-related language disruption. Although most common among dominant TLE, word-finding and language deficits are also observed in nondominant TLE, with a substantial portion of patients with nondominant TLE also experiencing worsening language difficulty after surgery. These language deficits are likely related to the prelexical object recognition and semantic association functions of the nondominant hemisphere.

- *Visuospatial* Deficits in visuospatial function are highly variable in epilepsy and are typically associated with primary generalized and generalized nonconvulsive epilepsy (e.g., CAE) and localization-related epilepsy involving the nondominant hemisphere. Specific deficits are more easily identified in lesional epilepsy (e.g., seizures associated with neoplasm in the nondominant hemisphere). Impaired object recognition, deficits in spatial organization, and lower performance on measures of visual-motor integration (drawing and copying), visuospatial learning, and complex perceptual processes (e.g., visual closure) have all been reported in patients with nondominant hemisphere epilepsy and in some studies of idiopathic generalized epilepsy (e.g., CAE, benign childhood epilepsy with centrotemporal spikes). However, the consistency of these findings is poor compared with language findings in dominant TLE and are likely due to a combination of factors including diversity in syndromes and individual presentation and the lower sensitivity of right-hemisphere cognitive tests.

  In some patients with large, early-onset epileptic lesions that provoke reorganization of language from the left to the right hemisphere or engage bilateral support of language, visuospatial deficits can be observed. This phenomenon has been referred to as the "crowding effect" and suggests that there are preferential neural resources allocated for language development. When there is an early injury to the primary language system, those resources are shifted to "back-up" systems in homologous areas in the contralateral hemisphere, but at a cost to functions that would have been mediated by those areas in the absence of injury. This is supported by a large body of literature that identifies relatively weak visuospatial function in epilepsy patients with early left-hemisphere injury and who are right-hemisphere dominant for language.

- *Learning and Memory* Memory is one of the most widely studied cognitive abilities in patients with epilepsy. Much of what we know about the neuroanatomical basis for learning and memory is attributable to studies of patients with epilepsy, particularly TLE. However, patients with other epilepsy syndromes also frequently exhibit memory deficits.

  Persons with TLE frequently have lateralized seizure onset, meaning that one temporal lobe is more extensively involved in seizure onset and propagation. Depending on the side of seizure onset, memory deficits may be "material specific" and involve mostly verbal information for dominant TLE or mostly nonverbal/visuospatial memory impairment for nondominant TLE. In patients with TLE and HS, the degree of memory impairment has been found to relate directly to the degree of cell loss in the hippocampus. Type 1 hippocampal sclerosis is most likely to be associated with impaired memory function. Although the relationship is robust across different verbal memory measures, the degree of sensitivity does vary somewhat depending on the measure used. List-learning measures tend to be the most sensitive to hippocampal pathology. However, as the degree of language processing increases, as with story/prose recall tasks, sensitivity to hippocampal pathology may decrease due to support from lateral neocortical language networks.

The association of nondominant TLE and visuospatial or nonverbal memory impairment is less robust. Although some studies have reported sensitivity of design reproduction and recall tasks to right TLE (assuming left-hemisphere language dominance), others have not. Multiple factors could help to explain this finding, including conceptual factors (e.g., poor models of nondominant hemisphere and TL function) and related methodological problems (lack of model-driven, sensitive, and specific tests for nondominant TL function).

Memory outcome following temporal lobectomy in persons with epilepsy is associated with a number of factors including baseline level of hippocampal function as determined by behavioral (e.g., performance on memory testing) and functional assessment (Wada testing and functional MRI). Assuming adequate task engagement, lower levels of baseline memory performance are associated with decreased risk of exacerbating existing memory impairments, while higher levels of performance are associated with risk of decline. Intracarotid amobarbital hemispheric suppression (Wada testing) is considered the gold standard for predicting catastrophic memory loss, but is also useful for predicting the more common declines associated with TL surgery by analysis of functional adequacy and functional reserve. More recently, accumulating evidence suggests that fMRI findings of increased activation ipsilateral to the seizure focus during memory testing can also predict memory declines. Assessing risk of memory decline is a critical component of preoperative assessment and allows the patient to more carefully consider the risk vs. benefit of various surgical treatment options including newer treatments that may minimize cognitive morbidity (e.g., laser ablation, RNS).

Although the specific relationship of memory deficits to TLE is well defined, memory deficits in other epilepsy syndromes can be more variable. There are many factors to consider, including the age of onset and the child's developmental stage when seizures and seizure risk factors occur, the epilepsy syndrome, frequency of seizures, treatment with anticonvulsant medications that may produce cognitive side effects indirectly affecting memory, and specific cognitive impairments related to localization outside the temporal lobe that adversely affect information processing and encoding. While TLE affects primary substrate associated with memory encoding and retrieval, other epilepsy syndromes may produce secondary memory deficits due to the impact on substrates of cognitive functions serving as a "gateway" to memory. For example, CAE is associated with attention problems that adversely affect encoding and storage of new information, with relatively greater impact on visuospatial and nonverbal memory. Memory deficits are also common in patients with frontal lobe epilepsy, related to poor organization and metacognitive strategies for learning and remembering.

- *Executive Functions* As with many other cognitive disturbances in epilepsy, early age of onset and longer duration of seizures is associated with greater levels of impairment. Involvement of frontal-subcortical systems that typically mediate executive function has also been identified as a risk factor for increased executive dysfunction.

  Seizures that specifically involve the frontal lobes can also have a wide range of clinical presentations, as well as diverse neuroanatomical underpinnings, making identification of a "frontal lobe epilepsy" cognitive phenotype difficult if not impossible. In children, a few studies report differences in verbal intellectual function, word finding/naming, and verbal conceptual reasoning in dominant frontal epilepsy. Children with frontal lobe epilepsy also demonstrate deficits in planning, mental flexibility/set shifting, impulse control, and motor coordination, although these deficits tend not to be associated with lateralization of frontal lobe seizures.

Lateralized deficits in frontal lobe epilepsy are not as common as in other forms of epilepsy, likely due to several factors. Frontal lobe seizures spread rapidly and frequently engage bilateral frontal structures. Frontal lobe epilepsy syndromes are also more commonly associated with malformations of cortical development, which typically indicates more widespread developmental abnormalities that involve both hemispheres. Also, tests of executive function may be less specific and lack sufficient sensitivity to identify subtle lateralized differences in frontal functions.

Temporal lobe epilepsy is also associated with deficits in executive function, although these deficits are highly variable and lack the consistency of memory deficits in TLE. The variability in cognitive expression of executive dysfunction in TLE may be associated with the significant variability in cortical morphometric variations in TLE that involve extratemporal structures including frontal and subcortical regions associated with executive function.

- *Sensorimotor Functions* Epilepsy that involves frontal or parietal sensorimotor cortex can result in problems with motor skills ranging from hemiparesis (e.g., in Rasmussen syndrome) to more subtle problems with strength and/or coordination.

- *Social Cognition* There is a high rate of comorbidity for epilepsy, intellectual disability, and autism. However, even among children who do not meet diagnostic criteria for autism, subtle impairments in social cognition are often present among individuals with epilepsy, which have a significant impact on quality of life.

    Functional deficits in social cognition are multidetermined in persons with epilepsy. From a neuroanatomical perspective, recent functional imaging studies on social cognition identify important networks that are also associated with epileptic networks in TLE and frontal lobe epilepsy. Social cognition engages medial frontal cortex including the anterior cingulate, temporal lobes, and amygdala. Epileptic disorders that disturb the development and function of these networks can impair development of social cognition.

    From a cognitive and behavioral perspective, social cognition involves the ability to quickly process and understand social cues, including understanding the intentions of others and anticipating behavioral and emotional responses based on cues such as facial emotion and situational factors. Social competence also depends on communication abilities that may be poorly developed in persons with epilepsy, affective issues such as social anxiety, attention (e.g., ability to sustain a lengthy conversation), and memory (e.g., ability to remember names, faces, shared experiences). From a psychosocial perspective, social competence and cognition is learned, and factors such as limited opportunities for social engagement due to seizures during formative years can interfere with development of social skills.

- *Emotion and Personality* Studies have identified higher rates of mood disorders, symptoms of anxiety/depression, and poorer quality of life in persons with epilepsy compared with the general population and children with other chronic diseases, such as diabetes. Similar findings have been observed in adult populations with epilepsy. More important, even among individuals who do not meet clinical criteria for diagnosis with an affective disorder, higher levels of associated symptoms and poor quality of life are reported, meaning subclinical presentations are even more common.

    Depression in epilepsy is common at all ages, but may manifest differently in children and adolescents than in adults. Children may exhibit more behavioral symptoms of depression, ranging from withdrawal and avoidance to anger, aggressive behavior, and acting out. Depression in persons with epilepsy at all ages is best viewed from a biopsychosocial perspective. Treatment of depression should be multimodal, and include optimization of seizure control, management of medications, addressing role restrictions and learning issues, social skills interventions, and psychotherapy. Medication management may be complicated by epilepsy, however management with commonly used medications for depression (e.g., SSRI, SNRI) is not contraindicated.

There have been some reports of increased suicidal thinking in persons with epilepsy using antiepileptic medications. However, despite the FDA requiring pharmaceutical companies to add a warning to AED labels regarding risk of suicide, subsequent studies have not confirmed an increased risk of suicide in persons with epilepsy taking antiepileptic medication compared with other groups (Bipolar, depression without epilepsy). Nonetheless, it is critical to monitor patients with epilepsy for symptoms of depression and suicidal thinking regardless of AED status.

- *Performance and Symptom Validity* There has been a recent increase in attention given to test-taking effort when evaluating persons with epilepsy, particularly in adults with TLE in whom surgical treatment is being considered. Although secondary gain may be present (e.g., disability benefits), of more concern is the validity of test results with respect to inferences about underlying neuropathological substrates associated with localized seizures and the ability to accurately assess the risk of cognitive morbidity associated with surgical treatment options. Early studies of test engagement have shown that as many as 20–25% of patients with epilepsy perform suboptimally on one or more performance validity tests.

Considerations when Treating Persons with Epilepsy and Seizure Disorders

Special considerations in treating individuals with epilepsy are age-related and dependent on disease-related variables such as seizure frequency, resistance to anticonvulsant medication treatment, whether a warning or aura is present, and the nature and extent of underlying neuropathology. Careful assessment of individual patient needs through comprehensive neuropsychological examination is crucial. Key issues are highlighted here.

- *Level of Supervision* Deficits in self-awareness and insight in children with epilepsy can increase the risk of injury. Atonic seizures can be associated with a high risk of falls, during which the reflexive self-protective mechanisms are absent. When seizures are reliably preceded by an aura, children can be taught to prevent injury by stopping activity and sitting or lying down. However, when there is no warning, seizures can occur suddenly and may even be precipitated by activities that are commonly sought out by children (e.g., video games in photosensitive seizures). While increased independence and normalization of activities is a desirable goal, role and activity restrictions are often a necessity due to increased risk of injury.

The need for increased supervision and monitoring, along with reduced independence and flexibility in choosing activities, may be factors in development of mood and behavior disturbances in children with epilepsy and should be explored when working with them and their families. However, a careful risk assessment may also lead to determination that the child is being unnecessarily restricted in his or her activities, and interventions targeting more realistic expectations may be helpful.

- *Driving* Rules regarding driving privileges and reporting of individuals with seizures to regulatory agencies vary from state to state. Generally, if a person with epilepsy has a sustained history of adequate seizure control, driving may be permitted. However, individuals with recurrent seizures despite therapeutic trials with anticonvulsants are typically not permitted to drive and should be discouraged from doing so. In patients who have been seizure free and whose physicians are contemplating discontinuation of AED treatment, driving is typically restricted during the drug withdrawal period and for a period afterward (often several months to a year). Driving restrictions are frequently cited as a factor in psychosocial issues in persons with epilepsy, including underemployment and reduced overall sense of independence and control.

- *Employment* Persons with epilepsy have a high rate of unemployment and underemployment due to multiple factors. Epilepsy that first emerges during childhood often results in educational problems related to cognitive difficulties or learning disabilities and, depending on the severity of the epilepsy, frequent absences and restricted educational opportunities, thus limiting occupational choices based on a lack of educational and training experiences. Work options are also reduced for safety reasons, particularly occupations that involve public safety (e.g., driving-related occupations). Finally, there may be limited work opportunities within a reasonable distance, particularly in rural regions. Restrictions on driving and limited public transportation options further reduce occupational choices. Treatment that includes educational interventions early in the course of the seizure disorder will have the best outcome. In adults, even when cognitive and vocational training is successful, practical limitations regarding transportation and medical issues may be significant.

- *School/Vocational Training* Early educational interventions with children who have seizures are an important component of treatment. Clinicians should be aware of resources available through multiple settings and encourage parents to work with an educational advocate whenever available. In some cases, simple accommodations in the classroom are sufficient. In more significant cases of epilepsy syndromes associated with communication or motor deficits, aggressive interventions with speech-language, occupational, or physical therapies are also often indicated. Clinicians also need to be able to clearly explain to school personnel and teachers how cognitive impairments in children with epilepsy differ from those in "run of the mill" attention and learning/reading disabilities in order to provide a stronger justification for costly school-based services. Interventions with peer education are also helpful for children with epilepsy. Providing age appropriate education and exposure to information about seizures and epilepsy can provide an important foundation for reducing psychosocial stigma and consequences of epilepsy.

- *Emotional and Psychological Issues* The preceding sections described briefly the complex nature of psychological and emotional disturbances in persons with epilepsy. The findings are similar in all ages and indicate that both biological and psychosocial factors play a role. Iatrogenic factors also need to be considered. Many medications used to treat seizures are associated with cognitive and behavioral side effects.

    While medical management of psychiatric and behavior symptoms can be effective, in many cases psychological intervention is also needed. Environmental and behavior interventions for children with comorbid ADHD symptoms, disruptive behaviors, and emotional dysregulation can be an important part of treatment. Cognitive behavior therapy is also recognized as among the most effective methods for managing symptoms of anxiety and depression in adolescents and adults, with some studies even showing larger effect sizes for CBT compared with medication for depression.

- *Medications* Medication management and an awareness of how medication side effects can create or exacerbate basic deficits in cognitive and emotional stability are important for both children and adults. Although there are some more common side effects of AED treatment (e.g., problems with psychomotor speed, attention, memory), certain medications are associated with more specific cognitive deficits. For example, language and memory impairments may be associated with some medications (e.g., topiramate). Although deficits are often reversible when treatment is discontinued, it is important to be aware of the side effects and to differentiate deficits associated with the epilepsy from iatrogenic deficits. Also, not all medication effects are negative, and many anticonvulsants have positive properties such as mood stabilization.

- *Interpersonal Relationships* Epilepsy may be associated with neurobehavioral conditions that interfere with social relationships. As noted above, social cognition is often affected in persons with epilepsy even in the absence of major developmental disorders (e.g., Autism spectrum disorder). However, persons with epilepsy frequently report social anxiety and withdrawal from social relationships, even when there is no neurobehavioral basis for impaired social interaction. The unpredictable nature of seizures, combined with the risk of embarrassing behaviors or loss of control, are often cited as factors in social withdrawal. Children and adults with epilepsy are often reticent to disclose their condition to others, resulting in further alienation from others and more difficulty forming intimate relationships. Overcoming these factors in persons with active epilepsy can be quite difficult. Not only are reluctance and withdrawal reinforced over years, but practical factors (e.g., not being able to drive) also limit social opportunities. Awareness of the complex interaction of neurobehavioral and psychological factors is key to improving quality of life with respect to interpersonal relations.

Relevant Definitions

Aura Typically, a subjective sensory phenomenon that precedes a seizure and may serve as a warning to the person with epilepsy that a seizure may be imminent. Not all auras are followed by observable seizures. When an aura occurs alone, it is considered a sensory seizure.

Febrile seizure A seizure brought on by a fever, typically higher than 102° F. Approximately 4–5% of children will have at least one febrile seizure. Febrile seizures do not constitute epilepsy and are not usually treated with AEDs. However, febrile seizures are a risk factor for later development of unprovoked seizures, particularly seizures arising from the temporal lobe.

Ictus A sudden neurological occurrence, such as a seizure. Ictal behaviors, or behavior changes that occur during a seizure, are often considered important lateralizing and localizing signs. "Interictal" refers to the period between seizures; for example, interictal EEG abnormalities are changes in the EEG pattern that occur between seizures and may be helpful in localizing regions of hyperexcitability and/or seizure onset. "Postictal" refers to the period of time after a seizure occurs, as in postictal confusion or drowsiness.

NMDAR N-methyl-D-aspartate receptor, one of three types of glutamate receptors in the brain. NMDAR encephalitis frequently (80% of patients) presents with new onset seizures. NMDA receptors are found throughout the brain with highest densities in the amygdala, hypothalamus, prefrontal cortex, and hippocampus.

Kindling The development of an epileptogenic network by exposure to recurrent seizures. Can occur in homologous areas of the contralateral hemisphere or within the same hemisphere as seizure onset through repetitive spread of seizures to areas of the brain functionally connected to the epileptogenic cortex.

Epilepsy and Seizure Disorders Questions

NOTE: Questions 9, 38, 53, 75, and 104 on the First Full-Length Practice Examination, Questions 12, 46, 79, and 119 on the Second Full-Length Practice Examination, Questions 14, 27, 57, 86, and 108 on the Third Full-Length Practice Examination, and Questions 7, 41, 46, 58, and 103 on the Fourth Full-Length Practice Examination are from this chapter.

1. Temporal lobe epilepsy is an example of ____.
   (a) catastrophic epilepsy
   (b) localization-related epilepsy
   (c) primary generalized epilepsy
   (d) psychogenic seizure

2. The most common underlying pathology in pediatric epilepsy is ____.
   (a) low-grade glioma
   (b) hippocampal sclerosis
   (c) malformation of cortical development
   (d) traumatic brain injury

3. Which of the following is considered to be a common cause of epilepsy?
   (a) concussion
   (b) history of chemotherapy
   (c) prenatal alcohol exposure
   (d) brain tumor

4. Which of the following is most important for classification of malformations of cortical development?
   (a) histological features
   (b) seizure type
   (c) syndromic presentation
   (d) familial history

5. Which of the following statements about persons with epilepsy is true?
   (a) Persons with epilepsy are typically intellectually disabled.
   (b) Persons with epilepsy are prone to violence and aggressive behavior.
   (c) Persons with epilepsy are likely to be under- or unemployed.
   (d) Persons with epilepsy typically have associated psychotic disorders.

6. Which of the following statements about IQ in persons with epilepsy is true?
   (a) Verbal IQ–Performance IQ (VIQ–PIQ) discrepancies are a lateralizing sign in children, but not adults.
   (b) IQ scores typically decline over time in persons with epilepsy.
   (c) Most persons with epilepsy have low IQ scores.
   (d) Age at seizure onset and pharmacoresistance are factors in how IQ is affected.

7. Epidemiological studies have shown an overall increase in early mortality for persons with epilepsy. Which of the following is considered a major risk?
   (a) motor vehicle accidents due to seizures while driving
   (b) injury (unintentional injury and suicide)
   (c) AED medication toxicity
   (d) socioeconomic status

8. Anxiety and depression are common comorbidities in epilepsy. Which of the following is true about treatment of depression in persons with epilepsy?

(a) Psychotherapy, particularly cognitive behavior therapy (CBT) is proven effective for treating depression in persons with epilepsy.

(b) Epilepsy is a neurological disorder, and as a result psychotherapy is less effective than treatment with antidepressant medications.

(c) Antidepressant medications are contraindicated due to interactions with epilepsy drugs.

(d) Treating symptoms of depression in persons with epilepsy is common due to the high comorbidity.

9. Which of the following is an important factor in impaired interictal attention and ADHD symptoms in persons with absence seizures?

(a) decreased cerebellar-frontal connectivity

(b) auditory processing deficits and auditory agnosia

(c) seizure frequency

(d) decreased medial frontal cortex activation

10. Which of the following is most accurate regarding language deficits in persons with epilepsy?

(a) language deficits only occur in left hemisphere seizures

(b) language deficits do not occur in adult onset epilepsy syndromes

(c) language deficits may be associated with impaired semantic association and lexical systems

(d) language deficits in Rasmussen syndrome will typically remit with speech-language intervention

11. The most common age of onset for newly diagnosed epilepsy is _____.

(a) before the age of 5 years   (c) during adulthood

(b) during adolescence   (d) over the age of 70

Epilepsy and Seizure Disorders Answers

1. **B—localization-related epilepsy** *Seizures that begin in a localized area, such as the temporal lobe, are by definition, localization related.*

   Reference: Berg, A. T., Berkovic, S. F., Brodie, M., Buchhalter, J., Cross, H., van Emde Boas, W. . . . Scheffer, I. E. (2010). Revised terminology and concepts for organization of seizures and epilepsies: Report of the ILAE Commission on Classification and Terminology, 2005–2009. *Epilepsia, 51*, 676–685.

2. **C—malformation of cortical development** *It is estimated that 25–40% of intractable or medication resistant epilepsy is attributable to malformations of cortical development, and that up to 75% of children with MCDs have epilepsy.*

   Reference: Leventer, R. J., Guerrini, R., & Dobyns, W. B. (2008). Malformations of cortical development and epilepsy. *Dialogues in Clinical Neuroscience, 10*, 47–62.

3. **D—brain tumor** *In patients with brain tumor, 20–40% will present with seizures as the first symptom. While traumatic brain injury that involves cerebral contusion, penetrating skull fracture, or other clear injury to the brain is associated with a substantial increased risk of later epilepsy, there is no evidence that concussion presents a risk factor for epilepsy.*

References:

(a) Maschio, M. (2012). Brain-tumor related epilepsy. *Current Neuropharmacology, 10,* 124–133.

(b) Wennberg, R., Hiploylee, C., Tai, P., & Tator, C. H. (2018) Is concussion a risk factor for epilepsy? *Canadian Journal of Neurological Science, 45,* 275–282.

4. **A—histological features**   *Although different malformations of cortical development (MCD) may be associated with different epilepsy syndromes, seizure type or epilepsy syndrome is not a basis for classification of MCD; classification is based on imaging studies, histological features when biopsy or resection is performed, and genetic and embryological principles.*

Reference: Desikan, R. S., & Barkovich, A. J. (2016) Malformations of cortical development. *Annals of Neurology, 80,* 797–810.

5. **C—Persons with epilepsy are likely to be under- or unemployed.**   *There are many myths and misconceptions about persons with epilepsy that contribute to the stigma associated with the disorder. It is important to acknowledge that there is an increased risk of psychiatric comorbidity associated with epilepsy, particularly depression and suicidality, but also including more severe psychiatric conditions including bipolar disorder and schizophrenia. However, it is not "typical" for persons with epilepsy to have psychotic disorders, intellectual disability, or aggressive/violent tendencies.*

Reference: England, M. J., Liverman, C. T., Schultz, A. M., & Strawbridge L. M. (Eds.). (2012). *Epilepsy across the spectrum: Promoting health and understanding.* Institute of Medicine (US) Committee on the Public Health Dimensions of the Epilepsies. Washington, DC: National Academies Press.

6. **D—Age at seizure onset and pharmacoresistance are factors in how IQ is affected.**   *Although large discrepancies between verbal and nonverbal abilities may have lateralizing significance, VIQ-PIQ discrepancies are not a consistent lateralizing sign, and research has indicated that the most important factor determining IQ is age at seizure onset, with earlier age of onset associated with lower IQ.*

References:

(a) Berg, A. T., Zelko, F., Levy, S., & Testa, F. (2012) Age at onset, pharmacoresistance, and cognitive outcomes: A prospective cohort study. *Neurology, 79,* 1384–1391.

(b) Blackburn, L. B., Lee, G. P., Westerveld, M., Hempel, A., Park, Y. D., & Loring, D. W. (2007). The verbal IQ/performance IQ discrepancy as a sign of seizure focus laterality in pediatric patients with epilepsy. *Epilepsy and Behavior, 10,* 84–88.

7. **B—injury (unintentional injury and suicide)**   *While AED toxicity and adverse reactions to medications used to treat epilepsy is a significant problem, there is no evidence that it is a factor in early mortality. Review of mortality studies in epilepsy has identified many factors linked to early mortality including SUDEP, unintentional injury (e.g., falls, drowning), intentional injury (suicide), comorbid brain disorders, and status-epilepticus. Mortality is higher in developing countries, but is also elevated in high-income developed countries. Early mortality is slightly greater for males, and is substantially greater in younger age groups.*

Reference: Thurman, D. J., Logroscino, G., Beghi, E., Hauser, W., Hesdorffer, D. C., Newton, C. R. . . . Epidemiology Commission of the International League Against Epilepsy (2017). The burden of premature mortality of epilepsy in high-income countries: A systematic review from the Mortality Task Force of the International League Against Epilepsy. *Epilepsia, 58,* 17–26.

8. **A—Psychotherapy, particularly cognitive behavior therapy (CBT) is proven effective for treating depression in persons with epilepsy.**   *Depression is one of the most common comorbidities with epilepsy, and is best seen through a biopsychosocial model. Despite the high prevalence, referrals for therapy and psychotherapy are underutilized by neurologists treating*

epilepsy. There have been several studies, including randomized controlled studies, showing the effectiveness of psychotherapy in treating depression in persons with epilepsy. Medical management along with psychotherapy is often essential, especially with psychotic depression and suicidal ideation and, although there are some potential drug interactions treatment with SSRI and other antidepressant medications is not contraindicated.

Reference: Elger, C., Johnston, S. A., & Hoppe, C. (2017). Diagnosing and treating depression in epilepsy. *Seizure, 44,* 184–193.

9. **D—decreased medial frontal cortex activation** *Absence seizures affect attention in a number of direct and indirect ways. Absence seizures are primary generalized nonconvulsive seizures that involve frontal and subcortical networks involved in regulating attention.*

Reference: Killory, B. D., Bai, X., Negishi, M., Vega, C., Spann, M. N., Vestal, M., . . . Blumenfeld, H. (2011). Impaired attention and network connectivity in childhood absence epilepsy. *Neuroimage, 56,* 2209–2217.

10. **C—language deficits may be associated with impaired semantic association and lexical systems** *Language deficits due to disruption of the semantic association and lexical systems can occur at any age regardless of lateralization. In progressive syndromes such as Rasmussen's, speech therapy can improve language outcome but when the dominant hemisphere is involved complete remission is unlikely.*

Reference: Fan, X., Yan, H., Shan, Y., Shang, K., Wang, X., Wang, P., . . . Zhao, G. (2016). Distinctive structural and effective connectivity changes of semantic cognition network across left and right mesial temporal lobe epilepsy patients. *Neural Plasticity.*

11. **A—before the age of 5 years** *The majority of epilepsy syndromes occur in childhood, before the age of 5 years. The second highest rate of new onset seizures occurs in the aging population, over 70 years old. Although seizures can occur at any age, new onset epilepsy in adolescents and adults is less common and more frequently associated with a new onset neurological risk factor (e.g., brain tumor).*

Reference: Banerjee, P. N., Filippi, D., & Hauser, W. A. (2009). The descriptive epidemiology of epilepsy: A review. *Epilepsy Research, 85,* 31–45.

Recommended Readings

Bien, C. G., & Scheffer, I. E. (2011) Autoantibodies and epilepsy. *Epilepsia, 52*(Suppl. 3), 18–22.

Blume, W. T., Luders, H. O., Mizrahi, E., Tassinari, C., van Emde Boas, W., & Engel, J. (2001). Glossary of descriptive terminology for ictal semiology: Report of the ILAE Task Force on Classification and Terminology. *Epilepsia, 42*(9), 812–818.

Desikan, R. S., & Barkovich, A. J. (2016) Malformations of cortical development. *Annals of Neurology, 80,* 797–810.

Fisher, R. S., Cross, J. H., French, J. A., Higurashi, N., Hirsch, E., Jansen, F. E., . . . Zuberi, S. M. (2017). Operational classification of seizure types by the International League Against Epilepsy: Position paper of the ILAE Commission for Classification and Terminology. *Epilepsia, 58,* 522–530.

Hermann, B. P., Loring, D. W., & Wilson, S. (2017) Paradigm shifts in the neuropsychology of epilepsy. *Journal of the International Neuropsychology Society, 23*(9–10), 791–805.

Jokeit, H., Eicher, M., & Ives-Deliperi, V. (2018) Toward social neuropsychology of epilepsy: A review on social cognition in epilepsy. *Acta Epilepsy, 1,* 8–17.

Orsini, A., Zara, F., & Striano, P. (2018) Recent advances in epilepsy genetics. *Neuroscience Letters, 667,* 4–9.

Scheffer, I. E., Berkovic, S., Capovilla, G., Connolly, M. B., French, J. A., Guilhoto, L., . . . Zuberi, S. M. (2017) ILAE classification of the epilepsies: Position paper of the ILAE Commission for Classification and Terminology. *Epilepsia, 58,* 512–521.

Wilson, S. J., Baxendale, S., Barr, W., Hamed, S., Langfitt, J., Samson, S., . . . Smith, M. L. (2015) Indications and expectations for neuropsychological assessment in routine epilepsy care: Report of the ILAE Neuropsychology Task Force, Diagnostic Methods Commission, 2013–2017. *Epilepsia, 56,* 674–681.

Websites

Epilepsy Information, Resources, and Publications: https://www.ilae.org/guidelines

Glossary of Descriptive Terminology for ictal semiology (Blume et al., 2001). https://onlinelibrary.wiley.com/doi/full/10.1046/j.1528-1157.2001.22001.x

23 Central Nervous System Infections

Lauren Krivitzky and Katherine Baum

Introduction

This chapter provides a review of central nervous system (CNS) infections with an emphasis on two of the most common types: meningitis, including both bacterial and aseptic meningitis, and encephalitis. Paraneoplastic and autoimmune encephalitis are specifically described. In the last section of the chapter, a brief review of several additional causes/types of CNS infection is provided, including brain abscesses, intrauterine infections, prion diseases, HIV encephalitis, progressive multifocal leukoencephalopathy (PML), cerebral toxoplasmosis, and acute disseminating *encephalomyelitis* (ADEM).

Section 1: Meningitis
Definition

Meningitis is an infection/inflammation that is confined to the meninges.

Neuropathology

The most common causes of meningitis are bacteria or viruses, although other causes also exist (e.g., fungal). Outcomes tend to be much worse when the etiology is bacterial as opposed to viral. The first part of this section will primarily include a discussion of bacterial meningitis, with comparisons to other forms when appropriate.

Bacterial Forms of Meningitis

Ninety-five percent of cases are caused by three primary agents:

- *Haemophilus influenzae type B* (Haemophilus meningitis)
- *Neisseria meningitides* (Meningococcal meningitis)
- *Streptococcus pneumoniae* (Pneumococcal meningitis)

Bacteria may spread to the meninges in several ways, including from an adjacent infected area, such as the ears or sinuses; from the environment through a penetrating injury or congenital defect; and through the bloodstream (hematogenous dissemination), which is the most common cause.

The primary cause of brain damage in bacterial meningitis is inflammation, which leads to tissue and vascular injury (vasculitis), septic thrombosis, and smaller infarcts. Other complications include brain (*cerebral*) *edema* and increased *intracranial pressure (ICP)*, which can lead to hypoxic ischemic encephalopathy (HIE). The pathophysiology of increased ICP is complex and may involve many proinflammatory molecules, as well as mechanical elements. Cranial nerve defects may also be present (although these are often reversible) and are more common in children (~5–11% of cases) than adults with bacterial meningitis. Although any of the cranial nerves can be affected in meningitis, the eighth cranial nerve (auditory nerve) is most often impacted, which can result in sensorineural hearing loss. When there is increased ICP, the most commonly involved nerve is the sixth cranial nerve (abducens nerve) because it has the longest intracranial route and is most vulnerable to compression. The third, fourth, and seventh cranial nerves may also be impacted.

Individuals with tuberculosis (TB) can also develop meningitis, which is caused by the bacteria *Mycobacterium tuberculosis*. The tuberculosis bacteria is spread to the brain and spine from another place in the body, usually the lung. Tuberculous granulomas (or Rich foci) release bacteria into the subarachnoid space, resulting in TB meningitis.

Epidemiology

Bacterial meningitis (see Table 23.1)

- 0.6–4 cases per 100,000 annually (all ages)
- Neonatal bacterial meningitis occurs in 0.25–1 cases per 1,000 live births.
- TB meningitis is rare in the United States. It occurs mainly in resource-poor regions with a high tuberculosis burden.

Mortality

Mortality from bacterial meningitis has been estimated to be 5–10% overall, which is a dramatic improvement relative to the 1950s (prior to the development of antibiotics), when rates were near 90%.

- *Age* Mortality rates are highest in the first year of life, decline in mid-life, and increase again in older adults.
- *Type* Mortality rates are highest in pneumococcal (10–30%) and lowest with meningococcal (4–5%).
- Mortality rates are also high in TB meningitis (15–30% in most studies, much higher rates in HIV positive individuals).

Morbidity

Long-term neurologic and/or neurobehavioral sequelae are seen in approximately 15–25% of survivors of bacterial meningitis. In developed countries, the most common long-term sequelae include hearing

TABLE 23.1 Incidence Rates for Bacterial Meningitis

Type	Incidence Rates
Pneumococcal Meningitis	• Most common cause, with approximately 6,000 cases reported in the United States each year • Children < age 2 years with compromised immune systems are at greatest risk
Meningococcal Meningitis	• Next most common cause, with ~2,600 cases in the United States per year or .9 to 1.5 per 100,000 • Occurs most frequently in children ages 2 to 18 years • Less frequent in adults >50 years • Crowding (e.g., college dorms) increases the risk of an outbreak
Haemophilus Meningitis	• Used to be the most common form of bacterial meningitis • Rates have dramatically decreased (particularly in newborns) since the discovery of the vaccine in the 1980s

loss (approximately 11%), intellectual disabilities (4%), spasticity/paresis (4%), and seizure disorders (4%). More broadly, approximately 50% of childhood survivors of bacterial meningitis have at least one negative sequelae more than 5 years after diagnosis, the most common of which (78%) fall in the category of cognitive/behavioral difficulties (e.g., cognitive impairments, academic limitations, ADHD). Data on outcomes from TB meningitis are limited. Early research has been mixed, but suggests that many survivors are left with mild to moderate disabilities.

Determinants of Severity

Age Factors

The highest prevalence of bacterial meningitis occurs in children (<5 years) and older adults (≥ 60). Meningococcal meningitis is also more common in college students, (freshmen in particular) who reside in dormitories. Children are also at higher risk of mortality than adults. The risk of death from bacterial meningitis is 15–20% in neonates and 3–10% in older children (non-neonates). Ranges are given because mortality risk also depends on the type of bacterial meningitis.

Medical Risk Factors

One of the biggest medical risk factors for contracting bacterial meningitis is immunosuppression because this leads to an increased risk for opportunistic infections. Individuals with HIV and other medical conditions with poor immune functioning (or who are immunosuppressed due to treatments they are undergoing) or presumed autoimmune etiologies are also at higher risk for bacterial meningitis; this includes individuals with cystic fibrosis, diabetes mellitus, hypoparathyroidism, and renal or adrenal insufficiency.

Cultural/Economic Risk Factors

Cultural/economic factors impact both the development and treatment of bacterial meningitis. Incidence and complication rates are higher in developing countries. It has been suggested that prevention through large scale vaccination programs is likely to be the most cost-effective strategy for improving the situation in these countries. These factors are also important to consider in TB, as the disease tends to impact countries and individuals with fewer resources. For example, one study in India found that 80% of the children with TB meningitis who underwent neurodevelopmental follow-up demonstrated deficits in locomotion, language, coordination, and personal, social, and executive function, despite many having made a good clinical outcome. These deficits are compounded by the fact that most of these children are reared in impoverished homes with limited child-caring options, and from communities with a shortage of schools able to provide adequate support.

Risk Factors That Influence Neuropsychological/ Neurological Outcomes

In some studies, individuals with pneumococcal meningitis have been shown to demonstrate greater cognitive impairments and neurological sequelae (such as hearing loss) than those with meningococcal meningitis. Poor outcomes from TB meningitis often relate to the neurological complications which include stroke, seizures, and hydrocephalus. Viral (aseptic) forms have better outcomes than bacterial forms.

Risk Factors in Children

- Acute-phase neurological complications including prolonged seizures, hemiparesis, coma, and bilateral hearing loss have been associated with worse outcomes.

- Low cerebrospinal fluid (CSF) glucose levels, Streptococcus pneumoniae infection, and two or more days of symptoms prior to admission have also been linked to worse outcomes in children.

- Younger age at the time of illness (particularly <1 year of age) contributes to worse language outcome. This is consistent with research in other pediatric disorders in which diffuse brain injuries in young children have been shown to be associated with delayed consequences in cognitive development, in this case reduced plasticity for language.

- Male gender may also be associated with worse behavioral outcome.

Presentation, Disease Course, and Recovery

Presenting Symptoms

- *Acute versus gradual*
  - Acute (several hours): Cardinal signs include (1) sudden fever, (2) severe headaches (due to inflammation of the meningeal blood vessels), and (3) nuchal rigidity (stiff neck).
  - Gradual (several days): Often nonspecific "flu-like" symptoms.

- Most common presenting symptoms in children include hyperthermia, lethargy, anorexia or vomiting, respiratory distress, convulsions, irritability, jaundice, bulging fontanelle (in infants), diarrhea, and nuchal rigidity.

Assessment Methods

- *Lumbar puncture* The diagnosis of bacterial meningitis is confirmed by the presence of bacteria in the CSF. Cerebrospinal fluid can also be examined for the presence of blood or white blood cells (elevations would suggest presence of an infection), high protein levels, and low glucose. CSF is also examined in TB meningitis.

- *Brain imaging* Although brain imaging studies may also be used in the work-up for meningitis, computed tomography (CT) scans of the head and magnetic resonance imaging (MRI) of the brain generally do not aid in the diagnosis of bacterial meningitis. Some patients may show meningeal enhancement, but its absence does not rule out the condition. MRI is used in TB meningitis to visualize leptomeningeal tubercles, to identify TB meningitis related cranial neuropathies, and to diagnose other complications of TB, such as stroke.

Treatment

- *Antibiotics* (oral and IV in more severe cases) for several types of bacterial meningitis.
- *Vaccine* for several types of meningococcal meningitis.
- *Corticosteroids* treat inflammation and brain swelling and may be helpful in preventing neurological sequelae and hearing loss in some types of meningitis. Several years ago, dexamethasone treatment was recommended as an adjunct to the standard of care treatment for adults with bacterial meningitis. Although several earlier studies suggested improved morbidity and mortality with adjunctive dexamethasone, more recent findings have not fully substantiated these claims, calling into question this recommendation.
- For TB meningitis, treatment includes *anti-tuberculosis drugs* and adjunctive corticosteroids

Recovery Course

After medical stabilization, children and adults with meningitis (and encephalitis) sometimes require inpatient or outpatient rehabilitation. The length of stay is variable depending on the severity of the illness. With the exception of cases in which there is also spinal cord involvement (e.g., *encephalomyelitis*), individuals with these conditions tend to show greater residual impairments in cognitive as opposed to physical domains.

Expectations for Neuropsychological Assessment Results

Table 23.2 outlines the research on neuropsychological functioning in both pediatric and adult meningitis.

TABLE 23.2 Pediatric and Adult Neuropsychological Findings in Meningitis

Domain	Adult Findings	Pediatric Findings
Intelligence & Achievement	Most studies have found average IQ scores in adults.	• Low average to average IQ with. relatively lower IQ in children with acute neurological complications. • ~4% of children in developed countries are diagnosed with intellectual disabilities. • Twice as likely as controls to require special education assistance. More likely to repeat a grade or be placed in special-needs school. • No consistent area of academic skill deficit is identified. Academic issues may be more related to problems in attention, speed, and executive functioning skills.
Attention	Studies have found attention problems (such as decreased performance on Trails B and Stroop) in adults (versus controls).	One large study with children infected with enterovirus (both meningitis and encephalitis) found parent/teacher reports of elevated ADHD symptoms including inattention and hyperactivity impulsivity (20% versus 3% in controls).
Processing Speed	Simple reaction time and other aspects of processing speed shown to be area of weakness in adults with a history of meningitis. Cognitive slowness has been suggested to be one of the main deficits.	
Language	Language problems have not generally been reported.	Language problems have been noted in children who contracted meningitis before the age of 1.
Visuospatial	No systematic findings, although a few studies have noted mild visuospatial processing weaknesses.	

(continued)

TABLE 23.2 Continued

Domain	Adult Findings	Pediatric Findings
Memory	Studies are mixed. Some findings suggest that adults with bacterial meningitis (pneumococcal) report the most significant cognitive deficit to be memory problems, whereas other studies have found no memory impairments.	
Executive Functions	Executive function problems are one of the more common problems reported after meningitis.	
	Subtle executive function problems are a relatively consistent finding in adult studies.	Studies have generally found that children are not severely impaired in executive functions but that their abilities are often below developmental expectations.
Sensorimotor	Sensorineural hearing loss is the most consistent sensory finding after meningitis (estimated about 11% overall, 5% with severe to profound deafness). It is more commonly reported following pneumococcal meningitis (rates in most studies are 15–26%, although some have reported even higher rates) versus meningococcal meningitis (9% of children, no prevalence rates found for adults). Meningitis is estimated to be the cause of about 3–6% of the deaf and hard-of-hearing youth population in the United States. Other acute-phase complications include hemiparesis (6–9%), cortical blindness (1–2%), and ataxia (2–6%), which typically resolve. Long-term spasticity or paresis occurs in approximately 4% of children with a history of bacterial meningitis.	
Emotion & Personality	No systematic findings in adults.	Behavioral changes (including ADHD) are one of the more commonly reported sequelae of pediatric meningitis. Adolescents with a history of meningitis have been shown to have poorer quality of life, greater fatigue, reduced social support, and reduced overall mental health 1–3 years post illness.
Symptom & Performance Validity	The issue of effort has not been systematically addressed in studies of meningitis.	
Work	Most adult survivors of bacterial meningitis are able to return to premorbid levels of functioning.	Adults who had meningitis as children are reported to have lower economic self-sufficiency.

Section 2: Aseptic Forms of Meningitis

Neuropathology

The term "aseptic" refers to nonbacterial forms of meningitis caused by viruses, fungi, and parasites. Enteroviruses (viruses transmitted through intestines) are by far the most common cause of aseptic meningitis (>85%). These viruses are a genus of single-stranded *RNA* associated with several human and mammalian diseases. The enteroviruses that occur in the United States include the coxsackieviruses and echoviruses. Polioviruses are also in the family of enteroviruses, but have generally been eradicated from the United States through vaccination.

There are several types of fungi that can cause meningitis including Cryptococcus, Histoplasma, Blastomyces, Coccidioides, and Candida. Candida is often acquired in a hospital, while the other types are typically acquired when fungal spores are inhaled from the environment.

Epidemiology

Viral forms of meningitis are more common than bacterial meningitis. More than 10,000 cases of viral meningitis are reported annually in the United States, but the actual incidence may be as high as 75,000. It occurs mostly in children and young adults and often presents in the summer months when enteroviruses are more common.

Fungal meningitis is rare and typically (but not always) occurs in individuals who are immune compromised, including those who are HIV positive. The most common cause of fungal meningitis for people with weak immune systems is *Cryptococcus*. This disease is one of the most common causes of adult meningitis in Africa. Premature babies with very low birth weights are also at increased risk for getting *Candida* blood stream infection, which may spread to the brain.

Mortality

With the exception of neonates, the rate of mortality for viral meningitis has been estimated to be less than 1%.

Morbidity

Long-term neurologic and/or neurobehavioral sequelae are far less common in viral (versus bacterial) meningitis. Most people recover within 7 to 10 days and have no residual neurologic deficits. When there are persistent deficits in viral meningitis, they tend to be mild (see "Expectations for Neuropsychological Assessment Results" section).

Presentation, Disease Course, and Recovery

Presenting Symptoms

Headaches (often severe) are the most common presenting symptom in viral meningitis. Fever is also common, often low-grade in the prodromal stage with higher temperature elevations at the onset of neurological signs. Other common symptoms include irritability, nausea, vomiting, stiff neck, rash, or fatigue. Younger children may not report headache and may simply be irritable. In terms of the timing, nonspecific flu-like symptoms and low-grade fever precede neurologic symptoms by approximately 48 hours.

Assessment Methods

- *Lumbar puncture/blood work* Primary assessment methods, are used to examine blood and CSF in an attempt to isolate the viral pathogen.

- *Other* Several of the other techniques mentioned later in the encephalitis section (CT, MRI, and electroencephalogram [EEG]) may be utilized to clarify the diagnosis of viral meningitis, particularly in more complex cases. These additional tests are often most relevant in cases where there is an additional suspicion of encephalitis (MRI with contrast enhancement) or subclinical seizures (EEG).

Treatment

- *Viral Meningitis* Antibiotics are ineffective. Treatment for viral meningitis is mostly supportive (i.e., rest, fluids, pain and anti-inflammatory medications), although patients may undergo additional treatments with antiviral medications (described further in encephalitis section later in the chapter).

- *Fungal Meningitis* Antifungal medication is the treatment of choice.

Recovery Course

Viral meningitis typically has a relatively benign course, with symptoms often resolving in one to two weeks. Long-term neurologic sequelae from uncomplicated viral meningitis are quite rare.

Expectations for Neuropsychological Assessment Results

Few long-term outcome studies have been conducted in adults and children with viral meningitis. Extant studies provide mixed results. Some studies have found no long-term neuropsychological problems, others have found subtle deficits. When neuropsychological impairments have been noted, they tend to be mild to moderate in nature and in the domains of attention and speed. Individuals with West Nile Virus "neuroinvasive" disease have been found to experience impairment in motor functioning, verbal learning and memory, and aspects of executive functioning.

Individuals with cryptococcal (fungal) meningitis have been shown to demonstrate broad deficits in cognition in the early stages of the disease, with improvements noted over the first year of recovery. Longer lasting deficits have been noted in motor speed, gross motor and executive functioning. Individuals with cryptococcal meningitis who require shunts have worse neuropsychological outcomes.

Section 3: Encephalitis

Definition

Encephalitis is a general term that refers to an infection of the brain tissue/parenchyma.

Neuropathology

Viruses are the most common cause of encephalitis, although it can also be caused by various bacteria, fungi, and parasites. Autoimmune encephalitis is also common and involves the body's own immune system attacking the brain (see "Section 4: Autoimmune and Paraneoplastic Encephalitis").

Primary Versus Secondary

- *Primary* (also known as acute viral encephalitis) refers to a direct infection of the brain through direct invasion of a pathogen.

- *Secondary* (also known as post-infective encephalitis) results from either a previous viral infection (most commonly chickenpox, mumps, or measles), or an immunization (measles vaccination) or via an immune response.

Etiology

- More than 100 viruses have been implicated. The most common include herpes simplex virus (HSV), varicella zoster virus, Epstein-Barr virus, adenoviruses, enteroviruses, *arboviruses* (e.g., ARthropod-BOrne viruses such as from ticks and mosquitoes), human parechovirus, and cytomegalovirus.

- Regional outbreaks occur, such as Japanese B and Lacrosse encephalitis in the Midwestern United States.

- Four types of mosquito-borne encephalitis exist in the United States: Lacrosse, Equine, St. Louis, and West Nile.

- Antibodies target neurons, either intra- or extracellular antigens, disrupting synaptic transmission. Creation of these antibodies is sometimes in response to a tumor or cancer in the body (termed paraneoplastic).

- Precise microbial etiology cannot be determined in approximately 50% of encephalitis cases.

Most viruses reach the CNS via the bloodstream. Some viruses (e.g., HSV) travel to the CNS along cranial nerves. Herpes simplex virus remains dormant in the trigeminal ganglia. If "activated," it is believed to travel along the trigeminal nerve into the brain. Viruses use cellular machinery for their replication and damage or kill the cells they infect. Brain damage is also caused by the cell-mediated immune reaction viruses and cancers elicit. Activation of T lymphocytes by viruses or cancers includes the release of potent cytokines and mobilization of macrophages that not only attack the viruses or cancer but assault the host, causing severe vascular and tissue injury. Some viruses and types of encephalitis have predilection for certain types of neurons or brain regions and may have a characteristic pattern on neuroimaging including involvement of the cerebellum (e.g., *cerebellitis*) brain stem and basal ganglia. Lesions in the thalamus, basal, ganglia, and midbrain are observed in eastern equine encephalitis while temporal lobe pathology and enhancement of orbitofrontal lobes are seen in HSV encephalitis. However, in neonates who develop HSV encephalitis, cortical lesions are seen within 48 hours but then often progress to subcortical white matter lesions within a week. Bilateral subcortical abnormalities are associated with poor cognitive and motor functioning.

Epidemiology

- 7.3 per 100,000 persons in the United States in 2000–2010

- Annual incidence of 20,000 cases per year, most of which are mild.

- In children aged 1 month to 15 years, incidence is 10.5 cases per 100,000. Highest incidence is in children younger than 1 year (18.4 per 100,000).

- Herpes simplex virus encephalitis is the most common cause of encephalitis in children and the most common severe form of encephalitis and is estimated at 2,000 cases per year in the United States (approximately 10% of all encephalitis cases in the United States).

- Incidence rates have increased in children over the past 10 years and show seasonal increases (summer and fall) due to arbo- and enteroviruses.

Mortality

Mortality rates for encephalitides are estimated to be 5% overall (3% in children), although the range is quite varied, depending on the specific type. Some factors include:

- *Age* Certain types have greater mortality in the elderly (e.g., Japanese B, St. Louis, and West Nile viruses)
- *Type* Highest mortality is for rabies virus encephalitis (virtually 100%) and HSV encephalitis if not treated (50% of children die if left untreated).

Morbidity

Approximately one third of individuals with encephalitis (all forms) have some ongoing neurological or cognitive difficulties at the time of their discharge from the hospital. Children who fully recover are most likely to do so within 6 to 12 months.

Determinants of Severity

Age Factors

- Severity is greatest in infants and the elderly.
- Prevalence rates are highest in children and young adults.

Risk Factors That Influence Neuropsychological/Behavioral Outcomes

Individuals with HSV encephalitis have been found to have more cognitive and psychiatric impairments than those with other etiologies, including two to four times the risk of cognitive impairment. Individuals with bilateral temporal lesions versus unilateral lesions are associated with worse cognitive and behavioral outcome in HSV encephalitis. Problems with daily living skills have been linked to changes in personality/mood, even in cases in which significant cognitive deficits are not present.

Risk Factors in Children

There are limited data on long-term neurologic outcomes in children, but those with longer hospital stays, confirmed infectious agent, and abnormal neuroimaging are less likely to fully recover and may report poorer quality of life. Outcomes also vary greatly by etiology. Children with HSV encephalitis often have long-term neurological impairment, particularly following a delayed start of acyclovir. Older infants and young children with encephalitis from enteroviruses usually recover fully, though neonates vary, some with significant long-term deficits.

Risk of Seizures

The 20-year risk for development of seizures is approximately 20% for those with early seizures and 10% without early seizures.

Presentation, Disease Course, and Recovery

Presenting Symptoms

- *Acute, Subacute, and Chronic*
  - *Acute* (hours to days): Presents with severe headache and fever (often resembling influenza) as well as altered consciousness, disorientation, behavioral and speech disturbances, and general and focal neurological signs.
  - *Subacute* (weeks): Presents with seizures and speech disturbance after a few weeks of altered behavior.
  - *Chronic*: Can present/progress over the course of years and produce acute symptoms only occasionally, such as HIV infection or untreated Lyme disease.
- *Behavioral Presentation* Encephalitis can initially present in the form of a behavioral or psychotic disorder (particularly in HSV) with symptoms ranging from delusions, hallucinations, and affective disorders (e.g., depression, aggression, and euphoria). A small number of HSV encephalitis cases present with symptoms of *Kluver-Bucy syndrome* due to bilateral damage to the amygdala.

Assessment Methods

- *Lumbar Puncture/Blood Work* Used to examine blood serum and CSF in an attempt to isolate the pathogen.
- *EEG* Used to assess brain wave activity and for the possibility of seizures. Findings on EEG tend to be nonspecific and have been reported to occur in upward of 90% of children with encephalitis. More specific temporal lobe focus has been noted in individuals with HSV encephalitis.
- *CT and MRI* Used to identify signs of swelling (*cerebral edema*), any localized infection (abscess), *mass effect*, and other signs of an inflammatory process. A CT or MRI scan with contrast is usually indicated to look for signs of infection, including meningeal enhancement in meningitis or ring-enhancing lesions in the case of a brain abscess. Magnetic resonance imaging with a diffusion sequence may be the preferred technique in these instances because it best differentiates among tumors, strokes, and abscesses.

Treatment

- *Antiviral drugs*, such as acyclovir and ganciclovir, are used to treat viral encephalitis.
- *Anticonvulsant drugs* May be prescribed to prevent future seizures.
- *Corticosteroid drugs* Are used to reduce swelling and brain inflammation.
- *Hemispherectomy* May be used to treat *Rasmussen's encephalitis* and often appears to slow down the neurological deterioration in pediatric cases.

Expectations for Neuropsychological Assessment Results

Caveat: With the exception of HSV encephalitis, limited large-scale studies on neuropsychological outcomes have been conducted. However, existing studies are outlined in Table 23.3.

TABLE 23.3 Pediatric and Adult Neuropsychological Findings in Encephalitis

Domain	Adult Findings	Pediatric Findings
Intelligence & Achievement	• Most studies find mean IQ scores in the low average to average range. • IQ scores tend to be lower than estimates of premorbid functioning by approximately 0.5–1 standard deviation (SD).	• Studies examining encephalitis from mixed etiologies have found overall IQs in the low average to average range. • Higher rate of learning disabilities • Studies of neonatal HSV encephalitis have found more variable outcomes, ranging from average IQ to intellectual disability.
Attention	Subtle attention problems (versus controls).	Higher prevalence of attention problems.
Processing Speed	Processing speed has been shown to be commonly affected following encephalitis.	
Language	Language is often reported to be unaffected. However, naming deficits (and sometimes more severe aphasias) have been observed in HSV encephalitis.	
Visuospatial	No consistent findings in the literature.	
Memory	Difficulty with memory (particularly anterograde) is a common sequelae of HSV encephalitis (estimated to occur in 25–75% of cases) and West Nile Virus encephalitis.	
Executive Functions	Executive function deficits are one of the most commonly reported problems following encephalitis and are estimated to occur in approximately 40% of cases of HSV encephalitis.	
Sensorimotor	No consistent findings in the literature for most types of encephalitis. Difficulties with motor functioning is the most common reported deficit in individuals with West Nile encephalitis.	
Emotion & Personality	• May see elevated psychiatric symptoms (e.g., mood and anxiety symptoms) • Individuals with HSV encephalitis more likely to show long term behavioral and personality changes and often show greater personality & emotional disturbance in early recovery.	• Children with a history of encephalitis are more likely to demonstrate behavioral difficulties than normal controls. • Higher likelihood of attention problems, hyperactivity-impulsivity, oppositional behavior, and, in some cases, psychiatric problems. • Case studies have noted symptoms of Kluver-Bucy syndrome in rare instances.
Symptom & Performance Validity	The issue of effort has not been systematically addressed in studies of encephalitis.	
Work/School	Good outcomes are generally reported for return to work, although this may take many months to a year.	Outcomes vary by etiology and treatment response. Children with HSV encephalitis are more likely to have long-term impairments.

Impact of Chronic Herpes Simplex Virus (HSV)

Recent literature has suggested a potential connection between chronic HSV and cognition, even in cases where there is no acute encephalitis episode. Although mild, in comparison to controls, individuals who are HSV positive have been found to have lower IQ scores (although still in the average range) and lower overall performance on broad neuropsychological batteries. Several studies have also found an increased risk for Alzheimer's disease (AD) in individuals with a history of HSV and presence of anti-HSV IgM antibodies- suggestive of re-activated infection. Several pathological processes have been proposed to explain the association between viral exposure and cognitive impairment. It has been suggested that re-activation of the virus may lead to cell death that has cumulative effects over the lifespan.

Section 4: Autoimmune and Paraneoplastic Encephalitis

Definition

Autoimmune encephalitis is an autoimmune syndrome associated with an attack of antibodies on neuronal cell-surface or synaptic receptors that can occur with or without a cancer association. When there is a cancer association, it is classified as a paraneoplastic neurologic disorder (PND) and in many cases, symptoms of the associated encephalitis often precede the diagnosis of cancer.

Neuropathology

Autoimmune encephalitis (AE) is often classified into groups:

- *Intracellular antibody disorders* PNDs generally fall into this group and the underlying disease mechanism seems to be an autoimmune reaction that is initiated in response to the tumor, which expresses neuronal antigens and is mediated by cytotoxic T-cell responses. Paraneoplastic limbic encephalitis (PLE) involves an inflammatory process related to cancers (small-cell lung is most common) and localized to structures of the limbic system. PNDs can be associated with specific antibody-related syndromes (e.g., anti-Hu, anti-Yo, anti-Ri, and anti-CV2 antibodies)

- *Synaptic and neuronal surface autoantibody disorders* Sixteen are known with syndromes classified based on the target antigen (e.g., N-methyl-D-aspartate, NMDA, α-amino-3-hydroxy-5-methyl-4-isoxazolepropionic acid receptor, AMPA, $GABA_b$, and glycine receptors). Antibodies disrupt the neuronal receptor or synaptic protein and prevent the post-synaptic electrical impulse causing the nerve cell and brain to stop working as it should.

Anti-NMDA receptor encephalitis (anti-NMDARE) is one of the most common AEs, second only to ADEM. It involves antibodies that decrease the number of cell-surface NMDA receptors and NMDA receptor clusters in postsynaptic dendrites. NMDA receptors are highly concentrated in the hippocampus as well as the forebrain and other parts of limbic system and, to a lesser extent, the frontal cortex. They play a primary role in synaptic excitatory transmission (glutamate). Anti-NMDARE can be associated with tumors (~50% of females over age 18 with this disease have ovarian teratomas, while only 15% of females <14 years do; carcinomas are seen in older men and women) but this is not always the case.

Epidemiology

- *Age* Classic PNDs are relatively rare and more often occur in older adults. While anti-NMDARE occurs across the age span (23 months–76 years; median age 19 years) other antibody-associated encephalitides (AMPA and $GABA_b$ receptors) occur only in adults (>24 years).

- *Gender* Certain autoimmune encephalitides more often affect females (NMDARE, 80%; AMPAR, 90%) while others affect men equally or more often.

- *Race* Ovarian teratomas occurred more often in African American patients with anti-NMDARE than in white patients.

Mortality

Rates vary with paraneoplastic being higher. Estimates for AE are around 6%, but some studies have shown higher rates in specific subgroups (i.e., one study in China of anti-NMDARE showed mortality was ~11% with GCS <8, number of complications, and admission to ICU being strongest predictors).

Morbidity

Though variable, PNDs and AEs are associated with significant morbidity, including secondary seizures, infections, and cognitive deficits. Rates vary based on associated cancer, specific antibody involvement, and access/response to treatment.

TABLE 23.4 Pediatric and Adult Neuropsychological Findings in anti-NMDARE

Domain	Adult Findings	Pediatric Findings* *Data are limited
Intelligence and Achievement	Majority of patients (74%) have favorable cognitive outcomes based on McKeon et al.'s 2018 meta-analytic study of 109 patients (ages 2–67)	
	• IQ is generally average long term, though impaired scores are seen soon after symptom onset	• IQ improves over time. About 1/3 show impairments (<9th %ile) acutely with most improving to the broad average range >12 months after symptom onset • Poor academic performance noted at follow-up in 36% of small pediatric sample
Attention	Attention and working memory deficits are seen at all points of recovery (averaging 42% and 38%, respectively)	
Processing Speed	Although it improves with time, deficits in processing speed persist for some.	
Language	Not consistently found to be impaired in adolescents/young adults	• Language problems (mutism) are often part of symptom presentation, but are generally intact at follow-up. • Verbal fluency impairments persist for a small percentage long-term.
Visuospatial	Visuospatial skills worse than controls in small samples. Majority show deficits initially, but this improves at follow-up	Visual motor integration is impaired in about 1/3 of patients initially, but most patients' scores are average at follow-up
Memory	• Episodic memory considered a core deficit (~55% of patients) • Inability to consolidate new memories is often last to recover • Verbal memory generally more affected, though visual memory impairment has also been reported	
Executive Functions	Persistent cognitive deficits seen in executive functions in ~50% of patients– disorganization, poor planning, disinhibition, and lack of impulse control.	
Emotion and Personality	Little data is reported specifically on psychological outcomes in this population	
	Higher levels of anxiety reported (compared to controls) though depression was not a noted issue	The vast majority of children (88%) present with behavior and personality changes, but show substantial or full recovery at follow-up
Social	Two studies document reports of impaired social cognition, with one based on objective testing.	Impaired social relationships were noted in about 1/3 of a small sample of pediatric patients at follow-up

Determinants of Severity

Factors That Influence Neuropsychological/Neurological Outcomes

Risk factors for poor outcomes include delayed initiation of immunotherapy or ineffective immunotherapy. In anti-NMDARE, age, gender, and MRI/EEG abnormality are not associated with cognitive outcomes, but surgical removal of associated tumor is associated with better outcomes and decreased risk for relapse. Presence of seizures during acute phase is associated with greater risk for development of seizures later but not with cognitive outcomes. See Table 23.4 for a summary of neuropsychological findings in this population.

PLE results in sleep disturbance, impairments of cognition (most notably anterograde amnesia) and psychiatric symptoms, such as depression, anxiety, agitation, and even hallucinations. The presenting symptoms of PLE often have a subacute onset of days or up to 12 weeks. Both herpes simplex virus and various autoimmune encephalitides affect the limbic system and have similar clinical characteristics.

Presentation, Disease Course, and Recovery

Presenting Symptoms

Paraneoplastic neurological syndromes have variable presentations including altered consciousness, behavioral and mood disturbance (in limbic encephalitis), sensory changes (in anti-Hu due to dorsal root involvement), cranial nerve palsies, rigidity, and cerebellar dysfunction (gait instability, apraxia, dysarthria).

Anti-NMDARE classically involves several phases, but varies by age. Varied presentations or phenotypes have been described, but the most common or "classic" type (seen in about 70% of adult patients) involves:

- *Prodromal phase* Includes flu-like illness with fever, malaise, headache, and fatigue, which lasts 5 to 14 days.

- *Psychotic phase* Patients may initially present to psychiatrists or are admitted to psychiatric units with a diagnosis of acute psychosis or schizophrenia.

- *Unresponsiveness phase* Patients stop following verbal commands, appear mute or akinetic, and may have a fixed gaze (like catatonia). Stereotyped athetotic movements and dyskinesias can also occur.

- *Hyperkinetic phase* Characterized by autonomic instability (hypo/hypertension, cardiac arrhythmia, and hypoventilation) though this is less common in children.

Children with anti-NMDARE more commonly present with behavioral changes, such as agitation, aggression, hyperactivity, and temper tantrums due, at least in part, to psychiatric symptoms being difficult to identify in young children. Speech, personality, and sleep changes are also more often seen in children along with movement disorders.

Assessment Methods

- *Labs/Lumbar puncture* The presence of specific antibodies in the blood serum and/or CSF can confirm an autoimmune or paraneoplastic process. CSF results are known to be more sensitive and specific. Inflammatory markers (oligoclonal bands, increased lymphocytes) are also seen. If known to be associated with a neoplastic process, a positive autoantibody test can dictate further imaging to search for a tumor.

- *Neuroimaging* Brain imaging (CT, MRI) findings vary widely. Some syndromes, like AMPAR, show medial temporal lobe abnormalities in 90% of cases where in other types findings are often normal. Abnormalities on T2 or FLAIR sequences are seen in about 50% of patients with anti-NMDARE encephalitis and these are often transient.

- *EEG* Focal or generalized slowing and occasional epileptiform activity (primarily in temporal lobes) is seen in anti-NMDARE and other encephalitides. In anti-NMDARE, patterns often return to normal a few months after disease onset.

Treatment

- *Cancer Treatment* If identified can include surgical removal of a tumor, chemotherapy/radiation, or immunotherapy with steroids or other immunosuppression.

- *Target Antibodies*

  - First Line Treatment: IVIg and steroids. Plasmapheresis is generally less effective in reducing CNS antibodies.

  - Second Line Treatment: Immune suppression (e.g., Rituximab and/or cyclophosphamide) are used in those with minimal response to initial treatment.

Recovery

In limbic encephalitis, seizures and behavioral issues often improve rapidly with treatment, but persistent deficits are seen in memory and new learning. In anti-NMDARE encephalitis, recovery is generally slow (can take up to 18 months), and patients are often hospitalized for several months; many go on to a rehabilitation hospital or even a psychiatric floor in a hospital. Despite significant improvement in the months following hospitalization, most patients with anti-NMDARE encephalitis (50–90%) show residual cognitive deficits at follow-up. Further, 20–25% of patients relapse and those without a tumor and no initiation of immunotherapy are most at risk.

Section 5: Other Infections and/or Causes of Encephalitis

Intracranial Abscess

Abscesses are infectious pus collections that occur in the brain or surrounding spaces. These infections can originate from nearby structures (e.g., ear infections, sinusitis, dental infections); can spread through the blood from a remote site; can occur after a depressed skull fracture, penetrating brain injury, or neurosurgery; or, in rare cases, following meningitis. They can cause brain damage by increasing ICP and by causing *mass effect* on the brain. There are two types:

- *Subdural or epidural empyema* Are found between the inner surface of the dura and outer surface of the arachnoid (subdural) or in the space between the dura and skull (epidural). Epidural abscesses are more common in the spinal cord than the brain.

- *Brain abscess* Is a cavity filled with pus in the brain parenchyma. These are typically marked by a ring enhancing lesion on CT with contrast.

Intrauterine and Intranatal Infections

The TORCH acronym (see Table 23.5) stands for a set of perinatal infections of viral, bacterial, and protozoal origins.

TABLE 23.5 Intrauterine and Intranatal Infections (TORCH)

Infection	Description
T oxoplasmosis / **T** oxoplasma gondii	A parasite that can pass from mother to fetus and cause necrotic lesions and cysts.
O ther infections	That can cross the placental barrier and enter fetal circulation including poliovirus, syphilis, western equine virus, and coxsackie virus.
R ubella	If it occurs in the first trimester of pregnancy can cause severe birth defects—interferes with CNS cell division. It is now relatively rare.
C ytomegalovirus	A virus that is typically unnoticed in healthy people but can cause significant problems in individuals who are immune compromised or in utero fetuses.
H erpes simplex virus-2	Can be transmitted from the mother in the birth canal.

Prion Diseases

Prion diseases are caused by infectious proteins called prions. These include Creutzfeldt-Jacob disease (CJD), Gerstmann-Sträussler-Scheinker syndrome (GSS), fatal familial insomnia (FFI), and kuru in humans.

Creutzfeldt-Jacob disease belongs to a family of human and animal diseases called transmissible spongiform encephalopathies. Brain tissue develops holes that give it a sponge-like appearance. It may be sporadic, hereditary, or caused by exposure of brain or nervous system (usually during a medical procedure). Creutzfeldt-Jacob disease is rapidly progressive and fatal (4 to 5 months for classic CJD and 14 to 15 months for variant CJD). Symptoms typically include rapidly progressive dementia, including memory issues, personality changes, and hallucinations and physical problems such as speech impairment and ataxia.

Human Immunodeficiency Virus (HIV)

Pathogenesis

Neurons do not appear to be directly impacted by HIV infection, but rather HIV infection leads macrophages and microglia to cause gradual destruction of neuronal integrity. Central nervous system pathology in HIV-positive individuals can often be related to both the HIV infection and associated opportunistic infections due to increased permeability of the blood-brain barrier.

MRI Findings

- Small areas of bilateral, subcortical signal hyperintensity
- Volume loss and metabolic changes (hyper- and hypo-) in basal ganglia
- Large hyperintensities consistent with discrete and generalized lesions
- Global and diffuse atrophy (sulcal and ventricular enlargement and reduced white matter volume)
- Isolated focal lesions
- MRI abnormalities have been found in asymptomatic individuals.

Two Key Syndromes

HIV-associated neurocognitive disorder (HAND) is common (up to 50% of infected individuals) and categorized by deficits in attention, executive function, fluency, memory, and psychomotor speed. Decreases in brain activation, particularly in left frontal attentional networks, contribute to those with HAND being unable to compensate for age-related decline.

More Severe: Dementia

The more severe form of cognitive impairment in HIV-infected individuals has been termed HIV-1 AIDS dementia complex (ADC) and HIV associated dementia. It is often described as a "subcortical" dementia because the pattern of deficits mimics disorders such as Parkinson's disease. The disruption of cortical connections, specifically fronto-striatal-thalamo-cortical loops, contribute to deficits in attention, working memory, executive functioning, and learning. Memory impairments are also seen likely due to hippocampal pathology and the interference of hippocampal neurogenesis while damage to cortical-striatal regions causes the psychomotor slowing and motor impairments commonly seen.

Less Severe: HIV-1-Associated Minor Cognitive/Motor Disorder

The less severe form of cognitive impairment has been termed HIV-1-associated minor cognitive/motor disorder. This has a similar "subcortical" profile to HIV dementia and is closely related to disease progression. This condition is found in approximately 2% of those with HIV and is associated with 0.5–1 SD impairment (relative to controls) in at least two cognitive domains. Similar to the more severe form, domains commonly impacted include speed of processing, attention, and psychomotor functioning. It is unclear if this is a precursor to HIV-associated dementia or a distinct syndrome.

Adolescents and adults who contract HIV infections may also fall into the group that is classified as "asymptomatic." This refers to individuals who do not show pronounced clinically significant or prominent sequelae of HIV infection (CDC Stage A). In this group, the evidence is less clear for a pattern of neuropsychological deficits. Although these individuals are considered asymptomatic as far as their HIV disease, there have been some studies that have documented abnormal MRI findings (particularly in subcortical structures) and evidence of correlation between neuropsychological abnormalities and neuroimaging abnormalities.

Children with Perinatally Acquired HIV-Infection

Children and adolescents who contract HIV perinatally tend to perform worse than controls and HIV-exposed but unaffected children in general cognition (IQ), though results vary. Poor working memory, slowed processing, and executive problems are most consistently reported with impaired visual memory, visuospatial reasoning and language skills also seen. Failure to acquire these cognitive abilities is due to potential effects of the virus, of ART and environmental and social factors. The high proportion of affected children with conductive hearing deficits (20% in higher-income countries; 38% in low-resource settings) is an important consideration when testing, especially given reported language problems in this population. Mental health problems are also pervasive (25% of HIV-infected children) and these problems (depression and conduct problems primarily) have a direct association with neuropsychological functioning. Medical factors like disease progression and severity factors (e.g., high plasma viral load, lower CD4 cell counts, and history of an AIDS defining illness) have also been associated with poorer neurocognitive performance

Treatment and Cultural Considerations

The addition of antiretroviral treatments (ART) has decreased the prevalence of HIV associated dementia from 17.1% in 1995–1996 to 11.2% in 1997–1998 though the ability of ART to minimize HAND symptoms or thwart the cognitive deficits in children is less clear. Despite widespread access to ART over the past 15 years, only about 28% of children with HIV worldwide have started it. Youth with more limited access to appropriate medical care and interventions are in Sub-Saharan Africa, where the burden of HIV disease is most prevalent. Further, individuals from this region are disproportionately underrepresented in studies of cognitive outcomes (estimated 13%) limiting the generalizability of findings.

Across all settings, patients and medical providers contend with issues of disclosure of HIV status. In the United States, less than half of children have been disclosed to despite World Health Organization (WHO) guidelines that recommend informing children of their HIV status between the ages of 6 to 12 years. The stigma associated with the disease and the possibility of exposing the HIV status of other family members (in the case of perinatally infected children) are influential factors.

Progressive Multifocal Leukoencephalopathy (PML)

Progressive multifocal leukoencephalopathy is a rare and usually fatal viral disease that results in progressive and multifocal damage of the white matter. It is caused by the JC (John Cunningham) virus and typically affects individuals who are immune compromised (e.g., transplant patients, HIV/AIDS patients). The JC virus is present in most individuals, but is kept under control by the immune system.

Cerebral Toxoplasmosis

Toxoplasmosis is an infection in the brain caused by the one-celled protozoan parasite *Toxoplasma gondii*. It is considered an opportunistic infection that typically affects patients with HIV/AIDS and is the most common cause of brain abscess in these patients.

Acute Disseminated Encephalomyelitis (ADEM)

Acute disseminated *encephalomyelitis* is an inflammatory demyelinating condition of the CNS (both brain and spinal cord are affected) that resembles multiple sclerosis (MS). The cause of ADEM is believed to be postinfectious or, less commonly postvaccination, typically occurring one to two weeks following the virus/infection or vaccination, although it can also occur without a known trigger. Acute disseminated *encephalomyelitis* can have a single occurrence or can be multiphasic in nature. The variant diagnosis of MDEM (multiphasic disseminated *encephalomyelitis*) is sometimes used when there is a recurrence of ADEM.

There are few epidemiologic studies of ADEM showing the highest incidence in early childhood (5 to 8 years). One study in Japan found a mean age of onset of 5.7 years, male-to-female ratio of 2.3:1, and incidence in children younger than 15 to be 0.64 per 100,000. Initial presentation often consists of confusion, cognitive impairment, and neurological deficits. Psychiatric symptoms (mood lability, then agitation, personality changes, and delusions/hallucinations) can present even prior to the neurological signs.

On brain MRI, ADEM may be associated with white matter hyperintensities in both hemispheres, subcortical regions, the cerebellum, and the spinal cord. Appearance characteristics of lesions on MRI can sometimes be used to differentiate between ADEM and MS, although controversy exists about whether or not ADEM and MS are distinct disorders or part of the same spectrum. Some studies have found that certain individuals initially diagnosed with ADEM later go on to be reclassified as having MS following a relapse. Acute disseminated *encephalomyelitis* is typically treated with high-dose steroids and plasmapheresis, and mortality is rare (80% of children fully recover with treatment).

Neuropsychological outcome following monophasic ADEM is better than pediatric MS. Subtle deficits in attention, information processing, and executive functioning have been noted.

Relevant Definitions

Arbovirus Refers to a group of viruses that are transmitted by arthropod vectors. The word *arbovirus* is an acronym (*AR*thropod-*BO*rne viruses).

Cerebral edema Describes brain swelling. Disorders that disrupt the blood-brain barrier (such as infections) can cause vasogenic edema, which refers to excessive extracellular fluid. Cytotoxic edema refers to excessive intracellular fluid collection within the brain cells, which often results from cellular damage (such as in the case of infarction).

Cerebellitis Infection of brain tissue localized to the cerebellum caused by a viral infection. Sudden onset of ataxia is often the presenting symptom.

Encephalomyelitis When both the brain and spinal cord are inflamed.

Intracranial pressure (ICP) Describes level of pressure within the brain. Elevated ICP can lead to brain damage as the result of reduced cerebral perfusion and brain ischemia. Common signs/symptoms of increased ICP include headache, altered mental status, nausea and vomiting, papilledema (engorgement and elevation of the optic disc), visual loss, diplopia, and Cushing's triad (hypertension, bradycardia, and irregular respiration). (See also Chapter 29, Traumatic Brain Injury.)

Kluver-Bucy syndrome Results from bilateral lesions to the medial temporal lobe and is associated with sexualized behaviors, hyperorality, visual agnosia, and memory loss among other impairments.

Leptomeningitis Inflammation of only the pia mater and subarachnoid space.

Mass effect Describes distortion of the normal brain geometry due to a mass lesion (such as an abscess or tumor).

Meningoencephalitis When patients with encephalitis also present with meningeal involvement.

Rasmussen's encephalitis (see also Chapter 22, Epilepsy and Seizure Disorders) Inflammatory disease characterized by frequent and severe seizures, loss of speech and motor skills, hemiparesis, and cognitive deficits.

Transverse myelitis Disorder caused by an inflammatory process in the spinal cord and results in demyelination of axons. It is not associated with neuropsychological dysfunction.

Central Nervous System Infections Questions

NOTE: Questions 16, 44, 83, and 109 on the First Full-Length Practice Examination, Questions 14, 50, and 82 on the Second Full-Length Practice Examination, Questions 32, 70, 89, and 119 on the Third Full-Length

1. Which of the following is not a typical impairment in individuals with successfully treated herpes simplex virus (HSV) encephalitis?

   (a) anterograde memory deficit

   (b) deficit in performance IQ

   (c) naming deficit

   (d) executive functioning deficit

2. Inflammation of the pia mater and the subarachnoid space is referred to as ____.

   (a) meningoencephalitis

   (b) subarachnoid hemorrhage

   (c) subdural empyema

   (d) leptomeningitis

3. Which of the following has not been associated with poorer cognitive or behavioral outcomes in bacterial meningitis?

   (a) acute neurological complications

   (b) male gender

   (c) treatment with dexamethasone

   (d) neonatal onset

4. Which of the following is true regarding encephalitis?

   (a) herpes simplex virus is the most common cause

   (b) viruses, fungi, parasites, and bacteria can be the cause

   (c) prevalence rates are highest in the elderly (>65)

   (d) positron emission tomography (PET) scans are typically used to confirm a diagnosis

5. Which of the following is true regarding HIV-associated dementia?

   (a) It cannot be caused by a CNS opportunistic infection.

   (b) It is most commonly seen in individuals in the CDC Stage A classification.

   (c) Cognitive symptoms often mimic those seen in Alzheimer's dementia.

   (d) Symptoms are typically reversible with treatment.

6. Anti-NMDARE ____.

   (a) rarely presents with psychiatric symptoms

   (b) typically has a benign course

   (c) is considered a prion disease

   (d) is considered a paraneoplastic disorder

7. A 14-year-old patient with a recent history of sinusitis presents to the hospital with acute onset headache, vomiting, right-sided weakness, and word-finding difficulties. Which of the following is most likely to be found on the MRI scan that was ordered on his arrival at the hospital?

   (a) a focal abscess

   (b) spongiform encephalopathy

(c) diffuse white matter changes in the cerebellum

(d) mesial temporal sclerosis

8. Rasmussen's encephalitis _____.

(a) affects both hemispheres in about 40% of cases

(b) typically affects adolescents/young adults

(c) is often treated with a hemispherectomy in children

(d) is characterized by multiple small infarcts in the basal ganglia

9. A previously healthy 60-year-old male patient presents with a recent (1–2 month) history of rapidly developing dementia, personality changes, speech disturbance, and hallucinations. Which of the following conditions should you most likely be concerned about?

(a) pneumococcal meningitis

(b) prion disease

(c) encephalitis caused by an adenovirus

(d) Parkinson's disease

10. Individuals with HIV infection _____.

(a) do not show MRI changes during the asymptomatic phases of the disease

(b) have been shown to have stable rates of HIV dementia since the introduction of highly active antiretroviral therapy (HAART) treatment

(c) often show signs of language impairments in the early stages of the disease

(d) may show CNS pathology not related to the HIV infection itself

11. What is the most common route for infections to be spread to the CNS?

(a) through the bloodstream

(b) along motor and sensory axons

(c) from infected cranial cavities (e.g., sinuses, middle ear)

(d) through direct access (e.g., from a skull fracture or penetrating wound)

12. A 16-year-old patient undergoes a work-up for new-onset deficits in attention and motor weakness and is found to have nonspecific CSF abnormalities and diffuse lesions in the white matter of the brain and spinal cord suggestive of an inflammatory demyelinating disorder. Which of the following disorders is least likely to be on the differential diagnosis list?

(a) ADEM

(b) multiple sclerosis

(c) transverse myelitis

(d) Devic disease

13. You are asked to evaluate a patient with language delays secondary to a history of mild to moderate hearing loss following a bout of bacterial meningitis in childhood. Based on this clinical presentation, which cranial nerve was most likely damaged as a result of the infection?

(a) 7th

(b) 8th

(c) 4th

(d) 10th

14. Your 56-year-old male patient presents with no changes in mood or behavioral functioning but clear Parkinsonian-type symptoms, including psychomotor slowing, motor weakness, memory

and learning problems, and poor executive function. The medical team has ruled out Parkinson's disease; which other diagnosis is more probable?

(a) HIV-associated AIDS dementia complex (ADC)

(b) Creutzfeldt-Jacob disease

(c) HSV encephalitis

(d) A paraneoplastic disorder

15. Which of the following is true about pediatric versus adult bacterial meningitis?

(a) Cranial nerve defects are more common in adults.

(b) Mortality rates are lower in young children compared to early adulthood.

(c) Adults who survive meningococcal meningitis generally have good outcomes.

(d) Language problems are not typically seen in very young children, but are often reported in adults.

Central Nervous System Infections Answers

1. **B—deficit in performance IQ** *Multiple studies of individuals with HSV encephalitis have documented that IQ scores typically fall within the average range. All of the other domains in the question have been found to be impacted in this condition.*

References:
(a) Hokkanen, L., & Launes, J. (1997). Cognitive recovery instead of decline after acute encephalitis: A prospective follow up study. *Journal of Neurology, Neurosurgery, and Psychiatry, 63*(2), 222–227.
(b) Hokkanen, L., & Launes, J. (2000). Cognitive outcome in acute sporadic encephalitis. *Neuropsychology Review, 10*(3), 151–167.
(c) Utley, T. F., Ogden, J. A., Gibb, A., McGrath, N., & Anderson, N. E. (1997). The long-term neuropsychological outcome of herpes simplex encephalitis in a series of unselected survivors. *Neuropsychiatry, Neuropsychology, and Behavioral Neurology, 10*(3), 180–189.

2. **D—leptomeningitis** *Meningo-encephalitis refers to inflammation of the brain and meninges, an empyema is an abscess or pus collection, and a subarachnoid hemorrhage refers to blood in the subarachnoid space.*

References:
(a) Blumenfeld, H. (2010). Chapter 5: Brain and environs, cranium, ventricles and meninges. In H. Blumenfeld (Ed.), *Neuroanatomy through clinical cases* (2nd ed., pp. 125–220). Sunderland, MA: Sinauer Associates.
(b) Loring, D. W. (2015). *INS dictionary of neuropsychology and clinical neurosciences* (2nd ed.). New York, NY: Oxford University Press.

3. **C—treatment with dexamethasone** *Treatment with dexamethasone has not been shown to lead to worse outcomes in studies with both adults and children with bacterial meningitis. Acute neurological complications, male gender, and neonatal meningitis have been associated with worse cognitive or behavioral outcomes.*

References:
(a) Anderson, V., Anderson, P., Grimwood, K., & Nolan, T. (2004). Cognitive and executive functioning 12 years after childhood bacterial meningitis: Effect of acute neurologic complications and age of onset. *Journal of Pediatric Psychology, 29*, 67–81.
(b) Bhimraj, A. (2018). Acute community-acquired bacterial meningitis. In J. C. Garcia-Monco (Ed.), *CNS infections: A clinical approach* (pp. 19–30). Switzerland: Springer International Publishing.

4. **B—viruses, fungi, parasites, and bacteria can be the cause**   *The cause of encephalitis is not identified in 1/3 to 2/3 of cases. HSV accounts for about 10% of cases. The prevalence rates are highest in children (not the elderly) and PET is not routinely used for diagnosis of encephalitis.*

   References:
   (a) Garcia-Monco, J. C. (2018), *CNS infections: A clinical approach* (pp. 19–30). Switzerland: Springer International Publishing.
   (b) Messacar, K., Fischer, M., Dominguez, S. R., Tyler, K. L., & Abzug, M. J. (2018). Encephalitis in US children. *Infectious Disease Clinics of North America, 32,* 145–162.
   (c) National Institute of Neurological Disorders and Stroke. (2011). *NINDS meningitis and encephalitis fact sheet.* http://www.ninds.nih.gov/disorders/encephalitis_meningitis/detail_encephalitis_meningitis.htm

5. **A—It cannot be caused by a CNS opportunistic infection**   *The other answers are all false, as HIV associated dementia is considered a more "subcortical" dementia—and thus does not mimic AD, it is typically seen in later stages of the disease (CDC-C) and it is not reversible.*

   Reference: Van Gorp, W., & Root, J. C. (2008). CNS infection: HIV associated neurocognitive compromise. In J. E. Morgan & J. H Ricker (Eds.), *Textbook of clinical neuropsychology* (pp. 508–520). New York, NY: Taylor and Francis.

6. **D—is considered a paraneoplastic disorder**   *Anti-NMDARE typically does not have a benign course. It is a paraneoplastic disorder and it often presents with psychiatric symptoms.*

   References:
   (a) Kayser, M. S., Kohler, C. G. & Dalmau, J. (2010). Psychiatric manifestations of paraneoplastic disorders. *American Journal of Psychiatry, 167,* 1039–1050.
   (b) Voltz, R. (2007). Neuropsychological symptoms in paraneoplastic disorders. *Journal of Neurology, 254 Suppl 2,* II84–II86.
   (c) Wandinger, K. P., Saschenbrecker, S., Stoecker, W., & Dalmau, J. (2011). Anti-NMDA-receptor encephalitis: A severe, multistage, treatable disorder presenting with psychosis. *Journal of Neuroimmunology, 231*(1–2), 86–91.

7. **A—a focal abscess**   *These symptoms would be suggestive of an acute focal lesion—likely in the left hemisphere. The history of sinusitis should raise concern about an infections process such as a brain abscess. The other answers suggest a more diffuse process (b and c) or a long-standing lesion (d).*

   Reference: Blumenfeld, H. (2010). Chapter 5: Brain and environs, cranium, ventricles and meninges. In H. Blumenfeld (Ed.), *Neuroanatomy through clinical cases* (2nd ed., pp. 125–220). Sunderland, MA: Sinauer Associates.

8. **C—is often treated with a hemispherectomy in children**   *Rasmussen's encephalitis typically impacts one hemisphere. It is most prevalent in young school age children (age 6), and is characterized by inflammation in the impacted hemisphere. Thus only answer C is correct.*

   Reference: Varadkar, S., Bien, C. G., Kruse, C. A., Jensen, F. E., Bauer, J., Pardo, C. A., . . . Cross, J. H. (2014). Rasmussen's encephalitis: Clinical features, pathobiology, and treatment advances. *Lancet Neurology, 13*(2), 195–205

9. **B—prion disease**   *That cluster of symptoms in a relatively short onset period would be suggestive of Creutzfeldt-Jacob disease (CJD), a rapidly progressive and fatal disease.*

   Reference: National Institute of Neurological Disorders and Stroke. (2012). *NINDS Creutzfeldt-Jacob disease fact sheet.* http://www.ninds.nih.gov/disorders/cjd/detail_cjd.htm

10. **D—may show CNS pathology not related to the HIV infection itself**   *Individuals with HIV infection may show CNS pathology related to opportunistic infections (e.g., toxoplasmosis) that is unrelated to the HIV infection itself. The other answers are all false. MRI abnormalities have*

been shown in some individuals in the earlier "asymptomatic" stages of the disease. Language impairments do not typically occur in HIV, particularly not in the early stages. HAART has actually decreased the rates of HIV dementia.

Reference: Van Gorp, W., & Root, J. C. (2008). CNS infection: HIV associated neurocognitive compromise. In J. E. Morgan & J. H Ricker (Eds.), *Textbook of clinical neuropsychology* (pp. 508–520). New York, NY: Taylor and Francis.

11. **A—through the bloodstream** *Although infections can be spread from all of the mentioned mechanisms, the most common mechanism is the bloodstream.*

Reference: Blumenfeld, H. (2010). Chapter 5: Brain and environs, cranium, ventricles and meninges. In H. Blumenfeld (Ed.), *Neuroanatomy through clinical cases* (2nd ed., pp. 125–220. Sunderland, MA: Sinauer Associates.

12. **C—transverse myelitis** *Although all of these diseases are considered demyelinating conditions, transverse myelitis is only associated with lesions in the spinal cord and thus not likely to cause cognitive symptoms (such as new onset attention problems). ADEM, MS, and Devic's disease can all be associated with lesions in both the brain and spinal cord.*

Reference: Deery, B., Anderson, V., Jacobs, R., Neale, J., & Kornberg, A. (2010). Childhood MS and ADEM: Investigation and comparison of neurocognitive features in children. *Developmental Neuropsychology, 35*(5), 506–521.

13. **B—8th** *Damage to the auditory nerve (8th nerve) can cause sensorineural hearing loss.*

Reference: Blumenfeld, H. (2010). Chapter 12: Brainstem I: Surface anatomy and cranial nerves. In H. Blumenfeld (Ed.), *Neuroanatomy through clinical cases* (2nd ed., pp. 493–564. Sunderland, MA: Sinauer Associates.

14. **A—HIV-associated AIDS dementia complex (ADC)** *ADC is often described as a "subcortical" dementia and involves disruption of fronto-striatal-thalamo-cortical loops as well as hippocampal pathology, contributing to the observed Parkinsonian symptoms.*

Reference: Van Gorp, W., & Root, J. C. (2008). CNS Infection: HIV associated neurocognitive compromise. In J. E. Morgan & J. H Ricker (Eds.), *Textbook of clinical neuropsychology* (pp. 508–520). New York, NY: Taylor and Francis.

15. **C—Adults who survive meningococcal meningitis generally have good outcomes.** *This is true. Adults who survive bacterial meningitis general have good outcomes. Children are more likely than adults to have cranial nerve problems and language issues, particularly if they had meningitis in the neonatal period.*

References:
(a) National Institute of Neurological Disorders and Stroke. (2017). *NINDS meningitis and encephalitis fact sheet.* https://www.ninds.nih.gov/Disorders/Patient-Caregiver-Education/Fact-Sheets/Meningitis-and-Encephalitis-Fact-Sheet
(b) Muralidharam, R., Mateen, F. J., & Rabinstein, A. A. (2014). Outcome of fulminant bacterial meningitis in adult patients. *European Journal of Neurology, 21*, 447–453.

Recommended Readings

Anderson, V., Anderson, P., Grimwood, K., & Nolan, T. (2004). Cognitive and executive functioning 12 years after childhood bacterial meningitis: Effect of acute neurologic complications and age of onset. *Journal of Pediatric Psychology, 29,* 67–81.

Dalmau, J., & Rosenfeld, M. R. (2014). Autoimmune encephalitis update. *Neuro-Oncology, 16*(6), 771–778.

Finke, C., Kopp, U. A., Prüss, H., Dalmau, J., Wandinger, K. P., & Ploner, C. J. (2012). Cognitive deficits following anti-NMDA receptor encephalitis. *Journal of Neurology, Neurosurgery, and Psychiatry, 83*(2), 195–198.

Hokkanen, L., & Launes, J. (2000). Cognitive outcome in acute sporadic encephalitis. *Neuropsychology Review, 10*(3), 151–167.

Hoogman, M., van de Beek, D., Weisfelt, M., de Gans, J., & Schmand, B. (2007). Cognitive outcome in adults after bacterial meningitis. *Journal of Neurology, Neurosurgery, and Psychiatry, 78*(10), 1092–1096.

McKeon, G. L., Robinton, G. A., Ryan, A. E., Blum, S., Gillis, D., Finke, C., & Scott, J. G. (2018). Cognitive outcomes following anti-N-methyl-D-aspartate receptor encephalitis: A systematic review. *Journal of Clinical and Experimental Neuropsychology, 40*(3), 234–252.

Messacar, K., Fischer, M., Dominiguez, S. R., Tyler, K. L., & Abzug, M. J. (2018). Encephalitis in children. *Infectious Disease Clinics of North America, 32*, 145–162.

Michaeli, O., Kassis, I., Shachor-Meyouhas, Y., Shahar, E., & Ravid, S. (2014). Long-term motor and cognitive outcome of acute encephalitis. *Pediatrics*, 133(3), e546–e552.

Van Gorp, W., & Root, J. C. (2008). CNS Infection: HIV associated neurocognitive compromise. In J. E. Morgan & J. H Ricker (Eds.) *Textbook of clinical neuropsychology* (pp. 508–520). New York, NY: Taylor and Francis

Website

National Institute of Neurological Disorders and Stroke. (2017). *NINDS meningitis and encephalitis fact sheet.* https://www.ninds.nih.gov/Disorders/Patient-Caregiver-Education/Fact-Sheets/Meningitis-and-Encephalitis-Fact-Sheet

24   Multiple Sclerosis

Lana Harder, Christine D. Liff, and William S. MacAllister

Definition

Multiple sclerosis (MS) is a chronic, progressive inflammatory autoimmune disorder of the central nervous system (CNS). In MS, the immune system response results in an attack on myelin sheathing in the brain and spinal cord, resulting in axonal damage and slowing axonal signal transmission.

Neuropathology

MS is an immune-mediated disease in which an individual's immune system becomes dysregulated and attacks the CNS. Brain biopsy studies show that MS lesions are characterized by perivascular inflammation and demyelination. Acutely, lesions show infiltrates of immune system T-cells, B-cells, and macrophages while chronically affected regions may show demyelination and associated gliosis, as well as axonal damage. Though previously considered a disease of the white matter only, it is now well established that gray matter can also be involved, even in the earliest stages.

Epidemiology

- MS primarily affects young adults between the ages of 20 and 40 (average age of onset about 30). However, it is recognized that MS can occur in younger individuals (i.e., pediatric MS) and as late as the 8th decade of life. About 2% to 5% of individuals with MS have an onset prior to the age of 18, with far fewer having onset prior to the onset of puberty (0.2–0.7% of cases).

- Genetics contribute to the development of MS; first degree relatives of patients with MS are 6 to 8 times more likely to develop the disease. Further, there is a 30% concordance rate in identical twins.

- More women develop MS in comparison to men (2.5 to 1). However, men are more likely to develop progressive disease associated with greater disability and cognitive impairment but less evidence of inflammation on MRI.

- In adult-onset MS, women experience onset about 5 years earlier than men.

- Adult-onset MS is more common in Caucasians of northern European heritage than it is in racial and ethnic minorities; however, this is not the case in pediatric-onset MS (see "Pediatric Considerations" section).

- Early work demonstrated that rates of MS are lowest near the equator and become increasingly more common as one moves farther north or south. However, recent work has shown that the latitude gradient may be lessening over time.

Environmental Factors

In addition to genetic factors, environmental factors clearly contribute to MS susceptibility in both children and adults. The onset of MS is thought to be a response to an environmental exposure that may have occurred many years prior to the actual clinical manifestation of the disease.

- Pediatric MS has been associated with an increased frequency of the Epstein Barr virus. Other pathogens implicated have included spirochetal bacterial infections, varicella zoster, and chlamydophila pneumoniae.
- Cigarette smoking may increase the risk of developing MS in adults and exposure to second-hand smoke may increase the risk of MS in children.
- Babies who are breastfed are less likely to develop MS later in life.
- Lower levels of vitamin D are associated with higher rates of MS. Likewise, vitamin D supplementation is recommended in pregnant women to reduce the likelihood of MS in their children.

Mortality

Approximately 90% to 95% of patients will experience an average life expectancy, but on average, life expectancy is about 5 to 10 years shorter in comparison to a healthy population.

Determinants of Severity

Disease severity varies widely across patients with MS, ranging from "benign MS" to very debilitating. Unfortunately, the determinants of disease severity are not well understood. This said, some factors have been identified.

- Younger age of onset has been associated with a lower relapse rate and slower overall rate of disease progression.
- Racial and ethnic minorities are less likely to contract MS. Unfortunately, however, these patients tend to have a more severe disease course.
- The role of vitamin D has been described in the MS literature with lower levels of serum vitamin D levels (25-hydroxyvitamin D) being associated with a higher relapse rate in MS patients.
- Pregnant women tend to experience fewer relapses and may even see improvement in neurologic function. Though the mechanism for this phenomenon is not entirely understood, hormonal factors are likely responsible. Unfortunately, upon giving birth some subsequently experience a rebound in relapse frequency.

Cognitive Reserve Theory and MS

The concept of cognitive reserve has been proposed as an explanatory model accounting for individual differences in the expression of cognitive impairments, with educational level, literacy, and enrichment activities having a protective effect in the face of neuropathology. In MS, intellectual enrichment has lessened the effect of disease burden on neuropsychological status. Further, cognitive processing speed declines may be moderated by high cognitive reserve in individuals with MS and those with high cognitive reserve may be able to withstand greater neuropathology (e.g., brain atrophy) without showing greater information processing speed deficits. For more information regarding cognitive reserve theory and the affiliated concept of cerebral reserve theory, please see Chapter 3, Important Theories in Neuropsychology: A Historical Perspective.

Diagnosis of Multiple Sclerosis

MS remains more or less a diagnosis of exclusion given the fact that its symptom presentation is quite heterogeneous in nature. Moreover, there is currently no definitive diagnostic laboratory test for MS, though the diagnostic criteria have evolved considerably in the past few decades, with the most recent revision occurring in 2017. The overarching goal of the latest revision was to improve diagnostic speed, but also to minimize false positives. As in the 2010 version of the McDonald Criteria, there must be evidence of CNS lesions that are disseminated across both space (i.e., implicating different regions of the CNS) and time.

- The patient must have two or more objective clinical attacks with positive MRI findings.
- Dissemination of lesions in space can be demonstrated in at least one T2 lesion in two of four areas in the CNS: periventricular, juxtacortical, infratentorial, and/or spinal cord.
- In prior criteria sets, clinical events had to be separated in time by 30 days or more. This is no longer true, and a new MRI lesion may establish dissemination in time regardless of time from baseline MRI.
- Other possible explanations for lesions and symptom presentation are excluded by additional testing.

Neuropsychological evaluation can assist in determining cognitive changes which may be present very early in the disease but progress in later stages, with declines in psychomotor processing speed, learning, and free recall (see "Expectations for Neuropsychological Assessment Results" section). As such, early assessment can help establish a baseline against which subsequent comparisons can be made. In addition, a neuropsychologist can determine the extent of strengths and weaknesses across cognitive domains for treatment purposes. When assessing a patient with MS, fatigue, slowed mental processing, and speech and upper extremity motor deficiencies need to be considered when selecting appropriate assessment instruments and determining the length of the testing session. Several brief batteries have been developed for the purposes of serially assessing cognition in individuals with MS over time. These include the *Brief Repeatable Battery of Neuropsychological Tests (BRB)* and the *Minimal Assessment of Cognitive Function in Multiple Sclerosis (MACFIMS)*. For pediatric patients with MS, neuropsychologists from the six National MS Society Centers of Excellence have established a core battery for use in the study of pediatric-onset MS. Each battery is described briefly in the "Relevant Definitions" section.

Presentation, Disease Course, and Treatment

Presentation

The clinical symptoms of MS are quite numerous given the fact that lesions can occur anywhere in the CNS. However, some symptoms tend to occur more frequently than others, with the most common initial symptoms being motor and sensory changes.

- *Optic Neuritis* Inflammation of the optic nerve results in blurring of vision. This is a common symptom and tends to occur unilaterally.

- **Somatosensory** Accounts for 21% to 55% of early symptomatology, climbing to 70% over the course of the disease. Includes paresthesias (i.e., sensation of numbness and tingling).

- **Corticospinal Tract** Accounts for 32% to 41% of early symptomatology, reaching up to 50% over the course of the disease. Corticospinal tract symptoms include bladder and bowel dysfunction.

- **Cerebellar/Brainstem** Symptoms of cerebellar and brainstem lesions may include ataxia, speech problems (e.g., dysarthria), or diplopia (i.e., double vision).

- **Fatigue** About 80% of adults and 50% of children with MS report fatigue over the course of the disease. This is often the most disabling symptom for many patients and is most frequently cited as the reason for unemployment in MS. This symptom is often exacerbated by heat.

- **Sleep** About half of adults with MS report sleep disturbance in comparison to about 26% of children and adolescents. For example, insomnia, sleep-disordered breathing, and restless legs syndrome are commonly seen in adults. Notably, sleep disturbance can also be secondary to pain and spasticity in MS.

Disease Course

Patients who have not yet met criteria for a definite diagnosis of MS but have had one episode of a neurologic event similar to MS have typically been diagnosed with a clinically isolated syndrome (CIS). CIS is used to describe the first episode that lasts at least 24 hours and results from inflammation or demyelination in the CNS. The first episode can consist of a single symptom (known as monofocal) such as numbness on one side of the body caused by a single lesion, or multiple symptoms (known as multifocal) such as numbness and optic neuritis caused by lesions in more than one location in the CNS. The likelihood that a patient diagnosed with CIS will develop MS in the future increases if he or she presents with brain lesions similar to those seen in MS as detected using MRI. It is worth noting that some may show a "radiologically isolated syndrome" (RIS), in which lesions are seen on imaging, but without clinical correlation. About a third of those with RIS convert to a diagnosis of MS within a 5-year period. Further, the term "tumefactive MS" refers to a presentation in which demyelinating lesions appear more "tumor-like" and the lesions can mimic tumors clinically and radiologically; tumefactive lesions are seen in only one or two of every 1,000 patients with MS.

Patients who have met criteria for a definite diagnosis of MS experience one of four types, which may be mild, moderate, or severe. The four types, or disease categories, are listed in Table 24.1.

- 85% of patients with MS initially present with a disease course consistent with relapsing-remitting MS (RRMS). Nearly all pediatric-onset patients present with RRMS.

- Of RRMS patients who remain untreated, about half will convert to secondary-progressive MS (SPMS) within 10 to 15 years after initial disease onset.

- Of the remaining patients with MS, 10% will be diagnosed with primary-progressive MS (PPMS), while 5% will be diagnosed with progressive-relapsing MS (PRMS).

Treatment

Treatment for MS involves three major components:

- treatment of acute relapses
- treatment of the overall disease progression
- treatments for specific symptoms of the disease

TABLE 24.1 Disease Courses in Multiple Sclerosis

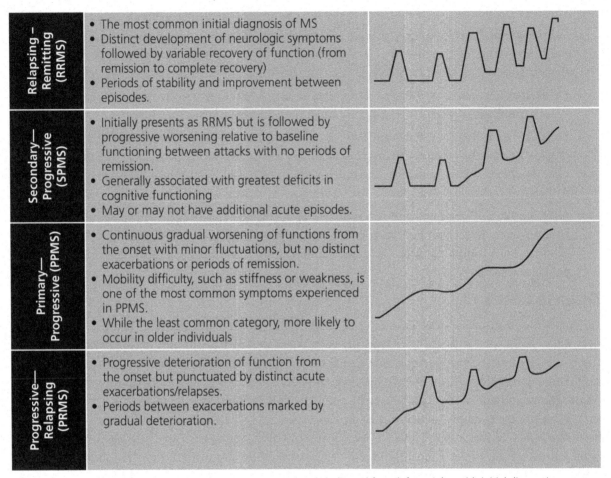

Relapsing – Remitting (RRMS)	• The most common initial diagnosis of MS • Distinct development of neurologic symptoms followed by variable recovery of function (from remission to complete recovery) • Periods of stability and improvement between episodes.	
Secondary— Progressive (SPMS)	• Initially presents as RRMS but is followed by progressive worsening relative to baseline functioning between attacks with no periods of remission. • Generally associated with greatest deficits in cognitive functioning • May or may not have additional acute episodes.	
Primary— Progressive (PPMS)	• Continuous gradual worsening of functions from the onset with minor fluctuations, but no distinct exacerbations or periods of remission. • Mobility difficulty, such as stiffness or weakness, is one of the most common symptoms experienced in PPMS. • While the least common category, more likely to occur in older individuals	
Progressive— Relapsing (PRMS)	• Progressive deterioration of function from the onset but punctuated by distinct acute exacerbations/relapses. • Periods between exacerbations marked by gradual deterioration.	

NOTE: In the four graphs above, disease progression across time is indicated from left to right, with initial diagnosis on the left.

The first two components are discussed here.

- *Acute Relapses*
  - Treated via intravenous corticosteroids followed by an oral prednisone taper. Notably, steroid treatment may have an impact on clinical presentation including mood and cognitive functioning; therefore, this should be taken into consideration when working with patients in and around acute treatment. Neuropsychology research often indicates that assessments were conducted at least 30 days from acute relapse and/or steroid use.
  - If steroids are ineffective, plasmapheresis or intravenous immunoglobulin (IVIG) may be used.
- *Disease Progression* The medications used to alter the overall progression of the disease are referred to as disease-modifying therapies (DMTs). These typically injectable drugs delay relapses, slow the disease progression, and have been used safely in both adults and children. Such medications include formulations of interferon (IFN) drugs such as IFN beta-1a (Avonex or Rebif), Peginterferon beta-1a (Plegridy), IFN beta-1b (Betaseron, Extavia) and glatiramer acetate (Copaxone, Glatopa) for injection.

- For those with very active disease that does not respond to the first-line treatments, mitoxantrone (Novantrone), an immunosuppressant, may be used, though this must be used cautiously given its potentially cardiotoxic effects.

- Natalizumab (Tysabri), a human monoclonal antibody, was the first of several second-line agents administered by infusion. Further, other infusible monoclonal antibodies used in the treatment of MS include rituximab (Rituxan), alemtuzumab (Lemtrada), and ocrelizumab (Ocrevus); ocrelizumab is the only medication approved by the FDA to treat both RRMS and PPMS. Of note, a similar agent, daclizumab (Zinbryta) was pulled from the market in March 2018 amid safety concerns involving several cases of inflammatory encephalitis and meningoencephalitis linked to this agent.

- Several oral agents have recently been introduced, including fingolimod (Gilenya; the first FDA-approved DMT for ages 10 years and up), teriflunomide (Aubagio), dimethyl fumerate (Tecfidera), and sphingosine 1-phosphate receptor (S1PR) modulator. Although patients often prefer these oral agents over injectable medications, these have been associated with serious side effects such as teratogenicity, hepatic failure, and leukopenia. Further, they may not provide as much benefit in terms of relapse frequency in comparison to traditional injectable agents.

Rule-Outs

There are a number of disorders that adversely impact white matter that may have symptom presentations similar to MS. These include (but are not limited to):

- Leukodystrophies
- Progressive multifocal leukoencephalopathy (PML)
- Acute disseminated encephalomyelitis (ADEM)
- Transverse myelitis
- Neuromyelitis optica (i.e., Devic's disease)
- Anti-MOG (Myelin oligodendrocyte glycoprotein) associated encephalomyelitis
- Systemic autoimmune diseases, such as systemic lupus erythematosus, Sjögren's syndrome, and sarcoidosis
- Guillain-Barré syndrome
- Toxic optic neuropathy
- Brain tumor

Expectations for Neuropsychological Assessment Results

In adults, cognitive impairment has been documented in 40% to 65% of patients with MS. Processing speed, sustained attention/concentration, learning and declarative memory impairments are the most common neuropsychological sequelae. Language, visuospatial perception, and remote memory are less affected. In general, adult-onset MS literature shows that deficits tend to progress over time, particularly with a progressive disease course. Whole-brain atrophy, with thalamic atrophy specifically implicated, accounts for significant variance in predicting cognitive dysfunction in adults with MS. Cognitive impairment gives rise to vocational disability, with some literature suggesting that verbal memory and executive function are the most predictive of vocational status. Evaluating cognitive status in patients with MS is often complicated by commonly observed emotional problems (e.g., depression), fatigue, and sleep problems. Please note, there are differences in cognitive presentation in adults compared to pediatric patients. Please see the "Pediatric Considerations" section.

- *Intelligence/Achievement* Intelligence and achievement are often unaffected in the early stages of illness. Processing speed problems may suppress perceptual reasoning and other index scores negatively affected by motor speed or speed of processing skill (e.g., time demands), however, select language-based performances such as fund of knowledge are rarely affected.

- *Attention/Concentration* Problems with sustained and complex attention (attentional shifting) are seen with relative sparing of simple attention span.

- *Processing Speed* Information processing speed and efficiency are the most commonly affected functions. It is important to rule out the potential contribution of problems with psychomotor speed. Reductions in processing speed often negatively affect new learning and executive functions. Thinning of the corpus callosum has been associated with decreased processing speed in MS.

- *Language* Language is not typically affected in the early stages. Aphasia is extremely rare. In the minority of patients who experience language problems, most common are mild dysfluency or naming difficulties. Primary speech difficulties are common (e.g., dysarthria, hypophonia). Some patients develop scanning speech, a speech disorder in which spoken words are broken up with interrupted syllables, noticeable pauses, and varying intonation. Scanning speech is typically caused by cerebellar lesions and is a common symptom of MS. There is some evidence that children with MS may show greater language impairments than do adults with the disease.

- *Visuospatial* Visuospatial skills, particularly timed visual scanning and visuospatial learning, are commonly affected.

- *Memory* Learning and memory (encoding and retrieval) are often among the earliest cognitive problems observed, although reduced memory is more reflective of a reduced learning curve, rather than impaired recall (forgetting). Explicit memory is affected early, whereas semantic and implicit memory are not affected until later in the disease course, if at all.

- *Executive Functions* Executive functions are commonly affected, especially executive aspects of attention and concentration or mental flexibility. Problems with word list generation, and concept formation and abstraction are also common. Further, reduced executive functioning typically affects job-related tasks and instrumental activities of daily living (e.g., planning and organizing). Frontal lesions have been associated with problems in executive function in MS.

- *Sensorimotor Functions* Sensorimotor functions are commonly affected. Motor speed may be affected bilaterally, whereas lateralizing signs may also be apparent depending on lesion location.

- *Emotion and Personality* Depression, anxiety, and emotional lability are common, especially in patients with frontal lobe white matter lesions. Literature suggests that depression may stem from immune-mediated insults to the brain, and evidence supports both lesions and cytokine effects as underlying causes for depression in MS. In addition, pseudobulbar episodes (uncontrollable laughing and crying) have occurred in select patients.

Considerations when Treating Select Populations with Multiple Sclerosis

Pediatric Considerations

It has been suggested that pediatric patients with MS may be at greater risk for cognitive dysfunction due to the consequences of the disease process on the developing brain during ongoing myelinogenesis. As is the case for adults with MS, evaluation of cognitive status in pediatric MS is complicated by factors associated with mood (i.e., anxiety, depression), increased fatigue, and sleep problems.

- *Prevalence* MS symptom onset occurs in approximately 2% to 5% of patients under the age of 18 years, most commonly in the teenage years. Much fewer have onset prior to puberty (0.2% to 0.7% of cases). Children almost exclusively present with RRMS. It has been suggested that pediatric MS may be more common in more racially and ethnically diverse populations when compared to adult-onset MS.

- *Gender* The female-to-male ratio varies with age, with girls generally outnumbering boys; however, prior to age 10, the ratio is generally equivalent.

- *Differential Diagnosis* Differential diagnosis is often a challenge, given that there are several pediatric conditions with common symptoms. For instance, ADEM is a CNS demyelinating condition that is more common in children and has a similar presentation to pediatric MS at onset. A discriminating clinical feature is the presence of encephalopathy (e.g., change in mental status, personality) observed in the early phases of ADEM. Neuromyelitis optica and anti-MOG associated encephalomyelitis are additional conditions that share common symptoms and require careful diagnostic workup to differentiate from pediatric MS.

- *Cognition* Research has been limited, and investigators have yet to identify a cognitive phenotype associated with pediatric MS. Nevertheless, research has revealed cognitive deficits in approximately one third of pediatric patients with MS. Regarding longitudinal neuropsychological outcomes, findings are quite mixed with some studies suggesting decline while others show no change or improvements over time. Similar to adult findings, pediatric patients with MS may show problems with memory, attention and executive functions, visual-motor skills, and processing speed. As compared to adults, children show more difficulty with language-based skills such as verbal knowledge, receptive/expressive language, and verbal fluency. Although findings are variable, some research suggests that IQ may be reduced in pediatric MS, in comparison to what is found in adult studies, which show this area is generally spared. For a review on cognitive outcomes associated with pediatric MS and other pediatric demyelinating conditions, see Tan et al., 2018.

- *Schooling* Pediatric patients with MS often require academic accommodations (Section 504 accommodations) or formal special education services with an Individualized Education Plan (IEP) to address medical and cognitive issues. Accommodations in the post-secondary setting are also frequently needed. Given the changing nature of the disease across time as well as the pediatric patient's developmental level and associated expectations, individual needs are expected to change, requiring serial assessments to determine the most appropriate support services. It is not uncommon for children with MS to have a significant number of medically related absences, and arrangements for the completion of work at home or in the hospital are often necessary to prevent the student from falling behind.

- *Psychological Functioning* Children with chronic illness are generally at higher risk for psychiatric problems. Existing literature on pediatric MS suggests that 30% to 50% of pediatric patients are at risk for internalizing disorders such as depression and anxiety. Pediatric MS patients experiencing mood disturbance may benefit from individual therapy and/or psychiatry consultation. Given the impact of chronic illness on families, a referral for family therapy may be indicated. Literature on support groups indicated that these may be useful for allowing teens and their families to communicate with others impacted by pediatric MS. Several pediatric centers have created therapeutic camp interventions that allow kids and teens with MS to connect with peers and receive education regarding the disease as well as its management.

- *Treatment Adherence* Given that DMTs are often administered through injection, pediatric patients with MS often struggle with treatment adherence. As such, patients may require intervention to address barriers to medication compliance (e.g., anxiety about needles, the desire to not appear "different" from peers) to promote medical regimen adherence. Fortunately, treatment is now available in other forms that eliminate the need for injections.

Adult Considerations

- *Level of Supervision* Typically not required until later stages of the illness. Exceptions include patients who have significant frontal system dysfunction.

- *Driving* Patients are often unable to continue to drive due to physical impairments and slowed reaction time. Problems with processing speed, visual scanning, and mental flexibility can also result in impaired driving ability.

- *Work* The majority of people diagnosed with MS are in the early or mid-stages of their employment history or career. Some are able to continue to work, but outcomes vary depending on impairments and the type of employment. People with more physical jobs often have to leave work earlier in the disease course than others. Those with significant fatigue are more likely to have reduced work hours or shorter work weeks, or cease working altogether.

- *Schooling* Patients diagnosed with MS may still be attending college and may find accommodations to be beneficial. Such services may include, but are not limited to, extended time for exams, note-taking assistance, preferential seating near the front of the classroom, and priority registration to maximize learning during periods of the day when the student is less prone to fatigue. It should be noted that college students are held to the same standards as other students and generally must follow attendance policies and may not have work modified. Vocational evaluations and/or retraining may be appropriate with select younger adults. However, the type of MS and the course of illness must be taken into consideration when making plans for educational and vocational intervention.

- *Capacity* Many patients retain the capacity to participate in instrumental activities of living (e.g., educational or career planning, medical and financial decision making), unless significant frontal system dysfunction develops. The ability to make more complex decisions can be limited by executive function deficits and reduced mental flexibility. With such changes, appointing durable power of attorney or conservator would be recommended.

- *Psychological and Emotional Issues* Depression is common, with a prevalence rate of 50%, which is greater than what is seen with most other neurologic conditions. Some studies suggest that depression can have a negative impact on disease course and outcome, although findings remain debatable. In addition, common symptoms of MS (e.g., fatigue, poor initiation) should not be confused with depression. Anxiety disorders are less common than depression in MS (about 25% of patients) but are more common in MS than in the general population and typically present in the early stages of the disease. Euphoria and apathy have both been associated with demyelination of frontal lobe systems. Adjustment issues relative to the lifestyle changes required of living with a chronic illness are also common. Literature on nonpharmacological intervention has shown promise for MS patients. In terms of treatment for psychological difficulties, cognitive-behavioral therapy appears to be equally as effective as antidepressant medication. Support groups are another effective strategy.

- *Severe Psychiatric Complications* Pathological crying or laughing (i.e., pseudobulbar affect) can occur when diffuse lesions interrupt the corticobulbar tracts. Some patients may develop hypomania or mania as a complication of treatment with corticosteroids. Psychosis is rare unless related to complications of steroid treatment.

- *Medications* In addition to medications to treat the actual disease course, individuals with MS may be on several adjunctive treatments for specific symptoms. Amantadine (Symmetrel) or modafinil (Provigil) are common medications for symptoms of fatigue. Antidepressants are often used to treat mood symptoms, such as clomipramine (Anafranil), which histologically also has an anti-inflammatory effect. Some stimulant medications (e.g., dextroamphetamine, methylphenidate) may show effectiveness in treating fatigue without modifying the patient's sleep cycle, and as a cognitive enhancer in treating MS-related attentional problems. Despite early studies that showed some promise in using acetylcholinesterase inhibitors (e.g., donepezil) for memory dysfunction, more recent, larger multicenter studies showed no effect from such interventions. Dalfampridine (Ampyra) may improve walking speed in those with mobility impairment.

- *Interpersonal Relationships* Patients may experience physical, cognitive, and emotional issues that can strain relationships. Marital distress due to financial issues or caregiver burnout is common. Patients with significant cognitive or physical impairment may become socially isolated or withdrawn.

- *Functional Issues and Rehabilitation* Above and beyond the use of canes, walkers, and wheelchairs, numerous treatments have been employed to improve mobility in those with MS. For example, electrical stimulators may improve toe drag, circumduction, energy expenditure, and walking speed. Exercise programs, including yoga and Pilates, have been shown to increase overall strength and improve stamina. Water exercise programs may allow for movement that some people with MS are not able to perform on land. However, information regarding cognitive rehabilitation remains limited. A recent meta-analysis of cognitive rehabilitation studies in MS concluded that, while substantial progress has been made identifying potentially effective cognitive treatments, further research is necessary to create a refined program that addresses the common cognitive changes experienced by patients with MS and meets "class I evidence in support of a given treatment strategy" (Goverover, Chiaravalloti, O'Brien, & Deluca, 2017).

Geriatric Considerations

Older patients with MS are more likely to have longer disease duration, which is associated with greater physical and cognitive disability. Although uncommon among the elderly, MS diagnosed at an older age typically presents with the progressive subtype, which often also leads to greater physical disability. As such, both of these patient populations are more likely to require a more substantial level of support. MS is not a fatal disease per se; rather, complications during the final stage of the illness are typically the cause of death. Patients with end-stage illness typically die from recurrent infections, such as pneumonia, pulmonary embolism, infections from decubitus ulcers, and, in some cases, suicide. Medical conditions (e.g., heart disease, hypertension, diabetes) can further complicate a patient's medical stability and shorten one's lifespan. Some of the physical complications seen with advanced MS include:

- Decubitus ulcers (i.e., pressure sores), due to lack of mobility

- Aspiration pneumonia due to swallowing problems

- Severe bladder or kidney infections and/or bladder control problems due to chronic urinary dysfunction

- Osteoporosis due to reduced mobility and corticosteroid treatment

Relevant Definitions

Brief Repeatable Battery of Neuropsychological Tests (BRB) Developed as a 40-minute battery administered to screen for cognitive dysfunction in adults. A short version of the BRB has been validated and includes three tests: Selective Reminding Test, Paced Auditory Serial Addition Test-3, and Symbol Digit Modalities Test.

Expanded Disability Status Scale (EDSS) One method of quantifying disability in MS. The EDSS quantifies disability based on eight functional systems including pyramidal, cerebellar, brainstem, sensory, bowel/bladder, visual, cerebral, other. Scores range from 0 to 10, with higher scores associated with greater disability.

Fatigue Severity Scale A method of evaluating severity of fatigue in MS. The scale consists of a brief questionnaire requiring the patient to rate his or her level of fatigue based on a 7-point scale indicating the rater's degree of agreement with the statement. This scale is available in multiple languages and has been used in multiple cultures.

Minimal Assessment of Cognitive Function in Multiple Sclerosis (MACFIMS) A 90-minute battery for adults including seven subtests targeting areas most commonly impacted in MS: Controlled Oral Word Association Test, Judgment of Line Orientation Test, California Verbal Learning Test (2nd Edition), Brief Visuospatial Memory Test—Revised, Symbol Digit Modalities Test, Paced Auditory Serial Addition Test, and Delis-Kaplan Executive Function System Sorting Test.

Multiple Sclerosis Functional Composite (MSFC) A screening battery validated in adults with MS; it includes 9-Hole Peg Test, Timed 25-Foot Walk, and the Paced Auditory Serial Addition Test (PASAT).

National MS Society (NMSS) Pediatric Centers of Excellence Neuropsychology Core Battery Researchers from six NMSS Centers of Excellence designed a core battery for use in studying pediatric MS. Measures include: Wechsler Abbreviated Scale of Intelligence; Wechsler Coding and Digit Span; Symbol Digit Modalities Test; California Verbal Learning Test, Children's Version; Beery Buktenica Test of Visual Motor Integration; Grooved Pegboard; Contingency Naming Test; Trail-Making Test; Conners' Continuous Performance Test; Expressive One-Word Picture Vocabulary Test; Controlled Oral Word Association; Behavior Rating Inventory of Executive Function; Behavior Assessment System for Children; PedsQL Multidimensional Fatigue Scale.

Multiple Sclerosis Questions

NOTE: Questions 4, 40, 80, and 105 on the First Full-Length Practice Examination, Questions 16, 58, 84, and 102 on the Second Full-Length Practice Examination, Questions 42, 92, and 122 on the Third Full-Length Practice Examination, and Questions 4, 37, and 82 on the Fourth Full-Length Practice Examination are from this chapter.

1. A common early sign of MS is _____.
   - (a) optic neuritis
   - (b) word-finding deficits
   - (c) hearing loss
   - (d) seizures

2. In patients with MS, depressive disorders have a lifetime prevalence of about _____.
   - (a) 15%
   - (b) 25%
   - (c) 50%
   - (d) 65%

3. The most common form of MS in pediatric patients is _____.
   - (a) PPMS
   - (b) SPMS
   - (c) PRMS
   - (d) RRMS

4. The prevalence rates of cognitive symptoms among adult patients with MS is approximately _____.
   - (a) 10–20%
   - (b) 25–35%
   - (c) 45–65%
   - (d) 70–80%

5. In terms of treatment of cognitive dysfunction in MS, the best support appears to be for _____.
   - (a) acetylcholinesterase inhibitors
   - (b) amphetamines
   - (c) Gingko biloba
   - (d) cognitive rehabilitation

6. Which of the following tests would be most sensitive in detecting cognitive impairment in an adult with MS?
   - (a) Symbol Digit Modalities Test
   - (b) Boston Naming Test
   - (c) Controlled Oral Word Association Test
   - (d) California Verbal Learning Test

7. MS is best described as which of the following?
   - (a) monophasic inflammatory demyelinating condition
   - (b) peripheral nervous system disease
   - (c) chronic autoimmune condition of the CNS
   - (d) inflammatory brain disease

8. In comparison to adult-onset MS, pediatric patients show greater _____.
   - (a) fatigue
   - (b) sleep disturbance
   - (c) memory impairment
   - (d) language impairment

9. Which of the following has been associated with increased risk for MS?

   (a) older age

   (b) exposure to cigarette smoke

   (c) history of drug abuse

   (d) living near the equator

10. Demyelinating lesions in MS are most likely to occur in the _____.

   (a) occipital lobe

   (b) thalamus

   (c) primary motor cortex

   (d) brainstem

Multiple Sclerosis Answers

1. **A—optic neuritis** *While all of these symptoms may occur in MS, optic neuritis is among the most common presenting concerns.*

   Reference: Brownlee, W. J., Hardy, T. A., Fazekas, F., & Miller, D. H. (2017). Diagnosis of multiple sclerosis: Progress and challenges. *The Lancet, 389*(10076), 1336–1346.

2. **C—50%** *The rate is estimated to be higher than for any other neurological disorder or chronic illness.*

   Reference: Feinstein, A., Magalhaes, S., Richard, J. F., Audet, B., & Moore, G. (2014). The link between multiple sclerosis and depression. *Nature Reviews Neurology, 10*(9), 507–517.

3. **D—RRMS** *RRMS is by far the most common type of MS observed in children and adolescents.*

   Reference: Dale, R. C., Brilot, F., & Banwell, B. (2009). Pediatric central nervous system inflammatory demyelination: Acute disseminated encephalomyelitis, clinically isolated syndromes, neuromyelitis optica, and multiple sclerosis. *Current Opinion in Neurology, 22*(3), 233–240.

4. **C—45–65%** *Rates are commonly cited between 45–65%, sometimes higher depending on the sample surveyed.*

   Reference: Rao, S. M., Leo, G. J., Bernardin, L., & Unverzagt, F. (1991). Cognitive dysfunction in multiple sclerosis. I. Frequency, patterns, and prediction. *Neurology, 41*(5), 685–691.

5. **B—amphetamines** *Research on medications to improve cognition in MS has been limited. It is known that those on DMTs do tend to have slightly better cognitive outcomes, but deficits remain. Studies have been mixed, but currently there is little support for natural substances such as Gingko biloba and the largest study of donepezil in MS failed to find an effect. Amphetamines, however, may improve attention.*

   Reference: Benedict, R. H., Munschauer, F., Zarevics, P., Erlanger, D., Rowe, V., Feaster, T., & Carpenter, R. L. (2008). Effects of l-amphetamine sulfate on cognitive function in multiple sclerosis patients. *Journal of Neurology, 255*(6), 848–852.

6. **A—Symbol Digit Modalities Test** *MS can result in widespread cognitive dysfunction, including memory impairment, but complex multifactorial tests of sustained attention and processing speed are most sensitive to neuropsychological impairment in these individuals.*

   Reference: Kim, S., Zemon, V., Rath, J. F., Picone, M., Gromisch, E. S., Glubo, H., . . . Foley, F. W. (2017). Screening Instruments for the Early Detection of Cognitive Impairment in Patients with Multiple Sclerosis. *International Journal of MS Care, 19*(1): 1–10.

7. **C—chronic autoimmune condition of the CNS** *MS is a condition that impacts the brain and spinal cord. While there are different clinical courses, MS is a chronic condition for which there is no cure.*

Reference: Lublin, F. D., Reingold, S. C., Cohen, J. A., Cutter, G. R., Sorensen, P. S., Thompson, A. J., . . . Bebo, B. (2014). Defining the clinical course of multiple sclerosis: The 2013 revisions. *Neurology, 83*(3), 278-286.

8. **D—language impairment** *A key difference in neuropsychological outcomes for pediatric-onset MS, compared to adult-onset MS, is greater language impairments. Researchers have posited that this finding may relate to disease onset during a time of active brain development creating vulnerability to language development, which occurs earlier in life.*

Reference: Tan, A., Hague, C., Greenberg, B. M., & Harder, L. (2017). Neuropsychological outcomes of pediatric demyelinating diseases: A review. *Child Neuropsychology, 24*(5), 575–597.

9. **B—exposure to cigarette smoke** *Genetic predisposition, exposure to cigarette smoke, and living at latitudes farther from the equator have all been associated with increased risk for MS. Although the condition may be seen in younger and older individuals, peak age for diagnosis of MS is around the third or fourth decade of life.*

Reference: Olsson, T., Barcellos, L. F., & Alfredsson, L. (2017). Interactions between genetic, lifestyle, and environmental risk factors for multiple sclerosis. *Nature Reviews Neurology, 13*, 25–36.

10. **D—brainstem** *The hallmark of MS is the demyelinated plaque or lesion secondary to the loss of myelin and formation of an astrocytic scar. Lesions have a predilection for the optic nerves, periventricular white matter, corpus callosum, brain stem, cerebellum, and spinal cord white matter; and they often surround larger blood vessels, and contrary to previous categorization, can also occur in gray matter. Lesions are least likely to occur in eloquent cortex, or areas that directly control functioning such as occipital lobes, primary motor cortex, and primary somatosensory cortex.*

Reference: Arnett, P. A., Meyer, Jessica, E., Merritt, V. C., & Strober, L. B. (2018). Multiple sclerosis and related disorders. In J. E. Morgan & J. H. Ricker (Eds.), *Textbook of clinical neuropsychology* (2nd ed., pp. 603–617). New York, NY: Taylor and Francis Group.

Recommended Readings

Arnett, P. A., Meyer, Jessica, E., Merritt, V. C., & Strober, L. B. (2018). Multiple sclerosis and related disorders. In J. E. Morgan & J. H. Ricker (Eds.), *Textbook of clinical neuropsychology* (2nd ed., pp. 603–617). New York, NY: Taylor and Francis Group.

Benedict, R. H., DeLuca, J., Enzinger, C., Geurts, J. J., Krupp, L. B., & Rao, S. M. (2017). Neuropsychology of multiple sclerosis: Looking back and moving forward. *Journal of the International Neuropsychological Society, 23*(9–10), 832–842.

Goverover, Y., Chiaravalloti, N. D., O'Brien, A. R., & DeLuca, J. (2018). Evidence-based cognitive rehabilitation for persons with multiple sclerosis: An updated review of the literature from 2007 to 2016. *Archives of Physical Medicine Rehabilitation, 99*(2), 390–407.

MacAllister, W. S., Christodoulou, C., Milazzo, M., Preston, T. E., Serafin, D., Krupp, L. B., & Harder, L. (2013). Pediatric multiple sclerosis: What we know and where are we headed? *Child Neuropsychology, 19*(1), 1–22.

Rosti-Otajarvi, E. M., & Hamalainen, P. I. (2011). Neuropsychological rehabilitation for multiple sclerosis. *Cochrane Database of Systematic Reviews (Online), 11*, CD009131.

Tan, A., Hague, C., Greenberg, B. M., & Harder, L. (2018). Neuropsychological outcomes of pediatric demyelinating diseases: A review. *Child Neuropsychology, 24*(5), 575–597.

Thompson, A. J., Banwell, B. L., Barkhof, F., Carroll, W. M., Coetzee, T., Comi, G., . . . Cohen, J. A. (2017). Diagnosis of multiple sclerosis: 2017 revisions of the McDonald criteria. *The Lancet, 17*(2), 162–173.

Website

Information from the National MS Society. https://www.nationalmssociety.org/

MEDICAL

25   Cancers

Celiane Rey-Casserly and Mary-Ellen Meadows

Introduction

Cancers that affect the nervous system can be grouped into two major areas: primary neoplasms of the central nervous system (CNS) and cancers of other organ systems that can affect CNS function either directly (i.e., brain metastases) or as a result of treatment (e.g., radiation, chemotherapy). These groups can be subdivided further into child and adult disorders. The types of cancers prevalent in adults and children are very different (see Table 25.1). This chapter first focuses on brain tumors and subsequently on non-CNS cancers.

Section 1: Brain Tumors

Brain tumors develop as a consequence of abnormal replication of cells inside the skull cavity due to genetic alterations that allow cells to circumvent normal cell regulatory functions and avoid immune system targeting.

Primary Brain Tumors

- Originate in the CNS
- Are more common in children than adults

Metastatic Brain Tumors

- Primary cancer is outside the nervous system and spreads to the brain
- Most common intracranial tumor in adults (occurs four times more frequently than primary brain tumors in adults)
- Occur in 20–40% of adults with cancer
- Malignancies that commonly spread to the brain: melanoma and cancer of the breast, colon, or lung
- 80% of metastatic tumors in the CNS seed in the cerebral hemispheres
- Most common location: gray and white matter junctions

Neuropathology

Marked heterogeneity exists in tumor types and their biological behavior; the incidence of specific tumor types varies by age group, and tumors with the same histology behave differently at different stages of development across the age span.

Classification of brain tumors has been conventionally based on the presumed cell of origin and proliferative potential. Current nosology incorporates molecular genetic features. Tumor grading ranges from I to IV and is based on the degree of histological malignancy and molecular genetic characteristics (see Table 25.2). In considering the impact of the tumor, the distinction between malignant and benign is less

TABLE 25.1 Adult and Childhood Cancers

	Adults (>19)	Children (0–19)
Most Common Cancers	Prostate, Breast, and Lung Cancer	Acute Lymphoblastic Leukemia, Brain Tumors
Incidence of Primary Brain and CNS Tumors	23.03 per 100,000 persons per year	5.94 per 100,000 persons per year
5 Year Survival Rate for Brain Tumors	35%	74%

useful in the context of primary brain tumors than in other body systems. Given the critical structures in the brain and the confined space within the skull, "benign tumors" can have a high morbidity. In the context of brain tumors, malignancy does not refer to capacity to metastasize to other regions of the body but is an indication of local growth pattern and capacity to spread to different areas in the CNS.

Major Categories of Primary Brain Tumors

- Brain tumors can be categorized by cell of origin: glial, neuronal, embryonal, mixed, or other. Within the category of gliomas, tumors can be more benign (pilocytic astrocytoma in children) or aggressive (glioblastoma in adults).

- Diffuse astrocytic and oligodendroglial tumors: glioblastoma, diffuse astrocytoma, anaplastic oligodendroglioma

TABLE 25.2 World Health Organization (WHO) Brain Tumor Grading

Grade	Characteristics	Histologic Types
I	Well-differentiated Non-infiltrative Low proliferative potential Slow growing Good possibility of cure with surgery	Pilocytic astrocytoma Ganglioglioma Craniopharyngioma Meningioma Pituicytoma
II	Moderately differentiated Somewhat infiltrative Low proliferative activity Can progress to higher grades	Diffuse astrocytoma, Isocitrate dehydrogenase (IDH) mutant Ependymoma Oligodendroglioma, IDH mutant and 1p/19-codeleted
III	Poorly differentiated Brisk mitotic activity Infiltrative Typically require adjuvant chemotherapy and/or radiation Tend to progress to higher grade	Anaplastic astrocytoma, IDH mutant Anaplastic ependymoma Choroid plexus carcinoma
IV	Undifferentiated Widespread infiltration, propensity for craniospinal dissemination High degree of anaplasia, mitotically active High degree of necrosis Require multi-modality treatment Rapid recurrence	Glioblastoma Medulloblastoma Pineoblastoma Atypical teratoid rhabdoid tumor

NOTE: Louis, D. N., Perry, A., Reifenberger, G., von Deimling, A., Figarella-Branger, D., Cavenee, W. K., . . . Ellison, D. W. (2016). The 2016 World Health Organization classification of tumors of the central nervous system: A summary. *Acta Neuropathologica*, 131(6), 803–820.

- Other astrocytic tumors: pilocytic astrocytoma
- Ependymal tumors
- Embryonal tumors: medulloblastoma, CNS embryonal tumor NOS, atypical teratoid rhabdoid tumor (AT/RT)
- Choroid plexus tumors
- Neuronal and mixed neuronal-glial tumors
- Tumors of the pineal region
- Tumors of cranial and paraspinal nerves
- Germ cell tumors
- Tumors of the sellar region: craniopharyngioma, pituicytoma
- Meningiomas

Epidemiology

Incidence Rates

- The overall incidence rate of primary brain and CNS tumors in the United States from 2010 to 2014 was 23.03 per 100,000 and age adjusted to the 2000 United States standard population and 5.65 for children and adolescents 0 to 14 years; highest incidence is among adults 85 and older.

- For primary brain tumors in the CNS the most common tumor site is the meninges (36.8%); 18.7% are in the lobes of the brain (frontal 8.2%, temporal 6%, parietal 3.5%, occipital 1%). Other sites include the cranial nerves, spinal cord, pituitary, craniopharyngeal duct, brainstem, and cerebellum.

- Different types of tumors are common at different periods over the lifespan (see Table 25.3).

TABLE 25.3 Distribution of Brain and Central Nervous System (CNS) Tumors by Age Group and Histology 2010 to 2014

Age Group (years)	Most Common Type	Second Most Common Type
0–4	Embryonal tumors	Pilocytic Astrocytoma
5–9	Pilocytic Astrocytoma	Malignant Gliomas
10–14	Pilocytic Astrocytoma	Malignant Gliomas
15–19	Pituitary	Pilocytic Astrocytoma
20–44	Pituitary	Meningioma
45–54	Meningioma	Pituitary
55–64	Meningioma	Glioblastoma
65–74	Meningioma	Glioblastoma
75 and older	Meningioma	Glioblastoma

NOTE: Ostrom, Q. T., Gittleman, H., Truitt, G., Boscia, A., Kruchko, C., & Barnholtz-Sloan, J. S. (2018). CBTRUS statistical report: Primary brain and other central nervous system tumors diagnosed in the United States in 2011–2015. Neuro Oncol, 20(suppl. 4), iv1–iv86.

- Gender/racial/ethnic differences
  - Overall incidence of primary brain tumors is higher in females.
  - Tumors of the meninges are twice as common in females.
  - Neuroepithelial tumors are 1.4 times more common in males.
  - Incidence of gliomas and germ cell tumors is higher in males.
  - Pituitary tumors are more common in females.
  - Incidence rates for all brain tumors are higher for whites than other groups; incidence rates for non-malignant tumors are highest in African Americans.
- Childhood brain tumors
  - Brain tumors are the second most common malignancy and the most common solid tumor in children.
  - Childhood brain tumors (age 0 to 19) account for 6% of all CNS tumors.

Mortality

- For primary malignant brain and CNS tumors, in adults 20 years and over, 5-year survival decreases with increasing age, from a high of 62% in young adults (age 20 to 44) to a low of 6% in adults diagnosed at age 75 and over.
- The highest proportion of adults diagnosed with primary brain tumors are aged 60 to 69 years with a 5-year survival rate of 6%.
- Poorest survival is in patients with *glioblastoma* for all age groups.
- For individuals with multiple brain metastases, the odds of survival beyond 6 months are low.
- Overall survival in children with primary brain tumor is lowest under 1 year of age.

Risk Factors

Several risk factors for developing brain tumors have been identified. These include exposure to ionizing radiation (therapeutic, diagnostic, or other sources) and various genetic cancer disposition syndromes (e.g., tuberous sclerosis, *neurofibromatosis types 1 and 2*, Li-Fraumeni syndrome, nevoid basal cell carcinoma syndrome, and Von Hippel-Lindau syndrome). An increased risk of CNS lymphoma is seen in those with human immunodeficiency virus (HIV).

Determinants of Severity

Severity of brain tumors is related to a number of factors. At diagnosis, tumor histology is determined and graded according to degree of malignancy (see Table 25.2). Location and mass effect are also very relevant, given the possibility of herniation caused by tumor growth. Some tumors (e.g., diffuse pontine glioma) are not resectable and affect vital brain structures.

Presentation, Disease Course, and Recovery

Presentation and Disease Course

- *Headaches* Most common presenting symptom in adults and children and are related to mass effect

- Persistent headaches are a presenting symptom in 35% of adults diagnosed with brain tumors.
- New-onset headaches associated with nausea and vomiting and increased severity in the mornings can also be associated with brain tumors.

- *Signs of increased intracranial pressure (ICP)* Headaches, nausea/vomiting.
- *Progressive neurologic deficits* Sensory and motor deficits, ataxia, cranial nerve palsies. Posterior fossa tumors, common in children, can present with nausea/vomiting and ataxia. Pineal tumors can present with Parinaud syndrome (lack of upward gaze, nystagmus) and double vision.
- *Endocrinopathies* Hormonal disruption, usually with hypothalamic/pituitary tumors. Tumors of the sellar region are associated with neuroendocrine dysfunction such as diabetes insipidus, hypogonadism, or growth delay.
- *Seizures* 15–20% of children present with seizures; 25–30% of adults present with seizures; 40–60% of adults have seizures at some time in the illness course.
- *Cognitive and behavioral changes* In adults, tumors can range from asymptomatic to causing major disturbances in cognition and behavior. Symptoms can be related to *increased ICP* from mass effect, cerebral edema, or obstruction of CSF flow (headache, nausea/vomiting) or local effect on a specific brain region (focal neurologic deficits, cognitive dysfunction).

Diagnosis

Computed tomography (CT) can show most tumors and can identify calcifications and hemorrhage but may not identify posterior fossa tumors or low-grade gliomas. Magnetic resonance imaging (MRI) with contrast is the imaging modality of choice for diagnosing and monitoring brain tumors and can delineate the location and characteristics of the tumor. Contrast enhancement can indicate breakdown of the blood-brain barrier, and enhancement patterns can provide information regarding the type and degree of malignancy of the tumor.

Treatment

Treatment for brain tumors includes surgery, radiation therapy, and chemotherapy; specific treatment protocols vary based on a range of factors related to the tumor type, location, age of patient, and treatment history. Current protocols are informed by molecular genetic factors such that treatments are individualized to target specific tumor types, minimize toxicity, and maximize effectiveness.

Surgery

Surgery is typically the first line of treatment for brain tumors. Surgery may not be feasible in the context of multiple metastases or sites. In addition, some tumors grow in locations where surgery is not an option (e.g., brainstem). The extent of resection is associated with more favorable prognosis in many tumor types. Surgery can be curative for low-grade tumors in children and for extra-axial tumors (e.g., meningioma, pituitary tumors). Brain tumors are often associated with hydrocephalus and edema, which need to be managed urgently. In children with posterior fossa tumors obstructing the fourth ventricle, surgical removal of the tumor can address the hydrocephalus. Steroids are often given to reduce edema. Of children with posterior fossa tumors, 10–35% require shunting to control hydrocephalus post-surgery. *Endoscopic third ventriculostomy* avoids complications associated with shunt placement and is used for management of hydrocephalus for tumors in the third ventricle (tectal gliomas) or pineal region.

- *Surgical Complications in brain tumor resection include:*
  - Perioperative stroke
  - Motor or sensory deficits

- Damage to pituitary/hypothalamic structures
- Posterior fossa or cerebellar mutism syndrome (complication of cerebellar tumor resection):
  - More common in children than adults after posterior fossa surgery
  - Presumably associated with brainstem involvement of the tumor and location in the vermis
  - In this syndrome injury to the inferior vermis and dentate nuclei and to the dentato-thalamo-cortical pathway from tumor or surgery affects cognitive and motor function.
  - Symptoms include mutism, emotional lability, cranial nerve deficits, and ataxia.
  - Mutism and motor deficits resolve over days/weeks, at times months; may require inpatient rehabilitation; some degree of impairment can persist in motor and speech function.

Radiation Therapy

Radiation therapy is an essential component of treatment for brain tumors. Whole-brain or craniospinal radiation is used to treat tumors with potential for dissemination in the neuroaxis (e.g., medulloblastoma) or for brain metastases. Radiation therapy targets rapidly dividing tumor cells by depositing high frequency energy in tissue, creating ionization and free radicals and damaging tumor DNA. Because cancer cells are preferentially involved in replication rather than cell maintenance and repair, they are more vulnerable to the effects of radiation. Radiation is often delivered in fractions to allow for tissue repair processes in healthy cells. Exposure to cranial irradiation can impair growth of normal tissue and subsequent brain development and function, consequently younger children (below 3 years of age) are most vulnerable, and radiation therapy is often deferred or contraindicated in this age group. Toxicity is also higher in the very old, due to less robust cellular repair mechanisms associated with aging. Innovations in radiation therapy hold promise for minimizing toxicity; these techniques include image guided three-dimensional conformal delivery to minimize impact on normal tissue and proton beam radiation therapy that reduces the exit dose.

- *Complications of radiation therapy*
  - Acute radiation encephalopathy develops early on (approximately 2 weeks after beginning treatment); characterized by headaches, somnolence, worsening of preexisting neurologic deficits; responds to treatment with corticosteroids.
  - Early radiation encephalopathy develops 1 to 6 months post radiotherapy treatment; presumably associated with reversible demyelination related to disruption of blood-brain barrier and neuroinflammation; return to baseline is typically seen in 12 months.
- *Late (more than 12 months) complications of radiation (adults)*
  - Typically not reversible
  - Can consist of local radionecrosis or diffuse *leukoencephalopathy*
  - Cognitive deficits range from mild to very severe (dementia)
  - Attention and short-term memory problems common in mild to moderately affected patients
  - Incontinence
  - Gait disturbance
  - MRI shows diffuse atrophy, ventricular enlargement, and white matter abnormalities in adults with severe late encephalopathy associated with radiation.
  - Sometimes treated with ventriculoperitoneal shunting in the context of hydrocephalus

- *Late (more than 12 months) complications of radiation (children)*
  - Neuropsychological deficits
  - Neuroendocrine dysfunction; infertility
  - Vascular complications
  - Hearing loss
  - Cataracts
  - Impaired growth and development
  - Secondary malignancy

- *Pathophysiology of Cognitive Dysfunction in Individuals Treated with Radiation* In children, radiation therapy is associated with damage to developing white matter, and younger children are more at risk for neurocognitive toxicity. Radiation injures oligodendrocyte precursor cells and brain microvasculature. Higher doses of radiation are associated with loss of normal-appearing white matter; white matter volume loss explains the relationship between age at diagnosis and neurocognitive function. Diffusion tensor imaging studies demonstrate reduced diffusivity in various regions of the brain, including the corpus callosum, internal capsule, and frontal white matter. Cranial radiation therapy also damages hippocampal progenitor cells, which presumably contributes further to problems with cognitive function over time. The synergistic role of other treatments (e.g., chemotherapy, glucocorticosteroids) needs to be considered as well. In adults, radiation therapy can cause focal demyelination and edema. Vascular injury can also emerge over the long term and contribute to necrosis. Radiation necrosis is important to distinguish from tumor recurrence and PET scanning is often used for this purpose.

Chemotherapy

Cytotoxic chemotherapy agents target rapidly dividing cells by disrupting DNA and interfering with transcription and replication. Chemotherapy has become increasingly important in the treatment of pediatric and adult brain tumors. For children, the addition of chemotherapy to treatment regimens has allowed for reduced doses of radiation. For example, children with medulloblastoma are treated with surgery, radiation therapy, and one year of maintenance chemotherapy; high-dose *intrathecal chemotherapy* and/or bone marrow transplant is used with very young children to avoid radiation therapy. Clinical trials and current protocols are including targeted therapies that selectively treat specific genetic mutations. Immunotherapy agents are also being incorporated into chemotherapy regimens.

Chemotherapy is sometimes given alone or combined with radiotherapy (termed chemoradiotherapy). Combined treatment may have a synergistic negative impact on late effects and has been associated with higher risk of cognitive impairments. Late effects of chemotherapy can be related to direct effects of the drugs on the CNS and/or indirect effects. Mechanisms of CNS damage due to chemotherapy are not well understood but include demyelination, inflammation (cytokine activation), oxidative stress, immune response, damage to progenitor cells, and microvascular injury.

- *Late effects and complications of chemotherapy (adults)*
  - Cerebral white matter damage—*leukoencephalopathy*, particularly with high-dose *methotrexate*)
  - Hearing loss, particularly with platinum agents (e.g., cisplatin)
  - Peripheral neuropathies—a frequent side effect, more severe during active treatment
  - Secondary cancers (damage to bone marrow stem cells may increase risk of blood cancers)
  - Fatigue
  - Neuropsychological deficits

- *Late effects and complications of chemotherapy (children)*
  - Cerebral white matter damage—*leukoencephalopathy*, particularly with antimetabolites (e.g., *methotrexate*)
  - Endocrine dysfunction; infertility
  - Cardiovascular problems, particularly with anthracyclines (e.g., Adriamycin)
  - Seizures
  - Hearing loss, particularly with platinum agents
  - Neuropathies, particularly with vinca alkaloids (e.g., vincristine)
  - Cerebellar symptoms
  - Organ dysfunction
  - Secondary cancers
  - Neuropsychological deficits

Inpatient Hospitalization

Recovery Course

- Children can recover quickly from surgery for brain tumors when surgical complications are absent or minimal. Some patients will require extended hospitalizations if intensive multimodality treatment or bone marrow transplant is required. If neurological complications develop, inpatient rehabilitation may be indicated.
- If radiation therapy is needed postsurgery, treatments are typically delivered in fractions over a 6-week period. Postradiation chemotherapy is delivered in cycles, and overall course of treatment can be a year or longer. Chemotherapy can be delivered on an inpatient or outpatient basis, depending on the type of protocol.

Assessment Methods

Neuropsychological assessment in adults after surgery and before additional tumor-directed therapy can provide useful information about functional status and the effects of tumor/surgery on cognition. Neuropsychological status assessed post-surgery has been shown to predict survival in adults with malignant gliomas, particularly measures of executive function and attention. Decline in cognitive function can also be an early sign of disease progression, and improvements in function can indicate positive response to treatment.

- *Issues to Consider in Assessing Neuropsychological Status During Treatment* Comprehensive neuropsychological assessment is often deferred until after radiation therapy or treatment is completed for several reasons.
  1. If the treatment period is protracted and involves extended time away from school or work, assessment may be most useful when return to school/work is approaching.
  2. Assessment during chemotherapy can be of limited benefit if patients are experiencing significant problems with fatigue or nausea or other functionally disruptive complications/symptoms.
  3. Assessment of mental status changes or other cognitive symptoms (e.g., memory problems, concentration issues) that develop during treatment may need to be addressed with a more targeted evaluation, with a plan for management and timing of ongoing follow-up.
  4. The assessment plan is guided by the referral questions, as well as by issues of patient age, stamina/fatigue, sensory/motor deficits, or cognitive limitations.

Treatment

During the treatment phase, individuals with brain tumors require multidisciplinary care and close monitoring of their medical condition and response to treatment. Psychological support during the treatment phase is a critical component of multidisciplinary care. Neurological complications and motor/sensory deficits may require specific rehabilitation efforts and/or supportive care. Neuroendocrine status needs to be monitored in patients who receive radiation to the pituitary-hypothalamus. Some patients may require additional surgery or treatment, such as stereotactic radiosurgery or a change in the chemotherapy regimen.

Outpatient Rehabilitation/Post-Treatment Care

Recovery Course

- The course of recovery from brain tumors and their treatment is quite variable. Disease progression is always a concern, and survival is poorest for adults, particularly older adults. In adults, care is dependent on pathology and location of tumor, age at treatment, treatment regimen, prognosis, and patient specific factors. Most patients are placed on anti-epileptic medication initially though this can be discontinued over time. Ongoing multidisciplinary follow-up is the standard of care for children. Neuropsychological monitoring and follow-up are structured according to patient status/needs, progression of disease, stage in rehabilitation, and developmental considerations.

- Residual complications of treatment, limited stamina, and physical deconditioning can compromise recovery and overall functioning.

- Adult survivors of childhood brain tumors are at increased risk of a number of medical and psychosocial problems including:

  - Neurological complications, including late occurring seizure disorder and *vasculopathy*
  - Neuroendocrine dysfunction
  - Sensory/motor deficits
  - Late-occurring stroke, particularly if treated with cranial radiation dose greater than 30 gray (Gy)
  - Secondary malignancy
  - Increased risk of death (13 times the rate of United States population)
  - Psychosocial complications, such as lower rates of employment and marriage

Assessment Methods

A thorough review of the history is critical in assessing outcomes, including specifics of disease and treatment (e.g., age at diagnosis, type of treatment, radiation dose, epoch of treatment), premorbid functioning, social-environmental context, and resources. Radiation therapy is associated with increased neurocognitive morbidity, but other complications also contribute to long-term neuropsychological functioning. Tumor location in the cerebral hemispheres can be associated with worse outcome. Neuropsychological assessment for children treated for brain tumors needs to be performed periodically (e.g., every 3 years or more frequently if specific issues arise or additional treatment is needed). An evaluation at completion of treatment provides a baseline for ongoing follow-up and develops a plan of intervention and school re-entry. Periodic follow-up is important because late effects can emerge over time, and some children are at risk for decline in neuropsychological functioning. Planning the transition to adulthood is also critical.

Treatment

Individuals treated for brain tumors can have a range of needs affecting physical, cognitive, psychological, and social functioning. Neuropsychologists develop a comprehensive treatment plan that outlines psychological interventions, school/vocational programming, rehabilitation plan, and direct therapies.

Medications can be helpful in many instances in addressing tumor-related neuropsychological deficits. Modafinil and other stimulants can be effective in addressing low arousal and fatigue. Stimulants can be helpful in some cases to manage attention and processing speed problems associated with treatment for childhood leukemia and brain tumors. Depression and anxiety can be treated with cognitive behavioral therapies and psychopharmacological agents. Preliminary studies have shown some role for donepezil for attention and processing issues related to cancer and its treatment, in both children and adults. Memantine has also been shown to delay cognitive dysfunction over time in patients with brain metastases treated with whole brain radiation.

Section 2: Non-CNS Cancers and Paraneoplastic Syndromes

Cognition can also be impacted by systemic cancers and the treatments used to treat the specific cancers. The incidence varies and depends on the specific cancer, type/dose of chemotherapy, and differences in individual susceptibility and biology. For those who develop cognitive problems following chemotherapy, patients coined the term "chemobrain" or "chemofog."

Adult Non-CNS Cancers and Paraneoplastic Syndromes

- It is expected that 1.7 million new cases of cancer will be diagnosed in 2018 in the United States.
- Overall 5-year survival for all non-CNS cancers is 70% (2008–2014).
- Cancer death rates are declining for both men and women.
- The most common cancer types in adults are breast (female), lung, prostate (male), colorectal, and melanoma of the skin.
- Cancer disparities
  - African American ethnicity has been found to be associated with increased mortality in early-stage pre-menopausal and post-menopausal breast cancer, advanced-stage ovarian cancer and advanced-stage prostate cancer despite enrollment in clinical trials with uniform treatment and follow-up.
  - African American males have a higher incidence rate and are more likely to die from lung cancer compared to white males.
  - Both African American men and women have a higher incidence rate of colorectal cancer compared to white men and women.
  - Worse outcomes among African Americans may be related to failure to provide optimal treatment, access to care, physician expertise (referred to less experienced surgeons, seen at low-volume medical centers).
- *Paraneoplastic syndromes*
  - Rare neurological complication of cancer; remote effects of cancer on the nervous system
  - Incidence: less than 5% of patients with systemic cancer
  - Causes severe neurological disability; can be focal or diffuse
  - Caused by indirect immune system reaction to cancer

TABLE 25.4 Specific Paraneoplastic Syndromes

Types	Possible Associated Cancer	Symptoms	Time Course	Brain Imaging
Progressive Encephalomyelitis	Lung; Hodgkin's disease	Seizures, amnesia, mental status changes, affective changes	Symptoms can precede diagnosis by up to 2 years	Usually normal; May show medial temporal lobe abnormalities
Cerebellar Degeneration	Lung; gynecologic cancer, Hodgkin's disease	Motor incoordination leading to progressive gait ataxia; dysarthria, nystagmus, vertigo, diplopia, cognitive changes	Symptoms can precede diagnosis up to 4 years	May be normal early in course; cerebellar atrophy and dilated 4th ventricle later
Opsoclonus Myoclonus	Neuroblastoma or chest/lung in children; lung cancer in adults	Arrhythmic, multidirectional involuntary conjugate saccades; may be accompanied by myoclonus of trunk, limbs, head, diaphragm, palate, larynx, pharynx	Symptoms manifested up to weeks/months before diagnosis	

- *Paraneoplastic syndromes* affecting CNS and neurological functioning (see Table 25.4):
  - Most common: Lambert-Eaton myasthenic syndrome, occurs in 3% of patients with small lung cancer
  - Progressive encephalomyelitis; can present with seizures, amnesia, and mental status changes
  - Cerebellar degeneration

Childhood Non-CNS Cancers

- Approximately 15,000 children and adolescents younger than age 20 years are diagnosed each year in the United States with non-CNS cancer. One in 350 individuals develops cancer before age 20 years.

- Cancer is the most common cause of disease-related mortality in children.

- Most common non-CNS cancers in children are leukemias, lymphomas, soft tissue sarcomas, neuroblastomas, and kidney tumors.

- In the United States overall 5-year survival is approximately 83% for all childhood cancers. One in 530 adults (20 to 39 years of age) is a childhood cancer survivor.

- Acute lymphoblastic leukemia (ALL) is the most common malignancy of childhood, and 5-year survival rates are 90% with treatment.

- ALL is a cancer of the blood and bone marrow in which precursors of lymphocytes proliferate and crowd out healthy and functional cells. It is most commonly diagnosed in the preschool years. Contemporary treatment protocols include systemic and intrathecal chemotherapy; very high risk patients are treated with cranial radiation therapy.

Recovery

Treatment

- *Effects of treatment for non-CNS cancers in adults*

    - The number of patients demonstrating cognitive dysfunction during chemotherapy varies widely (13–70%), though it has been observed in prospective studies that between 17–75% of patients prior to treatment can have cognitive dysfunction.

    - Some individuals may be more vulnerable to developing neurocognitive dysfunction with cancer therapy, presumably related to genetic variation in sensitivity to the effects of treatment, differences in inflammatory markers, and cognitive reserve.

    - It also important to assess the subjective report of the cognitive changes and the impact on their functioning at home or work/school, though the cognitive complaints may or may not be associated with the pattern of findings on testing. Collateral history can also be helpful in ascertaining impact of treatment on cognition. The patient's perception of deficits may be related to a number of factors, including need to expend more effort on tasks or emotional issues.

    - Complaints of learning and memory difficulties as well as attention, working memory, processing speed, and executive function problems are often reported during and after chemotherapy treatment.

    - Variability in impact of treatment across patients is related to differences in chemotherapy regimens, hormonal therapies, pretreatment cognitive reserve, and impact of other medical issues.

    - Most of the research on neurocognitive outcomes and etiology of "chemobrain" has been conducted in patients with breast cancer though studies have been conducted in populations with hematological malignancies, ovarian cancer, lung cancer, prostate cancer and colon cancer. Cognitive dysfunction following breast cancer therapy has been documented during and in the period immediately after treatment. Findings are more mixed with respect to longer periods post-treatment. Breast cancer studies have documented persistent cognitive changes in approximately a third of individuals at 1 year and more post-treatment. Longitudinal structural imaging studies in breast cancer survivors treated with chemotherapy have shown decreased gray matter densities and white matter changes.

    - Risk factors for neurocognitive impairment in patients with breast cancer include

        - Older age

        - Lower cognitive reserve

        - Genetic contributions (COMT-Val; ApoE ε4)

    - Treatment for non-CNS malignancies can have late effects that affect quality of life; these late effects vary by type of cancer and treatment. Late effects can include:

        - Cardiovascular problems, particularly with anthracyclines (e.g., Adriamycin, trastuzumab)

        - Endocrine changes (premature menopause in women <40, infertility)

        - Pulmonary problems (inflammation, difficulties breathing, thickening of lining)

        - Dental problems (treatment may impact tooth enamel)

- Increased risk of cognitive dysfunction is noted with higher doses, multiagent chemotherapy, *intrathecal* chemotherapy, and older age.

- Long-term effects can be apparent in selected patients though there are some patients whose difficulties resolve.

- Cognitive changes associated with cancer and cancer treatment have been hypothesized to affect the trajectory of normal aging by either accelerated aging or a parallel decline, and may vary depending on type of cancer and age at treatment. Recent findings note that survivors of breast cancer can experience health and cognitive problems characteristic of accelerated aging.

- **Bone marrow transplantation** The impact of bone marrow transplantation on neuropsychological functioning depends on a range of factors including type of underlying cancer, experience of previous therapy, autologous versus allogeneic transplant, full versus reduced intensity treatment, age of the patient (younger age at diagnosis and treatment is associated with more problems), cognitive reserve, and experience of complications of transplantation. Graft versus host disease can be a disabling condition in allogeneic stem cell transplant. The impact of prolonged immune dysfunction on children's development is unknown. Decline in executive functions and memory has been noted after bone marrow transplantation, but this may be related to the impact of treatment on other body systems affecting overall health status and stamina. Thus, assessments should include measures of memory and learning, processing speed, and executive function. Studies monitoring cognitive changes during treatment should include tests with alternate forms and should use reliable change or regression techniques to interpret changes over time.

- **Endocrine Therapy** Hormonal therapy is used to treat certain cancers (breast, prostate, thyroid) and to reduce the risk of recurrence. The therapy works to block, add, or remove hormones that can slow or stop the growth of cancer. Treatment includes surgical excision of the gland responsible for producing the hormone or taking medications that can prevent the cancer from using the hormones to grow. It may be used with other treatments (surgery, radiation, chemotherapy, immunotherapy). Side effects, including hot flashes, low libido, fatigue, nausea, and mood changes can affect quality of life. There is some evidence that tamoxifen, which is used in the treatment of certain breast cancers, can negatively impact word list generation and verbal memory. A decline in visuospatial skills was apparent in a study of patients with prostate cancer treated with androgen deprivation therapy.

- **Effects of treatment for non-CNS cancers in children**

  - Cancer treatment for non-CNS malignancies in children can have lasting effects on a range of body systems including brain development and function.

  - Approximately 60% of childhood cancer survivors experience at least one late effect of treatment.

  - Over 40% of childhood cancer survivors treated between 1960 through 1990s developed a chronic disease. Childhood cancer survivors are at increased risk for:

    - Reduction in life expectancy
    - Endocrine dysfunction and fertility problems
    - Neuropsychological impairments, particularly if treated with *intrathecal chemotherapy* or radiation
    - Cardiopulmonary dysfunction

- ◦ Sensory deficits (hearing loss, cataracts)
- ◦ Gastrointestinal disorders
- ◦ Secondary malignancies
- In children, the literature related to the neurocognitive effects of cancer treatment in non-CNS malignancies has focused primarily on leukemia. Central nervous system prophylaxis to avoid relapse in the CNS has contributed to dramatic improvement in survival. Central nervous system prophylactic treatment (either *intrathecal chemotherapy* or radiation) is associated with late neuropsychological effects that can emerge well after treatment (6–12 months later).
- Risk factors for neurocognitive impairment
  - ◦ Young age at treatment
  - ◦ Higher doses of radiation
  - ◦ Female gender; females less than 6 years of age at diagnosis are at highest risk

Expectations for Neuropsychological Assessment Results

Brain Tumors: Adults

Cognitive deficits are often present before treatment. Neuropsychological deficits can be related to the tumor, tumor progression, tumor-related neurological complications (e.g., edema), and seizures. Deterioration in cognitive function can indicate tumor progression, even before this is noted on imaging studies. Cognitive problems are generally more diffuse in adults with brain tumors than in patients with stroke. Increased intracranial pressure can cause structural shifts and can produce features suggestive of involvement of sites distant from the tumor. Focal effects can be apparent and dependent on tumor location. Neurocognitive late effects of radiation and chemotherapy implicate dysfunction in frontal-subcortical brain systems. Psychological symptoms, such as anxiety and depression, can also contribute to cognitive dysfunction. Assessment strategy and focus should be driven by the referral questions, risk of recurrence, and prognosis. The evaluation will typically focus on attention, executive functions, language, memory and learning, visuospatial skills, and psychological adjustment. Neuropsychological assessment can be requested to assess change in function following a particular treatment (e.g., radiation therapy, chemotherapy) or to assess the possibility of tumor progression or to plan a program of intervention or rehabilitation.

Brain Tumors: Children

Neuropsychological difficulties can be delayed and progressive in survivors of childhood brain tumors, particularly those receiving multimodality treatment. Cognitive deficits can range from fairly mild to very severe. Overall IQs of children treated for medulloblastoma with radiation tend to be in the low average range, and score declines are often noted over time. Children treated with only surgery typically have average cognitive ability, but the proportion of children scoring in the below average range is higher than expected in cohorts studied. A triad of cognitive processes appears particularly affected—attention, working memory, and information processing speed—because fluid cognitive skills are more vulnerable to disruption. Dysfunction in these areas is believed to contribute to later difficulties in intellectual ability and academic achievement. Social skills deficits are being increasingly identified and studied.

Non-CNS Cancers: Adults

Neuropsychologists can contribute to the ongoing care and management of patients being treated for non-CNS cancers. The areas to be assessed depend on the referral questions, stage of treatment, and other individual factors. During the treatment stage, neuropsychological consultation or assessment is relevant when significant cognitive symptoms or changes in functional status are noted. Consultation is particularly relevant when symptoms affect medical decision making, negatively impact quality of life, or impair functional capacity as the late cognitive effects can persist in some patients. In general, neuropsychological assessment should focus on the complaints and behaviors that prompted the referral. Evaluation of attention/concentration, learning and memory, executive functions, speed of processing, mood, and adaptive function should typically be included. In the post-treatment period, a more comprehensive evaluation may be important to develop a plan of treatment and recommend specific strategies and accommodations for work and daily living.

Childhood Leukemia

Children treated with chemotherapy only for leukemia typically have IQs within the normal range. Deficits in attention, verbal and visual memory, executive functioning, and processing speed have been found. Children experiencing cognitive or school difficulties should be referred for evaluation promptly because late effects become increasingly apparent over the course of development, and timely treatment and intervention are critical. Survivors treated at earlier epochs are more likely to have had more intense treatment that could include craniospinal radiation therapy at higher doses. Deficits in attention, visuospatial and visual motor skills, working memory, and processing speed have been documented.

Neuropsychological Assessment Findings: Specific Domains

- *Intelligence/Achievement* Cognitive dysfunction can be present in adults at presentation; for adults treated with chemotherapy for systemic cancers, overall IQ is generally preserved. In adults with brain tumors, significant decline in cognitive ability can be associated with relapse. Children treated with radiation (higher doses) and chemotherapy at an early age are at risk for decline in IQ with increased time from diagnosis. Loss in IQ can range from 2–4 points per year. Periodic follow-up to monitor intellectual development is critical for children receiving high-intensity multimodality treatment. Analysis of change in raw scores should be examined; it is estimated that children treated with craniospinal radiation therapy, particularly at higher doses, master new knowledge and skills at a reduced rate compared to same-age peers.

- *Attention/Concentration* Attention problems are quite common in adults and children. Treatment (radiation, chemotherapy) is associated with compromised attention, which can secondarily impact memory. Attention issues in childhood cancer survivors tend to be characterized by difficulties in sustaining attention rather than impulsive/hyperactive behaviors. Working memory is a common complaint of individuals during cancer treatment. In children treated for brain tumors, working memory problems emerge and can have a greater impact on functioning over time.

- *Processing Speed* Processing speed deficits are the most common finding across studies of adults and children treated for cancer. In children treated for primary brain tumors, slow processing speed is noted even in surgery-only groups. Processing speed is particularly affected in children treated with cranial radiation therapy. These problems contribute to difficulties keeping up with the pace and volume of material presented in the classroom and the need to devote additional time, energy, and resources to complete cognitive tasks. Adults treated for brain cancer with radiation therapy demonstrate declines in psychomotor speed. Rehabilitation strategies and vocational accommodations can be developed, informed by neuropsychological assessment.

- *Language* Children treated at a very young age can demonstrate language problems but, in general, foundational language skills are preserved, particularly in those diagnosed in later childhood and adolescence. Mild to moderate problems with retrieval may be an issue during cancer treatment and may persist. Adults with cortical brain tumors can present with language deficits/aphasia.

- *Visuospatial* Visuospatial and visual motor skills are often compromised in childhood cancer survivors. Ability to process and organize visuospatial materials can be significantly compromised. Children with *neurofibromatosis type 1* often demonstrate problems with visuospatial reasoning and constructive abilities. Visuospatial abilities may decline after treatment with androgen deprivation therapy in men with prostate cancer.

- *Memory* Memory problems can be more salient in patients treated for tumors in the third ventricle region. More severe learning and memory problems were documented in survivors of childhood leukemia who were treated in earlier decades with more intense treatment and are less commonly seen with current protocols that are more individualized, risk-adapted, and less likely to include cranial radiation. Problems with new learning can be seen in adults treated for brain tumors and other cancers.

- *Executive Functions* Deficits in executive functions can be seen in a range of conditions affecting different domains. Children treated for suprasellar tumors (craniopharyngioma) can develop problems with initiation, self-regulatory capacity, and organizational skills. Executive functions are very vulnerable in adults and children treated for cancer or brain tumors.

- *Sensorimotor Functions* Sensorimotor functions can be affected by neurological deficits associated with brain tumors and their treatment. Many chemotherapies have peripheral neuropathy as a side effect that can persist after treatment. Lymphedema can also impact motor speed. Reduced fine motor speed and output are common. Motor coordination, motor planning, and speed of output are affected in children with posterior fossa tumors, along with balance. Some children change handedness secondary to lateralized brain injury or postsurgical complications. Motor function can be affected by tumor location or neurological complications in adults and children treated for brain tumors.

- *Emotion and Personality* Psychosocial adjustment issues are expected in patients treated for cancer across age groups. Depression and anxiety issues are common. Increased risk of depression and suicidality has been reported in adolescents and young adults treated for brain tumors. In young children, problems adjusting to invasive medical procedures are common, and prompt psychological support and treatment are effective. Children may develop issues with increased dependency and compromised self-efficacy. Problems with regulation of emotion and behavior are seen in young children and are noted during treatment cycles of corticosteroids. Social skills problems are being reported more frequently in children and adolescents treated for brain tumors. Social adjustment, social competence, and integration with peer group are affected. Adult patients should be screened for symptoms of depression, anxiety, and fatigue because these are associated with self-report of cognitive limitations and can exacerbate any late cognitive effects.

- *Performance and Symptom Validity* Issues that can compromise test engagement are important to address. Cancer-related fatigue is a common problem, and persistent fatigue issues are noted in some childhood as well as adult cancer survivors. Nutritional problems and deconditioning during chemotherapy also compromise energy levels and the ability to put forth effort on cognitive tasks. Some adults may have preconceived notions and expectations about the cognitive effects of chemotherapy (misattribution bias), and this may compromise effort and interpretation of findings, especially if the individual is applying for long-term disability.

- *Achievement/Adaptive Functioning* Functional competence in school, work, and home setting is critical to assess for adults and children. Problems with mathematics are commonly seen in children treated for brain tumors or leukemia; these are also common in children with *neurofibromatosis type 1*. Speed and automaticity of academic skills need to be assessed due to slow processing speed. Early language and reading difficulties can be seen in children treated with intensive therapy at a young age. In children and adolescents treated for brain tumors, cognitive ability may be in the normal range, but adaptive skills can be seriously compromised. Assessment of functional and daily living skills is important in adults as well, particularly in patients with frontal tumors.

Interventions for Neuropsychological Late Effects of Cancer and Its Treatment

A range of interventions to address neuropsychological dysfunction are currently under study and many have demonstrated positive results. These include:

- Physical activity and exercise programs
- Cognitive training/rehabilitation programs targeting attention, speed or processing, working memory, and/or metacognitive strategies

Efforts to improve cognitive function in cancer survivors require further study and it will be important to determine which programs can be more effective for specific types of issues and when to intervene.

Considerations When Treating Select Populations with Cancer

Adults/Geriatric Considerations

Older patients treated for cancer are more vulnerable to cognitive dysfunction related to prior health problems and limited stamina. Radiation therapy in the older adult can be more toxic due to age-related decline in normal cell repair functions. Stress and anxiety related to complex treatment regimens, symptoms, and complications compromise integrity of cognitive function. In adults with metastatic brain tumors, treatments can be invasive and debilitating, exacerbating the effects of progressive disease. Careful attention to end-of-life issues and the patient's decision-making capacity is also important. Survivors may require work accommodations, reduced job responsibilities or a career change. Neuropsychologists need to consider carefully the timing and goals of an assessment, limiting the evaluation to answering referral questions and contributing to optimal adaptation of the patient and family.

Pediatric Considerations

Childhood cancer survivors are vulnerable to delayed effects of their disease and treatment. Late effects emerge as children face changing contextual demands and developmental challenges. Family system functioning and access to resources are critical variables related to the ability of the child to meet these challenges. In general, increased demands over the course of development for effective metacognitive skills and enhanced efficiency/speed of performance can overwhelm the compensatory capacity of many children treated for cancer. Consequently, eliminating supports if the child is adapting well needs to be carefully considered, particularly at times of transition to middle or high school.

- *School Re-entry* Both children and parents have unique concerns about school re-entry. Children can receive home tutoring during extended absences from school. Reintegration into the school environment needs to be carefully considered. Some children dealing with fatigue and complications may require a shorter school day at first. Many childhood cancer centers have specific programs to facilitate return to school after cancer treatment. Psychoeducation about cancer and treatment can help teachers and nurses understand the child's needs and reduce misconceptions. Academic accommodations may need to be made to facilitate the child's adaptation (reduced school day, compressed assignments, opportunities for rest, etc.).

- *Transition to Adulthood* This is a critical stage in the development of the young adult treated for childhood cancer. Social competence and integration can be undermined due to cancer and its late effects, so support for social development is important. Childhood cancer survivors have ongoing healthcare needs, and careful preparation for managing the transition to adult healthcare services needs to take place beginning in early adolescence. Preparation for transition needs to be gradual, risk-adapted, and individualized. The neuropsychologist can play an important role in multidisciplinary care, providing education and guidance about the impact of neuropsychological, psychological, and adaptive dysfunction on transition needs.

- *Guardianship/Supervision* A subgroup of young adults treated for childhood brain tumors have significant cognitive and adaptive function impairments and will continue to require supervision and support into adulthood. They may not be able to make sound decisions, exert appropriate judgment, or care for themselves to function independently. Families need counseling and guidance about these issues and appropriate planning for when adolescents turn 18 years of age. In addition, remaining in public school programs until age 22 years allows students to receive specialized programming and support toward developing optimal independence. Mental status and competence needs to be monitored carefully in adults with malignant brain tumors. Decision-making capacity can be compromised in the context of frontal lobe tumors and in patients with advanced disease.

Relevant Definitions

Endoscopic third ventriculostomy (ETV) Endoscopic third ventriculostomy is an alternative procedure to shunt placement to treat hydrocephalus. It involves using an endoscope and making a small perforation in the floor of the third ventricle, which allows CSF to flow out of the blocked ventricular system. (See also Chapter 20, Congenital and Acquired Hydrocephalus.)

Glioblastoma multiforme An aggressive glioma; its incidence increases over the course of middle age and older adulthood. It is called multiforme because it is composed of a heterogeneous mixture of neoplastic astrocytes.

Increased intracranial pressure Increased ICP is a rise in the pressure inside the skull; it can be caused by a rise in CSF pressure due to blockage of CSF flow or by increased pressure within the brain caused by a mass lesion, edema, or bleed. (See also Chapter 20, Congenital and Acquired Hydrocephalus, and Chapter 29, Traumatic Brain Injury.)

Intrathecal chemotherapy Intrathecal chemotherapy delivers therapeutic agents directly into the CSF surrounding the brain and spinal cord. This method of delivery is used to circumvent the blood-brain barrier and is administered via lumbar puncture.

Leukoencephalopathy Cerebral white matter injury that can be caused by radiation and/or chemotherapy.

Methotrexate An antineoplastic agent classified as an antimetabolite. It is a folic acid antagonist and causes folic acid deficiency in cancer cells, resulting in cancer cell death.

Neurofibromatosis type 1 (NF-1) An autosomal dominant genetic disorder and one of the most common inherited tumor predisposition syndromes. Individuals with NF-1 have a higher risk of developing brain tumors, particularly optic glioma. (See also Chapter 18, Chromosomal and Genetic Syndromes.)

Paraneoplastic syndrome or paraneoplastic neurological disorders Neurological complications of systemic cancer caused by immune reaction to antigens expressed by tumors and common to the nervous system; associated with several different antineural antibodies.

Vasculopathy A general term used to describe any disease affecting blood vessels and includes vascular abnormalities caused by a number of conditions and disorders (e.g., degenerative, metabolic and inflammatory conditions, embolic diseases, coagulative disorders).

Cancers Questions

NOTE: *Questions 15, 50, 61, and 82 on the First Full-Length Practice Examination, Questions 48, 86, and 124 on the Second Full-Length Practice Examination, Questions 35, 60, and 78 on the Third Full-Length Practice Examination, and Questions 18, 33, 76, and 118 on the Fourth Full-Length Practice Examination are from this chapter.*

1. Brain metastases occur most commonly in which region of the brain?

   (a) cerebellum

   (b) brainstem

   (c) cerebral hemispheres

   (d) meninges

2. Meningiomas are most common in _____.

   (a) adult females

   (b) children under six years of age

   (c) adolescents

   (d) adult males

3. A patient presents upon referral from a neuro-oncologist with memory problems status–post treatment for a glioblastoma multiforme. The patient is with her spouse and healthcare proxy and asks you what her prognosis is with respect to her survival time. You see in the note from the physician that this was discussed in the last appointment with the spouse and the note was shared with the patient. How should you proceed?

   (a) Read from the note what was discussed.

   (b) Tell the patient that this is best discussed with her physician.

   (c) State that the prognosis is variable from patient to patient.

   (d) Provide statistics on the survival rates.

4. Which of the following differences is most likely to account for the disparities in the higher mortality rates in African American versus Caucasian patients with cancer (breast, lung, colorectal)?

   (a) tumor biology

   (b) religious beliefs

   (c) tumor stage at presentation

   (d) access to optimal treatment

5. Children with NF-1 are at increased risk of which type of brain tumor?

   (a) embryonal tumors   (c) meningioma

   (b) optic glioma   (d) craniopharyngioma

6. Survival rates for an adult with a brain tumor are worse for which type of pathology?

   (a) pilocytic astrocytoma   (c) glioblastoma

   (b) oligodendroglioma   (d) meningioma with high MIB-1 Index

7. A patient has undergone allogeneic bone marrow transplantation for leukemia. Which of the following is a risk factor for cognitive impairment?

   (a) older age

   (b) absence of graft versus host disease

   (c) prolonged hospitalization

   (d) intensive chemotherapy or total-body irradiation

8. A neuropsychological evaluation of a young adult treated for acute lymphoblastic leukemia in early childhood with chemotherapy would most likely find ____.

   (a) general cognitive abilities in the average range

   (b) general cognitive abilities in the significantly below average range

   (c) evidence of speech articulation problems

   (d) evidence of combined surface dyslexia and deep dyslexia

9. Radiation therapy affects the developing brain by primarily causing ____.

   (a) hydrocephalus

   (b) compromise of white matter

   (c) cranial nerve dysfunction

   (d) hypoxic-ischemic injury in subcortical structures

10. The most common causes of structural damage to the frontal lobes are ____.

    (a) HIV encephalopathy, vascular disorders, Korsakoff's syndrome

    (b) vascular disorders, brain tumors, and traumatic injury

    (c) traumatic injury, encephalitis, brain tumors

    (d) vascular disorders, epilepsy, herpes encephalitis

Cancers Answers

1. **C—cerebral hemispheres** *Eighty percent of brain metastases occur in the cerebral hemispheres; common location is at the gray–white matter junction, where the vasculature changes in caliber and traps tumor emboli.*

   Reference: Quattrocchi, C. C., Errante, Y., Mallio, C. A., & Zobel, B. B. (2014). Non-uniform distribution of metastatic intracranial tumors in cancer patients. In M. Hayat (Ed.), *Brain metastases from primary tumors* (Vol. 1, pp. 37–51). Amsterdam, NL: Elsevier.

2. **A—adult females** *Meningiomas are twice as common in females and most common in females in their 60s to 70s.*

References:
(a) CBTRUS (2012, March 23). *CBTRUS statistical report: Primary brain and central nervous system tumors diagnosed in the United States in 2004–2008.* Retrieved from www.cbtrus.org
(b) Saraf, S., McCarthy, B. J., & Willano, J. L. (2011). Update on meningiomas. *The Oncologist, 16*(11), 1604–1613.

3. **B—Tell the patient that this is best discussed with her physician.** *While a clinical neuropsychologist likely has this information, and it is in the notes, this is best addressed with the treating physician. It may be tempting to provide the patient with some information, such as answer c. However, the discussion might evolve into more questions from the patient regarding medical treatment. Your role is to assess the cognitive issues and provide support/psychoeducation regarding any cognitive/behavioral changes and impact on quality of life, and ways/strategies to help the patient and family cope.*

General Principles and Ethical Standards: 2.01

Reference: American Psychological Association. (2017). *Ethical principles of psychologists and code of conduct.* Washington, DC: American Psychological Association.

4. **D—access to optimal treatment** *Research has documented disparities between individuals of African American and Caucasian descent with respect to mortality rates and treatment options. While there can be differences in tumor biology and stages at presentation, the limited treatment options appear to be a primary driver. These include access to specialized surgeons and underuse of evidence-based therapy.*

Reference: Esnaola, N. F., & Ford, M. E. (2012). Racial differences and disparities in cancer care and outcomes: Where's the rub? *Surgical Oncology Clinics of North America, 21*(3), 417–437, viii.

5. **B—optic glioma** *Children with NF-1 are at risk of developing brain tumors; optic glioma is the most common, representing 65–75% to tumors in children with NF-1.*

Reference: Khatua, S., Gutmann, D. H., & Packer, R. J. (2018). Neurofibromatosis type 1 and optic pathway glioma: Molecular interplay and therapeutic insights. *Pediatric Blood Cancer, 65*(3).

6. **C—glioblastoma** *Pilocytic astrocytomas have better survival rates. For oligodendrogliomas the survival rate is 55–93% with children conferring better survival rates. Most meningiomas (90%) are considered "benign" brain tumors; individuals with high MIB Index are considered at higher risk for recurrence though survival rates tend to be better.*

Reference: Ostrom, Q. T., Gittleman, H., Liao, P., Vecchione-Koval, T., Wolinsky, Y., Kruchko, C., & Barnholtz-Sloan, J. S. (2017). CBTRUS statistical report: Primary brain and other central nervous system tumors diagnosed in the United States in 2010–2014. *Neuro-Oncology, 19*(Suppl 5), v1–v88.

7. **D—intensive chemotherapy or total-body irradiation** *Younger age, intensive pre-treatment conditioning for bone marrow transplantation, and chronic graft versus host disease have been shown to be risk factors of neurocognitive dysfunction. Prolonged hospitalization has not been associated with neurocognitive impairment in the bone marrow transplantation population.*

Reference: Buchbinder, D., Kelly, D. L., Duarte, R. F., Auletta, J. J., Bhatt, N., Byrne, M., . . . Shaw, B. E. (2018). Neurocognitive dysfunction in hematopoietic cell transplant recipients: Expert review from the late effects and quality of life working committee of the CIBMTR and complications and quality of life working party of the EBMT. *Bone Marrow Transplant, 53*(5), 535–555.

8. **A—general cognitive abilities in the average range** *Mean IQ in children treated for leukemia with chemotherapy alone tends to be in the average range. These children tend to show more subtle cognitive issues, particularly problems with attention, processing speed, and mathematics.*

References:
(a) Janzen, L. A., & Spiegler, B. J. (2008). Neurodevelopmental sequelae of pediatric acute lymphoblastic leukemia and its treatment. *Developmental Disabilities Research Reviews, 14*(3), 185–195.
(b) Van Der Plas, E., Erdman, L., Nieman, B. J., Weksberg, R., Butcher, D. T., O'Connor D, L., . . . Spiegler, B. J. (2018). Characterizing neurocognitive late effects in childhood leukemia survivors using a combination of neuropsychological and cognitive neuroscience measures. *Child Neuropsychology, 24*(8), 999–1014.

9. **B—compromise of white matter** *Radiation induced damage to oligodendrocyte precursor cells is one of the mechanisms of CNS toxicity related to radiation. Damage to oligodendrocytes and precursors leads to demyelination and reduced normal appearing white matter.*

References:
(a) Brinkman, T. M., Reddick, W. E., Luxton, J., Glass, J. O., Sabin, N. D., Srivastava, D. K., . . . Krull, K. R. (2012). Cerebral white matter integrity and executive function in adult survivors of childhood medulloblastoma. *Neuro-oncology, 14*(Suppl. 4), iv25–iv36.
(b) King, T. Z., Wang, L., & Mao, H. (2015). Disruption of white matter integrity in adult survivors of childhood brain tumors: Correlates with long-term intellectual outcomes. *PLoS One, 10*(7), e0131744.

10. **B—vascular disorders, brain tumors, and traumatic injury** *Stroke and TBI commonly affect the frontal lobes. Additionally, 9% of primary brain tumors occur in the frontal lobes of the brain; 25% of primary malignant gliomas occur in the frontal lobes.*

References:
(a) CBTRUS. (2012). CBTRUS statistical report: Primary brain and central nervous system tumors diagnosed in the United States in 2004–2008 (March 23, 2012 revision). www.cbtrus.org
(b) Zada, G., Bond, A. E., Wang, Y. P., Giannotta, S. L., & Deapen, D. (2012). Incidence trends in the anatomic location of primary malignant brain tumors in the United States: 1992–2006. *World Neurosurgery, 77*(3–4), 518–524.

Recommended Readings

Buchbinder, D., Kelly, D. L., Duarte, R. F., Auletta, J. J., Bhatt, N., Byrne, M., . . . Shaw, B. E. (2018). Neurocognitive dysfunction in hematopoietic cell transplant recipients: Expert review from the late effects and quality of life working committee of the CIBMTR and complications and quality of life working party of the EBMT. *Bone Marrow Transplant, 53*(5), 535–555.

Cheung, Y. T., & Krull, K. R. (2015). Neurocognitive outcomes in long-term survivors of childhood acute lymphoblastic leukemia treated on contemporary treatment protocols: A systematic review. *Neuroscience Biobehavioral Review, 53*, 108–120.

Correa, D. D., & Root, J. C. (2018). Cognitive functions in adults with central nervous system and non-central nervous system cancers. In J. E. Morgan & J. H. Ricker (Eds.), *Textbook of clinical neuropsychology* (2nd ed., pp. 560–586). New York, NY: Routledge.

Donders, J., & Hunter, S. (Eds.). (2010). *Principles and practice of lifespan developmental neuropsychology.* Cambridge: Cambridge University Press.

Ferguson, K. E., Iverson, G. L., & Schoenberg, M. R. (2011). Brain tumors. In M. R. Schoenberg & J. G. Scott (Eds.). *The little black book of neuropsychology: A syndrome-based approach* (pp. 787–812). New York, NY: Springer.

Ris, D., & Abbey, R. (2010). Pediatric brain tumors. In K. Yeates, D. Ris, G. T. Taylor, & B. Pennington (Eds.), *Pediatric neuropsychology: Research, theory, and practice* (2nd ed., pp. 92–111). New York, NY: Guilford Press.

26   Stroke

Kathleen Y. Haaland and Keith Owen Yeates

Introduction

Historically, stroke has been an invaluable model to examine brain–behavior relationships, largely because damage can be focal and the patient's brain is in many cases relatively normal prior to stroke. A major purpose of this chapter is to summarize the various neurobehavioral syndromes that are seen with damage to different parts of the cerebral vasculature of the cerebral hemispheres. Therefore, the focus will be on ischemic rather than hemorrhagic stroke, and on large-vessel stroke rather than small-vessel stroke, *lacunar infarcts*, or periventricular white matter ischemic changes. However, the combination of large-vessel stroke and small-vessel ischemic events may interact to increase deficits. In addition, neuropsychologists most frequently consult after the patient with stroke has been medically stabilized, so we also focus on the postacute and chronic stages of stroke. We also highlight special considerations for pediatric populations throughout the chapter.

Definition

Stroke or cerebrovascular accident (CVA) is defined as a sudden onset of impairment in neurologic functioning due to severe decrease of blood supply to the brain. Stroke is caused by *ischemia*, which produces an *infarct* in the brain related to occlusion (thromboembolic), or *hemorrhage* of an artery in the brain. The acute symptoms depend on the location of the injury, duration of the effect (e.g., blood clot dissolves, collateral circulation compensation), associated physiological changes such as edema, more general changes in blood flow, and finally which blood vessel and therefore parts of the brain are damaged. Transient ischemic attack (TIA) has been redefined by neurovascular experts to decrease the probability of labeling mild strokes as TIAs. TIAs are brief episodes (most commonly < 1 hour but up to 24 hours in duration) of neurologic dysfunction resulting from focal cerebral *ischemia*. However, recent changes in the definition focus on the lack of evidence of permanent cerebral infarction based on neuroimaging rather than symptom duration. TIAs are considered to be a warning sign that a future stroke may be imminent since strokes are more common after TIAs, and thus typically prompt further workup to address the underlying problem (e.g., atrial fibrillation, carotid artery stenosis). In general, the chronic or persistent symptoms of a stroke depend on location and size of the stroke, as well as on age, hand preference, presence of previous stroke(s), time post stroke, and associated medical factors.

In children, the term "perinatal stroke" typically refers to strokes occurring between approximately 20 weeks gestation and the first 28 days of life. Presumed perinatal stroke refers to lesions that appear similar to those occurring during that period but that are not detected until later in life. Childhood stroke refers to strokes occurring after 1 month of life through age 18 years. Intraventricular *hemorrhages* in premature infants, and subdural and epidural *hemorrhages* arising from trauma, are typically excluded from definitions of pediatric stroke.

Neuropathology

Ischemic Stroke

As Table 26.1 shows, ischemic or thromboembolic stroke is most common in adults (about 88% of all stroke) and produces neuronal damage related to decreased cerebral blood flow due to an obstruction (e.g., plaque, blood clot), which can originate at the site of the occlusion (thrombus) or at a distance from the occlusion (embolus). The anterior circulation (anterior cerebral, middle cerebral, or anterior choroidal arteries) is affected most frequently, in about 80% of the cases, whereas the vertebrobasilar or posterior circulation, including the posterior cerebral artery, is affected in about 20% of cases. Importantly, the middle cerebral artery (MCA) territory encompasses about 50–60% of the brain. The damage or *infarct* is caused by inadequate blood supply to a particular part of the brain.

TABLE 26.1 Adult Stroke Etiologies

Thromboembolic Ischemic Stroke (88%)	
Direct/Primary	Embolic Thrombotic Vasospasm
Potential Mechanisms	Atherosclerosis Hypertension Atrial fibrillation Other (vasculitis, coagulopathy)
Hemorrhagic Stroke (12%)	
Direct/Primary	Intracerebral hemorrhage Subarachnoid hemorrhage
Potential Mechanisms	Hypertensive hemorrhage (50%) Amyloid angiopathy hemorrhage (15%) Aneurysm (30%) Arteriovenous malformation (3%) Other (anticoagulants, cocaine; 2%)

Hemorrhagic Stroke

Hemorrhagic stroke is much less common than ischemic stroke among adults (12% of all strokes, with 9% intracerebral *hemorrhages* and 3% subarachnoid *hemorrhages*) and is associated with higher mortality, especially for subarachnoid hemorrhage, which has a mortality of 50% in the first 6 months after stroke. Intracerebral *hemorrhages* are most frequently localized deep in the brain because they primarily affect small penetrating arteries, and they can begin as slow leaks so symptom onset may be more gradual than sudden. Etiology, especially for these deep intracerebral *hemorrhages*, is most commonly hypertension (50%). The two most common reasons for stroke in younger adults are aneurysm or arteriovenous malformation (AVM), which together account for about 33% of all *hemorrhages* (see Table 26.1). Aneurysm of the anterior communicating artery is the most common cause of subarachnoid *hemorrhage*.

Childhood Stroke

In contrast to adults, ischemic and hemorrhagic stroke are about equally common in children. The two major forms of infarction in children are arterial ischemic stroke (AIS) and cerebral sinovenous thrombosis (CSVT). AIS is far more common than CSVT. CSVT is more common in neonates than in older children.

The MCA territory is the most common location of AIS in children, and subcortical infarction (thalamus or basal ganglia) is also common. As in adults, ischemic stroke in the posterior circulation is less common in children than stroke in the anterior circulation.

Primary Injury

Decreased neuronal functioning after stroke is a result of both intracellular and extracellular damage. In the case of *ischemia*, lack of oxygen and nutrients can produce neuronal damage within 6 to 8 minutes if blood flow is below critical levels. Many metabolic changes occur in the intracellular space (e.g., elevated lactate levels, acidosis) and may result in cell death. Microscopic changes are not seen until about 6 hours after stroke, when swelling occurs. Glial proliferation begins about day 2, when there is new vascularization to supply the damaged region. Over months, the damaged tissue is resorbed and a cavity lined with glial cells can be seen. Typically, a center zone of ischemic damage or *infarct* does not recover, and a surrounding ischemic penumbra contains neurons that may recover if blood flow is restored within 6 hours (e.g., through collateral circulation, anticoagulant therapy) although there is general agreement that treatment efficacy increases with earlier treatment.

In adults, tissue plasminogen activator (tPA) has been shown to dissolve the occlusive clot and increase the probability of restoring blood flow to the surrounding ischemic penumbra. However, its use is limited by the need to provide such treatment within 3 to 4.5 hours of symptom onset. The use of tPA in children remains controversial because of the lack of a strong evidence base; the largest randomized controlled trial of tPA in pediatric AIS was stopped because of insufficient recruitment.

Secondary Injury

Secondary injury occurs directly or indirectly from a series of events that occur after brain tissue is injured or from the consequences of extracerebral events. Secondary injury can be gradual or accelerate quickly if not properly managed. For example, *brain herniation* and death can occur if intracranial pressure (ICP) is not managed properly following hemorrhagic stroke. Control or minimization of secondary injury is the focus of acute stabilization and intensive care unit (ICU) management.

Examples of secondary injury after ischemic stroke include vasospasm, which may result in additional infarction; enhanced collateral circulation, which can result in hemorrhagic transformation of an *infarct* due to bleeding into the *infarct* and additional cell death; swelling/edema resulting in deterioration due to mass effect (pressure on areas of the brain not directly involved in the stroke); and decreased blood flow in distant regions. Hemorrhagic stroke may be associated with increased ICP and, in the worst case, herniation of the brainstem through the tentorium, which is most often life threatening. Treatments to reduce pressure increase the potential for deterioration due to anesthesia and surgical side effects, as well as increased potential for infection. Other secondary problems include seizures.

Risk Factors

Many risk factors for stroke co-occur and interact to further increase risk largely due to their impact on vascular health (e.g., vascular narrowing due to atherosclerosis, deteriorated vessel wall due to hypertension, emboli of infarcted heart tissue). However, as noted in Table 26.1, although hypertension is an important risk for both ischemic and hemorrhagic stroke in adults, vascular abnormalities, such as AVM or aneurysm, are also important risk factors for hemorrhagic stroke. Some common risk factors for adult stroke:

- *Age* Relative risk doubles every decade after 55 years.
- *Hypertension* Three to six times the risk of age-matched sample.
- *Atrial Fibrillation* If untreated, three to five times the risk; on Warfarin, 1.5 times the risk.
- *Family History* Three times the risk if parent with ischemic stroke.

- *Prior TIA* Four times the risk of age-matched sample.

- *Cocaine* Two to five times the risk of age-matched sample.

- *Diabetes* Two to four times risk of age-matched sample.

- *Smoking* Current, two to four times the risk relative to nonsmokers or those who quit >10 years ago.

- *Sleep Apnea* Two times the risk of age-matched sample.

- *Serum Lipid Abnormalities* About 1.5 times risk of age-matched sample.

- *Obesity* Two times risk of age-matched sample.

The risk factors for stroke in childhood are quite different from those in adulthood:

- *Perinatal Ischemic Stroke* Common risk factors include maternal infertility, preeclampsia, prolonged rupture of membranes, chorioamnionitis, and prothrombotic states or thrombophilia. Congenital heart disease and bacterial meningitis are other risk factors for perinatal AIS. Infections are the primary cause of perinatal CSVT.

- *Childhood Ischemic Stroke* Common risk factors include cardiac disease, cerebral arteriopathies (including sickle cell disease), and infection.

- *Hemorrhagic Stroke* Trauma is the most common cause of intracranial *hemorrhage* in children. Nontraumatic hemorrhagic stroke in children is usually associated with intracranial vascular anomalies, such as AVMs, or medical disorders, such as brain tumors.

- A significant minority of children with strokes do not have any identifiable risk factors.

Epidemiology

Worldwide, stroke is the fourth leading cause of death after heart disease, cancer, and chronic lower respiratory disease when considered separately from other cardiovascular diseases (National Center for Health Statistics), and it is the leading cause of disability in the United States (Go et al., 2014).

- 795,000 new or recurrent strokes per year in the United States at a cost of $36.5 billion in 2010.

- There was a 35.8% decrease in mortality due to stroke from 2000 to 2010 due to improved early detection and better acute medical care as well as better long term management of risk factors, including hypertension, diabetes, and smoking.

- Stroke prevalence is predicted to increase by 23% by 2030 in the United States primarily due to an aging population.

- 26% of stroke survivors over age 64 are institutionalized, and 32% of those who return home use home healthcare services.

- Strokes are more common with increasing age, especially for females whose stroke incidence is greater than males only later in life.

- One-month fatality rate (1989–2000) over age 65 is 12.6% for all strokes (8.1% ischemic, 44.6% *hemorrhage*).

- Blacks have higher stroke incidence, morbidity, and mortality than whites, even after excluding for sickle cell disease in adults and children.

- Stroke is one of the top ten causes of death in childhood in the United States. Estimates of the annual incidence of childhood stroke (ischemic and hemorrhagic) range from 1.3 to 13.0 per 100,000 children. The incidence of perinatal stroke is closer to 1 per 5,000 live births.

- The incidence of childhood stroke is higher in boys than in girls, a difference that is not fully accounted for by trauma.

- Mortality rates for childhood stroke have decreased substantially during the past several decades but are still approximately 10% for ischemic stroke and around 25–35% for hemorrhagic stroke.

- Upward of 70% of survivors of childhood stroke have seizures or other neurological deficits. The occurrence of post-stroke epilepsy is associated with poorer outcomes after childhood stroke.

- Recurrence rates for childhood stroke (ischemic and hemorrhagic) are about 10–25%. Recurrence rates are much lower for perinatal stroke.

Determinants of Severity

The diagnosis of stroke severity is primarily based on parameters in the acute medical and postacute rehabilitation hospital record, as well as on demographic factors such as age and handedness. A variety of factors influence stroke severity: age of the patient, size and location of *infarct* or *hemorrhage*; acute treatment (e.g., tPA, neurosurgical intervention); medical comorbidities (e.g., previous stroke); secondary medical events, such as recurrent stroke, coma and its duration, infection, and whether surgery was necessary; and the success with which cardiovascular risk factors are treated to decrease the probability of recurrent stroke or cardiac events.

Presentation, Disease Course, and Recovery

Acute Hospitalization

Presentation

Physical symptoms, especially those that are life-threatening, are the initial focus after stroke. For example, *hemorrhage* is often associated with headache and, if extensive, with symptoms of nausea and vomiting that may reflect high ICP. Both ischemic and hemorrhagic stroke are commonly associated with poorly controlled hypertension and loss of or altered consciousness. Loss of consciousness or coma is more common after hemorrhagic stroke. Once such symptoms are under control, neurobehavioral symptoms, such as hemiparesis, hemianesthesia, aphasia, hemispatial inattention or neglect, and visuospatial deficits, are assessed. Table 26.2 summarizes the various syndromes associated with ischemic stroke and hemorrhagic stroke in particular artery distributions. Advances in anatomical and functional neuroimaging have led to increased controversy regarding the relationship between these syndromes and particular lesion loci. This change is largely related to an emphasis on the notion that complex behaviors are more often associated with damage to neural circuits rather than specific cortical loci. Regardless, these syndromes are usually more characteristic of adults than children.

- Given the higher frequency of anterior circulation strokes, those syndromes are most common and may include hemiparesis, hemianesthesia, aphasia, and visuospatial deficits, as well as visual field cuts if the visual pathway is affected. Visuospatial deficits are less commonly noticed by patients.

- Although hemiparesis is more common after involvement of the superior branch of the MCA, visual field cuts are more common with involvement of the inferior branch of the MCA as well as damage in the posterior cerebral artery (PCA) distribution that includes primary visual cortex.

TABLE 26.2 Major Clinical Syndromes of the Middle, Anterior, and Posterior Cerebral Artery Territories

Location Of Infarct	Affected Territory	Deficits
Left MCA *superior division*		Nonfluent, or Broca's aphasia and right face and arm weakness of the upper motor neuron type, impaired working memory and executive function deficits. In some cases there may also be some right face and arm cortical-type sensory loss. Visual field cut is usually absent. Limb apraxia may be seen in the right arm after resolution of paresis, and/or in the left arm.
Left MCA *inferior division*		Fluent, or Wernicke's, aphasia and a right visual field deficit. There may also be right face and arm cortical-type sensory loss, limb apraxia, and parts of Gerstmann's syndrome (agraphia, acalculia due to conceptual difficulty, right-left disorientation, finger agnosia). Motor findings are usually absent but mild right-sided weakness may be present, especially at onset.
Left MCA *deep territory*		Right pure motor hemiparesis of the upper motor neuron type. Larger infarcts may produce "cortical" deficits, such as aphasia as well, emphasizing the importance of larger circuits.
Left MCA *stem*		Combination of the above, with right hemiplegia, right hemianesthesia, right homonymous hemianopia, and global aphasia. There is often a left gaze preference, especially at the onset, caused by damage to left hemisphere cortical areas important for moving the eyes to the right.
Right MCA *superior division*		Left face and arm weakness of the upper motor neuron type, impaired working memory and executive functions. Left hemineglect is present to a variable extent. In some cases there may also be some left face and arm cortical-type sensory loss.
Right MCA *inferior division*		Profound left hemineglect. Left visual field and somatosensory deficits are often present; however, these may be difficult to test convincingly because of the neglect. Motor neglect with decreased voluntary or spontaneous initiation of movements on the left side can also occur. However, even patients with left motor neglect usually have normal strength on the left side, as evidenced by occasional spontaneous movements or purposeful withdrawal from pain. Some mild, left-sided weakness and right gaze preference may be present especially at stroke onset. There may also be anosognosia and visuospatial deficits characterized by impaired visuospatial skills (e.g., impaired figure drawing, 3-D construction, and dressing), and writing, reading and arithmetic problems due to neglect and spatial difficulties (e.g., misperceptions such as '6' for '9'). Patients may initially seem confused.

TABLE 26.2 Continued

Location Of Infarct	Affected Territory	Deficits
Right MCA *deep territory*	L / R brain section	Left pure motor hemiparesis of the upper motor neuron type. Larger infarcts may produce "cortical" deficits, such as left hemineglect and visuospatial deficits as well, emphasizing the importance of larger circuits.
Right MCA *stem*	L / R brain section	Combination of the above, with left hemiplegia, left hemianesthesia, left homonymous hemianopia, profound left hemineglect, visuospatial deficits, and anosognosia. There is usually a right gaze preference, especially at the onset, caused by damage to right hemisphere cortical areas important for moving the eyes to the left.
Left ACA	L / R brain section	Right leg weakness of the upper motor neuron type and right leg cortical-type sensory loss. Grasp reflex, executive function deficits, and transcortical motor aphasia can also be seen. Larger infarcts may cause right hemiplegia.
Right ACA	L / R brain section	Left leg weakness of the upper motor neuron type and left leg cortical-type sensory loss. Grasp reflex, executive function deficits, and left hemineglect can also be seen. Larger infarcts may cause left hemiplegia.
Left PCA	L / R brain section	Right homonymous hemianopia. Extension to the splenium of the corpus callosum can cause alexia without agraphia. Larger infarcts, including the thalamus and internal capsule, may cause transcortical sensory aphasia, right hemisensory loss, and right hemiparesis. Memory deficits (especially verbal) may be present if the lesion extends to the left medial temporal lobe, especially the hippocampus.
Right PCA	L / R brain section	Left homonymous hemianopia. Larger infarcts including the thalamus and internal capsule may cause left hemisensory loss and left hemiparesis. Memory deficits (especially spatial) may be present if lesion extends to the right medial temporal lobe, especially the hippocampus.

NOTE: Permission from Blumenfeld, H. (2010). *Neuroanatomy through clinical cases* (2nd ed.). Sunderland, MA: Sinauer Associates.

Seizures are the most common presentation of AIS in childhood. Other common presenting features include hemiparesis, altered mental status, and focal neurological signs. Stroke in the posterior circulation can present as ataxia, vertigo, or vomiting. Motor deficits are usually most apparent acutely, although the gradual appearance of signs of hemiparesis during later infancy is sometimes associated with a presumed earlier perinatal stroke. The progressive onset of symptoms can suggest an underlying arteriopathy. Large- and medium-sized vessel arteriopathy usually presents with acute neurological deficits and syndromes consistent with the occlusion of specific arteries. Small-vessel disease occurs less commonly in children and is more likely to present with a neurological deficit of gradual and variable onset.

Hemorrhagic strokes in infants and young children can present with very nonspecific features, such as altered mental status or convulsions. Focal neurological signs are less common. In older children, more specific clinical features usually raise concern about an underlying brain disorder, and may include sudden, severe headache and focal neurological signs. Hemorrhagic stroke in children usually involves the abrupt onset of several clinical signs followed by progressive neurological deterioration.

Recovery Course

Acute recovery is variable, depending on stroke severity; associated medical or neurologic problems, which require close monitoring; and any comorbid medical conditions, which can complicate recovery. These problems include dysphagia (swallowing difficulty), which may necessitate the insertion of a nasogastric tube or gastrostomy (i.e., feeding tube); incontinence, which may require catheterization and increases infection risk; mechanical ventilation, which is a risk for pneumonia; cardiac or metabolic abnormalities (e.g., arrhythmias or poorly controlled hypertension or diabetes); or deep vein thrombosis, especially in the paretic limb. Outcome after subarachnoid *hemorrhage*, even in the 50% of adults who survive, is guarded; 85% of adults with subarachnoid *hemorrhage* require supervision after discharge, and 6 months after stroke 33% continue to have cognitive impairment with impaired activities of daily living.

Assessment Methods

Laboratory tests on admission after stroke depend on individual characteristics but often include tests for clotting factor and blood sugar levels. Laboratory tests are performed routinely to identify metabolic changes in all types of stroke. For example, hyponatremia can occur after subarachnoid *hemorrhage* due to excessive antidiuretic hormone.

A computed tomography (CT) scan of the head is almost always conducted first to detect evidence of *hemorrhage*. Although the head CT is sensitive to acute intracerebral *hemorrhage*, it is not as sensitive to ischemic damage, especially in the first 24 hours after stroke. This is important because additional imaging is often not done, and the neuropsychologist who may be evaluating the patient in the postacute or chronic stage must be aware that a normal CT during that period is not a good indicator of whether the stroke produced damage. In contrast, although standard magnetic resonance imaging (MRI) can be normal for a few hours after stroke, diffusion-weighted MRI can detect *infarcts* within minutes of symptom onset. In a recent study of admissions to the emergency room for possible stroke (minutes to 8 days after symptom onset), CT and MRI (diffusion weighted and gradient echo) were equally able to identify acute intracerebral *hemorrhage*. They also both showed comparable specificity for ischemic stroke, but MRI sensitivity for ischemic stroke was better than CT (83% versus 26%). Such findings have led to the argument that MRI should be used for diagnosis of acute stroke, but it is not clear if such information would enhance outcome, and the practicalities of cost and rapid availability make routine use of MRI challenging. However, regardless of the imaging modality the size of the *infarct* acutely may be less than its size in the chronic stage. Magnetic resonance imaging is also more sensitive to *lacunar infarcts*, which frequently are clinically "silent" or "covert," but if these lacunae are extensive enough or strategically located, they may produce neurocognitive deficits that would not be predicted by the large-vessel stroke. Thus, this information may be important in making a differential diagnosis of the cause of cognitive deficits and especially their prognosis. See Chapter 31, Vascular Cognitive Impairment, for details regarding subcortical vascular ischemic disease or vascular cognitive impairment.

Other tests performed to identify the etiology of ischemic or hemorrhagic stroke and guide potential treatment include cerebral angiography, noninvasive magnetic resonance arteriography (MRA), or CT arteriography. These techniques can help identify aneurysms and AVMs in the case of *hemorrhage* or vessel narrowing in the neck or head for ischemic stroke. Extracranial Doppler ultrasonography can identify carotid artery narrowing in the neck. Finally, to identify cardioembolic sources of emboli, electrocardiograms can provide evidence of cardiac *ischemia* or arrhythmias, echocardiograms are used to identify thrombi, and cardiac ultrasound can identify stenosis of the cardiac vessels. In children, cranial ultrasound is safe and readily available, but may miss superficial and ischemic lesions. Transcranial Doppler can also be done to monitor vasospasm (see Chapter 6, The Neurologic Examination, Radiologic and Other Diagnostic Studies, for more thorough discussion regarding these techniques).

For adults, the NIH Stroke Scale (NIHSS) is commonly used to assess for symptoms especially when tPA is being considered for use. The scale is a quantitative neurologic exam with a maximum score of 42, which reflects severe impairment. The scale includes clinician ratings (0–4) of visual fields, facial, arm, and leg paralysis, limb ataxia, somatosensory sensation, language, dysarthria, and extinction. In children, the Pediatric Stroke Outcome Measure (PSOM) is a relatively new scale that is based on a structured neurological examination; it assesses impairment in sensorimotor, language, cognitive, and behavioral domains. It has been validated for assessing residual neurological impairment following stroke.

Brief neuropsychological assessments may be indicated during the acute, inpatient hospitalization to establish a baseline against which to track recovery and to assist with treatment and discharge planning. However, assessments are more commonly done in the postacute phase. Neuropsychological bedside exams can be done acutely in patients with more severe impairment for the purposes of providing an opinion regarding the utility of a more detailed evaluation. It is also used to provide recommendations for (1) cognitive rehabilitation, usually in collaboration with the speech and language pathologist or occupational therapist; and (2) management of behavioral problems and psychological issues, especially depression, which is common after adult stroke. Often, the neuropsychologist works with the speech and language pathologist if the patient is aphasic because evaluation of all cognitive domains can be influenced by aphasia, and speech pathologists are often the providers of more global cognitive rehabilitation and may address broad attention problems, hemispatial inattention, and memory deficits. In addition, the caregiver's needs should not be overlooked at this point in terms of expectations, coping strategies, and sensitivity to the possibility of post-stroke depression.

If the patient is alert and oriented, bedside evaluation focuses on level and type of neurocognitive deficits, after obtaining information from medical record regarding neurologic status (especially aphasia, presence of hemiparesis, visual field cut, cranial nerve abnormalities, and hemispatial inattention). If auditory comprehension deficits are significant after a left-hemisphere stroke, the value of formal neuropsychological evaluation may be limited, but the neuropsychologist, in concert with the rehabilitation team, should make this decision. In addition, the neuropsychologist, rehabilitation psychologist, or psychiatrist would ordinarily conduct an evaluation for depression, which is important because depression is present in 20% to 30% of adult patients with stroke and can be treated successfully with antidepressant medications. Regardless, an evaluation should begin with language assessment, which might be done by a speech and language therapist or by the neuropsychologist. If auditory comprehension deficits are not significant, the initial assessment is still usually quite brief because cognitive status often improves significantly over the first 6 months. However, if the patient is only mildly impaired, a more thorough assessment may be conducted.

Treatment

Ischemic Stroke

Any coagulant medications are discontinued and anticoagulant treatment is considered. Intravenous recombinant tPA, a powerful thrombolytic agent, has been shown to dissolve the occlusive clot, increase the probability of restoring blood flow to the surrounding ischemic penumbra, and improve outcome. It.is considered in adult stroke if the treatment can be initiated within three to 4.5 hours of symptom onset, and the patient has measurable deficits on the NIHSS with no evidence of brain *hemorrhage* on neuroimaging. The use of tPA is limited by the need to provide such treatment within 3 hours of symptom onset per FDA guidelines. However, recent data has supported the efficacy of extending the time window from 3 to 4.5 hours with better outcomes if treatment is initiated earlier in that time window. The 3- to 4.5-hour window is what most clinicians follow, but this change has not been approved by the FDA. Less than 6% of adult acute strokes are treated with tPA for a variety of reasons including the difficulty of meeting the time to treat guidelines, which must be preceded by a variety of assessments including imaging to rule out *hemorrhage*. Of the eligible patients who met these criteria, 82% received tPA in 2010. The use of tPA in children remains controversial because of the lack of a strong evidence base; the largest randomized controlled trial of tPA in pediatric AIS was stopped because of insufficient recruitment.

Other therapies, such as intra-arterial administration of thrombolytics or use of clot retrieval mechanical devices, can also be considered. The combined use of endovascular thrombectomy and tPA administration has been suggested as a way to further decrease occlusion in large vessel occlusions where tPA alone is less likely to dissolve the clot. However, well-designed randomized trials are needed. This need is especially acute in children, where the use of devices primarily designed for use with adults increases the risk of complications.

After the patient is medically stable, treatable reasons for the ischemic stroke must be considered. These include cardiovascular risk factors such as hypertension, diabetes, and hypercholesteremia, as well as cardiac abnormalities in the case of cardioembolic stroke, such as atrial fibrillation, myocardial infarction, or valvular disease. Atherosclerosis is particularly important in adults because it is frequently the mechanism of occlusion due to embolism or thrombosis. Carotid arteries are typically examined because in patients with severe stenosis, surgery (i.e., endarterectomy or angioplasty and stent) decreases future risk of stroke. For example, in symptomatic patients with stroke who have greater than 70% stenosis of the carotid artery, 2-year stroke rate decreased from 26% in patients treated medically to 9% in those treated with endarterectomy (North American Symptomatic Carotid Endarterectomy Trial). Angioplasty (temporary insertion and inflation of a tiny balloon to widen an artery) and stent (permanent placement of mesh device in artery to prop the artery open and decrease future narrowing) are recommended when endarterectomy is medically contraindicated.

Hemorrhagic Stroke

Acute medical treatment for hemorrhagic stroke first discontinues any anticoagulant medication. Because hypertension is the most common cause of *hemorrhage* in adults, anti-hypertensive medication is started as early as possible. *Hemorrhage* size, which influences ICP, is monitored (e.g., intracranial monitors, serial CT scan, neurologic status), and treated when necessary. *Hemorrhage* may require more intensive acute care due to its high mortality (50% in the first six months for subarachnoid *hemorrhage*). Treatments to reduce ICP include medications, as well as invasive procedures such as placement of an intraventricular catheter to drain excess fluid or surgical evacuation of the *hemorrhage*. Additional postacute surgical treatment may be necessary if the mechanism of the *hemorrhage* is identified and can be treated. This is frequently the case for aneurysm, which may be clipped at the neck or removed from the circulation by endovascular coil insertion into the aneurysm to cause clotting. Arteriovenous malformations can be treated surgically (direct removal or with precisely focused radiation that destroys the malformation over months) or with endovascular embolization, which entails threading a catheter to the malformation's feeder artery to block its blood flow with a glue-like substance.

Most patients with stroke participate in inpatient rehabilitation followed by outpatient rehabilitation, which may include speech and language therapy, occupational therapy, and physical therapy, as well as neuropsychology and/or rehabilitation psychology consultation.

Childhood Stroke

Approaches to the acute management of childhood stroke are largely based on those developed for adults and have only limited empirical support. Current recommendations include aggressive management of fever, extreme hypertension, seizures, and infection. In some cases, treatment of cerebral edema and increased ICP is needed. Immediate treatment of ischemic stroke with antithrombotic drugs (aspirin, heparin, and Warfarin) is commonly used to prevent recurrent events in the acute setting. The safety and efficacy of tPA for acute stroke in children have not been established.

The primary goal of long-term management of childhood stroke is to prevent recurrence. Because children who are untreated show high rates of recurrence, antithrombotic drugs are often used in children with ischemic stroke. Aspirin has been used for secondary stroke prevention in AIS, despite the absence of controlled trials in children. Chronic blood transfusion reduces the risk of secondary stroke in children with sickle cell disease. Cerebral arteriopathy is often treated with anti-inflammatory and immunosuppressive medications. Successful bone marrow transplantation also can stabilize or improve cerebral arteriopathy, especially in sickle cell disease, and thereby decrease stroke recurrence. Intracranial vascular anomalies increase the risk of recurrence of *hemorrhage* and should be corrected whenever possible. Occlusion of aneurysms should be attempted as early as possible.

Postacute Hospitalization

Presentation

See Table 26.2 for descriptions of various neurobehavioral symptoms after stroke affecting different arterial distributions, which are a focus at this stage of stroke recovery.

Recovery Course

Postacute recovery after stroke is generally agreed to reflect a negatively accelerating curve, such that the greatest degree of recovery occurs soon after stroke. For example, recovery between 1 and 3 months is typically greater than recovery between 4 and 6 months. In addition, the bulk of recovery is complete by 1 year, although significant individual variability can be seen in this pattern. Some evidence indicates that motor skills recover sooner than cognitive skills, though there are very few studies that examine both in the same sample. Regardless, the best predictor of outcome in the motor and cognitive realm is the extent of deficit in each domain immediately after stroke.

The cognitive deficits associated with stroke can complicate recovery, particularly if they influence the patient's ability to report problems accurately and follow instructions. Aphasia after left-hemisphere damage in right-handers and lack of awareness of deficits, as well as attention deficits, which are more frequent after right-hemisphere damage, can negatively influence treatment success.

Depression, which is more common after left frontal damage but can occur regardless of locus of damage, also influences other deficits and is important to assess. Depression peaks in the first 3 to 6 months after stroke, and while evidence suggests that psychotherapy or medication can be effective in managing depression, more studies have demonstrated the positive impact of medication. Poststroke depression is an independent risk factor for morbidity and mortality, and therefore its management is critically important for outcome. Neuropsychologists are often responsible for ensuring that depression is assessed in every patient and recommending treatment if present.

Motor weakness is a common complication of childhood stroke. Weakness is often succeeded by spasticity. Dystonia is another potentially disabling consequence of stroke. Chronic dystonia is most likely to occur following a stroke in the basal ganglia. Dystonia, weakness, and spasticity often occur in the same extremity. Dysphagia also can occur after stroke, as can aphasia and *dysarthria*. Many children with acute aphasia improve over time. The classic aphasia syndromes are less commonly observed in children, though, especially those who sustain strokes early in life.

Assessment Methods

Rehabilitation units commonly use the Functional Independence Measure (FIM), which is a clinician rating scale that assesses motor (13 items) and cognitive (5 items) abilities from dependent (1) to independent (7). Unfortunately, the FIM is poorly correlated with real-world functioning and is subject to examiner drift. It can also be very misleading with regard to degree and type of cognitive impairment, potentially resulting in errors in predicting the impact of cognitive impairment on actual function. More detailed neuropsychological evaluation may be appropriate at this point, or, depending on the patient's deficits and their severity, more complete assessment may be delayed until later.

Treatment

- Inpatient treatment typically consists of physical, occupational, and speech therapies.
- Although comprehensive neuropsychological evaluations are relatively rare at this stage, they are appropriate in some cases. For example, the neuropsychologist is consulted most commonly at this stage for patients who have minimal cognitive impairment, especially for those who want to return to cognitively demanding jobs as soon as possible. Despite the likelihood of continued improvement, the information from an evaluation at this point can be useful in providing education to patient and family, making decisions about outpatient rehabilitation, and working with the patient regarding the decision to return to work quickly. Early evaluation can also be used for tracking recovery after stroke. Finally, depending on the institution, neuropsychologists can also provide recommendations for cognitive rehabilitation, as well as for pharmacologic or behavioral treatment of emotional issues if indicated.

Outpatient Rehabilitation

Recovery Course

Recovery does not imply return to normal function. While significant improvement may occur compared to acute function, performance does not typically return to pre-stroke levels. For example, 70% of stroke survivors report persistent disuse or non-use of their paretic upper limb up to four years after their stroke.

Although many patients do not fully recover, most are independent for many activities of daily living. The mechanisms for recovery of function are not well understood, but several potential mechanisms have been proposed:

- Functional recovery of some neurons surrounding or in the infarcted region, such that neurons that were temporarily malfunctioning return to normal or near-normal functioning.
- Takeover of the infarcted region's functioning by the normal tissue surrounding the *infarct (penumbra)*, by homologous regions in the opposite hemisphere, or by subcortical regions; new synaptic connections are known potentially to develop, such that axons that normally connected to the infarcted region can connect to other areas.

- In addition, compensation strategies can be developed that utilize the functions of intact brain regions to compensate for the functions of the infarcted area. For example, a patient can use more proximal muscles to compensate for dysfunction in distal muscles.

Assessment Methods

- The outpatient neuropsychological assessment should be directed toward obtaining a more thorough assessment across all cognitive domains to inform rehabilitation and facilitate practical recommendations.

- Recommendations for treatment (e.g., for adults: individual or couples psychotherapy to cope with stroke, community resources such as support groups, medication and/or psychotherapy for depression; for children, parent training in behavior management, special education, medication for attention problems) should be based on the integration of neurocognitive and psychosocial aspects of the assessment.

- Depending on the patient's situation, the evaluation may need to include assessment directed toward determining the capacity to live independently and to manage finances and medications independently and to make healthcare decisions (or, for children, to perform in school). These recommendations are based upon direct assessment of these skills as well as a thorough assessment of all cognitive domains, motor skills, and psychosocial status. It should also provide realistic information to patient and family (or, for children, their parents) regarding current status and prognosis. This information is also useful for social workers who are typically involved with discharge planning.

- The pattern of deficits influences disability. For example, hemispatial inattention is particularly important for driving because it increases the risk of inattention to cars or pedestrians. Significant language deficits may also influence the patient's ability to manage personal finances or perform in school.

- Although ability to work is usually less important for adult patients with stroke than for those with other neurologic diagnoses, because they are often retired, stroke is occurring more frequently in younger adults. Neuropsychological evaluation is particularly important in these cases to characterize deficits and provide vocational recommendations if employment is an issue.

- In most cases, long-term definitive prognostic statements are unrealistic unless the stroke occurred at least 6 months and more ideally at least 1 year prior to evaluation because of the likelihood of some continued recovery. Of course, this will vary depending on severity of impairment in the postacute period; if impairment is minimal, then accurate recommendations can be made earlier. Neuropsychological evaluation and recommendations are particularly important for patients who may be able to return to previous high-level activities; for example, work, school, driving, and child care.

Treatment

The outpatient treatment needs of patients vary depending on individual characteristics, such as demographics, as well as on stroke etiology, location, and severity. Rehabilitation is typically interdisciplinary and includes neuropsychologists, physiatrists, occupational, physical, and speech and language therapists, with consultation from psychiatrists and neurologists. The patient's deficits will determine which provider may be most important. For example, for the patient who is aphasic, the speech and language therapist will be most influential, but if that patient also has significant motor deficits, the physical therapist will be important. Cognitive rehabilitation may be provided by neuropsychologists, rehabilitation psychologists, or occupational or speech and language therapists. The neuropsychological evaluation can be very useful in helping focus cognitive rehabilitation on critical areas and determining the degree of impairment in a particular cognitive domain, as well as determining available strengths that could be used to compensate for the deficits. The influence of anosognosia is of particular concern with regard to rehabilitation. A general lack of awareness of deficits has been elegantly demonstrated after traumatic brain injury but has been less methodically studied after stroke. Although general lack of awareness is quite common after anterior communicating aneurysm rupture associated with damage to the frontal lobe and its connections and in patients with hemispatial inattention associated with right parietal damage, patients with Wernicke's aphasia may also demonstrate lack of awareness specific to their comprehension deficits but not to any other deficits. Therefore, the mechanism of the lack of awareness reflects their inability to comprehend what they are saying, just as they have difficulty understanding what others say. Even though their lack of awareness is specific, it can influence aphasia rehabilitation. Finally, emotional status cannot be ignored, given the high incidence of depression after adult stroke, as well as significant changes in lifestyle with increased social isolation that can occur following adult or childhood stroke. In addition, clinicians often comment on the higher incidence of frustration and depression often seen in patients with Broca's aphasia relative to those with Wernicke's aphasia. Although this difference may be related to the higher incidence of depression after left frontal damage, clinicians also note that patients with Broca's aphasia have relatively intact comprehension, which means they are more likely to know when their verbal communication is poor. In contrast, patients with Wernicke's aphasia are less aware of their communication problems due to their comprehension deficits.

Despite the accepted practice of aphasia therapy for adults after stroke, empirical findings using randomized controlled trials have been variable, even when summarized in meta-analyses, given the large number of factors that influence therapeutic efficacy. Recent studies using theoretically motivated treatments have demonstrated somewhat promising results, but these findings are very preliminary, given their small sample sizes and lack of randomization.

Relatively little empirical evidence is available regarding rehabilitation specific to childhood stroke. Nevertheless, rehabilitation should start as soon as a child can tolerate therapies, to preserve mobility and strength and also to address cognitive and behavioral issues. Constraint-based therapies have generated considerable interest for treatment of motor deficits in children with stroke and hemiplegia, as well as for adults, and recently have been paired with non-invasive brain stimulation technologies to induce motor learning. However, these methods require further study to determine the optimal dosing and timing of intervention.

Expectations for Neuropsychological Assessment Results

As Table 26.2 shows, the pattern of neuropsychological deficits demonstrated after adult stroke varies significantly, largely as a function of the location of the damage, which is directly related to the part of the vascular bed involved. Table 26.2 summarizes the motor, sensory, and cognitive deficits that can be seen with involvement of the MCA, anterior cerebral artery (ACA), and PCA. However, in many cases, only certain branches of a particular vascular territory are involved, and the entire spectrum of deficits listed in the table is not present. The table is a reminder of what types of cognitive abilities should be examined to obtain a complete picture of the patient's deficits and abilities. Please see Chapter 5, Domains of Neuropsychological Function and Related Neurobehavioral Disorders, for a summary of the characteristics of the associated classic aphasia syndromes. The neuropsychologist, potentially in collaboration with the neurologist, must assess for the deficits listed in Table 26.2 for strokes affecting different parts of the vascular system. However, neuroimaging in combination with cognitive evaluation has shown that complex cognitive skills are more typically associated with damage to broader neural circuits rather than specific cortical regions alone. Therefore, a comprehensive assessment to determine the patient's deficits is important, usually with a somewhat greater focus on the cognitive skills detailed in this table.

Generally speaking, neuropsychologists begin by determining if deficits (e.g., aphasia, hemispatial inattention) exist that can affect performance in other cognitive domains. The domains assessed will vary depending on these deficits. For the patient with mild deficits, a typical assessment would likely include tests of premorbid functioning, attention/working memory, language, spatial skills, verbal and visual memory, processing speed, executive functions, motor skills, and psychosocial status. However, the neuropsychologist should select tests that minimize alternative explanations of deficits in a particular cognitive domain, and also should interpret test results based on both qualitative observation as well as quantitative scores, and with reference to other test performances. For instance, poor performance on a measure of auditory comprehension, which often requires the ability to carry out a set of actions, may not reflect language deficits per se, but instead may result from deficits in working memory. Given the deficits seen after stroke, the approach to evaluating patients with stroke may be somewhat different from what is typical in other neurological disorders because neuropsychologists frequently do not routinely assess all deficits that may occur based on the area of the damage. For example, several characteristics of Gerstmann syndrome, which is rarely seen in its entirety but is highly predictive of left parietal damage when it does occur, can be assessed using standardized tests developed by Arthur Benton.

As can be seen in Table 26.2, different patterns of symptoms are seen after left- or right-hemisphere stroke and after stroke in the different parts of each hemisphere. Importantly, these patterns of impairment may vary with hand preference. The left hemisphere is dominant for language in the majority of individuals, but less often for left-handers. Thus, left-hemisphere damage produces language deficits or aphasia in about 99% of right-handers but in only 60–70% of left-handers, and focal language deficits occur somewhat less often in children overall, especially when the stroke occurs in infancy or early childhood. However, again the neuropsychologist should be aware that both hemispheres typically contribute to language abilities, as shown by neuroimaging studies in healthy individuals and more detailed examination of patients with unilateral damage.

Another important consideration is how tests of premorbid functioning, such as vocabulary or reading recognition, may be confounded after stroke that causes aphasia; in that instance, premorbid status would be best predicted by demographic factors. Consultation with speech and language therapists can be helpful for assessing how influential aphasia is likely to be, and their evaluation may suffice for assessing language skills.

- *Attention/Concentration* Attention, such as hemispatial inattention, must also be assessed, especially in patients with right-hemisphere damage. This assessment is often qualitative, based upon the character of their writing samples or drawing of geometric forms. Measures such as line bisection, letter cancellation, or double simultaneous visual stimulation if the patient does not have a visual field cut are also commonly used.

- *Language* Regardless of stroke location, language skills must be assessed with consideration of aphasia type, although this is often difficult to specify (See also Chapter 5, Domains of Neuropsychological Function and Related Neurobehavioral Disorders). Assessment should include measures of auditory comprehension for simple one-step commands (e.g., point to the wall), multistep sequential commands (e.g., point to the floor, the ceiling, and the window), and syntactically more complex commands (e.g., before pointing to the table, point to the wall). Testing the limits can provide useful qualitative information about what techniques improve auditory comprehension and can thereby aid in planning rehabilitation and providing additional information to the family. Furthermore, qualitative information about spontaneous speech, such as presence of hesitations, neologisms, or paraphasic errors, is important for classifying the type of aphasia; at the same time, the neuropsychologist should note whether, despite qualitative speech deficits that affect communication efficiency, content is intact enough to produce functional communication. In addition, because dysnomia is common in many patients who are mildly aphasic, confrontation naming should be examined routinely in such patients.

- *Visuospatial* Spatial and form perception skills can be assessed with well-known tests of visual perception and simple and complex two- and three-dimensional constructions.

- *Memory and Executive Functions* Memory and executive function assessment can be especially problematic in patients with language deficits after left-hemisphere damage or visuospatial and attentional deficits after right-hemisphere damage, because deficits on measures of these more complex functions may reflect impairment in either memory or executive functions or the more primary language, visuospatial, or attentional problems.

- *Sensorimotor Functions* Motor deficits should also be examined using measures such as grip strength, finger tapping, and grooved pegboard because contralesional deficits are common after unilateral stroke, and ipsilesional deficits can be seen on more complex tasks, such as the grooved pegboard. This information can be used to emphasize the importance of motor rehabilitation of both arms because both hemispheres appear to be critical for the more complex movements that comprise most real-world activities.

- *Emotion and Personality* Although not mentioned in detail in Table 26.2, emotional distress must be examined, especially because depression is commonly reported after stroke in adults, is treatable, and is an independent risk factor for morbidity and mortality.

- *Symptom and Performance Validity* Formal evaluation of effort and test engagement is less common after stroke, but can be an issue, especially when evaluation is for determination of disability. Again, however, the same cautionary notes apply here as to other neuropsychological domains. Namely, the examiner must consider the impact of primary deficits frequently associated with the stroke, such as language, visuospatial, and attentional impairment.

In children, the issue of plasticity in the face of early focal lesions has been a significant focus of research. The relationship of age at the time of stroke to outcome does not appear to be linear, although the poorest outcomes are often seen after perinatal stroke. In general, younger children are less likely to demonstrate the classic syndromes outlined in Table 26.2 or aphasia syndromes discussed in Chapter 5, Domains of Neuropsychological Function and Related Neurobehavioral Disorders, and are more likely to show patterns of neuropsychological functioning that change over time as they grow older. Focal lesions are not necessarily more benign in younger children, but may result in a less localizing and more diffuse pattern of impairment. Early focal lesions also can lead to differences in the usual adult organization of brain–behavior relationships. For example, language skills may be lateralized to the right hemisphere after an early focal left-hemisphere lesion. Controversy continues about whether such changes leads to "crowding" of functions traditionally linked to the right hemisphere (e.g., visuospatial skills). Such reorganization of the brain is more often apparent for cognitive functions. In the majority of cases, sensory and motor functions retain their usual lateralization, although "pathological" left-handedness can occur.

Relevant Definitions

Amyloid angiopathy hemorrhage Intracranial hemorrhage due to cerebral amyloid angiopathy, which refers to the deposition of beta-amyloid in small and mid-sized arteries (and, less frequently, veins) of the brain (especially cerebral cortex and the leptomeninges). Although often asymptomatic, intracranial hemorrhage is the most recognized result of cerebral amyloid angiopathy.

Cerebral vasospasm Acute narrowing of a cerebral blood vessel that reduces the blood flow and therefore increases risk for stroke.

Dysarthria A speech articulation disorder caused by impaired muscular control due to damage to the central or peripheral nervous system. There are several types of dysarthria including spastic, hyperkinetic, hypokinetic, and ataxic dysarthria, each of which is seen after damage to different regions of the brain. Dysarthria is distinct from verbal or oral apraxia, which is always due to CNS damage and is a higher order speech problem characterized by impaired sequencing of the muscles used in speech (tongue, lips, jaw muscles, vocal cords).

Brain herniation Life-threatening brain displacement from the cranial vault through the tentorial notch or foramen magnum; usually caused by brain edema or hemorrhage with increasing ICP.

Infarct Area of necrotic tissue resulting from obstruction of local blood supply or ischemia (e.g., by thrombus or embolus).

Ischemia Insufficient blood supply to an organ, usually due to a blocked artery.

Lacunar infarct Small subcortical cerebral infarct (<1.5 cm cavities) related to occlusion or stenosis of small penetrating branches of the MCA, PCA, or basilar artery including the lenticulostriate arteries. Lacunes are frequently associated with chronic hypertension.

Paraphasias Linguistic speech errors seen in individuals with aphasia. Characterized by use of the wrong word or senseless combinations of words, which includes neologisms (nonwords, such as "forbis" for "pencil"), phonemic or literal paraphasias (phonemic errors, such as "spoot" for "spoon"), and semantic or verbal paraphasias (confusing words within a semantic category, such as "orange" for "apple").

Tissue plasminogen activator (tPA) is the only acute, anticoagulant treatment recommended by the FDA for adult ischemic stroke if the patient can be treated within 3 to 4.5 hours of symptom onset, has significant deficits on the NIH Stroke Scale, and has no evidence of hemorrhage on neuroimaging. As noted previously, although clinical practice typically uses the 3- to 4.5-hour time frame, FDA guidelines endorse the 3-hour time window.

Vasculitis Inflammation of blood vessels, which can lead to narrowing of the vessel, blood clot formation, or aneurysm formation due to weakening of the vessel wall, all of which increase the probability of stroke.

Stroke Questions

NOTE: Questions 22, 47, and 107 on the First Full-Length Practice Examination, Questions 40, 47, 85, and 122 on the Second Full-Length Practice Examination, Questions 18, 33, 63, and 99 on the Third Full-Length Practice Examination, and Questions 12, 36, 85, and 116 on the Fourth Full-Length Practice Examination are from this chapter.

1. What is the most likely vascular distribution of a stroke in a left-handed man with Broca's aphasia?

    (a) right superior MCA

    (b) left superior MCA

    (c) right inferior MCA

    (d) left inferior MCA

2. The frequency of ischemic and hemorrhagic stroke in adults is about ____, respectively.

    (a) 60% and 40%

    (b) 40% and 60%

    (c) 88% and 12%

    (d) 12% and 88%

3. The most common single reason for hemorrhagic stroke in adults is ____.

    (a) hypertension

    (b) atherosclerosis

    (c) aneurysm

    (d) AVM

4. Ischemic strokes in adults are most common in what vascular distribution?

    (a) vertebral artery

    (b) MCA

    (c) basilar artery

    (d) PCA

5. The most important limitation(s) of CT scans when used for diagnosis of stroke are insensitivity to ____.

    (a) acute intracerebral hemorrhage

    (b) lacunar infarcts

    (c) ischemia, especially chronically

    (d) ischemia, especially acutely

6. Which of the following treatments would be least likely in a case of ischemic stroke in an adult?

    (a) tissue plasminogen activator

    (b) endarterectomy

    (c) endovascular embolization

    (d) antithrombotic drugs

7. A 65-year-old patient with ischemic stroke received tPA acutely. Further medical workup identified greater than 70% stenosis of the right carotid artery. What is the most common recommended treatment to decrease future strokes?

    (a) carotid angioplasty

    (b) carotid stent

    (c) endovascular thrombectomy

    (d) endarterectomy

8. Three months after an ischemic stroke a 55-year-old man is diagnosed with depression. What treatment has the greatest empirical support in clinical trials?

    (a) pharmacologic treatment

    (b) psychotherapy

    (c) combined psychotherapy and pharmacologic treatment

    (d) neither psychotherapy nor pharmacologic treatment

9. A 6-year-old child with a history of arterial ischemic stroke is referred for a neuropsychological evaluation. Which lesion location is likely to be associated with the worst cognitive outcome?

    (a) left parietal and temporal lobes

    (b) right temporal and frontal lobes

    (c) left temporal lobe and basal ganglia

    (d) right thalamus and basal ganglia

10. The new definition of a transient ischemic attack requires _____.

(a) abnormal brain imaging

(b) normal brain imaging

(c) no residual deficits

(d) symptoms for < 24 hours

Stroke Answers

1. **B—left superior MCA** *The left hemisphere is dominant for language in 60–70% of left-handers, and it is the superior MCA that damages the suprasylvian region and Broca's area (Brodmann area 44) to produce Broca's, nonfluent, or expressive aphasia.*

   References:
   (a) Cullum, C. M., Rossetti, H. C., Batjer, H. Festa, J., Haaland, K. Y., & Lacritz, L. (2017). Cerebrovascular disease, In J. Morgan & J. Ricker (Eds.), *Textbook of clinical neuropsychology* (2nd ed., pp. 350–386). New York, NY: Taylor & Francis.
   (b) Swanda, R. M., & Haaland, K. Y. (2017). Clinical neuropsychology. In B. J. Sadock, V. A. Sadock, & P. Ruiz (Eds), *Comprehensive textbook of psychiatry,* (10th ed., pp. 976–993). Philadelphia, PA: Lippincott Williams & Wilkins.

2. **C—88% and 12%** *The incidence of ischemic stroke is higher than that of hemorrhagic stroke.*

   Reference: Cullum, C. M., Rossetti, H. C., Batjer, H. Festa, J., Haaland, K. Y., & Lacritz, L. (2017). Cerebrovascular Disease, In J. Morgan & J. Ricker (Eds.), *Textbook of clinical neuropsychology* (2nd ed., pp. 350–386). New York, NY: Taylor & Francis.

3. **A—hypertension** *Intracerebral hemorrhage is most common in small vessels within the brain, because hypertension particularly weakens their thin-walled vessels causing rupture.*

   Reference: Mohr, J. P., Wolf, P. A., Grotta, J. C., Moskowitz, M. A., Mayberg, M. R., & von Kummer, R. (2011). *Stroke: Pathophysiology, diagnosis and management* (5th ed.). Philadelphia, PA: Saunders.

4. **B—MCA** *The MCA, which, along with the ACA, is part of the internal carotid anterior circulation.*

   Reference: Mohr, J. P., Wolf, P. A., Grotta, J. C., Moskowitz, M .A., Mayberg, M. R., & von Kummer, R. (2011). *Stroke: Pathophysiology, diagnosis and management* (5th ed.). Philadelphia, PA: Saunders.

5. **D—ischemia, especially acutely** *A CT scan is not sensitive to ischemic changes in the first 24 hours after stroke; it is highly sensitive to intracerebral hemorrhage (as sensitive as diffusion weighted MRI) but less sensitive than MRI to lacunar infarcts.*

   Reference: Blumenfeld, H. (2010). *Neuroanatomy through clinical cases* (2nd ed.). Sunderland, MA: Sinauer Associates.

6. **C—endovascular embolization** *This is a treatment for aneurysms.*

   Reference: Lo, W. D. (2011). Childhood hemorrhagic stroke: An important but understudied problem. *Journal of Child Neurology, 26,* 1174–1185.

7. **D—endarterectomy** *This is the recommended treatment for greater than 70% stenosis of the carotid stenosis artery. It has been shown to decrease future stroke incidence relative to patients who are medically treated.*

   Reference: Furie, K., Kasner, S., Adams, R., Albers, G., Bush, R., Fagan, S., . . . Wentworth, D. (2011). Guidelines for the prevention of stroke in patients with stroke or transient ischemic attack: A guideline for healthcare professionals from the American Heart Association/American Stroke Association. *Stroke, 42*(1), 227–276.

8. **A—pharmacologic treatment** *The greatest number of studies have shown the efficacy of antidepressant medications for depression after stroke. The use of medication treatment has been supported in a meta-analysis such that in 2010 the American Heart Association recommended assessment of depression after stroke and pharmacological treatment for diagnosed depression.*

A limited number of studies have also supported the use of psychotherapy for depression after stroke, but the evidence is limited at this point.

References:
(a) Adams, H. P., & Robinson, R. G. (2012). Improving recovery after stroke: A role for antidepressant medications? *Stroke, 43*, 2829–2832.
(b) Miller, E. L., Murray, L., Richards, L., Zorowitz, R. D., Bakas, T., Clark, P., . . . Billinger, S. A. (2010). Comprehensive overview of nursing and interdisciplinary rehabilitation care of the stroke patient. *Stroke, 41*, 2402–2448.

9. **C—left temporal lobe and basal ganglia** *Several studies have shown that combined cortical-subcortical lesions are associated with worse cognitive outcomes than cortical or subcortical lesions alone.*

Reference: Fuentes, A., Deotto, A., Desrocher, M., deVeber, G., & Westmacott, R. (2016). Determinants of cognitive outcomes of perinatal and childhood stroke: A review. *Child Neuropsychology, 22*, 1–38.

10. **B—normal brain imaging** *This is a change in the definition of TIA, which was previously defined as any focal cerebral ischemic event typically lasting less than 1 hour but no more than 24 hours. However, studies have shown that 30% to 50% of patients meeting that criterion had evidence of ischemic damage on diffusion-weighted magnetic resonance imaging. Therefore, TIA is now defined as a transient episode of neurologic dysfunction caused by focal brain, spinal cord, or retinal ischemia, without acute infarction. This definitional change has been accepted by the American Heart Association and other organizations focused on cerebrovascular health. This is an important issue because such episodes are risk factors for additional strokes and require detailed assessment to minimize the risk of future stroke.*

Reference: Mohr, J. P, Wolf, P. A., Grotta, J. C., Moskowitz, M. A., Mayberg, M. R., & von Kummer, R. (2011). *Stroke: Pathophysiology, diagnosis and management* (5th ed.). Philadelphia, PA: Saunders.

Recommended Readings

Blumenfeld, H. (2010). *Neuroanatomy through clinical cases* (2nd ed.). Sunderland, MA: Sinauer Associates.

Cullum, C. M., Rossetti, H. C., Batjer, H., Festa, J., Haaland, K. Y., & Lacritz, L. (2017). Cerebrovascular disease, In J. Morgan & J. Ricker (Eds.), *Textbook of clinical neuropsychology* (2nd ed., pp. 350–386). New York, NY: Taylor & Francis.

Fuentes, A., Deotto, A., Desrocher, M., deVeber, G., & Westmacott, R. (2016). Determinants of cognitive outcomes of perinatal and childhood stroke: A review. *Child Neuropsychology, 22*, 1–38.

Greenham, M., Gordon, A., Anderson, V., & Mackay, M. T. (2016). Outcome in childhood stroke. *Stroke, 47*, 1159–1164.

Kirton, A., & deVeber, G. (2015). Paediatric stroke: pressing issues and promising directions. *Lancet Neurology, 14*, 92–102.

Roach, E. S., Golomb, M. R., Adams, R., Biller, J., Daniels, S., Deveber, G., . . .Smith, E. R. (2008). Management of stroke in infants and children: A scientific statement from a special writing group of the American Heart Association Stroke Council and the Council on Cardiovascular Disease in the Young. *Stroke, 39*, 2644–2691.

MEDICAL

27   Delirium and Disorders of Consciousness

Kirk J. Stucky and Christine D. Liff

Definition

Delirium is a reversible, acute-onset condition that typically develops over a short period of time and results in fluctuating and transient global cognitive dysfunction. The disturbance represents an acute change from baseline that is not solely attributable to another neurocognitive disorder and does not occur in the context of severely reduced arousal or coma. Given the many causes of delirium, it is considered a syndrome rather than a specific disease process or disorder. In the DSM-5 delirium is classified as a neurocognitive disorder. Core diagnostic criteria are outlined and described below:

A. *Disturbance of attention and awareness* The patient has a reduced ability to direct, focus, sustain, or shift attention with reduced orientation to the environment. These changes can profoundly impact other cognitive domains. Patients are often unable to maintain a coherent stream of thought or action and can be highly distractible and inattentive.

B. *Acute onset and fluctuation* These are the hallmark features of delirium. The disturbance develops over a short period of time (usually hours to a few days), represents a change from baseline attention and awareness, and tends to fluctuate in severity during the course of a day. Disturbances in mood and the sleep–wake cycle are common. Periods of somnolence may be counterbalanced by excessive alertness, intense agitation, and frenzied excitement. Three distinct subtypes are recognized—hyperactive, hypoactive, or a mixture of both. Increased motor activity, restlessness, stereotyped behaviors, and psychomotor agitation are hyperactive examples, whereas lethargy, lack of initiation, and slow reaction time represent hypoactive symptoms. Certain types of delirium are more prone to hyperactive or hypoactive states (e.g., alcohol withdrawal delirium is typically marked by hyperactive psychomotor behavior and sympathetic arousal).

C. *Other cognitive impairments* An additional disturbance in cognition (e.g., memory impairment, visuospatial and or perceptual impairments). This may include disorders of perception such as misperceptions and sensory *illusions*, which range from simple to complex. Delusions and/or hallucinations in delirium are often erratic and nonsystematic and are most commonly visual (see Table 27.1). Psychotic symptoms are not required for the diagnosis of delirium, but when present they are clinically distinct from what is typically observed in chronic psychiatric conditions (see the "Expectations for Neuropsychological Assessment Results" section that follows for more detail).

D. The disturbances in Criteria A and C are not better explained by a pre-existing, established or evolving neurocognitive disorder and do not occur in the context of a severely reduced level of arousal. Thus, delirium cannot be diagnosed in individuals who are in coma, deeply sedated, or a minimally responsive state.

E. There is evidence from the history, physical examination, and laboratory findings that the disturbance is a direct physiologic consequence of a medical condition (see Table 27.1 for various potential etiologies.).

In some cases, delirium can be confused with a number of psychiatric or chronic neurologic conditions because there can be considerable symptom overlap. Additionally, delirium has been used synonymously or in conjunction with multiple terms including acute confusional state (ACS) and *encephalopathy*. It is important to recognize that *encephalopathy* is a nonspecific term used to describe any medical condition impacting the brain's function. Thus, *encephalopathy* has been used to describe both acute and chronic conditions, which is not the case with delirium. Although still employed by some, the term "intensive care unit (ICU) psychosis" should be avoided because there is no cause-and-effect relationship between ICU admission and the development of delirium. Alternatively, the conditions that commonly result in ICU admission frequently cause delirium. Furthermore, the term ICU psychosis places a disproportionate emphasis on psychiatric symptoms that are not present for the vast majority of patients with delirium in the ICU.

TABLE 27.1 Delirium Differential Diagnosis: I WATCH DEATH

Infection	CNS infections (e.g., encephalitis, vasculitis, meningitis, syphilis, HIV), sepsis, systemic infections.
Withdrawal	Alcohol, benzodiazepines, sedative-hypnotics, opiates
Acute metabolic	Acidosis (e.g., diabetic ketoacidosis—DKA), alkalosis, electrolyte imbalances (sodium, glucose, calcium, magnesium), organ failure (hepatic, renal)
Trauma	Traumatic brain injury, burn injury, postoperative confusion, exsanguination (i.e., extensive blood loss)
CNS pathology	Abscess, tumor, metastases, inflammatory or autoimmune disorders (e.g., paraneoplastic syndromes), postictal states
Hypoxia	Pulmonary/respiratory failure, cardiac arrest, hypotension, strangulation, near drowning, carbon monoxide poisoning, anesthesia accident, anemia
Deficiencies (Nutritional)	Vitamin B_{12}, folate, thiamine, cobalamine, niacin
Endocrinopathies	Hyper/hypoadrenocorticism, hyper/hypoglycemia, hypothyroidism, hyperparathyroidism, adrenal hyper- or hypofunction
Acute vascular	Stroke, hypertensive encephalopathy, posterior reversible encephalopathy syndrome (PRES), arrhythmia, shock, microembolism/embolic shower
Toxins or drugs	Medications (sedative hypnotics, antihistamines, anticholinergics, antiparkinsonian agents, gastrointestinal agents (e.g., H_2 blockers), analgesics, general anesthetics, corticosteroids), illicit substances, toxic chemicals
Heavy Metals	Lead, manganese, mercury

NOTE: Adopted from Wise, M. G., & Trzepacz, P. T. (1996). Delirium (confusional states). In J. R. Rundell & M. G. Wise (Eds.), American Psychiatric Press textbook of *Consultation-liaison psychiatry* (p. 268). Washington DC: American Psychiatric Press.

Neuropathology

A myriad of pathophysiological causes can lead to the development of delirium, but their unique contributions vary depending on the underlying predisposing and precipitating factors. Generally accepted pathological contributors include but are not limited to the following:

- neurotransmitter system dysfunction
- CNS response to inflammatory processes
- hypothalamic pituitary adrenal axis dysregulation
- direct cerebral insult/injury (e.g. diffuse brain injury, hypoxia)

Discussion of the wide variety of possible conditions and substances contributing to delirium are beyond the scope of this chapter. However, the mnemonic I WATCH DEATH is a useful tool to assist clinicians in the systematic differential diagnosis of delirium. Table 27.1 outlines this approach and lists common causes of delirium.

Although some medical conditions that result in delirium have unique laboratory or exam features, clinical presentations overlap considerably. For example, *hepatic encephalopathy* often coincides with elevated ammonia levels and, in some cases, *asterixis*. However, these features can be observed in other types of delirium as well. Thus, there are no specific "text book" behavioral, cognitive, or medical features that reliably differentiate one type of delirium from another. Consequently, once a delirium diagnosis has been established via clinical examination, the etiologic determination is often based on the integrated review of the patient's unique history in light of current laboratory and radiologic studies.

Neurochemical Features of Delirium

Delirium results in an impairment of general attentional systems most likely due to the disruption of mechanisms affecting the interaction and connections among the reticular activating system, subcortical regions, and cortex. Regardless of etiology, in most cases, dysfunction occurs at the cellular/neurotransmitter level. Dopamine and acetylcholine systems are considered primarily involved, but serotonergic systems most certainly play a role in some types of delirium as well.

- Acetylcholine plays a role in attention, memory, and arousal. Decrease in acetylcholine, known as the cholinergic deficiency hypothesis, most likely contributes to impairments in attention and memory disturbance. The hypothesis was based on the observation that delirium occurs with drugs and toxins that impair cholinergic function. Furthermore, delirium caused by anticholinergic drug overdose is reversed via administration of physostigmine (eserine). Serum anticholinergic activity (SAA) at a high level is also strongly associated with delirium, while low levels often correspond with resolution of delirium.

- Excess dopamine or enhanced receptor site sensitivity is thought to be the cause of hallucinations. For example, bupropion can exacerbate delirium because it acts as a dopamine reuptake inhibitor, and can cause hallucinations, paranoia, and/or confusion. Additionally, levodopa can cause hallucinations, agitation, and bradykinesia or akinesia, the latter of which can result in falls. Conversely, dopamine antagonists and antipsychotics which target dopaminergic systems are often used to treat delirium.

- Disruption or over excitation of serotonergic systems may cause hallucinations and emotional lability (e.g., hallucinogen intoxication). Additionally, overdose with or the use of multiple serotonergic agents can result in mental status changes, agitation, myoclonus, hyperreflexia, diaphoresis, tremor, diarrhea, incoordination, and fever (i.e., *serotonin syndrome*). If left untreated and medications continue, death can occur. Treatment requires the discontinuation of all serotonergic drugs and close monitoring with an expectation for improvement within 24 hours.

Risk Factors

Delirium typically develops in patients who are vulnerable due to predisposing factors and then subsequently experience noxious events or precipitating factors. As a general rule, when a number of predisposing factors are present, even minor precipitating factors (e.g., addition of a medication) can trigger delirium. Studies have identified a wide variety of predisposing and precipitating risk factors. It is unlikely that the exam will require the memorization of all possible contributors, but neuropsychologists are expected to know the primary risk factors, outlined here.

- **Predisposing Factors** Older age, dementia, severity of physical/chronic illness, polypharmacy, metabolic disturbances, depression, sensory loss or dysfunction, respiratory failure or myocardial infarction, and infections.
  - Preexisting brain disease or cognitive impairment resulting in reduced cerebral reserve lowers the patient's tolerance threshold, which explains why individuals with preexisting neurocognitive disorders are at much higher risk for developing delirium following relatively minor medical events or surgery. Similarly, patients who have experienced a delirious episode may subsequently be diagnosed with an evolving dementing disorder that was previously unrecognized.
  - Age is an independent risk factor most likely due to normal age-related variables, such as changes in vasculature, decreased cholinergic activity, and/or increased monoamine oxidase activity. The aging brain is less able to tolerate or adapt to physiologic perturbations. For example, although the reason(s) remain unclear, healthy older adults are more prone to developing delirium after contracting a urinary tract infection (UTI), whereas this complication is uncommon in younger adults or children. With perhaps the exception of urosepsis, delirium in older patients with UTI is more likely related to the physiologic effects and response to infection as opposed to the infection directly affecting the brain.
  - Comorbid physical problems, such as sleep deprivation, sensory impairment, immobility, functional decline, dehydration, and untreated or poorly managed pain, can also increase susceptibility.
  - Medical comorbidities and chronic or poorly controlled medical conditions can have a systemic impact when left untreated (e.g., hepatic or renal disease, diabetes, hypertension).
- **Precipitating Factors** Surgery, drug side effects, drug withdrawal, infections, iatrogenic complications, metabolic derangements, and pain.
  - Postoperative states and complications such as *hyponatremia*, infections, and/or iatrogenic medication effects can promote persistent confusion. Post-transplant patients are also at high risk for complications that cause delirium, such as infection, transplant rejection, or drugs given to reduce risk of transplant rejection (e.g., calcineurin inhibitors like Prograf).
  - Acute injuries (e.g., burn injury, polytrauma) or medical/surgical procedures that do not directly affect the central nervous system (CNS) but result in metabolic or other complications can lead to acute confusion. For example, heart valve surgery, coronary artery bypass graft (CABG), and the surgical repair of long bone fractures have been associated with embolic shower and or cerebral fat emboli (i.e., microembolism) leading to delirium and, in some, cases permanent cognitive impairments.

Epidemiology

- Prevalence with hospitalized older patients increases with age, with up to 14% of individuals 85 years and older experiencing delirium. Approximately 60% of patients in post-acute care and/or nursing homes experience an episode of delirium.

- For patients in critical care settings mixed type delirium is most common (50–60%), followed by hypoactive (35–45%), and hyperactive (less than 5%).
- In noncritical care settings hypoactive delirium is more common in the elderly than hyperactive or mixed type delirium.
- In the elderly, the most common cause is infection.
- Illicit and licit drug abuse and/or withdrawal is the most common cause of delirium in young adults.
- In children, iatrogenic medication side effects can lead to delirium.

Specific Medical Population Incidence Rates

- Higher base rate in certain medical populations (e.g., end-stage renal disease, burn injury, diabetes, stroke, *sepsis*)
- 60–80% of patients requiring intensive or critical care
- 22–70% of patients in long-term care settings, 40–50% in hospice settings
- Post-stroke delirium occurs in 13–48% of patients

Surgical Population Incidence Rates

Delirium risk varies between 10–50% depending on the type of surgery. Higher rates have been noted in patients who have neurocognitive disorders, are medically fragile, or require more complicated surgeries (e.g., 35% rate in the elderly after vascular operations). Delirium has also been associated with longer hospital stays, higher risk of nursing home placement, and greater morbidity and mortality.

Morbidity

- Longer length of hospitalization and ICU admission, higher rate of reintubation, and increased cost of care
- Up to 50% experience permanent cognitive impairments following resolution
- Higher complication rates relative to other patients
- High rates of impulsivity, picking at clothes or skin, and agitation lead to unintentional injury (e.g., falls, self-extubation, pulling at intravenous lines, tubes, catheters, or other medical equipment)

Mortality

- Approximately 80% of patients experience delirium in the stages prior to death.
- Of hospitalized patients with delirium, 20–25% eventually expire as a result of the underlying medical condition and/or subsequent complications. Mortality rates for patients with delirium are similar to mortality rates for patients with acute myocardial infarction or *sepsis*.
- For those who survive an episode of delirium, there is an increased likelihood of death within one year relative to other patients who have been treated and discharged from the hospital (approximately 35–40%).

Determinants of Severity

Delirium is a life-threatening condition. If not identified or treated properly, patients can die or sustain permanent, debilitating medical or cognitive outcomes. Thus, all types of delirium are treated seriously, and patients typically require 24-hour monitoring such as that provided on the ICU or specialized hospital units. Generally speaking, the following causes and/or associated features of delirium increase both mortality rates and the risk for permanent debilitating injury:

- Multisystem organ failure

- Sustained autonomic hyperarousal and/or storms despite treatment

- Status epilepticus or multiple treatment-resistant seizures

- Wernicke's *encephalopathy* and/or persistent delirium tremens (DTs), the latter of which is characterized by global confusion, hallucinations (typically visual and/or tactile), and autonomic hyperactivity

- Chronic, uncorrected metabolic disturbance or physiologic condition (e.g., renal failure, diabetic ketoacidosis). For example, vitamin B_{12} deficiency can result in permanent CNS damage resulting in reduced pressure and vibration perception, fatigue and weakness, gait dysfunction, and paresthesias.

Presentation, Disease Course, and Recovery

Acute Hospitalization Recovery Course

Delirium onset has two potential general courses:

- *Abrupt/immediate onset* can occur, such as with moderate to severe traumatic brain injury (TBI) or stroke. In these cases, a sudden neurologic event results in immediate confusion and behavioral change. If managed properly, survivors typically experience a period of steady recovery, although many do not return to baseline levels of function.

- *Slow onset/fluctuating course* with a prodromal period in which symptoms develop over hours or days (e.g., developing metabolic disturbance such as vacillating *hyponatremia* as the result of small-cell lung cancer). In these cases, subsyndromal symptoms often wax and wane, with islands of lucidity. Mild to moderate cognitive impairments (e.g., memory, divided and complex attention, visual tracking, psychomotor speed) are often easily identified via formal evaluation even during these "lucid" periods. In delirium related to metabolic or chronic medical conditions, a prodromal stage can often be historically identified during interviews with collaterals. Clinicians and researchers are hopeful that proactive detection in patients who are at risk might facilitate prompt intervention and or pre-emptive efforts at prevention. There is some evidence to suggest that subsyndromal symptoms are easier to detect or anticipate in patients with chronic or developing conditions (e.g., systemic illness, organ failure, worsening infection), but research is minimal at this time.

Once hospitalized, delirium can result in a wide variety of potential outcomes and courses of recovery. Some patients have a clearly identified singular etiology that, once addressed, results in steady recovery, often with return to baseline function (e.g., development of *serotonin syndrome* with full recovery after multiple antidepressants are discontinued). In other patients, there may be multiple possible etiologies that, once addressed, result in steady recovery although the primary cause of delirium remains unclear (e.g., alcohol withdrawal delirium with *sepsis* and/or withdrawal seizures). Despite identification and treatment, some individuals with delirium do not return to baseline function or expire despite clinician efforts.

Assessment Methods

Although neuropsychologists do not perform physical examinations or order laboratory and radiologic tests, they should have a basic understanding and appreciation of their purpose and utility in differential diagnosis. The approach to a delirium assessment will vary to some extent by case circumstance and clinician preference but, in general, neuropsychologists should:

- Monitor confusion with periodic reassessment. Various measures have been developed, including but not limited to the Intensive Care Delirium Screening Checklist, Delirium Rating Scale, Cognitive-Log, and the Confusion Assessment Method for the ICU (CAM-ICU). It should be noted that formal assessment measures are often difficult to administer to the delirious patient and thus a flexible approach to assessment is often required. Furthermore, a good clinical interview including reliable collateral report and basic mental status examination is often sufficient to diagnose delirium. That said, the recording of objective scores over time can be helpful in tracking a patient's clinical course and/or response to treatment (e.g., daily Cognitive-Log scores in a patient with severe TBI).

- Many patients are unable to complete more detailed screening measures (e.g., MoCA, MMSE, RBANS). Tools that assess basic, sustained, and divided attention should be stressed. Brief assessment at different times of day is recommended to track waxing and waning confusion.

- Assume that the delirious condition is reversible and work collaboratively with colleagues to identify all probable or possible etiologies.

- Determine if physicians have reviewed all medications and potential interaction effects.

- Determine if physicians have investigated the possibility of infection and/or other medical causes (e.g., neurologists may conduct a lumbar puncture when CNS infection or subarachnoid hemorrhage is suspected).

- Review clinician and collateral reports with regard to the onset of and/or patterns of confusion. Attempt to identify trends and determine if they coincide with treatment delivery, time of day, or other external factors.

- In collaboration with physicians, carefully review all laboratory studies—renal and liver function, oxygen saturation, complete blood count (CBC), electrolytes, creatinine, glucose, thyroid function tests, urinalysis, and toxicology screens.

- Neuroimaging or additional neurodiagnostic studies may or may not be ordered. However, review of neuroimaging and electroencephalography (EEG) studies past and present, if available, can be helpful. In delirium caused by metabolic factors, *sepsis*, or systemic medical issues, neuroimaging is often negative or serves only to rule out acute or space-occupying lesions. Electroencephalography (EEG) is typically abnormal in delirium, often revealing nonfocal, generalized slowing or fast activity, especially in metabolic delirium, but in patients with seizures the EEG may reveal focal findings (see also Chapter 6, The Neurologic Examination, Radiologic and Other Diagnostic Studies).

- *Differential diagnosis* Delirium typically can be differentiated from dementia and other psychiatric disorders using features such as onset, time course, fluctuating mental status, and inattention. Unlike delirium, dementia and psychiatric disorders tend to be insidious, developing over months to years, vital signs in patients are typically normal, and there is little fluctuation in cognitive impairment over time. Please see Table 27.2 for more detail on clinical features that can assist in the differential diagnosis between dementia, delirium, and depression.

TABLE 27.2 Differential Diagnosis of Delirium, Dementia, and Depression in the Hospitalized Patient

		Dementia	Delirium	Depression
Clinical Course / History	Symptom Onset	Onset often indistinct / gradual	Onset often sudden	Onset fairly well defined
	Symptom History	History of decline apparent before consultation	Often come to medical attention soon after symptoms arise	History may be short or have previous episodes
	Deficits	Evidence of early / unnoticed deficits	Deficits apparent to lay people	Deficits may be rapidly progressive
	Psychiatric	Uncommon occurrence of previous psychiatric problems or emotional crisis	Often seen in patients with chronic medical/substance use issues	History of previous psychiatric conditions or recent crisis
	Diagnosis	Historical data often required for diagnosis	Historical data may not be required for diagnosis	Historical data often required for diagnosis
Clinical Presentation	Cognitive Complaints	Little complaint of cognitive loss; may hide or make excuses for deficits	Little complaint or awareness of cognitive loss	Detailed / elaborate complaints of cognitive loss
	Attention	May or may not have pronounced attentional difficulties	Arousal / attention deficits always central and primary barrier to cognitive tasks	Attention normal. With encouragement often perform within expectation or improve considerably
	Arousal	Arousal is typically constant	Variable arousal; may vacillate from agitated to stuporous state	Consistency in arousal and attention
	Behavioral Change	Behavior compatible with cognitive loss	Behavior bizarre or out of proportion to cognitive loss	Behavior does not reflect cognitive loss
	Confabulation	May confabulate (more often with certain dementias)	May confabulate	Do not confabulate
	Sleep/Wake Cycle	Night time exacerbation of cognitive difficulties common (e.g., sundowning)	Exacerbation may occur any time of day	Night time exacerbation rare
	Neurologic Exam	Focal neurologic deficits not often seen until late stages (exception—Vascular dementia)	Focal neurologic deficits sometimes seen	Focal neurologic deficits not seen

Common Neuropsychological Findings	**Test Engagement**	Usually tries items presented, good effort. All except severe dementia are able to participate in full neuropsychological testing	• May be cooperative or remain belligerent in their refusal. • Attention/behavior often barrier to full assessment. • Wide range of behaviors.	Motivation a barrier to assessment not arousal. Frequently answers, "I don't know" before trying.
	Memory and Memory Gaps	• Memory loss for recent information worse than for remote information. May have storage and/or retrieval deficits. Often disoriented • No specific memory gaps exist	• Variable memory patterns. Storage / retrieval deficits vary depending upon when tested. Always disoriented at some level • May have specific memory gaps daily	• Inconsistent memory loss for recent and remote information. Retrieval deficits common. Not typically disoriented • May have specific memory gaps (emotional events)
	Consciousness	Consciousness not clouded. Consistently impaired performance throughout the day, week, month.	Consciousness clouded. Variable performance throughout day, week, month.	Consciousness not clouded. Inconsistent performance not explained by cognitive impairment
	Executive Function	Tend to be concrete in thought	May or may not be concrete	Often abstract, not concrete
	Awareness	In early stages patient may recognize changes; in later stages often lack insight	Typically unaware of changes in cognition	Demonstrate insight and or awareness of problems.
	Sensitive Measures	Memory performance patterns and impact on daily function often most sensitive indicators	Attentional performance or dysgraphia among the most sensitive indicators	Motivational inconsistency and lack of comparative impact on function may be the most sensitive
Affective/ Neurovegetative symptoms	**Mood**	• Emotional lability uncommon • May appear dysphoric and lack initiation, but status remains stable • Mood often apathetic with shallow emotions	• Emotional lability frequently seen • May vacillate between paranoia, euphoria, and dysphoria (hyper- and hypoactive states) • Mood marked by high levels of anxiety, fear, and depression alone or in combination often seen.	• Affective change often remains stable, but lability can be seen • Often dysphoric. Atypical mood features often occur in the elderly (e.g., irritability, anxiety) • Mood symptoms often profound and patient able to describe psychological pain or distress
	Hallucinations	Hallucinations not typically present in early or middle stages (exception—Lewy body dementia)	Hallucinations common and more often visual	Hallucinations not typically present (exception—major depression with psychosis—often auditory)
	Delusions	Delusions rare and if occur not present until later stages (e.g. Capgras syndrome)	Delusions commonly seen and may vacillate or be inconsistently present	Delusions seen in some cases of severe depression but typically remain stable over time
	Sleep	Sleep typically stable (exception—Lewy body dementia, sundowning)	Often have disrupted sleep wake cycles, night terrors but unable to express or describe content	Sleep cycle often disrupted. Initial insomnia due to worry common. Nightmares with themes of loss common
	Appetite	Appetite typically stable (exception dementia with depression)	Appetite often absent, poor, or variable. May be a history of malnutrition.	Appetite often low but in some cases over eating can be seen as well.

For patients with chronic psychiatric conditions, hallucinations and delusions are typically consistent and systematic. In delirium and other neurologic conditions (e.g., Lewy body dementia), hallucinations and delusions are often unsystematic, variable, and may come and go throughout the day. Hallucinations can be both formed and unformed in delirium whereas in psychosis they are typically formed (e.g., formed = distinctive shapes, objects, people, or scenes; unformed = simple images, flashing lights, spots, colored lines). Types of hallucinations commonly and uncommonly observed in delirium have been listed in Table 27.3.

TABLE 27.3 Hallucinations and Delusions That May Be Associated with Delirium

Formication Hallucinations	The perception or feeling that bugs are crawling over the skin. Often reported by patients during drug withdrawal delirium but when unilateral suggests focal parietal or thalamic lesions.	
Hypnagogic Hallucinations	Hallucinations that occur in the process of falling asleep.	
Hypnopompic Hallucinations	Hallucinations that occur in the process of awakening. Often coincide with sleep paralysis (i.e., inability to move or speak despite being awake).	
Lilliputian Hallucinations	A type of formed visual hallucination in which people, animals, and/or objects are seen and perceived as smaller than they would be in real life. Occurs in individuals with neurologic and psychiatric conditions.	
Metamorphopsia	The perception that one's body is changing in size or shape. A component symptom within the so-called Alice in Wonderland syndrome.	
Misidentification Syndromes	A fixed delusional belief that objects, people, or places have been duplicated	**Capgras Syndrome** A delusional belief that a person has been replaced by an imposter or duplicate. Often associated with frontal system dysfunction such as that seen in schizophrenia and progressive dementias. Rarely observed in delirium.
		Reduplicative paramnesia A delusional belief that a place has been replaced or duplicated. Typically associated with conditions causing severe and persistent neurocognitive dysfunction (e.g., dementia).
Peduncular Hallucinations	Vivid, motion-filled hallucinations that include the perception of small objects, animals, people, or familiar landscapes. Unlike other hallucinations, they are often experienced as pleasant or entertaining, but can become anxiety provoking. Typically associated with lesions involving the posterior circulation and structures (e.g., occipital regions, cerebral peduncles, midbrain, middle thalamic nuclei). One symptomatic component of the so called "top-of-the-basilar-syndrome."	
Release Hallucinations	Occur as a consequence of sensory loss and subsequent disengagement of higher cerebral systems. For example, palinopsia is a condition in which a visual image continues to appear or be re-experienced hours or days after it is no longer present. Other examples include phantom limb sensations (post amputation) and Charles Bonnet syndrome following complete or partial loss of vision (e.g., macular degeneration).	
Visceral Hallucinations	Sensations that are believed to stem from internal organs. They are typically unpleasant and are difficult to localize. Can occur in both neurologic and psychiatric conditions.	

Treatment

Emergency Care and Acute Hospitalization

- In some cases, the primary etiology of delirium is not identified, but all concerning conditions are treated simultaneously. Treatment always begins with the correction of all possible causative factors. Due to the dangers inherent in delirium, physicians do not typically treat one problem at a time and wait to see results. Consequently, some patients improve, and the true etiology remains unclear or undetermined.

- In the emergency room, patients with delirium of unknown etiology often receive IV fluids and thiamine followed by glucose. These treatments are safe, relatively easy to administer, and cover a host of potential problems, which, if left untreated prior to full workup, could result in more serious consequences.

- Adequate hydration, nutrition, and airway management are often the primary focus of acute care specialists. Physical restraints and medical safety devices are sometimes necessary as a last resort to maintain safety and prevent unintentional injury.

- Vitals and medical status must be monitored closely. All nonessential medications should be placed on hold. If a probable etiology has not been identified, further workup should be conducted.

- During acute hospitalization, management also includes prevention of complications such as pressure sores, contractures, and deep vein thrombosis (DVT).

Sleep–Wake Cycle Disturbances

The diurnal rhythm is often reversed, with pronounced lethargy during the day and agitated arousal at night. The promotion of normal, proper, and uninterrupted sleep–wake schedules via medication, environmental modifications, mobilization, structured daytime activities, and out-of-bed schedules during the day should be emphasized.

Psychological and Behavioral Interventions

- These can be effective interventions in any setting but are never curative for delirium. Various environmental and systematic interventions have been associated with improved safety, shorter lengths of stay, and reduced complication rates. Interventions include frequent orientation, cueing, and reassurance; use of large clocks and calendars; placing familiar objects in the room; quiet, well-lit surroundings; night lights; windows to help with time of day; having glasses and hearing aids available to improve sensory quality; avoidance of restraints and preference for one-on-one safety observers; removal of Foley catheters; the presence of familiar faces and use of collateral support.

- Early mobility, out of bed schedules, and range of motion exercises have also been associated with reduced risk of complications during and after resolution of delirium.

- Delirium can be confusing and frightening for visitors and family members. In fact, a sizable percentage of family members will report symptoms of acute stress disorder, depression, and anxiety. Thus, collateral education and support are also important. Psychologists who work in the hospital setting are often in a unique position to provide these value-added services.

Medications

Physicians may employ a variety of medications to manage delirium:

- Neuroleptics to address hallucinations and sleep disturbances.

- Patients with substance intoxication may receive drugs that counteract their effects (e.g., naloxone in narcotic overdose).
- Benzodiazepines are often used for alcohol withdrawal syndrome (AWS), but should be avoided in the elderly and patients with acute neurologic injury.
- Mood stabilizing agents and drugs that target gamma-aminobutyric acid (GABA) are sometimes used in specific types of delirium (e.g., divalproex [Depakote] for agitated patients with TBI).

Physicians may eliminate medications known to cause or promote delirium. Additionally, some patients may experience a toxic or allergic reaction to certain drugs.

- Some drugs commonly used with the elderly can lead to delirium due to less recognized anticholinergic or other effects. Examples include digoxin, warfarin, codeine, ranitidine, and prednisolone. The Beers Criteria, developed by the American Geriatrics Society (AGS) is an excellent resource regarding potentially harmful medications for older adults (AGS 2018 Beers Criteria). Additionally, the STOPP (Screening Tool of Older Persons' potentially inappropriate Prescriptions) and START (Screening Tool to Alert doctors to Right Treatment) address similar concerns.
- The medication classes commonly associated with delirium include tricyclic antidepressants, anticholinergics, benzodiazepines, corticosteroids, H_2-receptor antagonists, sedative hypnotics, anticonvulsants, antiparkinsonian drugs, sympathomimetics, anti-inflammatories, and antineoplastic drugs.
- Ideal medications for use with patients experiencing or predisposed to delirium include medications with low toxicity, minimal anticholinergic effect, short half-life, minimal effect on cardiovascular and respiratory systems, and no or negligible effect on seizure threshold.

Expectations for Neuropsychological Assessment Results

A wide variety of medical conditions can lead to the development of delirium. Additionally, individuals with reduced cognitive reserve are typically more susceptible. Consequently, in addition to formal bedside examination, whenever possible, the clinician should also obtain historical information regarding symptom development and collateral reports regarding premorbid functioning and prior neurologic/ medical history.

- *Intelligence/Achievement* Patients typically display significant declines in intellectual function during delirium. After resolution, some patients return to baseline whereas others may experience substantial decline in fluid aspects of intelligence due to persistent cognitive impairments.
- *Attention/Concentration* Patients have significant difficulty sustaining attention but may have moments of clarity with intact basic attention. Patients are often highly distractible. Concentration is typically moderate to severely impaired, whereas with dementia basic attention is often unaffected or less of a factor in causing cognitive impairments.
- *Processing Speed* Moderate to severely impaired. Patients may experience periods of lucidity in which they are able to carry on conversations and perform overlearned tasks and activities with no apparent difficulty. However, deficits are often obvious during formal examination.

- *Language* Fluent aphasia may be present in some forms of delirium. Some patients may become mute or display pronounced dysnomia with paraphasic errors. Large or strategic lesions that cause specific language syndromes may also contribute to delirium. Consequently, it can be difficult to rule out or rule in delirium in patients who are aphasic post stroke. Thus, assessment of sleep-wake cycle, arousal consistency, and behavior is often more informative.

- *Visuospatial* Commonly affected. Patients often have difficulty copying complex figures, clock drawings, and the like. Due to the severity of attentional impairments and executive dysfunction, it is often difficult to discern if a true spatial or form perception impairment exists.

- *Memory* Disorientation to time and place is common, although orientation to self is rarely affected. Memory is typically impaired and compounded by the consequences of severe impairments in attention and concentration. Memories may become mixed up or blend with transient delusional beliefs resulting in confabulation. Following resolution of delirium, some patients are completely amnestic whereas others may have "islands" of intact memory for specific experiences.

- *Executive Functions* Always impaired, commonly with obvious impairments in mental flexibility, reasoning, and judgment. Thought patterns are typically disorganized, difficult to follow, and may follow linear or literal patterns. Patients often display confabulation, circumstantiality, flight of ideas, concrete reasoning, perseveration, poor initiation, and are often unaware of their difficulties (i.e., anosognosia).

- *Sensorimotor Functions* Changes in reflexes and muscle tone may be apparent on physical examination. Some patients are so impaired that they are unable to coordinate pencil and pen use. Intention tremor is often observed, whereas resting tremor is less common but not unusual. Patient lethargy, somnolence, distractibility, impulsivity, and or irritability often make it difficult or impossible to complete a reliable motor and sensory examination. Perceptual disturbances are quite common, including misperceptions and *illusions*. Visual hallucinations are most common in delirium, but auditory, tactile, and visceral hallucinations can occur as well. Gustatory and olfactory hallucinations are less common but can occur with focal lesions or seizures.

- *Emotion and Personality* Emotional lability and dramatic changes in personality or emotional expression are common. Patients may be hyperactive or hypoactive or may vacillate between the two. Individuals with hypoactive delirium sometimes go unnoticed or may be mislabeled as unmotivated, depressed, lazy, or intentionally uncooperative. Hallucinations and delusions may not be present, but when present, they will typically be fragmented, non-systematic, and fluctuating during the course of hours or days. This is unlike schizophrenia, in which symptoms remain more consistent over time. The severity of thought disturbance can range between tangentially and circumstantiality to loose associations.

- *Symptom and Performance Validity* It can be extremely difficult to examine and reliably test a patient with delirium. Although this does not reflect an intentional attempt by the patient to mislead or obfuscate, the neuropsychologist will often recognize that scores are unreliable and may change dramatically from one assessment session to the next. Because of this, brief evaluations and basic screening measures are typically employed. It is rarely, if ever, appropriate to administer longer testing batteries to a patient with delirium. Assessment should primarily be used to track symptoms and monitor the effectiveness of interventions.

Considerations When Treating Patients with Delirium

- *Safety* Patients require 24-hour supervision and monitoring. Many are on an ICU or have one-on-one observers. Restraints and medical safety devices may be employed as a last resort when the patient represents a danger to self or others.

- *Driving* Patients are obviously unable to work or drive during a period of delirium. Typically, these activities are restricted even after resolution of the delirium, because persistent cognitive impairments and functional decline may still be present.

- *School/Vocational Training* Following the resolution of delirium, patients can be phased back into various activities depending on the residual impact of the medical event that caused the delirium. For example, an adolescent who recovers from delirium following substance intoxication may be able to return to normal activities whereas a peer with severe TBI may experience lifelong symptoms that require an Individualized Education Plan (IEP) and specific accommodations.

- *Capacity* Capacity concerns are common in patients with delirium. Some patients may remain capable of expressing basic preferences or desires, but they are often incapable of making complex, informed decisions while delirious. A temporary guardian and conservator or activation of a durable power of attorney is often recommended or required. It should be noted that formal documentation endorsed by the patient prior to the delirium remains legally binding, including advanced directives such as "do not resuscitate" requests.

- *Medications* Physicians typically eliminate anticholinergic and dopaminergic agents. Antipsychotic medications may decrease agitation, hallucinations, and promote normal sleep-wake cycles but should be avoided in acute neurologic injury such as stroke or brain injury due to the potential negative impact on long-term recovery. Anticonvulsants are sometimes helpful in withdrawal, seizure, and acute injury.

- *Family and Collateral Considerations* Dramatic changes in behavior and emotional lability can place tremendous strains on the patient's family and loved ones. Collaterals may not understand the reason for behavioral changes and confusion. They may argue with the patient or one another. Additionally, families may become understandably frustrated with medical providers when an etiology cannot be determined, or different clinicians provide varying or contradictory information. Patients are often amnestic for the delirium episode, which can also make it difficult for families to resolve conflicts or misunderstandings that occurred during the hospitalization and once the delirium has resolved.

- *Functional Issues* Patients are typically dependent on others for basic self-care and activities of daily living (ADLs). They are often unaware of functional declines and may make claims that they are ready to return to work, leave the hospital, or perform other advanced ADLs without assistance or oversight.

- *Rehabilitation Considerations* After medical stabilization, some patients meet criteria for inpatient rehabilitation, although they still remain delirious or acutely confused (e.g., TBI, stroke, polytrauma). If the delirium and ICU admission was lengthy, debility is common. Rehabilitation treatment consists of environmental management, as outlined previously. Nursing care, as well as physical, occupational, and speech therapy typically establish a structured daily routine in a controlled environment. Progressive improvement is often observed, but significant cognitive impairments may persist for weeks and months even after the primary medical conditions have been addressed (e.g., posttraumatic amnesia following severe TBI).

Considerations When Treating Select Populations with Delirium

Pediatrics

Children and/or adolescents who display uncooperative behavior or immature/poorly developed language skills may be misidentified as delirious. Evaluation of baseline functions should include the assessment of play/social interaction, as well as interview of parents and caregivers. Neuropsychologists should remain mindful that information from collateral sources may minimize behavioral and/or cognitive changes due to fear regarding the implications of the patient's condition. Children who require or have undergone transplant, are in treatment for cancer, have ongoing seizures, are on multiple medications, or have reduced cognitive and cerebral reserve are often at higher risk for delirium. Serial assessment is often helpful in identifying fluctuations in level or arousal, behavior, and sleep patterns.

Patients in Minimally Conscious States

By definition patients in coma or minimally conscious states cannot be diagnosed with delirium and a sizable percentage of patients who remain in these states eventually die. However, for those patients who do emerge a period of delirium is quite common and should be anticipated. As these states evolve the patient may display an unresponsiveness wakefulness syndrome in which they display some arousal but there is no evidence of environmental awareness. Patients may open their eyes, yawn, and regain fairly normal appearing sleep wake cycles which may give collaterals the impression that the patient has regained some level of conscious awareness despite the contrary (e.g., coma vigil). It is also important to note that while in these states underlying electrochemical and brain related activity often evolves although it may not be apparent on clinical exam. For example, patients in coma do not show evidence of sleep/wake cycles on EEG but after several days to weeks surviving in this condition changes in EEG patterns often occur. Psychologists are sometimes consulted during this period of recovery to (1) provide family support and education, (2) facilitate treatment as part of an interdisciplinary treatment team, and (3) track recovery. Common assessment scales used in this patient population include the Glasgow Coma Scale (see also Chapter 29, Traumatic Brain Injury), Coma Recovery Scale-Revised, Coma near Coma Scale, and Sensory Modality Assessment and Rehabilitation Technique. Physicians will often employ EEG, event-related potentials (ERPs), and neurologic examination to assess an individual's level of consciousness, whether there is seizure activity, and or to determine if brain death has occurred. The potential utility of functional neuroimaging in this patient population is still under study.

Overlapping Conditions That Are Forms of or Mimic Delirium

There are common terms used to describe specific types of delirium or conditions that mimic delirium but may not meet all criteria (e.g., AWS, posttraumatic amnesia, sundowning, postictal confusion). For example, during the postictal period, one patient may experience confusion, agitation, and emotional and cognitive changes reflective of a postictal delirium, whereas another patient may display only mild confusion and thus would not meet full delirium criteria. Not surprisingly, individuals with Lewy body dementia can be misdiagnosed with delirium as they sometimes experience hallucinations, sleep-wake cycle disturbances, and fluctuating attention and concentration. Furthermore, some, but not all patients with posttraumatic amnesia/confusion following moderate to severe TBI will meet full criteria for delirium.

Collateral Education and Support

Family education and support is especially critical because collaterals are often heavily relied on to provide reassurance and structure for the patient. In addition, helping collaterals understand and use techniques that increase the patient's participation with various treatments can often help staff avoid the use of more aggressive management methods (e.g., heavy sedation, restraints). Educating the family/ collaterals about environmental interventions can also facilitate and improve the overall quality and consistency of treatments aimed at modifying things that can exacerbate delirium or delay recovery.

Relevant Definitions

Asterixis A wrist tremor noticeable when the hands and arms are extended. Often referred to as a hand flapping tremor. Can be observed in liver failure but has been observed in other types of delirium as well (e.g., Wilson disease, metabolic encephalopathy).

Autonomic storms (aka autonomic hyperreflexia) A reaction of the autonomic nervous system to severe injury, metabolic disturbance, or overstimulation. Symptoms include high blood pressure, tachycardia, diaphoresis, and other signs of sympathetic hyperarousal. The most common cause is a spinal cord injury above T5, during which stimulation perceived as normal in a healthy individual may generate an excessive autonomic response in the patient. Other causes of autonomic storms include illicit substance use, medication side effects, and severe brain injury.

Charles Bonnet Syndrome A term used to describe visual release hallucinations that occur in some people who have partial or complete loss of sight. Hallucinations can be vivid, complex, and well formed. The perception of faces, small objects or people (Lilliputian), patterns, images, and cartoons are common. Patients are aware that these are "not real," which helps distinguish them from other types of hallucinations.

Encephalopathy A disorder or disease of the brain characterized by significant global cognitive dysfunction. The term can be used to describe both reversible/acute and chronic/permanent conditions. Consequently, in medical literature, it has been used to describe a wide variety of brain disorders with very different etiologies, prognoses, and implications (see also Chapter 23, Central Nervous System Infections.).

Hepatic encephalopathy A type of delirium that occurs as the result of liver failure/dysfunction. When left untreated, it typically leads to coma and then death. When the liver begins to fail, toxic substances such as ammonia accumulate in the bloodstream. This condition is commonly treated with lactulose or other drugs that suppress the production of toxic substances in the intestine.

Hypernatremia An electrolyte disturbance in which sodium concentration in the serum is abnormally high (above 145 mmol/L). Typically caused by dehydration or conditions that result in excessive water loss (e.g., diarrhea, gastroenteritis), hypernatremia can cause cerebral dehydration resulting in subsequent delirium.

Hyponatremia An electrolyte disturbance in which sodium concentration in the serum falls below 135 mmol/L. It commonly occurs when water accumulates in the body at a faster rate than it can be excreted (e.g., polydipsia, congestive heart failure, syndrome of inappropriate antidiuretic hormone [SIADH]). The condition can lead to cerebral edema. Approximately 25% of cases are postoperative.

Illusions (misperceptions) Misinterpretations of real stimuli.

Neuroleptic malignant syndrome (NMS) A rare complication following neuroleptic use marked by muscle rigidity, pallor, dyskinesia, hyperthermia, incontinence, unstable blood pressure, tachycardia, and pulmonary congestion. Treatment requires discontinuation of neuroleptics, intravenous hydration, and close monitoring of vital signs and mental status.

Sepsis A broad term used to describe a serious infection in the bloodstream or body tissues. It can be caused by many types of microscopic disease-causing organisms (e.g., bacteria, viruses, fungi). Sepsis is sometimes referred to as bacteremia, septicemia, and/or septic syndrome. Severe sepsis refers to a systemic infection coupled with organ dysfunction and has been most commonly associated with white matter and blood-brain barrier compromise. Ischemic and hemorrhagic lesions are observable on MRI in approximately 10% of patients, whereas postmortem studies have revealed ischemic lesions in the majority of cases.

Serotonin syndrome Typically caused by the conjoint use of multiple serotonergic agents. In the early stages, it can be marked by mental status changes, agitation, myoclonus, hyperreflexia, diaphoresis, tremor, diarrhea, incoordination, and fever. If left untreated and medications continue, death can occur. Treatment requires the discontinuation of all serotonergic drugs and close monitoring with an expectation for improvement within 24 hours.

Delirium and Disorders of Consciousness Questions

NOTE: Questions 17, 77, and 125 on the First Full-Length Practice Examination, Questions 35, 75, and 114 on the Second Full-Length Practice Examination, Questions 7, 28, 84, and 125 on the Third Full-Length Practice Examination, and Questions 19, 44, 87, and 109 on the Fourth Full-Length Practice Examination are from this chapter.

1. Which of the following represent the most common features of serotonin syndrome?

   (a) tremor, diarrhea, diaphoresis   (c) tremor, confusion, visual impairments

   (b) rigidity, hyperthermia, confusion   (d) metallic taste, hyperthermia, confusion

2. A physician's note indicates that the patient you have been consulting on is currently displaying signs of delirium tremens (DTs). What combination of primary clinical features would you specifically expect to observe on exam?

   (a) resting tremor, agitation, diaphoresis

   (b) hallucinations, tachycardia, tremor

   (c) confusion, autonomic hyperactivity, hallucinations

   (d) delusions, severe anxiety, intention tremor

3. You are consulted to evaluate a 10-year-old boy recently admitted to the inpatient rehabilitation unit. Acute medical history indicates that he was originally admitted to the hospital following a bicycle accident in which he sustained a compound femur fracture. He also developed severe sepsis following wound infection that resolved after two weeks and prior to the rehabilitation admission. On examination, he displays impairments in sustained attention and memory, but is appropriately

oriented for his age. Assuming that the child was cognitively normal prior, what is the most likely reason for these persistent impairments?

(a) sepsis-related meningitis

(c) cerebral edema

(b) sepsis-related encephalitis

(d) ischemic lesions

4. An agitated 45-year-old patient who experienced a ruptured aneurysm one week ago is still on the ICU. He develops new symptoms of fever, increased blood pressure, and stiffness in his extremities over the weekend. Which of the following would you want to explore first?

(a) hyponatremia

(c) changes in medication

(b) stroke extension

(d) increased intracranial pressure

5. A patient with a known history of dementia is admitted to the hospital with sudden-onset hallucinations, agitation, and recent falls. What medication could result in these types of symptoms?

(a) levodopa

(c) Aricept

(b) Namenda

(d) Ritalin

6. You are assessing a 54-year-old woman who underwent embolization of an anterior communicating artery aneurysm nine months ago. Family is reporting numerous safety concerns due to impulsivity and poor safety awareness. During the interview she indicates that she had a surgery but that she is fine now and her family is being overprotective. She wants to get back to living on her own, working, and driving as soon as possible. Assuming that neuropsychological assessment confirms the presence of moderate to severe executive dysfunction, what type of intervention/approach to treatment would not be indicated?

(a) activity based

(c) self-evaluation based

(b) Rogerian based

(d) adaptation based

7. You are consulted to evaluate a 17-year-old girl who sustained multiple pelvic and leg fractures as the result of being hit by a car. She was described as alert and oriented at the scene. A CT scan of the head was normal in the emergency room, and there was no evidence of confusion during neurologic examination. However, on the day following orthopedic surgery for repair of long bone and pelvic fractures, the patient clearly displays symptoms consistent with delirium. Among the following which is the most likely etiology?

(a) cerebral fat emboli

(c) sepsis

(b) undiagnosed brain injury

(d) hypernatremia

8. What is the primary difference between hallucinations due to delirium versus hallucinations due to schizophrenia?

(a) Hallucinations in schizophrenia are more often visual.

(b) Hallucinations in schizophrenia are more bizarre.

(c) Hallucinations in delirium vacillate between visual, tactile, and auditory.

(d) Hallucinations in delirium are typically nonsystematic.

9. A patient presents to your outpatient office with a shuffling gait and slow body movements. The neuropsychological profile reveals rapid forgetting, pronounced dysnomia, and executive dysfunction. The patient's wife also reports that for the past 6 months, at different times of day, the patient has been seeing people who have been long dead or animals running in the house that are not actually there. Despite these symptoms, she denies significant fluctuations in arousal. This presentation raises the highest concern regarding what possible condition?

(a) sundowning

(c) dementia with delirium

(b) Lewy body dementia

(d) medication side effects

10. One hour after experiencing a grand mal seizure, a 10-year-old boy continues to display agitation, impulsivity, inattention, emotional lability, and confusion. This is best described as ____.

(a) encephalopathy due to kindling

(c) postictal delirium

(b) delirium due to kindling

(d) interictal dementia

11. Delirium following discontinuation of long-term benzodiazepines is most similar to withdrawal from ____.

(a) cocaine

(c) opiates

(b) alcohol

(d) narcotics

12. Subsyndromal delirium is more likely to develop over several weeks in a patient ____.

(a) status post hip surgery

(c) on peritoneal dialysis

(b) on CPAP

(d) with a history of seizures

13. You are consulted to see an 8-year-old boy on the neuro ICU. He sustained a near drowning with severe hypoxic brain injury three weeks ago. Medical records and examination indicate that he is able to open his eyes and will sometimes visually track things in the room. However, he does not follow commands, respond to pain, or display environmental awareness. This is most accurately referred to as ____?

(a) delirium

(c) locked-in syndrome

(b) akinetic mutisim

(d) coma vigil

14. A 35-year-old woman presents to your office with complaints of persistent memory problems after a hospitalization three months ago. No records are available but she explains that she developed a bad headache, visual hallucinations, and increasing confusion over several days. She does not recall being taken to the hospital. She denies any other medical issues with the exception of high blood pressure while she was on birth control and smoking regularly (she has quit since the hospitalization). She denies any changes in motor or sensory function currently. Based on this limited information, which condition is most likely to have resulted in this hospitalization?

(a) partial complex seizures

(b) posterior reversible encephalopathy syndrome

(c) anterior communicating artery aneurysm rupture

(d) normal pressure hydrocephalus

15. A 67-year-old woman is hospitalized with distractibility, sleep-wake cycle disturbances, and frequent falls. What other clinical features or historical information would be most useful in the differential diagnosis of delirium versus Lewy body dementia?

(a) Parkinsonian gait

(c) Capgras syndrome

(b) Lilliputian hallucinations

(d) visuospatial impairments

Delirium and Disorders of Consciousness Answers

1. **A—tremor, diarrhea, diaphoresis** *In the early stages, serotonin syndrome is often marked by tremor and diarrhea. As it continues, diaphoresis, confusion, and increased anxiety can occur. Cognitive and visual impairments are more representative of anticholinergic side effects, along with dry mouth, constipation, and urinary retention. Marked rigidity, hyperthermia, and confusion are signs of possible NMS. A side effect of some medications is a metallic taste in the mouth, but this does not often occur along with confusion.*

   Reference: Perry, P. G., & Wilborn, C. A. (2012). Serotonin syndrome versus neuroleptic malignant syndrome: A contrast of causes, diagnoses, and management. *Annals of Clinical Psychiatry, 24*(2), 155–162.

2. **C—confusion, autonomic hyperactivity, hallucinations** *Despite overuse in the literature and medical records, DTs only occur in 5–10% of patients with AWS. Although all of the symptoms listed can be observed in DTs, C is the best answer because they are the primary symptoms required for a diagnosis of DTs.*

   Reference: Eyer, F., Schuster, T., Felgenhauer, N., Pfab, R., Strubel, T., Saugel, B., & Zilker, T. (2011). Risk assessment of moderate to severe alcohol withdrawal—Predictors for seizures and delirium tremens in course of withdrawal. *Alcohol and Alcoholism, 46*(4), 427–433.

3. **D—ischemic lesions** *Severe sepsis has been most commonly associated with white matter and blood-brain barrier compromise. Ischemic and hemorrhagic lesions are observable on MRI in approximately 10% of patients, whereas postmortem studies have revealed ischemic lesions in the majority of cases.*

   References:
   (a) Bridges, E., McNeill, M. M., & Munro, N. (2017). Research in review: Advancing critical care practice. *American Journal of Critical Care, 26*(1), 77–88.
   (b) Iwashyna, T.J ., Ely, E. W., Smith, D. M., & Langa, K. M. (2010). Long-term cognitive impairment and functional disability among survivors of severe sepsis. *Journal of the American Medical Association, 304*(16), 1787–1794.
   (c) Sobbi, S. C., & van den Boogaard, M. (2014). Inflammation biomarkers and delirium in critically ill patients: New insights? *Critical Care, 18*(3).

4. **C—changes in medication** *These are signs of NMS. There should be concern that a neuroleptic may have been started to address agitation, thus leading to these new symptoms. Hyponatremia would not be expected to cause stiffness or rigidity in all four extremities. Stroke extension and/ or increased intracranial pressure (ICP) alone would not be expected to result in this specific symptom cluster.*

   Reference: Perry, P. G., & Wilborn, C. A. (2012). Serotonin syndrome versus neuroleptic malignant syndrome: A contrast of causes, diagnoses, and management. *Annals of Clinical Psychiatry, 24*(2), 155–162.

5. **A—Levodopa** *As the condition progresses, patients with Parkinson's disease often require higher and higher doses of dopaminergic agents to obtain symptom relief. In some cases, this can result in delirium marked by hallucinations, confusion, and increased agitation. Although Namenda and Aricept are used to treat dementia, they do not result in these side effects. Ritalin could increase agitation, but hallucinations are uncommon, and this medication is not often used in the treatment of dementia.*

Reference: Kennedy, K. A., & Ryan, M. (2009). Neurotoxic effects of pharmaceutical agents III: Neurological agents. In M. R. Dobbs (Ed.), *Clinical neurotoxicology: Syndromes, substances, environments* (pp. 358–371). Philadelphia, PA: Saunders and Elsevier.

6. **B—Rogerian based** *For individuals with anosagnosia interventions aimed at improving the patient's intellectual, emergent, and anticipatory awareness have the best potential for benefit. However, depending on the severity of self-awareness deficits these interventions have variable success. Rogerian based methods are person centered and nondirective, which would be unlikely to help someone who does not recognize their own impairments and is not motivated to learn or change behavior.*

Reference: Bechtold, K. T., & Hosey, M. M. (2018). Consciousness: Disorders, assessment, and intervention. In Morgan, J. E., & Ricker, J. H. (Eds.). *Textbook of clinical neuropsychology* (2nd ed., pp. 332–350). New York, NY: Taylor and Francis.

7. **A—cerebral fat emboli** *Can occur following long bone fracture and joint arthroplasty, often resulting in delirium or mental status changes. Considering the injury parameters provided, an undiagnosed brain injury is unlikely in this case. Additionally, several days would be required for sepsis to develop. Finally, hyponatremia can occur following surgery, whereas hypernatremia is uncommon postoperatively.*

References:
(a) Banerjee, A., Girard, T. D., & Pandharipande, P. (2011). The complex interplay between delirium, sedation, and early mobility during critical illness: Applications in the trauma unit. *Current Opinion in Anaesthesiology, 24*(2), 195–201.
(b) Cox, G., Tzioupis, C., Calori, G. M., Green, J., Seligson, D., & Giannoudis, P. V. (2011). Cerebral fat emboli: A trigger of post-operative delirium. *Injury, International Journal of the Care of the Injured, 42*(Suppl 4), S6–S10.

8. **D—Hallucinations in delirium are typically nonsystematic.** *In schizophrenia, hallucinations are more often auditory. Bizarre hallucinations can occur in both schizophrenia and delirium. Although a variety of hallucinations can occur in delirium and schizophrenia, it is rare for them to vacillate between visual, tactile, and auditory in one individual.*

Reference: Trzepacz, P. T., & Meagher, D. J. (2009). Neuropsychiatric aspects of delirium. In S. C. Yudofsky & R. E. Hales (Eds.), *Textbook of neuropsychiatry and behavioral neurosciences* (pp. 445–518). Washington, DC: American Psychiatric Publishing.

9. **B—Lewy body dementia** *Patients with Lewy body dementia often experience recurrent visual hallucinations which can assist in differentiating the condition from Alzheimer's disease. Sundowning can occur in patients with dementia but is typically a night time or near night time phenomena. There is no evidence in the case report regarding fluctuations in the patient's level of arousal or a pattern as to when the hallucinations occur. Thus, delirium and/or iatrogenic medication side effects is less likely.*

References:
(a) Finney, G. R. & Rusovici, D. (2011). Lewy body dementia. In C. Noogle, R. S. Dean, & A. M. Horton (Eds.), *The encyclopedia of neuropsychological disorders* (pp. 426–427). New York, NY: Springer Publishing Company
(b) Trzepacz, P. T., & Meagher, D. J. (2009). Neuropsychiatric aspects of delirium. In S. C. Yudofsky & R. E. Hales (Eds.), *Textbook of neuropsychiatry and behavioral neurosciences* (pp. 445–518). Washington, DC: American Psychiatric Publishing.

10. **C—postictal delirium** *Also referred to as postictal confusion, the delirium typically lasts 5–30 minutes following seizure but can persist for longer periods depending on the seizure type and severity. Interictal refers to the period of time between seizures but would not apply here. Kindling may indeed occur following seizure but A and B would not be good descriptions of this phenomena.*

References:
(a) Kaufman, D. M. (2007). *Epilepsy: Clinical neurology for psychiatrists.* Philadelphia, PA: Saunders Elsevier.
(b) Luders, H., Amina, S., Bailey, C., Baumgartner, C., Benbadis, S., Bermeo, A., . . . Tsuji, S. (2014). Proposal: different types of alteration and loss of consciousness in epilepsy. *Epilepsia, 55*(8), 1140–1144.

11. **B—alcohol** *Benzodiazepines and alcohol target similar receptors. Not surprisingly, discontinuation of long-term benzodiazepines results in withdrawal symptoms similar to withdrawal from alcohol. This is also why long-acting benzodiazepines are typically used to treat AWS.*

References:
(a) Clegg, A., & Young, J. B. (2011). Which medications to avoid in people at risk of delirium: a systematic review. *Age and Aging, 40,* 23–29.
(b) Rothberg, M. B., Herzig, S. J., Pekow, P. S., Avrunin, J., Lagu, T., & Lindenauer, P. K. (2013). Association between sedating medications and delirium in older inpatients. *Journal of the American Geriatrics Society, 61,* 923–930.

12. **C—on peritoneal dialysis** *Slow onset subsyndromal delirium is more likely to develop in patients with systemic illness and chronic medical conditions such as renal disease. As the disease progresses or if it is managed improperly complications ensue. Delirium can occur in patients shortly after surgery but not typically weeks later unless other complications occur (e.g., fall injury, pain medication side effects). Seizures can result in postictal confusion but rarely if ever result in persistent delirium unless there are complications (e.g., status epilepticus, respiratory arrest with hypoxic brain injury). Individuals with sleep apnea are at higher risk for developing cognitive impairment, but CPAP is not associated with risk for delirium.*

References:
(a) Meagher, D., Adamis, D., Trzepacz, P., & Leonard, M. (2012). Features of subsyndromal and persistent delirium. *British Journal of psychiatry: the journal of mental science, 200*(1), 37–44.
(b) Meagher, D., O'Regan, N., Ryan, D., Connolly, W., Boland, E., O'Caoimhe, R., . . . Timmons, S. (2014). Frequency of delirium and subsyndromal delirium in an adult acute hospital population. *British Journal of Psychiatry, 205,* 478–485.
(c) O'Regan, N. A., Fitzgerald, J. M., Molly, D. W., & Timmons, S. (2014). Early detection of delirium: Prodromal features. In Alonso, R. (Ed.). *Delirium diagnosis, management, and prevention* (pp. 35–67). New York, NY: Nova Science Publishers.

13. **D—Coma vigil** *Patients in coma or minimally conscious states cannot be diagnosed with delirium. Vegetative state is an older term that is fading from use secondary to its potential for misinterpretation and anxiety-provoking impact on families. Locked in syndrome occurs when there is focal injury to the brainstem (usually vascular lesion in the ventral pons due to basilar artery occlusion) and the patient cannot move but retains conscious awareness and volitional vertical gaze and eyelid movement. As coma and minimally conscious states evolve the patient may move into what some refer to as an unresponsiveness wakefulness syndrome in which they display some arousal but there is no evidence of environmental awareness. Patients may open their eyes, yawn, and regain fairly normal appearing sleep wake cycles, which may give the impression that the patient has regained some level of conscious awareness despite the contrary. This is commonly referred to as coma vigil.*

Reference: Bruno, M., Vanhaudenhuyse, A., Thibault, A., Moonen, G., & Laureys, S. (2011). From unresponsive wakefulness to minimally conscious PLUS and functional locked-in-syndromes: Recent advances in our understanding of disorders of consciousness. *Journal of Neurology, 258*(7), 1373–1384.

14. **B—posterior reversible encephalopathy syndrome** *PRES is presumed to be due to vasogenic edema secondary to hypertension and dysregulation of the cerebral vasculature. If it is identified promptly some patients have experienced good overall recovery while others complain of persistent symptoms. Aneurysm rupture does not develop over several days and is typically associated with a "thunderclap" type headache. Individuals with NPH often present with complaints of headache, confusion, urinary incontinence, and gait disturbance but not hallucinations. Additionally, NPH is uncommon in young adults and hypertension is not a significant risk factor. Finally an individual with a history of partial complex seizures would likely report auras and confusion would likely occur following seizures as opposed to progressively worsening over several days.*

References:

(a) Fischer, M., & Schmutzhard, E. (2017). Posterior reversible encephalopathy syndrome. *Journal of Neurology, 264*(8),1608–1616.

(b) Gao, B., Lyu, C., Lerner, A., & McKinney, A.M. (2018). Controversy of posterior reversible encephalopathy syndrome: what have we learnt in the last 20 years? *Journal of Neurology, Neurosurgery & Psychiatry, 89*(1),14–20.

15. **A—Parkinsonian gait** *Lilliputian hallucinations are more common following acute neurologic events impacting posterior structures (e.g., brainstem, occipital lobes, cerebral peduncles, medial thalamus). Capgras syndrome is relatively rare but can occur in both delirium and dementia and thus would not assist with the differential. Visuospatial disturbances are common in both delirium and Lewy body dementia (LBD). Although parkinsonian symptoms can occur in both LBD and delirium, its presence in this case should raise more concern regarding the latter.*

References:

(a) Ferman, T., Boeve, B., Smith, G., Lin, S., Silber, M., Pedraza, O., . . . Dickson, D. (2011). Inclusion of RBD improves the diagnostic classification of dementia with Lewy Bodies. *Neurology, 77*(9), 875–882.

(b) Ferman, T. J., Smith, G. E., Kantarci, K., Boeve, B. F., Pankratz, V. S., Dickson, D. W., . . . Uitti, R. (2013). Nonamnestic mild cognitive impairment progresses to dementia with Lewy bodies. *Neurology, 81*(23), 2032–2038.

Recommended Readings

American Psychiatric Association. (2013). *Diagnostic and statistical manual of mental disorders* (5th ed.). Arlington, VA: American Psychiatric Publishing.

Bechtold, K. T. & Hosey, M. M. (2018). Consciousness: Disorders, assessment, and intervention. In Morgan, J. E., & Ricker, J. H. (Eds.). *Textbook of clinical neuropsychology* (2nd ed.). New York, NY: Taylor and Francis.

McCoy, T. H., Jr., Hart, K. L., & Perlis, R. H. (2017). Characterizing and predicting rates of delirium across general hospital settings. *General Hospital Psychiatry, 46*, 1–6.

Turco, R., Bellelli, G., Morandi, A., Gentile, S., & Trabucchi, M. (2013). The effect of poststroke delirium on short-term outcomes of elderly patients undergoing rehabilitation. *Journal of Geriatric Psychiatry and Neurology, 26*(2), 63–68.

28 Hypoxic and Ischemic Brain Injury

William Garmoe and Sid Dickson

Definition

Broadly, anoxic/hypoxic damage in the brain results secondary to conditions that affect the cardiac and/or respiratory systems, reducing or preventing oxygen delivery to the brain. Deficient oxygen supply to the brain can result from a reduced amount or concentration of oxygen in the blood or from deficient perfusion of blood to the brain. For the purposes of this chapter, anoxia/hypoxia is defined as a lack of or insufficient supply of oxygen circulating to tissue in the presence of adequate blood flow (see Table 28.1).

These terms may be confusing because they are used variably in the literature. Anoxia and hypoxia are often used interchangeably. Further, conditions such as hypoxemia can lead to hypoxia, and they are not always distinguished from one another by authors. In their purest presentations, anoxia/hypoxia and ischemia may produce somewhat different neuropathology, but, for most cases in which the brain sustains marked disruption of oxygen supply, both processes become involved and thus the term *ischemic-hypoxic encephalopathy* is often used. In this chapter, anoxia/hypoxia and ischemia are considered together unless otherwise noted.

A range of medical conditions can result in hypoxic/ischemic damage to the brain, including but not limited to the conditions listed in Table 28.2. It is important not to equate the medical condition with anoxic/hypoxic damage. For example, out-of-hospital cardiac arrest results in much higher rates of brain damage and death than when arrest occurs in the hospital and receives rapid medical response. Rapid medical response for many of the conditions listed in 28.2 may ameliorate damage to the brain.

TABLE 28.1 Key Terms and Definitions Related to Anoxia and Hypoxia

Anoxia	Most typically defined as a complete lack of oxygen in arterial blood, due to a profound and sudden medical event such as cardiac arrest or loss of perfusion pressure (e.g., attempted suicide by hanging, strangulation).
Hypoxia	A deficient amount of oxygen availability in the blood supply to the brain. It is distinguished from anoxia, but the two are often used interchangeably in the literature and medical reports.
Hypoxemia	Another term commonly used to refer to reduced *partial pressure of oxygen* in arterial blood (below 60 mm Hg). Hypoxemia can lead to hypoxia.
Ischemia	The failure of perfusion of blood through the cerebral vessels to tissue (e.g., lack of blood supply). Both ischemia and anoxia are usually involved in cases of profound and sudden cardiac arrest.

Neuropathology

Prevalence estimates of cognitive impairment following conditions such as cardiac arrest range widely (e.g., 6–100%). Several factors complicate attempts to characterize patterns of neuropathology and cognitive dysfunction due to hypoxic/ischemic conditions. These include:

- the broad range of conditions that can cause hypoxic-ischemic damage (see Table 28.2)
- multi-system/multi-organ complications that often occur and that may exacerbate encephalopathy
- comorbid medical conditions that may result in compromised cardiovascular and cerebrovascular functioning prior to the major anoxic/hypoxic event
- cognitive impairment from milder hypoxic/ischemic states that may not always be recognized in the hospital setting
- methodology and operational definitions of key terms such as hypoxia that vary across studies

The brain is highly dependent on a consistent supply of blood, oxygen, and glucose and consumes these at levels disproportionate to its mass relative to other parts of the body. Additionally, neurons lack the capacity to store energy and oxygen in ways similar to cells in other parts of the body. Oxygenation of the blood is the result of a complex process involving hemoglobin concentration and oxygen saturation.

- Partial pressure of arterial oxygen (PaO_2) in healthy adults at sea level is typically 95–100 mm Hg.
- When this level rapidly drops, complex cognitive processes such as memory and judgment become impaired.
- Homeostatic protective mechanisms are triggered when PaO_2 or perfusion is disrupted, and these are effective within certain parameters:
  - The nervous system responds to hypoxic states by increasing cerebral blood flow up to as much as 400%.
  - Autoregulatory response to a reduction or loss of perfusion pressure involves several mechanisms, including dilatation of blood vessels to maintain flow.
- Beyond a certain point, protective measures are insufficient to prevent central nervous system (CNS) injury.
- The brain depletes energy sources within several minutes of onset of complete ischemia, although conditions such as hypothermia can extend that period.

These processes seem to differ for chronic obstructive pulmonary disease (COPD) and other types of advanced pulmonary illness, which are characterized by persistent, gradual reduction in arterial oxygen levels and elevated carbon dioxide levels. In such individuals, arterial oxygen partial pressure may

TABLE 28.2 Medical Conditions That May Cause Hypoxic-Ischemic Brain Damage

Acute Conditions	• Cardiac Arrest (especially out-of-hospital events) • Acute respiratory distress syndrome (ARDS) (especially onset out of hospital) • Carbon monoxide poisoning • Suffocation, drowning, hanging • Massive blood loss due to trauma • Prolonged seizures • Anesthesia accidents in surgical procedures
Chronic Conditions	• Chronic obstructive pulmonary disease (COPD) • Obstructive sleep apnea (OSA) • Asthma • Conditions that paralyze the respiratory system (e.g., amyotrophic lateral sclerosis, myasthenia gravis, etc.)

gradually decline to levels which, if sustained acutely, produce rapid onset of coma or marked cognitive impairment. Similarly, high-altitude climbers can acclimate (e.g., through gradual acclimatization to increasing altitudes) to lower oxygen saturation, although not necessarily without physiologic and cognitive effects.

Neuropathological changes from hypoxia/ischemia are consistent with the mechanism of insult; brain regions with high metabolic demands and those at the distal end of cerebral arteries (in particular, *watershed regions*) are more vulnerable. Brain regions that show high vulnerability to hypoxia/ischemia include:

- neocortex (layers 3, 5, 6)
- hippocampus (especially pyramidal cells in CA1)
- basal ganglia (striatum, globus pallidus)
- cerebellar regions (Purkinje cells)
- visual cortex
- thalamus

There are additional more generalized processes, which lead to damage throughout the brain. A common response of the brain following anoxic/hypoxic insult is edema. Additionally, when neurons are damaged a complex cascade of metabolic events can ensue. These can lead to *Wallerian degeneration*, accelerated *apoptosis*, and ultimately atrophy. For example, a major output destination for the hippocampus is the fornix. When hippocampal axons degenerate, the fornix atrophies. Atrophy and degeneration are post-acute processes that evolve over the course of many weeks and months.

Neuroimaging also shows time-dependent vulnerability to damage in specific regions, and lesions often evolve over weeks or months.

- Early neuroimaging studies are variable, sometimes showing loss of distinction between white and gray matter in the cortex, but also often appearing normal.
- Basal ganglia and neocortex regions may show damage on neuroimaging soon after onset.
- Hippocampal damage may not be evident on imaging studies until days, weeks, or even months later.
- Diffuse atrophy may appear chronically but would not be expected acutely.
- White matter tracts appear to be generally preserved in hypoxia/ischemia, but they are vulnerable to carbon monoxide poisoning.

Hippocampal damage has historically been considered the hallmark feature of hypoxic damage, but reviews of published cases with neuroimaging data have shown that (a) hippocampal damage is frequently not noted and (b) when damage is visible, it is usually present in multiple brain regions. One review showed that watershed cortex and the basal ganglia were both more frequently damaged than the hippocampus (Caine & Watson, 2000). The hippocampus was the sole affected structure in only 18% of reported cases.

Hypoxia/ischemia triggers a cascade of neuronal cellular processes that are multifaceted, time-dependent, and neurotoxic.

- Most energy required by neurons is derived from hydrolysis of *adenosine triphosphate (ATP)*.

- The brain has almost no inherent energy stores (in contrast to other tissue) and thus is critically dependent on uninterrupted flow of oxygen and glucose.
- A sudden loss of cerebral perfusion or anoxia/hypoxia causes a critical shortage of the oxygen and glucose supply to neurons and, if not rapidly reversed, initiates processes that result in neuronal death.
- A series of secondary toxic processes are also triggered:
  - Sodium and calcium pumps fail, resulting in depolarization of the neuronal membrane and release of excessive levels of *glutamate*.
  - *Glutamate* is the most common excitatory neurotransmitter, but at excessive levels it becomes excitotoxic to neurons.
  - A further series of toxic effects are triggered that involve lactic acidosis from anaerobic metabolism, cytotoxic edema, free radical production, and others.
  - *Necrosis, Wallerian degeneration*, and *apoptosis* become factors as the pathology evolves.

Once circulation is effectively restored, there are additional potential sources of damage to the brain. The processes are not fully understood but include:

- *Secondary hypoxia* Following return of circulation, cerebral blood flow may go through a period of 30–50% reduction, resulting in a mismatch of oxygen requirements and blood flow.
- *Reperfusion Injury* Following reperfusion, several processes ensue that can cause further damage, including free radical formation, nitric oxide toxicity, additional *glutamate* release, edema and microhemorrhages, and impaired ability to remove toxic metabolites.

Carbon monoxide (CO) poisoning shows many of the same effects as other forms of hypoxia/ischemia, but there are notable differences in the pathologic process.

- Carbon monoxide is a gas that is present naturally in the environment but also results from combustion of man-made fuel (e.g., gasoline engine and furnace exhaust).
- Carbon monoxide has a very high affinity for binding with hemoglobin, forming carboxyhemoglobin (COHb).
- The effect is to displace oxygen binding sites on the red blood cells, resulting in hypoxia and acidosis.
- Once carboxyhemoglobin rises above 20–30% of total hemoglobin in the blood, acute effects are seen, and levels above 50% will result in coma and other severe CNS effects.
- It is not clear whether CO is directly toxic to neurons, but the most significant effects are very similar to what is seen following cardiac arrest.
- Carbon monoxide poisoning often results in delayed neurologic deterioration, which may occur 1 to 3 weeks after severe exposure. This is thought to be likely related to CO-mediated oxidative stress and cumulative toxic effects although the exact mechanisms are not well understood.
- Basal ganglia damage is common, contributing to the extrapyramidal features often seen following severe CO poisoning.
- Hippocampal atrophy and generalized brain atrophy (as measured by ventricle-to-brain ratio) may be seen months following injury.
- Neuropsychological deficits include attention, information processing, executive functioning, and verbal and nonverbal memory.

Epidemiology

Incidence rates for hypoxia/ischemia are extremely difficult to estimate, and reliable estimates are lacking. There are a range of conditions, both acute and chronic, that can result in hypoxia/ischemia. For example, approximately 356,000 individuals in the United States annually are treated by emergency personnel for out-of-hospital cardiac arrest (OHCA) with greater than 200,000 additional patients experiencing in-hospital cardiac arrest. While survival rates for OHCA are still low, improvements in emergency personnel training, larger numbers of individuals trained in CPR and use of defibrillators, and post-resuscitation protocols have resulted in significant gains in mortality and functional outcome in cases where effective circulation is rapidly restored. Nonetheless, large percentages of individuals continue to sustain anoxic/hypoxic injury, with up to 50% of survivors experiencing permanent brain damage. Additionally, it is not clear how many survivors of anoxia/hypoxia experience milder forms of cognitive impairment that go undetected in the hospital but may have functional implications at home and in the community.

Determinants of Severity

The effects of hypoxia/ischemia vary depending on the nature of the underlying condition that produced the disruption of oxygen supply to the brain and how rapidly the pathological process can be reversed. Hypoxia that does not involve collapse or cessation of functioning of the circulatory system will typically result in less neurocognitive and neurologic damage. It should also be noted that if hypoxia is not severe enough to disrupt consciousness, CNS damage is unlikely. Mild hypoxia that does not lead to loss of consciousness (for example, high-altitude climbing) may induce mild cognitive and motor impairment that would not be expected to have lasting effects, although some studies suggest possible persistence of mild changes (Ropper & Samuels, 2009). In general, the most severe cases result from sudden cardiac arrest or *acute respiratory distress syndrome* (ARDS). Loss of consciousness occurs very rapidly. Once the brain is deprived of oxygen for several minutes, damage progresses rapidly and, if the underlying condition is not quickly reversed, brain death or a persistent vegetative or minimally conscious state may result. Those who emerge from prolonged coma typically have lasting cognitive and functional disability (e.g., varying degrees of major neurocognitive disorder) and may also show extrapyramidal syndromes such as parkinsonism. Alternatively, when cardiac arrest or ARDS occurs in a hospital setting and receives rapid effective resuscitation and intense management there is much greater likelihood of preventing permanent damage to the brain.

Severity of chronic hypoxic/ischemic conditions from chronic disease states differs from that due to sudden onset events. Many individuals with chronic pulmonary disease may function, albeit in a compromised fashion, with blood oxygen levels that would produce rapid onset of coma were they to occur suddenly. *Obstructive sleep apnea* (OSA) and COPD are two examples of conditions in which hypoxia may result in neuropathological changes and cognitive impairment. However, these conditions also are often accompanied by other comorbidities such hypertension and cardiovascular disease, which complicate a clear understanding of the etiology of cognitive impairment.

Chronic Obstructive Pulmonary Disease

- Examples include emphysema, neuromuscular weakness, fibrosing lung disease
- Results in persistent respiratory acidosis with reduced arterial oxygen saturation and elevated carbon dioxide
- Cognitive deficits may not occur in mild cases that do not produce persistent hypoxia.

- Severe COPD often results in cognitive impairment, with lower scores on objective measures relative to less severely affected individuals.
- Positive-pressure ventilation with oxygen may improve cognitive functioning but not necessarily lead to a better quality of life or meaningful functional gains.

Obstructive Sleep Apnea

- Involves recurrent episodes of blood oxygen desaturation due to total (apnea) or partial (hypopnea) breathing cessation.
- Disrupts normal sleep architecture. Repeated hypoxic periods may result from drops in blood oxygen saturation.
- Oxygen desaturation may occur up to 100 times per hour.
- Neuroprotective vasodilatory response to hypoxia may be lacking.
- Severe sleep apnea has been associated with greater risk for white matter hyperintensities and cognitive impairment (learning and recent memory, executive abilities, psychomotor impairments associated with severe sleep apnea), but results are not consistent across studies.
- Older adults are more vulnerable to sleep-disordered breathing.
- Community-dwelling elderly women with sleep-disordered breathing show increased risk of cognitive impairment.
- Nasal continuous positive airway pressure (CPAP) for OSA
  - reduces episodes of breathing disruption
  - reduces oxygen desaturation during sleep
  - improves daytime sleepiness
  - may lead to improvement in only select areas of cognition presentation, disease course, and recovery

Presentation, Disease Course, and Recovery

Acute Hospitalization

Recovery Course

The recovery course from a hypoxic/ischemic event can be quite variable. More favorable outcomes are generally seen in patients who have had only a short period of impaired consciousness, regain purposeful motor movements, and have preserved memory within a few hours following resuscitation. Poor outcome has been associated with the following factors (when not accounted for by effects of intentional sedation):

- total Glasgow Coma Scale (GCS) score of 3–5 after 24 hours post-onset
- no pupillary response on day 3 post-injury
- sustained abnormal eye functions (e.g., nystagmus, dysconjugate gaze)
- lower cranial nerve/brainstem dysfunction (e.g., absent cough and gag reflexes)
- seizures or myoclonus
- alpha coma electroencephalogram pattern
- bilateral absence of somatosensory evoked potential on median nerve stimulation

In evaluating the patient in the acute recovery phase, it is important to be mindful of interventions, medications, and comorbid conditions, each of which can cause or contribute to encephalopathy, thus confusing or complicating the overall presentation. In adults, older age has been shown to negatively correlate with recovery. Inpatient rehabilitation is appropriate and can improve functioning and reduce subsequent care requirements; however, recovery curves in patients with severe hypoxic/ischemic injury are fairly flat, and return to independence is rarely achieved.

An uncommon but important syndrome sometimes seen following anoxia/hypoxia is delayed post-hypoxic leukoencephalopathy (DPHL). This is most commonly seen following CO poisoning but may occur due to any etiology producing prolonged hypo-oxygenation. The individual initially makes a good recovery from a neurologically impaired state and may even return home and back to work quickly. There then is abrupt onset of progressive neurologic decline typically involving parkinsonism or akinetic mutism with prominent cognitive impairment. A majority who survive show significant improvement but are left with lasting neurologic and cognitive impairment. Imaging studies typically show prominent white matter demyelination particularly in the frontal and parietal regions.

Assessment Methods

Assessment of the patient during acute, inpatient recovery will vary depending on the patient's level of functioning, ranging from base assessment of sensory and motoric responsiveness to more comprehensive neuropsychological screening and assessment. Instruments useful for evaluating individuals early in recovery (in acute care or early inpatient rehabilitation) and that focus on basic functioning include:

- GCS
- Coma Recovery Scale-Revised
- Coma–Near Coma Scale
- Rancho Los Amigos Levels of Cognitive Functioning

Instruments useful for structured basic assessment of mental status:

- Mini-Mental State Examination
- Orientation Log (O-Log)
- Cognitive Log (C-Log)
- Montreal Cognitive Assessment (MoCA)
- Cognistat

Assessment of individuals with higher cognitive functioning early in their recovery will typically include the Repeatable Battery for the Assessment of Neuropsychological Status (RBANS) as a standalone measure, or with supplemental measures added as part of a brief test battery.

Treatment

For comatose patients or those in a minimally responsive state, serial assessment of responsiveness and coma stimulation are indicated. Once a patient has emerged from the minimally responsive state, early behavioral and pharmacological management will need to be focused on addressing confusion and agitated behavior if present. During this phase, it is important to put emphasis on:

- frequent reorientation
- establishment of consistent daily routines
- use of short treatment sessions

- attending carefully to basic physiologic needs (e.g., nutrition, toileting, sleep, etc.)
- maintaining a quiet treatment environment and avoiding overstimulation

As recovery progresses, the attention deficits, distractibility, severe anterograde amnesia, and executive dysfunction that often emerge need to be addressed in order to ameliorate functional consequences in daily life. Rehabilitation generally involves focus on family training/education, teaching compensatory strategies, and or attempting to directly address areas of cognitive deficit.

Outpatient Rehabilitation

Recovery Course

Several studies have compared patterns of recovery from hypoxia/anoxia to traumatic brain injury (TBI). Recognizing that it is not possible to equate levels of severity between hypoxia/anoxia and TBI, some group patterns emerge:

- Amount of tissue loss is more critical in determining outcome than etiology (e.g., anoxia vs. TBI).
- Measures of memory correlate with hippocampal atrophy in both hypoxia/anoxia and TBI.
- Intelligence correlates with whole brain volume in both conditions.
- Individuals with hypoxia/anoxia have similar lengths of inpatient stay compared to TBI but show slower progress and poorer outcomes.
- Individuals with hypoxia/anoxia are more likely to be referred to residential care.
- Individuals with hypoxia/anoxia perform worse on all measures of functional outcome than those with TBI.
- Individuals with hypoxia/anoxia have significantly lower Functional Independence Measure (FIM) motor and cognitive gains relative to those with TBI.

Outpatient and post-acute brain injury rehabilitation is appropriate and may extend treatment gains from the inpatient setting. Treatment focuses on compensatory strategies, skill acquisition and building, independence in the home, and community reintegration. Family training and support is critical. There may be very significant differences between patient and family perspectives on how the individual with anoxic injury is functioning. Family members may experience feelings of isolation and caregiver burnout due to the lasting cognitive and behavioral changes that follow moderate and severe hypoxia/anoxia. Periods of respite care for the family can be crucial.

Assessment Methods

Initial computed tomography (CT) or magnetic resonance imaging (MRI) of the brain often does not reveal significant changes. Follow-up radiologic studies at a later date may reveal white matter changes, corpus callosum atrophy, cortical edema, cerebellar lesions, basal ganglia lesions, thalamic lesions, and/or hippocampal atrophy. These abnormalities often take weeks or months before they can be visualized on traditional scans.

Neuropsychological assessment during this phase will vary in breadth and depth, depending on the individual's level of functioning, and may serve multiple purposes, including:

- characterizing strengths and deficits and linking such patterns to daily functioning
- helping identify target goals for continued rehabilitation
- identifying the presence and severity of psychological disturbance (e.g., depression, anxiety) that may impact recovery and rehabilitation

- determining decisional capacity and need for supervision
- identifying areas for which accommodations will be needed in return to school and employment

Treatment

Appropriate treatment interventions will vary depending on the individual's level of functioning. For lower functioning patients, orientation, attention, and memory impairment are the major focus of cognitive rehabilitation. Physical and occupational therapy are often indicated for motor impairment due to damage to cerebellar and basal ganglia structures. Speech-language therapy will likely focus more on pragmatics and basic cognitive abilities because aphasia is less likely with anoxic injury. For higher functioning patients, an emphasis on evidenced-based treatments for attention, memory, processing speed, visuospatial deficits, and executive dysfunction is appropriate.

Outcomes

Outcome following hypoxia/ischemia depends on multiple factors, including initial severity, brain regions most severely damaged, age, and medical comorbidities.

- The most catastrophic cases may result in brain death or persistent minimally responsive states.
- Less severe cases show variable periods of coma, marked confusion in early recovery phase, and lasting significant cognitive impairment and/or dementia.
- High percentage of survivors (>30%) of sudden cardiac arrest and ARDS show generalized cognitive impairment. A higher percentage show specific/focal deficits in memory, attention, or processing speed.
- Changes in memory have been reported in more than 50% of survivors of severe hypoxia/ anoxia, and personality changes have been reported in nearly one third.
- Individuals with lasting cognitive and functional deficits often require extensive rehabilitation. Studies show that less than 50% of those who require rehabilitation regain full independence of daily functioning, but there is a great deal of variability in outcomes.
- Even when there is seemingly rapid and full neurologic recovery, a significant percentage of individuals display persistent mild cognitive deficits.

Expectations for Neuropsychological Assessment Results

Neuropsychological deficits following hypoxic/ischemic injury include impaired attention and memory, executive dysfunction, visuospatial deficits, and overall cognitive decline. Memory is the most commonly affected cognitive domain, but most individuals experience deficits in other areas as well.

- *Intelligence/Achievement* Hold tests are not typically affected, but overall scores may be reduced due to impairments in processing speed and efficiency, especially in pediatric populations.
- *Attention/Concentration* Gross confusion is often present very early in recovery. Impaired attention and concentration continue to be significant problems even as recovery progresses and may be a long-term issue. Distractibility is also often observed both early in recovery and over the long term.
- *Processing Speed* Often impaired, both cognitively and motorically.

- *Language* Formal language disorders are rarely seen, although in cases involving severe watershed damage transcortical aphasia or higher order language syndromes may be present.

- *Visuospatial* If watershed zones are affected, deficits can be noticeable. Cortical blindness or other severe visuospatial impairment variants have occurred following hypoxic/anoxic injury to posterior *watershed regions*. Lower performance on visuospatial tasks may also, in part, reflect slowed information processing.

- *Memory* Impairments in storage, capacity, and retrieval are common. In severe cases with bilateral hippocampal damage, a marked amnestic state may be evident. Pure amnestic syndromes are rare following anoxia/hypoxia, as cognitive impairment is typically more extensive due to diffuse cerebral injury. A subset of patients may have no identifiable memory impairment, but display motor or cognitive impairments in other domains (e.g., functions associated with *watershed regions*).

- *Executive Functions* May be minimally affected in milder cases, with the exception of executive aspects of attention or concentration. However, executive deficits are common and often very disabling in more severe cases. Many patients display orbitofrontal system dysfunction because this is a watershed region.

- *Sensorimotor Functions* The basal ganglia and cerebellum are at high risk for injury. Severe hypoxic injury can cause spastic quadriparesis, ataxia, parkinsonism syndromes, and other motor impairments/dysfunction, along with the cognitive changes associated with damage to those regions.

- *Emotion and Personality* Anosognosia (impaired self-awareness) is common early post injury and may persist as a long-term feature. Depression is commonly observed. Changes in self-regulation of emotions may occur due to medial temporal and frontal system injury. Behavioral dysregulation may be seen in more severe cases and may become a chronic feature.

- *Symptom and Performance Validity* Both performance and symptom validity measures should always be employed in the assessment of adults and school-aged children, regardless of injury severity, because reduced test engagement or response bias can occur in any individual patient.

Considerations when Treating Patients with Hypoxic and Ischemic Brain Injury

- *Level of Supervision* Varies but patients will likely have high supervision needs early in recovery due to memory and/or motor impairment.

- *Driving* Prognosis for return to driving is not good in severe cases, but may be possible with mild to moderate injuries and good recovery.

- *Work* Prognosis for return to prior type and level of work is unlikely in severe cases, but may be possible with mild injuries and good recovery. For individuals unable to return to competitive employment, alternative vocational or volunteer placements may be appropriate.

- *School/Vocational Training* Unlikely, but may be possible with mild injuries and good recovery. For students in grammar, middle, and high school, it is critical to involve the school and educational specialists as early as possible to plan for academic re-entry. This is both an important aspect of recovery and a legally mandated requirement (e.g., the schools are required to provide appropriate education for disabled students).

- *Capacity* Decisional capacity for medical, financial, and legal affairs will likely be severely limited early in recovery. Despite recovery, capacity may remain compromised due to memory impairment and executive dysfunction. Assessment of capacity is an important clinical and ethical matter. Legal standards for assessing capacity and the legal processes involved to determine competence vary across jurisdictions. It is important for neuropsychologists to understand the regulations that govern their respective institutions and jurisdictions and to become comfortable performing such assessments.

- *Psychological and Emotional Issues* Personality disturbance, agitation, and impaired self-awareness occurs frequently following severe anoxia/hypoxia; patients may be at risk for depression.

- *Severe Psychiatric Complications* Major psychiatric issues are common in severe cases, which may include behavioral dysregulation, major depression, and anxiety. Posttraumatic stress disorder (PTSD) may also be seen following milder hypoxia/anoxia and ARDS if there is recall of the traumatic event or critical care experience. PTSD is uncommon following severe hypoxia/anoxia/ARDS, unless the person regains consciousness and awareness during acute trauma care. New onset of frank psychotic disorders is less common.

- *Medications* Medications focusing on improving attention and memory may be administered, such as methylphenidate (e.g., Ritalin) other neurostimulants, or acetylcholinesterase inhibitors (e.g., Aricept), and N-methyl-D-aspartate (NMDA) receptor antagonists (e.g., Namenda). Selective serotonin reuptake inhibitors (SSRIs) or anticonvulsants may be used for mood stabilization. Evidence for support of these in anoxia/hypoxia is anecdotal more than evidence-based.

- *Risk Factor Modification* Increased supervision for safety, external and environmental structures, assistance with decision-making (e.g., power of attorney, guardianship), and family training/support are needed.

- *Interpersonal Relationships* Can be very challenging due to persistent memory impairment, poor insight, executive dysfunction, and changes in premorbid role functioning.

- *Functional Issues* Changes in memory, executive, and motor functioning can be debilitating:
  - Select patients can experience persistent anterograde amnesia.
  - However, a number of patients are able to develop routines and compensatory strategies that allow them to live semi-independently as long as they adhere to a rigid daily structure with some level of external monitoring.
  - Severe injuries often result in dystonia, spastic hemiparesis, or quadriparesis due to basal ganglia involvement. Ataxia may persist due to cerebellar involvement. Many of these patients remain unemployable and require some level of attendant care for the remainder of their lives.

- *Rehabilitation Considerations* Compensatory strategy training is critical for patients with memory or other cognitive impairments. Patients who display progressive cognitive improvement within the first month of injury may benefit more relative to other patients who make limited cognitive gains. Emphasis should be placed on errorless learning, procedural learning, attention process training (APT), and evidenced-based cognitive rehabilitation treatment. Some studies show that individuals with severe anoxic injury have poorer cognitive and functional recovery compared to those with severe traumatic brain injury or hemorrhagic cerebrovascular events, though when the latter two conditions result in prolonged coma this may not be the case.

Considerations when Treating Select Populations with Hypoxic and Ischemic Brain Injury

Pediatric Considerations

The brains of infants and children require a higher percentage of oxygen than adults (requiring over 30% total body oxygen consumption from infancy to 4 years of age). The impact of hypoxia/anoxia will depend in part on the developmental period in which it occurs. Perinatal hypoxia-ischemia may contribute to later development of ADHD. Neonatal hypoxia may contribute to major developmental disorders and impaired cognition, depending on the severity and pattern of the damage sustained. A recent meta-analysis demonstrated an increased risk for intellectual disabilities and, to a lesser extent, autism spectrum disorders when impaired gas exchange occurred at birth. Cerebral palsy was once thought to be a frequent result of acute intrapartum hypoxia which led to unnecessarily high caesarean births; however, more recent research has found an increased risk of cerebral palsy due to other factors as well (i.e., preterm delivery, congenital malformations, intrauterine infection, fetal growth restrictions, multiple pregnancy, and placental abnormalities). The predominant pattern of brain injury in neonates found to be most strongly associated with long-term outcome, more so than the severity of injury in any given region, is injury to the basal ganglia and thalamus. Congenital heart disease and sleep-disordered breathing have also been found to have a relationship with cognitive, academic, and behavioral functioning. A significant correlation has been demonstrated between decreased diffusion of the left dentate gyrus and lower verbal learning and memory scores in children with OSA. In addition to the importance of treating the specific cognitive, psychosocial, and behavioral deficits that may be seen in the pediatric patient, special consideration also needs to be given to disruption in development of academic skills and accommodations that will be needed in the school setting. Visuospatial deficits tend to be less severe in children with hypoxic brain injury, whereas intellectual abilities, attention, memory, and behavioral impairments tend to be more pronounced in that population. It is also important to note that some cognitive and behavioral effects may not emerge or be recognized until later developmental periods (e.g., when a child begins to attend school). The individual with lasting changes in brain functioning may not derive the same maturational benefits from normal childhood and adolescent developmental experiences.

Geriatric Considerations

Older brains are less able to recover from an hypoxic brain injury and are more likely to experience permanent and severe cognitive deficits due to reduced cerebral reserve. For many older adults, there may have been preexisting mild cognitive and functional impairments, particularly if anoxia/hypoxia was related to a chronic cardiovascular condition. Further, many older adults who were healthy will have experienced age-related changes in sensory and physical functioning that can exacerbate the effects of anoxia/hypoxia. Although questions of ability to return home safely and capacity to manage one's affairs are important for all age groups, they can be particularly challenging in older adults who may not have the same support systems in place as younger adults.

Relevant Definitions

Acute respiratory distress syndrome (ARDS) A severe, often life-threatening medical condition in which the lungs are compromised or damaged and are unable to supply sufficient oxygen to the arterial blood (e.g., hypoxemia). It can result in anoxic/hypoxic damage to the brain, among many other systemic problems.

Apoptosis In the strictest sense refers to programmed cell death. Apoptosis is part of normal regulation and turnover of cells, but can also result from pathologic processes such as ischemia.

Adenosine Triphosphate (ATP) A chemical compound that provides energy for cells/neurons. Under anoxic/hypoxic conditions, less ATP becomes available in the neuron, leading it to catabolize itself.

Chronic obstructive pulmonary disease (COPD) A term that encompasses several conditions of pulmonary disease (e.g., emphysema, bronchitis) in which there is progressive obstruction of expiration; COPD can produce chronic hypoxia and, depending on the severity, may result in cognitive impairment.

Delayed Post-Hypoxic Leukoencephalopathy (DPHL) An uncommon condition following anoxia/hypoxia in which there is initially good recovery and return to near or full independence, followed days or weeks later by abrupt onset of marked neurologic and cognitive decline.

Glutamate The most common excitatory neurotransmitter in the brain. Under conditions of anoxia/hypoxia, excessive amounts of glutamate are released into the synaptic cleft, and it becomes excitotoxic, as well as contributing to further deleterious processes in the neuron.

Ischemic-hypoxic encephalopathy Refers to the encephalopathy resulting from the combined effects of anoxia/hypoxia and ischemia. In their purest presentations, anoxia/hypoxia and ischemia may produce somewhat different neuropathology, but most cases in which the brain sustains marked disruption of oxygen supply involve both processes.

Necrosis Refers to the death of tissue or neurons, typically due to insufficient blood supply.

Obstructive sleep apnea (OSA) A disorder that involves recurrent episodes of blood oxygen desaturation and also disrupts normal sleep architecture. During episodes of total breathing cessation (apnea) or partial (hypopnea), blood oxygen saturation can fall to harmfully low levels, resulting in repeated hypoxic periods.

Partial pressure of oxygen (PaO$_2$) Partial pressure refers to the pressure exerted independently by a specific gas within a larger mix of gases. The partial pressure of arterial oxygen (PaO$_2$) in healthy adults at sea level is typically 95–100 mm Hg. When this level rapidly drops, complex cognitive processes, memory, and judgment show impairment.

Reperfusion injury A complex process ensuing following restoration of cerebral circulation which results in further damage to neurons. Reperfusion injury involves multiple processes such as edema and microhemorrhages, free radical formation and nitric oxide toxicity, further glutamate release, and others.

Watershed region In the brain, this refers to overlapping border zones between the distal supplies of two arteries. For example, the region supplied by the distal branches of the middle and anterior cerebral arteries is a watershed region. Watershed regions are particularly vulnerable to the effects of hypoxia/ischemia.

Hypoxic and Ischemic Brain Injury Questions

NOTE: Questions 6, 23, 56, and 95 on the First Full-Length Practice Examination, Questions 21, 66, and 125 on the Second Full-Length Practice Examination, Questions 22 and 91 on the Third Full-Length Practice

Examination, and Questions 70 and 119 on the Fourth Full-Length Practice Examination are from this chapter.

1. Which of the following regions of the brain would likely be the least sensitive to the effects of anoxia/hypoxia?

    (a) hippocampus

    (b) globus pallidus

    (c) Broca's area

    (d) cerebellar Purkinje cells

2. Ischemia is defined as ____.

    (a) a total lack of oxygen in the arterial blood

    (b) failure of perfusion of blood through the cerebral vessels to tissue

    (c) excessive carbon dioxide in the blood

    (d) insufficient expiration through the pulmonary system

3. In severe cases of anoxic/hypoxic injury involving basal ganglia and cerebellar structures, you would be least likely to observe ____.

    (a) homonymous hemianopsia

    (b) ataxia

    (c) spastic quadriparesis

    (d) dystonia

4. Which of the following is a poor prognostic indicator for functional recovery from an anoxic/hypoxic incident?

    (a) amnesia for the first day of hospitalization

    (b) coma longer than 6 hours

    (c) GCS 9–12

    (d) seizure on day of admission

5. In perinatal hypoxic-ischemic conditions, there is a significant correlation with later development of what disorder?

    (a) Alzheimer's disease

    (b) aphasia

    (c) epilepsy

    (d) ADHD

6. A 58-year-old male presents with rapid onset of neurocognitive impairment and parkinsonian-like tremor. A clinical history reveals that he was recently hospitalized for carbon monoxide poisoning but responded to treatment quickly, made a rapid recovery and returned to work and family responsibilities. Which of the following is the most likely etiology for his current presentation?

    (a) early symptoms of frontotemporal dementia

    (b) hemorrhagic subcortical stroke

    (c) delayed post-hypoxic leukoencephalopathy

    (d) persistent subclinical hypoxia

7. Reperfusion injury refers to which of the following processes?

    (a) Additional neuronal damage due to toxicity, glutamate release, edema, and microhemorrhages

    (b) Subarachnoid hemorrhage caused by restoration of cerebral circulation

    (c) Onset of temporal lobe seizures during the early recovery period

    (d) Rapid neurologic decline following a period of increased lucidity

8. As a neuropsychologist you are designing an outpatient rehabilitation program for adults recovering from severe anoxia/hypoxia caused by cardiac arrest or carbon monoxide poisoning. Which of the following areas of intervention is least likely to be needed as part of your program?

(a) strategies to improve attention functioning

(b) treatment for language disorders

(c) improving self-awareness

(d) training compensatory strategies for memory impairment

9. Which of the following is generally true when comparing recovery from severe hypoxia/anoxia to TBI?

(a) Severity of memory impairment correlates with extent of hippocampal atrophy following anoxia but not TBI.

(b) Individuals with TBI tend to have significantly longer inpatient rehabilitation stays compared to those with anoxia.

(c) Individuals with anoxia tend to show poorer functional recovery and return to independence.

(d) Total amount of brain atrophy is critical in predicting TBI outcome but not anoxia.

10. Which of the following neuropsychiatric syndromes is least likely to be seen following severe hypoxia/anoxia and ARDS?

(a) Bipolar Disorder

(b) Major Depressive Disorder

(c) Generalized Anxiety Disorder

(d) Schizophrenia

Hypoxic and Ischemic Brain Injury Answers

1. **C—Broca's area**   *Brain regions most sensitive to anoxia/hypoxia include those with the highest metabolic demand and those in watershed or distal regions of the cerebral vascular system. Although all brain regions are vulnerable if anoxia/hypoxia is severe, in general, regions with robust vascular supply (e.g., Broca's area) are less vulnerable.*

Reference: Hopkins, R. O. (2018). Hypoxia of the central nervous system. In J. E. Morgan & J. H. Ricker (Eds.), *Textbook of clinical neuropsychology* (2nd ed., pp. 494–506). New York, NY: Taylor & Francis.

2. **B—failure of perfusion of blood through the cerebral vessels to tissue**   *Ischemia results from loss of blood supply perfusion, in contrast to when there is adequate supply but low or lack of oxygen content (anoxia/hypoxia). In most severe cases, both ischemia and anoxia/hypoxia exist.*

Reference: Victor, M., Ropper, A. H., & Samuels, M. A. (2009). *Adams and Victor's principles of neurology* (9th ed.). New York, NY: McGraw Hill.

3. **A—homonymous hemianopsia**   *Severe hypoxic injury can cause spastic quadriparesis, ataxia, and other motor impairments/dysfunction. A homonymous hemianopsia (visual field defect) would be least likely in this case. Visuospatial impairments may be observed when injury involves watershed zones.*

Reference: Blumenfeld, H. (2010). *Neuroanatomy through clinical cases* (2nd ed.). Sunderland, MA: Sinauer Associates.

4. **B—coma longer than 6 hours**   *Howard, Holmes, and Koutroumanidis (2011) report the following as poor prognostic indicators, in the absence of sedation effects: patient is in coma more than 6 hours, no spontaneous limb movements or localization of pain stimuli, prolonged loss of pupillary responses, sustained conjugate eye deviation, abnormal eye movements (e.g., nystagmus), presence of myoclonic seizures, and lower cranial nerve dysfunction (e.g., absent cough and gag reflexes). A syncopal episode would suggest a very brief loss of consciousness that would be unlikely, in and of itself, to cause any lasting injury.*

Reference: Howard, R. S., Holmes, P. A., & Koutroumanidis, M. A. (2011). Hypoxic-ischaemic brain injury. *Practical Neurology, 11*, 4–18.

5. **D—ADHD**   *There is a significant correlation between perinatal hypoxic-ischemia and attention deficit/hyperactivity disorder.*

Reference: Zhu, T., Gan, J., Huang, J., Li, Y., Qu, Y., & Mu, D. (2016). Association between perinatal hypoxic-ischemic condition and attention-deficit/hyperactivity disorder. *Journal of Child Neurology, 31*(10), 1235–1244.

6. **C—delayed post-hypoxic leukoencephalopathy**   *A small percentage of individuals who display good early recovery following anoxic/hypoxic events experience delayed rapid onset of neurologic and neurocognitive decline, typically within days or weeks. Additionally, individuals who sustain hypoxic injury following carbon monoxide poisoning are at higher risk of delayed decline.*

Reference: Shprecher, D., & Mehta, L. (2010). The syndrome of delayed post-hypoxic leukoencephalopathy. *NeuroRehabilitation, 26*, 65–72.

7. **A—additional neuronal damage due to toxicity, glutamate release, edema, and microhemorrhages**   *Following restoration of cerebral circulation after a anoxic/hypoxic event free radical formation, other toxic processes, edema, and microhemorrhages often develop. While the other options are sometimes seen they are not part of reperfusion injury.*

Reference: Busl, K. M., & Greer, D. M. (2010) Hypoxic-ischemic brain injury: Pathophysiology, neuropathology mechanisms. *NeuroRehabilitation, 26*, 5–13.

8. **B—treatment for language disorders**   *Residual neurocognitive impairment following anoxia/hypoxia commonly includes attention, memory, executive functions, and self-awareness, and a well-designed rehabilitation program will need to address all these areas. Prominent aphasia syndromes are not commonly seen following anoxia/hypoxia. It is possible that transcortical language syndromes may be seen due to damage to watershed regions, but prominent aphasias such as Wernicke's or Broca's are uncommon.*

References:
(a) Anderson, C. A., & Arciniegas, D. B. (2010). Cognitive sequelae of hypoxic-ischemic brain injury: A review. *NeuroRehabilitation, 26*, 47–63.
(b) Haskins, E. C. (2012). *Cognitive rehabilitation manual: Translating evidence-based recommendations into practice.* Reston, VA: ACRM Publishing.

9. **C—Individuals with anoxia tend to show poorer functional recovery and return to independence.**   *When comparing outcomes with individuals who sustained severe anoxia versus TBI, those with TBI achieved greater functional outcome and likelihood of returning home following rehabilitation.*

Reference: Smania, N., Avesani, R., Roncari, L., Ianes, P., Girardi, P., Varalta, V., . . . Gandolfi, M. (2013). Factors predicting functional and cognitive recovery following severe traumatic, anoxic, and cerebrovascular brain damage. *The Journal of Head Trauma Rehabilitation, 28*(2), 131–140.

10. **D—Schizophrenia**   *Survivors of anoxia and ARDS are at significantly elevated risk for major psychiatric conditions including depression, anxiety, and PTSD, but frank psychotic syndromes, while sometimes seen following the most severe cases, are uncommon.*

Reference: Herridge, M. S., Moss, M., Hough, C. L., Hopkins, R. O., Rice, T. W., Bienvenu, O. J., . . . Azoulay, E. (2016). Recovery and outcomes after the acute respiratory distress syndrome (ARDS) in patients and their family caregivers. *Intensive Care Medicine, 42*, 725–738.

Recommended Readings

Blumenfeld, H. (2010). *Neuroanatomy through clinical cases* (2nd ed.). Sunderland, MA: Sinauer Associates

Caine, D., & Watson, J. D. G. (2000). Neuropsychological and neuropathological sequelae of cerebral anoxia: A critical review. *Journal of the International Neuropsychological Society, 6*, 86–99.

Cullen, N., & Weisz, K. (2011). Cognitive correlates with functional outcomes after anoxic brain injury: A case-controlled comparison with traumatic brain injury. *Brain Injury, 25*(1), 35–43.

Haskins, E. C. (2012). *Cognitive rehabilitation manual: Translating evidence-based recommendations into practice.* Reston, VA: ACRM Publishing.

Hopkins, R. O. (2018). Hypoxia of the central nervous system. In J. E. Morgan & J. H. Ricker (Eds.), *Textbook of clinical neuropsychology* (2nd ed., pp. 494–506). New York, NY: Taylor & Francis.

Hopkins, R. O., & Bigler, E. D. (2012). Neuroimaging of anoxic injury: Implications for neurorehabilitation. *NeuroRehabilitation, 31*, 319–329.

Ropper, A. H., & Samuels, M. A. (2009). The acquired metabolic disorders of the nervous system. In *Adams and Victor's principles of neurology* (9th ed.). New York, NY: McGraw Hill.

MEDICAL

29   Traumatic Brain Injury

Kirk J. Stucky, Michael W. Kirkwood, and Jacobus Donders

Definition

Moderate to severe traumatic brain injury (TBI) results from damage to brain tissue caused by an external mechanical force, as evidenced by loss of consciousness, *post-traumatic amnesia* (PTA), positive neuro-imaging, or objective neurological findings attributed to TBI on physical or mental status examination.

Uncomplicated mild traumatic brain injury (mTBI), often referred to as concussion, involves a traumatically induced physiological disruption of brain function that results in a graded set of clinical symptoms that most often resolve spontaneously. Alteration or loss of consciousness and other transient neurologic signs are typically used to define mTBI. Relative to moderate and severe TBI, mTBI has a different recovery course.

Neuropathology

The pathological effects of TBI can be roughly classified as either anatomical or metabolic/biochemical. Effects may occur immediately following injury (primary injury) or days to weeks following injury (secondary injury).

- *Primary Injury* Occurs immediately upon impact and results from linear and/or rotational forces. Examples of primary injury include skull fracture, contusion, *subarachnoid hemorrhage*, and mechanical injury to axons and blood vessels. Because of the anatomical arrangement of the brain and skull, focal injury is most common in the frontal and temporal lobes. *Diffuse axonal injury* tends to be most prominent at the gray–white matter junctions. Prevention of TBI is the only way to address primary injury.

- *Secondary Injury* Secondary injury occurs directly or indirectly from a cascade of events that occur after brain tissue is injured or from the consequences of extracerebral events. Examples of secondary injury include hypoxia, ischemia, swelling/edema, hypotension, mass lesions, increased *intracranial pressure* (ICP), and poor *cerebral perfusion pressure*. Secondary injury can be gradual or accelerate quickly if not properly managed. For example, brain herniation and death can occur if ICP is not managed properly. Control or minimization of secondary injury is the focus of acute stabilization and ICU management (also see *neurometabolic cascade*).

Risk Factors

- Age is an independent risk factor for TBI, but the causes vary within each group. For example, the risk for *severe* TBI is higher at both ends of the age spectrum, but for different reasons:
  - 0–7 years: falls and child abuse
  - 15–19 years: motor vehicle related injuries
  - 65 and older: falls
- Motor vehicle related injuries were the leading cause of TBI in late adolescents (15–19) and younger adults (20–24)

- Other TBI risk factors include alcohol and/or substance abuse, high-risk behavior, male gender, history of prior TBI, psychiatric illness, ADHD, lower socioeconomic status and/or education, and unemployment.
- When symptomatic complaints persist beyond 3 months after mTBI, the diagnostic and treatment challenges are formidable due to the fact that symptom persistence is often multifactorial and typically not primarily associated with brain injury. Risk factors that increase the likelihood of persistent problems after mTBI include:
  - Medical factors
    - polytrauma and/or chronic pain
    - prior history of neurologic injury/reduced cerebral reserve
    - history of recent or multiple mTBIs
    - history of chronic medical condition
  - Demographic factors (e.g., female, less education)
  - Mental health/Psychological factors
    - history of psychopathology (depression, anxiety, etc.)
    - high degree of psychosocial stress or distress
    - substance abuse
    - beliefs/expectations (e.g., *misattribution bias*)
  - Potential for *secondary gain*
    - litigation
    - disability incentives or seeking disability
    - financial disincentives for recovery
    - overt or covert incentives for persistent impairments

Incidence Rates, Morbidity, and Mortality

According to a CDC report and surveillance summary regarding TBI in the United States and other resources (Taylor et. al., 2017):

- Annually, approximately 2.8 million TBI-related ED visits, 282,000 hospitalizations, 56,000 deaths.
- The majority of injuries are mild (70–80%), but it has been estimated that around 25% of individuals do not seek care following mild TBI. Thus an unknown number of people with mTBI are not seen in hospital settings. Of the remaining injuries approximately 20% are moderate and 15–20% severe although the incidence rate varies between studies based on injury classification criteria
- The most common principal mechanisms of injury for all age groups included falls, motor-vehicle related incidents, being struck by or against an object, and assaults.
- TBI rates vary by age, with the highest rates in those ≥75 years, 0–4 years, and 15–24 years.
- 80,000–90,000 new onset disability due to TBI/year (about 43% of hospital survivors). Odds of long term disability increase as a function of injury severity and age.

- mTBI mortality rates are negligible. However, a small number of patients initially present with injury parameters consistent with mTBI but later regress (e.g., due to *epidural* [EDH] or *subdural* [SDH] *hematoma*). These cases are then no longer considered uncomplicated mild injuries.

- Relative to younger adults, individuals older than age 60 are four times more likely to develop chronic subdural hematoma. This is most likely due to widening of the cortical sulci with aging and thus increased bridging vein vulnerability.

- A minority of patients with mTBI injury parameters will have positive neuroimaging. These injuries are now commonly referred to as "complicated mTBI." Functional outcome after such injury tends to be similar to moderate TBI.

Determinants of Severity

The diagnosis of TBI is primarily based on parameters in the medical/historical record and not the neuropsychological examination. In other words, brain injury severity cannot typically be determined without accurate and objective information obtained during the acute injury period. Classification of TBI severity can be accomplished using a combination of various indicators including *Glasgow Coma Scale* (GCS) score, *time to follow commands* (TFC), and length of PTA. Additionally, radiologic findings can be used to further differentiate injury severity. A computed tomography (CT) scan is currently the imaging method of choice in acute care because it is widely available and is sufficient for identifying intracranial findings that require urgent intervention (e.g., surgical evacuation of an *epidural hematoma*). However, other radiologic techniques are becoming more available and affordable which may ultimately lead to changes in acute assessment (e.g., fast sequence MRI). Magnetic resonance imaging (MRI) in the subacute (> 3 months) period is more reliable than CT in identifying structural changes and correlates better with longer term outcomes. Focal neurologic signs, such as pupillary reflex abnormalities, may indicate the presence of TBI but are not consistently related to injury severity because they may or may not be transient. Despite these challenges, researchers have proposed various classification systems, but currently, no universally accepted TBI classification system exists given that:

- Injuries tend to be heterogeneous

- The use of one injury severity marker without consideration of other variables such as acute intoxication, sedating or paralytic medications, complications, and other injuries can result in under or overestimates of injury severity.

- Injury severity estimation from admission through the entire hospitalization may change substantially depending on variables that the emergency medicine or trauma physician cannot possibly know or reliably predict (e.g., length of PTA, length of coma, medical complications)

- Radiologic studies in individuals who have sustained obvious TBI are not always positive. Moreover, relative to other indicators, radiologic studies are poor predictors of actual injury severity and long-term functional outcome except perhaps at the severe end of the TBI spectrum (e.g., obliteration of the third ventricle or basal cisterns).

- Focal neurologic signs indicate the presence of brain dysfunction but are not as predictive of injury severity because they may or may not be transient (e.g., posturing, seizures).

When determining TBI severity, neuropsychologists must appreciate these complexities and know how to accurately integrate all available data, particularly objective information collected in the first hours, days, or weeks post-injury. Subjective information gathered months or years later is often misleading.

Presentation, Disease Course, and Recovery

Acute Hospitalization

Recovery Course

- Acute recovery is often idiosyncratic and quite variable depending on the severity of injury and the presence or nature of complications such as internal injuries, multiple fractures, or infection.

- Non-TBI related factors such as developmental immaturity, intoxication, internal or peripheral injuries, medications, metabolic disturbances, substance withdrawal, and infection can influence common markers of severity such as GCS, TFC, and PTA.

- Common complications following TBI include cranial nerve injury and sensory changes causing anosmia, dizziness, balance disorders, tinnitus, and visual disturbance (e.g., diplopia, photophobia). A large percentage of patients with moderate to severe TBI will have additional injuries, such as long-bone fractures and internal injuries, which cause complications such as chronic pain, deep vein thrombosis, and internal bleeding. The risk for secondary injury must be closely monitored. Additionally, patients who require mechanical ventilation are at higher risk for pneumonia and urinary tract infections are common for patients with Foley catheters.

Assessment Methods

- Patients with severe TBI typically spend some period of time in a minimally responsive state. Validated measures exist to determine whether a patient displays subtle responsiveness to stimuli (e.g., Coma Recovery Scale-Revised, Coma/Near Coma Scale).

- Individuals with moderate to severe TBI will typically experience a period of PTA for days, weeks, or even months post-injury. Exceptions to this can occur with *penetrating TBI*, in which some patients sustain severe injuries but may not lose consciousness nor experience any persistent PTA. While patients are in PTA, brief cognitive measures are effective and typically include basic tests of orientation, attention, and speed of information processing (e.g., Cognitive Log, Orientation Log).

Treatment

- Treatment in the acute period includes medical stabilization, emergent surgical intervention when indicated, and efforts to minimize secondary injury.

- Maintaining a low-stimulation environment and structured/predictable routine are important in that they can reduce cerebral metabolism and modify the impact of factors that may contribute to secondary injury.

- Research regarding potentially neuroprotective agents (e.g., progesterone) has not resulted in sufficient evidence to support any specific evidence-based guidelines for incorporation into treatment.

- The regular use of neuroleptics, benzodiazepines, and certain anticonvulsants (e.g., Dilantin) should be avoided due to the deleterious effect they can have on cognition and recovery. However, in some cases, when severe agitation or delirium does not respond to other interventions, these agents may be used on a short-term basis.

Inpatient Hospitalization

Recovery Course

After medical stabilization, many patients with moderate to severe TBI require inpatient rehabilitation. The length of stay varies and is often influenced by the patient's available resources, level of care required, projected severity of disability, and progress in response to rehabilitation interventions.

Assessment Methods

When the patient demonstrates a measurable level of continuous memory for 2 to 3 consecutive days, it is typically appropriate to perform a relatively brief neuropsychological examination to establish a postinjury baseline and to assist with rehabilitation treatment and discharge planning. However, studies have demonstrated that a brief neuropsychological battery administered one month following complicated mild to severe TBI (regardless of PTA resolution) provided incremental value and was predictive of outcome above and beyond functional and injury severity variables.

Treatment

- Inpatient treatment typically consists of specialized nursing, as well as physical, occupational, and speech therapies. Psychologists, physicians, and other health professionals are also involved.
- Discharge planning should be consistent with patient and family needs, preferences, and available resources.

Outpatient Rehabilitation

Recovery Course

- Long-term recovery following moderate to severe TBI is variable, with more severe injuries resulting in a progressively higher probability of long-term impairments and persistent disability. Despite this, many patients with moderate to severe TBI eventually experience good overall functional recoveries following outpatient rehabilitation, and, although residual cognitive deficits may persist, some patients are able to return to independent living, driving, gainful employment, and/or adequate school functioning.
- Persistent symptoms 3 months following uncomplicated mild TBI are uncommon and typically represent the influence or impact of non-TBI related factors.

Assessment Methods

The outpatient neuropsychological assessment should be directed toward fine-tuning the treatment plan and making practical recommendations for future care. Assessment is rarely helpful if it only outlines the nature of the patient's cognitive impairments and psychological issues. Examples of important issues an assessment may address include but are not limited to:

- the need for supervision, guardianship, conservatorship, and attendant care
- restrictions or accommodations regarding school, work, leisure activities, driving, child care, and the like

- the appropriateness of current treatment and need for additional services, including psychological and behavioral interventions
- assisting in decisions about returning to military duty, school, work, and sports

Neuropsychological assessment should also add positive incremental value and improve patient outcomes by:

- predicting clinical outcome beyond what can be ascertained on the basis of conventional medical variables
- objectively measuring cognitive and psychological changes
- monitoring the effects of repeated injury
- identifying malingering and other noncredible presentations
- differentiating the effects of injury from developmental and psychiatric conditions like depression, posttraumatic stress, and ADHD

The neuropsychologist must also integrate the assessment findings with the patient's unique demographics, developmental level, estimated premorbid functioning, suspected cognitive reserve, and injury parameters. Interpretation of test scores without considering these variables often leads to over or underestimates with regard to TBI-related impairments.

- **Ecologic Validity** Some patients with moderate to severe TBI will appear to have a relatively good cognitive recovery on lab-based tests whereas family members, treatment providers, and collaterals continue to complain of changes in personality, behavior, social skills, and the like. The neuropsychologist needs to be aware of assessment tool limitations and the risk for false-positive or false-negative errors.

Treatment

The needs of patients can vary significantly depending on injury severity, the unique combination of physical, cognitive, behavioral, and emotional impairments, and available resources. Patients often receive a combination of speech, occupational, and physical therapies depending on their unique needs. Ideally, the neuropsychologist should be a member of an integrated team of professionals.

- **Stage of Recovery** Recovery after moderate to severe TBI often takes more than 12 months, although the majority of recovery typically occurs during the initial months post injury, with a less steep curve afterward. Over time, social support and access to resources tend to have more influence on functional recovery than injury severity (especially in children). Typically, rehabilitation then shifts toward compensatory strategy training. Pediatric patients injured during the first few years of life may display declines in test performance relative to same-age peers over time (i.e., delayed consequences or growing into deficits).

- **Cognitive rehabilitation** There are two general approaches to cognitive rehabilitation: restorative and compensatory skills training. Restorative approaches focus on treatments intended to reinforce or directly improve specific cognitive domains, whereas compensatory approaches teach patients strategies to compensate and adapt to cognitive impairments. Neuropsychological assessment can be critical in determining what types of rehabilitation will be most effective. It should be noted that despite widespread advertising and use, computer-based cognitive rehabilitation has very limited utility in improving function. Instead, broad-based, real-world training in problem solving and compensatory techniques tends to be the

MEDICAL

most effective treatment. Many direct retraining techniques during the acute phase of recovery do not have sufficient evidence to support real-world generalization. Possible exceptions include process-specific approaches that address cognitive functions such as attention and concentration, visual scanning, and spatial organization. The true effects of cognitive rehabilitation are sometimes unclear when factoring in natural recovery.

- *School* Neuropsychologists are often central in assisting patients, parents, and school professionals in the timing and manner of educational reentry and needed supports at school. Individual Education Programs (IEPs) and accommodations often hinge on the neuropsychologist's recommendations.

- *Vocational Rehabilitation* This treatment is directed at returning an individual to gainful employment. Some patients return to their former level of employment, but many others require retraining, accommodations, or additional supports to work successfully. Neuropsychologists often assist in planning, implementing, and monitoring the process.

- *Psychotherapy Services* Neuropsychologists and rehabilitation psychologists often provide adjustment to disability counseling, behavioral management, family therapy, marital therapy, psychotherapy, and social skills training. These services often complement other rehabilitation efforts.

Expectations for Neuropsychological Assessment Results

Due to the heterogeneity in moderate to severe TBI, no single pathognomonic neurobehavioral profile exists. Even so, there are common patterns within neuropsychological assessment which are briefly outlined below. There are also common neuropsychological patterns in mTBI immediately following injury. However, the majority of patients with mTBI experience rapid improvement on performance-based tests within days to weeks.

- *Intelligence/Achievement* Performance on "hold tests" that primarily measure overlearned skills, such as the patient's general fund of information or vocabulary, are unlikely to be affected. Performance on tasks requiring speed and novel problem solving are more often affected. Exceptions to this rule can occur in patients who sustain focal or penetrating injuries within language centers. Moderate to severe injury in infancy and very early childhood also often results in broad-based long-term intellectual and academic consequences. Although academic problems might not be apparent on formal achievement tests in older children, poor everyday classroom functioning is common, as seen in increased rates of failing grades and need for special education services.

- *Attention/Concentration* Problems with attention and concentration are ubiquitous while patients are in PTA. After resolution of PTA, patients often display a decreased ability to multitask, as well as to sustain or divide attention. Progressive recovery in basic attention and concentration should be anticipated once PTA resolves, but it may or may not return to baseline for patients with moderate to severe injury. More complex aspects of attention can remain impaired indefinitely. Children who sustain moderate to severe TBI may develop secondary ADHD.

- *Processing Speed* This is the most commonly affected cognitive ability, especially during early stages of recovery, likely due in large part to the diffuse nature of most TBI and its broad impact on the integrity of white matter pathways. Thus, measures in this domain are highly sensitive to the effects of TBI (e.g., Coding, Symbol Digit Modalities Test, Trail Making Test).

- *Language* Persistent aphasia 6 to 12 months post-injury is uncommon unless there has been a focal or penetrating injury. However, dysnomia and phonological processing deficits can be observed following diffuse injury, and language pragmatics are often affected. Many commonly used neuropsychological measures may not be sensitive enough to identify mild impairments or inefficiencies in higher level aspects of language.

- *Visuospatial* In adults, visuospatial skills may be affected with more focal injuries, but in children deficits in this domain can occur following focal or diffuse injury. Due to the planning and organizational requirements of many tests tapping this domain, the neuropsychologist often has to tease out the impact of executive function deficits before concluding that spatial or form perception are primarily impaired.

- *Memory* Frontal and temporal lobe system dysfunction is common following TBI, resulting in reduced processing speed, learning capacity, and organizational skills, thus leading to faulty encoding, storage, and retrieval. Deficits may persist into the later stages of recovery and or indefinitely.

- *Executive Functions* Problems with organization, planning, mental flexibility, and judgment are common due in part to the high probability of injury to frontal systems. These impairments often act as a major barrier to functional recovery, social skills acquisition, community re-entry, and return to school and work. More difficult to determine are a TBI's effect on frustration tolerance, personality, social skills, social judgment, risk tolerance, humor, and interpretation of contextual, interpersonal, or nonverbal cues.

- *Sensorimotor Functions* In adults, motor and sensory deficits are more likely to result from focal injuries. However, reduced psychomotor speed and coordination is common following moderate to severe TBI. In children, more diffuse injuries can lead to general and long-standing declines in psychomotor speed. Patients with significant right-left differences may have sustained peripheral injuries or may have obvious spasticity or increased muscle tone related to significant motor system damage or dysfunction (e.g., basal ganglia, internal capsule).

- *Emotion and Personality* Depression and anxiety are common following TBI. Additionally, patients with initiation disorders and executive dysfunction may be misdiagnosed as depressed. In some cases, frontal system injuries can result in the development of psychological problems that mimic bipolar disorder, obsessive-compulsive disorder, and other psychiatric conditions. Patients may also display poor deficit awareness, reduced self-control, impulsivity, apathy, excessive fatigue, and deficient social skills. Due to poor deficit awareness, some patients do not develop adjustment related mood symptoms for weeks or months.

- *Symptom and Performance Validity* Both performance and symptom validity measures should always be employed in the assessment of adults and school-aged children, regardless of injury severity, because reduced test engagement or response bias can occur in any individual patient.

Considerations when Treating Select Populations with TBI

Generally speaking, patients at the extremes of age (very young or very old) are more vulnerable to the effects of moderate to severe TBI.

Pediatric Considerations

Children have developing brains that, in certain ways, respond differently to TBI. The Kennard principle suggested that younger brains had more "plasticity" and therefore a better prognosis following injury. Researchers have failed to confirm this in the context of diffuse brain injuries such as TBI. In fact, strong evidence indicates that neurobehavioral outcomes are worse following severe TBI in infancy and the preschool years.

- *Delayed Consequences* Essentially, in a young child, the full impact of an injury may not be apparent until the patient reaches developmental stages in which more demands are made on general intelligence, memory, executive skills, higher level communication, and social problem solving. This process also interacts with normal brain maturation (e.g., myelination of the prefrontal regions normally continues into adolescence).

- *Family and Social Support* There is clear evidence that access to resources and strong social support can lead to better functional outcomes in children regardless of injury severity. This further emphasizes the importance of the neuropsychologist's role as a clinician, educator, advocate, and family resource.

Geriatric Considerations

Older patients more commonly sustain TBI as the result of falls, and fall risk increases significantly in people older than 75. Not surprisingly, increasing age is also a risk factor for increasing TBI morbidity and mortality, especially after more severe injuries. The vast majority of older patients experience a relatively good recovery following mTBI unless they have preexisting neurologic issues.

- *Complications* Elderly patients who are hospitalized have much higher complication rates relative to younger adults (e.g., ventilator complications, infection, metabolic disturbances). Elderly patients on anticoagulant and antiplatelet medication are more prone to SDH and can develop significant complications due to increased bleeding and pressure effects.

- *Past Medical History* The neuropsychologist must be attentive to other comorbid variables in this population as well. For example, some patients have a prior history of cerebrovascular disease, substance abuse, or significant prior brain injury.

- *Outcome* Relative to younger adults, elderly patients are more likely to require prolonged supervision, attendant care, and/or placement in an extended care facility. Patients with severe TBI are at somewhat higher risk for developing dementia later in life. The literature is inconsistent about the degree to which this risk is moderated by other factors (e.g., genetics, hypertension, substance abuse).

Sport-Related Considerations

- *Chronic Traumatic Encephalopathy (CTE)* Some researchers have suggested that, as the direct result of repetitive concussive or even sub-concussive injuries (particularly in those who played contact sports), a unique distribution of p-tau accumulates in the depths of the cortical sulci, which in turn is associated with severe behavioral, cognitive and mood changes in older adulthood. These conclusions have been based largely on methodologically weak case series data. Recent comprehensive literature reviews suggest that the neuropathological changes described in CTE are not unique to that condition, and that a sizable percentage of persons who have such changes will *not* develop dementia or commit suicide. Future higher quality research needs to determine to what extent factors other than concussive injuries (e.g., substance abuse, depression) interact with p-tau load or contribute independently to prediction of long-term outcomes after repetitive concussive injuries.

Relevant Definitions

Acceleration/deceleration injuries These occur following unrestricted movement of the head creating tensile, shear, and compressive strains that often follow high-speed events.

Brain reserve hypothesis (BRH) and cognitive reserve hypothesis (CRH) These are related but not synonymous hypotheses. The BRH (also called cerebral reserve hypothesis) maintains that there is variability across individuals with regard to resilience and susceptibility to brain injury and/or poor outcome. Individuals who have a prior history of neurologic illness or injury are at higher risk for complicated outcome following TBI. For example, elderly patients with dementia may not recover as expected following mTBI. Children with preexisting ADHD or other learning problems are also at higher risk for complications in recovery following TBI. The Cognitive reserve hypothesis is similar but emphasizes the potentially protective effects of higher premorbid intelligence and better quality of education prior to injury (also see Chapter 3, Important Theories in Neuropsychology: A Historical Perspective).

Cerebral perfusion pressure (CPP) A measure of the amount of blood flow through the brain. It is calculated by subtracting the ICP from the mean systemic arterial blood pressure. The level and duration of reduced CPP is a main determinant in the severity of cerebral damage. By regulating blood pressure, adequate CPP can be maintained even when ICP is high. However, when ICP is too high or blood pressure is too low, CPP may drop resulting in diffuse ischemic damage. In acute care management the goal is to lower ICP and keep CCP at or around 60–70 mm Hg to optimize the rate of blood flow to the brain.

Concussion grading Multiple grading systems for mTBI have been proposed, but there is controversy regarding their value because they do not significantly assist the clinician in predicting outcome or necessarily modifying the treatment plan. For example, presence/absence of loss of consciousness was initially included in several grading systems but has been de-emphasized in recent years because of its inconsistent relationship with outcome.

Diffuse axonal injury (DAI) or traumatic axonal injury Caused by the stretching of myelinated axons between brain tissues of differing densities (e.g., gray–white matter junction). DAI is strongly related to the effects of secondary injury, such as deleterious biochemical and metabolic cascades, and not just the primary injury. In other words, DAI evolves over time. Advanced MRI techniques (e.g., diffusion tensor and weighted susceptibility imaging) show some promise in evaluating the extent of DAI, although they are not available in all settings and no cross-validated criteria have yet been established for their use in TBI. DAI is not observable on conventional MRI or CT because axons cannot be viewed with neuroimaging. Technically speaking, DAI is a neuropathological diagnosis confirmed via microscopic analysis on autopsy.

Dose–response fallacy An erroneous assumption based on the concept of the magnitude of a stressor (the dose) and the subsequent response of the receptor, which leads to the false conclusion that mTBI results in permanent mild to moderate cognitive impairments because moderate to severe TBI often results in persistent moderate to severe impairments.

Epidural (extradural) hematoma (EDH) Caused by rupture of arteries between the skull and dura. Because of the high pressure in arteries, bleeding into the epidural space can result in a rapidly expanding hematoma that causes compression of brain tissue, which in turn can lead to tentorial herniation and death. Outcome from EDH has a somewhat binomial distribution, with some patients recovering similar to mild TBI if the EDH is evacuated quickly versus high morbidity and mortality if the patient does not receive timely neurosurgical management.

Glasgow Coma Scale (GCS) A scale that assesses responsiveness in patients who have sustained brain injury. There are three parameters: eye opening, motor response, and verbal response. The scale ranges from 3 to 15, with scores of 8 or less indicating severe injury and scores over 13 associated with mild injuries. It is common to use the term "complicated mild" with GCS over 13 in the context of positive acute neuroimaging findings. In severe TBI, lower GCS (3 to 5) is clearly associated with increased mortality rates. GCS is not very robust in the prediction of long-term outcome following TBI, in part because it can be affected by non-brain injury related factors such as intoxication, intubation, patient age, iatrogenic medication effects, and polytrauma.

Intracranial pressure The intact cranium, vertebral canal, and dura are relatively inelastic. Thus, an increase in the size of any of its contents (brain tissue, blood, or cerebrospinal fluid [CSF]) will increase the ICP. The ICP is measured by recording the subarachnoid fluid pressure.

Misattribution bias In mTBI, patients may assume that persistent bothersome symptoms are due to the injury, thus increasing anxiety and reinforcing the belief that they have "permanent brain damage." These same individuals may become preoccupied with minor physiological symptoms that can result in a vicious cycle of escalating somatic dysfunction and emotional arousal. Misattribution bias can be seen in patients with a variety of medical conditions, not just mTBI.

Neurometabolic cascade Following TBI, a process of ionic shifts, impaired neuronal function and connectivity, altered brain metabolism, disruption of normal brain function/signal transmission, and indiscriminate neurotransmitter release can occur. In mTBI, a gradual reversal to normal function typically occurs within days or weeks following injury. In moderate to severe TBI, this cascade often leads to secondary injury.

Nonpenetrating TBI (aka closed-head injury) Refers to injuries in which the dura and skull remain intact (also see acceleration/deceleration injuries).

Penetrating TBI (aka open-head injury) Refers to injuries in which there is a breach of the dura mater. Examples include depressed skull fracture or gunshot wound to the head. Patients who sustain penetrating injuries are often at higher risk for certain complications, such as seizures and infection, due to blood–brain barrier compromise.

Postconcussion syndrome (PCS) Although still commonly used, the World Health Organization (WHO) has discouraged use of this term because PCS does not meet the formal criteria for a syndrome and significant scientific questions remain with regard to definition, etiology, pathophysiology, and incidence. The symptoms typically ascribed to PCS are also nonspecific and overlap a great deal with other variable symptom constellations that occur in patients with other conditions (e.g., fibromyalgia, depression, anxiety, chronic fatigue syndrome, individuals in litigation).

Posttraumatic amnesia PTA has been defined differently by various researchers. The original definition stated that PTA is the amount of time following brain injury that an individual remains confused and is not able to demonstrate continuous memory (e.g., anterograde amnesia), including any time spent in coma. Newer definitions include the period of confusion following TBI, but do not count any period of unconsciousness or coma. This second iteration has been frequently called posttraumatic confusion (PTC). Either definition can be used. PTA is best tracked prospectively via serial testing with instruments like the Orientation Log or Children's Orientation and Amnesia Test. Relative to other outcome predictors in TBI, such as the GCS or TFC, length of PTA is considered to be the most robust. Even so, there is no consensus regarding injury severity classification based on PTA alone. For example, some early methods classified one to seven days of PTA as severe, but more recent studies have revealed that adult patients with less than 14 days of PTA often experience good functional outcomes one year post injury.

Posttraumatic seizures (PTS) Seizures following nonpenetrating TBI are relatively uncommon (5%) although more frequent in children than adults. There are three types: immediate occur within 24 hours, early occur within one to seven days, and late occur more than one week following injury. Regardless, seizures in the first week following nonpenetrating TBI are not predictive of long-term risk for epilepsy, and thus continued anticonvulsant prophylaxis is not typically recommended. Alternatively, penetrating brain injury and direct injury to the cortex is a significant risk factor for seizure (30–50%).

Secondary gain This refers to external advantages (e.g., social, financial, interpersonal) gained indirectly from illness or injury. A high percentage of adults with persistent subjective symptoms following mTBI are also involved in litigation. Multiple studies have demonstrated that more than 30% of these individuals exhibit insufficient test engagement, response bias, suboptimal effort, and/or other behaviors suggestive of symptom magnification or fabrication during formal neuropsychological assessment.

Subarachnoid hemorrhage (SAH) Caused by multiple sources, including brain injury, cerebral aneurysm, arteriovenous malformation, and high blood pressure, SAH is often associated with poorer long-term outcome in moderate to severe TBI. Generally speaking, when blood directly contacts brain tissue, there are higher risks for complications and worsening secondary injury effects.

Subdural hematoma (SDH) Caused by rupture of bridging veins between sulci on the upper surface of the brain. In high-speed injuries, hematomas are commonly found in the frontal and anterior temporal lobes due to the skull and brain's anatomical arrangement. Elderly and pediatric patients are often at higher risk for SDH although for different reasons (i.e. widening of the sulci in the elderly versus unique anatomical features of the head, brain, and neck in young children).

Time to follow commands (TFC) Refers to the amount of time following TBI in which the patient is unable to follow simple motor commands and is unable to maintain arousal or awareness. It is also referred to as length of coma, although this is problematic because after several days or weeks surviving in coma individuals typically progress to a different level of consciousness (e.g., sleep-wake cycles reemerge, may open eyes but remain minimally responsive, EEG patterns change or evolve). Clinicians are now using other terms to describe this state such as minimally responsive, minimally conscious, and unresponsive wakefulness syndrome. The assessment of TFC can be challenging because it must take into account the impact of sedation and paralytics. Emergence from a minimally responsive state corresponds to a score of 6 on the Motor subscale of the GCS.

Traumatic Brain Injury Questions

NOTE: Questions 14, 48, 73, 101, and 118 on the First Full-Length Practice Examination, Questions 18, 34, 41, 81, and 105 on the Second Full-Length Practice Examination, Questions 21, 45, 67, 80, and 106 on the Third Full-Length Practice Examination, and Questions 13, 27, 51, 79, 81, 110, and 125 on the Fourth Full-Length Practice Examination are from this chapter.

1. The most common cause of severe TBI in infants is ____.
   - (a) child abuse
   - (b) falling down stairs
   - (c) penetrating injuries
   - (d) vehicle collisions

2. Persistent cognitive complaints > 3 months post uncomplicated mild TBI are ____.
   - (a) sufficient to change the diagnosis to complicated mild TBI
   - (b) a reason to follow up with specialized neuroimaging, such as DTI
   - (c) typically representative of factors other than TBI on functioning
   - (d) almost never seen outside of malingering for financial or other gain

3. In the management of severe TBI in the Intensive Care Unit, the goal is typically to keep ____.
   - (a) ICP up and cerebral perfusion down
   - (b) cerebral perfusion up and ICP down
   - (c) both ICP and cerebral perfusion up
   - (d) both cerebral perfusion and ICP down

4. What is true about chronic traumatic encephalopathy?
   - (a) It often develops in mid to late adulthood when a person has had > two concussions.
   - (b) The build-up of p-tau in the subcortical areas is fueled by impaired glucose metabolism.
   - (c) Not all persons with CTE pathology demonstrate a progressive neurodegenerative process.
   - (d) It is a disease, not a syndrome, and it is unique to those who played violent contact sports.

5. What is the primary role for neuroimaging in the acute phase following moderate to severe TBI?
   - (a) determine prognosis
   - (b) determine injury severity
   - (c) identify diffuse axonal injury
   - (d) neurosurgical planning

6. Low stimulation protocols are commonly implemented during the acute phases of recovery following moderate to severe TBI primarily to ____.
   - (a) reduce the cerebral metabolic rate
   - (b) lower ICP
   - (c) reduce the risk of infection
   - (d) prevent posttraumatic seizures

7. Which of the following is most likely to be affected after a moderate to severe TBI in a pre-teen?
   - (a) single word reading
   - (b) oral vocabulary
   - (c) math calculation
   - (d) classroom performance

8. Following mild TBI in children and adults, postconcussive symptoms persisting beyond a month have been found to benefit most from interventions aimed at:

(a) diet

(c) school/work scheduling

(b) physical exercise

(d) medications

9. Which combination of factors would generally have the most impact on long-term outcome following traumatic brain injury in a pediatric patient?

(a) injury severity and injury location

(c) injury lateralization and injury age

(b) injury age and injury location

(d) injury severity and psychosocial support

10. Compared to acceleration-deceleration brain injury, penetrating brain injury carries a higher risk for ____.

(a) edema and infection

(c) seizure and subarachnoid hemorrhage

(b) seizure and infection

(d) infection and subarachnoid hemorrhage

Traumatic Brain Injury Answers

1. **A—child abuse** *In infants, child abuse and falls account for the majority of brain injuries. Injuries from falling down stairs can occur but not as frequently as abuse. Penetrating injuries are rare in infants. As children grow older the incidence rates of TBI from vehicle crashes steadily increases.*

References:
(a) Taylor, C. A., Bell, J. M., Breiding, M. J., & Xu, L. (2017). *Traumatic brain injury-related emergency department visits, hospitalizations and deaths-United States 2007 and 2013.* US Department of Health and Human Services.
(b) Yeates, K. O., & Brooks, B. L. (2018). Traumatic brain injury in children and adolescents. In J. E. Morgan & J.H. Ricker (Eds.), *Textbook of clinical neuropsychology* (2nd ed., pp. 141–157). New York, NY: Taylor and Francis.

2. **C—typically representative of factors other than TBI on functioning** *The injury severity is based on the history and medical records, not the course of recovery. While secondary gain and litigation must be considered in individuals with persistent complaints this is certainly not the only plausible explanation for continued problems. Specialized neuroimaging is contraindicated and if done may sometimes inadvertently reinforce the patient's erroneous belief that their brain injury is more serious than is actually the case.*

Reference: Cassidy, J. D., Canelliere, C., Carroll, L. J., Côté, P., Hincapié, C. A., Holm, L. W., . . . Borg, J. (2014). Systematic review of self-reported prognosis in adults after mild traumatic brain injury: Results of the International Collaboration on Mild Traumatic Brain Injury Prognosis. *Archives of Physical Medicine and Rehabilitation, 95,* S321–S151

3. **B—cerebral perfusion up and ICP down** *Cerebral perfusion pressure is calculated by subtracting the ICP from mean arterial pressure (CPP = MAP – ICP). In acute care management the goal is to lower ICP and keep CCP at or around 60–70 mm Hg to optimize the rate of blood flow to the brain.*

Reference: Haddad, S. H., & Arabi, Y. M. (2012). Critical care management of severe traumatic brain injury in adults. *Scandinavian Journal of Trauma Resuscitation and Emergency Medicine, 20,* 1–15.

MEDICAL

4. **C—Not all persons with CTE pathology demonstrate a progressive neurodegenerative process.** *The number or severity of concussions that are definitively sufficient to cause CTE has not been established. Glucose metabolism is unrelated to p-tau distribution. The neuropathology described in CTE is neither universal in those who have played contact sports, nor is it unique to those with such a history. Even when the neuropathology of CTE is present, it may not be clinically progressive in a substantial proportion of persons.*

References:
(a) Iverson, G. L., Keene, C. D, Perry, G., & Castellani, R. J. (2018). The need to separate chronic traumatic encephalopathy neuropathology from clinical features. *Journal of Alzheimer's Disease, 61,* 17–28.
(b) Solomon, G. (2018). Chronic traumatic encephalopathy in sports: A historical and narrative review. *Developmental Neuropsychology, 43,* 279–311.

5. **D—neurosurgical planning** *Neuroimaging provides valuable information but its primary role in the acute phase is determining whether neurosurgical intervention is required (e.g., epidural or subdural hematoma causing significant midline shift). Initial neuroimaging is sometimes normal in patients who have clearly sustained moderate to severe TBI. Thus, neuroimaging is not used to determine or classify injury severity like GCS, TFC, and PTA. Neuroimaging cannot definitively identify DAI although certain findings are associated with a higher probability of DAI (e.g., gliding contusions at the gray–white mater junction, hemorrhages in the corpus callosum). At the very severe end of the TBI spectrum certain neuroimaging findings can predict a grim prognosis (e.g., obliteration of the basal cisterns, large midline shift with uncal herniation), but this does not apply to most cases.*

Reference: Pasquine, P., Kirtley, R., & Ling, G. (2014). Moderate-to-severe traumatic brain injury. *Seminars in Neurology, 34,* 572–583.

6. **A—reduce the cerebral metabolic rate** *Even when severely injured the brain will expend energy when exposed to external stimulation (e.g., noise, bright light, tactile stimuli). Critical care specialists sometimes pharmacologically induce a coma to reduce ICP, achieve a burst-suppression EEG pattern, and reduce the cerebral metabolic rate. Low stimulation protocols also result in less sensory processing demands on the individual and thus are primarily employed to reduce the cerebral metabolic rate.*

Reference: Pasquine, P., Kirtley, R., & Ling, G. (2014). Moderate-to-severe traumatic brain injury. *Seminars in Neurology, 34,* 572–583.

7. **D—classroom performance** *Answers A, B, and C all represent academic skills or abilities that are over-learned in older school-aged children and are thus often more resilient following TBI. In contrast, studies have suggested that declines are frequently seen in classroom functioning, in part because everyday school performance is more reliant on abilities that are known to be affected by TBI such as attention, executive control, processing speed, and new learning/memory.*

Reference: Yeates, K. O. & Brooks, B. L. (2018). Traumatic brain injury in children and adolescents. In J. E. Morgan & J. H. Ricker (Eds.), *Textbook of clinical neuropsychology* (2nd ed.). New York, NY: Taylor and Francis.

8. **B—physical exercise** *Studies in both children and adults with prolonged symptoms after mild TBI have found that physical exercise that does not worsen symptoms reduced postconcussive symptoms in "active rehabilitation" models. Although the other interventions listed may be helpful, exercise has been shown to be the most beneficial.*

References:
(a) Hung, R., Carroll, L. J., Cancelliere, C., Cote, P., Rumney, P., Keightley, M., . . . Cassidy, D. (2014). Systematic review of the clinical course, natural history, and prognosis for pediatric mild traumatic brain injury: Results

of the International Collaboration on Mild Traumatic Brain Injury Prognosis. *Archives of Physical Medicine & Rehabilitation, 95*, S174–191.

(b) Kirkwood, M. W., & Yeates, K. O. (Eds.). (2012). *Mild traumatic brain injury in children and adolescents: From basic science to clinical management.* New York, NY: Guilford Press.

9. **D—injury severity and psychosocial support** *Increasing severity of TBI is associated with progressively lower probability of good functional outcome. Additionally, the degree of psychosocial support available also has a significant influence on long-term recovery, especially in children. With some exceptions, injury location is not predictive of long-term recovery.*

References:

(a) Ponsford, J., Draper K., & Schonberger, M. (2008). Functional outcome 10 years after traumatic brain injury: Its relationship with demographic, injury severity, and cognitive and emotional status. *Journal of the International Neuropsychological Society, 14*(2), 233–242.

(b) Yeates, K. O., & Brooks, B. L. (2018). Traumatic brain injury in children and adolescents. In J. E. Morgan & J. H. Ricker (Eds.), *Textbook of clinical neuropsychology* (2nd ed., pp. 141–157). New York, NY: Taylor and Francis.

10. **B—seizure and infection** *Penetrating head trauma typically results in blood-brain barrier compromise and the introduction of foreign matter into brain parenchyma (e.g., bullet fragments, bone shards, hair). These factors significantly increase the risk for infection and seizure relative to nonpenetrating injuries.*

Reference: Levin, H., Shum, D., & Chan, R. (Eds.). (2014). *Understanding traumatic brain injury: Current research and future directions.* New York, NY: Oxford University Press.

Recommended Readings

Cassidy, D., Cancelliere, C., Carroll, L., Cote, P., Hincapie, C., Holm, L., . . . Borg, J. (2014). Systematic review of self-reported prognosis in adults after mild traumatic brain injury: Results of the International Collaboration on Mild Traumatic Brain Injury Prognosis. *Archives of Physical Medicine and Rehabilitation, 95*(Suppl 3), S132–S151.

Donders, J., & Hunter, S. (Eds.). (2018). *Neuropsychological conditions across the lifespan.* Cambridge: Cambridge University Press. [Particularly chapter 8].

Hung, R., Carroll, L. J., Cancelliere, C., Cote, P., Rumney, P., Keightley, M., . . . Cassidy, J. (2014). Systematic review of the clinical course, natural history, and prognosis for pediatric mild traumatic brain injury: Results of the International Collaboration on Mild Traumatic Brain Injury Prognosis. *Archives of Physical Medicine & Rehabilitation, 95*, S174–191.

Kirkwood, M. W. ,& Yeates, K. O. (Eds.). (2012). *Mild traumatic brain injury in children and adolescents: From basic science to clinical management.* New York, NY: Guilford Press.

Levin, H., Shum, D., & Chan, R. (Eds.). (2014). *Understanding traumatic brain injury: Current research and future directions.* New York, NY: Oxford University Press.

McCrea, M. (Ed.). (2008). *Mild traumatic brain injury and postconcussion syndrome: The new evidence base for diagnosis and treatment.* New York, NY: Oxford University Press.

Roebuck-Spencer, T., & Sherer, M. (2018). Moderate and severe traumatic brain injury, In J. E. Morgan & J. H. Ricker (Eds.), *Textbook of clinical neuropsychology* (2nd ed., pp. 387–410). New York, NY: Taylor and Francis.

Taylor, C., Bell, J., Breiding, M., & Xu, L. (2017). Traumatic brain injury–related emergency department visits, hospitalizations, and deaths—United States, 2007 and 2013. *Morbidity & Mortality Weekly Report, 66*(9), 1–16.

Yeates, K. O., & Brooks, B. L. (2018). Traumatic brain injury in children and adolescents. In J. E. Morgan & J. H. Ricker (Eds.), *Textbook of clinical neuropsychology* (2nd ed., pp. 141–157). New York, NY: Taylor and Francis.

30 Mild Cognitive Impairment and Alzheimer's Disease

C. Munro Cullum and Christine D. Liff

Introduction

Alzheimer's disease (AD) is a progressive, degenerative brain disorder with no known cure that results in generalized cerebrocortical dysfunction and dementia, typically characterized by *anterograde amnesia* that is eventually accompanied by deficits in other cognitive domains such as language, executive function, attention, processing speed, and visuospatial skills. Importantly, for a diagnosis of AD, these neuropsychological deficits must reflect a significant decline from premorbid functioning and must interfere with an individual's ability to perform activities of daily living (ADLs).

Usually considered a prodromal phase prior to AD onset, mild cognitive impairment (MCI) consists of relatively isolated cognitive impairment beyond that seen in normal aging. Several subtypes of MCI have been described, including amnestic, nonamnestic, and multiple-domain (see Table 30.1).

In the most common presentation of amnestic MCI, verbal episodic memory is usually impaired first, although some cases show greater visual memory impairment. In nonamnestic MCI, a nonmemory impairment predominates (e.g., executive function), and in multiple-domain MCI, several areas of impairment are present. By definition, the cognitive impairments in MCI do not dramatically interfere with an individual's everyday functioning and therefore do not reach a clinical level to warrant a diagnosis of dementia. MCI is a clinical diagnosis that requires memory or other cognitive complaints from the patient and psychometric evidence of impairment. This is sometimes delineated as a performance of 1.5 standard deviations below the normative mean on formal neuropsychological tests, although there are no universally accepted psychometric criteria for this, as MCI is a clinical diagnosis. Obviously, the determination of "impairment" may vary according to individual patient profiles in terms of domains involved as well as patients' medical and demographic backgrounds. Roughly 10% of MCI cases per year develop or "convert" to dementia, with the amnestic subtype most commonly progressing to AD. Although we are using the term MCI for this chapter, the term "mild neurocognitive disorder" (MND) is a diagnostic and billing classification reflective of MCI.

TABLE 30.1 Mild Cognitive Impairment (MCI) Classifications

Amnestic MCI, Single Domain	Most common presentation and most likely to progress to AD; focal memory impairment in the absence of other gross cognitive impairments
Amnestic MCI, Multiple Domain	Impairment in memory plus at least one other cognitive domain such as language, executive function, or visuospatial skills.
Non-Amnestic MCI, Single Domain	Impairment in a cognitive domain other than memory, such as executive function, visuospatial processing, or language.
Non-Amnestic MCI, Multiple Domain	Impairment in several cognitive domains other than memory, but not to the extent that meets criteria for dementia.

Definitions of Preclinical AD and DSM-5 Definition of "Neurocognitive Disorder Due to Alzheimer's Disease"

The original criteria for preclinical AD were based on a hypothetical model of stages of progression, ranging from cognitively normal to MCI to dementia, with the earliest pathological biomarkers being accumulation of a-beta42, a buildup of aggregated *tau*, then hippocampal volume loss, followed by the later emergence of clinical symptoms (Sperling et al., 2011). Initial validation of the National Institute on Aging - Alzheimer's Association (NIA-AA) criteria for preclinical AD has shown promise, and the criteria represent an advance in our thinking about preclinical disease modeling, although many operational challenges and definitions must be addressed (e.g., criteria for "abnormality" and how to handle cases with discrepant data) before the criteria can be fully validated and applied clinically. An important issue in this model is the use of maximally sensitive neuropsychological measures to detect abnormal cognitive decline at an early stage because cognitive screening and limited testing will not provide maximum sensitivity. Nevertheless, the latest research criteria for the biological/research diagnosis of AD from NIA-AA relies heavily on biomarker data. As such, this diagnostic approach (which is to be used in research and **not** applied to clinical care settings) does not consider clinical signs or symptoms of disease and instead rests on the presence of abnormal protein deposits. The criteria states that "The term 'Alzheimer's disease' refers to an aggregate of neuropathologic changes and thus is defined in vivo by biomarkers and by postmortem examination, not by clinical symptoms." The biomarker classification system that was proposed is based on *amyloid, tau*, and other measures of neurodegeneration (i.e., currently based upon structural MRI, PET, and/or CSF *amyloid/tau*), collectively referred to as the "AT(N)" (*amyloid, tau*, neurodegeneration) system (Jack et al., 2018). From a clinical perspective, the workgroup proposed a cognitive staging continuum that includes cognitively unimpaired, MCI, and dementia.

In addition to the NIA-AA research criteria for AD, the American Psychiatric Association's *Diagnostic and Statistical Manual of Mental Disorders* (DSM-5) Neurocognitive Disorders Work Group updated the DSM-5 clinical criteria for dementia to focus on "major" and "minor" neurocognitive disorders, with the following criteria relating specifically to AD:

- The individual meets criteria for mild or major neurocognitive disorder:
  - There is insidious onset and gradual progression of impairment in one or more cognitive domains (for major neurocognitive disorder, two domains must be impaired). (See also Chapter 5, Domains of Neuropsychological Function and Related Neurobehavioral Disorders, for a listing of cognitive domains.)
  - Memory impairment is an early and prominent feature.
  - The syndrome as a whole is not better attributed to any concurrent active neurological or systemic illness.

Under the proposed cognitive staging scheme associated with the biomarker-based definition of AD (Jack et al., 2018), MCI is defined as "cognitive performance below expected range for that individual based on all available information." What constitutes "below expected range" was purposely left rather vague and may or may not include formal neuropsychological test results, and it is noted that this interpretation may or may not include the use of population-based norms as a reference. Beyond the presence of cognitive impairment, it is stated that the criteria for MCI include evidence of decline from premorbid status, which may be based upon the clinician's impressions from the patient, a caregiver or family member, and/or longitudinal neuropsychological test results.

Thus, the definition of MCI will no doubt continue to evolve, along with the controversy over the biomarker-based diagnosis of AD and secondary consideration of clinical symptoms and disease staging. In clinical practice, however, at the time of this writing, MCI and AD remain clinical diagnoses (with support of biomarker findings to the extent possible), placing a high level of importance on the neuropsychological evaluation for early detection and documentation of functional decline and analysis of the neuropsychological profile.

Neuropathology

- The lesions of AD consist of synaptic and neuronal loss associated with progressive deposition of *amyloid* in the form of diffuse *neuritic plaques*, along with the accumulation of *tau* in the form of *neurofibrillary tangles* and neuropil threads.

- During disease progression, there is cell atrophy, loss, and subsequent reduction in the production and function of various neurotransmitters, including choline acetyltransferase, as well as serotonin and norepinephrine.

- The neuropathological/functional progression of the disease follows a temporal-to-frontal spread and eventually involves multiple brain systems (see Figure 30.1). Specifically, the hippocampus and entorhinal cortex are implicated in the early stage of the disease, followed by frontal, temporal, and parietal association areas with disease progression. It is in the temporal lobe and association areas where most atrophy occurs in many cases.

- Primary motor, visual, auditory, and somatosensory cortices, as well as aspects of subcortical structures, tend to be relatively unaffected until quite late in the disease process.

  - Other conditions that may present with clinical symptoms of MCI and AD include a condition known as *Suspected Non-Alzheimer Pathophysiology* (SNAP), which is characterized by biomarker evidence of neurodegeneration without prominent presence of *amyloid*. Primary age-related tauopathy (PART) is another recently described condition that is associated with cognitive impairment and can present with an AD-like onset but may show slower clinical progression.

Risk Factors

Currently age (typically over 65) is the single largest known risk factor for AD. Although most AD cases appear sporadic, having a first-degree family member with AD increases risk. Early-onset familial

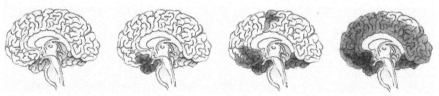

FIGURE 30.1 Cortical Progression of Alzheimer's Disease

NOTE: On the left is a normal brain (right temporal lobe is shaded at bottom; cerebellum has been removed) with progression of the disease state moving to the far right brain, which depicts advanced Alzheimer's Disease.

AD has been implicated with a mutation in identified genes on chromosomes 1 (Presenilin 2 gene), 14 (Presenilin 1 gene), and 21 (APP gene). Chromosome 21 is also involved in Down syndrome, and older individuals with Down syndrome typically develop plaques consistent with AD. In addition, individuals with the *Apolipoprotein ε4* (ApoE ε4) genotype (carried on chromosome 19) have a heightened risk of developing AD. At present, several dozen other genetic mutations have been associated with AD, although none of them are completely predictive of risk in most individual cases. In addition to known and as-yet unknown genetic factors that may elevate risk, other potential risk factors include, but are not limited to the following:

- Cardiovascular risk factors such as elevated blood cholesterol in midlife
- Concurrent small vessel/cerebrovascular disease (can accelerate or independently contribute to cognitive decline)
- Diabetes mellitus, particularly if poorly controlled
- Moderate to severe traumatic brain injury
- History of major depression (reported in some cases)
- Lower education and/or lower cognitive reserve (see also the section "Cognitive Reserve Hypothesis" in Chapter 3, Important Theories in Neuropsychology: A Historical Perspective)

Epidemiology

Incidence

- Estimates vary, but up to 10% of people over age 65 have symptoms consistent with AD. Current National Institutes of Health (NIH) and Alzheimer's Association estimates place the prevalence of AD in the United States around 5.7 million, with prevalence rates doubling approximately every 4 to 5 years.
- Recent figures from the NIH suggest that the average age at diagnosis is approximately 75 years, with most patients being diagnosed between the ages of 70 and 79. While less common, AD can occur in much younger individuals, sometimes with an onset between age 50 and 65.
- It is estimated that up to 50% of individuals over age 85 meet criteria for AD.
- African Americans are approximately twice as likely and Latin/x about 1.5 times more likely than Caucasians to develop AD or other forms of dementia. The relationship between ethnicity and dementia is believed to be moderated by increased prevalence of related medical conditions (e.g., cardiovascular risks) and other factors such as quality of education and access/utilization of healthcare.
- Less than 5% of patients with AD are believed to have a familial variant of the disease. Such cases are typically early-onset and have more rapid decline, with symptoms presenting between the ages of 40 and 60.

Mortality

Alzheimer's disease is currently listed as the 5th and 6th leading cause of death among individuals aged 65 and older, and affected patients typically die as a result of related complications or illnesses (e.g., aspiration, cardiovascular failure, pneumonia, etc.). Once a clinical diagnosis of AD is made, life expectancy varies widely depending on a number of factors, but averages around 5 to 10 years.

Presentation, Disease Course, and Recovery

Although there are many causes of dementia, AD accounts for the majority (i.e., 70%) of cases. The length of illness typically ranges from 2 to 20 years, with a mean duration of around 7 to 10 years. When AD strikes later in life, it tends to progress at a slower rate. The early stages of AD are typically marked by insidious deficits in episodic memory, involving acquisition and storage. Sometimes in the early stage, patients are initially unaware of or downplay their memory problems, a finding that can be helpful in differential diagnosis (e.g., patients with depression or anxiety often complain extensively about memory deficits). Whereas gross personality changes are less common early in the AD process (and may suggest another etiology, such as frontotemporal lobar degeneration), changes in behavior such as progressive social withdrawal and apathy/decreased interest in hobbies and usual activities may be seen, as well as problems with sequencing and problem solving in the work and/or home environment. By the time most patients with AD present to a neuropsychologist, the illness has been present for some time, with clinician-estimated age of onset of symptoms usually several years prior to clinic presentation.

Diagnosis

The presence of AD pathology can only be ascertained by neuropathologic examination of brain tissue, although clinical diagnosis is 85–90% accurate when based on comprehensive evaluation. The neurodiagnostic workup of patients with suspected AD should include MRI, biomarker/blood chemistry studies, neurologic exam, and neuropsychological evaluation, in addition to a careful clinical history. Positron emission tomography imaging has been approved as a clinical tool to aid in the diagnosis of AD in some cases, as well as assist in the differential diagnosis of AD from frontotemporal dementia (FTD). *Amyloid* imaging has shown promise in the identification of AD pathology, and *tau* imaging is beginning to be used, although some individuals with normal cognition may have abnormal PET findings. CSF analysis for *amyloid* and *tau* is another useful tool for diagnostic confirmation. The clinical diagnosis of AD requires the integration of information from a variety of sources but is often characterized by the history and nature of presenting symptoms, in addition to the need to rule out other potential causes of dementia. Of note, there is now a biologic definition of AD that has been proposed that is currently distinguished from the clinical syndrome of AD. The stages of normal aging through the progression of severe AD are outlined below.

Normal Aging, Mild Cognitive Impairment, and Alzheimer's Disease

Normal Aging/Unimpaired Cognition

Declines in certain aspects of cognition and neurobehavior are typically seen with normal aging. However, the effects of aging on the brain and cognitive functions is quite variable across individuals. Below are some of the changes commonly observed in normal aging.

- Sensory and motor loss are common:
    - hearing is decreased in up to 70% of persons over age 70
    - decreased visual acuity, scanning efficiency, and light–dark adaptation
    - reduced olfactory sensitivity
    - decreased motor speed, coordination, and strength
- Sleep patterns change with age, with nighttime sleep shorter and more fragmented (which may result in more daytime naps) and sleep onset and awakening occurring earlier.

- Brain volume declines, as reflected by increased cortical atrophy and ventricular size.
- Some cognitive abilities are sensitive to aging effects whereas others are more resistant. Cognitive abilities typically resistant to aging include:
  - vocabulary and verbal skills; reading ability; macrolevel processing
  - simple attention and concentration
  - basic arithmetic problem solving
  - recognition memory and recall of the gist of stories
  - remote memory (i.e., recall from many years ago)
- Examples of common cognitive changes with aging include:
  - decreased sustained and divided attention
  - less efficient and slower rates of learning new information (may require more practice, time, and rehearsal)
  - reduced recall of detailed information presented recently (episodic memory)
  - reduced cognitive flexibility

Prestage: Mild Cognitive Impairment

Despite various definitions and proposed nomenclature, common diagnostic guidelines for MCI include the original Petersen Criteria (2008), which consist of memory complaints, demonstration of abnormal memory for age on formal memory tests, intact general cognitive functioning, essentially intact ADLs, and absence of dementia. In practice, MCI classifications have been divided into subtypes, including amnestic single domain, amnestic multiple domain, nonamnestic single domain, and nonamnestic multiple domain (see Table 30.1).

- Prevalence rates for MCI increase with age, occurring in at least 10% of 70- to 79-year-olds and 25% of 80- to 89-year-olds. Studies suggest that around 10% to 15% of patients with MCI progress from MCI to dementia annually.
- Not all patients diagnosed with MCI will develop dementia. However, the initial severity of the patient's cognitive impairment is most predictive of progression to AD, and the extent to which the neuropsychological profile of a patient with MCI appears similar to that seen in AD suggests more likely progression.
- Given the limited sensitivity of clinical interview or even brief neurocognitive screening instruments, such as the Mini-Mental State Examination (MMSE) or Montreal Cognitive Assessment (MoCA), the diagnosis of MCI can best be made based on comprehensive neurodiagnostic evaluation that includes a detailed clinical history, neurologic examination, blood chemistry and biomarker studies, MRI, and importantly, formal neuropsychological evaluation.
- PET *amyloid* imaging may be useful in the identification of AD, with posterior cingulate and parietal regions in particular demonstrating increased tracer uptake in many patients with MCI and AD. PET has been approved as a clinical tool in challenging neurodiagnostic cases, although, as with other biomarkers, false-positive findings do occur. Amyloid and *tau* obtained through cerebrospinal fluid, as well as *tau* imaging, are also promising tools that may aid in diagnosis.
- MRI and CT results often show cortical atrophy and ventricular enlargement, but, in many cases, are unremarkable for age. The correlation between degree of atrophy and level of

cognitive impairment across studies is typically in the range of 0.5 to 0.6, suggesting a significant, but imperfect association. Standard EEG may show diffuse slowing as the disease progresses but is often normal, particularly in early-stage cases.

Stage 1 (1–3 years): Memory Impairment, Dysnomia, and Lack of Awareness

- Patients are typically able to function relatively independently in familiar environments, although they may experience some difficulty in novel settings.

- Common early changes include impairment and worsening of recent memory, learning problems, and declining initiative (possibly accompanied by apathy, which can be misinterpreted as depression).

- Patients may start to shy away from new situations, preferring isolation or familiar routines.

- Structural neuroimaging results may continue to remain unremarkable, although atrophy (particularly hippocampal) may develop.

- Although some individuals may not be aware of their cognitive changes and deny problems, others will become aware and may develop symptoms of apathy, depression, or anxiety in response.

Stage 2 (2–10 years): Amnesia, Aphasia, Visuospatial Difficulties, and Personality/ Emotional Changes

- Patients may be able to function adequately in familiar settings and on overlearned tasks, but begin to show difficulty with more complicated tasks, such as operating appliances and managing finances.

- Increasingly poor episodic memory and rapid forgetting becomes quite apparent in the context of relatively intact remote memory.

- Word-finding deficits typically emerge, along with slower speech patterns. Sustained attention may suffer, and patients may lose their train of thought during conversation.

- Visuospatial deficits can occur, commonly topographical disorientation and poor visuoconstructional ability. In conjunction with episodic memory impairment (particularly nonverbal), misplacing things may become commonplace.

- Mood changes may include guardedness or suspiciousness, as well as irritation and agitation, sometimes as a result of forgetfulness.

- Some patients display apathy and lack of initiation, which may be misperceived as depression.

- Later, many require assisted living arrangements, particularly when behavioral problems arise.

- MRI results often reveal progressive sulcal enlargement and ventricular dilation.

- When obtained, PET/single photo emission computed tomography (SPECT) results often reveal bilateral parietal hypometabolism/ hypoperfusion.

- EEG, though rarely done for clinical purposes in such cases, may demonstrate diffuse slowing of background rhythm.

Stage 3 (8–12 years): Severe Dementia, Global Aphasia, and Mutism

- In the later stages of AD, cognitive impairment becomes profound, involving all aspects of cognition. Patients often require 24-hour assistance/supervision and/or nursing home care and are clearly disabled and dependent on others.

- Sleep disturbance and behavioral abnormalities may develop, including hallucinations and nighttime wandering.
- MRI and CT show progressive atrophy in most cases, and EEG reveals global diffuse slowing.

Stage 4: Severe Dementia and Complete Dependence

- Patients are often disoriented and no longer capable of following basic routines.
- Psychotic symptoms may emerge (e.g., hallucinations).
- Patients may become increasingly sedentary and may become incontinent.

Stage 5: Severe Disability

- Patients may become noncommunicative. Others may develop difficulty chewing and swallowing.
- Patients are often nonambulatory at this stage, leading to progressive muscle wasting and weight loss prior to death.
- An increased vulnerability to pneumonia and other illnesses develops.

Typical Hospital/Acute Course

Patients with AD are rarely hospitalized for the condition in the early stages. More often, patients are identified by primary care physicians or internists during their outpatient treatment or examination as part of the annual wellness exam, or after family members become concerned and seek neurologic evaluation. This often leads to subsequent referral for neuropsychological evaluation, which is an important part of the neurodiagnostic evaluation for suspected dementia. In some cases, patients with AD are identified after they have been admitted to the hospital for a different reason (e.g., surgery, hip or knee replacement, infection, injuries, cardiac or other illnesses). Initially, these patients may experience episodes of increased or prolonged confusion following surgery, anesthesia, or urinary tract infection, and they are commonly diagnosed with delirium. Moreover, family members occasionally raise concerns about memory with physicians or nursing staff after their loved one has been admitted. Whether based on inpatient or outpatient evaluations, medical staff often subsequently request neuropsychological consultation, seeking differential diagnosis regarding dementia, depression, and normal aging.

Rule-Outs

Vascular cognitive impairment (VCI), Lewy body disease (LBD), FTD, Parkinson's disease, and other less common forms of dementia (e.g., normal pressure hydrocephalus (see also Chapter 20, Congenital and Acquired Hydrocephalus), as well as delirium, should be ruled out before a diagnosis of AD is considered.

- Delirium can occur due to causes such as urinary tract infections, iatrogenic effects of medications, and metabolic issues. Stabilizing the patient through treatment of acute medical conditions and/or medication changes should be completed prior to more detailed neuropsychological assessment.
- If patients have (a) a rapid onset of symptoms, (b) demonstrate stepwise symptom progression, or (c) their symptom onset occurred within 3 months of an identified cerebrovascular event, alternative diagnoses should be considered such as VCI (see also Chapter 31, Vascular Cognitive Impairment). Contrary to previous guidelines, it is now recognized that vascular dementia does not always present in a stepwise fashion, and that vascular disease and AD pathology often coexist.

- If personality or behavioral changes are most prominent early, alternative diagnoses should be considered, such as FTD (see also Chapter 32, Frontotemporal Dementias). The behavioral variant of FTD initially presents with more pronounced behavioral disturbances, whereas the language variant of FTD presents with pronounced deficits in language and semantic knowledge. Interestingly, while most patients with FTD demonstrate cognitive impairments, the behavioral variant of FTD may present with profound behavioral/personality change in the absence of striking neuropsychological deficits on formal testing.

- Whereas it is often difficult or impossible to distinguish AD from LBD clinically, the finding of mild memory deficits in the face of more prominent visuospatial impairment, along with other clinical features such as extrapyramidal symptoms, visual hallucinations, rapid eye movement (REM) sleep behavior disorder, and/or fluctuating symptoms, may suggest LBD (see also Chapter 33, Movement Disorders).

Expectations for Neuropsychological Assessment Results

In MCI, as well as the early stages of AD, neuropsychological assessment tends to be the most sensitive and specific for detection. Tests of declarative/episodic memory (i.e., verbal learning and delayed recall), language (e.g., confrontation naming, word list generation), and executive function (e.g., cognitive flexibility) have demonstrated the greatest sensitivity in differentiating AD from both normal aging and other forms of dementia. Brief mental status examinations and neurocognitive screening often miss MCI and early stages of AD. Additionally, standard neurological examination, neuroimaging, and other laboratory tests have not outperformed the diagnostic or predictive accuracy of neuropsychological tests. Blood-based biomarkers (often related to indices of inflammation) have shown promise in terms of sensitivity and specificity at the group level, although their utility in individual cases and relation to neuropsychological function is only beginning to be explored. At this point, the combination of thorough clinical history, neurologic examination, neuropsychological evaluation, and genetic and biomarker data (i.e., measures of *amyloid, tau,* and neuroimaging) provide the best diagnostic and prognostic accuracy. Regardless of their use in neurodiagnosis, neuropsychological techniques remain the only means of objectifying and characterizing relative cognitive strengths and weaknesses in individuals with known or suspected cognitive compromise due to MCI or AD. A thorough neuropsychological examination may be needed to detect subtle neurobehavioral deficits and changes, and the quantitative data afforded by formal assessment may be very useful in providing feedback to patients, families, and physicians regarding an individual patient's cognitive capabilities and limitations, as outlined here, by cognitive domain.

- *Intelligence or "G"* Patients with MCI and early AD often earn normal scores on tests of crystallized cognitive abilities (e.g., sight word reading, vocabulary/word definitions) during early stages. Although unaffected early-on, even more basic sight-word reading ability and vocabulary also show declines in later stages.

- *Attention/Concentration* Patients may display early problems with divided attention and complex concentration. General alertness and basic attention (e.g., digit span forward) tend to remain relatively intact until later stages.

- *Language* Patients often display problems with word finding and may make phonemic or semantic paraphasic errors on confrontation naming tests early in the illness. Other symptoms of aphasia may emerge with disease progression (middle to late stages). Echolalia and mutism typically occur in the later stages.

- *Visuospatial Abilities* Some patients display early impairments in geographical orientation, spatial perception, and design copy tasks. Other visuospatial abilities, such as visual attention and scanning and visual discrimination, remain relatively intact until the middle to late stages.

- *Memory* Episodic memory impairments are typically the first observable symptom. This is usually characterized by limited learning, rapid forgetting, intrusion errors during recall of word lists, heightened recency recall effects, and impaired recognition. Delayed verbal recall tends to be the most sensitive measure. Decline is further delineated by greater anterograde than retrograde memory loss and greater explicit than implicit learning impairment. However, retrograde memory loss will develop and typically has a temporal gradient, with older autobiographical memories better preserved than newer ones. Remote autobiographical memory remains relatively intact until later stages.

- *Executive Functions* Problems with mental flexibility, reasoning, and judgment are common. Patients may lack insight or awareness as to the severity and impact of their cognitive or functional decline. Assessment of this domain requires objective evaluation, with neuropsychological tasks requiring cognitive flexibility and a detailed clinical interview, including interview of reliable collateral sources when feasible.

- *Sensorimotor Functions* Sensorimotor abilities may decline in later stages, although typically only after cognitive dysfunction is more pronounced. Ideomotor apraxia or dyspraxia may occur. Limb rigidity can occur in the late stages, as opposed to early, as in parkinsonian and other extrapyramidal syndromes.

- *Emotion and Personality* Changes in personality typically do not become an issue until middle to later stages of AD. Patients may become apathetic, lack initiation, and/or become withdrawn and less talkative, which may be misperceived as depression. Symptoms of anxiety, suspiciousness, and/or irritability may develop, which can increase caregiver distress. Hallucinations, paranoia, suspiciousness of loved ones/caregivers, and delusions occur with higher frequency in the later stages.

- *Symptom and Performance Validity* Whereas clinicians should be aware that reduced effort/engagement can occur in patients with neurological illness, symptom validity testing may be less necessary in cases of known or suspected dementia in routine situations outside of litigation or disability evaluations. It should also be noted that individuals with more advanced dementia may perform poorly on performance validity testing secondary to cognitive impairment rather than effort issues.

Considerations when Treating Patients with MCI and AD

- *Level of Supervision* During MCI and in early AD stages, patients often do not require increased supervision and often continue to drive, manage ADLs, and function relatively independently. Patients steadily require more and more supervision or attendant care with disease progression. Neuropsychologists should address supervision needs in reports and treatment plans, with an understanding that a given patient's needs will change with time.

- *Functional Issues* To meet criteria for a dementia diagnosis, the patient must have evidence of functional decline. The rate and type of functional decline can vary considerably. Typical early functional limitations may manifest at work first, followed by hobbies, and then other daily activities. Routine, overlearned abilities tend to remain more intact and may help hide insidious functional decline. Specific testing of instrumental ADLs may be a useful adjunct to neuropsychological evaluation (e.g., Texas Functional Living Scale [TFLS]).

- *Behavioral Interventions* Patients require stepwise increases in monitoring and assistance from caregivers as the disease progresses. Environmental management and compensatory memory strategies can help patients remain in the home longer. Relatively intact implicit or procedural memory functioning typically continues well into the disease course and may be assistive in providing structure and routine for the patient. A regular daily routine, healthy diet, and exercise can improve a patient's and family's overall quality of life, as well as help prevent secondary complications and safety issues. There is also growing evidence suggesting that physical exercise is beneficial in maintaining and promoting cognitive efficiency. Formal behavioral programs can help minimize caregiver burnout and reduce the frequency of undesirable behaviors. It is important for caregivers to take good care of themselves so that they can optimally assist their loved ones.

- *Driving* The ability to operate a motor vehicle safely may continue for patients diagnosed with MCI and the early stages of AD but should be a consideration and queried. However, assessment of driving skills may be indicated as memory impairment, visuospatial deficits, and slowed reaction times worsen. Restrictions to driving in familiar or light traffic locations, on short trips, and/or during daytime hours may be advisable, depending on cognitive deficits. As symptoms progress, periodic on-the-road driving evaluations are commonly recommended. Neuropsychological test results may be particularly helpful in assisting physicians and advising patients regarding the need for a driving evaluation or identifying individuals who should not be driving, although driving is such an overlearned behavior, prediction of driving skills can be challenging in patients until neurobehavioral impairments become obvious.

- *Employment* For those patients with MCI or early-onset AD who are employed, many may continue to work, although increasing assistance with aspects of work may be needed and transition to retirement or long-term disability should be considered or recommended with greater cognitive deterioration.

- *Capacity* Many patients retain the capacity to participate in medical and financial decision-making during the early stages of AD. The ability to make more complex decisions is often limited by the memory impairment and executive function deficits characteristic of the middle and later stages. Recommendation for durable power of attorney, and a conservator and/or guardian may become necessary.

- *Emotional and Psychological Issues* Early in the course of AD, patients may develop symptoms of anxiety or depression, particularly as awareness of impairments sets in. Patients may also be perceived as depressed when they have problems with initiation. Family members may report that the patient has become progressively less interactive and socially isolated, with reduced interest in hobbies and activities. Antidepressant medications such as SSRIs can reduce emotional distress without the anticholinergic side effects that may accompany tricyclic antidepressants. In addition, maintaining a healthy lifestyle with adequate exercise and cognitive stimulation is important. Activities that promote heart health are generally good for the brain, and engagement in pleasurable activities and social interaction can improve mood functioning and enhance quality of life.

- *Other Psychiatric Complications* Hallucinations and delusions (the latter typically paranoid), may emerge in middle and later stages of AD, occurring in approximately 50% of cases at some point. Many patients develop personality changes in later stages, which may strain caregivers. *Sundowning* may occur relative to acute or chronic issues associated with AD.

- *Medications* Early treatment may slow disease progression in some patients, although most experience continued progression. Acetylcholinesterase inhibitors, such as donepezil (Aricept), rivastigmine (Exelon), and galantamine (Razadyne), can be used to treat AD symptoms, and N-methyl-D aspartate (NMDA) receptor antagonists such as memantine (Namenda) are often used in combination with other cognitive enhancers. Stabilization in functioning is the desired outcome when treating symptoms with acetylcholinesterase inhibitors. The efficacy of these medications varies across individuals, and currently there is no way to indicate which patients will respond to what extent, or to which treatment. Nevertheless, these medications have demonstrated modest benefit in helping to stabilize and delay disease progression for 12 to 18 months or even more for a small percentage of patients. There is also evidence that a combination of medications may result in potentially greater benefit through synergic effects for some patients. However, none of these medications treat the cause of the cholinergic degeneration, and most clinical trials (e.g., those involving anti-*amyloid* drugs) have failed, although research continues to explore pharmaceutical interventions that may show benefits.

Relevant Definitions

Amnestic Disorder Disorder in which an individual loses the ability to transfer new information to long-term memory, whereas long-term memories already created remain intact. Anterograde amnesia can be caused by AD, as well as by other dementias, alcohol or substance abuse, traumatic brain injury, neoplasms, brain surgery, or other disorders affecting the memory systems.

Amyloid Protein fragments that the body produces normally. In healthy brains, these protein fragments are broken down and eliminated. In AD, the fragments accumulate to form hard, insoluble plaques. The "amyloid hypothesis" regarding its causative role in AD remains dominant in the field, although whether amyloid represents a cause or a byproduct of the disease remains a question.

Apolipoprotein ε4 (ApoE ε4) genotype Apolipoprotein E combines with fats (lipids) in the body to form molecules called low-density lipoproteins (LDLs). Lipoproteins are responsible for packaging cholesterol and other fats and carrying them through the bloodstream. There are three major but slightly different versions (alleles) of the APoE gene: ε2, ε3, and ε4. The most common allele is ε3, which is found in more than half of the general population. The second most common allele is ε4, which increases an individual's risk for developing AD. People who inherit one copy of the ApoE ε4 allele have an increased chance of developing the disease; those who inherit two copies of the allele are at even greater risk. ApoE ε4 acts as a regulator of lipid metabolism that has an affinity for the beta-amyloid protein. This allele is associated with an increased number of protein clumps, called amyloid plaques. A buildup of toxic amyloid beta peptide and amyloid plaques may lead to the death of neurons and the progressive signs and symptoms of this disorder. Conversely, research suggests that there may be a protective effect of having ApoE ε2 and ApoE ε3 alleles. Research from the Alzheimer's Disease Neuroimaging Initiative (ADNI) suggests that individuals with the ε2 allele have biomarker signatures indicating less AD pathology, lower hippocampal atrophy rates, and slower rates of cognitive decline.

Neuritic plaques Extracellular deposits of amyloid that consist of beta-amyloid protein mixed with branches of dying nerve cells, found in the brains of patients with AD. The presence of neuritic plaques and neurofibrillary tangles (see below) are used to diagnose AD at autopsy.

Neurofibrillary tangles Insoluble twisted fibers found inside the brain's cells that consist primarily of the tau protein. This protein typically forms part of a microtubule, a cellular structure that transports nutrients and other important substances from one part of the nerve cell to another. In AD, the tau protein becomes abnormal and the microtubule structures collapse. The neurofibrillary tangles are aggregates of this hyperphosphorylated tau protein and are recognized as a hallmark feature of AD pathology.

Sundowning (aka Sundown syndrome) Behavioral changes that can occur in the late afternoon or evening in people with dementia. These changes can include increased confusion, agitation, aggression, hallucinations, paranoia, increased disorientation, or pacing/wandering. Individuals with sundowning do not always meet full criteria for delirium. Also, in select cases, sundowning may be confused with delirium superimposed on dementia, which is more severe and leads to adverse events such as accelerated cognitive and functional decline, hospitalization, institutionalization, and increased mortality.

Tau abnormalities The microtubule-associated tau protein is situated on chromosome 17 and serves to stabilize microtubules. Abnormal phosphorylation of tau protein destabilizes microtubules, which causes degenerative change. Pathological tau protein inclusions occur in a range of neurodegenerative disorders called the tauopathies; these include FTD, progressive supranuclear palsy, corticobasal syndrome, some Parkinson's disease spectrum disorders, and AD.

Mild Cognitive Impairment and Alzheimer's Disease Questions

NOTE: Questions 45, 67, 94, and 116 on the First Full-Length Practice Examination, Questions 9, 43, 72, 91, and 103 on the Second Full-Length Practice Examination, Questions 26, 29, 51, 58, 66, 85, and 107 on the Third Full-Length Practice Examination, and Questions 14, 42, 63, 96, 113, and 117 on the Fourth Full-Length Practice Examination are from this chapter.

1. A 50-year-old woman comes to you with concerns that she might develop AD after age 65. What combination of risk factors would carry the greatest risk for AD later in life?

   (a) prior concussion and migraine headaches

   (b) vascular disease and anxiety

   (c) family history of AD and prior severe brain injury

   (d) exposure to toxic chemicals and family history of AD

2. A patient who has all the neurocognitive features of AD on formal neuropsychological evaluation but also displays parkinsonian symptoms most likely _____.

   (a) has frontotemporal dementia
   (c) is in the late stages of AD
   (b) has a Lewy body variant of AD
   (d) does not have AD

3. All of the following memory functions are typically impaired in early stage AD, except _____.

   (a) episodic memory
   (c) visual memory
   (b) semantic memory
   (d) procedural memory

4. A patient with AD who has been treated with acetylcholine inhibitors _____.

   (a) may show memory improvement initially, but then decline rapidly
   (b) may improve initially and decline at a slower pace
   (c) typically shows no improvement or deceleration of decline
   (d) typically shows significant functional improvement

5. AD has been described as a disease of _____.

   (a) subcortical and limbic systems
   (c) the primary cortices
   (b) the association cortices
   (d) the heteromodal cortices

6. A 67-year-old woman presents to your office with family concerns of increasing memory difficulties. She has gotten lost driving home and has forgotten to pay her bills. She is often anxious and has accused family members of stealing items from her home. Based on this information, what is her most likely diagnosis?

   (a) Mild Neurocognitive Disorder
   (c) Parkinson's dementia
   (b) Alzheimer's disease
   (d) frontotemporal dementia

7. You receive a referral for a 68-year-old woman who was found wandering outside at 2:00 am by her daughter. During clinical interview, the daughter also reports that her mother has become more aggressive, requires constant, daily reminders to perform activities of daily living (including taking her medications), and rarely initiates conversations with others. Based on this information, what is her most likely diagnosis?

   (a) Mild Neurocognitive Disorder
   (c) Major Depressive Disorder
   (b) Major Neurocognitive Disorder
   (d) Brief Psychotic Disorder

8. Which of these mild cognitive impairment subtypes most often progresses to AD?

   (a) non-amnestic multi-domain
   (c) non-amnestic single domain
   (b) amnestic single domain
   (d) frontal variant

9. A 65-year-old man and his wife present to your office due to his memory issues. The man explains that he began noticing memory problems about 4 weeks ago, which seem to be increasing significantly. He noted that he often forgets appointments, forgets where he has left his keys and other personal items, and has trouble remembering names when he meets a new person. His wife reported that she is concerned about the significant change in his memory, which she indicated

has affected his day-to-day activities. She reported current relief that he retired from his job as an attorney about 4 months earlier, because she is certain he would not have been able to function at the his job with his current memory issues. Based on this information, what is your initial hypothesis prior to formal neuropsychological assessment?

(a) Major Depressive Disorder

(c) Lewy body dementia

(b) Mild Neurocognitive Disorder

(d) frontotemporal dementia

10. Why might a clinician avoid recommending tricyclic antidepressants for a patient with dementia?

(a) They may exacerbate the dementing process.

(b) They do not effectively treat mood disorders in patients with dementia.

(c) They may cause hallucinations.

(d) They may cause side effects which negatively affect memory.

Mild Cognitive Impairment and Alzheimer's Disease Answers

1. **C—family history of AD and prior severe brain injury** *Additional risk factors include elevated blood cholesterol, diabetes mellitus, concurrent small-vessel disease, and a history of chronic major depression.*

References:
(a) Alzheimer's Association. (2015). 2015 Alzheimer's disease facts and figures. *Alzheimer's & Dementia: The Journal of the Alzheimer's Association, 11*(3), 332.
(b) Li, J. Q., Tan, L., Wang, H. F., Tan, M. S., Tan, L., Xu, W., . . . Yu, J. T. (2016). Risk factors for predicting progression from mild cognitive impairment to Alzheimer's disease: A systematic review and meta-analysis of cohort studies. *Journal of Neurology, Neurosurgery, and Psychiatry, 87*(5), 476–484.
(c) National Institutes of Health (NIH) State-of-the-Science Conference: Preventing Alzheimer's Disease and Cognitive Decline. April 26–28, 2010, Bethesda, Maryland. Retrieved from http://consensus.nih.gov/2010/alzstatement.htm

2. **C—is in the late stages of AD** *Changes such as rigidity, gait disturbance, and bradykinesia are parkinsonian signs that occur with later progression of AD. Additionally, ideational and ideomotor apraxia typically occur in the middle to late stages of the disease. Lewy body dementia is an unlikely choice as visuospatial impairment is more significant than memory dysfunction, the latter of which is the cardinal symptom of AD, and patients with Lewy body dementia also experience early extrapyramidal symptoms and visual hallucinations, whereas patients with AD typically do not.*

References:
(a) Donaghy, P. C., O'Brien, J. T., & Thomas, A. J. (2015). Prodromal dementia with Lewy bodies. *Psychological Medicine, 45*(2), 259–268.
(b) Ismail, Z., Smith, E. E., Geda, Y., Sultzer, D., Brodaty, H., Smith, G., . . . ISTAART Neuropsychiatric Symptoms Professional Interest Area. (2016). Neuropsychiatric symptoms as early manifestations of emergent dementia: Provisional diagnostic criteria for mild behavioral impairment. *Alzheimer's & Dementia, 12*(2), 195–202.

3. **D—procedural memory** *Research and rehabilitation programs have found that patients with AD can still benefit from implicit or procedural learning methods, during which skills can be learned and subsequently revived without conscious awareness.*

References:

(a) Beaunieux, H., Eustache, F., Busson, P., de la Sayette, V., Viader, F., & Desgranges, B. (2011). Cognitive procedural learning in early Alzheimer's disease: Impaired processes and compensatory mechanisms. *Journal of Neuropsychology, 6*(1), 31–42.

(b) Giebel, C. M., Challis, D., & Montaldi, D. (2015). Understanding the cognitive underpinnings of functional impairments in early dementia: A review. *Aging & Mental Health, 19*(10), 859–875.

4. **B—may improve initially and decline at a slower pace** *Most patients do not show objective evidence of memory improvement, but may experience a slower course of decline when treated pharmacologically.*

References:

(a) Eyjolfsdottir, H., Eriksdotter, M., Linderoth, B., Lind, G., Juliusson, B., Kusk, P., . . . Westman, E. (2016). Targeted delivery of nerve growth factor to the cholinergic basal forebrain of Alzheimer's disease patients: Application of a second-generation encapsulated cell biodelivery device. *Alzheimer's Research & Therapy, 8*(1), 30.

(b) Howard, R., McShane, R., Lindesay, J., Ritchie, C., Baldwin, A., Barber, R., . . . Jones, R. (2015). Nursing home placement in the Donepezil and Memantine in Moderate to Severe Alzheimer's Disease (DOMINO-AD) trial: Secondary and post-hoc analyses. *The Lancet Neurology, 14*(12), 1171–1181.

5. **B—the association cortices** *Neuronal degeneration has been found to be greatest in the medial temporal lobe and heteromodal association areas, with sparing of the primary sensory and motor cortices until later in the disease process. Most vulnerable are the cortico-cortical projections, disruption of which can contribute to degradation of the hippocampal formation and subsequent memory impairment.*

References:

(a) Dubois, B., Hampel, H., Feldman, H.H., Scheltens, P., Aisen, P., Andrieu, S., . . . Broich, K. (2016). Preclinical Alzheimer's disease: Definition, natural history, and diagnostic criteria. *Alzheimer's & Dementia, 12*(3), 292–323.

(b) Jack, C. R., Bennett, D. A., Blennow, K., Carrillo, M. C., Feldman, H. H., Frisoni, G. B., . . . Petersen, R. C. (2016). A/T/N: an unbiased descriptive classification scheme for Alzheimer's disease biomarkers. *Neurology, 87*(5), 539–547.

(c) Schoenberg, M. R., & Duff, K. (2011). Dementias and mild cognitive impairment in adults. In M. R. Schoenberg & J. G. Scott (Eds.), *The little black book of neuropsychology: A syndrome-based approach* (pp. 357–403). New York, NY: Springer Publishing.

6. **B—Alzheimer's disease** *Patients with moderate AD present with increasing memory difficulties with rapid forgetting, and typically begin to demonstrate declines in visuospatial ability. Topographical disorientation is more common at this stage, and given both the propensity to misplace personal objects and mood changes which may include suspiciousness, accusing family and/or friends of stealing personal items can occur.*

References:

(a) Cullum, C. M., & Lacritz, L. H. (2012). Neuropsychological assessment. In M. Weiner & A. M. Lipton (Eds.), *Clinical manual of Alzheimer's disease and other dementias* (pp. 65–88). Arlington, VA: American Psychiatric Publishing.

(b) Smith, G., & Butts, A. (2018). Dementia. In J. E. Morgan & J. H. Ricker (Eds.), *Textbook of clinical neuropsychology* (2nd ed., pp. 717–741). New York, NY: Taylor & Francis Group.

7. **B—Major Neurocognitive Disorder** *This patient is demonstrating moderate to late stage AD. All aspects of cognitive functioning are affected, and physical changes are now more common, such as changes in sleep patterns with nighttime wandering. Patients also demonstrate significant language dysfunction and may also develop mutism. Twenty-four hour supervision and/or nursing care are often necessary.*

References:

(a) Cullum, C. M., & Lacritz, L. H. (2012). Neuropsychological assessment. In M. Weiner & A. M. Lipton (Eds.), *Clinical manual of Alzheimer's disease and other dementias* (pp. 65–88). Arlington, VA: American Psychiatric Publishing.

(b) Smith, G., & Butts, A. (2018). Dementia. In J. E. Morgan & J. H. Ricker (Eds.), *Textbook of clinical neuropsychology* (2nd ed., pp. 717–741). New York, NY: Taylor & Francis Group.

8. **B—amnestic single domain** *Amnestic subtypes of mild cognitive impairment (MCI) reflect a relatively singular deficit (amnestic single domain) or primary deficit (amnestic multidomain) in episodic memory as reflected by impaired performance on measures of delayed verbal recall in particular. Those with amnestic multidomain MCI have an impairment in episodic memory in addition to other impaired cognitive domains. Patients with amnestic MCI (single or multidomain) are more likely to develop AD than nonamnestic MCI types.*

Reference: Petersen R. C. (2016). Mild Cognitive Impairment. *Continuum, 22*(2 Dementia), 404–418.

9. **A—Major Depressive Disorder** *While it may seem logical to consider cognitive impairment in a 65-year-old person, the recent and acute nature of his memory changes are not typical of a neurogenerative disorder without an accompanying change in medical status, such as a stroke. Further, he had no difficulty performing in his position as an attorney as recently as 4 months ago, and the wife reported a significant increase in his memory problems within a few weeks, neither of which suggests a progressive decline. It is more likely that he is experiencing symptoms of emotional distress secondary to his retirement and major lifestyle change. However, it remains salient that in some patients, even after symptoms of depression have remitted or been effectively treated, select cognitive deficits may still be present with an increased risk of developing dementia.*

References:
(a) Bieliauskas L. A., & Drag L. L. (2013). Differential diagnosis of depression and dementia. In L. Ravdin & H. Katzen (Eds.), *Handbook on the neuropsychology of aging and dementia* (pp. 257–270). Clinical Handbooks in Neuropsychology. New York, NY: Springer Publishing.
(b) Kang, H., Zhao., F, You., L., Giorgetta, C., Venkatesh, D., Sarkhai., S., & Prakash, R. (2014). Pseudo-dementia: A neuropsychological review. *Annals of Indian Academy of Neurology, 17*(2), 147–154.

10. **D—They may cause side effects which negatively affect memory** *In addition, SSRIs are often the preferred antidepressant for people with AD and depression because they have a lower risk of causing interactions with other medications.*

Reference: Hort, J., O'Brien, T., Gainotti, G., Pirttila, T., Popescu, B.O . . . Scheltens, P. (2010). EFNS guidelines for the diagnosis and management of Alzheimer's disease. *European Journal of Neurology, 17*(10), 1236–1248.

Recommended Readings

Albert, M .S., DeKosky, S. T., Dickson, D., Dubois, B., Feldman, H. H., Fox, N. C., . . . Phelps, C. H. (2011). The diagnosis of cognitive impairment due to Alzheimer's disease: Recommendations from the National Institute on Aging-Alzheimer's Association Workgroups on diagnostic guidelines for Alzheimer's Disease. *Alzheimers Dementia, 7*(3), 270–279.

Bondi, M. W., Salmon, D. P., & Kaszniak A. W. (2009). The neuropsychology of dementia. In I. Grant & K. M. Adams (Eds.), *Neuropsychological assessment of neuropsychiatric and neuromedical disorders* (3rd ed., pp. 159–198). New York, NY: Oxford University Press.

Jack, C. R., Bennett, D. A., Blennow, K., Carrillo, M. D., Dunn, B., Haeberlein, S. B., . . . Sperling, R. (2018). NIA- AA Research Framework: Toward a biological definition of Alzheimer's disease. *Alzheimers Dementia, 14*(4), 535–562.

Jack, C. R., Knopman, D. S., Jagust, W. J., Shaw, L. M., Aisen, P. S., Trojanowski, J. Q., . . . Trojanowski, J. Q. (2010). Hypothetical model of dynamic biomarkers of the Alzheimer's pathological cascade. *The Lancet Neurology, 9*(1), 119–128.

Jack, C. R., Knopman, D. S., Weigand, S. D., Wiste, H. J., Vemuri, P., Lowe, V., . . . Petersen, R.C. (2012). An operational approach to National Institute on Aging–Alzheimer's Association criteria for preclinical Alzheimer's disease. *Annals of Neurology, 71*(6), 765–775.

McKhann, G. M., Knopman, D. S., Chertkow, H., Hyman, B. T., Jack, C. R., Kawas, C. H., . . . Phelps, C. H. (2011). The diagnosis of dementia due to Alzheimer's disease: Recommendations from the National Institute on Aging–Alzheimer's Association workgroups on diagnostic guidelines for Alzheimer's disease. *Alzheimer's & Dementia, 7,* 263–269.

Petersen. R. C. (2016). Mild cognitive impairment. *Continuum, 22*(2 Dementia), 404–418.

Petersen, R. C., & Nagash, S. (2008). Mild cognitive impairment: An overview. *CNS Spectrum, 13*(1), 45–53.

Smith, G., & Butts, A. (2018). Dementia. In J. E. Morgan & J. H. Ricker (Eds.), *Textbook of clinical neuropsychology* (2nd ed., pp. 717–741). New York, NY: Taylor & Francis Group.

Sperling, R. A., Aisen, P. S., Beckett, L. A., Bennett, D. A., Craft, S., Fagan, A. M., . . . Phelps, C. H. (2011). Toward defining the pre- clinical stages of Alzheimer's disease: Recommendations from the National Institute on Aging-Alzheimer's Association workgroups on diagnostic guidelines for Alzheimer's disease. *Alzheimer's Dementia, 7,* 280–292.

Websites

An overview of MCI, both original publication and recent update: https://www.researchgate.net/publication/5648026_Petersen_RC_Negash_S_Mild_cognitive_impairment_an_overview_CNS_Spectr_13_45-53

https://www.drperlmutter.com/wp-content/uploads/2018/01/Practice-guideline-update-summary-Mild-cognitive-impairment.pdf

Alzheimer's disease and neuroimaging: https://pubs.rsna.org/doi/pdf/10.1148/radiol.2018180958

Alzheimer's disease, disease information, treatment considerations, and caregiver resources: www.alz.org

MEDICAL

31 Vascular Cognitive Impairment

Andrew A. Swihart

Definition

Vascular cognitive impairment (VCI) is an umbrella term referring to the full range of severity of cognitive impairments attributable, in part or in whole, to cerebrovascular disease (CVD). Hence, it does not refer to a specific disease state but, rather, labels a syndrome with multiple potential neuropathologic bases. Vascular mild cognitive impairment (VaMCI) has been used when the pathophysiological basis of the prodromal dementia syndrome of mild cognitive impairment is presumed to be vascular in nature. Vascular cognitive impairment, no dementia (VCIND) has also been used to describe this early stage of milder cognitive decline not yet broad or severe enough to meet diagnostic criteria for dementia. Vascular dementia (VaD) is the diagnostic term applied when the patient's cognitive impairment and daily functioning meet current criteria for all-cause dementia and CVD is the known or presumed etiology of the dementia.

Vascular dementia (VaD) is a clinico-radiological syndrome defined by the presence of significant cognitive impairment that, in turn, produces significant impairment in fundamental daily activities (e.g., vocational, home management, social) attributable to ischemic and/or hemorrhagic CVD. Multiple schemes for specific diagnostic criteria for VaD have been offered; however, a lack of consensus remains regarding how best to define this disorder. First, agreement is lacking on the specific nature of the cognitive deficits necessary to constitute dementia. Second, there is no consensus on what pathophysiologic abnormalities suffice to explain the presence of the cognitive and functional impairment in VaD. Hence, VaD remains a construct lacking both pathognomic neuropsychological and biological diagnostic marker(s). Similar conceptual problems prevent consensus in defining VaMCI/VCIND.

Among the most widely cited diagnostic criteria for VaD are the National Institute of Neurological Disorders and Stroke and Association Internationale pour la Recherché et l'Enseignement en Neurosciences (*NINDS-AIREN*) criteria. The diagnosis of probable VaD requires the following:

1. Dementia, characterized by the presence of memory impairment and impairment in at least two additional cognitive domains.

2. Interference in activities of daily living (ADLs) not attributable to the physical effects of stroke alone, delirium, major psychiatric disorders, or other dementias such as Alzheimer's disease (AD).

3. Evidence of CVD, as manifest in focal neurologic signs consistent with stroke and neuroimaging evidence of CVD.

4. Presumed causal relationship between dementia and CVD, as suggested by:

   (a) onset of dementia within 3 months of recognized stroke event and/or
   (b) abrupt deterioration of, or stepwise progression of, cognitive impairment.

Although the *Diagnostic and Statistical Manual of Mental Disorders* (DSM-IV) has been supplanted by the DSM-5, most available research regarding VaD citing the DSM has utilized the diagnostic criteria set forth in DSM-IV and, hence, understanding those criteria remains necessary for understanding this literature. The DSM-IV diagnostic criteria require (a) memory impairment and impairment in at least one additional cognitive domain, (b) co-occurrence of focal neurologic signs and symptoms or neuroimaging evidence of causally related CVD, and (c) impairment producing significant social and/or occupational dysfunction.

The State of California Alzheimer's Disease Diagnostic and Treatment Centers (ADDTC) criteria for VaD are also often cited. In defining dementia, the ADDTC criteria do not require memory impairment; they only require that more than one cognitive domain be affected. The severity of the cognitive deficits must result in impairment in the conduct of fundamental everyday affairs.

The DSM-5 uses the terms major and mild neurocognitive disorder when referring to dementia and MCI, respectively. The diagnosis of major neurocognitive disorder requires (a) significant cognitive decline in one or more cognitive domains, (b) which, at a minimum, interfere with independence in instrumental activities of everyday living (e.g., bill paying, home financial management), and (c) these symptoms and decline are documented by observations of the patient, knowledgeable informants, or the clinician and also through neuropsychological assessment. The DSM-5 notes that major and mild neurocognitive disorders differ only in where they fall on a continuum of cognitive and ADL symptom severity and, therefore, identifying the threshold differentiating the two is necessarily arbitrary. To specify a major or mild neurocognitive disorder as a vascular neurocognitive disorder, the DSM-5 adds the following criteria: (a) documentation of a temporally concurrent relationship between symptom onset and one or more cerebrovascular events, (b) prominent evidence of decline in complex attention and executive functions and (c) evidence of CVD sufficient to explain the observed cognitive impairments. Further criteria are provided that differentiate probable from possible vascular neurocognitive disorder (i.e., neuroimaging evidence of CVD, a temporal relationship between the onset of the cognitive symptoms and the cerebrovascular events, and clinical and genetic evidence of CVD permit the application of the "probable" label).

Each of these diagnostic criteria sets has well-recognized research and clinical diagnostic shortcomings. First, the *NINDS-AIREN* and DSM-IV criteria exclude dementia syndromes lacking significant memory impairment. Second, the *NINDS-AIREN* criteria require evidence of impairment in at least three cognitive domains; the DSM-IV and ADDTC require only two affected domains; DSM-5 requires only one. Hence, patients meeting *NINDS-AIREN* criteria must be more diffusely cognitively impaired than patients meeting DSM-IV, ADDTC, or DSM-5 criteria. Third, all of these criteria sets are inconsistent with the reality that pure VaD and pure AD are the opposing anchors of a commonly occurring spectrum of disease, with many patients experiencing dementia due to the additive effects of co-occurring CVD and AD (i.e., *mixed dementia*). Fourth, none of these diagnostic sets adequately defines what constitutes CVD of a severity sufficient to account for the observed dementia. Fifth, the presence of a clearly established temporal relationship between cognitive symptom onset and causative cerebrovascular events has proven to be the exception, not the rule. Finally, the differences in how these classification systems operationally define dementia, and their failure to adequately define CVD sufficient to explain observed dementia, result in very poor diagnostic agreement at the individual case level, as well as marked variation in incidence and prevalence estimates for VaD.

In light of the conceptual problems and inconsistencies characterizing current diagnostic criteria for VaD, the American Heart Association/American Stroke Association released a statement that proposes specific diagnostic criteria for probable VaD, possible VaD, probable VaMCI, possible VaMCI, and unstable VaMCI (Gorelick et al., 2011). These criteria are intended to resolve the conceptual and terminological problems that have arisen as research on vascular contributions to cognitive impairment and dementia has proliferated. The AHA/ASA criteria for probable VaD include (a) impairment in two or more cognitive domains (without a requirement for impairment in memory), (b) impairment in ADLs that are not attributable to purely motor or sensory deficits, (c) neuroimaging evidence of CVD, (d) a clear temporal relationship between a cerebrovascular event and cognitive impairment or a clear relationship between the pattern/severity of subcortical CVD and cognitive impairment, and (e) the absence of a gradual cognitive decline preceding the onset of the CVD. See Gorelick et al. (2011) for the criteria sets for possible VaD, as well as for probable, possible, and unstable VaMCI. Shortcomings remain, however. First, "a clear temporal relationship" between a cerebrovascular event and cognitive impairment is not operationally defined. In like manner, "a clear relationship" between the pattern/severity of subcortical CVD and cognitive impairment is also left undefined. Furthermore, the criterion requiring "the absence of a gradual cognitive decline preceding the onset of the CVD" could very well exclude *Binswanger's disease* as a cause of VCIND.

Neuropathology

Vascular cognitive impairment is a uniquely heterogenous syndrome, with multiple differing pathophysiological routes from normal cognitive functioning through VaMCI/VCIND to VaD. Attempts have been made to define specific subtypes of VaD based on pathophysiological differences, but consensus on such is absent. In general, the underlying pathogenesis may involve cardioembolic, atherosclerotic, ischemic, hemorrhagic or genetic processes resulting in:

- multiple small vessel disease (occlusive or nonocclusive) resulting in microinfarction, leukoencephalopathy and/or lacunar infarctions
- large-vessel occlusive disease
- microhemorrhagic lesions
- macrohemorrhagic lesions
- any combination of these processes

Attempts to understand the specific nature and extent of vascular disease necessary to produce VCI are complicated by multiple factors. First, CVD is present in a large proportion of community-dwelling, non-demented older adults. Community-based neuropathology studies identify parenchymal ischemic lesions in >75% of adults aged 70+. One third to one half of older adults have macroscopic infarcts, and an undoubtedly larger proportion have microscopic infarcts. White matter lesions have been reported to occur in most individuals over the age of 30. Hence, the mere presence of CVD in individuals with cognitive impairment does not constitute evidence of vascular compromise as a causal factor for the cognitive impairment. Second, the co-occurrence of AD, Lewy body disease, and/or other neuropathology with CVD is very common, complicating confident causal attribution for cognitive impairment. Third, individual differences in factors such as depression and cognitive reserve influence the effects of CVD on cognition. Acknowledging the above, it remains clear that greater burden of CVD is associated with greater risk of cognitive impairment, with larger volume and larger number of infarcts and white matter hyperintensities (WMH) associated with increasing probability of VCI. The presence of extensive WMH volume (>1 SD above 5-year age group mean) is associated with a more than doubling of risk of VaD and VaMCI in individuals ≥60 years of age.

Specific Neuropathophysiological Subtypes

- ***Binswanger's Disease*** Prior to contemporary use of the term "vascular dementia," dementia occurring in the context of significant vascular disease burden was conferred a variety of labels, depending on the specific nature of the observed or presumed CVD. *Binswanger's disease* was diagnosed in the context of cognitive impairment co-occurring with increased periventricular white matter signal on neuroimaging; lacunar infarcts occurring in subcortical structures such as the thalamus, basal ganglia, and the periventricular white matter; and sparing of subcortical U fibers, all occurring in the context of a slowly progressing clinical course. However, with the advent of routine neuroimaging studies in the aged, it has become evident that white matter abnormalities abound in the elderly in the absence of significant cognitive impairment (such as WMH and silent brain infarcts [SBI]) and, consequently, the validity of *Binswanger's disease* has been called into question and the term is not commonly used today.

- *Leukoaraiosis* The term *leukoaraiosis* was introduced by Hachinski as a label for the apparently more benign white matter abnormalities commonly observed in the elderly and not associated with dementia (see above). *Leukoaraiosis* refers to nonspecific loss of density of subcortical white matter, presumably due to diffuse microvascular ischemia (but not occlusion) and is generally synonymous with periventricular white matter disease and WMH.

- *Multi-Infarct Dementia (MID)* The label MID is typically applied in cases involving dementia in the context of multiple cerebral infarctions with subsequent cerebral volume loss and a temporally concurrent, stepwise progression of cognitive impairment. Unlike *Binswanger's disease*, MID often involves lesions of the cerebral cortex, as well as subcortical white matter and deep gray matter structures.

- *Strategic Infarct* Vascular dementia can occur secondary to a single *strategic infarct*. For example, lesions of the vasculature supplying the left angular gyrus region, the caudate nucleus, the globus pallidus, and the thalamus are often cited as locations of strategic infarctions resulting in symptoms meeting criteria for VaD. Each such *strategic infarct* has been associated with a particular constellation of neuropsychological deficits. In brief, see Table 31.1.

- *Lacunar Infarcts* Multiple lacunar states can produce dementia. The pathophysiology underlying such states involves multiple, diffuse lacunar infarcts, frequently involving the perforating arteries (e.g., lenticulostriate branches of the MCA) supplying the thalamus and/or other subcortical and brainstem structures (e.g., the basal ganglia, pons). Lacunae are typically defined as areas of ischemic necrosis of no more than 15 mm diameter. There is no consensus on the precise number, volume, or location of lacunae required to explain a co-occurring dementia.

- *Cerebral amyloid angiopathy (CAA)* is caused by a pathophysiologic process involving amyloid deposition in blood vessels and resulting in repeated hemorrhage (typically lobar), ischemic infarction, and cognitive loss. The amyloid deposition usually has its onset after age 55, is present in varying degrees in the vast majority of non-demented older adults, occurs in both sporadic and hereditary forms, and can lead to hemorrhages and VaD as it progresses.

- *Cerebral autosomal dominant arteriopathy with subcortical infarcts and leukoencephalopathy (CADASIL)* is a hereditary nonatherosclerotic arteriopathy affecting the cerebral small vessels and resulting in diffuse white matter disease and small lacunar infarctions. Pathologically, CADASIL is characterized by the presence of granular osmiophilic material (GOM) in both cerebral and extracerebral vascular smooth muscle, leading to the arteriopathy of CADASIL. Clinically, individuals with CADASIL often present with migraine, seizures, depression, recurrent transient ischemic attacks (TIA), and stroke. Onset is typically early to middle adulthood, and stroke events may occur in the absence of other known risk factors for stroke. The dementia reflects the frequently frontal and subcortical focus of the stroke events. CADASIL is a rare disease, with prevalence estimated at 5 per 100,000.

- *Subcortical ischemic vascular disease (SIVD) or small vessel disease* These terms are used to refer to a variety of processes and can encompass *Binswanger's disease*, lacunar states, CAA, and CADASIL, as well as other subcortical microvascular infarcts and ischemia that may result in VCI of any severity. Small-vessel disease may occur secondary to atherosclerosis (subendothelial accumulation of atheromatous plaque within the blood vessel) or lipohyalinosis (reduced diameter of small-vessel wall lumen secondary to vessel wall thickening) and may result in hypoperfusion, microinfarction, or lacunar infarction of the subcortical white matter. Small-vessel disease affects the subcortical white matter and nuclei via pathology of the penetrating arteries (e.g., the lenticulostriate branches from the middle cerebral artery and the thalamic branches of the posterior cerebral artery), as well as the smaller vessels of the white matter more generally.

- *Metabolic and Toxic States* Cerebral white matter disease can also result from metabolic disorders (e.g., folate deficiency, vitamin B_{12} deficiency, hypoxia), as well as from toxin exposure (e.g., chemotherapy, radiation therapy, drug abuse, solvent exposure, carbon monoxide poisoning). All of these can result in cognitive impairment or frank dementia.

- *Mixed Dementia* This term is applied to cases in which coexisting pathophysiology of CVD and another dementing disorder (most commonly AD or Lewy body disease) is observed, leading to uncertainty as to the causal attribution for the cognitive impairment. Cerebrovascular disease and AD have additive and independent effects in producing dementia, resulting in an earlier expression of cognitive impairment and dementia than would be seen in patients with either AD (i.e., amyloid plaques and neurofibrillary tangles) or CVD alone. Cerebrovascular disease and AD pathology may actually be intertwined through impaired beta-amyloid clearance secondary to hypoperfusion. The resulting beta-amyloid accumulation may exacerbate CAA, with subsequent areas of bleed. Cerebrovascular disease may also result in microvascular disease with consequent neuronal damage and loss. However, the precise relationship between the varied pathological processes observed in *mixed dementia* and the associated cognitive impairments remains unsettled.

TABLE 31.1 Strategic Infarct Syndromes

Area of Infarct	Neuropsychological Deficits
Left angular gyrus	Characteristic symptoms of Gerstmann syndrome, as well as constructional dysfunction (i.e., difficulty drawing or copying figures due to visuospatial deficits)
Caudate nucleus, globus pallidus, and thalamus	May disrupt critical dorsolateral prefrontal-subcortical circuits underlying various executive and motor functions
Thalamus	A broad range of cognitive and behavioral disturbances that manifest as executive dysfunction, language impairment, memory dysfunction, and/or disorders of initiation, inhibition and modulation of mood, and emotional behavior
Single infarctions in branches of posterior cerebral artery (PCA)	Specific deficits produced are determined by laterality of lesion and the specific PCA branch(es) occluded. Memory deficits are common
Single infarctions in branches of anterior cerebral artery (ACA)	Specific deficits produced are determined by laterality of lesion and the specific ACA branch(es) occluded. Neurobehavioral syndromes are common

Risk Factors

Biological risk factors for VCI include:

- hypertension
- hypercholesterolemia
- hyperhomocysteinemiae
- chronic hyperglycemia, diabetes mellitus and metabolic syndrome (i.e., the presence of any three of the following: hypertension, hyperglycemia, hypertriglyceridemia, low serum high-density lipoprotein and abdominal obesity)
- inflammation (as reflected in levels of C-reactive protein levels)
- cardiac disease (including coronary artery disease and cardiac arrhythmias such as atrial fibrillation)
- congestive heart failure
- coronary artery bypass grafting (CABG; via embolism and hypoperfusion)
- obstructive sleep apnea
- chronic kidney disease
- obesity, as reflected in a high waist-hip ratio or BMI $\geq$ 30
- underweight, defined as a BMI <18.5
- transient ischemic attacks
- recurrent stroke
- ApoE ε4 genotype is associated with increased risk of cerebral amyloid angiopathy and, subsequently, VCI

Behavioral risk factors for VCI include:

- cigarette smoking
- sedentary lifestyle
- maladaptive dietary habits (e.g., diets high in fats and sodium).

Demographic risk factors for VCI include:

- advancing age
- African American, Native American, and Latin/x ethnicity

Epidemiology

The presence of multiple differing, but commonly used criteria for the diagnosis of VCI and VaD adds significant variance to occurrence estimates. The requirement of significant impairment of memory as a diagnostic criterion in the *NINDS-AIREN* and DSM-IV-TR criteria results in a systematic underestimation of VaD frequency. The insensitivity to significant cognitive impairment of standard screening instruments (e.g., the Mini-Mental State Examination [MMSE]), as well as the use of differing cut points for defining impairment with these instruments, may result in both underestimates of VaD incidence and prevalence, as well as increased variance in such estimates across studies. Finally, the specific age range sampled will significantly affect estimates of both incidence and prevalence. Methodological issues are even more problematic in regards to estimating incidence and prevalence of *mixed dementia*. As a consequence, all estimates of VCI, VaD, and *mixed dementia* incidence and prevalence must be viewed with caution.

With this acknowledged, VCI has been cited as second only to AD as a cause of cognitive impairment in late life. The prevalence of VaD has been reported to be 2.4% in persons older than 70, with prevalence rates doubling every 5.3 years. Incidence of VaD in the United States, derived from large and nationally representative samples, range from 6.2 to 14.6 cases per 1,000 person years in individuals older than 70. In sum, despite variance in estimates across studies and the probable systematic underestimation of VaD due to limitations in diagnostic criteria, it appears certain that VaD and *mixed dementia* represent significant public health problems. Autopsy series reveal pathology consistent with a diagnosis of VaD in 18% of all dementia cases, behind only AD (77%) and Lewy body disease (26%). However, only 3% of all dementia cases had "pure" VaD (no co-occurring pathology sufficient to explain the dementia). Mixed pathology was found in 77% of the VaD cases, with AD + VaD being, by far, most common. Such mixed pathology accounts for 11% of all dementia cases. However, WMH and SBI are observed upon MRI imaging in approximately 20% to 30% of non-demented, community-residing, aged adults. Furthermore, microinfarctions are observed at autopsy in approximately 25% of aged adults without dementia. Therefore, uncertainty remains when drawing conclusions regarding causation of impairment in *mixed dementia* cases.

Presentation, Disease Course, and Recovery

The symptoms and clinical course characterizing VCI are, of necessity, heterogeneous, reflecting the many differing pathophysiologic processes and lesion location(s) underlying this syndrome.

Data from the Aging, Demographics, and Memory Study (ADAMS) reveal that VaD accounts for approximately 17.4% of all dementia in individuals aged 71 years and older in the United States. The prevalence of VCIND in United States residents age 71 and older is approximately 5.7%. Of individuals meeting criteria for VCIND in ADAMS, 6.1% progress to dementia in 1 year. Data from the Canadian Study of Health and Aging revealed that 44% of individuals with VCIND meet criteria for dementia at 5-year follow-up. Of those cases progressing to dementia, 43% met criteria for VaD, 35% for AD, 13% for *mixed dementia*, and 9% were demented without a specific classification determined. Deficits in memory and category word-list generation at baseline predicted progression to dementia.

Symptoms most commonly reported as occurring early in VCI include deficits in executive functions attention, and slowing of processing speed. The fact that VCI pathology commonly disrupts the deep frontal white matter, frontal-subcortical circuitry, the basal ganglia, and the thalamus is thought to explain the common and early presence of these specific cognitive impairments. Positive correlations among WMH, executive function deficits, and slowing of processing speed have been reported in multiple studies.

Subcortical vascular dementia attributable to SVID, and affecting the anterior and/or dorsomedial thalamus, has been described as presenting with predominant apathy, impaired attention, and memory dysfunction. Recent research on *mixed dementia* with subcortical ischemic vascular disease (i.e., lacunes and WMHs) and AD reveals that the association between AD pathology and cognitive impairment is significantly stronger than the association between subcortical ischemic disease and cognitive impairment, and that memory is disproportionately more impaired than executive functioning in these cases with mixed pathology. Lacunar states affecting predominantly the basal ganglia, thalamus and related white matter may have disproportionate dysarthria, impaired gait, pseudobulbar palsy (i.e., disinhibition of emotional display, such as uncontrollable crying or laughing, in response to stimuli that would otherwise be of insufficient intensity to elicit such) and loss of initiation.

Intuitively, VaD may be expected to have a relatively abrupt onset when the underlying pathology involves a single *strategic infarct*. Alternatively, when the dementia occurs in the context of MID, a more stepwise progression may be expected. Finally, in the context of SVID, an insidious onset and a progressive course of impairment may be observed. However, despite the intuitive logic of this, research to date has not produced strong or consistent support for these relationships. This may be due to the facts that (a) VaD frequently involves mixtures of the just-described pathophysiological processes, (b) *mixed dementia*, combining the pathology of AD and VaD, is commonly present and (c) longitudinal studies with 1-year (or longer) follow-up assessment points cannot determine whether cognitive decline observed at follow-up occurred in a stepwise or smoothly progressive manner.

Consensus is lacking regarding the rate of progression of VaD. Some studies report that VaD, AD, and Lewy body dementia (LBD) have similar rates of cognitive decline. Other studies have reported a shorter survival time relative to AD and LBD. None of these findings have been consistently replicated. Again, the heterogeneity of VaD, and a failure to separate pure VaD from *mixed dementia* cases, may explain some of this inconsistency in the literature. Furthermore, comparisons of survival time for these dementias are rendered difficult by differential rates of comorbid health problems, such as hypertension, diabetes mellitus, and coronary artery disease.

Expectations for Neuropsychological Assessment Results

VaMCI and VaD are heterogeneous syndromes and, hence, no uniform pattern of neuropsychological performance will characterizes all patients with VCI. Furthermore, the pattern and severity of neuropsychological impairment will change across time as VaMCI and VaD progress, further rendering expectations for an invariant pattern inappropriate. Attempts to differentiate VCI from AD on the basis of neuropsychological assessment results have been quite mixed, and are complicated by the common co-occurrence of VCI and AD (*mixed dementia*) as well as the heterogeneous nature of the pathology underlying VCI itself. Consequently, although general statements regarding neuropsychological assessment results may accurately characterize aggregate groups of patients with VaMCI or VaD, such statements may not hold true at the individual case level.

The 2006 NINDS-Canadian Stroke Council VCI harmonization standards (Hachinski et al., 2006) provide suggestions for a standard neuropsychological test battery for assessment of VCI. The recommended test battery emphasizes assessment of executive, visuospatial, language, memory, mood, and premorbid cognitive status and can serve as a foundation for constructing an assessment protocol of adequate breadth to assess the full range of impairments possible in VCI.

Research to date suggests that expectations for neuropsychological assessment results may reasonably include the following:

- *Intelligence/Achievement* Typically, problem-solving and reasoning tasks dependent on speed of processing, and executive functions will show the earliest declines. In VaD with a primarily subcortical, diffuse white matter locus of pathology, the so-called hold tests of intellect and achievement (such as Information and Vocabulary, or Spelling and Word Reading) may be relatively spared. However, in cases of *strategic infarct* affecting left perisylvian regions or thalamic nuclei, performance on these tests may be quite adversely affected. However, as the dementia progresses, deficits in all measures of intellectual functioning can eventually be expected.

- *Attention/Concentration* Deficits in attention and concentration have their onset early in VCI and can be expected to result in poor performance on relevant tasks (e.g., Digit Span).

- *Processing Speed* Processing speed deficits are ubiquitous in VCI, particularly in those patients with pathology predominantly affecting subcortical white matter and nuclei. Hence, performance on timed measures (e.g., Trail Making Test A, Symbol Search, Symbol Digit Modalities Test) may be disproportionately affected early on.

- *Language* Unlike the typical patient with AD, patients with VaD often lack early disruption of language functions. However, early declines in word list generation (letter) tasks (i.e., Controlled Oral Word Association) performance are reported in VaD, possibly reflecting underlying problems in speed of processing and executive functions. Semantic and letter word list generation have been said to be roughly equally affected in VaD. Confrontation naming performance is often affected in VaD, but not as markedly as in AD. In the absence of focal language cortex infarct, frank aphasia is not common.

- *Visuospatial* Visuoconstructional task performance is often affected, with deficits to be expected on figure copy tasks or clock drawing. More fundamental problems in executive functions may also account for impaired visuoconstructional task performance.

- *Memory* Unfortunately, inclusion of memory impairment as a requirement for the diagnosis of VaD by two widely used criteria sets leads to the tautological finding of memory impairment as typical of VaD. However, if the criteria for all-cause dementia proffered by the *NIA-AA* work group are applied to patients with CVD, it is likely that memory impairment will be seen to be a later occurring deficit in most patients with VaD, appearing only after significant declines in speed of processing, word-list generation, and executive functions are observed. This pattern can be expected to typify patients with primarily white matter involvement; *strategic infarcts* in posterior cerebral artery branches supplying the mesial temporal lobe, or in perforating vessels supplying thalamic nuclei, may produce exceptions.

- *Executive Functions* In addition to declines in speed of processing, impairment on tasks tapping executive functions (e.g., Trail Making Test B, Wisconsin Card Sorting Test) are often cited as among the earliest deficits observed in VCI. This is presumed to reflect disruption of frontal-subcortical circuits consequent to the pervasive white matter involvement characterizing many such patients.

- *Sensorimotor* In patients with VaD who have a primarily subcortical focus of pathology, sensorimotor deficits, gait disturbance, dysarthria, extrapyramidal signs, and urinary incontinence are common. Consequently, given the overlap in presenting symptoms, care must be taken in differentiating between VaD and normal pressure hydrocephalus. Furthermore, cortical infarction can produce visual field deficits, motor impairment, somatosensory loss, and other focal symptoms that can aid in differentiating VaD from other dementias. Because of the more common and earlier presence of impaired mobility, urinary incontinence, and depression in VaD, VaD may have greater functional impairment associated with it than does AD when level of cognitive impairment is equated across patient groups.

- *Emotion and Personality* Psychomotor slowing and depression are frequently reported in patients with VaD and may be present from the earliest stages. Pseudobulbar palsy may also occur. Psychotic symptoms, including delusions and visual hallucinations, occur in a sizable minority. Anxiety also commonly occurs.

Considerations when Treating Patients with VCI

Patient Lifestyle Considerations

Recommendations for treatment begin with reduction of the known risk factors for VCI. Unlike other dementing disorders, VCI offers many routes for effective treatment (although not reversal) and, hence, accurate and early diagnosis is of unique importance here. Ideally, actions to reduce or eliminate these risk factors should begin in healthy individuals before the onset of VCI (primary prevention). Primary targets for treatment should include hypertension, hypercholesterolemia, diabetes mellitus, atrial fibrillation, and other CVD risk factors. Life-style modification is important, including smoking cessation, weight reduction, dietary modification (both calorie reduction and reduction of saturated fats), limiting alcohol consumption, and increasing physical exercise. Exercise has positive benefits, both through risk-factor reduction and, possibly, through direct effects on cognition.

Randomized double-blind, placebo-controlled trials of the cholinesterase inhibitors donepezil (Aricept) and galantamine (e.g., Razadyne, Reminyl) have shown effectiveness in delaying cognitive decline in VaD and *mixed dementia*, respectively. Relative to placebo, donepezil produces a statistically significant but quite modest benefit in scores on the cognitive subscale of the Alzheimer Disease Assessment Scale (the mean change from baseline was −1.99) and also on the MMSE (mean change from baseline of +1.53) over a 24-week trial. Rivastigmine and the NMDA receptor antagonist memantine (Namenda) have performed similarly in some trials, but benefits are less well established.

Addressing comorbidities that may worsen clinical symptoms in VCI is also important. Targets for such intervention include depression, sleep disruption, and physical pain.

Caregiver Considerations

Interventions directed at reducing caregiver burden are important in maintaining maximal functioning and independence for the patient with VaD. Such interventions should include increasing caregiver self-efficacy through education and coping skill training, increasing caregiver activity, maintaining/ improving the quality of social support (including family, peer, and community resource support), and training in effective coping strategies (e.g., confronting problems) versus ineffective strategies (e.g., avoiding, venting, self-distracting through unrelated activity involvement). Maintaining sleep quality has been shown to be of particular importance. Pharmacological and psychotherapeutic intervention for caregiver depression and anxiety is often indicated. Evaluating and treating the patient for depression, anxiety, and aggressive/ disruptive behavior has beneficial effects both directly and indirectly through a reduction in caregiver burden.

The patient's family may require guidance in how to plan for eventual loss of capacity issues, both through referral to appropriate resources (e.g., family lawyer) and through direct assessment of capacity as the severity of VCI progresses. Driving will eventually become unsafe, and the neuropsychologist should assess factors predicting driving safety early and regularly. Follow-up assessment with an on-the-road evaluation is indicated if frank contraindications to such are not obtained during neuropsychological evaluation. Safety in the home should be assessed and environmental modifications recommended as needed (e.g., fall risk precautions, door alarms to aid in preventing wandering, lifeline personal medical alert systems, etc.). Referral to appropriate community resources will be essential (e.g., the county commission on aging). Utilization of available community options for respite care is important in reducing caregiver burden. Discussion of and planning for the possibility of increasing impairment and concomitant need for assistance in the home, residence in assisted living, and skilled nursing home placement are important. As severity of VaD worsens, referral for palliative care may also be appropriate.

Acknowledgments

The critical comments of Frederick W. Unverzagt, Department of Psychiatry, Indiana University School of Medicine, are gratefully acknowledged.

Relevant Definitions

Binswanger's disease Ischemia affecting the small vessels of the periventricular regions, but sparing subcortical U (arcuate) fibers, resulting in leukoencephalopathy and dementia. First described by Otto Binswanger (1894).

Cerebral amyloid angiopathy (CAA) Amyloid deposition in blood vessels; can result in repeated hemorrhage, ischemic infarction, and cognitive loss.

Cerebral autosomal dominant arteriopathy with subcortical infarcts and leukoencephalopathy (CADASIL) Nonatherosclerotic arteriopathy of the cerebral small vessels resulting in diffuse white matter disease and lacunar infarctions. Presents as migraine, seizures, recurrent TIA, stroke, and depression. Onset is typically early to middle adulthood. The eventually occurring dementia often reflects the frequently frontal and subcortical focus of the stroke events.

Lacunae Subcortical areas of ischemic necrosis of less than 15 mm in diameter.

Lacunar state The occurrence of VaD secondary to the cumulative effect of recurrent subcortical lacunar infarctions, often involving the perforating arteries supplying the thalamus and basal ganglia.

Leukoaraiosis Nonspecific loss of density of subcortical white matter presumably due to diffuse microvascular ischemia. Generally synonymous with periventricular white matter disease and WMH.

Mixed dementia Dementia occurring in the presence of both CVD and the AD or other neurodegenerative disease (e.g., Lewy body disease). The dementia is attributed to the combined effects of these comorbid processes.

Multi-infarct dementia Dementia occurring in the context of repeated, relatively large-vessel strokes (e.g., affecting the branches of the anterior cerebral artery [ACA], middle cerebral artery [MCA], or posterior cerebral artery [PCA]), cortical and/or subcortical in location. An older term, falling into disuse.

NIA-AA National Institute on Aging-Alzheimer's Association. The NIA-AA charged a work group to revise the criteria for Alzheimer's dementia, resulting in the publication of new criteria for all-cause dementia as well as for Alzheimer's dementia (see McKhann et al. in the section "Recommended Readings").

NINDS-AIRENS National Institute of Neurological Disorders and Stroke and Association Internationale pour la Recherché et l'Enseignement en Neurosciences (see Román et al. (1993) in the section "Vascular Cognitive Impairment Answers").

Silent brain infarct Cerebral infarction occurring in the absence of temporally concurrent new clinical symptoms. The accrual of infarcts, each individually clinically silent, may collectively result in VCI and frank VaD.

Strategic infarct An infarct whose anatomical location is more critical than its volume for determining its symptom presentation. Infarcts affecting single branches of the ACA, MCA, or PCA, as well as infarcts disrupting frontal-subcortical pathways, are often termed strategic infarcts.

Vascular cognitive impairment (VCI) Cognitive loss attributable to CVD. VCI is used in reference to any degree of cognitive impairment secondary to CVD (including dementia).

Vascular Cognitive Impairment Questions

NOTE: Questions 18, 60, 110, and 120 on the First Full-Length Practice Examination, Questions 28, 64, 93, 101, and 107 on the Second Full-Length Practice Examination, Questions 43, 69, 88, and 112 on the Third Full-Length Practice Examination, and Questions 22, 24, 65, and 106 on the Fourth Full-Length Practice Examination are from this chapter.

1. The term vascular cognitive impairment (VCI) refers to _____.
   (a) the prodromal state of vascular dementia (VaD)
   (b) vascular mild cognitive impairment(VaMCI)
   (c) the full spectrum of cognitive impairment due to CVD
   (d) pure VaMCI and VaD

2. The threshold between major and mild vascular neurocognitive disorder as defined by DSM-5 occurs when _____.
   (a) the patient progresses from modest to substantial cognitive impairment and can no longer independently complete complex IADLs
   (b) the patient displays impairment in three or more cognitive domains regardless of degree of dependence in IADLs
   (c) functioning falls ≥1.5 SD below the patient's age group in two or more cognitive domains
   (d) the onset of cognitive deficits is demonstrated to be temporally related to one or more neuroradiologically documented cerebrovascular events

3. Which of the following statements is false in regard to VaD?
   (a) The precise nature of CVD sufficient to produce VaD is unknown.
   (b) Leukoencephalopathy is found in all VaD subtypes.
   (c) VaD can be diagnosed in the absence of memory impairment.
   (d) There is no pathognomic biological marker for VaD.

4. A stepwise decline in cognitive functioning associated with temporally concurrent vascular brain injury is _____.
   (a) required for a diagnosis of major vascular neurocognitive disorder
   (b) common in VaD but not VaMCI
   (c) most commonly observed in CADASIL
   (d) a relatively uncommon finding in VCI

5. An effective caregiver coping strategy is ____.
    (a) confronting problems
    (b) venting about problems
    (c) journaling about problems
    (d) self-distraction in response to chronic problems

6. Which of the following is true?
    (a) The AHA/ASA diagnostic criteria are now universally used to define VaD.
    (b) VaMCI and VCIND refer to different subtypes of VCI.
    (c) The AHA/ASA criteria were developed to resolve previously existing differences in diagnostic criteria for VCI.
    (d) The DSM-5 criteria for major and mild vascular neurocognitive disorder are now the standard criteria.

7. A relatively rare phenomenon leading to VaD is ____.
    (a) cerebral amyloid angiopathy
    (b) CADASIL
    (c) Binswanger's disease
    (d) leukoaraiosis

8. An 80-year-old male presents with pronounced impairments in memory and word-finding difficulty, periventricular white matter hyperintensities, and a single basal ganglia lacunar infarct. Mood, motor functions, speed of processing, and behavior are normal. The symptoms are relatively invariant within and across days. The most likely dementia associated with this pattern is ____.
    (a) vascular dementia
    (b) diffuse Lewy body disease
    (c) frontotemporal dementia
    (d) Alzheimer's disease

9. Vascular dementia is often associated with early pronounced ____.
    (a) depression and executive dysfunction
    (b) fluctuations in alertness and arousal
    (c) paresthesias and memory loss
    (d) language deficits and personality change

10. What percent of vascular cognitive impairment without dementia progresses to dementia within 1 year?
    (a) approximately 2%
    (b) approximately 12%
    (c) approximately 6%
    (d) this is not yet known

Vascular Cognitive Impairment Answers

1. **C—the full spectrum of cognitive impairment due to** CVD *The phenomena of VaMCI, VCIND, and VaD are all examples of VCI, differing only in breadth and severity of impairment.*

References:
(a) Chui, H. C., & Ramirez-Gomez, L. (2018). Vascular cognitive impairment: Executive dysfunction in the era of the human brain connectome. In B. L. Miller & J. L. Cummings (Eds.), *The human frontal lobes: Functions and disorders* (3rd ed., pp. 357–367). New York, NY: Guilford Press.
(b) Gorelick, P. B., Scuteri, A., Black, S. E., Decarli, C., Greenberg, S. M., Iadecola, C., . . . Seshadri, S. (2011). Vascular contributions to cognitive impairment and dementia: A statement for healthcare professionals from the American Heart Association/American Stroke Association. *Stroke, 42,* 2672–2713.
(c) Stephan, B. C., Matthews, F.E ., Khaw, K. T., Dufouil, C., & Brayne, C. (2009). Beyond mild cognitive impairment: Vascular cognitive impairment, no dementia (VCIND). *Alzheimer's Research & Therapy, 1*(1), 4.

2. A—the patient progresses from modest to substantial cognitive impairment and can no longer independently complete complex IADLs *Neither "modest" nor "substantial" impairment are operationally defined and, hence, the threshold separating the two remains ambiguous.*

Reference: American Psychiatric Association. (2013). *Diagnostic and statistical manual of mental disorders* (5th ed.). Arlington, VA: American Psychiatric Association.

3. B—Leukoencephalopathy is found in all VaD subtypes *Cerebrovascular disease occurs in many forms, and leukoencephalopathy is not necessary for CVD to result in VaD. It may be absent in MID, CADASIL, and strategic infarcts, for example.*

Reference: Iadecola, C. (2013). The pathobiology of vascular dementia. *Neuron, 80,* 844–866.

4. D—a relatively uncommon finding in VCI *First, VaD frequently occurs in the context of mixed dementia, combining the pathology of AD and VaD, therefore obscuring a possible temporal association between cerebrovascular events and onset of greater cognitive decline. Second, VaD may be caused by progressively worsening subcortical small vessel disease with the gradually progressive white matter impairment underlying the cognitive decline. Third, longitudinal studies with 1-year (or longer) follow-up assessment points cannot determine whether cognitive decline observed at follow-up occurred in a stepwise or smoothly progressive manner. For these, as well as other reasons, documentation of stepwise cognitive decline attributable to discrete cerebrovascular events is not common.*

Reference: Gorelick, P. B., Scuteri, A., Black, S. E., Decarli, C., Greenberg, S. M., Iadecola, C., . . . Seshadri, S. (2011). Vascular contributions to cognitive impairment and dementia: A statement for healthcare professionals from the American Heart Association/American Stroke Association. *Stroke, 42,* 2672–2713.

5. A—confronting problems *Increasing caregiver self-efficacy through education in effective coping strategies has been shown to effective in reducing overall caregiver burden.*

Reference: Tremont, G., Davis, J. D., & Spitznagel, M. B. (2005). Understanding and managing caregiver burden in cerebrovascular disease. In R. H. Paul, R. Cohen, B. R. Ott, & S. Salloway. (Eds.), *Vascular dementia: Cerebrovascular mechanisms and clinical management* (pp. 305–321). Totowa, NJ: Humana Press.

6. C—The AHA/ASA criteria were developed to resolve previously existing differences in diagnostic criteria for VCI. *However, no single criteria set is yet used universally. Gorelick et al. (2011) addresses these issues in full, as well as the use of VCIND and VaMCI.*

Reference: Gorelick, P. B., Scuteri, A., Black, S. E., Decarli, C., Greenberg, S. M., Iadecola, C., . . . Seshadri, S. (2011). Vascular contributions to cognitive impairment and dementia: A statement for healthcare professionals from the American Heart Association/American Stroke Association. *Stroke, 42,* 2672–2713.

7. B—CADASIL *CADASIL has an estimated prevalence of 5 per 100,000 and, hence, is relatively rare in the general population and in the population of individuals experiencing dementia. See Choi (2010) for a review.*

Reference: Choi, J. C. (2010). Cerebral Autosomal Dominant Arteriopathy with Subcortical Infarcts and Leukoencephalopathy: A genetic cause of cerebral small vessel disease. *Journal of Clinical Neurology (Seoul, Korea), 6*(1), 1–9.

8. D—Alzheimer's disease *Memory impairment and dysnomia are very common presenting symptoms in AD. Periventricular hyperintensities and isolated subcortical lacunar infarctions are commonly found in cognitively normal aged adults and, alone, do not indicate vascular causation of cognitive decline. Motor and psychomotor slowing, as well as depression, would be more common in VaD than AD. Diffuse Lewy body disease is more often characterized by*

fluctuations in cognition, as well as visual hallucinations and motor symptoms. FTD is more often characterized by early and pronounced behavioral changes.

References:
(a) Gorelick, P. B., Scuteri, A., Black, S. E., Decarli, C., Greenberg, S. M., Iadecola, C. . . . Seshadri, S. (2011). Vascular contributions to cognitive impairment and dementia: A statement for healthcare professionals from the American Heart Association/American Stroke Association. *Stroke, 42*, 2672–2713.

(b) Smith, G.E ., & Bondi, M. W. (2008). Normal aging, mild cognitive impairment, and Alzheimer's disease. In J. E. Morgan & J. H. Ricker (Eds.), *Textbook of clinical neuropsychology* (pp. 762–780). New York, NY: Taylor and Francis.

9. **A—depression and executive dysfunction** *Fluctuations would be more common with delirium. Memory loss can be present early but paresthesias would be uncommon. Early language deficits would be more common in Alzheimer's disease. Depression is more common than personality change, at least in the early stages.*

References:
(a) Jefferson, A. L., Brickman, A. M., Aloia, M. S., & Paul, R. H. (2005). The cognitive profile of vascular dementia. In R. H. Paul, R. Cohen, B. R. Ott, & S. Salloway (Eds.), *Vascular dementia: Cerebrovascular mechanisms and clinical management* (pp. 131–143). Totowa, NJ: Humana Press.

(b) Kumar, A., Lavretsky, H., & Haroon, E. (2005). Neuropsychiatric correlates of vascular injury. In R. H. Paul, R. Cohen, B. R. Ott, & S. Salloway (Eds.), *Vascular dementia: Cerebrovascular mechanisms and clinical management* (pp. 157–168). Totowa, NJ: Humana Press.

10. **B—approximately 12%** *The Aging, Demographics, and Memory Study (ADAMS) presents a nationally representative sample of 856 individuals assessed for cognitive impairment and dementia attributable to AD, VCI, and other conditions and also followed longitudinally.*

Reference: Plassman, B. L., Langa, K. M., Fisher, G. G., Heeringa, S. G., Weir, D. R., Ofstedal, M. B., . . . Wallace, R. B. (2008). Prevalence of cognitive impairment without dementia in the United States. *Annals of Internal Medicine, 148*, 427–434.

Recommended Readings

Arvanitakis, Z., Leurgans, S. E., Barnes, L. L., Bennett, D. A., & Schneider, J. A. (2011). Microinfarct pathology, dementia, and cognitive systems. *Stroke, 42*, 722–727.

Benisty, S., Hernandez, K., Viswanathan, A., Reyes, S., Kurtz, A., O'Sullivan, M., . . . Chabriat, H. (2008). Diagnostic criteria of vascular dementia in CADASIL. *Stroke, 39*, 838–844.

Chui, H. C., & Ramirez-Gomez, L. (2015). Clinical and imaging features of mixed Alzheimer and vascular pathologies. *Alzheimer's Research & Therapy, 7*(1), 21.

Chui, H. C., & Ramirez-Gomez, L. (2018). Vascular cognitive impairment: Executive dysfunction in the era of the human brain connectome. In B. L. Miller & J.L. Cummings (Eds.), *The human frontal lobes: Functions and disorders* (3rd ed., pp. 357–367.). New York, NY: The Guilford Press.

Cullum, C. M., Rossetti, H. C., Batjer, H., Festa, J. R., Haaland, K. Y., & Lacritz, L. H. (2018). Cerebrovascular disease. In J. E. Morgan & J. H. Ricker (Eds), *Textbook of clinical neuropsychology* (2nd ed., pp. 350–386). New York, NY: Routledge.

Gorelick, P. B., Scuteri, A., Black, S. E., Decarli, C., Greenberg, S. M., Iadecola, C., . . . Seshadri, S. (2011). Vascular contributions to cognitive impairment and dementia: A statement for healthcare professionals from the American Heart Association/American Stroke Association. *Stroke, 42*, 2672–2713.

Iadecola, C. (2013). The pathobiology of vascular dementia. *Neuron, 80*, 844–866.

Lopez, O. L., & Wolk, D. A. (2009). Clinical evaluation: A systematic but user-friendly approach. In L.-O. Wahlund, T. Erkinjuntti, & S. Gauthier (Eds.), *Vascular cognitive impairment in clinical practice* (pp. 32–45). Cambridge, UK: Cambridge University Press.

McKhann, G. M., Knopman, D. S., Chertkow, H., Hyman, B. T., Jack, C. R., Kawas, C. H., . . . Phelps, C. H. (2011). The diagnosis of dementia due to Alzheimer's disease: Recommendations from the National Institute on Aging-Alzheimer's Association workgroups on diagnostic guidelines for Alzheimer's disease. *Alzheimer's & Dementia, 7,* 263–269.

Santiago, C., Herrmann, N., Swardfager, W., Saleem, M., Oh, P. I., Black, S. E., & Lanctôt, K. L. (2015). White matter microstructural integrity is associated with executive function and processing speed in older adults with coronary artery disease. *American Journal of Geriatric Psychiatry, 23,* 754–763.

MEDICAL

32   Frontotemporal Dementias

Shane S. Bush and Dominic A. Carone

Introduction

Frontotemporal dementias (FTDs) are a group of neurodegenerative disorders that share overlapping pathologies and clinical features. The term FTLD stands for frontotemporal lobar degeneration and is used to refer to the underlying neuropathology (e.g., neural cell loss, astrocytic gliosis) in the frontal and temporal lobes that cause these disorders. In FTDs, progressive deterioration of the anterior temporal and/or frontal lobes results in behavioral changes, language dysfunction, and/or motor deficits. The progressive deterioration ultimately causes significant functional decline. Although about 40% of all FTDs are caused by an abnormal accumulation of tau protein, more than half of FTDs are tau negative and are caused by an abnormal accumulation of TDP-43 protein. The abnormal accumulation of these proteins interferes with neuronal functioning. About 40% of patients with FTD have a family history of dementia, indicating a genetic component in many instances. In about 10% of FTD cases, first-degree relatives across two generations have developed dementia.

Known for being a younger-onset dementia syndrome, FTDs should be especially considered in the differential diagnosis when cognitive and behavioral changes begin in the mid 40s to 50s. This can be a useful clinical distinction from Alzheimer's disease (AD), which is typically not diagnosed until after age 65. FTD is also known for having a shorter survival time and more rapid progression compared to AD. Although a frontal variant of AD exists, it is rare and is characterized by more executive dysfunction than would typically be seen in the early stages of FTD. In addition to neurological comorbidities, clinicians need to consider that FTD can either overlap with or initially mimic many psychiatric conditions such as major depressive disorder and obsessive-compulsive disorder.

FTDs are commonly divided into three variants according to the symptom pattern: Behavioral variant, language variant, and motor variant. The motor variant is particularly important to identify early because it progresses rapidly, with death normally occurring in the late 50s. There are other ways of characterizing FTDs, such as by neuropathology, which can typically only be determined with certainty by means of biopsy or at autopsy. This chapter focuses on symptom variants. Each variant consists of specific disorders with unique characteristics. This chapter is organized according to the three variants, with a common section for definitions, questions, and references.

Section 1: FTD Behavioral Variant

Definition

The behavioral variant is variously referred to behavioral variant FTD (bvFTD), frontal variant FTD, *Pick complex*, or Pick's disease (PiD). It is referred to as the behavioral variant because the initial changes involve declines in social behavior as well as personality. PiD, named for Arnold Pick, who first described the disorder in 1892, is caused by progressive, focal degeneration of the frontal and temporal brain regions, and/or the presence of *argyrophilic* globular inclusions (Pick bodies) and swollen, achromatic neurons

(Pick cells). Pick's descriptions of cerebral pathology in a series of patients with progressive aphasia and behavioral changes were based on gross examinations without the benefit of microscopic analysis. Alois Alzheimer later described PiD on the basis of histology, noting the presence of the Pick bodies and Pick cells, and the absence of the amyloid (senile) plaques and neurofibrillary tangles that characterize the disease that bears his name. The straight, fibrous appearance of tangled tau proteins found in Pick bodies differs markedly from the paired and coiled construction of the neurofibrillary tangles found in AD.

Neuropathology

Tau protein, when mutated, affects the microtubules to which it binds and produces the toxic inclusions that characterize PiD. The *argyrophilic*, circular inclusions are known as Pick bodies and co-occur with balloon-shaped Pick cells in neuronal cytoplasm. Pick's disease is associated with three microtubule repeats. Common cerebral locations include:

- frontal and temporal neocortex
- amygdala
- dentate gyrus
- pyramidal cells of the CA1 section and subiculum of the hippocampus
- hypothalamic lateral tuberal nucleus
- dorsomedial region of the putamen
- globus pallidus
- locus ceruleus
- mossy fibers and monodendritic brush cells in the granule cell layer of the cerebellum

Histopathological evidence (Pick cells and Pick bodies) of the disease, besides having an affinity for fairly specific anatomical locations, is found in the layers II and IV of the neocortex, which project within the cortex and to thalamic synapses, respectively. Explaining why it is sometimes referred to as frontal variant FTD, PiD is characterized by prominent bilateral frontal lobe atrophy. Fifty percent of patients with PiD present with greater left hemisphere involvement, while 20% have greater right hemisphere pathology. Structural neuroimaging (MRI) commonly shows atrophy of the orbitofrontal, mesial frontal, and anterior insular cortices. Functional neuroimaging shows frontal hypoperfusion (SPECT) and frontal hypometabolism (FDG-PET). There is also evidence that neuroinflammation may play a role in the underlying pathology of FTD. The rates of non-thyroid spectrum autoimmune disorders are twice as common in people with the semantic variant of FTD (also known as the temporal variant of semantic dementia, where there is distinct loss of individual word knowledge), indicating that certain auto-immune disorders may pose a risk for FTD.

Although frontotemporal regions are the most common areas of neuropathology in PiD, lesions can occur in other areas, with corresponding clinical manifestations. Neurotransmitters also seem to be affected by bvFTD, including altered metabolism of serotonin and lower levels of CSF dopamine, although functioning of the cholinergic system appears to be unaffected.

Epidemiology

Of the three FTD variants, bvFTD is the most common (about half of all FTD cases) and occurs more frequently in men than women. The average age of onset is younger than with AD. The onset of PiD typically occurs between the ages of 40 and 65, with an average age of 54 years. Compared to the incidence of AD, which increases significantly with age, the onset of FTD is very rare after age 75. Adults between ages 45 and 64 are diagnosed with FTD at a rate of approximately 15 to 22 per 100,000, which reflects the second most common cause of early-onset dementia.

The reported median survival rates (from diagnosis to death) for bvFTD vary considerably, from 3 to more than 8 years. Compared to the other variants, patients with bvFTD have a shorter average life expectancy. Patients with semantic dementia have lived as long as 12 years.

Determinants of Severity

Functional neuroimaging and neuropsychological test results can serve as indicators of disease severity. FDG-PET reveals frontal hypometabolism early in the disease process, before changes are evident on structural imaging. Despite significant personality changes and behavioral problems, patients with bvFTD perform well on cognitive tests early in the disease process. The presence, breadth, and severity of neuropsychological dysfunction increases as the disease progresses. Currently, there are no rating systems for severity.

Presentation, Disease Course, and Recovery

The onset of bvFTD is insidious. It begins with changes in personality, interpersonal conduct, and emotional regulation, reflecting progressive disintegration of the underlying neural circuits. There are generally two subtypes. The first is an apathetic subtype, characterized by reduced social cognition, reduced motivation, inertia, lack of interest in prior activities, progressive social isolation, decreased empathy, increased pain response latency, and poor decision-making. The second is a disinhibited subtype characterized by disinhibition (e.g., overspending), impulsivity (e.g., inappropriate comments in public), hyperorality (especially for sweet foods), stereotyped motor movements, and perseverative behaviors. The changes in diet and spending behaviors are partly due to deficits in reward processing. Hyper-religiosity can also occur, but this is not as common as the other disinhibition signs. Embarrassing social behaviors often occur in the disinhibited subtype. Obsessive-compulsive behaviors, ritualistic behaviors, and psychosis can also occur in bvFTD, which in younger patients can be a sign of early bvFTD. This can result in bvFTD being misdiagnosed as schizophrenia. Unlike schizophrenia, however, bvFTD rarely presents with hallucinations and delusions. Due to the presence of emotional and behavioral disturbances, bvFTD may also initially be misdiagnosed as a psychiatric condition.

Individuals with bvFTD often lack insight into their deficits, which makes friends and family critically important in identifying onset and progression. The pathologic course of bvFTD varies among patients, so disease duration is often best estimated by early clinical features. Diagnostic criteria for bvFTD using probabilistic language (i.e., possible, probably, definite) were provided by an international consensus panel in 2013 and are commonly referred to as the Rascovsky criteria. The criteria for *possible* bvFTD consist of the general categories listed in Table 32.1 and can be useful for reducing misdiagnosis as a psychiatric condition.

For *probable* bvFTD, the patient must meet criteria for possible bvFTD, exhibit significant functional decline, *and* have structural or functional neuroimaging results that are consistent with the disorder (i.e., frontal and/or anterior temporal lobe atrophy on MRI of CT, or frontal and/or anterior temporal hypoperfusion or hypometabolism on PET or SPECT). Criteria for *definite* bvFTD require the patient to meet criteria for possible or probable bvTFD *and* have histopathological evidence of FTLD on biopsy or at postmortem examination or have a known genetic mutation (typically involving the microtubule-associated protein tau [MAPT], charged multi-vesicular body protein 2B [CHMP2B], valosin-containing protein [VCP], and progranulin [PGRN]).

Individuals with bvFTD typically experience a progressive decline in cognitive, behavioral and functional abilities over time. However, there are a subset of patients who have behavioral features characteristic

TABLE 32.1 The Criteria for *Possible* bvFTD (3 of the 6 must be present)

CORE Criteria	Symptom
Early behavioral disinhibition (a hallmark feature of bvFTD)	1. Socially inappropriate behavior 2. Loss of manners or decorum 3. Impulsive, rash or careless actions
Early apathy or inertia (the most common symptom in bvFTD)	
Early loss of sympathy or empathy	1. Diminished responsiveness to other people's needs and feelings 2. Diminished social interest, interrelatedness, or personal warmth
Early perseverative, stereotyped or compulsive/ritualistic behavior	1. Simple repetitive movements 2. Complex, compulsive, or ritualistic behaviors 3. Stereotypy of speech
Hyperorality and dietary changes	1. Altered food preferences 2. Binge eating, increased consumption of alcohol or cigarettes 3. Oral exploration or consumption of inedible objects
Neuropsychological Profile	Executive/generation deficits with relative sparing of memory and visuospatial functions

of possible FTD but who do not progress to dementia and have non-progressive neuroimaging results (i.e., no atrophy or minimal atrophy; normal PET scan findings). This subset is classified as the bvFTD phenocopy syndrome. The cause of bvFTD phenocopy syndrome varies and is typically unknown, but it has been associated with the presence of mood disorders, autism spectrum disorders, and psychological decompensation due to psychosocial stressors.

Expectations for Neuropsychological Assessment Results

Neuropsychological performance is typically unaffected early in the disease process. Cognitive screening measures, such as the Mini-Mental State Exam (MMSE), are insensitive to cognitive deficits early in the course of PiD. Although there is no prototypical cognitive profile early in the disease process, deficits with executive functions and episodic memory may be found. Later in the course of the disease, the cognitive profile reflects more global impairment and is similar to that seen with other advanced dementias. Because of the difficulty identifying a modal bvFTD profile, examiners have turned to social cognition theory (theory of mind), emotion recognition, complex problem-solving, and use of naturalistic tasks that resemble daily activities. In bvFTD phenocopy syndrome, memory is intact and executive functioning is normal to mildly impaired.

- *Intelligence/Achievement* Typically preserved until late in the disease course, although problems with emotional intelligence may be evident. That is, while scores on intelligence and achievement tests usually do not decline substantially until late in the disease process, the application of those abilities in daily life can be affected.

- *Attention/Concentration* Preserved until late in the disease course.

- *Processing Speed* Preserved until late in the disease course.

- *Language* Preserved until late in the disease course.

- *Visuospatial* Preserved until late in the disease course.

- *Memory* Typically preserved until late in the disease course, although 10% to 15% of patients present with severe amnesia.

- *Executive Functions* A source of controversy. Some tasks have been found to differentiate patients with bvFTD from healthy controls, including digit repetition backward, the Iowa Gambling Task (choosing options with a high risk of rewards despite a high risk of monetary loss), the Hayling Test to measure rapid verbal response inhibition, set shifting tasks (e.g., Trail Making Test part B), rapid generative fluency tasks (e.g., figural fluency, word list generation), and the Executive and Social Cognition Battery (short form). Patients with bvFTD tend to have problems with self-monitoring and make perseverative errors as a result. However, some patients, especially early on in the disease, may perform well on laboratory-based tasks that are administered in a structured environment, while displaying executive difficulties in daily life.

- *Sensorimotor Functions* Preserved until late in the disease course.

- *Emotion and Personality* Emotional distress is typically absent, in part because of a lack of awareness of changes (i.e., anosognosia). However, frustration and anger may emerge in response to reactions from, or limits set by, family members. Personality changes are the cardinal feature of bvFTD. Changes that reflect decreased drive and withdrawal and/or disinhibition may or may not be reflected on measures of personality traits, but very little research has been done in this area. Deficits in sympathy and empathy are often present, especially as the disease progresses. Patients also often have difficulty recognizing emotionally salient stimuli, especially negative emotions.

- *Performance and Symptom Validity* Patients with bvFTD commonly lack awareness of the changes that others observe and therefore do not understand the reason for neuropsychological evaluation. They may not fully engage in the evaluation process, or they may comply at the request or insistence of family members. Intentional exaggeration or fabrication of problems is extremely uncommon.

Considerations when Treating Select Populations with bvFTD

There are no specific treatments for bvFTD. Interventions need to be symptom-focused or palliative.

Functional Independence

The ability to live independently without supervision, work, make decisions regarding finances and other personal matters, and drive all depend on the nature and severity of the presenting problems. Because interpersonal problems, poor motivation, and impaired problem-solving typically emerge early in the course of the disease, multiple aspects of life are usually affected to the point that patients begin to require increasing levels of supervision. Importantly, this includes driving, particularly in cases of bvFTD due to impaired social cognition and disinhibited behavior that can result in hit-and-run accidents, speeding, and traffic violations (e.g., not stopping at red lights). Behavior modification and environmental modifications approaches are often needed. Family education and support is usually essential. Ultimately, increased supervision and assistance and end-of-life planning are needed. Patients with bvFTD are generally more functionally impaired than patients with AD or the language variant of FTD.

Medications

Because the cholinergic system appears to be unaffected, acetylcholinesterase inhibitors, which are commonly prescribed for patients with AD, have little value for patients with bvFTD. Similarly, little empirical evidence exists to support the use of glutamate antagonists such as Namenda. Symptom-focused treatment may be of value, although compliance with mediations may require assistance from family or others. Despite limited research, SSRIs/SNRIs are typically the treatment of choice for the emotional and behavioral symptoms of bvFTD.

Section 2: FTD Language Variant

Definition

The language variant of FTD, commonly referred to as primary progressive aphasia (PPA), is divided into three subtypes: nonfluent/agrammatic variant (also called progressive nonfluent aphasia [PNFA]), semantic dementia (also called temporal variant FTD or semantic variant FTD), and logopenic variant (also called logopenic progressive aphasia and phonological variant PPA). Technically, some do not consider the logopenic variant a form of FTD due to the high preponderance of AD associated with this syndrome. Detailed diagnostic guidelines for these three subtypes were published by Gorno-Tempini and colleagues in 2011 with specific criteria provided for clinical diagnosis, imaging supported diagnosis (based on structural or functional neuroimaging), and pathologically confirmed diagnosis (based on genetic testing or pathology results). In general, PPA is characterized by initial and prominent language deterioration with relative preservation of other cognitive abilities until late in the disease process. PPA commonly presents with marked word-finding difficulty, decreased performance on word list generation tasks, problems with verbal comprehension, and dysarthria. Reading and writing abilities typically remain preserved longer than speech. Additionally, swallowing problems commonly co-occur. With regard to PPA subtypes, PNFA is characterized by syntax difficulties, paraphasic errors, pitch distortions, and flawed grammar in writing and speech (e.g., mostly content words with few function words). It is sometimes associated with apraxia of speech (a motor speech disorder resulting in interrupted speech and inconsistent speech sounds and distortions) and difficulty comprehending complex sentences. Semantic dementia is characterized by naming deficits with loss of single word knowledge (typically for objects) and eventually progresses to loss of person recognition. In the logopenic variant, there is anomia without loss of word knowledge, but there is also difficulty with sentence/phrase repetition and often phonologic errors.

After establishing the presence of PPA, determining the extent to which various speech and language features exist helps to determine the specific variant. The features to examine include the following: grammar, motor speech, sound errors, word-finding problems or delays, repetition, single-word and syntax comprehension, confrontation naming, semantic knowledge, reading, and spelling.

Neuropathology

PPA is a clinical syndrome with heterogeneous neuropathological etiologies, with each variant resulting from different pathological processes. Most cases of PPA have tau-positive, *ubiquitin*/TDP-43-positive frontotemporal lobar degeneration (FTLD) pathology or AD pathology. Neuroanatomic deterioration in the left posterior frontal and insular regions is associated with the nonfluent forms of the disease; deterioration in the bilateral anterior temporal region results in semantic dementia; and pathology involving the left temporoparietal regions results in the logopenic variant. Like PiD, most patients with semantic dementia present with more left hemisphere atrophy, but about 25% have initial right anterior temporal lobe atrophy. Almost all semantic dementia cases are caused by an abnormal accumulation of TDP-43. TDP-43 inclusions are also common to amyotrophic lateral sclerosis (ALS), partly explaining the association between ALS and FTD.

PPA can be inherited in an autosomal dominant manner, most commonly from mutations in the progranulin (*GRN*) gene. However, semantic dementia is the least likely to be inherited. PNFA is strongly associated with tau pathology and predominant left posterior frontal-insular pathology. The

TABLE 32.2 FTD Language Variants

Nonfluent/ Agrammatic Variant	**Core Features**	Agrammatism in language production Effortful, halting speech with inconsistent speech sound errors (apraxia of speech)
	Common Features	Impaired comprehension of syntactically complex sentences Spared single-word comprehension Spared object knowledge
Semantic Dementia	**Core Features**	Impaired confrontation naming Impaired single-word comprehension
	Common Features	Impaired object knowledge, particularly for low frequency or low-familiarity items Surface dyslexia or dysgraphia Spared repetition Spared speech production (grammar and motor speech)
Logopenic Variant	**Core Features**	Impaired single-word retrieval in spontaneous speech and naming Impaired repetition of sentences and phrases
	Common Features	Speech (phonologic) errors in spontaneous speech and naming Spared single-word comprehension and object knowledge Spared motor speech Absence of frank agrammatism

microtubule-associated protein tau (*MAPT*), which in AD and other dementias aggregates to form neurofibrillary tangles within cells, may also be present in PPA.

Epidemiology

The incidence rates for PPA alone (without the other FTD variants) in the United States are unknown. Approximately 20% to 25% of patients with FTD have semantic dementia. Males are more likely to have semantic dementia, whereas females are more likely to have PNFA. There is an increased number of non-right-handedness in semantic dementia compared with the general population suggesting that atypical brain lateralization could be a risk factor for this form of FTD. Patients with learning disabilities have also been found to be at increased risk for the language variant of FTD. For the language variant, the average length of time from onset to death is 12 years.

Determinants of Severity

Severity of the clinical syndrome is determined by the progression of language impairments and the onset and progression of additional neuropsychological problems, including behavior problems, impaired motor functions, more global cognitive deficits, and functional declines. Structural neuroimaging reveals increasing cerebral atrophy, beginning in the frontal and temporal regions. There are no rating systems for severity.

Presentation, Disease Course, and Recovery

The disease begins with disordered language and progressively worsens to include more widespread neuropsychological problems. Semantic dementia is also known to be associated with emotional processing deficits and compulsive behaviors due to deterioration of the temporal lobes. Initial left anterior temporal involvement is associated with worse language impairment. Patients with semantic dementia with initial right anterior temporal lobe atrophy are known to have worse insight, problems with facial recognition, more obsessive-compulsive behaviors, work difficulties, dietary changes, rigid thinking, lack of empathy, and social awkwardness. Disinhibition and apathy can occur in semantic variant FTD as in behavioral variant FTD, but typically not until 5 to 7 years after symptoms began. The language deficits in language variant FTD can significantly impair communication and social engagement early in the disease.

In PNFA, it is common to observe stuttering, slurring, and/or pausing within words due to motor speech difficulties. As PNFA progresses, the language problems become more severe and the patient may become mute and immobile. Behavioral problems can occur as well. Because visuospatial deficits tend to occur later in the disease process, driving is typically not affected until dementia severity is moderate. Basic activities of daily living are generally preserved for many years. In the logopenic variant, there is minimal verbal output, word retrieval deficits, simple utterances, impaired sentence repetition, intermittent interruptions of verbal fluency, and relatively spared grammar. The relatively spared grammar, object knowledge, and single word comprehension, helps distinguish the logopenic from the semantic variant. Spared motor speech helps to distinguish the logopenic variant from the PNFA variant.

There is little evidence that the progression of PPA can be slowed, and there is no cure. However, the progression of semantic dementia is generally slower than the behavioral variant and PNFA subtype.

Expectations for Neuropsychological Assessment Results

Neuropsychological assessment reveals clear evidence of impairment on language-based measures, with relatively strong performance in other domains. Patients with semantic variant of FTD are known to do extremely poorly on naming to confrontation whereas patients with PNFA are more known for having problems with word list generation. In semantic dementia, deficits in object knowledge begin with loss of the ability to finely distinguish between types of objects (e.g., types of animals such as a tiger and a lion), progresses to a broader difficulty making such distinctions (e.g., the difference between a tiger and an alligator), and ultimately progresses to a loss of knowledge of the word and the category (e.g., a loss of knowledge of what tigers are and what animals are). For this reason, patients with semantic dementia will usually also perform very poorly on word list generation for animal names and on tasks such as the Palms and Pyramids Test. Semantic paraphasic errors are common. A phonemic approach to reading irregular words often occurs, leading to errors. On the latter test, patients are shown a stimulus (a picture or a word) and must chose a related picture or word from two choices.

As the disease progresses, greater impairment becomes evident on language-based measures, and more widespread cognitive (e.g., executive dysfunction), motor, and behavioral problems may also become evident. Episodic memory, visuospatial memory, visuospatial processing, and executive functions tend to be relatively preserved early on but can deteriorate as the disease progresses. Social-emotional deficits tend to be worse in semantic dementia compared to PNFA and can be related to deficits in face and emotion recognition (especially negative emotions).

Considerations when Treating Patients with PPA

Pharmacologic or psychological treatment of behavioral symptoms may be appropriate. Family education and support are often important components of treatment because caregiver burnout and family distress frequently mounts as the disease progresses.

Section 3: FTD Motor Variant

Definition

The FTD motor variant is characterized by progressive deterioration of motor functions, with cognitive and psychological symptoms. The FTD motor variant consists of three subtypes: progressive supranuclear palsy (PSP), corticobasal syndrome (CBS), and FTD with motor neuron disease (FTD-MND). PSP is the most common motor variant. Motor neuron disease (MND), FTD-MND, and frontotemporal lobar degeneration (FTLD) are thought to represent a clinical continuum, with MND on one end of a spectrum, FTD-MND in the middle, and FTLD on the other end. Despite considerable overlap of signs and symptoms of the three variants, differences exist.

TABLE 32.3 FTD Motor Variants

Progressive Supranuclear Palsy (PSP)	**Core Features**	Supranuclear vertical gaze palsy (impaired downward gaze) Bradykinesia Rigidity Swallowing problems Frequent falls
	Additional Features	Behavioral and cognitive changes, particularly executive dysfunction
	Age of Onset	Typically in the 60s
Corticobasal Syndrome (CBS)	**Core Features**	Limb apraxia (asymmetric presentation initially) Alien limb syndrome Cortical reflex myoclonus Cortical sensory impairment
	Additional Features	Asymmetric ideomotor and limb kinetic apraxia (poor spatial organization, timing, and sequencing) Executive dysfunction (including disinhibition, apathy, perseveration, and inattention).
	Age of Onset	Typically ranges from the 50s to the 70s
FTD with Motor Neuron Disease (FTD-MND)	**Core Features**	Dementia (impaired memory and executive functions) Speech production deficits Significant disinhibition Personality changes
	Additional Features	Slowed vertical saccades Muscle atrophy, weakness, cramps, and clumsiness Weak respiratory muscles Hyperflexia Fasciculations Dysphagia and dysarthria

Neuropathology

PSP is characterized by astrocytic lesions, tau-positive neurofibrillary tangles, and neuropil threads within the brainstem and basal ganglia. CBS is characterized by asymmetrical atrophy of the bilateral premotor cortex, superior parietal lobules, and striatum. Both PSP and CBS are associated with four microtubule repeats. FTD-MND is characterized by *ubiquitin*-based pathology rather than tau pathology, involving the frontal and temporal lobes.

Epidemiology

The estimated prevalence of PSP in the United States is 5.3 cases per 100,000 for ages 50–99 years. Clinically significant motor problems typically emerge about 4 years after disease onset, and the average life expectancy after diagnosis is 5 years. The epidemiology of CBD and FTD-MND has not been well established. With FTD-MND, the average age at onset is 55 years, there is an equal male to female ratio, and there is a rapid progression from diagnosis to death, with death typically occurring when patients are in their late 50s.

Determinants of Severity

The severity of the FTD motor variant is characterized by the extent of motor problems and the onset and severity of cognitive and psychological problems. There are no rating systems for severity.

Presentation, Disease Course, and Recovery

The FTD motor variants are characterized clinically by decreased gait and balance and tend to overlap clinically with neurodegenerative disorders such as Parkinson's disease (PD). PSP is the most common of the subtypes. Persons with PSP often initially present with difficulty coordinating eye movements; specifically, they cannot look up or down (supranuclear vertical gaze palsy), which may be perceived as blurred vision. This symptom can be particularly useful in distinguishing PSP from PD, although it is not always an early symptom. Slowed saccades are also characteristic of PSP. Additionally, bradykinesia and rigidity develop, and falls are common. Problems with motor skills also involve speech, swallowing, and facial affect. Inappropriate emotional expression, such as forced laughing or prolonged crying, also occurs. The disease is progressive and often fatal within 5 years.

CBD presents clinically as clumsy, rigid, and slow movements of the left arm and leg, followed by impairment of the right limbs, as well as extreme impairment of voluntary movements, and resting tremor. Cognitive symptoms may include impaired visuospatial skills, impaired ability to perform calculations, apraxia, and alien hand syndrome.

FTD should also likely be considered as a comorbidity of ALS as frontotemporal dysfunction is known to occur in 50% to 60% of patients with ALS and about 9% of individuals with ALS/MND will meet diagnostic criteria for FTD. Approximately 15% of patients with bvFTD cases eventually also develop ALS. When FTD is associated with ALS, the survival rate declines by about 1 year. Additionally as opposed to ALS with spinal onset, bulbar onset of ALS is associated with a greater risk for FTD.

Expectations for Neuropsychological Assessment Results

Neuropsychological profiles are characterized by impaired executive functions, including impaired mental flexibility, planning, problem-solving, judgment, and impulse control. Progressive problems with language and memory also occur. Apathy, indifference to others, and lack of insight into their problems are often noted.

Considerations when Treating Patients with the FTD Motor Variant

There is still no treatment to address the underlying neurodegenerative disease directly. As such, the focus is on treating the signs and symptoms, typically the behavioral manifestations. There is some research literature supporting the use of SSRIs and certain antipsychotic medications in FTD. There is not strong evidence supporting the use of acetylcholinesterase inhibitors in the treatment of FTD, and they can actually worsen the psychiatric symptoms. Memantine use in FTD has not been shown to lead to significant improvement. Patient safety is paramount in managing FTD, especially the risk of frequent falls, which may result in traumatic injury to the brain. Appropriate assistive devices should be used, and all clinicians should reinforce their use. Instruction in the use of compensatory strategies as well as use of adaptive equipment and environmental modifications may help maintain independence with cognitive tasks. Psychological problems can be addressed with medications and psychotherapy.

Family education and support (including counseling) are also essential aspects of patient care, given:

- the lack of awareness that patients have about their limitations
- the need for family members to provide supervision of their loved ones
- the emotional toll that dealing with and managing patients' changes can have on family members, especially with regard to the behavioral variant of FTD.

Cultural Considerations

As with all neuropsychological assessments, neuropsychologists must make sure that they have the training, experience, consultation, or supervision necessary to ensure the provision of competent services to individuals from culturally diverse backgrounds. This is especially important in the neuropsychological assessment of dementia in which language assessment plays a prominent role. For example, a patient could be mistaken as having a semantic processing impairment after struggling to find words in English during conversation and during testing when the problem is actually due to limited English proficiency. Neuropsychologists should monitor the research periodically for cross-cultural articles pertaining to FTD. Neuropsychologists working in other countries need to have increasing awareness of the behavioral signs of FTD. This is especially true in Greece and Turkey, where patients have been found to be diagnosed with FTD at a later age than patients in the United States, presumably because medical systems in Greece and Turkey have more difficulty detecting it. Support for this notion is that symptom onset in FTD in Greece and Turkey was reported later than for patients in the United States despite patients from Greece and Turkey being more impaired than their United States counterparts.

Relevant Definitions

Agrammatism The inability to speak grammatically, typically because of simplified sentence structure and errors in tense, number, and gender. Speech may include omission of function words (known as telegraphic speech).

Alien Limb Syndrome Unintended but purposeful and autonomous movements of the upper limb.

Argyrophilic Having an affinity for silver; binding to silver salts.

Fasciculation A small, local, involuntary muscle contraction and relaxation (twitch).

Pick Complex Includes PiD and overlapping clinical syndromes such as primary progressive aphasia, frontal lobe dementia and FTD, semantic dementia, corticobasal syndrome and other related conditions.

Stereotypy of speech Persistent, inappropriate mechanical repetition of phrases or themes.

Surface dyslexia An inability to recognize words as a whole, resulting in failure to read irregularly spelled words that cannot be sounded out phonetically. Also known as dyseideic dyslexia, surface dyslexia is often contrasted with phonological dyslexia.

Ubiquitin A small regulatory protein which, among its functions, directs protein recycling.

Vertical Saccades Very short, rapid vertical movement of both eyes at the same time. Saccades are the fastest movements produced by the human body. Once they are underway, they cannot be altered by will.

Frontotemporal Dementia Questions

NOTE: Questions 27, 64, 91, and 122 on the First Full-Length Practice Examination, Questions 13, 55, and 83 on the Second Full-Length Practice Examination, Questions 24, 49, and 72 on the Third Full-Length Practice Examination, and Questions 47 and 99 on the Fourth Full-Length Practice Examination are from this chapter.

1. FTDs are commonly divided into three variants according to the symptom pattern. Which of the following is not an FTD variant?

   (a) motor variant

   (b) behavioral variant

   (c) language variant

   (d) visuospatial variant

2. The behavioral variant of FTD is commonly referred to by other names. Which of the following is a commonly used name for the behavioral variant of FTD?

   (a) progressive supranuclear palsy

   (b) Binswanger's disease

   (c) Pick's disease

   (d) temporal variant FTD

3. Pick bodies are ____.

   (a) swollen, achromatic neurons

   (b) argyrophilic globular inclusions

   (c) amyloid plaques

   (d) neurofibrillary tangles

4. A very challenging aspect of bvFTD is that patients often ____.

   (a) become depressed by their personality changes

   (b) blame their parents for the genetic contribution

   (c) intentionally act out to demonstrate control

   (d) lack awareness of their personality changes

5. Because of the difficulty identifying a bvFTD profile, examiners have turned to social cognition theory (theory of mind), emotion recognition, complex problem solving, and which of the following?

   (a) use of naturalistic tasks that resemble daily activities

   (b) prolonged semi-structured clinical interviews

   (c) flexible test batteries that emphasize executive functions

   (d) comprehensive standardized measures of personality

6. Which of the following is typically the treatment of choice for patients with bvFTD?

   (a) atypical antipsychotic medications

   (b) acetylcholinesterase inhibitors

   (c) family education and support

   (d) SSRIs and/or SNRIs

7. Neuroanatomic degeneration in the left posterior frontal and insular regions is associated with what form of the language variant of FTD?

(a) semantic

(c) nonfluent

(b) logopenic

(d) dysarthric

8. The FTD motor variant consists of three subtypes: progressive supranuclear palsy (PSP), FTD with motor neuron disease (FTD-MND), and which of the following?

(a) frontotemporal degeneration

(c) precentral gyrus atrophy

(b) striatal degeneration

(d) corticobasal syndrome

9. Progressive supranuclear palsy (PSP) is characterized by astrocytic lesions, tau positive neurofibrillary tangles, and neuropil threads, primarily within which brain regions/structures?

(a) brainstem, basal ganglia, and cerebellum

(c) bilateral premotor cortex

(b) hippocampus and amygdala

(d) frontal lobes

10. Corticobasal syndrome (CBS) is characterized by asymmetrical atrophy of ____.

(a) brainstem, bilateral premotor cortex, thalamus, and cerebellum

(b) bilateral premotor cortex, superior parietal lobules, and striatum

(c) brainstem, cerebellum, thalamus, hypothalamus, and striatum

(d) basal ganglia, thalamus, posterior temporal lobe, and striatum

11. For individuals with FTD with motor neuron disease (FTD-MND), the average age at onset is ____.

(a) 55 years

(c) 65 years

(b) 59 years

(d) 69 years

12. A patient with dementia obtains a raw score of 5 out of 60 on the Boston Naming Test-II. This patient most likely has ____.

(a) Alzheimer's disease

(b) progressive non-fluent aphasia

(c) semantic dementia

(d) logopenic variant primary progressive aphasia

13. A 50-year-old patient presents with a 2-year history of disinhibited and embarrassing social behaviors, normal memory, no brain atrophy on repeat neuroimaging, and has not advanced to dementia over several years. This patient is best described as having ____.

(a) factitious disorder

(c) intermittent explosive disorder

(b) bvFTD phenocopy syndrome

(d) adult ADHD combined type

14. For a patient to meet definite criteria for bvFTD according to the Rascovsky criteria, the patient must have three core behavioral/cognitive changes, ____.

(a) along with frontal and/or temporal atrophy on structural neuroimaging, and no family history of dementia

(b) frontal and/or temporal atrophy on structural neuroimaging, and at least three cognitive test scores at or below the 1st percentile

(c) frontal and/or temporal hypoperfusion on functional neuroimaging, and at least three cognitive test scores at or below the 1st percentile

(d) frontal and/or temporal degeneration/hypoperfusion on neuroimaging, and genetic or pathological evidence

15. Which type of tests would likely show low to extremely low performance in semantic dementia?

(a) tests assessing sentence repetition

(b) tests assessing receptive language

(c) tests assessing word knowledge and object knowledge

(d) tests assessing organization and planning

Frontotemporal Dementia Answers

1. **D—visuospatial variant**   *The three FTD variants are behavioral variant, language variant, and motor variant. Thus, visuospatial variant is not an FTD variant.*

   Reference: Han, D. Y., Pyykkonen, B. A., Shandera-Ochsner, A. L., & Schmitt, F. A. (2012). Frontotemporal dementias. In C. A. Noggle, R. S. Dean, S. S. Bush, & S. Anderson (Eds.), *Neuropsychology of cortical dementias* (pp. 221–247). New York, NY: Springer.

2. **C—Pick's disease**   *The behavioral variant of FTD is commonly referred to as behavioral variant FTD (bvFTD), Pick's disease (PiD), and frontal variant FTD (fvFTD). PiD is named for Arnold Pick, who discovered the disorder and described it in 1892.*

   Reference: Bush, S. S., & Myers, T. (2010). Pick disease. In J. E. Morgan, I. S. Baron, & J. H. Ricker (Eds.), *Casebook of clinical neuropsychology* (pp. 606–618). New York, NY: Oxford University Press.

3. **B—argyrophilic globular inclusions**   *Pick bodies are argyrophilic globular inclusions, clumps of protein that build up within brain cells. They are toxic and are circular in shape. Cellular inclusions stain positive for tau protein. Tau protein is involved in stabilizing microtubules, which supports the structure and shape of neurons. A second type of cellular inclusion that occurs with FTD is comprised of two other proteins (ubiquitin and TDP-43), which are tau-negative.*

   Reference: Takeda N., Kishimoto Y., & Yokota O. (2012). Pick's disease. *Advances in Experimental Medicine and Biology, 724,* 300–316.

4. **D—lack awareness of their personality changes**   *Because they lack awareness, it can be very difficult to help patients understand the impact of their changes on family members and others and to devise behavioral treatment plans to control problematic or dangerous behavior.*

   Reference: Piguet, O., Hornberger, M., Mioshi, E., & Hodges, J. R. (2011). Behavioral-variant frontotemporal dementia: Diagnosis, clinical staging, and management. *The Lancet Neurology, 10,* 162–172.

5. **A—use of naturalistic tasks that resemble daily activities**   *Such tasks provide more ecologically valid information about functional abilities and limitations than is available from many traditional neuropsychological measures.*

   Reference: Han, D. Y., Pyykkonen, B. A., Shandera-Ochsner, A. L., & Schmitt, F. A. (2012). Frontotemporal dementias. In C. A. Noggle, R. S. Dean, S. S. Bush, & S. Anderson (Eds.), *Neuropsychology of cortical dementias* (pp. 221–247). New York, NY: Springer.

6. **D—SSRIs and/or SNRIs** *Despite limited empirical support for their efficacy, SSRIs/SNRIs are typically the treatment of choice for bvFTD.*

   Reference: Rabinovici, G. D., & Miller, B. L. (2010). Frontotemporal lobar degeneration. *CNS Drugs, 24,* 375–398.

7. **C—nonfluent** *Neuroanatomic degeneration in the left posterior frontal and insular regions is associated with the nonfluent forms of the disease; deterioration in the anterior temporal region results in semantic dementia; and pathology involving the left temporo-parietal regions result in the logopenic variant.*

   Reference: Gorno-Tempini, M. L., Hillis, A. E., Weintraub, S., Kertesz, A., Mendez, M., . . . Grossman, M. (2011). Classification of primary progressive aphasia and its variants. *Neurology, 15,* 1006–1014.

8. **D—corticobasal syndrome** *The FTD motor variant consists of progressive supranuclear palsy (PSP), corticobasal degeneration (CBD), and FTD with motor neuron disease (FTD-MND).*

   Reference: Al-Sarraj, S. (2008). Dementia and motor neuron disease. In P. J. Vinken & G. W. Bruyn (Eds.), *Handbook of clinical neurology (89)* (pp. 431–441). Amsterdam, NL: Elsevier.

9. **A—brainstem, basal ganglia, and cerebellum**

   Reference: Golbe, L. (2014). Progressive supranuclear palsy. *Seminars in Neurology, 34,* 151–159.

10. **B—bilateral premotor cortex, superior parietal lobules, and striatum**

    Reference: Boxer, A. L., Geschwind, M. D., Belfor, N., Gorno-Tempini, M.L., Schauer, G. F., Miller, B. L., . . . Rosen, H. J. (2006). Patterns of brain atrophy that differentiate corticobasal degeneration syndrome from progressive supranuclear palsy. *Archives of Neurology, 63,* 81–86.

11. **A—55 years** *With FTD-MND, the average age at onset is 55 years, there is an equal male-to-female ratio, and there is a rapid progression from diagnosis to death, with death typically occurring when patients are in their late 50s.*

    Reference: Mitsuyama, Y., & Inoue, T. (2009). Clinical entity of frontotemporal dementia with motor neuron disease. *Neuropathology, 29,* 649–654.

12. **C—semantic dementia** *although naming deficits commonly occur in AD and logopenic variant PPA, the effect is most pronounced in semantic dementia due to extensive atrophy of the lateral and inferior temporal cortex that profoundly impairs both multimodal conceptual representations and modality-specific visual association cortex. Thus, naming tests with a visuospatial component (such as the BNT-II) will be particularly affected.*

    Reference: Reilly, J., Peelle, J. E., Antonucci, S. M., & Grossman, M. (2011). Anomia as a marker of distinct semantic memory impairments in Alzheimer's disease and semantic dementia. *Neuropsychology, 24,* 413–426.

13. **B—bvFTD phenocopy syndrome** *When possible bvFTD does not progress to dementia and neuroimaging findings remain stable over time, it is known as bvFTD phenocopy syndrome.*

    Reference: Gossink, F.T ., Dols, A., Kerssens, C. J., Krudop, W. A., Kerklaan, B. J., Scheltens, P., . . . Pijnenburg, Y. A. (2016). Psychiatric diagnoses underlying the phenocopy syndrome of behavioural variant frontotemporal dementia. *Journal of Neurology, Neurosurgery, and Psychiatry, 87,* 64–68.

14. **D—frontal and/or temporal degeneration/hypoperfusion on neuroimaging, and genetic or pathological evidence** *These are the diagnostic criteria for bvFTD. Although neuropsychological profiles are considered as part of the cognitive profile criteria, percentile range criteria are not.*

    Reference: Rascovsky, K., & Grossman, M. (2013). Clinical diagnostic criteria and classification controversies in frontotemporal lobar degeneration. *International Review of Psychiatry, 25,* 145–158.

15. **C—tests assessing word knowledge and object knowledge**   *Due to loss of word knowledge and object knowledge, performance on tests of semantic knowledge would be expected to be particularly affected in semantic dementia.*

    Reference: Finger, E. C. (2016). Frontotemporal dementias, *Continuum, 22*, 464–489.

Recommended Readings

Bott, N. T., Radke, A., Stephens, M. L., & Kramer, J. H. (2014). Frontotemporal dementia: Diagnosis, deficits and management. *Neurodegenerative Disease Management, 4*, 439–454.

Gorno-Tempini, M. L., Hillis, A. E., Weintraub, S., Kertesz, A., Mendez, M., . . . Grossman, M. (2011). Classification of primary progressive aphasia and its variants. *Neurology, 15*, 1006–1014.

Kirshner, H. S. (2010). Frontotemporal dementia and primary progressive aphasia: An update. *Current Neurology and Neuroscience Reports, 10*, 504–511.

Miller, Z. A., Rankin, K. P., Graff-Radford, N. R., Takada, L. T., Sturm, V. E., Cleveland, C. M., . . . Miller, B. L. (2013). TDP-43 frontotemporal lobar degeneration and autoimmune disease. *Journal of Neurology, Neurosurgery, and Psychiatry, 84*, 956–962.

Perry, D. C., & Miller, B. L (2018). Clinical aspects of Frontotemporal dementia, In B. L. Miller & J. L. Cummings (Eds.), *The human frontal lobes* (3rd ed., pp. 239–252). New York, NY: Guildford Press.

Piguet, O., Halliday, G. M., Reid, W. G. J., Casey, B., Carman, R., Huang, Y., . . . Kril, J. J. (2011). Clinical phenotypes in autopsy-confirmed Pick disease. *Neurology, 76*, 253–259.

Piguet, O., Hornberger, M., Mioshi, E., & Hodges, J.R. (2011). Behavioral-variant frontotemporal dementia: Diagnosis, clinical staging, and management. *The Lancet Neurology, 10*, 162–172.

Rascovsky, K., & Grossman, M. (2013). Clinical diagnostic criteria and classification controversies in frontotemporal lobar degeneration. *International Review of Psychiatry, 25*, 145–158.

33   Movement Disorders

Laura Lacritz and Dixie J. Woolston

Introduction

Movement disorders are a group of diseases that primarily involve subcortical brain structures that are part of the extrapyramidal motor system, including the basal ganglia (caudate, putamen, and globus pallidus), subthalamic nucleus, and substantia nigra, and their interconnections to each other, thalamic nuclei, and the cortex. The extrapyramidal motor system regulates movement and maintains muscle tone and posture. Dopamine (inhibitory), acetylcholine (excitatory), and gamma-aminobutyric acid (GABA; inhibitory) are the three primary neurotransmitters of the basal ganglia that contribute to symptomatology (due to decreased or increased levels). This chapter describes four disorders in detail that share some clinical features, but are also distinguishable by particular classic symptoms, genetic features, or response to treatment, in addition to other movement disorders you should know. Each of the disorders discussed has cognitive impairment as a primary or secondary aspect of the disease.

Section 1: Parkinson's Disease

Definition

Parkinson's disease (PD) is an alpha-synucleinopathy characterized by parkinsonism, neuronal loss in the substantia nigra, dopamine depletion in the striatum, responsiveness to dopaminergic treatment (typically), presence of Lewy bodies, and frontal subcortical circuitry dysfunction. Diagnostic criteria of clinically established PD includes:

- Parkinsonism, defined as bradykinesia, in combination with either rest tremor and/or rigidity.
  - *Bradykinesia* is a slowness of movement and reduced amplitude in continuous movement.
  - *Rigidity* involves stiffness and velocity independent resistance to passive movement that may include cogwheeling.
  - *Rest tremor* is usually described as slow (4–6 Hz) tremor in a limb at rest that is suppressed with movement initiation.

According to the Movement Disorder Society's diagnostic criteria for PD, once parkinsonism has been diagnosed, clinically established PD requires at least *two supportive criteria* (clear and dramatic beneficial response to dopaminergic therapy, presence of levodopa-induced *dyskinesia*, rest tremor of a limb, and the presence of either olfactory loss or cardiac sympathetic denervation) and *absence of absolute exclusion criteria*, with no "red flags" (see Table 33.1). A diagnosis of clinically probable PD allows for presence of no more than two "red flags" as long as they are counterbalanced with supportive criteria.

TABLE 33.1 Elements of the Movement Disorders Society's Diagnostic Criteria for Parkinson's Disease

Essential Criteria: Parkinsonism

- Bradykinesia
- Rest Tremor OR
- Rigidity

Supportive Criteria

- Clear and dramatic beneficial response to dopaminergic therapy
- Presence of levodopa-induced *dyskinesia*
- Rest tremor of a limb, documented on clinical examination
- The presence of either olfactory loss or cardiac sympathetic denervation on *MIBG scintigraphy*

Absolute Exclusion Criteria (The presence of any of these features rules out PD)

- Unequivocal cerebellar abnormalities, such as cerebellar gait, limb ataxia, or cerebellar oculomotor abnormalities
- Downward vertical supranuclear gaze palsy, or selective slowing of downward vertical saccades
- Diagnosis of probable behavioral variant frontotemporal dementia or primary progressive aphasia within the first 5 years of disease
- Parkinsonian features restricted to the lower limbs for more than 3 years
- Treatment with a dopamine receptor blocker or a dopamine-depleting agent in a dose and time-course consistent with drug-induced parkinsonism
- Absence of observable response to high-dose levodopa despite at least moderate severity of disease
- Unequivocal cortical sensory loss (i.e., graphesthesia, stereognosis with intact primary sensory modalities), clear limb ideomotor apraxia, or progressive aphasia
- Normal functional neuroimaging of the presynaptic dopaminergic system
- Documentation of an alternative condition known to produce parkinsonism

Red Flags

- Rapid progression of gait impairment requiring regular use of wheelchair within 5 years of onset
- A complete absence of progression of motor symptoms or signs over 5 or more years unless stability is related to treatment
- Early bulbar dysfunction: severe dysphoria, dysarthria, or dysphagia
- Severe autonomic failure in the first 5 years of disease (e.g., orthostatic hypotension, severe urinary retention or urinary incontinence)
- Recurrent (>1/year) falls because of impaired balance within 3 years of onset
- Disproportionate anterocollis (dystonic) or contractures of hand or feet within the first 10 years
- Absence of any of the common nonmotor features of disease despite 5 years of disease duration. These include sleep dysfunction (sleep-maintenance insomnia, excessive daytime somnolence, symptoms of REM behavior disorder), autonomic dysfunction (constipation, daytime urinary urgency, symptomatic orthostasis), hyposmia, or psychiatric dysfunction (depression, anxiety, or hallucinations)
- Otherwise-unexplained pyramidal tract signs, defined as pyramidal weakness or clear pathologic hyperreflexia (excluding mild reflex asymmetry and isolated extensor plantar response)
- Bilateral symmetric parkinsonism at onset.

NOTE: Adapted from Postuma, Berg, Stern, et al. (2015)

Other classic signs of PD that are not part of formal diagnostic criteria but may be part of the clinical presentation include:

- masked facies
- hypophonia
- *micrographia*
- shuffling gait

- dysphagia
- postural instability (usually manifests later in the disease)

Neuropathology

- Pigmented, dopaminergic neuronal loss in the substantia nigra with dopaminergic denervation of the striatum. Preferentially affects the ventrolateral cell group that projects to the posterolateral putamen.

- Lewy bodies and Lewy neurites (abnormal aggregates of protein) in the brainstem.

- Alpha-synuclein pathology outside the nigro-striatal system affecting the autonomic nervous system, structures of the lower brainstem, the limbic system, and the olfactory bulbs, as well as mesocortical and neocortical regions, likely contributes to the nonmotor symptoms of the disease, including psychiatric problems (especially depression and anxiety), autonomic dysfunction, sensory disturbances, pain, sleep problems, and cognitive deficiencies.

- Potential contributions from brain-gut axis (using the microbiome or gut biopsy).

Risk Factors for PD

Risk factors for PD and/or *parkinsonism* include viral encephalitis, drugs with dopamine antagonistic properties such as neuroleptics, toxic substances, exposure to MPTP (a contaminant of synthetic heroin), herbicides, pesticides (especially Rotenone), heavy metals such as manganese and cadmium, elevated iron levels, and drinking of contaminated well water. Gut dysfunction frequently precedes motor symptoms, and has been recently hypothesized as the starting point for PD pathology. Other risk factors include gender (more common in males), age, ethnicity (more common in Hispanics followed by non-Hispanic whites, Asians, and then blacks), history of brain injury, and genetics. While the 90% of cases are sporadic PD, positive family history of PD is found in 10% of patients. Autosomal dominant genes in Parkinson's disease include mutations in SNCA, which provides coded instructions for alpha-synuclein, and LRRK2. Autosomal recessive genes in Parkinson's disease include Parkin, PINK1, DJ-1, and ATP13A2.

Risk Factors for PD Dementia

Approximately 30% of patients with PD in cross sectional studies meet criteria for dementia, while longitudinal studies have found that 75% or more will develop dementia over time. Risk factors for dementia in PD include:

- older than age 70
- greater severity of motor symptoms with higher scores on the *Unified Parkinson's Disease Rating Scale* (UPDRS III)
- diagnosis of Parkinson's disease mild cognitive impairment
- past or comorbid depression
- levodopa side effects of mania, agitation, disorientation, or psychosis
- increased sensitivity to medications (e.g., hallucinations)
- excessive daytime sleepiness or *REM sleep behavior disorder,*

- postural instability and gait disturbance predominant symptoms
- cerebrovascular disease, including risk factors of hypertension and history of smoking
- low socioeconomic status (SES—for various reasons including environmental exposures and lack of access to high-quality healthcare)

Imaging Findings

- *Magnetic resonance imaging (MRI)* Typical brain MRI protocols are non-diagnostic for PD, but can be helpful in differentiating PD from other parkinsonian syndromes (described below)
- *Positron emission tomography (PET)* Preserved striatal metabolism on FDG-PET and normal or increased postsynaptic dopaminergic uptake on raclopride PET.
- *Single proton emission computed tomography (SPECT)* Dopamine transporting (DaT) imaging using SPECT differentiates between patients with and without a dopaminergic deficit. Preservation of the caudate nucleus compared with putaminal uptake is suggestive of PD. Cardiac iodine-123*MIBG scintigraphy* can also separate PD from atypical conditions.

Epidemiology

Incidence

- Parkinson's disease is the second most common neurodegenerative disease.
- Incidence rate is approximately 1–2 per 1000, and increases with age.
- Many individuals may go undiagnosed.
- Men are 1.5 times more likely to develop PD than women.

Morbidity

- Depression is present in up to 40%
- Dementia (30% in cross-sectional studies, up to 75% in longitudinal studies)
- Medication side effects (e.g., hallucinations, *dyskinesias*, motor fluctuations) are seen with high doses, and behavioral side effects with dopamine agonists (e.g., gambling, hypersexuality, other compulsive behaviors)
- Fall risk is increased
- Genitourinary system diseases such as prostatic hypertrophy and increased urinary infection
- Constipation
- Olfactory dysfunction
- Rapid eye movement *(REM) sleep behavior disorder*
- Swallowing problems (dysphagia)

Mortality

The Centers for Disease Control and Prevention rates complications from PD as the fourteenth leading cause of death in the United States; however, with advances in medications, mortality in treated PD is almost the same as in age-matched controls.

Determinants of Severity

Age Factors

Onset before age 40–45 has slower progression with fewer cognitive difficulties. Later onset is associated with a more rapid progression of disease and is more likely to be accompanied by cognitive deficits.

Motor-Predominant, Intermediate, and Diffuse Malignant Subtypes

When tremor and motor symptoms predominate, the course of PD is more likely to be benign. Patients with the diffuse/malignant subtype are more likely to have mild cognitive impairment, orthostatic hypotension, and *REM sleep behavior disorder* at baseline and show a more rapid progression of cognitive decline and other non-motor symptoms.

Presentation, Disease Course, and Recovery

Presenting Symptoms

Initial complaints in early PD include a subtle decrease in motor dexterity that may be experienced as clumsiness in one hand, decreased arm swing, soft voice, reduced facial expression, sleep disturbance, diminished sense of smell, and autonomic dysfunction (constipation, excessive sweating, sexual dysfunction). Tremor is the symptom that generally leads to a PD diagnosis and is observed in approximately 70% of patients. At disease onset, patients typically report one side of the body to be more affected. This motor symptom asymmetry is associated with asymmetric dopaminergic degeneration in the brain. Typical tremor progression is from a single hand, to the ipsilateral leg, and then contralateral limbs.

Stages of Parkinson's Disease

Individuals progress at different rates, and may never progress to stage five (see Table 33.2).

Treatment

There is no cure for PD; the focus of treatment is generally on reducing individual symptoms.

- *Early to middle stages treatment considerations*
  - *Medications* The most common forms of treatment for PD include levodopa, dopamine agonists, and MAO-B inhibitors. Treatment choices are dependent on age, stage of disease,

TABLE 33.2 Stages of Parkinson's Disease

Stage 1	• Signs and symptoms on one side only, typically, presentation involves tremor of one limb • Symptoms mild, inconvenient but not disabling • Minor changes in posture, locomotion and facial expression
Stage 2	• Symptoms are bilateral • Minimal disability • Posture and gait affected
Stage 3	• Slowing of movements, reduced balance, decreased reflexes • Generalized dysfunction that is moderately severe
Stage 4	• Severe symptoms, can still walk to a limited extent but may require an assistive device • No longer able to live independently
Stage 5	• Requires 24/7 nursing care

and presence of non-motor symptoms (e.g., cognitive impairment). Anticholinergic drugs are useful in patients under 70 with disturbing tremor who do not have significant bradykinesia or gait disturbance. Amantadine can be used in younger patients or later when *dyskinesia* becomes problematic. The most common side effects are nausea, vomiting, low blood pressure, an increase in involuntary movements (*dyskinesias*), vivid dreaming, visual hallucinations, and impulse control symptoms (with dopamine agonists). Antidepressants, cognitive enhancing medication and/or prescription supplements, may also be useful pharmacological agents to treat PD symptoms. Atypical antipsychotics may be used for the treatment of psychosis in PD (e.g., Nuplazid).

- *Nonpharmacological Interventions* Physical exercise (especially exercises designed to improve balance, flexibility, and strength), cued exercises with visual (mirror), auditory (metronome), and tactile feedback, voice therapy, speech/swallowing therapy, and biofeedback; fall risk may be reduced by balance-related exercises such as Tai Chi. Cognitive therapy and light therapy may be useful in treating excessive daytime sleepiness. Nutrition is also important. A high fiber diet and adequate hydration help reduce constipation. Large, high-fat meals that slow gastric emptying can interfere with medication absorption and should be avoided.

- *Advanced stages treatment considerations*
  - Medication combinations to maximize symptomatic relief; reduce "wearing off" periods (a loss of the beneficial drug effect before the next dose is due).
  - Surgical interventions
    - *Deep brain stimulation (DBS)* Best candidates have severe motor symptoms in the off-medication condition; targets include subthalamic nucleus or globus pallidus as the most common sites, although ventrointermedius (VIM) thalamic nucleus has clear effect on tremor; dementia is usually a contraindication for DBS.
    - Other surgical techniques include pallidotomy, thalamotomy, and subthalamotomy; these are no longer commonly used.
  - Levodopa-carbidopa intestinal gel pumped into the duodenum is a possibility for patients who are not candidates for or decline DBS.
  - Treat freezing and falls with physical therapy; consider assistive devices (canes, walkers); modify the patient's environment to decrease obstacles.
  - Treat patient's individual nonmotor symptoms; make sure symptoms are not side effects from PD medication.

Expectations for Neuropsychological Assessment Results

Most individuals with PD will develop cognitive difficulties at some point in their disease course. See Table 33.3 for more details.

TABLE 33.3 Neuropsychological Assessment Results Across Disorders

Domain/Disorder	Parkinson's Disease	Huntington's Disease	Lewy Body Dementia	Progressive Supranuclear Palsy
Intelligence/Achievement	Largely intact except for reduced processing speed	Relative preservation until later stages	Nonverbal IQ subtests may show mild impairment	Declines related to impaired processing and psychomotor speed
Attention/Concentration	Complex attention slow or impaired; working memory usually impaired	Impaired early, especially visual attention.	Impaired early, particularly working memory and vigilance	Simple attention preserved early; complex attention impaired
Processing Speed	Impaired, due in part to motor slowing, but also bradyphrenia	Impaired early	Impaired early	Impaired early
Language	Speech output reduced, dysarthria and hypophonia are common; naming intact early, may become impaired later; comprehension, grammar, and syntax remain intact	Slowed speech that can progress to complete mutism	Variable deficits in word list generation and confrontation naming early on with progression over time; hypophonia may be present	Impaired word list generation, slow response latencies
Visuospatial	Micrographia common; trouble with perceptual judgment, angular orientation, and constructional praxis	Impaired; especially spatial integration, complicated by interference of motor symptoms	Early, marked impairment in visuospatial and constructional abilities common	Impairment related to slow responding
Learning and Memory	Initial learning of new material is impaired; can benefit from cues, recognition, and recall aids, but have difficulty initiating/generating the strategies	Significant deficits in learning, but recognition memory remains intact in middle stages; Semantic memory and delayed recall preserved until later stages	Learning and memory reduced but not as impaired as other domains (e.g., executive functioning) early on, though memory becomes more impaired as disease progresses (similar to Alzheimer's disease)	Impaired learning, better recognition than free recall
Executive Functions	Impaired, particularly with reduced mental flexibility	Severely impaired, especially working memory (e.g., N-back test)	Impaired early	Impaired early
Sensorimotor Functions	Impaired, though pattern varies by individual tremor pattern and other PD symptoms	Impaired motor programming, involuntary movements, reduced odor identification, inefficient visual tracking & abnormal saccadic eye movements, speeded tapping impaired in prodromal stage	Micrographia, -parkinsonism (tremor less common than gait problems, rigidity, and bradykinesia)	Downward gaze palsy affects visual scanning, gait disturbance, falls, rigidity, bradykinesia, ideomotor dyspraxia possible, "applause sign" (impaired motor control leading to perseveration due to frontal dysfunction), blepharospasm
Emotional Functioning	Depression and anxiety are common, medication-induced hallucinations	Depression, anxiety, psychosis, behavioral disturbance, obsessive-compulsive symptoms, difficulty recognizing negative emotions on emotional recognition tasks	Well-formed visual hallucinations early that can become more disruptive as disease progresses; delusions (e.g., *Capgras syndrome*) can occur	Can see *pseudobulbar affect*, depression, anxiety, disinhibition, apathy
Performance and Symptom Validity	Not usually an issue	Psychiatric features such as avolition may interfere with test engagement	Cognitive fluctuations and poor attention can result in reduced engagement in testing and trouble switching tasks	Not usually an issue

Considerations when Treating Patients with PD

- *Level of Supervision* Depends on the level of impairment/stage of the disease; ranges from fully independent to 24/7 nursing home placement.

- *Driving* Problematic with more severe disease due to problems with processing speed, reaction time, executive functioning, complex attention, visuospatial abilities, and motor control.

- *Work* Motor and cognitive difficulties can interfere with employment as disease progresses; see the following website for some ideas for job accommodations for individuals with PD: https://askjan.org/disabilities/Parkinson-s-Disease.cfm?cssearch=1966211_1

- *Capacity* Individually varies depending on presentation of disease, dementia development, and how responsive symptoms are to medication.

- *Psychological/Emotional* Depression and anxiety are commonly comorbid with PD and should be treated (must distinguish masked facies, apathy, and poor initiation from depression); hallucinations can develop as side effect of medication.

- *Interpersonal Relationships* Increasing caregiver burden as disease progresses. Refer spouse/family to support groups.

- *Functional Issues* Refer patient for specialized speech therapy, physical therapy, and occupational therapy for improved symptom management; teach compensatory/environmental modification strategies such as using lined paper to improve handwriting, focusing on one aspect of movement (e.g., walking with long strides or speaking with a big voice), performing activities with visual or auditory cues, install touchless faucets, good lighting, grab bars, and handrails where needed, and remove environmental hazards; refer for adaptive equipment (shower chairs, canes, walkers, toilet chairs with arms) if indicated.

- *Risk Factor Modification* Fall precautions (at higher risk for fractures, traumatic brain injury, and other injuries due to falls with lack of protective reflexes); monitor medication side effects (e.g., gambling and hypersexuality with dopamine agonists), cognition, and need for assistance.

- *Rehabilitation Considerations* Physical therapy can help with gait, balance, and transition to assistive devices; voice training can help with hypophonia, speech therapy helps with swallowing.

Section 2: Huntington's Disease

Definition

Huntington's disease (HD) is a fatal autosomal dominant neurodegenerative disorder. It is defined genetically as CAG (cytosine-adenine-guanine) trinucleotide repeats (36 or more) on chromosome 4 that codes for huntingtin protein and can be definitively diagnosed with genetic testing. Earlier onset is inversely associated with CAG repeats. Huntington's disease is characterized by motor, cognitive, and psychiatric (depression, obsessive-compulsiveness, apathy, psychosis) disturbances. It is currently characterized as a multisystem degenerative disease. Core motor symptoms include:

- chorea
- hypokinesia

- dystonia (sustained muscle contractions leading to torticollis (neck turning) and opisthotonos (back arching)
- tic
- incoordination

Other features of HD include unintended weight loss, sleep and circadian rhythm disturbances, and autonomic nervous system dysfunction.

Neuropathology

- Loss of medium spiny cells, with sparing of interneurons, is seen in the caudate nucleus and putamen.
- Indirect basal ganglia thalamocortical circuitry is most affected, explaining why chorea and motor impersistence occur early in the disease course. However, neurodegeneration also includes the cerebral cortex, thalamus, pallidum, brainstem, and cerebellum.
- As the disease progresses, further degeneration is observed in areas connected to striatal circuits, including frontal and temporal neocortical regions.
- At death, brain volume can be decreased by as much as 25%.

Risk Factor

Affected parent

Imaging Findings

Magnetic resonance imaging (MRI) shows caudate and putamen atrophy, resulting in "box car" ventricles. Other imaging modalities have potential as HD biomarkers such as DTI (abnormalities in neuronal fiber orientation and integrity in white matter and subcortical gray matter structures), FMRI, FDG PET, and MRS (abnormal metabolic activity indicative of neuronal health).

Epidemiology

Incidence

- Mean age at onset between 30–50, with a range of 2 to 85 years
- Prevalence in Caucasian population is four to 12 per 100,000
- Geographical variations (e.g., much lower prevalence in Japan, whereas Venezuela has one of the highest prevalence rates)
- No differences between men and women

Morbidity

- Psychiatric problems (depression has 40% prevalence in HD) and high suicide rate (even before symptoms begin)
- Behavioral problems that interfere with functioning, relationships, and employment
- Other associated risks include choking, physical injury from falls, and malnutrition
- Heart failure occurs in 30% of patients with HD (versus 2% of age-matched controls)
- Severe weight loss can lead to cachexia

Mortality

Disease duration is 15–20 years. Causes of death include pneumonia (related to dysphagia), heart disease, and suicide (7.3% completion rate, second most common cause of death in HD).

Determinants of Severity

CAG Repeats

Number of CAG repeats determines age of onset. CAG of less than 27 is normal, 27 to 35 is intermediate, 36 to 40 is reduced penetrance (+/– affected), more than 40 is full penetrance. Once onset occurs, the clinical course is divided into three stages (see Table 33.4). Around 1% of patients with suspected HD test negative and have different genetic mutations known as HD phenocopies.

TABLE 33.4 Stages of Huntington's Disease

I: Early Stage (0 to 8 years after disease onset)	• Mostly functional at home and work • Maintain pre-disease levels of independence • May experience mild cognitive symptoms and psychiatric changes, motor symptoms typically do not affect ADLs • Death rare but suicide contemplation possible
II: Early intermediate stage (3 to 13 years after disease onset)	• Work becomes more difficult or unable to work • Requires slight to mild assistance with daily functions • Chorea may develop at this stage
III: Late intermediate stage (5 to 16 years after disease onset)	• Can no longer work or manage household responsibilities • Requires substantial help with daily financial affairs, household responsibilities, and ADLs • Cognitive, psychiatric, and motor symptoms worsen
IV: Early Advanced Stage (9 to 21 years after disease onset)	• No longer independent, but still capable of residing at home with help; needs may be better met at extended care facility • Requires substantial assistance in financial affairs, household responsibilities, and most ADLs
V: Advanced Stage (11 to 26 years after disease onset)	• Need total support from professional/skilled nursing care • Patients often die due to pneumonia, heart failure, or infection

Rating Scales for Severity

The most common scales to measure HD severity are the Unified Huntington's Disease Rating Scale (UHDRS), Shoulson and Fahn capability scale, and Problem Behavior Scale.

Presentation, Disease Course, and Recovery

Motor changes in HD include involuntary, unwanted movements. Initially, they occur in distal extremities such as fingers and toes or small facial muscles. Gait is unstable, and the person may look slightly intoxicated. Unwanted movements spread to all other muscles from distal to more proximal and axial. Choreatic movements are present continuously during waking hours. Talking and swallowing become more problematic. Dysarthria and dysphagia become prominent. All patients eventually develop hypokinesia, akinesia, and rigidity, leading to slower pace of all activities and difficulty starting movements.

Behavioral and psychiatric symptoms and signs include irritability (retrospectively commonly identified as the very first sign), depression (40–50%), anxiety (34–61%), and obsessive-compulsive features, as well as psychosis. Apathy has been identified as a core neuropsychiatric feature of HD and can manifest very early. Suicide occurs more frequently in early symptomatic individuals and in premanifest gene carriers. Psychiatric changes can be present many years before motor signs become visible. Cognitive decline is the other main sign and can be present before the first motor symptoms. Executive functioning is particularly affected.

All patients with HD report an unintended weight loss, which has been historically attributed to chorea. Weight loss is correlated with longer CAG repeat. Practical issues, such as slowed functioning, appetite loss, and trouble swallowing and manipulating food certainly play a role, as does reduced hypothalamic neurons. Sleep and circadian rhythm disturbances are common in HD, and dysautonomia can have major effects on cardiac health.

Treatment

There is no cure for HD; death is inevitable, and there is no known way to slow progression. Treatment is focused on assisting the individual to live as long and as comfortably as possible, mitigating individual symptoms. Disease modifying therapies under investigation include "gene suppression" or reduction of Huntington expression, but to date, there have been no successful outcomes in completed Phase 3 clinical trials.

Expectations for Neuropsychological Assessment Results

Cognitive changes can be detected up to 15 years prior to clinical onset. Measures that appear most sensitive in the prodromal period are psychomotor performance and attention/working memory measures. Please refer to Table 33.3.

Considerations when Treating Patients with HD

Quality of life in HD is greatly impacted by cognitive and motor symptoms. Chorea may be treated with tetrabenazine (TBZ), a dopamine-depleting agent. Atypical neuroleptics can also be useful. In later stages, medications to reduce rigidity and spasticity such as tizanidine and baclofen may be useful, or botulinum toxin injections for muscle spasms. SSRIs may be helpful for depression and anxiety, though careful observation of suicide risk in the HD population is warranted.

Non-pharmacological treatments to reduce symptoms include physical therapy to optimize gait and balance, speech and language therapy with an emphasis on functional communication, and dietary consultation to help maintain adequate nutrition. Cognitive behavioral therapy can reduce anxiety, depression, and OCD symptoms. Social workers can help arrange home care and coordinate moving into a residential or nursing home. End-of-life care specialists will also be helpful in the later stages of the disease course.

Several ethical issues have been raised regarding genetic testing in HD, such as whether genetic test results can be used to determine eligibility for employment or life insurance, selective abortion following prenatal genetic testing, and preimplantation genetic diagnosis during in vitro procedures to ensure the embryo is not a disease carrier. Of note, children less than 18 years of age cannot consent to genetic testing as they have a right not to know their genetic status until they are adults.

- *Level of Supervision* Depends on the level of impairment/stage of the disease, ranges from fully independent to 24/7 nursing home placement.

- *Driving* Restrictions based on processing speed, executive functioning, attention, and visuospatial deficits, as well as motor symptoms.

- *Work* See the following website for some ideas for job accommodations for individuals with HD: https://askjan.org/disabilities/Huntington-s-Disease.cfm?cssearch=1966212_1

- *Capacity* Individually varies depending on stage of disease.

- *Psychological/Emotional* Pharmacological treatment recommended for psychiatric/ emotional symptoms.

- *Medications* There is no cure for HD; chorea is treated with dopamine receptor blocking or depleting agents; treatment for depression and aggressive behavior may be required.

- *Interpersonal Relationships* Refer spouse/family to support groups and genetic counseling if appropriate.

- *Functional Issues* Weight loss and eating difficulties are common; nutrition management is important (referral to dietitian, feeding tube placement, etc. may be necessary); genetic counseling may also be beneficial. Refer the patient for specialized speech therapy, physical therapy, and occupational therapy to improve coping with functional loss.

Considerations when Treating Select Populations with HD

Pediatric Considerations

Antenatal diagnosis is possible, but usually only initiated if parents know their own genetic status. Preimplantation diagnostics are also offered in several countries—embryos without elongated CAG repeats are used in in vitro fertilization.

Juvenile HD is rare and involves disease onset before the age of 20. The CAG repeats are generally greater than 55. The first signs of juvenile HD are often behavior disturbances and learning difficulties, and because juvenile HD is uncommon, these children are often misdiagnosed with psychiatric problems. Interestingly, frequent epileptic seizures are observed in individuals with juvenile HD. In 75% of these cases, the father is the affected parent.

Section 3: Lewy Body Dementia

Definition

Lewy body disease (LBD) or dementia with Lewy bodies (LB) is a progressive neurodegenerative disorder that is characterized by *parkinsonism* and cognitive decline/dementia. It is actually thought to include three types of dementia:

- Parkinson's disease with dementia (PDD)

- Diffuse Lewy body disease (DLBD)

- Lewy body variant of Alzheimer's disease (LBV)

Diagnosis is clinically based and can be hard to distinguish from related disorders (e.g., Alzheimer's disease [AD]) when cardinal symptoms are not present. Lewy body–related dementia is the second most common form of dementia (after AD), and 20–30% of patients with a neurodegenerative dementia have comorbid AD and LBD pathology. With primary LBD, dementia typically occurs concurrently or within 1 year of parkinsonian symptoms.

Neuropathology

- Lewy bodies (abnormal aggregates of protein that form within nerve cells and displace other cell components; alpha-synuclein is the primary component) and Lewy neuritis (LN; alpha-synuclein cytoplasmic inclusion bodies) in the cortex (cingulate gyrus, insular cortex, and parahippocampal gyrus most concentrated) and brainstem, with or without Alzheimer-type neuropathologic changes (neuritic plaques and neurofibrillary tangles) and can be classified as follows depending on location of LBs and LNs:
  - olfactory bulb only = low likelihood of LBD
  - amygdala-predominant = low likelihood of LBD
  - brainstem-predominant = low likelihood of LBD
  - limbic (transitional) = low to high likelihood of LBD depending on severity of AD pathology
  - diffuse neocortical = intermediate to high likelihood depending on severity of AD pathology
- Pallor of the substantia nigra (black appearance of the substantia nigra fades in association with cell loss and dopamine depletion).
- Neuronal loss in hippocampus is variable.
- Depletion of cholinergic neurons in the nucleus basalis of Meynert.

Risk Factors

Compared to controls, patients with LBD are more likely to have a history of anxiety, depression, stroke, family history of PD, and be an APOε4 allele carrier.

Imaging Findings

- *MRI* Nondiagnostic, atrophy may be present but relative preservation of medial temporal lobe structures
- *PET* Diffuse glucose hypometabolism, including disproportionate involvement of the occipital lobes
- *SPECT* Low dopamine transporter (DaT) uptake in the basal ganglia
- *Iodine-123 MIBG scintigraphy* Reduced uptake on metaiodobenzylguanidine myocardial scintigraphy

Epidemiology

Incidence

- Responsible for 20% or more of all dementias, second to AD.
- Mean age of onset for DLBD is late 50s, whereas onset of LBV varies from 50s to 80s.
- Incidence/prevalence data are lacking but estimates include up to 5% of general population, with yearly incidence of 0.1% a year for the general population and 3.2% a year for all new dementia cases.
- Males have a higher incidence.

Morbidity

- *Neuroleptic sensitivity* can result in development or worsening of extrapyramidal motor symptoms.
- Treatment of motor symptoms with levodopa can aggravate hallucinations.
- Treatment with dopamine agonists can result in compulsive behaviors
- Motor problems increase risk of falls that can cause orthopedic injury and head trauma.

Mortality

Survival time (average of 8 years) is typically shorter than with AD, but with a wide range (2 to 20 years). Those with greater LB pathology have shorter life expectancy.

Determinants of Severity

Homozygous APOε4 allele carriers have greater neuritic plaques and cerebral amyloid angiopathy, which is associated with shorter disease duration.

Presentation, Disease Course, and Recovery

Dementia with Lewy bodies presents with onset of motor and cognitive symptoms in close proximity (usually within 1 year), although *parkinsonism* can occur before or after cognitive deficits are evident (more often occurs after). Diagnostic criteria according to the new McKeith et al. criteria (2017) include the following core clinical features:

- Fluctuating cognition with marked variations in attention and alertness (almost like a delirium in some cases)
- Recurrent visual hallucinations that are usually well formed
- *REM sleep behavioral disorder* (may precede cognitive deficits)
- One or two features of *parkinsonism*

Supportive clinical features include *neuroleptic sensitivity*, postural instability, repeated falls, syncope, severe autonomic dysfunction, hallucinations in other modalities, systematized delusions, apathy, anxiety, and depression. Supportive biomarkers include low dopamine transporter uptake in the basal ganglia on SPECT/PET imaging, abnormal (low uptake) on myocardinal *iodine-123 MIBG scintigraphy* and polysomnographic confirmation of REM sleep without atonia.

- *Probable dementia with Lewy bodies*: Presence of two or more core clinical features, or only one core clinical feature but with one or more indicative biomarkers
- *Possible dementia with Lewy bodies*: Only one core clinical feature, with no biomarker evidence, or one or more biomarkers (but no core clinical features)

The overall course is one of slow progression, but with frequent fluctuations whereby the patient may have episodes of marked confusion interspersed with periods of complete lucidity. See Table 33.5.

TABLE 33.5 Stages of Lewy Body Dementia

Early Stage (1–3 years)	• Mild *parkinsonism* • Cognitive deficits present but still fairly functional • Confusion, if present, is mild • Insight largely preserved • Hallucinations, if present, are usually benign and the patient has insight they are not real • REM behavioral symptoms may or may not be present
Middle Stage (3–6 years)	• Motor symptoms cause greater difficulty with mobility • Dementia more pronounced and causing functional problems such that assistance with medications, finances, and driving likely needed • Insight slipping • Confusion more frequent
Late Stage (>7 years)	• Severe dementia • Increasingly dependent with even basic activities of daily living • Eventually immobile without assistance

Expectations for Neuropsychological Assessment Results

Please refer to Table 33.3.

Considerations when Treating Patients with LBD

Older adults often have a variety of health issues, and dementia can interfere with medical compliance, necessitating oversight of medications and medical decision-making. Furthermore, awareness and reporting of physical symptoms diminishes with worsening of dementia and can lead to treatable medical issues going undetected until they become severe.

- *Level of Supervision* Increases as disease progresses, ultimately requires 24/7 care.

- *Driving* Should be monitored early as visuospatial deficits and slowed processing speed can pose safety risks.

- *Work* Able to work in early stages, but not as disease progresses; may often need help to know when to stop working.

- *School and Vocational Training* Transition to disability.

- *Capacity* Incapacity is inevitable; affairs should be put in order early including living will, trust, advanced directives, and power of attorney.

- *Psychological and Emotional Issues* Assess for hallucinations and depression to determine need for treatment; sleep disturbance is common.

- *Severe Psychiatric Complications* Psychosis can become more disturbing to the patient as the disease progresses and potentially leads to agitation and behavioral acting out.

- *Medications* Dementia can be treated with cholinesterase inhibitors (e.g., donepezil [Aricept], rivastigmine [Exelon]), which may have beneficial effects on apathy and visual hallucinations as well; patients with LBD may actually respond better than those with AD. Hallucinations can be treated with low-dose antipsychotics, but due to mortality risk in patients with dementia and *neuroleptic sensitivity* (leading to a worsening of motor symptoms), antipsychotics are often avoided. Treatment of motor symptoms with levodopa could exacerbate psychosis. SSRIs and SNRIs can be used to treat depression.

- *Interpersonal Relationships* Dependence on caregiver(s) can put a strain on relationships; caregiver burnout is common.

- *Functional Issues* Driving often has to be addressed early given visuospatial deficits and cognitive fluctuations; other limitations will depend on severity of cognitive and motor symptoms.

- *Risk Factor Modification* Closely monitor use of antipsychotic and levodopa agents for side effects; take fall precautions.

- *Rehabilitation Considerations* Physical therapy can help with gait and transition to assistive devices; cognitive compensation strategies may help maximize functioning; voice training can help with hypophonia.

Section 4: Progressive Supranuclear Palsy

Definition

Progressive supranuclear palsy (PSP), also known as Richardson syndrome (PSP-RS), is a progressive neurodegenerative disorder that represents the most common Parkinson's plus syndrome. The disease involves erosion of subcortical structures, as well as of subcortical-cortical connections (primarily to the prefrontal cortex) leading to a triad of motor, cognitive, and emotional/personality symptoms. Core diagnostic symptoms include:

- *vertical gaze palsy* (particularly downward gaze)
- axial rigidity
- postural instability with falls (often backward)

Other common symptoms include:

- dysarthria
- dysphagia
- bradykinesia
- gait disorder (apraxia)
- cognitive impairment
- behavioral changes (apathy, depression, anxiety, *pseudobulbar affect*, neurobehavioral symptoms)

Neuropathology

- Mostly a sporadic disease, with very rare familial forms, although polymorphisms in the microtubule-associated protein tau (MAPT) gene may be associated with some cases of PSP.
- Insoluble 4-repeat tau protein deposits.
- Dopamine depletion in the substantia nigra, caudate, and putamen.

- Neuronal loss and gliosis in the globus pallidus, subthalamic nuclei, red nuclei, dentate nucleus, superior colliculi, and periaqueductal gray matter.
- Neurofibrillary tangles and neuropil threads in the basal ganglia, brainstem, dentate, and nucleus basalis of Meynert.
- Dopaminergic, cholinergic, and adrenergic neurotransmitter systems are affected.

Risk Factors

No clear risk factors have been identified.

Imaging Findings

- *MRI* Atrophy of the midbrain tegmentum (i.e., hummingbird sign) and cerebellar peduncles.
- *PET* Fluorodeoxyglucose hypometabolism in frontal cortex, caudate, midbrain, and thalamus. Tau ligands in development.
- *SPECT* Scans of the presynaptic dopamine transporter (DaT) show reduced uptake bilaterally; rCBF hypoperfusion of cingulate and medial frontal cortex.

Epidemiology

Incidence

- Onset typically in the 60s, can occur in 40s.
- Age-adjusted prevalence of 1.4 per 100,000.
- Average annual incidence (for age 50–99) of 5 per 100,000, with marked increase with age (up to 14.7 per 100,000 for ages 80–99).
- Possibly higher incidence in males, but not a consistent finding.

Morbidity

- Dementia occurs in 50–80% of cases.
- Brain injury and fractures related to falls.
- Choking or aspiration related to swallowing problems.

Mortality

- Survival time 6 to 9 years from symptom onset.
- Most common cause of death is respiratory arrest due to pneumonia or degeneration of brainstem respiratory centers.

Determinants of Severity

Older age at diagnosis has consistently been associated with shorter survival time. Although impaired downward gaze is a cardinal diagnostic feature of PSP, it may not be present until later in the course of the disease, often delaying diagnosis. Presence of dementia at diagnosis, executive function deficits, and early dysphagia have been associated with shorter survival.

Presentation, Disease Course, and Recovery

Presenting symptoms of PSP can vary, but most frequently include postural instability and falls (typically backward). Other *parkinsonian* symptoms can be present, including rigidity, bradykinesia, and gait problems, although tremor is usually absent. Oculomotor dysfunction, primarily involving downward gaze, is a hallmark feature of the disease and distinguishes it from other movement disorders, although this occurs later in the course of the disease (up to 3 or 4 years after symptoms begin). This involves an inability to look down on command, whereas spontaneous gaze may be intact since the associated lesion is at the level above the eye gaze nuclei in the brainstem (hence the name "supranuclear"). Cognitive dysfunction can occur early in the disease process and is typically present within 2 years of symptom emergence. Onset of gait problems occurs early, and gait assistance is typically needed by 3 years into the disease, with ultimate progression to wheelchair. At the late stage of the disease, patients are typically dependent on a wheelchair and many become mute. A subgroup of patients with PSP present with prominent language or behavioral symptoms and may be misdiagnosed with primary progressive aphasia or a behavioral variant of frontotemporal dementia. The subtypes listed in Table 33.6 reflect the disparate

TABLE 33.6 Progressive Supranuclear Palsy (PSP) Subtypes

PSP—Richardson Syndrome (RS)*	• Postural instability (with falls), bradykinesia, and unsteady gait • Subtle personality changes (apathy, disinhibition) • Executive dysfunction • Slow, ataxic, and hypophonic speech • Dysphagia • Impaired ocular movements (with vertical supranuclear gaze palsy up to 3–4 years after disease onset)
PSP—Parkinsonism*	• Features more consistent with Parkinson's disease (asymmetric onset of limb symptoms, tremor) • Some response to levodopa
PSP—Progressive gait freezing*	Progressive gait disturbance with freezing of gait, speech or writing, but without tremor, rigidity, dementia or eye movement abnormality during the first 5 years of disease
PSP—Speech language	• Present with language features of a nonfluent primary progressive aphasia: effortful, halting speech, phonemic errors, dyspraxic speech, and agrammatism • Later development of gait and balance problems • Rarer presentation and overlaps clinically with primary progressive aphasia (PPA), but histopathology is PSP not PPA
PSP—Predominant cerebellar ataxia	Cerebellar ataxia as the initial and main symptom
PSP—Frontal presentation	Clinical features of behavioral variant frontotemporal dementia (deterioration of personality social compartment, behavior [apathy, disinhibition, hypo-orality], and cognition) years before PSP-RS symptoms
PSP—Corticobasal syndrome	• Progressive, asymmetric rigidity • Dyspraxia, typically begins asymmetric onset then spreads • Cortical sensory loss • Alien limb • Bradykinesia • Unresponsive to levodopa • Rarer presentation and overlaps clinically with corticobasal degeneration (CBD) as a separate disorder, but histopathology is PSP not CBD

NOTE: * Most common subtypes

presentations of PSP that illuminate why clinical diagnosis can be difficult in some cases. Furthermore, there is much overlap between some of these syndromes, blurring the presentations even more. In particular, the subtypes of progressive nonfluent aphasia, behavioral variant, and corticobasal syndrome are rare, but reflect a small percentage of patients who present with symptoms that essentially mimic those found in primary progressive aphasia, frontotemporal dementia or corticobasal degeneration, respectively, but histopathologically are actually PSP. Stages of PSP are listed in Table 33.7.

TABLE 33.7 Stages of Progressive Supranuclear Palsy (PSP-RS)

Early Stage (1–2 years)	• Postural instability • Falls • Bradykinesia
Middle Stage (3–5 years)	• Ophthalmoplegia (impaired downward gaze) • Cognitive impairment • Rigidity • Dysphagia • Gait problems and increased falls • Dysarthria • Apathy
Late Stage (6–9 years)	• Wheelchair needed • Worsening cognitive impairment • Speech increasingly slow and slurred • Significant visual problems • Death

Expectations for Neuropsychological Assessment Results

Please refer to Table 33.3.

Considerations when Treating Patients with PSP

Older patients may have other comorbid conditions that can slow early diagnosis (e.g., orthopedic problems or neuropathy contributing to falls).

- *Level of Supervision* Close supervision is needed secondary to falls and poor judgment.

- *Driving* Restrict early due to impact of vertical gaze disorder and cognitive deficits on safety.

- *Work* Usually unable to work soon after diagnosis given impact of motor symptoms and cognitive deficits.

- *School and Vocational Training* Transition to disability.

- *Capacity* Can be an issue given high rate of dementia and language problems; affairs should be put in order early, including will, advanced directives, and power of attorney.

- *Psychological and Emotional Issues* Emotional incontinence needs to be distinguished from depression to be treated appropriately; masked facies, slow response latencies, and apathy can be mistaken for signs of depression.

- *Severe Psychiatric Complications* Not typically an issue; some patients can develop neurobehavioral symptoms that may result in management issues and alienation of caregivers.

- *Medications* Only limited response to dopaminergic or anticholinergic agents; emotional symptoms can be treated with antidepressants; tau therapies are in development.

- *Interpersonal Relationships* Dependence on caregiver(s) can put a strain on relationships.

- *Functional Issues* Ambulation, speech, and gaze problems contribute to functional limitations; poor judgment may lead to risky behaviors that can result in falls or accidents.

- *Risk Factor Modification* Fall precautions are paramount, particularly in those with impulsivity; swallowing problems can result in aspiration, and food choices may need monitoring.

- *Rehabilitation Considerations* Assistive devices can help with gait problems but do not address falls; physical therapy may help with balance and gait, but evidence-based research on efficacy is lacking; speech pathology is needed for management of dysphagia and dysarthria.

Section 5: Other Movement Disorders

Essential Tremor

This chapter did not review in detail essential tremor (ET; manifest as a postural or action tremor), which is the most commonly occurring movement disorder and is hereditary (autosomal dominant) in 50% of cases. It has typically been thought of as benign, but can be debilitating in severe cases. Patients with ET are at increased risk for cognitive deficits, including mild cognitive impairment and dementia. *Dopamine transporter (DaT)* SPECT imaging can be used to help with differential diagnosis between ET and PD, multiple system atrophy, PSP, and corticobasal degeneration. In severe cases, ET may be treated with DBS, focused ultrasound thalamotomy, or radio-surgical gamma knife thalamotomy, and botulinum toxin injections for disabling head or vocal cord tremor.

Cortical Basal Syndrome

Cortical basal syndrome (CBS) is another important movement disorder to be aware of, as it is often in the differential diagnosis when evaluating patients with motor symptoms. Cortical basal degeneration (CBD) is a tauopathy with distinct neuropathological features, although clinical presentation can overlap with PSP, frontotemporal dementia, PD, and AD. As such, CBD is often reserved to characterize the pathological diagnosis and corticobasal syndrome to describe the clinical presentation, which includes asymmetric motor symptoms involving (1) limb rigidity or akinesia, limb dystonia, and/or limb myoclonus, plus (2) limb apraxia, cortical sensory loss, and/or alien limb phenomenon.

Recent diagnostic criteria for CBS recognizes the presentation of overlapping syndromes associated with this disease and have characterized five different phenotypes:

- Probable corticobasal syndrome
- Possible corticobasal syndrome
- Frontal behavioral-spatial syndrome
- Nonfluent/agrammatic variant of primary progressive aphasia
- PSP syndrome

Patients can present with either cognitive symptoms, motor symptoms, or both. Early motor symptoms may present as "clumsiness" of the affected limb. The apraxia typically begins in one limb and spreads to other limbs within 2 years, though some continued degree of asymmetry is common. Early cognitive symptoms typically include impairment in language production, executive functioning, and attention/concentration. Onset usually occurs in the 60s but ranges from the 50s to the 70s and is insidious and progressive, with death occurring 6 to 8 years following onset. The prevalence of CBS is 4.9–7.3 cases/100,000. Neuroimaging may reveal focal, asymmetric cortical atrophy (particularly in the frontal/parietal areas contralateral to the clinically most affected side), and similar asymmetric hypoperfusion/hypometabolism can be seen on SPECT/PET imaging. There is no cure for CBS, and the focus of treatment is generally on reducing individual symptoms. Psychiatric symptoms can include depression, apathy, anxiety, irritability, disinhibition, and other neurobehavioral symptoms.

Multiple System Atrophy

Multiple system atrophy (MSA) is a synucleinopathy with overlapping, but distinct clinical features from other movement disorders that can include a combination of cerebellar ataxia, autonomic dysfunction, and both pyramidal and extrapyramidal motor signs due to abnormal alpha-synuclein depositions in both the central and peripheral autonomic nervous systems. Classification of MSA subtypes has changed over time, with the previously described distinct conditions of striatonigral degeneration, Shy-Drager syndrome, and olivopontocerebellar atrophy now combined into one disorder, MSA. However, two motor subclassifications have been identified that correspond to initial symptomatology and neuropathology: parkinsonism (MSA-P; 80% of cases) and cerebellar ataxia (MSA-C; ~20% of cases). Early symptoms can involve genitourinary dysfunction, autonomic hypotension, and REM behavioral disorder (~80% or more of cases) that may progress fairly rapidly to include balance, speech, and coordination problems. Motor symptoms (parkinsonism) are typically symmetrical and generally do not respond to L-dopa or improvements are short-lived. Mean age of onset is 55–60 with duration approximately 8 to 9 years from onset of motor symptoms. Annual incidence is approximately 3 per 100,000 in those over age 50 and prevalence estimates range from 2 to 5 per 100,000. Consensus criteria from 2008 do not include cognitive impairment and dementia is less likely in MSA, though deficits can be seen in executive functioning, attention, visuospatial abilities, and aspects of memory, typically later in the course of the disease. Neuroimaging abnormities can be seen on standard MRI, including atrophy of the putamen, pons, middle cerebellar peduncles, cerebellum, and medulla oblongata, as well as a dilation of the fourth ventricle. Cardiovascular autonomic testing is often performed to further evaluate orthostatic hypotension, which is seen in 70% of MSA cases. Sleep study, DaT scan, and dysphagia evaluation may also be performed to help with differential diagnosis.

Tourette Syndrome

Tourette syndrome (TS) is characterized by repetitive, stereotyped involuntary movements and vocalizations called tics, generally proceeded by a premonitory urge or sensation. The presence of multiple motor and one or more vocal tics for at least 1 year is required for diagnosis. Age of onset is usually between 5 to 7 years, with symptoms peaking around 10–12 years of age, and prevalence three to four times higher in males than females. Tics can be simple (e.g., eye blinking, grimacing, shoulder shrugging, head or shoulder jerking, throat clearing, sniffing, barking, or grunting sounds) or complex (e.g., facial grimacing combined with a head twist and a shoulder shrug, or words or phrases, such as swearing or echolalia). Simple tics are sudden, brief, and repetitive, and involve a limited number of muscle groups, whereas complex tics are distinct, coordinated movement patterns involving several muscle groups. Tics vary in type, frequency, and severity and may worsen during periods of illness, stress, fatigue, or excitement. Tics usually progress from simple to complex and worsen during the teenage years, followed by improvement in adulthood, although 10% have a progressive course that continues to worsen over time. Type of tics may evolve over time and can often be temporarily controlled with great effort for short periods of time. Tics are thought to be a disorder of the basal ganglia/cortical brain circuitry, though the exact pathophysiology is unknown. Brain MRI and CT scans are usually within normal limits. Dopamine, serotonin, and norepinephrine are thought to play a role. Tourette syndrome is frequently comorbid with ADHD, learning disabilities, obsessive-compulsive disorder, rage attacks, depression, generalized anxiety, panic attacks, sleep disorders, and migraines, thus requiring multimodal interventions. Because TS occurs during childhood, involvement of the educational system to help meet individual needs is common (e.g., specialized tutoring, smaller or special classes, individualized accommodations, and classroom modifications depending on tic expression). One of the most influential factors in a child's experience with TS is whether a supportive teacher at the school is involved.

Relevant Definitions

Capgras syndrome Well-formed delusional disorder in which a person believes that a spouse, parent, friend, or other close family member has been replaced by an identical-looking "imposter." In some instances, the delusion may carry over to their home, believing that they have "two houses." This latter phenomenon is also referred to as reduplicative paramnesia.

Deep brain stimulation (DBS) Surgical treatment that is effective for certain individuals with advanced PD and other movement disorders, which involves implantation of a medical device similar to a pacemaker that sends electrical impulses to specific parts of the brain (subthalamic nucleus, global pallidus, and ventrointermedius nucleus are the most common targets).

Dopamine transporting (DaT) imaging Defines the integrity of the dopaminergic system and has its main clinical application in differentiating patients with/without a parkinsonian disorder (e.g., essential tremor from PD, LBD vs. AD).

Dyskinesias Impairment in the ability to control movements, characterized by spasmodic or repetitive motions or lack of coordination.

Iodine-123 meta-iodobenzylguanidine (MIBG) scintigraphy A nuclear medicine scan involving an injection of a radioactive medication called iodine-123 MIBG used in movement disorders to evaluate cardiac sympathetic denervation. MIBG scintigraphy can show low uptake of MIBG in Lewy body-related disorders, including PD, LBD, pure autonomic failure and REM sleep behavior disorder.

Micrographia Handwriting that decreases in size from normal to minute, seen in parkinsonism.

Neuroleptic sensitivity Oversensitivity to side effects of neuroleptic medications with particular vulnerability to developing extrapyramidal symptoms.

Parkinsonism A constellation of neurological symptoms marked by the features of PD (e.g., hypokinesia, bradykinesia, tremor, and muscular rigidity) but do not meet criteria for PD. Drug-induced parkinsonism is the most common condition causing secondary parkinsonism. Neuroleptics and antipsychotic drugs are the most frequent medications that can cause drug-induced parkinsonism, and symptoms can take up to 1 year to resolve after medications have been discontinued.

Pseudobulbar affect Involuntary or uncontrollable episodes of crying and/or laughing that do not necessarily coincide with the underlying emotion being experienced. Can be seen in PSP as well as in other neurological disorders (e.g., stroke, multiple sclerosis, amyotrophic lateral sclerosis, head injury), presumably related to disruption of the corticobulbar pathways involved in the voluntary control of emotions.

REM sleep behavioral disorder The paralysis that normally occurs during REM sleep is incomplete or absent, allowing the person to "act out" his or her dreams. Dream-enactment behaviors include talking, yelling, punching, kicking, sitting, jumping from bed, arm flailing, and grabbing.

Unified Parkinson's Disease Rating Scale (UPDRS) A measure of severity of Parkinson's disease, based on a scale with a 0–160 total score and 0–44 motor section score.

Vertical gaze palsy Impaired ability to voluntarily move the eyes up or down. Downward gaze deficits are associated with lesions above the eye gaze nuclei in the brainstem, hence the name "supranuclear" in PSP, in which downward gaze deficits are a core diagnostic feature.

Movement Disorders Questions

NOTE: Questions 25, 52, and 98 on the First Full-Length Practice Examination, Questions 57, 87, and 112 on the Second Full-Length Practice Examination, Questions 8, 31, 34, 93, 101, and 114 on the Third Full-Length Practice Examination, and Questions 9, 32, 40, 59, and 102 on the Fourth Full-Length Practice Examination are from this chapter.

1. Onset of Parkinsonism and cognitive dysfunction in close proximity occurs in which of the following disorders?
   - (a) Parkinson's disease
   - (b) progressive supranuclear palsy
   - (c) Lewy body dementia
   - (d) multiple system atrophy

2. Which of the following would be most helpful with differential diagnosis of Huntington's disease from other movement disorders?
   - (a) dopamine transporting imaging
   - (b) neuropsychological assessment
   - (c) quantitative EEG
   - (d) genetic testing

3. What is the most prominent MRI finding in individuals with Huntington's disease?
   - (a) hippocampal sclerosis
   - (b) depigmentation of the substantia nigra
   - (c) caudate atrophy
   - (d) global cortical atrophy

4. Which of the following is the most common side effect of levodopa?
   - (a) auditory hallucinations
   - (b) constant daydreaming
   - (c) tardive dyskinesia
   - (d) compulsive behavior

5. The cognitive fluctuations that can be seen in Lewy body dementia most resemble which of the following?

(a) freezing

(b) delirium

(c) sundowning

(d) psychosis

6. Dementia is a central diagnostic feature for which of the following?

(a) corticobasal syndrome

(b) Parkinson's disease

(c) Lewy body dementia

(d) Huntington's disease

7. Which of the following is NOT an accepted etiology for parkinsonism?

(a) vascular disease

(b) traumatic brain injury

(c) toxic exposure

(d) aspartame

8. What is a core psychiatric symptom in individuals with Huntington's disease?

(a) visual hallucinations

(b) depression

(c) anxiety

(d) apathy

9. A patient arrives with a constellation of recent onset of motor and non-motor symptoms. Which of the following would help most in distinguishing multiple system atrophy from Parkinson's disease:

(a) presence of rapid eye movement behavioral symptoms

(b) daytime sleepiness

(c) orthostatic hypotension

(d) minimal response to L-dopa

10. Cognitive dysfunction in Parkinson's disease tends to be higher in individuals who ____.

(a) have early age of onset (< 70 years old)

(b) do not have tremor at initial presentation

(c) eventually develop bilateral tremor

(d) have comorbid restless leg syndrome

Movement Disorders Answers

1. **C–Lewy body dementia**   *Co-occurring (within 1 year) cognitive and motor symptoms are most common in LBD and are, in fact, part of the diagnostic criteria. Dementia is inevitable in LBD. Cognitive impairment in PSP can occur before, simultaneous with, or after motor symptoms and may not eventually progress to dementia. Dementia in PD can occur, but tends to be much later in the course of the disease, although milder deficits can be seen earlier. Cognitive and personality symptoms may represent the initial stages of HD, although the motor symptoms are not the typical parkinsonian symptoms seen in PD, LBD, or PSP.*

Reference: McKeith, I. G., Boeve, B. F., Dickson, D. W., Halliday, G., Taylor, J.-P., Weintraub, D., . . . Kosaka, K., (2017). Diagnosis and management of dementia with Lewy bodies. *Neurology, 89,* 88–100.

2. **D—genetic testing**   *Huntington's disease is one of a few movement disorders that can definitively and consistently be diagnosed using genetic testing because it is a hereditary, autosomal dominant disorder.*

   Reference: Quaid, K. A. (2017). Genetic testing for Huntington disease. In A. S. Feigin & K. E. Anderson (Eds.), *Handbook of Clinical Neurology*, Vol. 144: *Huntington Disease*). Amsterdam, NL: Elsevier.

3. **C—caudate atrophy**   *Ventricular enlargement due to caudate atrophy can often be seen in HD. Significant reductions in caudate as well as putamen volume are often seen in symptomatic and presymptomatic HD gene carriers.*

   Reference: Niccolini, F., & Politis, M. (2014) Neuroimaging in Huntington's disease. *World Journal of Radiology, 6, 301–312.*

4. **D—compulsive behaviors**   *Side effects of levodopa agents include hallucinations, dyskinesias, and vivid dreaming: Dopamine agonists are especially implicated in the impulse control disorders (ICDs) that can be seen in PD, including hypersexuality, overeating, compulsive spending, and gambling, in addition to hobbyism and punding behaviors. Risk factors for the development of both medication addiction and compulsive behaviors in PD are sex (males at greater risk for gambling; females for shopping), younger age at the PD diagnosis, a premorbid history of drug or alcohol abuse, depression, and elevated scores on the personality measure of novelty seeking.*

   Reference: Voon, V., Mehta, A. R., & Hallett, M. (2011). Impulse control disorders in Parkinson disease: Recent advances. *Current Opinions in Neurology, 24, 324–330.*

5. **B—delirium**   *When cognitive fluctuations are pronounced, the transient confusion can be mistaken for delirium. Presence of cognitive fluctuations is more likely to be associated with dementia and clinical ratings of impairment.*

   Reference: Escandon, A., Al-Hammadi, N., & Galvin, J. E., (2010). Effect of cognitive fluctuation on neuropsychological performance in aging and dementia. *Neurology, 74, 210–27.*

6. **C—Lewy body dementia**   *Dementia is a central feature, essential for a diagnosis of possible or probable LBD.*

   Reference: McKeith, I. G., Boeve, B. F., Dickson, D. W., Halliday, G., Taylor, J.-P., Weintraub, D., . . . Kosaka, K., (2017). Diagnosis and management of dementia with Lewy bodies. *Neurology, 89, 88–100.*

7. **D—aspartame**   *Toxins, vascular disease, structural brain damage (including TBI, tumors, hydrocephalus, Wilson's disease), drugs (neuroleptics, dopamine depleting agents), and infections can cause secondary PD. To date, research does not support aspartame as a cause of PD.*

   Reference: Hou, J.-G. G., & Lai, E. C. (2008). Overview of Parkinson's disease. In M. Trail & E. J. Protas (Eds.), *Neurorehabilitation of Parkinson's disease* (pp. 1–40). Thorofare, NJ: SLACK,.

8. **D—apathy**   *Apathy is the most prevalent neuropsychiatric feature of HD, and is primarily associated frontal-striatal circuit damage.*

   Reference: Martínez-Horta, S., Perez-Perez, J., Sampedro, F., Pagonabarraga, J., Horta-Barba, A., Carceller-Sindreu, M., . . . Kulisevsky, J. (2018), Structural and metabolic brain correlates of apathy in Huntington's disease. *Movement Disorders, 33, 1151–1159.*

9. **D—minimal response to L-dopa**   *Patients with both MSA and PD can have REMBD, daytime sleepiness, and orthostatic hypotension, though these may be more common in MSA than PD. Non-responsiveness to L-dopa in combination with these symptoms may be most helpful in differentiating the two conditions.*

Reference: Palma, J.-A., Norcliffe-Kaufmann, L., & Kaufmann, H. (2018). Diagnosis of multiple system atrophy. *Autonomic Neuroscience, 211*, 15-25.

10. **B—do not have tremor at initial presentation** *Older age of onset and initial symptoms other than tremor are risk factors for dementia in PD*

> **Reference:** Uc, E. Y., McDermott, M. P., Marder, K. S., Anderson, S. W., Litvan, I., Como, P. G., Auinger, P., Chou, K., L., and Growdon, J. C., (2009). Incidence of and risk factors for cognitive impairment in an early Parkinson disease clinical trial cohort. *Neurology, 73*, 1469–1477.

Recommended Readings

Armstrong, M. J., Litvan, I., Lang, A. E., Bak, T. H., Bhatia, K. P., Borroni, B., . . . Weiner, W. J. (2013). Criteria for the diagnosis of corticobasal degeneration. *Neurology, 80*, 496–503.

Boxer, A. L., Yu, J. T., Golbe, L. I., Litvan, I., Lang, A. E., & Hoglinger, G. U. (2017). Advances in progressive supranuclear palsy: New diagnostic criteria, biomarkers, and therapeutic approaches. *Lancet Neurology, 16*, 552–563.

Chen, W., Hopfner, F., Becktepe, J. S., & Deuschl, G. (2017). Rest tremor revisited: Parkinson's disease and other disorders. *Translational Neurodegeneration, 6*, 16. http://doi.org/10.1186/s40035-017-0086-4

Ghosh, R., & Tabrizi, S. J. (2018). Clinical features of Huntington's disease. In C. Nóbrega & L. Pereira de Almeida (Eds.), *Polyglutamine disorders* (pp. 1–28). New York, NY: Springer.

McKeith, I. G., Boeve, B. F., Dickson, D. W., Halliday, G., Taylor, J. P, Weintraub, D., . . . Kosaka, K. (2017). Diagnosis and management of dementia with Lewy bodies. *Neurology, 89*, 88–100.

Palma, J. A., Norcliffe-Kaufmann, L., & Kaufmann, H. (2018). Diagnosis of multiple system atrophy. *Autonomic Neuroscience, 211*, 15-25.

Parmera, J. B., Rodriguez, R. D., Neto A. S. Nitrini, R., & Dozzi Brucki, S. M. (2016). Corticobasal syndrome: A diagnostic conundrum. *Dementia and Neuropsychologia, 10*, 267–275.

Pizzolato, G., & Mandat, T. (2012). Deep brain stimulation for movement disorders. *Frontiers in Integrative Neuroscience, 6*, 1–5.

Postuma, R. B., Berg, D., Stern, M., Poewe, W., Olanow, C. W., Oertel, W, . . . Deyschl, G. (2015). MDS clinical diagnostic criteria for Parkinson's disease. *Movement Disorders, 30*, 1591–1601.

Schoenberg, M. R., & Scott, J. G. (Eds.). (2011). *The little black book of neuropsychology: A syndrome-based approach.* New York, NY: Springer.

Stout, J. C., Paulsen, J. S., Queller, S., Solomon, A. C., Whitlock, K. B., Campbell, J. C., . . . Aylward, E. H. (2011). Neurocognitive signs in prodromal Huntington disease. *Neuropsychology, 25*, 1–14.

Troster, A. I., & Garrett, R. (2018). Parkinson's disease and other movement disorders. In J. Morgan & J. Ricker (Eds.), *Textbook of clinical neuropsychology* (2nd ed., pp. 507–559). New York, NY and London, UK: Taylor & Francis Group.

Section III Disorders and Conditions: Psychiatric

34　Mood Disorders: Depression, Mania, and Anxiety

Mark T. Barisa

Introduction

Mood and anxiety disorders are characterized by somatic, emotional, cognitive, and behavioral signs and symptoms that result in difficulties in usual life functions, including work or social activities and relationships with others (Table 34.1). This chapter reviews epidemiological, neuropathological, and nosological aspects of these disorders, as well as their specific manifestations in pediatric and elderly populations. While specific diagnostic updates will be reviewed, the focus will be on mood and anxiety disorders in a broad perspective.

Section 1: Mood Disorders

Definition

The two main mood disorders are depression and mania. These occur on a continuum from clearly normal to clearly pathological. A third abnormality, bipolar disorder, includes a pathological fluctuation of mood. Depressive signs and symptoms include sad mood, *anhedonia*, loss of appetite and weight, sleep disturbance, *psychomotor retardation*, agitation, fatigue and low energy, feelings of worthlessness, excessive or inappropriate guilt, and suicidal ideation. Manic signs and symptoms include elevated or expansive mood, inflated self-esteem or grandiosity, decreased need for sleep, increased verbal output or pressured speech, flight of ideas or racing thoughts, distractibility, increase in goal-directed activity, and excessive involvement in pleasurable activities that have a high potential for negative consequences.

Neuropathology

Neuroanatomical Factors

- In general, neuroanatomical changes associated with mood disorders include disturbances of the limbic system, as well as neurochemical changes.
- Functional neuroimaging studies in patients with depression have shown increased activity in ventral limbic regions (the genu of the cingulate gyrus, the amygdala, and the ventral striatum), and functional abnormalities in these limbic regions are thought to reflect the emotional and autonomic symptoms of mood disorders.
- Atrophy of select areas of the brain has been associated with depression including the amygdala, hippocampus, prefrontal cortex, striatum, nucleus accumbens, and the cerebellum. Specifically, hippocampal volume loss among persons with major depressive disorder was found to be as high as 19%, and the number of days an individual had untreated depression had a direct effect on hippocampal size.

TABLE 34.1 Clinically Recognized Mood Disorders and Specifiers

Major Depression	A medical illness of general emotional demoralization and withdrawal or sadness greater and more prolonged than that warranted by any objective reason.
Mania	A state of excitement manifested by mental and physical hyperactivity, disorganization of behavior, and elevation of mood.
Bipolar Affective Disorder	• *Bipolar I Disorder* Presence of both depression and mania in a cycling pattern • *Bipolar II Disorder* Presence of depression and *hypomania* in a cycling pattern with no history of full manic episodes
With Mixed Features	Allows for the presence of manic symptoms as part of the depression diagnosis in patients who do not meet the full criteria for a manic episode.
With Anxious Distress	Allows for the acknowledgment of anxiety in patients with depression that may affect prognosis, treatment options, or response.

- Cortical thinning and surface area reductions in the frontal lobe, somatosensory, and motor areas have been shown in adults and adolescents with recurrent depression, with additional cortical thinning of the temporal lobe in adults.

- The neurobiological substrates of mania and bipolar disorder have been less thoroughly explored, but similar brain regions are implicated.

  - Reductions in brain volume and blood flow in the dorsal medial and dorsal lateral prefrontal cortices have been among the most consistent findings in unipolar and bipolar disorders.

  - The ventral prefrontal cortex has been shown to be compromised and functionally abnormal with reduced engagement and atypical connectivity with the anterior cingulate cortex and medical temporal structures, including the amygdala and hippocampal gyrus.

  - It has been suggested that disruption of white matter connectivity within brain networks that modulate emotional behavior in early development leads to decreased connectivity among ventral prefrontal networks and limbic brain regions, especially amygdala. This was hypothesized to cause developmental failure in healthy ventral prefrontal–limbic modulation resulting in the onset of mania and ultimately, with progressive changes throughout these networks over time and with affective episodes, a bipolar course of illness.

Neurochemical Factors

The neurochemical basis of depression is complex and not the result of any one specific deficit. Mood disorders have been linked to a deficit or imbalance in monoamine neurotransmitters, notably serotonin, norepinephrine, and dopamine. Glutamate has been studied more recently regarding its role in depression and mood stability. Antidepressants may also act on other neurotransmitters, such as acetylcholine and *gamma-aminobutyric acid* (GABA).

- *Serotonin*

  - Serotonergic neurons arise from the median and dorsal raphe nuclei in the brainstem and project throughout the forebrain. Serotonin is involved in regulating many important physiological functions, such as sleep, aggression, eating, sexual behavior, impulse control, and mood.

  - Research suggests that a decrease in the production of serotonin can cause depression. Two major theories exist:

- A deficit of serotonin activity may directly cause depression.
- A serotonin deficit serves as a risk factor for depression, but is not a direct cause.
- *Norepinephrine* (also called noradrenaline)
  - Norepinephrine helps the brain recognize and respond to stressful situations. Research suggests that people who are vulnerable to depression may have a norepinephrinergic system that does not handle the effects of stress very efficiently. A deficiency of norepinephrine in certain areas of the brain has been found to result in depressed mood.
  - Autopsy studies show that people who have experienced multiple depressive episodes have fewer norepinephrinergic neurons than people who have no depressive history.
  - Recent studies suggest that, in some people, low levels of serotonin trigger a drop in norepinephrine levels, which then leads to depression.
- *Dopamine*
  - Dopamine plays an important role in regulating drives to seek out rewards, as well as the ability to obtain a sense of pleasure, but has not been fully established as having a direct role in depression.
  - Low dopamine levels may, in part, explain why people with depression don't derive the same sense of pleasure out of activities or people that they did before becoming depressed.
  - Neuroimaging studies of medication-free patients with depression have found decreased ligand binding to the dopamine transporter and increased dopamine binding potential in the caudate and putamen, suggesting a functional deficiency of synaptic dopamine.
- *Glutamate*
  - Glutamate is the major excitatory neurotransmitter in the brain that acts on both metabotropic and ionotropic receptors. Multiple lines of evidence suggest that glutamate and its receptors have an impact on depression and antidepressant activity.

Epidemiology

Incidence and prevalence rates for mood and anxiety disorders are somewhat variable by specific disorder classification (Table 34.2). For more details and more updated information over time, please refer to the websites listed in recommended readings.

Presentation and Disease Course

Major Depression and Persistent Depressive Disorder (Dysthymia)

Some people experience only a single episode of depression within their lifetime, but individuals with depressive disorders will typically have multiple episodes (see Table 34.3 for symptoms of depression). Depression is caused by a combination of factors including biological, environmental, psychological, and genetic factors.

- Neurochemical changes, including reductions in serotonin, noradrenalin, and dopamine have been associated with depression.
- Structural and metabolic changes in the brain have been noted in patients with depression.
- Psychosocial and environmental factors or events often precede depressive episodes.

TABLE 34.2 Prevalence and Incidence Rates of Mood Disorders

	Adults	Children and Adolescents
All Mood Disorders Combined	• Affects about 16.2 million adult Americans. • Lifetime prevalence: 21.4% • 12 mo. prevalence: 9.7% • Prevalence of "severe" mood disorder is 4.3% • Prevalence is higher for females (11.6%) than males (7.7%). • Average age of onset is 30 • Prevalence by age: 　▪ 18–29 years old 12.9% 　▪ 30–44 years old 11.9% 　▪ 45–59 years old 9.4% 　▪ 60+ years old 3.6%	• Less likely in children • Lifetime prevalence of adolescents is14.3% • Prevalence of "severe" mood disorder is 11.2% • Prevalence increases with age: 　▪ 13–14 years old: 10.5% 　▪ 15–16 years old: 15.5% 　▪ 17–18 years old: 18.1% • Females more likely than males (18.3% to 10.5%, respectively).
Major Depressive Disorder	• One of the most common disorders in the United States • Lifetime prevalence: 16.5% • 16.2 million adults in the United States had at least one major depressive episode in 2016 representing 6.7% of all United States' adults • Of adults with major depression, 64% had severe impairment • Prevalence of major depressive episode was higher among adult females (8.5%) compared to males 4.8% • Prevalence of adults with a major depressive episode was highest among individuals aged 18–25 (10.9%). • Racial Prevalence 　▪ American Indian/Alaskan Native 8.7% 　▪ White 7.4% 　▪ Native Hawaiian or Pacific Islander 7.3% 　▪ Hispanic or Latin/x 5.6% 　▪ African-American 5.0% 　▪ Asian American 3.9% 　▪ Mix of two or more races 10.5%	• 2.2 million of adolescents aged 12–17 years old had at least one major depressive episode with severe impairment representing 9.0% of the United States population aged 12–17 • Of adolescents with a major depressive episode in 2016, 70% had severe impairment • Prevalence rates for children increase with age • Prevalence rates for girls are nearly three times higher than boys
Bipolar Disorder	• Lifetime prevalence 4.4% • 12-month prevalence 2.8% • In 2016, past year prevalence was similar for males (2.9%) and females (2.8%) • Average age of onset is 25 years old • Prevalence rates decrease with age • 82.9% of people with bipolar disorder had serious impairment, the highest percent serious impairment among mood disorders	• Prevalence of childhood-onset bipolar disorder is not well established due to variations in definitions and characteristics. • Lifetime prevalence is estimated to be 2.9% among adolescents, and 2.6% had severe impairment • Prevalence among adolescents was higher for females (3.3%) than for males (2.6%) • Onset is typically in late adolescent or early adulthood, but children can have the disorder with prevalence increasing with age • Children with a parent or sibling with the disorder are four to six times more likely to develop the illness.

TABLE 34.3 Signs and Symptoms of Depression

Mood Symptoms	• Feelings of sadness, despondency, worry, pessimism, etc. • Loss of interest in previously enjoyed activities, social activities, sex, etc.
Behavioral Symptoms	• Feeling tired, fatigued, or slowed down • Restless or irritable behaviors or reactions • Psychomotor slowing • Changes in eating, sleeping, or other habits • Problems with concentration, memory, problem solving • Indecisiveness • Thoughts of death or suicide, with suicidal behavior in severe cases

- Trauma, death of a loved one, relationship difficulties, or any stressful event or situation can trigger a depressive episode, resulting in some of the biological and neurochemical changes described.
- Genetic risk factors also play a role in depressive reactions in the context of environmental and other factors.
- *Demographic Features:*
  - *Women:*
    - Depression is more common among women than men.
    - Biological, lifecycle, hormonal, and psychosocial factors are all thought to be linked to the higher depression rate in women.
    - As women age, the transition into menopause has been shown to increase the risk for depression.
    - Women with depression tend to present with feelings of sadness, worthlessness, and excessive guilt.
    - More women attempt suicide, but more men die from suicide.
  - *Men:*
    - Men tend to present with complaints of feeling very tired, irritable, lost interest in activities, and sleep disturbance.
    - Men are more likely than women to abuse alcohol or other substances when depressed.
    - Behaviorally, men often become more frustrated, discouraged, irritable, and angry, and often increase work activities while avoiding family and friends.
  - *Elderly:*
    - Contrary to common beliefs, depression is not a normal part of the aging process. Most elderly report being very satisfied with their lives, even in the context of medical illnesses or physical limitations.
    - Depressive signs and symptoms in the elderly are often overlooked:
      - They are less likely to endorse specific feelings of sadness or grief, and instead tend to report more physical manifestations of depression.
      - It is difficult to distinguish depression from normal grief and bereavement over the loss of a loved one.

- Older adults may have medical conditions that result in depressive symptoms (e.g., low testosterone, vitamin B_{12} deficiency, thyroid abnormalities, cardiac conditions, various dementias, cerebrovascular disease).

- Medication side effects may present as, or contribute to, depression.

  o Elderly patients with depression, particularly males, have the highest rate of completed suicide in the United States. Many of these patients had been seen by their physicians within 1 month of their deaths. Elderly individuals with severe depression, prior history of suicide attempts, and poor social support are most likely to have suicidal ideation and should be targeted for urgent interventions.

- *Children and Adolescents:*

  o Children who develop depression often continue to have episodes throughout adulthood and are more likely to have other more severe medical and psychiatric illnesses in adulthood.

  o Young children tend to report physical illness, avoid school and other activities, become overly attached to a parent, or express worry that a parent or family member may die.

  o Older children and adolescents tend to sulk, develop behavioral problems at school, become more negative and irritable, and feel misunderstood or unappreciated.

  o Many of the signs and symptoms are overlooked as being mood and personality changes associated with normal development.

  o Depression in adolescence frequently co-occurs with other disorders such as anxiety disorders, eating disorders, and substance abuse, as well as increased risk of suicide.

Bipolar Disorder

Bipolar disorder is a lifelong disorder with symptoms varying across the full continuum of mood from severely depressed to extremely elated or manic states. In addition to the depression signs and symptoms just described, patients with bipolar disorder also have signs and symptoms of mania (Table 34.4).

- Depressive and manic cycles vary in terms of the type, duration, and intensity of these specific symptoms. Between episodes, many patients are free of obvious symptoms, but some have lingering, albeit milder, symptoms.

- At times, a mood episode may include symptoms of both depression and mania referred to as a "mixed state.

TABLE 34.4 Signs and Symptoms of Mania

Mood Symptoms	• Long period of elevated mood • Extended feelings of happiness, excitement, and being "high" • Extreme irritability, agitation, hypervigilance, tension
Behavioral Symptoms	• Rapid, pressured speech • Tangential or circumstantial thought processes with flight of ideas • High distractibility • Restlessness and psychomotor agitation • Limited need for sleep • Unrealistic/grandiose belief in one's abilities • Impulsive, pleasure-seeking behaviors without regard for consequences such as spending sprees, sexual behavior, financial investments, etc.

- Psychotic symptoms, including delusions and hallucinations, can develop in the context of severe bipolar disorder. The presenting psychotic symptoms typically reflect the person's extreme mood. Patients with bipolar disorder that includes psychotic features are often misdiagnosed as having schizophrenia or schizoaffective disorder.

- Some patients are diagnosed with rapid-cycling bipolar disorder. This is diagnosed when a person has four or more episodes of major depression, mania, *hypomania*, or mixed symptoms within a 1-year period. Patients can experience one or more episodes over the course of a month, week, or even a day. Rapid cycling is more common in patients with a severe form of bipolar disorder or in those who have their first episode at a younger age.

- Patients with bipolar disorder are at higher risk for thyroid disease, migraine headaches, heart disease, diabetes, obesity, and other physical illnesses:

  - These physical illnesses may cause symptoms of depression or mania.

  - Treatment of bipolar disorder can lead to the development of some of these physical illnesses as well (e.g., lithium treatment has a negative impact on thyroid function).

Section 2: Anxiety Disorders

Definition

Anxiety is defined as a state of apprehension, uncertainty, and fear resulting from the anticipation of a realistic or fantasized threatening event or situation, often impairing physical and psychological functioning. Anxiety is experienced as a part of everyday life and can be viewed along a continuum. At one end of the scale, mild anxiety improves motivation and productivity. At the other end, intense anxiety promotes survival in response to danger through a *"fight or flight" response*. When occurring at inappropriate times, or when the anxiety becomes excessive or interferes with normal life functions, it may fall under the classification of an anxiety disorder. Common signs and symptoms of anxiety include muscle tension, heart palpitations, tremors, restlessness, sweating, being easily fatigued, gastrointestinal discomfort, headaches, dizziness, shortness of breath, sleep disturbance, irritability, and cognitive complaints (Table 34.6). In the recent revision of the American Psychiatric Association DSM-5, several new disorders were added to the anxiety disorders section, and these are included in Table 34.5. Additionally, posttraumatic stress disorder (PTSD) and obsessive-compulsive disorder (OCD) were removed from the anxiety disorder category and placed in new categories specific to these disorders. Given the fact that anxiety is typically associated with these disorders, PTSD and OCD are included in the current section of the chapter for completeness, but are addressed separately in terms of disorder characteristics and related information.

Obsessive-Compulsive Disorder (OCD)

No longer included with anxiety disorders in the DSM-5, OCD is now a section in its own right. Diagnoses included in this new section of the DSM-5 include OCD, body dysmorphic disorder, hoarding disorder, trichotillomania, excoriation disorder, and other secondary or unspecified variants (Table 34.6).

Trauma- and Stressor-Related Disorders

This reflects a new disorder classification section of the DSM-5 that includes PTSD and acute stress disorder, but is expanded to include other disorders as well. Trauma- and stressor-related disorders involve exposure to a traumatic or stressful event resulting in anxiety and other psychological, behavioral, and cognitive changes. These disorders were previously considered anxiety disorders, but they are now viewed as being distinct due to the fact that many individuals with these disorders have symptoms of anhedonia

TABLE 34.5 Clinically Recognized Anxiety Disorders in the DSM-5

Separation Anxiety Disorder	Characterized by persistent and excessive anxiety beyond that expected for a child's developmental level related to separation or impending separation from an attachment figure (e.g., primary caretaker, close family member). Occurs in youth younger than 18 years (persistent and lasting for at least 4 weeks) and in adults (typically requiring a duration of 6 months or more). Separation anxiety disorder can also be associated with panic attacks that can occur with comorbid panic disorder.
Selective Mutism	Characterized by consistent failure to speak in specific social situations (in which there is an expectation for speaking, e.g., at school) despite speaking in other situations.
Specific Phobia	Characterized by avoidance behavior mediated by fear and capable of interfering in a significant way with the normal activities of an individual.
Social Anxiety Disorder	Characterized by persistent fear of one or more social or performance situations in which the person is exposed to unfamiliar people or to possible scrutiny by others. The individual fears that they will act in a way (or show anxiety symptoms) that will be embarrassing and humiliating.
Agoraphobia	Characterized by a disproportionate fear of public places, often perceiving such environments as too open, crowded or dangerous.
Panic Disorder	Characterized by experience of recurring, unexpected panic attacks in a person's lifetime. Panic attacks are characterized by an abrupt surge of intense fear or physical discomfort, reaching a peak within a few minutes, including a number of physical and anxious symptoms.
Generalized Anxiety Disorder	Characterized by chronic feelings of excessive worry and tension that is unfounded or much more severe than the normal anxiety most people experience given the circumstances.

TABLE 34.6 Clinically Recognized Obsessive-Compulsive Disorders in the DSM-5

Obsessive-Compulsive Disorder (OCD)	Characterized by recurrent, persistent, unwanted, and intrusive thoughts, urges, or images (obsessions) and/or by repetitive behaviors or mental acts that patients feel driven to do (compulsions) to try to lessen or prevent the anxiety that obsessions cause.
Body Dysmorphic Disorder	Characterized by preoccupation with one or more perceived defects in physical appearance that are not apparent, or only minimally apparent to other people. The preoccupation causes clinically significant distress or impairment in social, occupational, academic, or other aspects of functioning. At some point during the course of the disorder, patients must repetitively and excessively perform one or more repetitive behaviors such as mirror checking, comparing their appearance with that of other people, weighing themselves, or other activities) in response to the preoccupation with appearance.
Hoarding Disorder	Characterized by persistent difficulty discarding or parting with possessions, regardless of their actual value, resulting in the accumulation of possessions that congest and clutter living areas to the point that the intended use of the areas is significantly compromised
Trichotillomania	Characterized by repeated urges to pull out scalp hair, eyelashes, eyebrows, or other body hair. This may occur with or without awareness.
Excoriation Disorder	Characterized by recurrent picking of one's skin resulting in skin lesions. This may include picking or scratching for cosmetic or noncosmetic reasons, including picking at healthy skin. This may occur with or without awareness.

TABLE 34.7 Clinically Recognized Trauma- and Stressor-Related Disorders in the DSM-5

Posttraumatic Stress Disorder (PTSD)	PTSD is characterized by anxiety, tension, and fear that develops after exposure to a terrifying event or ordeal in which grave physical harm occurred or was threatened. Symptoms must be present for greater than 1 month and characterized by experiencing the event, avoidance of reminders of the event, and hypervigilance in response to anxiety-provoking stimuli.
Acute Stress Disorder	Similar to post traumatic stress disorder, in that in both cases, the victim experiences a traumatic event involving death or a threat of death or serious physical injury to themselves or to others. In acute stress disorder, duration varies from just a few days to about one month. Acute stress disorder may also include dissociative symptoms such as dissociative amnesia, dissociative fugue, depersonalization, and derealization.
Reactive Attachment Disorder	Characterized by a consistent pattern in children of inhibited, emotionally withdrawn behavior toward adult caregivers, manifested by the child rarely or minimally seeking comfort when distressed and rarely or minimally responding to comfort when distressed. This also includes persistent social or emotional disturbance, and patterns of extremes of insufficient care.
Disinhibited Social Engagement Disorder	Characterized by a pattern of behavior in which a child actively approaches and interacts with unfamiliar adults including reduced or absent reticence in approaching and interacting with unfamiliar adults, overly familiar verbal or physical behavior, diminished or absent checking back with adult caregiver after venturing away, and/or a willingness to go off with an unfamiliar adult with little or no hesitation
Adjustment Disorders	Characterized by markedly distressing and impairing emotional and/or behavioral symptoms caused by an identifiable stressor. In contrast to normal reactions to stressful events, reactions in adjustment disorders are more intense than what would typically be expected or when the person's ability to function is significantly impaired.

or dysphoria, anger, aggression, or dissociation that are more prominent than specific anxiety-based symptoms. In addition to PTSD and acute stress disorder, additional diagnoses in this new DSM-5 category include reactive attachment disorder, disinhibited social engagement disorder, adjustment disorders, and unspecified trauma- and stressor-related disorder (Table 34.7)

Neuropathology

Neuroanatomical Factors

There is heterogeneity in the phenotypic presentation of anxiety disorders, yet structural and functional imaging studies suggest that the cingulate gyrus, prefrontal cortex, and anterior temporal cortices are involved in most anxiety disorders. Anxiety does not appear to depend on specific areas performing unique functions but should instead be viewed as networks of interacting brain regions.

- Although the neural networks are very complex, limbic structures have specific roles and relationships in the anxiety process:
  - The amygdala is one of the most consistently identified regions of hyperactivity in anxiety. The central nucleus of the amygdala senses and identifies fear and anxiety-laden stimuli and initiates the emotional response.
  - The hypothalamus, pituitary, and adrenal gland respond to heighten sympathetic responses to the stressful stimuli.

- The cingulate and orbitofrontal cortex are responsible for feelings associated with the anxiety.
  - The interconnected frontal cortex is responsible for control of the reactions to anxiety-producing stimuli.
- The insular cortex shows hyperactivity in anxiety disorders such as post-traumatic stress disorder (PTSD), social anxiety disorder, and specific phobias:
  - The insula has been proposed, in combination with the amygdala, hypothalamus, periaqueductal gray, parabrachial nucleus, and nucleus tractus solitarius, as part of the *circuit of Papez*, to be part of an internal regulation system that controls the visceromotor, neuroendocrine, and pulmonary system, as well as pain sensations.
  - It is activated by negative emotions, regulates the autonomic nervous system activity, and has been implicated in the recognition and experience of disgust, sadness, and fear.
- These neural networks in combination create two primary responses:
  - A "defense system" making immediate responses to threatening stimuli.
  - A behavioral inhibition system responsible for the suppression of behaviors that could enhance danger.
- These circuits are under modulatory influence of several other systems such as serotonergic, noradrenergic, and dopaminergic inputs from the raphe nuclei, locus coeruleus, and ventral tegmental area.

Obsessive-Compulsive Disorder (OCD)

In OCD, a specific neural network is implicated with abnormally increased activity in the basal ganglia (especially the head of the caudate), as well as in the anterior cingulate gyrus and orbitofrontal cortex. Given the involvement of these structures, some have compared it to a hyperkinetic movement disorder, but with unwanted thoughts or compulsions instead of movements.

- Overlap is noted in other neurological conditions:
  - Obsessive-compulsive disorder is present in about 50% of patients with Tourette syndrome.
  - Trichotillomania has been associated with increased gray matter densities in the left striatum, left amygdalo-hippocampal formation, and multiple cortical regions bilaterally.
  - Obsessive-compulsive tendencies are also associated with Huntington's disease, Sydenham's chorea, and other disorders involving the basal ganglia.

Posttraumatic Stress Disorder (PTSD)

Three general areas of brain dysfunction have been described in PTSD, including the prefrontal cortex, amygdala, and hippocampus. The amygdala has been shown to be strongly involved in the formation of emotional memories, especially fear-related memories. The amygdalocentric model proposes that PTSD is associated with hyperarousal of the amygdala and insufficient top-down control by the medial prefrontal cortex and the hippocampus, particularly during extinction. Decreased activation of Broca's area has been associated with the difficulty patients have in labeling their experiences.

Neurochemical Factors

The neurochemical factors associated with anxiety disorders are similar to those noted in the "Mood Disorders" section, including the monoamine neurotransmitters serotonin, norepinephrine, and, to a lesser extent, dopamine. Changes in GABA levels are also associated with anxiety. Research regarding the neurochemical basis of anxiety has been challenging, with initial research being driven by the chance discovery of drugs with anxiety-reducing properties. As a result, the just-named neurotransmitters have dominated the field, based on evidence that effective anxiolytics interact with these systems.

GABA

Gamma-aminobutyric acid is the major inhibitory neurotransmitter in the central nervous system (CNS), playing a role in helping to induce relaxation and sleep, and in preventing overexcitation. Depletion of GABA results in a reduction in the normal inhibitory regulation of emotion and the sympathetic nervous system, thus heightening the anxious response.

Serotonin

Although serotonin has been implicated in anxiety disorders via its role in the regulation of appetite, energy, sleep, mood, libido, and cognitive functioning, identification of the precise relationship of the serotonin system to anxiety disorders has been difficult.

In anxiety disorders, decreased activity of serotonin is felt to limit the inhibition of stress responses, increasing the susceptibility to panic states. More recent research suggests that abnormalities in the serotonin system are just one part of the complex brain chemistry involved in anxiety disorders and are not a primary cause.

Norepinephrine

Norepinephrine is an excitatory neurotransmitter and also a stress hormone. It helps maintain alertness and preparation to respond to external threats, such as the *"fight or flight" response.* Stressful events, including emotional stress, cause a marked increase in norepinephrine release in several brain regions, especially the hypothalamus, amygdala, and locus coeruleus.

- Increased activity in the norepinephrine systems produces physical symptoms of anxiety, such as blushing, sweating, and palpitations.
- Norepinephrine has also been linked to the production of flashbacks in people with PTSD.

Corticotropin-Releasing Hormone (CRH)

Similar to norepinephrine, CRH acts as both a stress hormone and a neurotransmitter. Increased secretion of CRH helps the body mobilize energy for the *"fight or flight" response,* and increased CRH secretion levels have been found in individuals with anxiety disorders.

Epidemiology

Incidence and prevalence rates for anxiety disorders are somewhat variable by disorder classification (Table 34.8). For more details and more updated information over time, please refer to the websites listed in recommended readings.

Presentation and Disease Course

Generalized Anxiety Disorder (GAD)

- Individuals with GAD experience excessive anxiety and worry (apprehensive expectation), throughout the day even though there is little or no reason for it or the response is beyond what would be expected or warranted.
- Symptoms must be present for at least 6 months to meet criteria for the disorder.
- When symptoms are mild, individuals with GAD can function socially, maintain work activities, and complete daily life activities in an appropriate manner. When severe, these individuals have difficulty completing even basic daily activities because they become overwhelmed by their anxious symptoms.

TABLE 34.8 Prevalence and Incidence Rates of Common Anxiety Disorders

	Adults	Children And Adolescents
All Anxiety Disorders Combined	• Affects about 19 million adult Americans. • Lifetime prevalence 31.1% • 12-month prevalence 19.1% • Of those with anxiety disorder, the prevalence of "serious" impairment is 22.8%. A majority experienced "mild" impairment (43.5%) • Prevalence is higher for females (23.4%) than males (14.3%) • Prevalence is 21–23% for ages 18–59, with a prevalence of 9% for those 60+ • African Americans are 20% less likely • Latin/x are 30% less likely	• Anxiety disorders are the most common form of psychopathology in children • Lifetime prevalence in adolescents is 31.9% • Of adolescents with any anxiety disorder, an estimated 8.3% had severe impairment • The prevalence of anxiety disorder among adolescents was higher for females (38%) than for males (26%) • No significant differences in prevalence across adolescent age groups (31–32%)

Generalized Anxiety Disorder	• Affects about 6.8 million adult Americans.
	• Lifetime prevalence 5.7%
	• 12-month prevalence 2.7%
	• Prevalence is higher for females (3.4%) than males (1.9%)
	• Prevalence by age:
	  ▪ 18–29 years old 2.0%
	  ▪ 30–44 years old 3.5%
	  ▪ 45–59 years old 3.4%
	  ▪ 60+ years old 1.5%
	• Impairment is distributed evenly among adults with GAD with 32.3% with serious impairment
	• Average age of onset is 31 years old
		• Less likely in children than adults
		• Lifetime prevalence of 2.2% with 0.9% experiencing severe impairment
		• Prevalence rate was higher for girls (3.0%) than males (1.5%)
		• Prevalence increases with age:
		  ▪ 13–14 years old 1.0%
		  ▪ 15–16 years old 2.8%
		  ▪ 17–18 years old 3.0%

Obsessive-Compulsive Disorder	• Affects about 2 million adult Americans • Lifetime prevalence 2.3% • 12-month prevalence 1.2% • Among adults with OCD, approximately one half (50.6%) had had serious impairment • Prevalence of OCD is higher for females (1.8%) than for males (0.5%) • Prevalence is 1.1–1.5% for ages 18–59, with a prevalence of 0.5% for those 60+ • Average age of onset is 19 years old • 1/3 of adults report having first symptoms as children.	• Affects about 1 million children and adolescents • Twice as many boys than girls. • Average onset in children is 10 years old • 20% of children and adolescents with OCD also have another family member with OCD

Panic Disorder	• Affects about 6 million adult Americans
	• Lifetime prevalence 4.7%
	• 12-month prevalence 2.7%
	• Prevalence is higher for females (3.8%) than males (1.6%)
	• Prevalence by age:
	  ▪ 18–29 years old 2.8%
	  ▪ 30–44 years old 3.7%
	  ▪ 45–59 years old 3.1%
	  ▪ 60+ years old 0.8%
	• Serious impairment is noted in 44.8% of individuals with Panic Disorder
	• *Panic attacks* typically develop in late adolescence to early adulthood
	• Average age of onset is 24 years old
		• Lifetime prevalence for United States adolescent population is 2.3%
		• Prevalence rates slightly higher for girls (2.6%) than boys (2.0%)
		• Prevalence increases with age:
		  ▪ 13–14 years old 1.8%
		  ▪ 15–16 years old 2.3%
		  ▪ 17–18 years old 3.3%

(continued)

TABLE 34.8 Continued

	Adults	Children And Adolescents

Post traumatic Stress Disorder	• Affects about 7.7 million adult Americans
	• Lifetime prevalence 6.8%
	• 12-month prevalence 3.6%
	• Prevalence of PTSD is higher for females (8.0%) than for males (2.3%)
	• Prevalence by age:
	  ▪ 18–29 years old 4.0%
	  ▪ 30–44 years old 3.5%
	  ▪ 45–59 years old 5.3%
	  ▪ 60+ years old 1.0%
	• Impairment is distributed evenly among adults with PTSD; 36.6% with serious impairment
		• Percent of United States population for ages 13–18 years is 5.0%, and an estimated 1.5% had severe impairment
		• Prevalence rates higher for girls (8.0%) than boys (2.3%)
		• Prevalence increases with age:
		  ▪ 13–14 years old 3.7%
		  ▪ 15–16 years old 5.1%
		  ▪ 17–18 years old 7.0%

MOOD DISORDERS

Panic Disorder

• Panic disorder is characterized by sudden attacks of fear or panic, accompanied by multiple physical symptoms including heart palpitations, chest pain, nausea, sweating, shakiness, weakness, fainting, flushing or chills, or other symptoms. Symptoms vary widely across individuals and may even be variable from event to event in the same person.

• *Panic attacks* usually produce a sense of unreality, a fear of impending doom, or fear of losing control. During panic attacks, people often feel that they have a severe medical problem (e.g., heart attack) and may seek acute medical treatment. Events typically peak within 10 minutes, but symptoms may last much longer.

• Without treatment, people with panic disorder develop a pattern of increasing frequency and intensity, ultimately becoming severely impaired in their ability to maintain daily social and functional activities. In very severe cases, *agoraphobia*, or fear of open spaces or leaving home, can develop.

Obsessive-Compulsive Disorder

• Obsessive-compulsive disorder is characterized by persistent, upsetting thoughts (obsessions) and rituals (compulsions) that are maladaptive coping behaviors to manage anxiety, but symptoms are extremely variable across individuals with OCD.

• Common rituals include repetitive hand washing, avoiding contact with public objects (e.g., doorknobs), or other behaviors to avoid germs.

• Performance of these behaviors is not pleasurable and can be an additional source of anxiety. At best, these behaviors provide a temporary relief from the anxiety created by obsessive thoughts.

• Healthy individuals may have rituals at times but not to the point that it interferes with daily life.

• Most adults with OCD recognize that what they are doing is irrational, but some adults and most children do not believe their behaviors are abnormal.

651

- People with OCD will attempt to avoid situations that trigger their obsessions and compulsive behaviors, or they may use alcohol or other substances to minimize symptoms. Both of these behaviors can worsen the overall severity of the illness.

Posttraumatic Stress Disorder

- Posttraumatic stress disorder develops after a traumatic event that involved physical harm, the potential for physical harm, or being a witness or involved in a situation in which others were harmed. It can result from a variety of traumatic events including war, robbery, rape, assault, torture, kidnapping, child abuse, accidents, or natural disasters.
- People with PTSD present with multiple symptoms characterized by reexperiencing the traumatic event, avoidance of places or situations that remind them of the event, and hyperarousal in response to related stimuli.
- During a flashback or reexperience of the event, the person may lose touch with reality and believe that the traumatic event is happening again.
- Symptoms of PTSD tend to be worse if the event triggering them was a deliberate act initiated by another person.
- Symptoms typically begin within 3 months of the traumatic event, but occasionally emerge years later.
- Course of the illness is variable, with some recovering within 6 months, whereas others have symptoms for years. In some individuals, the disorder becomes chronic, with only limited benefit noted from treatment.

Social Phobia Disorder

- Social phobia (social anxiety disorder) is diagnosed when people become overwhelmingly anxious and/or excessively self-conscious in everyday social situations. Individuals experience an intense, persistent, and chronic fear of being watched and judged by others or of doing things that will embarrass them. Affected individuals are aware that the fears and anxiety are unreasonable or excessive.
- Physical symptoms are often present, including blushing, profuse sweating, trembling, nausea, and difficulty speaking.
- When able to participate in a social activity, these individuals experience anticipatory anxiety beforehand, are intensely uncomfortable during the event, and ruminate about how they were perceived or judged afterward for extended periods of time (hours to days).
- Presentation of symptoms is variable across individuals with the disorder:
  - Limited to a specific type of situation (e.g., public speaking).
  - Limited to settings outside of their immediate family.
  - May cross multiple settings, situations, and social groups.

Specific Phobia Disorder

- Intense or irrational fear of a specific object, person, place, or situation that actually poses little or no threat. Some of the most common specific phobias include fear of heights, elevators, tunnels, escalators, driving, closed-in spaces, water, flying, dogs, spiders, and bleeding (self or others).

- At times, the fears are inconsistent with a person's behaviors—a person may be able to rappel down a high cliff, but be unable to go in an elevator in a high-rise building.

- If a person is able to avoid the source of their fear(s), there is typically no effort made to obtain treatment for the condition.

Comorbid Conditions

- Mood and anxiety disorders often accompany each other with one or the other serving as the primary diagnosis. People with PTSD are particularly vulnerable to comorbid depression. Alcohol and other substance abuse is commonly present in patients with depressive and anxious disorders, undertaken as a means of self-medication, but ultimately worsening the symptom presentation.

- Depression and anxiety are often associated with serious medical conditions. People who have comorbid medical conditions and depression/anxiety tend to have more severe symptoms of both conditions. Treating the mental disorder has been shown to improve the outcome of treatments involving the co-occurring medical condition.

Section 3: Mood and Anxiety Disorders: Severity, Assessment and Treatment

Determinants of Severity

In addition to the specific symptoms associated with each disorder classification, the *Diagnostic and Statistical Manual of Mental Disorders, Fifth Edition* (DSM-5) specifies that the symptoms and severity of the disorder must represent a change from previous functioning and cause clinically significant distress or impairment in social, occupational, or other important areas of functioning. As such, severity level is determined by the level of impairment in daily life functions. The identification, assessment, and treatment of mood and anxiety disorders are complicated by variability noted across the type, duration, and severity of symptoms, even when the specific disorder has been identified. Additionally, the extent of treatment does not provide a good indication of severity. Symptoms can range from normal reactions to daily life stressors to more pathological and persistent symptoms. Patients typically seek treatment only when they are actively experiencing symptoms at a level causing significant distress. As a result, regular assessment is required to monitor the severity of symptoms and the effectiveness of treatment(s).

Assessment Methods

A large number of biomarkers are being considered that have the potential to guide the diagnosis and treatment of depression and anxiety. In addition to neurotransmitter and neuroendocrine markers which have been subject to widespread study for many decades, recent studies exploring inflammatory response, the immune system, metabolic and growth factors, and other factors are being studied in terms of their role in depression. However, no consensus has been established in the research, and there are a number of challenges that need to be addressed before biomarker research can be applied to improve the management of depression and anxiety. Thus far, mood and anxiety disorders cannot be identified through typical medical evaluations such as blood tests or neuroimaging studies, but these tests are used to rule out other causal or contributing medical factors. If no medical abnormalities are identified, these individuals are typically referred to mental health professionals for a complete diagnostic evaluation. Any evaluation of mood or anxiety disorders should include a number of methods:

- Comprehensive diagnostic interview
- Review of family history for the suspected disorder or other mental illness.
- Collateral information from relatives or others.
- Psychological assessment techniques (see also Chapter 10, Personality Assessment and Self-Report Instruments).
  - Brief self-report measures of depression and anxiety (e.g., Beck Depression Inventory II, Geriatric Depression Scale, PHQ-9, etc.).
  - Objective measures of emotional functioning, personality, and psychopathology (e.g., Minnesota Multiphasic Personality Inventory-2 RF).
- Regular assessment during the course of treatment via interview, observation, and objective testing to monitor symptom presentation and the effectiveness of treatment(s) and to determine outcomes.

Expectations for Neuropsychological Assessment Results

No definitive pattern of neuropsychological deficits is viewed as diagnostic for mood and anxiety disorders. There are, however, definite trends in terms of neuropsychological performance. Many of these trends reflect qualitative or style of performance factors as much as quantitative differences. The most consistent neurocognitive findings in mood and anxiety disorders include deficits in attention, working memory, executive functions, and retrieval-based memory (with sparing of recognition memory). Increased cognitive dysfunction is associated with greater symptom severity. However, residual persisting cognitive deficits have been found in a subset of some euthymic and recovered depressive patients.

- *Intelligence* Patients with mood and anxiety disorders do not exhibit reductions in intellectual or achievement scores. When declines are noted, they typically relate to lowered scores on specific subtests/subscales associated with sustained attention and working memory, task persistence, and speeded performance.
- *Attention/Concentration* In the acute phase of their illness patients with depressive disorders often exhibit inefficiencies in sustained attention, working memory, processing efficiency, and overall speed of performance. The level of impairment in these areas is strongly related to the severity of the illness. Milder difficulties in sustained attention and concentration may persist during nonsymptomatic periods.
- *Processing Speed* Patients with depression tend to lack a sense of urgency on tasks requiring speeded performance and exhibit diminished reaction times. This is not to say that their ability to perform quickly is impaired, but instead this often reflects limitations in motivation, engagement, and persistence. Anxious patients may demonstrate this same pattern, but, in some cases, they attempt to overperform, resulting in impulsive and error-prone performance in conjunction with attempts to complete tasks in rapid fashion.
- *Language* Expressive and receptive language deficits are not associated with mood and anxiety disorders. In severe depression or anxiety, patients may lack the initiative to interact (depressive) or appear "paralyzed" by their fear (anxious), but this does not reflect an underlying language disturbance.

- *Visuospatial Abilities* There is evidence to suggest that right-hemisphere dysfunction is associated with bipolar illness and OCD, with greater impairments seen in visuospatial functioning. This is also seen in the organization and structure of reproduction and memory of complex figures such as the Rey Complex Figure Test. Unipolar depression and other anxiety disorders do not demonstrate this pattern of performance.

- *Memory* Memory and learning functions can be impaired in patients with depression or anxiety, but the pattern of deficits is notably stereotypic. Patients with both disorders typically show difficulties in the acquisition of new material, with limited benefit noted from repeated presentations. Delayed recall is marked by deficits in retrieval (spontaneous recall), with relative sparing in recognition memory. Although patients with depression tend to provide limited responses on spontaneous recall tasks, patients with anxiety will often exhibit poor consolidation and organization of the new material with multiple perseverative or intrusive errors. Memory deficits are not as apparent when information is presented in a structured format. As the presentation structure is disrupted, however, memory inefficiencies increase. This is noted in better performance on narrative recall tasks in the context of poor performance on the learning and spontaneous recall of an unrelated word list. Visual memory deficits are variable depending on the tasks used but, in general, are lower for patients with bipolar or OCD, whereas relative sparing is noted in other mood and anxiety disorders. It is important to note that the memory inefficiencies associated with mood and anxiety disorders are less consistent and are typically not at the severity level observed in neurologic conditions.

- *Executive Functions* Executive functioning, including planning, abstract concept formation, set shifting, and higher-level problem solving may be compromised in symptomatic patients, but are typically normal in fully recovered patients.

- *Sensorimotor Functions* Sensory deficits are uncommon. Patients with depression have been shown to demonstrate deficits on speeded motor tasks (e.g., tapping) and on skills requiring sustained effort (e.g., pegboard), but in general, motor functions are spared.

- *Emotion and Personality* Emotional and personality difficulties are inherent in these disorders. This has been addressed in detail in previous sections.

- *Performance and Symptom Validity* Failure on free-standing tests of effort and engagement is not expected. However, patients with mood and anxiety disorders may underperform relative to actual ability levels, with disengagement noted on lengthy measures and/or on tasks that are perceived to be difficult or challenging. This is not necessarily a reflection of cognitive symptom exaggeration, but instead may reflect limited motivation and persistence, or a lack of urgency on timed tasks.

Treatment

Early intervention has been shown to improve outcomes in the treatment of all mood and anxiety disorders. The most common treatment options for mood and anxiety disorders include medications, psychotherapy, and combination treatment, with the latter typically shown to be the most effective intervention for most of the disorders.

Major Depression and Dysthymia

- *Medications*
    - Psychotropic medications can take up to 4 to 5 weeks before they are fully effective. In recent years, the FDA approved three new antidepressants; vilazodone (Viibryd),

levomilnacipran (Fetzima), and vortioxetine (Trintellix and Brintellix), that have shown some promise for more rapid effectiveness and increased tolerability. One of the biggest developments in depression treatment has been the use of augmenting agents, such as atypical antipsychotics (e.g., Abilify), as a common strategy in depression management. Antidepressant medications primarily target the neurotransmitters serotonin and norepinephrine. Other antidepressants target dopamine.

- Selective serotonin reuptake inhibitors (SSRIs):
  - Examples: fluoxetine (Prozac), sertraline (Zoloft), vilazodone (Viibryd), vortioxetine (Trintellix and Brintellix)
- Serotonin and norepinephrine reuptake inhibitors (SNRIs):
  - Examples: venlafaxine (Effexor), duloxetine (Cymbalta), desvenlafaxine (Pristiq), levomilnacipran (Fetzima)
- Norepinephrine-dopamine reuptake inhibitors:
  - Have some mild psychostimulant effects.
  - Increases a person's risk of seizures.
  - Example: bupropion (Wellbutrin).
- Tricyclics (older class of antidepressants):
  - Used less frequently due to more serious side-effect profile.
  - Examples: imipramine, nortriptyline.
- Monoamine oxidase inhibitors (MAOIs; oldest class of antidepressants):
  - Used less frequently, but can be particularly effective in cases of atypical depression and depression accompanied by anxiety and panic symptoms.
  - Should not be combined with SSRIs due to risk of developing serotonin syndrome.
  - Examples: isocarboxazid (Marplan), phenelzine (Nardil).
- N-methyl-D-aspartate (NMDA) receptor antagonists:
  - May reflect a new line of treatments in the management of depression, but research in this area is limited.
  - Memantine (Namenda) has been considered in this regard.
  - Recent studies have explored the use of ketamine in treating treatment-resistant depression and acute suicidal ideation. Ketamine has a long history in analgesia and anesthesiology, and its use for acute depression is relatively new.

- *Psychotherapy*
  - Psychotherapy has been shown to be effective in reducing depressive signs and symptoms and increasing overall level of functioning. For mild to moderate depression, psychotherapy has been shown to be the best option. For more severe depression, a combination of medication and psychotherapy is most effective.
  - Two main types of psychotherapy are used in the treatment of depression: cognitive-behavioral therapy (CBT) and interpersonal therapy (IPT).

- *Electroconvulsive therapy and other brain stimulation techniques*
  - Electroconvulsive therapy (ECT) is typically used in moderate to severe cases in which medications and psychotherapy were not effective in relieving symptoms. In recent years,

ECT has regained acceptance and increased use because it has been shown to provide relief for patients with severe depression that has been nonresponsive to medication management. It has been associated with temporary side effects including confusion, disorientation, and memory loss, but with newer approaches to ECT, these have been reduced and research has shown fewer adverse cognitive effects one-year post treatment.

- Vagal nerve stimulation (VNS) and repetitive transcranial magnetic stimulation (rTMS) are newer treatment methods that are increasing in terms of use. Research shows some promise, but more studies need to be completed.

Bipolar Disorder

It is important to note that there is no cure for bipolar disorder, but appropriate treatment results in better control of the cycling moods and related symptoms for most patients regardless of the severity of illness. Combination therapy is the most effective approach to symptom management, but treatment must be maintained on a continuous basis to appropriately manage bipolar disorder. Patients with bipolar disorders respond to medications differently. As such, patients with this disorder require regular monitoring and medication adjustments to maintain mood stability.

- *Mood stabilizing medications*
  - Mood stabilizing medications are the initial treatment for bipolar disorder and are typically maintained for many years.
  - Aside from lithium (Eskalith, Lithobid), most of these medications are anticonvulsants:
    - Lithium has multiple side effects requiring regular monitoring of blood levels to avoid toxicity.
    - Valproic acid or divalproex (Depakote) is a common alternative to lithium in terms of safety and side-effect profile but is not recommended for females due to the side effects associated with increased levels of testosterone.
    - Other anticonvulsant medications are used less frequently including lamotrigine (Lamictal), gabapentin (Neurontin), topiramate (Topamax), carbamazepine (Tegretol), and oxcarbazepine (Trileptal).
- *Atypical antipsychotic medications*
  - These medications are often used to treat symptoms of bipolar disorder in both acute settings for severe manic episodes or for more chronic symptom management. They are typically used in combination with an antidepressant medication to manage symptoms of severe mania or psychosis and are available in an injectable form to quickly manage agitation associated with a manic or mixed episode.
  - Examples: olanzapine (Zyprexa), aripiprazole (Abilify).
- *Antidepressant medications* (*see "Mood Disorders" section for details*)
  - Antidepressant medications are sometimes used to treat the depressive symptoms in bipolar disorder in combination with other mood stabilizers.
  - Antidepressants alone can increase the risk of mania, *hypomania*, or more rapid cycling.
- *Psychotherapy*
  - As with the other depressive disorders, psychotherapy has been shown to be an effective treatment for bipolar disorder. This is also useful in the provision of support, education, and guidance to patients and families to increase understanding and insight regarding the illness.

- *Electroconvulsive therapy and other brain stimulation techniques*
  - As described in the depressive disorders section, ECT, VNS, and rTMS are also used to manage symptoms of bipolar disorder.

Anxiety Disorders

As with mood disorders, anxiety disorders are typically treated with medications, psychotherapy, and/or a combination of the two. Combination therapy has been found to be the most effective approach. Early intervention is crucial in treating any anxiety disorder but is often delayed due to the search for medically based etiologies prior to correct diagnosis. Any comorbid conditions, such as depression or substance abuse, are considered in the identification of the most appropriate mode of treatment.

Medications do not cure anxiety disorders, but instead help manage the symptoms and severity while the person receives psychotherapy. These typically include antidepressants, antianxiety medications, and beta-blockers.

- *Antidepressant medications*
  - Selective serotonin reuptake inhibitors are the most commonly prescribed antidepressants in anxiety disorder (see previous discussions for medication details).
  - Tricyclics are used occasionally, but typically not for OCD.
  - Monoamine oxidase inhibitors may be used with close monitoring, which is required to minimize risk for *serotonin syndrome.*
- *Benzodiazepines*
  - High-potency benzodiazepines are effective for the management of anxiety with few side effects aside from drowsiness. However, patients tend to develop a tolerance for these medications and require higher doses over time to maintain benefit.
  - These are typically prescribed for short periods of time, and withdrawal symptoms can develop if they are stopped abruptly.
  - These medications are commonly associated with cognitive slowing and memory loss if chronically used or abused.
  - Examples: lorazepam (Ativan), alprazolam (Xanax), diazepam (Valium)
- *Beta-blockers*
  - Beta-blockers are used to treat heart conditions, but are effective in managing the physical symptoms that accompany certain anxiety disorders, particularly social phobia.
  - *Example*: propranolol (Inderal).
- *Other Medications*
  - Buspirone (BuSpar) is an azaperone, and is used to treat GAD. Unlike benzodiazepines, BuSpar must be taken consistently for 2 weeks to be effective.
- *Psychotherapy*
  - Psychotherapy is an effective treatment for anxiety disorders, particularly in combination with medications, with CBT being one of the more well studied forms of psychotherapy. Other examples include exposure-based therapy and manualized CBT.
  - Eye movement desensitization and reprocessing (EMDR) is a psychotherapy treatment that was originally designed to alleviate the distress associated with traumatic memories, and is used in treatment of PTSD and other trauma induced disorders. EMDR is typically used in conjunction with CBT.

Considerations when Treating Select Populations with Mood and Anxiety Disorders

Pediatric Considerations

Many adult psychiatric disorders have their origins or first manifestations during childhood or adolescence. Fryers and Brugha (2013) examined childhood determinants of adult psychiatric disorders through an extensive review of longitudinal studies to determine contributing factors to the onset of psychiatric disorders and the association of childhood psychiatric issues with psychiatric disturbance later in life. Specifically, they assessed these relationships based on ten factors including psychological disturbance, genetic influences, neurological deviance, neuroticism, behavior, school performance, adversity, child abuse or neglect, parenting and parent–child relationships, and disrupted and dysfunctional families. While this study was not specific to mood and anxiety disorders, these conditions represented a large portion of the studies reviewed. There was evidence for the association with later mental illness or mental health problems for each of the ten factors with varying degrees of significance. The strongest predictors of psychiatric disorder in adult life was psychological disturbance, psychiatric symptoms, or diagnosable psychiatric disorder during childhood and adolescence. In some specific studies, anxiety, depression, delinquency, and aggressive behaviors were core predictors of adult psychiatric difficulties. Additionally, childhood depression and anxiety were predictive of earlier diagnoses of these conditions in adulthood. In summary, there was evidence of transition from psychological problems in early and mid-childhood, to psychological symptoms and well-defined disorder in adolescence, to psychiatric disorder in adults. This highlights the need to understand these disorders in childhood and their relevance to adult psychiatric difficulties.

Diagnosis of childhood depression typically follows the same criteria as noted for adults. However, research consistently shows that children present differently than adults, including variations across age groups. An allowance made by the DSM-5 included the substitution of irritability for depressed mood in diagnosing major depressive disorder in children. This along with other distinctions is critical in identifying depressive disorders in children.

- For younger children, irritability and sadness remain the most sensitive predictors of depression, but anhedonia was noted to be the most specific.

- Younger children often present with somatic complaints and behavior problems, and may demonstrate a persistent engagement in activities or play with themes of death or suicide.

- Adolescents more commonly display hypersomnia and have an increased risk for suicide in comparison to younger children.

- Girls tend to display changes in appetite or weight, increased frequency of crying, and feelings of guilt or low self-esteem.

- Boys are more likely to endorse anhedonia, social withdrawal, and variation in mood or energy.

In studies of incidence rates, anxiety and depression were highly correlated in each age group and in both boys and girls, suggesting that although they can be measured independently, there is significant overlap. Anxiety often appears earlier, whereas depression tends to develop as children age. There are a number of specific anxiety disorders associated with childhood:

- *Separation anxiety disorder (SAD)* is characterized by anxiety of even temporarily separating from loved ones and is frequently associated with various fears, nightmares, and nonspecific physical complaints.

- *Social Anxiety Disorder* (*social phobia*) is characterized by an intense fear of interacting with others.

- *Overanxious disorder* is characterized by excessive anxiety, unrealistic worries, and fearfulness not related to a specific object or situation.
- *Disinhibited social engagement disorder* is a childhood attachment disorder that may develop when a child lacks appropriate nurturing and affection from parents. As a result of unfulfilled needs, the child is not closely bonded to parents and is as comfortable with strangers as they are with their primary caregivers. They are not afraid of adult strangers and not shy of meeting new people for the first time. Instead, they may be overly friendly, very talkative, and may even begin hugging or cuddling unknown adults.
- *Obsessive-compulsive disorder:*
  - Although adults with this disorder may have insight into the irrational nature of their obsessions and compulsions, children often view these thoughts and behaviors as normal.
  - Children with OCD may develop *trichotillomania*, which involves urges to pull out hair, eyelashes, and/or eyebrows, or *excoriation disorder*, which involves repeated picking at the skin resulting in skin lesions.
  - Other medical conditions in which OCD symptoms are common include:
    - Tourette syndrome, characterized by motor and phonic tics and often also comorbid with ADHD.
    - Pediatric autoimmune neuropsychiatric disorders associated with streptococcal infections (PANDAS), a controversial diagnosis involving rapid-onset OCD and tics after streptococcal infection.

Few medications have been FDA approved for the management of depressive and anxiety disorders in pediatric populations. SSRIs and SNRIs were shown to be more beneficial than placebo in children and adolescents, but the benefit was small and disorder specific. There was a larger difference in drug-placebo difference for children with anxiety disorders in comparison to mood disorders. There is limited FDA approval for SSRIs and SNRIs for the treatment of depressive disorder and obsessive-compulsive disorder. It is important to note that severe adverse events are significantly more common with these medications than placebo. Given the potential for life-threatening events in young children and adolescents, understanding the extent to which these medications pose a genuine risk to youth is critical.

Comorbid depression and anxiety are common for children with ADHD and autism spectrum disorder (ASD). Anxiety and depression, in and of themselves, can cause ADHD-like symptoms including concentration deficits and restlessness. The presence of these comorbid disorders complicates accurate diagnosis and creates challenges when determining the appropriate treatment of both the primary and the comorbid conditions. Estimates of the prevalence of depression among patients with ADHD range from 13% to 27% in research studies and as high as 60% in a clinical sample. Comorbid anxiety has been shown to be as high as 33% in girls and 28% in boys. Depression and anxiety can arise as a consequence of the chronic frustration and disappointment of living with untreated or poorly managed ADHD, but can also present distinct comorbidities and must be managed accordingly.

Depressive syndromes can represent a disabling comorbidity for children with high-functioning ASD, however the differentiation of depression can be complicated by the overlap between the two conditions and the atypical presentation of depression in children with ASD. Children with ASD may have significant impairments in communication that limit their ability to express subjective states of sadness, hopelessness, or disinterest. Identification and diagnosis of depression for children with ASD relies on observation of outward behaviors or changes in mental state rather than the traditional subjective reporting. Observable behaviors include increased sadness, tearfulness, apathy, or an increasingly negative affect. Additional signs of anhedonia, sleep and appetite changes, vegetative signs, and regression in daily functional skills have also been noted in children and adolescents with ASD.

Geriatric Considerations

- *Depression versus dementia* (*pseudodementia*)

  - Depression is frequently accompanied by cognitive problems, and this is especially true in older persons. Identifying depression in someone with dementia can be difficult, since dementia can cause some of the same symptoms. Conversely, identifying dementia in a patient with depression can be equally difficult.

  - Late-onset depression, particularly in patients with no prior psychiatric history, can be related to an underlying neurologic condition or illness.

  - Cognitive difficulties can rise to a level of severity that results in a misdiagnosis of dementia when, in fact, these symptoms improve with proper treatment of the mood disorder. This presentation of dementia-like symptoms in patients with depression or other mental disorders has been called *pseudodementia*. In recent years, many have gravitated to "dementia syndrome of depression" or "dementia of depression" because depression is the most common cause.

  - Cognitive declines associated with depression typically clear, or at least improve, if the depression is treated, although the rate of dementia in these patients is still 20% per year even after full recovery of intellectual function following depression treatment.

  - Overlap of symptoms is seen in a variety of areas including:

    - Depressed mood or agitation.
    - A history of psychiatric disturbance.
    - *Psychomotor retardation.*
    - Impaired immediate memory and learning abilities.
    - Defective attention, concentration, and tracking.
    - Impaired orientation.
    - Poor quality of cognitive products.
    - Listlessness with loss of interest in one's surroundings.
    - Limitations in self-care activities.

  - Depression in the context of dementia includes some differing characteristics relative to primary depression:

    - Patients with dementia have difficulty understanding their mood-related problems and may have difficulty articulating their sadness, helplessness, hopelessness, fears, and other feelings associated with depression.
    - Symptoms may appear less severe due to limited affective expression
    - Depressive symptoms may be sporadic based on situational/environmental factors
    - Patients with dementia are less like to discuss, plan, or attempt suicide

- *Anxiety versus dementia*

  - Dementia-like symptoms are also noted in elderly patients with anxiety disorders, but this distinction is not as prevalent in the literature.

- These patients present with similar cognitive deficits as seen in dementia of depression, although their test performance is characterized by more erratic responses or indecisiveness.

- Disordered thought patterns, including paranoid thinking, suspiciousness, excessive worry about unlikely threats or benign concerns, false accusations, or ideas of reference are sometimes noted in elderly patients with severe anxiety. This can lead to a misdiagnosis of a late-onset psychotic disorder or a frontotemporal variant of dementia.

- When elderly patients with anxiety disorders are treated with sedating medications (e.g., benzodiazepines) further cognitive declines or, in some cases, delirium may occur.

- *Differential diagnosis*

  - In many cases, it is difficult to determine where a psychiatric disorder stops and a neurological disorder begins. Such a distinction is not required as long as it can be established that the course is nonprogressive.

  - Accurate differential diagnosis is important because many of the causes of *pseudodementia* are both treatable and reversible.

  - When uncertain, the least serious diagnosis (i.e., depression or dementia) should be given, and the appropriate treatment prescribed, with further monitoring for improvements or declines over time.

Functional Implications

Mood and anxiety disorders are two of the leading causes of disability in the United States. However, if managed appropriately, the level of functional disability can be minimized. In most cases, intervention is necessary in only the acute phases of the illness, with resolution of functional impairments occurring with mood and behavioral stability. In severe cases, medicinal and therapeutic interventions are required in accordance with the level of severity at the time. This may mean additional assessments to address questions related to capacity, driving, level of disability, need for acute hospitalization/suicide risk assessment, and disposition planning.

Relevant Definitions

Affect A psychological term for an observable expression of emotion. It is the expression of emotion or feelings displayed through facial expressions, hand gestures, voice tone, and other emotional signs such as laughter or tears.

Agoraphobia Comes from two Greek words that mean "fear" and "marketplace." The anxiety associated with agoraphobia leads to avoidance of situations that involve being outside one's home alone, being in crowds, or traveling by car or public transportation.

Anhedonia The inability to experience pleasure from activities usually found enjoyable.

Circuit of Papez One of the major pathways of the limbic system that is chiefly involved in the cortical control of emotion, as well as in memory storage. See additional details in the chapter covering the limbic system (see also Chapter 4, Functional Neuroanatomy and Essential Neuropharmacology).

Corticotropin-releasing hormone (CRH) A hormone produced by the hypothalamus that stimulates the anterior pituitary gland to release adrenocorticotropic hormone. Similar to norepinephrine, CRH acts as both a stress hormone and a neurotransmitter, and increased secretion of CRH helps the body to mobilize energy for the fight or flight response.

Disinhibited social engagement disorder A childhood attachment disorder that may develop when a child lacks appropriate nurturing and affection from parents. As a result of unfulfilled needs, the child is not closely bonded to parents and is as comfortable with strangers as they are with their primary caregivers. They are not afraid of adult strangers and not shy of meeting new people for the first time. Instead, they may be overly friendly, very talkative, and may even begin hugging or cuddling unknown adults. DSED is also known as disinhibited attachment disorder.

Excoriation disorder Also referred to as skin picking or dermatillomania. Involves repeated picking at the skin resulting in skin lesions. This is sometimes seen in children with OCD.

Fight or flight response A physiological reaction in response to stress, characterized by an increase in heart rate and blood pressure, elevation of glucose levels in the blood, and redistribution of blood flow to prepare muscles for activation. These changes are caused by activation of the sympathetic nervous system by noradrenaline, which prepares the body to challenge or flee from a perceived threat.

Hypomania A condition similar to mania but less severe. The symptoms are similar, but do not cause significant distress or impair one's work, family, or social life in an obvious way whereas manic episodes do.

Postpartum depression Depression experienced by women after giving birth in relation to hormonal and physical changes, along with new responsibilities associated with having a child. Misrepresented as "baby blues" or benign adjustment difficulties. Approximately 10–15% of women experience postpartum depression after giving birth.

Pseudodementia (dementia syndrome of depression) A condition that resembles dementia but is actually due to depression. In pseudodementia, a person may present with significant cognitive deficits, appear confused, exhibit depressive symptoms, and complain of memory impairment and other cognitive problems. However, on careful testing, the cognitive difficulties are not reflective of those typically seen in dementia or other neurologic disorders. Instead, the cognitive inefficiencies represent functional cognitive declines representing a symptom of depression.

Psychomotor agitation Increase in activity brought on by mental tension including, but not limited to, restlessness, pacing, tapping fingers or feet, abruptly starting and stopping tasks, and meaninglessly moving objects around.

Psychomotor retardation A visible slowing of physical activity such as movement and speech; has a mental, not organic, cause.

Psychotic depression Occurs when severe depression or bipolar disorder is accompanied by some form of psychosis, such as hallucinations or delusions.

Serotonin syndrome A potentially life-threatening drug reaction caused by too much serotonin availability or sensitivity. This most often occurs when two or more drugs that affect the body's level of serotonin are taken together at the same time. The excess serotonin activity produces a spectrum of specific symptoms including cognitive, autonomic, and somatic effects. The symptoms may range from barely perceptible to fatal.

Trichotillomania Repeated urge to pull out scalp hair, eyelashes, eyebrows, or other body hair. Sometimes seen in children with OCD.

Mood Disorders: Depression, Mania, and Anxiety Questions

NOTE: Questions 24, 58, 93, 113, and 114 on the First Full-Length Practice Examination, Questions 23, 27, 53, 61, 89, and 98 on the Second Full-Length Practice Examination, Questions 13, 55, 81, and 111 on the Third Full-Length Practice Examination, and Questions 15, 28, 43, 56, 68, and 90 on the Fourth Full-Length Practice Examination are from this chapter.

1. During morning rounds the psychiatrist on your team indicates that the patient you are discussing requires a medication that will help them relax, sleep better, and potentially prevent overexcitation. Which neurotransmitter system is this medication most likely going to target?

   (a) serotonin

   (b) norepinephrine

   (c) GABA

   (d) dopamine

2. What unique neuropsychological findings are often seen in patients with bipolar disorder and obsessive-compulsive disorders that are not typically seen in other mood and anxiety disorders?

   (a) visuospatial deficits

   (b) language deficits

   (c) executive deficits

   (d) recent memory deficits

3. A 29-year-old man presents with a long-standing history of Tourette syndrome and obsessive and compulsive behaviors. Which neuroanatomical structure is likely involved in the maintenance of these symptoms?

   (a) insula

   (b) amygdala

   (c) caudate nucleus

   (d) prefrontal cortex

4. Which of the following most represents a lifelong disorder?

   (a) Bipolar Disorder

   (b) Major Depressive Disorder

   (c) Generalized Anxiety Disorder

   (d) Posttraumatic Stress Disorder

5. In assessing memory complaints in a patient who presents with depression, which of the following characteristics best characterizes the difficulties associated with mood problems rather than a neurologic based memory disorder?

   (a) better recall of unrelated material, with poor recall of narrative material

   (b) poor attention, procedural learning, and autobiographical memory

   (c) poor visual memory in the context of sparing of verbal memory

   (d) limited acquisition and retrieval, with spared recognition memory

6. A 65-year-old man had a long standing history of dysthymia with periodic bouts of major depression. He has gone long periods without treatment or has been sporadically adherent to treatment recommendations. Due to increasing memory complaints the psychiatrist requests an MRI of the brain. Atrophy in which area of the brain might be anticipated?

   (a) caudate nucleus

   (b) hippocampus

   (c) frontal lobe

   (d) raphe nuclei

7. Disruption of white matter connectivity within brain networks that modulate emotional behavior in early development leads to decreased connectivity among ventral prefrontal networks and limbic brain regions, especially amygdala, contributing to the onset of what disorder?

    (a) Major Depression

    (b) Generalized Anxiety Disorder

    (c) Bipolar Disorder

    (d) Posttraumatic Stress Disorder

8. A 51-year-old divorced woman has a prior history of epilepsy that has been controlled with anticonvulsants for over 10 years. However, in the past 5 years she has been hospitalized five separate times following suicide attempts. She has received inpatient psychiatric treatment, combination therapy in various outpatient settings, and multiple medication trials. What type of alternative treatment might be considered next?

    (a) ketamine

    (b) propofol

    (c) etomidate

    (d) amytal

9. An 11-year-old girl was referred for an evaluation due to difficulties with attention in school and possible mood problems. She is noted to have sores on her arms and hands and pulls at her hair, eyebrows, and sores during interview and testing. This presentation is associated with which of the following disorders?

    (a) Generalized Anxiety Disorder

    (b) Posttraumatic Stress Disorder

    (c) Bipolar 1 Disorder

    (d) Obsessive-Compulsive Disorder

10. When initially evaluating a 6-year-old girl who was referred for an evaluation due to attention difficulties and behavioral distractibility in school, she gives you a hug, and repeatedly attempts to sit in your lap or hold your hand during the interview. Her parents apologize and say that she is like this with all new people she meets, and has had the same behavior with her teachers. This is a characteristic of what disorder?

    (a) Separation Anxiety Disorder

    (b) Disinhibited Social Engagement Disorder

    (c) Bipolar Disorder

    (d) Autistic Spectrum Disorder

Mood Disorders: Depression, Mania, and Anxiety Answers

1. **C—GABA** *GABA is the primary inhibitory neurotransmitter in the CNS. Medications targeting this system often result in mood stabilization, relaxation, and improved sleep or lethargy.*

References:
(a) Kandel, E. R. (2013). Disorders of mood and anxiety. In E. R. Kandel, J. H. Schwartz, T. M. Jessell, A. A. Siegelbaum, & A. J. Hudspeth (Eds.), *Principles of neural science* (5th ed., pp. 1402–1424). New York, NY: McGraw-Hill.
(b) Stein, M. B., & Steckler, T. (2010). *Behavioral neurobiology of anxiety and its treatment.* New York, NY: Springer.

2. **A—visuospatial deficits** *There is evidence to suggest that right-hemisphere dysfunction is associated with bipolar illness and OCD, with greater impairments seen in visuospatial functioning. Unipolar depression and other anxiety disorders do not demonstrate this pattern of performance.*

References:
(a) Sahu, A., Das, B., & Gupta, P. (2017). Visuospatial memory in patients with obsessive-compulsive disorder. *Journal of Mental Health and Human Behavior, 22*, 1, 55–60.

(b) Tsitsipa, E., & Fountoulakis, K. N. (2015). The neurocognitive functioning in bipolar disorder: A systematic review of data. *Annals of General Psychiatry, 14*, 42, 1–29.

3. **C—caudate nucleus** *The caudate nucleus has been found to be dysfunctional in persons with OCD, as well as in Tourette syndrome, PANDAS, and other disorders. It is thought that poor functioning of the caudate results in an inability to properly regulate the transmission of information regarding worrying events or ideas between the thalamus and the orbitofrontal cortex.*

References:
(a) Felling, R. J., & Singer, H. S. (2011). Neurobiology of Tourette syndrome: Current status and need for further investigation. *Journal of Neuroscience, 31*, 35, 12387–12395.
(b) Menzies, L., Chamberlain, S. R., Laird, A. R., Thelen, S. M., Sahakian, B. J., & Bullmore, E. T. (2008). Integrating evidence from neuroimaging and neuropsychological studies of obsessive-compulsive disorder: The orbitofrontostriatal model revisited. *Neuroscience & Biobehavioral Reviews, 32*, 525–549.

4. **A—Bipolar Disorder** *Bipolar disorder is thought to be a lifelong disorder with symptoms varying across the full continuum of mood from severely depressed to extremely elated or manic states. There is no cure for bipolar disorder, but appropriate treatment results in better control of the cycling moods and related symptoms for most patients regardless of severity of the illness.*

References:
(a) American Psychiatric Association. (2013). *Diagnostic and statistical manual of mental disorders* (5th ed.). Washington, DC: American Psychiatric Publishing.
(b) Kandel, E. R. (2013). Disorders of mood and anxiety. In E.R. Kandel, J. H. Schwartz, T.M. Jessell, A. A. Siegelbaum, & A. J. Hudspeth (Eds.), *Principles of neural science* (5th ed., pp. 1402–1424). New York, NY: McGraw-Hill.

5. **D—limited acquisition and retrieval, with spared recognition memory** *In general, patients with depression show difficulties in the acquisition of new material with limited benefit from repeated presentations. They show better recall with contextually based information as opposed to unrelated word lists and tend to perform better when recognition cues are provided. See detailed discussion in the "Expectations for Neuropsychological Assessment Results" section.*

Reference: Chamberlain, S. R., & Sahakian, B. (2006). Cognition in depression and memory. In C. G. Cruse, H. Y. Meltzer, C. Sennef, & S. V. van de Witte (Eds.) *Thinking and cognition: Concepts, targets and therapeutics* (pp. 39–49). Fairfax, VA: IOS Press.

6. **B—hippocampus** *Atrophy of select areas of the brain has been associated with depression including the amygdala, hippocampus, prefrontal cortex, striatum, nucleus accumbens, and the cerebellum. Specifically, hippocampal volume loss among persons with major depressive disorder was found to be as high as 19%, and the number of days an individual had untreated depression had a direct effect on hippocampal size.*

Reference: Oakes, P., Loukas, M., Oskouian, R. J., & Tubbs, R. S. (2017). The neuroanatomy of depression: A review. *Clinical Anatomy, 30*(1), 44–49.

7. **C—Bipolar Disorder** *It has been suggested that disruption of white matter connectivity within brain networks that modulate emotional behavior in early development leads to decreased connectivity among ventral prefrontal networks and limbic brain regions, especially amygdala. This was hypothesized to cause developmental failure in healthy ventral prefrontal-limbic modulation resulting in the onset of mania and ultimately, with progressive changes throughout these networks over time and with affective episodes, a bipolar course of illness.*

Reference: Strakowski, A. M., Adler, C. M., Almeida, J., Altshuler, L. L., Blumberg, H. P., Chang, K. D., . . . Townsend, J. D. (2012). The functional neuroanatomy of bipolar disorder: A consensus model. *Bipolar Disorder, 14*(4), 313–325.

8. **A—ketamine** *Ketamine, via intravenous infusions, has emerged as a novel therapy for treatment-resistant depression, given rapid onset and demonstrable efficacy in both unipolar and bipolar depression. A reduction in suicidality has been shown as well, and preliminary studies with ketamine in the treatment of severe depression have been promising.*

Reference: Ryan, W. C., Marta, C. J., & Koek, R. J. (2014). Ketamine and depression: A review. *International Journal of Transpersonal Studies, 33*(2), 40–74.

9. **D—Obsessive-Compulsive Disorder** *Excoriation (repetitive skin picking) and trichotillomania repetitive pulling of hair, eyelashes, eyebrows, or other body hair) are associated with children with OCD.*

Reference: American Psychiatric Association. (2013). *Diagnostic and statistical manual of mental disorders* (5th ed.). Washington, DC: American Psychiatric Publishing.

10. **B—Disinhibited Social Engagement Disorder** *This is a childhood attachment disorder that may develop when a child lacks appropriate nurturing and affection from parents. As a result of unfulfilled needs, the child is not closely bonded to parents and is as comfortable with strangers as they are with their primary caregivers. They are not afraid of adult strangers and not shy of meeting new people for the first time. Instead, they may be overly friendly, very talkative, and may even begin hugging or cuddling unknown adults. Autistic spectrum disorder is a developmental disorder that is not precipitated by limited nurturing and affection from parents. In contrast, patients with autistic spectrum disorder have limitations in social communication/ interaction, limiting their ability to receive or benefit from parental contact.*

Reference: American Psychiatric Association. (2013). *Diagnostic and statistical manual of mental disorders* (5th ed.). Washington, DC: American Psychiatric Publishing.

Recommended Readings

American Psychiatric Association. (2013). *Diagnostic and statistical manual of mental disorders* (5th ed.). Washington, DC: American Psychiatric Publishing.

Fryers, T., & Brugha, T. (2013). Childhood determinants of adult psychiatric disorder. *Clinical Practice and Epidemiology in Mental Health, 9,* 1–50.

Kandel, E. R. (2013). Disorders of mood and anxiety. In E. R. Kandel, J. H. Schwartz, T. M. Jessell, A. A. Siegelbaum, & A. J. Hudspeth (Eds.), *Principles of neural science* (5th ed., pp. 1402–1424). New York, NY: McGraw-Hill.

Oakes, P., Loukas, M., Oskouian, R. J., & Tubbs, R. S. (2017). The neuroanatomy of depression: A review. *Clinical Anatomy, 30*(1), 44–49.

Schmidt, C. K., Khalid, S., Loukas, M., & Tubbs, R. S. (2018, January 12) Neuroanatomy of anxiety: A brief review. *Cureus, 10*(1), e2055. https://doi.org/10.7759/cureus.2055

Strakowski, A. M., Adler, C. M., Almeida, J., Altshuler, L. L., Blumberg, H. P., Chang, K. D., . . . Townsend, J. D. (2012). The functional neuroanatomy of bipolar disorder: A consensus model. *Bipolar Disorder, 14*(4), 313–325.

Strawbridge, R., Young, A. H., & Cleare, A. J. (2017). Biomarkers for depression: Recent insights, current challenges and future prospects. *Neuropsychiatric Disease and Treatment, 13,* 1245–1262.

Wright, S. L., & Persad, C. (2007). Distinguishing between depression and dementia in older persons: Neuropsychological and neuropathological correlates. *Journal of Geriatric Psychiatry and Neurology, 20*(4), 189–198.

Websites

https://www.cdc.gov/mentalhealth/data_publications/index.htm
http://www.nimh.nih.gov/statistics/index.shtml

35 Schizophrenia Spectrum and Other Psychotic Disorders

Robert M. Bilder, Amy M. Jimenez, Vidyulata Kamath, and Paul J. Moberg

Definition

The *Diagnostic and Statistical Manual of Mental Disorders, Fifth Edition* (DSM-5) groups together schizophrenia, other psychotic disorders, and schizotypal personality disorders based on their shared clinical characteristics, and acknowledges that there is a broad range of severity in the associated symptoms, which may include abnormalities in one or more of the following domains: *delusions, hallucinations,* disorganized thinking (speech), grossly disorganized or abnormal motor behavior (including *catatonia*), and negative symptoms. Schizophrenia, which requires that continuous signs of the disturbance persist for a 6-month period, is a chronic and disabling psychiatric disorder that is marked by significant disruptions in perception, cognition, mood, and behavior. Clinical features are broadly classified in at least three categories including positive symptoms (e.g., *delusions, hallucinations*), negative symptoms (e.g., affective flattening or blunting, anhedonia-asociality, avolition-apathy, physical anergia, alogia), and disorganized symptoms (e.g., disorganized speech and behavior). Schizophreniform disorder has the same symptoms as schizophrenia but does not last 6 months and for formal diagnosis does not require a decrement in functioning. Brief psychotic disorder lasts 1 day to 1 month. There are two syndromes that are limited to a single domain of symptoms: delusional disorder and *catatonia.* Cognitive disturbances are increasingly recognized as core features of schizophrenia spectrum disorders and the cognitive deficits are stronger correlates of real-world outcomes than are positive symptoms. Based on current criteria, a diagnosis of schizophrenia is warranted when two or more of the following symptoms (*delusions, hallucinations,* disorganized speech, disorganized behavior or *catatonia,* and negative symptoms) have been present for a 1-month period (or less if treated successfully), and there are some signs of the disturbance lasting at least 6 months, resulting in impairment in interpersonal, social, or occupational functioning. If the total duration of illness does not last 6 months, the correct diagnosis is schizophreniform disorder. Other psychiatric diagnoses such as schizoaffective disorder and major depression with psychotic features, as well as psychotic symptoms due to substance abuse disorders, dementias, stroke, and brain injury must be ruled out prior to making the diagnosis of schizophrenia. *Catatonia* may occur in the context of other disorders (including neurodevelopmental, psychotic, bipolar, depressive and other mental disorders).

There is significant heterogeneity in the clinical presentation of the schizophrenia syndrome. Traditionally, diagnostic subtypes were used in an attempt to classify individuals based on the predominant symptom profile including paranoid type, disorganized type, catatonic type, undifferentiated type, and residual type. However, given a lack of empirical support and clinical utility, revisions to the DSM-5 removed these subtypes, and instead listed a single optional specifier "with *catatonia*" to describe cases marked by motoric immobility, excessive nonpurposeful motor activity, extreme negativism, peculiarities of voluntary movement, echolalia, or echopraxia.

Neuropathology

The neuropathology of schizophrenia has not been fully elucidated, but it is currently conceptualized as a multifactorial neurodevelopmental disorder with genetic *diathesis* or vulnerability. The genetic basis of the illness is supported by family, twin, and adoption studies showing increased probability for the disorder proportional to the percentage of genes shared with an affected individual, and by genome-wide association studies (GWAS) showing strong associations of schizophrenia spectrum disorders with genetic variation. Furthermore, parents, siblings, and off-spring of persons with schizophrenia show similar, yet attenuated, intermediate phenotypes of the illness. Nevertheless, the manner of inheritance is complex and heterogeneous across different people diagnosed with these syndromes, likely involving many common genes of small effect, some rare mutations with larger effects, and complex interactions of genes with other genes, and the interaction of genes with the environment (i.e., with genetic vulnerability or *diathesis* interacting with environmental stressors).

Neurodevelopmental models of schizophrenia have been proposed to account for the role of environmental stressors as these interact with genetic vulnerability (sometimes referred to as the *diathesis*-stress model). These models generally postulate that genes underlying neurodevelopment and brain maturation, along with others involved in signal transduction, are most likely responsible for the heritable risk observed in individuals with schizophrenia. These genetic variants could disrupt key central nervous system (CNS) signaling pathways during embryogenesis (e.g., those that govern cell migration and/or adhesion) leading to the development of faulty neurocircuitry during maturation. These models suggest that deficient circuitry is particularly susceptible to later environmental stressors, with the degree and scope of early susceptibility factors potentially commensurate with an individual's vulnerability to later insults. Additionally, predisposing genotypes may interact with normal developmental periods that occur later, resulting in, for example, abnormal or excessive synaptic pruning processes during late adolescence and early adulthood. Indeed, there is substantial evidence for neurodevelopmental abnormalities in schizophrenia, including premorbid behavioral and neurological signs, adverse prenatal and perinatal events, reduced dendritic complexity and lower spine and synapse density on cortical pyramidal neurons in individuals with schizophrenia. In addition, individuals with schizophrenia show cortical and subcortical reductions in gray matter volume, as well as decreased white matter integrity, as measured by histology, structural magnetic resonance imaging (MRI), and diffusion tensor imaging (DTI).

There have been multiple hypotheses about schizophrenia being due to specific neuroanatomic deficits in frontal, fronto-temporal, fronto-limbic, cortico-striato-pallido-thalamic, or cortico-limbic-cerebellar circuits, but so far none of these hypotheses has been well validated and the emerging consensus is that the most characteristic anatomic deficits are widespread, relatively non-specific, and marked by considerable heterogeneity. Neuroimaging findings including widespread prominence of the cortical sulci and ventricular enlargement have been considered among the most robust findings in schizophrenia, yet the causes of these abnormalities remain unknown. Among the clearest neuropathological findings is reduced "neuropil," presumably reflecting reductions in synaptic processes, and this appears to be widespread. Some hypotheses suggest this may be due to excessive "pruning" of synaptic processes during adolescence but his has not been confirmed. There has been recent excitement about complex genetic variation affecting complement component four genes, which are linked to excessive synaptic pruning that may cause neuropathologic features of reduced neuropil. Overall, the neurodevelopmental model considers the heterogeneity of schizophrenia and suggests that the etiology of this disorder is influenced by the complex interaction of genetics, brain development, and environmental factors. In summary, current evidence suggests:

- Schizophrenia is marked by widespread changes in the cortex, with cortical thinning, decreased neuropil, reductions in white matter integrity, ventricular enlargement, and abnormalities in subcortical structure.

- Multiple neurodevelopmental factors are suspected, including possible flaws in cell migration, establishment and/or pruning of synapses.

- A combination of genetic and early developmental risk factors probably serve as a substrate, increasing vulnerability to stressors, that may precipitate decompensation and further dysregulation of brain function.

Risk Factors

- *Genetic Liability* Family history of schizophrenia is believed to increase the risk of developing the disorder, and this risk increases with the degree of genetic relationship (so the identical twin of a person with schizophrenia has about a 50% chance of having schizophrenia, while a sibling has about a 9% chance, and a cousin only about a 2% chance). Established heritability estimates range from 80% to 85%, and researchers continue to search for specific associations with genetic variants. Large-sample GWAS of common genetic variants already have revealed significant associations with schizophrenia for more than 100 genetic loci. These risk loci, however, are thought to account for only a portion of the liability for schizophrenia overall, and many published claims about "candidate genes" (for example, that polymorphisms in the gene for catechol-O-methyl-transferase (COMT) may cause schizophrenia or cognitive impairment in schizophrenia) may well be false positive findings, so it is important to be skeptical when surveying literature on genetic associations. Hundreds, if not thousands, of common genetic variants, each with small effects, are probably involved in multiple pathogenic pathways to disorder. In addition, research has revealed rare genetic variants and de novo mutations, some of which have larger effects; but, because they are so rare, these account for relatively few cases of schizophrenia overall. Large-scale sequencing studies, studies of gene–gene interactions, and epigenome-wide association studies may soon contribute further to our understanding of the genetic vulnerability to schizophrenia. The Whole Genome Sequencing in Psychiatric Disorders (WGSPD) Consortium already has more than 25,000 individuals including people with schizophrenia and other psychiatric syndromes, in whom the DNA will be sequenced and associations sought with both diagnostic categorical and dimensional phenotypes. The most recent findings highlight that the genetic risks for schizophrenia spectrum disorders are largely shared with a wide range of other psychiatric syndromes, including ADHD, major depressive disorder, bipolar disorder, and autism spectrum disorders (ASDs).

- *Obstetric Complications* Maternal infection during pregnancy, maternal malnutrition, labor and delivery complications, prematurity, and low birth weight all increase the risk of schizophrenia.

- *Premorbid Intelligence and Pervasive Developmental Disorders* The presence of intellectual disability (ID) and ASDs are considered risk factors for the development of schizophrenia, although these may be better characterized as coincident symptoms of shared biological risks. Retrospective studies of individuals who later develop schizophrenia have documented increased rates of IDs and ASDs in childhood, as well as evidence of language, motor, and social abnormalities.

- *Substance Abuse* Substance abuse, including frequent cannabis use during adolescence, has been associated with increased schizophrenia risk.

- *Age* Although schizophrenia can occur at any age, it tends to develop during late adolescence and young adulthood, with earlier onset generally associated with poorer prognosis. Research suggests that reducing the gap between onset of psychosis and treatment initiation improves outcomes, highlighting the value of early detection and intervention.

- *Sex* Schizophrenia is observed in both men and women; however, women with schizophrenia tend to have later illness onset, lower negative symptom severity, greater affective symptoms, and better social, cognitive, and premorbid functioning than men with schizophrenia. There is also evidence for a bimodal age of onset distribution in women, with a second peak occurring after age 40.

- *Socioeconomic Status* Schizophrenia occurs at higher rates in families in which the parents are unmarried or divorced when compared to those in which the parents are married or widowed. In addition, low income and increased poverty increase the illness risk.

Epidemiology

- Schizophrenia affects more than 24 million individuals worldwide, occurring in 0.5–2% of the world population. According to the World Health Organization (WHO), schizophrenia predominantly impacts individuals between the ages of 15 and 35 years. Although the incidence rate of schizophrenia is low, prevalence is high due to the chronicity of the illness. Indeed, schizophrenia contributes significantly to the global burden of disease, with a total cost estimate of $94 to $102 billion. It is ranked within the top ten causes of disability worldwide.

- Medical comorbidities are a common complicating factor. Individuals with schizophrenia have greater cardiovascular morbidity, owing to increased prevalence of cigarette smoking, obesity, diabetes mellitus, hypertension, and hyperlipidemia that collectively results in a 20% reduction in the lifespan of an individual with schizophrenia. The increased risk of developing metabolic syndromes substantially raises the risk for myocardial infarction and cerebrovascular accidents, and long-term use of *antipsychotic* medication is known to increase the occurrence of weight gain and metabolic syndromes, thus compounding cardiovascular risks. Other risk factors that contribute to the increased risk of cardiovascular disease in persons with schizophrenia include malnutrition, sedentary lifestyle, and markers of abnormal coagulation or inflammation. Finally, chronic obstructive pulmonary disease and tuberculosis are also a source of medical morbidity in the illness, at least in part associated with high rates of smoking among people with schizophrenia.

- Individuals with schizophrenia have a two- to threefold increased mortality rate, which is attributed to increased risk of suicide, high-risk behaviors, accidents, and substance abuse. Notably, the rate of suicide in schizophrenia is twelve times higher than that of the general population. There is a substantial mortality gap between schizophrenia and the general population, one that has widened over the past three decades, suggesting that persons with schizophrenia have not experienced improved health outcomes such as those observed in the population at large.

Determinants of Severity

Schizophrenia is diagnosed based on the presence and duration of symptoms, as determined by clinical observation and interview, review of medical/psychological records, and collateral reports from caregivers. Diagnosis using a well-validated structured or semistructured interview (e.g., Structured Clinical Interview for DSM-IV [SCID] or WHO Composite International Diagnostic Interview [CIDI]) is the standard for research, but these schedules are seldom utilized in clinical settings. Similarly, illness severity may be assessed using rating scales such as the Brief Psychiatric Rating Scale, Positive and Negative Syndrome Scale, Scale for the Assessment of Positive Symptoms, and the Scale for the Assessment of Negative Symptoms, which have all demonstrated sound psychometric properties. These scales allow for the derivation of scores on different dimensions, including positive, negative, disorganized, and mood symptoms (e.g., depression, mania). The DSM-5 includes freely available rating scales to enable screening for psychiatric syndromes broadly (the "Level 1 Cross-Cutting Symptom Measure") and psychosis specifically (see "Clinician-Rated Dimensions of Psychosis Symptom Severity") that may be useful for clinical assessment. It should be noted that amelioration of positive symptoms does not appear to be associated with major benefits in interepisode functioning, including occupational attainment, independent living, or social relations. However, cognitive impairment and other symptoms (negative, disorganized) appear to be stronger determinants of functional outcome in schizophrenia. Other correlates of poor prognosis include younger age of onset, insidious onset, family history, greater number of relapses, poor social support, and trauma history (Box 35.1).

BOX 35.1 Risk Factors for Poor Outcome in Schizophrenia

- Neuropsychological impairments
- Early age of onset
- Insidious onset with poor premorbid social function (compared to acute onset following relatively typical social and cognitive development)
- Positive family history of schizophrenia
- Predominantly negative and disorganization symptoms
- Lack of social support
- Poor compliance with prescribed treatments
- History of trauma

Presentation, Disease Course, and Recovery

Premorbid

Early pre- and perinatal neurodevelopmental anomalies are thought to occur in schizophrenia. Retrospective studies in schizophrenia cohorts suggest evidence of cognitive, emotional, and behavioral changes prior to the prodromal phase of the illness. Studies have also shown significantly poorer social adjustment and intelligence in the premorbid phase. Behavioral signs include increased shyness and learning difficulties in elementary school, poor social interaction, withdrawn behavior, clumsiness, and depressed mood.

Prodromal or Attenuated Psychosis Syndrome

During this stage, the adolescent or young adult is often experiencing attenuated or "subthreshold" positive psychotic symptoms or brief intermittent psychotic symptoms. These attenuated symptoms are typically milder than those seen in patients with psychosis. For example, a prodromal individual may report "perceptual abnormalities" or a milder experience of *hallucinations* that can be characterized by hearing noises or sounds that are not really there—but not actual voices. Along this same line, as opposed to unshakable *delusions*, prodromal individuals may experience unusual thought content which may include wondering if it is possible that others could hear their thoughts as opposed to clear endorsement of thought broadcasting. According to the Yale PRIME Psychosis Prodrome Research Clinic, the following behaviors of concern could be indicative of prodromal syndromes in adolescents or young adults: (1) withdrawal/isolation, (2) social difficulties, (3) poor hygiene, (4) bizarre behavior/appearance, (5) increased difficulty at school or work, (6) falling asleep in class repeatedly, (7) sadness/tearfulness, (8) excessive anxiety, (9) absenteeism/ staying in room, (10) poor concentration/spacing-out/difficulty thinking clearly, (11) hypervigilance, (12) decrease in work performance/activity level, (13) becoming neglectful and unfeeling, (14) suspiciousness or mistrust of others, (15) changes in the way things look or sound, and (16) emotional outbursts/emotional flatness. Often, the prodromal individual may have a diagnosis of anxiety, mood, or substance use disorder. During this stage, impairments in social, occupational, and academic functioning are frequently observed. Neuropsychological impairment is consistently observed in youths at risk for schizophrenia or psychotic disorders, including deficits in verbal and visual memory, attention and working memory, verbal fluency, emotion recognition, and olfactory processing.

First-Episode Psychosis

During this stage, the appearance of full-threshold psychotic symptoms occurs. Severe neuropsychological deficits are already clearly apparent, with most prominent impairments in memory, attention, and executive functions. These impairments are paralleled by problems with social and academic or occupational functioning. The cognitive impairments tend to persist despite resolution of florid psychotic symptoms.

Acute

The *acute* phase describes any period (including the first episode) in which an individual is actively experiencing symptoms of psychosis, including thought disorder, *hallucinations*, and *delusions*. An acute period can last several weeks or months if left untreated and can require inpatient hospitalization for psychiatric stabilization. Psychotic symptoms tend to fluctuate from states of acute exacerbation to relative stability or remission. Cognitive symptoms are also often apparent.

Residual

The residual phase describes a period in which psychotic symptoms have largely remitted and the individual is stable. Individuals may continue to experience negative symptoms, odd beliefs, and poor social functioning during a residual phase. Of note, cognitive impairment tends to persist throughout all phases of the illness.

Expectations for Neuropsychological Assessment Results

It is widely acknowledged that the heterogeneous functional outcomes are better correlated with neurocognitive and social cognitive deficits than with specific psychotic symptoms. In addition to this association with real-world outcomes, characterization of neuropsychological deficits in schizophrenia is important to treatment and educational or vocational planning. Although the DSM-5 does not include cognitive impairment as one of the diagnostic criteria for schizophrenia, assessment of cognitive function is considered helpful. The DSM-5 suggests that brief assessment of cognition, without formal neuropsychological assessment, can be sufficient for diagnostic purposes, and a single-item, clinician rating of cognitive impairment on a 5-point scale is included in Section III: Emerging Measures and Models.

Several comprehensive batteries with sound psychometric properties have been used to assess cognition in schizophrenia in clinical research settings. The Measurement and Treatment Research to Improve Cognition in Schizophrenia (MATRICS) project led to development of the MATRICS Consensus Cognitive Battery (MCCB), and the Battery for the Assessment of Cognition in Schizophrenia is a briefer assessment developed specifically to measure cognitive deficits in schizophrenia. Meta-analyses reveal that patients with schizophrenia show moderate to severe deficits across almost all neuropsychological functions, with memory, attention, and executive functioning demonstrating the most robust impairments. The severity of impairments estimated from large-scale and/or meta-analytic studies tends to vary from 1.0 to 1.5 standard deviation units below the average scores of demographically matched control groups.

- *Intelligence/Achievement* Data from twin studies has suggested both global premorbid cognitive deficits and cognitive decline accompanying the onset of frank illness. Fluid intellectual abilities demanding attention, working memory, abstraction, and processing speed are reliably more impaired than crystallized intellectual abilities. Paralleling this finding, people with schizophrenia tend to have smaller relative deficits on academic achievement tests than on tests of fluid intellectual abilities. Following resolution of the first episode, intellectual ability tends to show relative stability through later phases of illness.

- *Attention/Concentration* Attention deficits are considered a fundamental feature of schizophrenia. During attentional tasks, patients often demonstrate slowed reaction time (to even simple stimuli), poor vigilance (selectively attending to relevant information while ignoring distractors), and impaired selective attention (sustained concentration in continuous effort-demanding situations). Several possible explanatory mechanisms have been proposed, including ineffective filtering, information loss in working memory, disordered control and maintenance of selective processing strategies, reduced processing capacity, and impaired effortful or controlled processing. The extensive interaction of the attentional system with working memory and executive control systems (and, indeed, blurring of conceptual boundaries between these domains) results in difficulty parsing out the relative role of each in observed impairments.

- *Processing Speed* Evidence for reduced information processing speed has been consistently observed in individuals diagnosed with schizophrenia and recent meta-analytic findings identify this as among the most significant deficits (in terms of effect size) observed in the disorder.

- *Language* Basic abilities acquired early in life (e.g., reading, spelling, or vocabulary tests) tend to be relatively preserved. In contrast, higher level language processing, such as comprehension of complex syntax or ease of semantic access, show moderate levels of impairment. Measures of language that emphasize initiation, generation, and speed of processing (i.e., word-list generation tasks) often reveal marked impairments. There are also measures of formal thought disorder that index disruptions in speech, language, and communication skills that are often not as fully assessed in the typical neuropsychological assessment of expressive and receptive language functions (e.g., idiosyncratic word usage, incongruous combinations). Usually history helps differentiate the diagnoses of schizophrenia spectrum disorders from other neurological syndromes causing disruptions of speech and language, but the ultimate neural circuit-level causes of these disturbances remains unclear in schizophrenia and may overlap with mechanisms that cause similar disturbances in certain aphasias.

- **Visuospatial Abilities** Basic visuospatial skills, although sometimes impaired, are typically among the better-preserved functions in this disorder. Timed tasks relying on good attentional and psychomotor skills typically show the greatest deficits, whereas those of a more purely visual perceptual nature tend to be better preserved. Some refined experimental tasks may nevertheless be used to detect perceptual anomalies in schizophrenia.

- **Memory** Deficits in declarative memory are also among the most severe neuropsychological impairments seen in the disorder. Impairments are mostly characterized by deficits in encoding, consolidation, organization, and retrieval. In young individuals at risk for schizophrenia, deficits in memory appear to predict a more rapid conversion to psychosis.

- **Executive Functions** Given the similarities between many of the clinical features of schizophrenia and those associated with frontal system dysfunction (e.g., reduced spontaneity, avolition, mental rigidity, and lack of social judgment), along with functional neuroimaging findings suggesting either a lack of engagement or excessive engagement of prefrontal cortex, a considerable amount of research has focused on executive dysfunction in schizophrenia. Executive deficits are severe in schizophrenia, but, as noted earlier, the boundaries between impairments in executive functions and other domains (i.e., working memory, attention, and cognitive control) are typically blurred.

- **Sensorimotor Functions** Several movement disorders are due to treatment with *antipsychotic* drugs (particularly higher doses of "typical" *antipsychotic* drugs). These include parkinsonian symptoms (tremor, bradykinesia, bradyphrenia) and akathisia (motor restlessness and agitation) that are usually reversible if treatment is discontinued or doses lowered, and which may be mitigated by adjunctive anticholinergic treatments (which in turn, may cause adverse effects on cognition, especially memory functions). There is further a potentially irreversible iatrogenic movement disorder—*tardive dyskinesia*—associated with long-term exposure to conventional *antipsychotic* drugs. Finally, the syndrome of *catatonia*, which may include abnormal stereotyped repetitive movements, waxy flexibility, or immobility and negativism, used to be highly prevalent (20–50%) but today is less prevalent (<20% among most inpatient samples), and the reason for this decrease is unclear. In addition to motor function, studies of olfaction in schizophrenia indicate robust deficits that appear to be related to the severity of negative symptoms.

- **Emotion and Personality** Patients with schizophrenia show significant and persistent impairments in a variety of social cognitive domains, including emotion processing, social perception, attributional bias, and *theory of mind*. Impaired social cognition has been shown to be a key determinant of functional disability in people with schizophrenia. Indeed, social cognition appears to explain additional variance in the prediction of functional outcome that cannot be accounted for by neuropsychological function alone, such that social cognition may mediate the relationship between neuropsychological measures and functional outcome.

- **Performance and Symptom Validity** The use of performance and symptom validity measures is always valuable in the assessment of patients with psychosis. Reduced test engagement or response bias can be seen for a variety of reasons, and some empirical studies of people with schizophrenia show very high rates of failure on performance validity tests, even when secondary gain is extremely unlikely to be an explanatory factor. Examiners should exercise special effort to monitor individuals with psychotic disorders, attempt to maximize their engagement in assessment, and be alert to lapses in attention or engagement. While neuropsychological screening may be of value in acute psychosis, detailed neuropsychological characterization is often better deferred until the individual is not in an acute phase of illness.

Considerations when Treating Patients with Schizophrenia

- *Level of Supervision* Independent living among individuals with schizophrenia is often challenging, and many patients require some degree of supervision. Patients capable of living more independently report higher quality of life, and identifying the least restrictive placement is an important goal for clinicians working with people who have chronic schizophrenia. Negative symptoms in particular have been associated with poorer outcomes in multiple domains of functioning, including independent living. In addition to negative symptoms, depressive symptoms, particularly among men, have been associated with lower levels of independence and increased need for supervised living.

- *Rehabilitation Considerations* Cognitive remediation strategies have been shown to produce reliable improvements in multiple domains of cognition regardless of symptom severity. These changes are independent of changes in clinical status and may be better predictors of functional outcome than are symptoms, especially in more chronic cases of the disease. However, cognitive improvements alone are insufficient for improvement in daily living skills. When used in conjunction with targeted strategy-based interventions for adaptive behaviors, cognitive remediation may improve functional outcomes over skills training alone and help maintain these functional improvements over time.

- *Driving* The extant literature has generally shown that most patients with schizophrenia who are stable (not in acute episodes of illness) and receiving treatment for their illness are relatively safe drivers. Indeed, a person's accident history and record of violations is likely a better predictor of driving risk than a diagnosis of schizophrenia. That being said, the presence of significant cognitive deficits may, in some cases, raise concerns about driving. Similar to the driving literature in healthy controls, impairments in cognitive flexibility and attention may add additional risk to safe driving in patients. Review of medication regimen may also be important to assure adverse side effects do not affect skills required for safe driving. Close attention to these factors can help establish the threshold for safe driving in any given patient.

- *Employment* Although findings are mixed, research generally supports that helping individuals with schizophrenia return to work is associated with reduced symptoms, better overall functioning, and a generally higher reported quality of life. These considerations must be balanced against the risks of engagement in stressful settings for the patient who may not possess adequate coping skills. Following recent-onset schizophrenia, cognitive functioning, specifically working memory, memory for verbal information, and information processing speed, reliably predicts return to work or school. However, additional factors including social cognition also play a significant role. In addition to psychiatric symptoms, comorbid substance use can be a barrier to obtaining employment, as are multiple environmental factors including, most notably, access to supportive employment services.

- *School/Vocational Training* In the absence of specific interventions targeting work-related functioning, typical outpatient interventions generally do not adequately address issues of employment and return to work. Individual placement with supportive services (IPS) is one method that increases the likelihood of securing competitive employment as compared to conventional vocational rehabilitation services, and it also reduces the number of days of psychiatric hospitalization.

- *Capacity* Considerable attention has been paid to decision-making capacity in individuals with schizophrenia, particularly in treatment research, where informed consent is so important. The majority of people with schizophrenia have been found to possess adequate capacity for most decision-making roles, but there is enormous variation. For some individuals, the illness does interfere with decision-making to a significant degree, requiring intervention and identification of guardians, conservators, or other surrogates. The issues are complex and understandably have been associated with significant controversy and deliberation, including multiple Supreme Court decisions, which most frequently have upheld individual rights to refuse treatment or set high standards for involuntary treatment. Neuropsychologists must be familiar with relevant mental health laws and their application in the area in which they practice. There is evidence that the presence or absence of capacity may be more clearly related to cognitive function than other symptoms of the syndrome.

- *Emotional and Psychological Issues* Comorbid mental illness is a common problem in schizophrenia, and there may be syndromal overlap with other diagnostic entities including depression, obsessive-compulsive, and anxiety disorders. It can be particularly challenging to distinguish schizophrenia from schizoaffective disorder and mood disorders with psychotic features. The primary bases of differential diagnosis come from interview and history taking (to document whether depressive, manic, or mixed episodes have occurred together with active-phase symptoms and, if so, how their duration compares to active and residual periods). In some cases, objective personality testing or projective testing can highlight psychotic processes that may not emerge during interview. Significant problems are posed by comorbid substance use disorders. Cigarette smoking, for example, is extremely common among individuals with schizophrenia and includes all the associated health risks, which may be a contributing factor in the overall reduced life expectancy. Alcohol and illicit drug use also frequently complicate the diagnosis and management of people with schizophrenia. The question remains, however, as to whether the presence of comorbid disorders results in a unique presentation of schizophrenia and, furthermore, whether the comorbid disorders are a viable target of separate intervention.

- *Medications* Antipsychotic medications ameliorate positive symptoms of schizophrenia such as *hallucinations* and *delusions*, but do not usually yield cognitive benefits beyond limited normalization of certain attentional and receptive language skills. Higher doses of conventional *antipsychotic* drugs may be associated with some adverse effects on cognition, but a major clinical trial comparing newer *antipsychotic* agents (risperidone, olanzapine, aripiprazole) with a conventional *antipsychotic* drug (perphenazine) did not show any differences in cognitive functioning between groups, so it may be that only high doses, not widely used in clinical practice today, are responsible for the research findings of treatment-associated adverse effects. The use of lower doses of conventional *antipsychotic* agents is also associated with lower incidence of adverse effects on motor function including extrapyramidal symptoms (which are clearly dose-related), *tardive dyskinesia*, and tardive dystonia. There is a reliable adverse effect on cognitive function from overall anticholinergic burden, which is prominent in patients being treated with anticholinergic agents (e.g., cogentin, artane) for *extrapyramidal side effects*, and this is potentiated by benzodiazepine-like drugs. It should be noted that some *antipsychotic* drugs themselves have a significant impact on the cholinergic system (e.g., clozapine).

- Medications used to treat neuropsychological deficits in other cognitive disorders (e.g., cholinesterase inhibitors, modafinil, and stimulants) have yielded inconsistent results and/ or poor benefit–risk ratios. It should be noted that stimulants including amphetamines and methylphenidate are sometimes prescribed to address cognitive complaints for people with schizophrenia despite lack of evidence for efficacy. This may be particularly problematic because these agents may increase vulnerability to the development of psychotic episodes, given the body of literature showing that stimulants may precipitate psychosis in vulnerable individuals.

- People with schizophrenia often receive a range of other medications in addition to an *antipsychotic* agent. The most common additions are: (1) mood stabilizers and/or antidepressants, usually added to address treatment-nonresponsive mood disorders or affective lability; (2) sedatives, usually added to address agitation; (3) anticholinergic, to address iatrogenic movement disorders; and (4) soporifics, to address sleep disturbances. Because there is a high incidence of polypharmacy, it is important that the neuropsychologist pay attention to possible adverse effects of adjunctive treatments and in conjunction with physician colleagues carefully consider drug–drug interactions as possible contributors to cognitive impairment.

- Neuroleptic malignant syndrome (NMS) is an uncommon (with incidence about 0.01% to 0.02%) but potentially life-threatening reaction to antipsychotic drug treatment that involves fever, altered mental status, muscle rigidity, and autonomic dysfunction. If a patient receiving *antipsychotic* drugs presents with fever and mental status changes, it is important to recognize this syndrome rapidly. NMS usually occurs within hours or days and nearly all cases occur within 30 days of exposure to the drug.

- Serotonin syndrome is another relatively rare and also life-threatening adverse reaction to drugs that overstimulate 5-HT_{1A} receptors in the central gray nuclei and medulla, and possibly also overstimulation of 5-HT_2 receptors. It usually occurs more rapidly (within 24 hours of introduction of the causative serotonergic agent), and is sometimes confused with NMS because they both involve alterations in mental status, fever, muscle rigidity, and autonomic changes. While serotonin syndrome is usually linked to agents used as antidepressants or mood stabilizers, some *antipsychotic* agents, notably the atypical *antipsychotics*, may have substantial serotonergic effects, and patients with movement disorders or sleep problems may receive drugs that impact serotonin metabolism (e.g., L-dopa, selegiline for movement disorders, trazodone for insomnia) and can trigger serotonin syndrome.

- Finally, agranulocytosis is another rare and potentially fatal adverse reaction involving an acute lowering of white blood cells, that may arise among patients treated with a variety of agents, including antiepileptics, antidepressants, and *antipsychotics* but is particularly noteworthy among patients treated with clozapine. Agranulocytosis may also present with sudden fever, and the diagnosis is made after a complete blood count.

- *Other Novel Treatment Strategies* In addition to medication management, there have been recent advances in development of non-invasive neurostimulation methods designed to target specific symptoms and cognitive deficits in schizophrenia. Several approaches in development include transcranial pulsed ultrasound (TPU), transcranial direct current stimulation (tDCS), transcranial alternating current stimulation (tACS), and transcranial magnetic stimulation (TMS). These methods provide non-invasive regional brain stimulation to varying degrees of specificity, including both cortical and subcortical regions. So far, however, these interventions remain experimental.

- *Risk Factor Modification* A number of risk factors have been identified in schizophrenia epidemiology, although most show small effects. But some—such as advanced paternal age and winter or urban birth—may have a relatively large impact in the population. Stressors may play a role in both precipitating psychosis onset and increasing the likelihood of relapse, but, so far, intervention strategies focused on reducing stress or increasing stress coping skills have had at best mixed efficacy. Drug abuse may be a modifiable risk factor. The most well established risk factor for relapse is discontinuation of *antipsychotic* medication. Consequently long-acting *antipsychotic* agents have been introduced to promote compliance with prescribed treatments and reduced recidivism rates.

- *Interpersonal Relationships* Deficits in social cognition are considered one of the causes of poor functional outcomes and lower quality of life in schizophrenia, the effects of which may be significant over and above the impact of cognitive dysfunction. Social cognition is more strongly associated with positive community integration and social functioning than other neuropsychological functions, with the best outcomes obtained from a combination of social skills training and cognitive remediation.

Considerations when Treating Select Populations with Schizophrenia

Pediatric Considerations

Childhood-onset schizophrenia is defined as onset prior to the age of 13, and estimated prevalence rates approximate 1 in 10,000; early-onset schizophrenia is defined as development of psychotic symptoms between the ages of 13 and 17. Presentation of schizophrenia in children and adolescents is similar to that seen in young adults, and, moreover, similar diagnostic criteria may be employed with adequate reliability and diagnostic efficiency. *Antipsychotic* medications should be used cautiously with children, based on low rates of remission and frequent adverse effects, mainly metabolic syndrome.

Geriatric Considerations

There have been hypotheses that in late life, there may be a subgroup of people with schizophrenia who show unusually rapid cognitive decline, but recent reviews and meta-analyses indicate that the evidence so far is inconclusive, and more prospective longitudinal research is needed. It remains a high priority for clinicians to be alert to possible rapid decline in older people with schizophrenia, particularly to help rule out other treatable causes of impairment. It is clear that people with chronic schizophrenia have increased morbidity and mortality relative to age peers, and a range of preventable causes have been identified (smoking, obesity, hypercholesterolemia, diabetes mellitus, hypertension, and suicide), and long-term use of *antipsychotic* agents may contribute to the risks for abnormal lipid profiles (see "Epidemiology" section).

It is also important to recognize that late-onset schizophrenia (LOS), with onset after age 40) is relatively uncommon in men, but is observed more often in a subset of women, possibly related to hormonal changes after menopause. In older individuals (e.g., after age 60), the syndrome is sometimes referred to as "Very-Late-Onset Schizophrenia-like Psychosis" or VLOSLP). In LOS and VLOSLP special attention should be paid to ruling out mood disorders with psychotic features, psychotic disorders due to another medical condition and substance/medication-induced psychotic disorders. Both LOS and VLOSLP have been linked to lower genetic risk, suggesting that other environmental risks may predominate.

Cultural and Individual Differences

There is substantial heterogeneity of symptom presentation in schizophrenia, yet our understanding of individual differences and cultural factors which may contribute to that heterogeneity is incomplete. In addition, cultural and ethnic disparities exist in terms of treatment access and patient outcomes, with disadvantages consistently reported for minority populations in countries such as the United States and Great Britain. Culturally adapted psychosocial interventions are increasingly being validated for use with such populations to address these concerns. It is also important to consider cultural and socioeconomic background factors before making a diagnosis, as these may play a role in determining presence of *delusions* and *hallucinations* (certain beliefs and perceptions, for example experiences involving communications with God or deceased relatives, are culturally normative). Further, anomalies in speech and language, eye contact, and other aspects of emotional expression may vary markedly across cultural contexts. The DSM-5 Cultural Formulation (pp. 749–659) includes background on relevant concepts and a Cultural Formulation Interview that is valuable.

Relevant Definitions

Antipsychotic A medication used in the treatment of psychotic symptoms; they are most often used to alleviate positive symptoms. Traditional or "first-generation" antipsychotic medications include chlorpromazine (Thorazine), haloperidol (Haldol), and fluphenazine (Prolixin), all of which are thought to have their antipsychotic efficacy mediated by action at D_2-type dopamine receptors. These drugs were once called neuroleptic drugs due to their tendency to produce parkinsonian motor symptoms. Second-generation antipsychotic agents also have activity at D_2-type receptors, but also tend to have more complex pharmacological profiles; these agents include clozapine (Clozaril), olanzapine (Zyprexa), aripiprazole (Abilify), and risperidone (Risperdal).

Catatonia A state characterized by significant motoric disturbance including symptoms such as (1) motor immobility or stupor, (2) excess motor activity that has no apparent purpose, (3) extreme negativism or mutism, (4) peculiar movements (posturing, stereotyped movements), and (5) echolalia or echopraxia.

Delusion A strongly held personal conviction that is often firmly maintained despite compelling evidence that it is false.

Diathesis A predisposition that serves as the background upon which environmental effects cause disease. The "diathesis-stress" model suggests that schizophrenia is caused by the combination of pre-existing vulnerabilities (from genetic, perinatal, and possibly subsequent alterations in brain development) upon which stressors act, causing symptoms to appear.

Dopamine A catecholamine neurotransmitter (or messenger) involved in pleasure, sexual functioning, interest, and apathy. It is found in the mesolimbic, tuberoinfundibular, mesocortical, and nigrostriatal pathways in the brain.

Extrapyramidal side effects Signs and symptoms that occur following the use of antipsychotic medication; can be acute or chronic. The acute symptoms include parkinsonism, dystonia, and akathisia. Chronic signs include tardive dystonia and tardive dyskinesia.

Hallucination A false sensory distortion in an individual's experience of reality that occurs in the absence of an external sensory stimulus. A hallucination can involve any of the five senses or a combination of them.

Tardive dyskinesia A neurological syndrome of involuntary movements of the head, tongue, trunk, or extremities associated with the long-term use of antipsychotic medications or drugs that block dopamine receptors. Signs of tardive dyskinesia include chorea, facial grimacing, dystonia, tics, tongue protrusion, and rapid eye blinking.

Theory of mind An ability to recognize the thoughts of others as distinct from one's own thoughts, to recognize others' intentions, and to take another individual's perspective. These abilities develop rapidly in healthy individuals over the first few years of life and are usually impaired in schizophrenia and ASDs, and more rarely in other brain disorders.

Schizophrenia Spectrum and Other Psychotic Disorders Questions

NOTE: Questions 21, 29, 69, 92, and 103 on the First Full-Length Practice Examination, Questions 5, 31, 63, and 111 on the Second Full-Length Practice Examination, Questions 10, 39, 62, 98, and 117 on the Third Full-Length Practice Examination, and Questions 1, 17, 52, 97, and 115 on the Fourth Full-Length Practice Examination are from this chapter.

1. A major benefit of second-generation antipsychotic drugs is amelioration of _____.
   (a) cognitive deficits
   (b) positive symptoms
   (c) extrapyramidal symptoms
   (d) social skills deficits

2. Which of the following treatments has shown consistent benefits for cognitive functioning in schizophrenia?
   (a) cognitive remediation
   (b) inhibiting glycine reuptake
   (c) acetylcholinesterase inhibition
   (d) aerobic exercise

3. Early-onset schizophrenia is defined as development of symptoms _____.
   (a) between the ages of 13 and 17
   (b) prior to age 12
   (c) after age 18 but before 21
   (d) prior to age 6

4. The DSM-5 retains which of the following diagnostic specifiers?
   (a) disorganized
   (b) paranoid
   (c) undifferentiated
   (d) with catatonia

5. According to most definitions, negative symptoms include ____.

   (a) formal thought disorder and bizarre behavior

   (b) delusions and hallucinations

   (c) flat affect and avolition/apathy

   (d) attention and memory impairments

6. The genetic risk for schizophrenia is ____.

   (a) probably explained by five to ten genetic polymorphisms

   (b) probably explained by thousands of genetic variations, each of which has a small effect

   (c) probably explained by a few rare mutations affecting dopamine metabolism (e.g., the dopamine transporter, COMT, and MAO)

   (d) probably largely the byproduct of epigenetic changes

7. Current recommendations for evidence-based practice in the treatment of schizophrenia include all but which of the following psychosocial interventions?

   (a) assertive community treatment (ACT)

   (b) supported employment

   (c) cognitive behavioral therapy

   (d) dialectical behavior therapy

8. The DSM-5 diagnosis of schizophrenia requires continuous signs of disturbance lasting for at least what period of time?

   (a) 1 month   (c) 6 months

   (b) 3 months   (d) 12 months

9. How is schizophrenia best distinguished from schizophreniform disorder?

   (a) symptoms and symptom duration   (c) symptoms and decrement in functioning

   (b) symptom duration and decrement in functioning   (d) symptom duration only

10. Men with schizophrenia tend to have ____ illness onset, ____ negative symptom severity, and ____ affective symptoms.

   (a) earlier; higher; lower   (c) later; higher; greater

   (b) earlier; lower; greater   (d) later; higher; lower

Schizophrenia Spectrum and Other Psychotic Disorders Answers

1. **B—positive symptoms** *The major action of both conventional and atypical antipsychotic medications is reduction of frequency and severity of positive symptoms; neither yield consistent, significant cognitive or social cognitive benefits. Extrapyramidal motor symptoms are side effects of conventional antipsychotics.*

Reference: Leucht, S., Corves, C., Arbter, D., Engel, R. R., Li, C., & Davis, J. M. (2009). Second-generation versus first-generation antipsychotic drugs for schizophrenia: A meta-analysis. *Lancet, 373*(9657), 31–41.

2. **A—cognitive remediation**   *The positive effect of medication on cognition in schizophrenia has been inconsistent; in contrast, cognitive remediation strategies have been shown to produce reliable improvements in multiple domains of cognition regardless of symptom severity. There have been some small studies suggesting that exercise may be beneficial, but the evidence so far is not consistent.*

Reference: Wykes, T., Huddy, V., Cellard, C., McGurk, S., & Czobor, P. (2011). A meta-analysis of cognitive remediation for schizophrenia: Methodology and effect sizes. *American Journal of Psychiatry, 168*(5), 472–485.

3. **A—between the ages of 13 and 17**   *Early-onset schizophrenia is characterized by development of the disorder in childhood or early adolescence, generally between the ages of 13 and 17.*

Reference: American Psychiatric Association. (2013). *Diagnostic and statistical manual of mental disorders* (5th ed.). Washington, DC: American Psychiatric Publishing.

4. **D—with catatonia**   *The criteria for the DSM-5 no longer include specification of subtypes, but retain this one specifier; there is also an optional severity specifier.*

Reference: American Psychiatric Association. (2013). *Diagnostic and statistical manual of mental disorders* (5th. ed.). Washington, DC: American Psychiatric Publishing.

5. **C—flat affect and avolition/apathy**   *Negative symptoms, originally referred to as "negative" to signify a loss or decrease of normal function in contrast to positive symptoms, is a term that was first applied to the "five A's," affective flattening, alogia, anhedonia, avolition-apathy and attentional impairment. Alogia and attentional impairment, however, may better be considered part of the disorganization syndrome.*

Reference: American Psychiatric Association. (2013). *Diagnostic and statistical manual of mental disorders* (5th ed.). Washington, DC: American Psychiatric Publishing.

6. **B—probably explained by thousands of genetic variations, each of which has a small effect**   *There may be some sporadic cases of schizophrenia spectrum disorders that are caused by rare mutations, but most of the risk is better understood as reflecting thousands of small contributions across the genome, affecting many different systems.*

Reference: Anttila, V., Bulik-Sullivan, B., Finucane, H. K., Walters, R.K., Bras, J., Duncan, L., . . . Patsopoulos, N. A. (2018). Analysis of shared heritability in common disorders of the brain. *Science, 360*(6395), 1–15.

7. **D—dialectical behavior therapy**   *Evidence-based practices for schizophrenia that address symptom management and psychosocial functioning based on randomized controlled trials research include all of the interventions listed, except dialectical behavior therapy.*

Reference: Dixon, L. B., Dickerson, F., Bellack, A. S., Bennett, M., Dickinson, D., Goldberg, R. W., . . . Kreyenbuhl J. (2010). The 2009 Schizophrenia PORT Psychosocial Treatment Recommendations and Summary Statements. *Schizophrenia Bulletin, 36*(1), 48–70.

8. **C—6 months**   *The diagnosis of schizophrenia requires that continuous signs of the disturbance persist for a 6-month period.*

Reference: American Psychiatric Association. (2013). *Diagnostic and statistical manual of mental disorders* (5th ed.). Washington, DC: American Psychiatric Publishing.

9. **B—symptom duration and decrement in functioning**   *Schizophreniform disorder has the same symptoms as schizophrenia but does not last 6 months and does not require a decrement in functioning for diagnosis.*

Reference: American Psychiatric Association. (2013). *Diagnostic and statistical manual of mental disorders* (5th ed.). Washington, DC: American Psychiatric Publishing.

10. **A—earlier; higher; lower**   *Men with schizophrenia tend to have earlier illness onset, higher negative symptom severity and lower affective symptoms when compared to women. In addition, women with schizophrenia tend to have better social, cognitive, and premorbid functioning than men with schizophrenia.*

Reference: Hanlon, M. C., Campbell, L. E., Single, N., Coleman, C., Morgan, V. A., Cotton, S. M., . . . Castle, D. J. (2017). Men and women with psychosis and the impact of illness-duration on sex-differences: The second Australian national survey of psychosis. *Psychiatry Research, 256*, 130–143.

Recommended Readings

American Psychiatric Association. (2013). *Diagnostic and statistical manual for mental disorders* (5th ed.). (DSM-5). Washington, DC: American Psychiatric Press.

Degnan, A., Baker, S., Edge, D., Nottidge, W., Noke, M., Press, C. J., . . . Drake, R. J. (2018). The nature and efficacy of culturally-adapted psychosocial interventions for schizophrenia: A systematic review and meta-analysis. *Psychological Medicine, 48*(5), 714–727.

Marcopulos, B. A., & Kurtz, M. M. (2012). *Clinical and neuropsychological foundations of schizophrenia*. New York, NY: Psychology Press.

Seidman, L., & Mirsky, A. (2017). Evolving notions of schizophrenia as a developmental neurocognitive disorder. *Journal of the International Neuropsychological Society, 23*(9–10), 881–892.

Wykes, T., Huddy, V., Cellard, C., McGurk, S., & Czobor, P. (2011). A meta-analysis of cognitive remediation for schizophrenia: Methodology and effect sizes. *American Journal of Psychiatry, 168*(5), 472–485.

36 Substance Use Disorders

Robin C. Hilsabeck and Eileen M. Martin

Introduction

Misuse of alcohol or licit or illicit drugs is often neurotoxic. Neurocognitive impairment and disruption of daily function are common among individuals who meet criteria for a *substance use disorder* (SUD). The *Diagnostic and Statistical Manual of Mental Disorders, Fifth Edition* (DSM-5) broadly defines SUDs as a cluster of behavioral, physiological, and cognitive symptoms indicating persistent use of a given substance despite significant associated problems. Three severity levels, mild, moderate, and severe, are determined based on the number of criteria met. These criteria apply to ten separate classes of substances, including alcohol, opioids, cannabis, hallucinogens, sedative/hypnotics, and stimulants. DSM-5 diagnostic criteria for SUDs do not distinguish "substance abuse" from "substance dependence" as was the case in DSM-IV. The National Institute on Drug Abuse (NIDA) and many researchers define *"addiction"* as a chronic, relapsing disease that includes compulsive substance seeking and use despite full knowledge of harmful consequences. For purposes of clarity, this chapter employs "SUD" and *"addiction"* interchangeably.

Patients with known or suspected SUDs are often referred for neuropsychological evaluation, especially in Veterans Administration (VA) or correctional settings, and a working knowledge of common and uncommon neurocognitive effects of SUDs is essential for effective clinical assessment. The focus of this chapter is SUDs most commonly encountered by clinical neuropsychologists in the United States. Websites for NIDA, the National Institute on Alcohol Abuse and Alcoholism (NIAAA), and the Substance Abuse and Mental Health Services Administration (SAMHSA) are excellent resources for understanding the scope of the problem and changes over time. Below are some introductory facts about SUDs:

- The 12-month prevalence of DSM-5 alcohol use disorder (AUD) is approximately 14%; lifetime prevalence is about 29%. Mild AUD is twice as prevalent as moderate and severe (i.e., approximately 7% vs. 3% and 3%, respectively) within the past 12 months while lifetime prevalence of mild and moderate AUD is less common than severe AUD (i.e., approximately 9%, 7%, and 14%, respectively).

- The 12-month prevalence of other drug use disorders (DUDs) is about 4% while lifetime prevalence is approximately 10%. Mild and moderate to severe DUDs occur at equal rates of approximately 2% when considering the past 12 months but lifetime prevalence of moderate to severe DUD is almost twice as common as mild DUD. Cannabis, opioids, and cocaine are more prevalent than other DUDs.

- There are sex differences in essentially every aspect of SUDs. For example, women become addicted more rapidly, experience more severe withdrawal, and relapse more readily with stimulants. Additionally, functional neuroimaging studies have shown sex differences in the pattern and type of neural activity in response to drug cues.

- Motor vehicle accidents, brain injury, suicide, psychiatric disorders, chronic diseases such as liver cirrhosis and diabetes, neonatal conditions such as fetal alcohol syndrome, and infections with *human immunodeficiency virus* (HIV) or *hepatitis C virus* (HCV) are more prevalent among individuals with SUDs compared with the general population.

- Consequences of SUDs for the community include lost work hours, domestic violence, demands on law enforcement, legal and correctional facilities, and service agencies; and costs of emergency room visits and detoxification.

Section 1: Commonalities Across SUDs

Demographic Risk Factors

The following are key demographic risk factors for SUDs according to DMS-5 criteria as determined by face-to-face semi-structured interviews with over 36,000 civilian non-institutionalized adults aged 18 and over as part of the 2012–2013 National Epidemiologic Survey on Alcohol and Related Conditions III (NESARC-III) (Grant et al., 2015, 2016).

- *Male sex* Men are nearly twice as likely to meet criteria for an AUD in the past 12 months and severe AUD in their lifetimes (about 18% vs. 10% for women). For DUDs, approximately 5% of men compared to 3% of women will meet criteria in the past 12 months and about 12% of men compared to 8% of women will meet criteria for DUDs in their lifetimes.

- *Age 18-29 years* The average age of onset of SUDs is early- to mid-20s. However, SUDs typically begin during adolescence, and poorer outcomes are related to earlier initiation of substance use. Alcohol is the most common substance used during youth, followed by cannabis.

- *Native American ethnicity* Individuals of Native American ethnicity have a lifetime prevalence of 43% for AUDs and 17% for DUDs. In comparison, lifetime prevalence rates of other ethnicities range from 15%–33% for AUD and 4%–11% for DUDs. Individuals of Asian or Pacific Islander ethnicities have the lowest lifetime prevalence rates of 6% for AUD and 4% for DUDs.

- *Education ≤ 12 years* 12-month and lifetime prevalence rates of AUDs are approximately 26% and 51%, respectively, in individuals with a high school education or less compared to 12-month and lifetime prevalence rates of 14% and 31%, respectively, for individuals with at least some college. For DUDs, 12-month and lifetime prevalence rates are nearly 10% and 22%, respectively, for individuals with a high school education or less compared to 3% and 9%, respectively, for individuals with some college education.

- *Income < 20,000/year* 12-month prevalence of AUDs tends to decrease as annual income increases, and for DUDs, the prevalence is approximately double that of the next two income categories (i.e., $20,000–$34,999 and $35,000–$69,999) and nearly four times as prevalent as that of individuals who make $70,000/year or more.

Comorbidities

Interpretation of neuropsychological test data from individuals with SUDs is not always straightforward. In the United States, most individuals with SUDs misuse multiple substances: "pure" use of one substance is uncommon, and it can be difficult or impossible to distinguish neurocognitive effects of one substance from another. To make matters more difficult, multiple medical and neuropsychiatric conditions are comorbid with SUDs and can further confound neurocognitive findings.

Medical

Multiple medical comorbidities of chronic substance use arise from chronic drug exposure, high-risk sexual and injection practices and consequences of chaotic social and environmental factors, such as domestic violence and trauma. Below are a few of the most common medical comorbidities in people with SUDs, all of which may affect neurocognitive performance:

- infections such as HIV, HCV, and endocarditis
- myocardial infarction and stroke
- cirrhosis and other liver diseases
- hyperthermia, dehydration
- traumatic brain injury

Neuropsychiatric

Neuropsychiatric conditions are also highly prevalent in people with SUDs and often predate substance use. Premorbid characteristics associated with increased risk for SUDs include emotional dysregulation, impulsivity, risk-taking, and poor judgment. Frequent co-occurring neuropsychiatric comorbidities include:

- *Mood disorders*, especially major depressive disorder (MDD) and bipolar disorder (BD). Prevalence of SUDs in persons with BD range from 20% to 70% and from 10% to 30% in persons with MDD. AUD is the most common SUD in individuals with BD, occurring in about 42%, and cannabis use disorder is the next most common at about 20%.

- *Schizophrenia* Lifetime prevalence of SUDs in people with schizophrenia is approximately 50%. Alcohol, cannabis, cocaine, and amphetamines are the substances most commonly used following nicotine, and many individuals engage in polysubstance use.

- *Posttraumatic stress disorder (PTSD)* Approximately one third of individuals with SUD have co-occurring PTSD.

- *Anxiety disorders* 12-month prevalence rates of SUDs in people with anxiety disorders range from 33% to 45%

- *ADHD* Prevalence rates of ADHD in individuals with SUDs range from 10–33%. AUD and cannabis use disorder are higher in persons with ADHD compared to the general population.

- *Obsessive-compulsive disorder (OCD)* Approximately one fourth of individuals with OCD will meet criteria for SUD in their lifetime.

- *Personality disorders*, particularly borderline and antisocial. Up to 62% of individuals treated for SUDs meet criteria for personality disorder, with over one fourth meeting criteria for more than one personality disorder. Borderline and antisocial personality disorders are most common, occurring in approximately 15% and 14%, respectively.

- *Neuropsychiatric disorders*, especially depression, are more highly prevalent among women with SUDs.

- A positive family history of one or more of these disorders is common and should be queried in any interview.

Suicidality

A special note should be made about SUDs and suicidality. Substance use, particularly alcohol use, is present in a substantial number of suicides and suicide attempts. Blood alcohol levels (BACs) over the legal limit are present in approximately 22% of completed suicide and in 30%–40% of suicide attempts. Multiple substances are often present on toxicology screens with completed suicides, most often opioids and marijuana at 20% and 10%, respectively. It is hypothesized that the strong link between substance use and suicide is due in part to the disinhibiting effects of substances during intoxication.

Neurobiology of Addiction

Conceptualization of *addiction* as a disease of the brain is still somewhat controversial, but mounting evidence has characterized the underlying neural circuitry contributing to the chronic, relapsing nature of SUDs as well as pre-existing neural risk factors for initiating and escalating substance use during adolescence. While profiles of neural and behavioral effects of different substances are not identical, certain neurobehavioral abnormalities are observed with all SUDs, reflecting disruption of common mesolimbic and prefrontal cortical pathways and dopaminergic systems. Physiological effects and associated neurotransmitter systems for nine substances commonly used in North America are summarized in Table 36.1.

Neurobiologic Circuitry

- Dopaminergic projections of the *mesocorticolimbic* system are considered the neural substrates mediating motivation and reward.
- Intoxicating doses of many substances, including alcohol, cannabis, opioids, cocaine, and methamphetamine, release dopamine into the *ventral striatum*, primarily the nucleus accumbens, where a large number of dopamine receptors are present. The degree of subjective euphoria is dependent in part on the rate of dopamine release.
- Repeated episodes of substance use paired with rewarding subjective experience results in the association of reward with environmental stimuli or cues that precede actual substance use. Thus, people and places associated with frequent use may become triggers that elicit craving and substance-seeking behaviors, resulting in additional use.
- Over time, release of dopamine in response to the substance and its cues becomes attenuated and blunts rewarding feelings to all stimuli, including non-substance-related stimuli that used to be rewarding. Prefrontal brain systems underlying decision-making, self-regulation, mental flexibility, and error monitoring are affected by dopamine down-regulation. Impaired glutamate signaling in prefrontal systems also contributes to craving and decreased motivation to avoid further drug use.
- Other neuroadaptations associated with repeated, heavy substance use include decreased capacity to tolerate stress or negative emotions mediated by the amygdala and basal forebrain. This decrease in "distress tolerance" can precipitate substance use with the goal of "self-medication" through negative reinforcement or fuel further substance use to avoid symptoms of withdrawal. This withdrawal response is associated with decreases in dopaminergic, serotonergic, and gamma-aminobutyric acid (GABA)ergic transmission and increases in glutamatergic transmission. Dysregulation of the hypothalamic-pituitary-adrenal (HPA) axis is also evident as indicated by elevations in corticotropin-releasing factor in the amygdala.
- In general, neuroimaging findings consistently reveal reductions in cortical volume, particularly in the frontal lobes, functional disturbances to frontostriatal circuitry, and changes in anterior white matter. However, a great deal of heterogeneity is evident across imaging studies

TABLE 36.1 Effects of Licit and Illicit Substances

Substance	Physiological Effect	Primary Immediate Neurocognitive Effect	Chronic Neurocognitive effect	Primary Neurotransmitter System Affected
Alcohol	Sedation, including muscle relaxation, slurred speech, and somnolence	Loss of inhibitions, poor decision-making, and slowed reaction times	Small effects on processing speed, learning, and working memory	Dopamine, serotonin, glutamate, GABA
Cannabis	Sedation, mood elevation, and hallucination	Adverse effects on learning and memory	No serious neurotoxicity	Binding to endogenous cannabinoid receptor (CB1)
Cocaine	Euphoria, increases in energy and motor activity	Improved attention, processing speed, and inhibition	Decreased attention, working memory, and visual memory	Increased dopamine availability in limbic system
Methamphetamines	Increased neural firing, euphoria, vasoconstriction, appetite suppression, increases in respiration, energy, and libido	Enhanced attention and speed of information processing, paranoid psychosis	Decreased verbal episodic memory, complex information processing speed, working memory, response inhibition, novel problem solving, and decision-making	Mesolimbic-mesocortical and nigro-striatal dopaminergic pathways
Barbiturates	Reduced neural firing Sedation, euphoria, anxiolytic, respiratory depression, decreased blood pressure	Decreased concentration, confusion, impaired coordination, and impaired decision-making	Risk of cognitive impairment Risk of depression	GABA receptor
Benzodiazepines	Reduced neural firing Sedation	Mental slowing Anterograde amnesia	Memory and motor deficits	GABA receptor
Opioids	Decreased pain perception, sedation, respiratory depression, constipation, and euphoria	Attention, working memory, psychomotor speed, problem solving, and decision-making	Deficits in executive functioning, working memory, and impulsivity	Binding to endogenous opioid receptors
Hallucinogens	Marked alteration in sensory gating, perception, mood, and thought Acute psychosis Dreamlike states Pseudohallucination	Heightened response to internal stimuli, reduced effectiveness responding to external stimuli	Studies of chronic cognitive effects not available	Serotonin
Ecstasy	Euphoria, extroversion, elevated mood, Hallucination, confusion	Few studies to warrant generalization. Possible memory deficits	Decreased short and long term memory, and attention	Serotonin

due to comorbid disorders; additionally, abnormalities observed with different drug classes (e.g., methamphetamine) are more frequent and severe than others.

- Individuals who relapse show persistent increases in activation to substance-related cues/rewards, reduced activation to non-substance-related cues, and reduced connectivity in mesocortical and striatal regions after cessation of use compared to individuals who remain abstinent.

- Neuroimaging studies provide compelling evidence of sex differences in responsivity to cue-induced cocaine cues, including decreased amygdala activity among women but increased activation among men.

Pre-Existing Neural Risk Factors

- Maturation of brain regions involved in reward systems (e.g., *mesocorticolimbic* areas) occurs before brain regions responsible for cognitive control and inhibition (e.g., prefrontal areas), which may play a role in decisions to engage in risky behaviors, such as substance use, during adolescence.

- Rapid development of the brain during adolescence may increase its vulnerability to persistent effects of excessive substance use. For example, heavy drinking in adolescence results in accelerated gray matter volume loss in frontal and temporal brain regions and attenuated increases in white matter volume compared to non-users.

- Structural brain differences and alterations in neural response patterns during tasks requiring inhibition, working memory, and reward processing are markers for vulnerability to substance use initiation and escalation. For example:

  - Both longitudinal, prospective studies and cross-sectional studies suggest that poor inhibitory functioning and altered working memory are risk factors for initiating and escalating substance use during adolescence.

  - Less brain volume in regions involved in impulsivity (prefrontal cortex-subcortical circuitry), reward sensitivity (nucleus accumbens) and decision-making (anterior cingulate) and altered white matter integrity are associated with increased likelihood of initiation of substance use during adolescence.

Expectations for Neuropsychological Assessment Results

It is important to note that while there is extensive literature on neurocognitive effects of substance use, methodological variations and inconsistencies, including participant characteristics, measures utilized, and inclusion/exclusion criteria applied, contribute to contradictory findings and conclusions. Further, variables such as age of onset, patterns of use (e.g., amount, type, frequency, polysubstance), severity and duration of use, number of episodes of withdrawal, and duration of abstinence are typically not addressed in a systematic way, if at all. However, some general conclusions can be drawn:

- Neuropsychological functioning is globally affected in individuals with SUDs, with executive functions most commonly affected and language/verbal intellectual functions least affected.

- Neurocognitive impairment is more common and severe among persons with AUD or stimulant use disorder, especially methamphetamine.

- Milder neurocognitive impairment is not uncommon among individuals with heavy substance use that does not meet DSM-5 criteria for SUD.

Although neurocognitive effects of different SUDs are not identical since each substance exerts "idiomatic" effects on certain brain pathways, *all* substances of abuse result in some degree of impairment in executive functions, particularly:

- Decision-making, the ability to choose a delayed but optimal outcome over an attractive immediate reward, as indexed by measures such as the Iowa Gambling Task and Delay Discounting (a questionnaire about the amount of time the patient is willing to wait for different amounts of money, e.g., "Would you prefer $10 today or $25 next week?").

- Capacity to suppress a prepotent but incorrect behavior (e.g., Stroop and Go/No Tasks).

- Difficulty with set switching, i.e., ability to adapt ongoing behavior in response to a change in context (e.g., Wisconsin Card Sorting Test).

- Ability to form strategies to enhance performance on memory or other neurocognitive tasks (e.g., semantic clustering component of the California Verbal Learning Test [CVLT] or the Hopkins Verbal Learning Test).

Other neurocognitive domains frequently affected by SUDs are:

- Sustained attention/concentration (e.g., Digit Vigilance Test).

- Processing speed, particularly speeded tasks with a cognitive component (e.g., Trail Making Test–Part B).

- *Verbal and spatial episodic memory* Impaired performance on memory tasks, such as the CVLT and Rey-Osterreith Complex Figure Test (RCFT) is common; however, deficits in non-memory functions, particularly executive impairment that interferes with acquisition and encoding, often account for poor performance on memory tasks rather than impairment in free recall, retention, or recognition. For example, individuals with AUDs typically produce a poorly organized, spatially distorted RCFT copy trial that may be mistaken for evidence of structural or functional abnormalities in the nondominant hemisphere.

- Visuoperception/visuospatial abilities, by measures such as WAIS-IV Block Design or RCFT although executive impairment frequently affects performance on these tasks as well.

- Working memory, indexed by performance on the WAIS-IV Letter-Number Sequencing subtest or other tasks requiring mental activity with no external cues provided.

For a high-level summary of immediate and chronic neurocognitive effects for substances commonly used in North America, refer to Table 36.1.

Longitudinal data in heavy substance-using youth in treatment at age 16 and followed approximately 10 years have shown that learning and memory, visuospatial functioning, and attention and working memory were performed more poorly by heavy substance users compared to non-users and persisted even in youth whose SUD had remitted. Studies suggest a dose-dependent relationship between worse cognitive functioning and heavier use patterns and greater hangover and withdrawal symptoms over time.

Longitudinal studies of adults with SUDs are limited but results of meta-analyses reveal medium to large effect sizes in most neurocognitive domains for most substances except cannabis, which tends to affect fewer domains at smaller magnitudes. Attenuation of deficits over time with longer periods of abstinence also is suggested. It is hypothesized that neural repair or regeneration and/or reorganization of neural networks may account for improved cognitive performance. Neuroimaging studies also show recovery in brain volume, neurochemistry, and microstructure following periods of abstinence, which have been associated with improved performance on neuropsychological measures. Potential reasons for recovery of neural tissue include remyelination, rehydration, and/or neurogenesis.

Evidence-Based Treatment and Outcomes

Relapse, defined as a return to substance use following a period of abstinence, is common among individuals with SUDs and occurs at similar frequencies to other chronic diseases, such as type 1 diabetes, asthma, and hypertension. Three or four treatment admissions are usually needed before at least 50% of individuals are able to remain abstinent for a year or longer. Fortunately, relapse rates become more stable over time, and relapse is rare in individuals who remain abstinent for 5 years. Better outcomes are associated with more intense treatment, less severe substance use problems, less cognitive impairment, higher self-confidence about outcome, and fewer comorbid psychiatric conditions.

Due to the chronicity of relapse and the many aspects of life it affects, treatment approaches are long-term and multimodal, aimed at reducing length, frequency, and severity of substance use while simultaneously improving health and quality of life. A comprehensive treatment program typically includes medical and psychiatric care, counseling, case management, and peer support groups, as well as access to support for vocational, legal, financial, housing, transportation, and child care needs. Treatment for SUDs often involve:

- assessment,
- management of intoxication and withdrawal symptoms,
- treatment of comorbid psychiatric and medical conditions, and
- development of a long-term treatment plan focused on abstinence or reducing use and associated harms, relapse prevention, and improved psychosocial functioning.

Unfortunately, there is limited research elucidating which individuals benefit from which treatment approaches (or components) at which frequencies and for how long. Notably, only about 20–25% of persons with SUDs receive treatment. Another significant limitation in understanding outcomes is that a large majority of potential study participants—between 64–96%–are excluded from treatment research, which limits the external validity of findings. In alcohol studies, for example, severity of alcohol problems and psychiatric problems are the top two most common exclusion criteria applied, with individuals with more several substance and psychiatric problems excluded from treatment studies. African Americans and individuals with low incomes have also been disproportionately excluded from treatment studies.

Treatment for neuropsychological deficits associated with SUDs is an emerging area of interest. Rehabilitative efforts have focused on executive dysfunction and working memory deficits and typically employ computerized training approaches. However, this research is in its early stages, and important details about frequency and breadth of training, which individuals are most likely to benefit, duration of treatment effects, and generalization are unknown.

Psychosocial Interventions

Psychosocial approaches primarily target motivation and cognitive bias. Cognitive-behavioral therapies in a variety of formats have been shown to have small to moderate treatment effects in SUDs. There has been a growing interest in developing psychosocial treatments for specific conditions that commonly co-occur with SUD, such as BD, PTSD, and ADHD. Early work has been promising but additional research is needed before wide adoption can be recommended. In 2015, the VA and Department of Defense (DoD) updated their clinical practice guideline for SUDs and after an extensive review, they reported good evidence for the following psychosocial interventions within the first 90 days of recovery:

- Behavioral Couples Therapy (alcohol)
- Cognitive Behavioral Coping Skills Training (alcohol, stimulants, cannabis)
- Community Reinforcement Approach (alcohol, stimulants)

- Motivational Enhancement Therapy (alcohol, cannabis)
- 12-step support groups such as Alcoholics Anonymous and Narcotics Anonymous provide a useful adjunct to treatment but have not been formally reviewed by clinical practice guidelines and are not considered a stand-alone treatment.

Pharmacotherapy

Pharmacological interventions aim to reduce craving, increase cognitive control, and/or decrease stress reactivity and negative moods. Pharmacotherapy for SUDs is an understudied area with few FDA-approved treatments available (i.e., disulfiram, acamprosate, and naltrexone for AUD and methadone, buprenorphine, and naltrexone for opioid use disorder). Medication management strategies supported by research include:

- medications that reduce distress during acute withdrawal, such as benzodiazepines (BZDs),
- agonists that mimic drug effects, resulting in reduced withdrawal symptoms and cravings (e.g., nalmefene),
- antagonists that block drug rewards (e.g., naltrexone),
- medications that produce adverse reactions to a substance (e.g., disulfiram), and
- medications that treat psychiatric symptoms during recovery (e.g., antidepressants).

The 2015 VA/DoD clinical practice guidelines for SUDs indicate there is good evidence for use of acamprosate, disulfiram, naltrexone (oral or extended release), and topiramate for AUD. For opioid use disorder, there is good evidence for the combination of buprenorphine/naloxone and methadone in the context of an opioid treatment program. Buprenorphine alone and extended-release injectable naltrexone were recommended with good evidence in certain circumstances.

Neuromodulation

An emerging area of research is electrophysiological treatment of SUDs, particularly repeated transcranial magnetic stimulation (rTMS) and deep brain stimulation (DBS). The options are being explored primarily in patients with treatment refractory SUDs. Areas targeted in DBS are the nucleus accumbens and the subthalamic nucleus. Areas targeted in rTMS are dorsolateral prefrontal cortex and orbitofrontal cortex, which are involved in inhibitory control of substance use. It may also reduce cravings through modulation of the HPA and dopaminergic systems. It is important to note that both pharmacological and electrophysiological treatments are always used in combination with psychosocial approaches, and these treatment approaches are still in the early stages of study and require additional validation.

Section 2: Specific Substances

Alcohol

Key Terms and Definitions

NIAAA, SAHMSA, and Alcoholism and Dietary Guidelines from the United States Department of Health and Human Services and United States Department of Agriculture provide the following definitions:

- *Moderate alcohol use* Up to 1 drink per day for women and 2 drinks per day for men.
- *Low-risk drinking* ≤ 3 drinks per day and ≤ 7 drinks per week for women and ≤ 4 drinks per day and ≤ 14 drinks per week for men.

- *Binge drinking* ≥ 4 drinks for women and ≥ 5 drinks for men within about 2 hours, which brings BAC levels to 0.08 g/dL for most individuals, which is the point at which one is considered legally impaired or intoxicated in most states in the United States.

- *Heavy drinking* ≥ 8 drinks for women and ≥ 15 drinks for men in a week or binge drinking on ≥ 5 days in the past month.

- *Excessive alcohol use* Includes both binge and heaving drinking

Primary Mechanism of Action

There is no specific alcohol receptor or molecular target; the neurobiologic circuitry described earlier applies to AUD. Genes explain 40–60% of risk of AUD, and the rest is explained by gene–environment interactions.

Clinical Presentation, Disease Course, and Recovery

The usual age of first drinking is 15 years old, with variations across cultural groups. However, this age does not predict who will develop AUD. Earlier age of regular drinking is more strongly associated to risk of AUD. Heaviest drinking is usually between the ages of 18 and 22, although this also is not necessarily predictive of who will develop AUD. Repeated heavy drinking is associated with 40% risk of temporary depressive episodes and associated suicidal ideation and attempts, severe anxiety, and insomnia. These episodes can be considered substance-induced and typically improve with 2 to 4 weeks of abstinence. Polysubstance use is common, particularly for individuals with very early-onset AUD and antisocial personalities.

Clinically relevant symptoms of withdrawal occur in about 50% of individuals with AUD. Withdrawal symptoms begin about 6 to 8 hours after significant decreases in BAC levels, peak on day 2 or 3, and are substantially reduced by day 4 or 5. Fewer than 5% of individuals with AUD experience grand mal seizures or delirium tremens (DTs), which is a severe agitated state characterized by confusion, disorientation, hallucinations, and/or seizures. In rare cases DTs can last up to 2 weeks but usually subside within 5 days. For a more detailed discussion of delirium, see Chapter 27.

AUD has a fluctuating course like other chronic medical diseases characterized by days to months of sobriety, often precipitated by a crisis, followed by a period of temporary controlled drinking, which usually then gives way to increasing intake and heavy drinking. Treatment is effective at decreasing heavy drinking, with about 50–60% of individuals with AUD achieving abstinence or showing substantial improvements in functioning in the year after treatment. Long periods of non-problematic drinking occur in fewer than 10% of individuals, which is one of the reasons abstinence is the usual goal of treatment. Of individuals with AUDs, 20–30% are able to achieve long-term remission without treatment or involvement in self-help programs. Remission in these circumstances is usually prompted by a new life partner, parenthood, new job, deteriorating health, and/or maturation over time. Women are more likely to seek help sooner than men and are less likely to be violent or arrested.

Early death is increased in AUD by three or four times, typically due to heart disease, stroke, cancer, and high risk of cirrhosis, suicide, and accidents. Cancer is the second leading cause of early death in AUD; almost 75% of individuals with head and neck cancers have AUD and the risk of esophagus, rectum, and breast cancers are doubled in people with AUD. Women with AUD develop cognitive deficits after shorter drinking histories and more medical problems than men, which may be related to different pharmacokinetics, effects of alcohol on brain functioning, and sex hormone levels. Psychosocial and cultural factors also play a role in gender differences in AUD, such as lower levels of consumption and behavioral problems in women.

Wernicke-Korsakoff Syndrome (WKS)

Individuals with AUD are at risk for thiamine deficiency due to poor nutrition and reduced metabolism of thiamine. Thiamine deficiency can lead to Wernicke's encephalopathy (WE), which is an acute neurological disorder characterized by oculomotor abnormalities, cerebellar dysfunction (e.g., gait ataxia), and altered mental status. Altered mental status is present in about 82% of individuals with WE, but the complete triad is present in < 20% of cases of WE. Thus, only two of these symptoms are needed for diagnosis of WE. WE is typically accompanied by neuronal loss and hemorrhagic lesions in the paraventricular and periaqueductal gray matter.

In 56–84% of cases of WE, development of profound anterograde amnesia known as Korsakoff syndrome (KS) occurs. Because KS shares similar pathological substrates and often follows an episode of WE, it is usually referred to as WKS. WKS occurs in < 1% of individuals with AUD but can also occur in individuals with thiamine deficiency from other causes such as gastrointestinal disease, acquired immunodeficiency syndrome, and anorexia nervosa. In addition to severe anterograde amnesia, individuals with WKS often show some degree of retrograde amnesia and executive dysfunction and milder deficits in visuospatial skills and processing speed. Confabulation, anosognosia, lack of empathy, and a detached, apathetic demeanor are often present as well. Neuroimaging shows atrophy in mammillary bodies, thalamus, and cerebellum.

Cannabis

Cannabis is a commonly used psychoactive substance, both in the United States and worldwide. In 2011 prevalence of marijuana use in the United States was estimated at 17.4 million, and most common among males and young adults.

Because effects of cannabis include sedation, mood elevation, and hallucinations, it is not readily categorized within a single class of substances. Central nervous system (CNS) effects of cannabis occur through binding of *tetrahydrocannabinol* (THC) to cannabinoid (CB) receptors (particularly the CB1 subtype), which are distributed across multiple cortical regions as well as in hippocampus, striatum and cingulate. Cannabis stimulates release of dopamine, GABA, and glutamate, and neuroimaging reveals decreased activity of cortical frontal, limbic, and cerebellar cortical regions.

Acute cannabis use typically affects attention, learning, and memory functioning, which dissipates over several hours. Notably, the half-life of cannabis is much longer than other substances of abuse and the lipophilic properties of THC means it is stored in fat tissue, which results in urine toxicology screens that can remain positive for several weeks following cessation of use. For most individuals use of cannabis alone is not thought to have severe lasting neurotoxic effects (though alterations in functional neuroimaging are frequently reported), and persistent impairment in memory and psychomotor functions is typically limited to heavy, active users. In general, measurable adverse neurobehavioral effects typically resolve about a month after abstinence. Current research is directed toward identifying risk factors for longer term neurocognitive impairment among cannabis users. By contrast, few studies to date have investigated neurocognitive effects of medical marijuana.

Stimulants

In general, neurocognitive, and psychiatric effects and abnormal neuroimaging findings are more frequent and severe with methamphetamine ("ice," "Tina," "crystal") than those of cocaine or prescription stimulants such as dextroamphetamine (Dexedrine) and methylphenidate (Ritalin), used to treat ADHD and narcolepsy. Stimulants produce vasoconstriction, accelerated heart rate, and increased blood pressure, and increase dopamine, serotonin, and norepinephrine availability in limbic, prefrontal, and striatal regions. Chronic heavy use of methamphetamine is neurotoxic; evidence for neurotoxicity of cocaine is less consistent. The effects of a single dose of cocaine generally last about 20 to 30 minutes. Intensity of the initial rush, or peak feeling of euphoria will vary according to method of administration; injected cocaine or methamphetamine crosses the blood-brain barrier most rapidly with peak plasma levels within 5 minutes, followed by smoked cocaine (rock or freebase), with slowest absorption by intranasal (snorting) ingestion. The half-life of cocaine is approximately one hour. Peak levels of injected methamphetamine are also reached within a few minutes, but its half-life (10–11 hours) is longer than cocaine. Decreasing blood levels of either drug triggers an intense craving for more drug; continuous use (binging or "on a run") for several days is very common. Stimulant misuse is associated with increased risk of seizure, cerebrovascular accident, or myocardial infarction, which all have the potential to produce additional cognitive compromise.

Controlled administration of cocaine, methamphetamine, or methylphenidate (Ritalin) under laboratory conditions results in improved attention and processing speed. Initially, stimulant intoxication results in increased energy, motor activity, euphoria, and hypersexuality. Psychomotor *sensitization*, a progressive increase in the psychomotor activating response, has been reported to occur with repeated stimulant use, while tolerance develops to the euphoria and sexual effects.

Long-term misuse of stimulants is most likely to adversely affect sustained attention, working memory, episodic memory, and executive functioning, including decision-making and inhibitory control, although impairment in speed of information processing and psychomotor functions has been reported. Functional neuroimaging studies have typically revealed disruption of frontal-striatal and frontal-parietal activity. Abnormal findings on neuroimaging and neurocognitive deficits can persist for several years following cessation of methamphetamine use. Impairment in executive functions and attention are most commonly reported by studies of cocaine use, but in general studies of cocaine's neurocognitive effects have yielded inconsistent results. Misuse of prescription stimulants has been studied primarily among college students, and their long-term neurocognitive effects have not been investigated in detail.

Women are more vulnerable to the development of stimulant *addiction* compared with men: their progression from initial use to *addiction* is more rapid ("*telescoping*"), withdrawal symptoms are more severe, and relapse rates are higher.

Sedative/Hypnotics

Benzodiazepines (BZDs) and barbiturates are classified as sedative/hypnotics. BZDs such as diazepam (Valium), alprazolam (Xanax) and lorazepam (Ativan), are among the most commonly misused (defined as using without a prescription and/or solely for the drug's psychoactive effects) prescription drugs and have largely replaced barbiturates for both medical and recreational use, due to less severe side effects and lower risk of overdose. They are typically used for anxiety disorders but are also employed for management of seizure disorders and alcohol withdrawal.

Sedative/hypnotics act on GABA receptors, hyperpolarizing neurons by opening chloride channels and closing calcium channels. A corresponding reduction in neural firing reduces performance across neuropsychological tasks and produces mental slowing, anterograde amnesia, and attentional lapses. Memory, attention, and motor deficits can persist even with lengthy abstinence from chronic benzodiazepine use.

Barbiturates such as secobarbital (Seconal) and pentobarbital (Nembutal) have been typically prescribed for sleep or occasionally for seizure disorders (phenobarbital) or migraine headaches (butalbital with aspirin and caffeine [Fiorinal]). Acute effects of barbiturates are relatively more prominent than those of BZDs, and include respiratory depression, confusion, poor coordination, and impaired decision-making; long-term barbiturate use is associated with increased risk of depression and cognitive impairment. Notably, withdrawal from either BZDs or barbiturates increases risk of seizures, may require an inpatient setting, and must be managed by an experienced physician (preferably board certified in *addiction* psychiatry).

Opioids

Heroin is the most commonly used illicit opioid, while acetaminophen with codeine (Vicodin) and oxycodone (OxyContin) are the primary misused prescription opioids. Over the last 10 to 15 years, misuse of both prescription opioids and heroin has increased exponentially in the United States. Some individuals will transition from prescription opioid to heroin use, often for practical reasons; federal and state regulations on prescribing and dispensing opioids are steadily increasing, and heroin is considerably cheaper and more readily obtainable. However, the practice of "cutting" heroin with fentanyl, which is 50 to 100 times more potent than morphine, or with carfentanil, which is <u>100 times</u> more potent than fentanyl, has resulted in a significant increase in fatal heroin overdose. The demographic characteristics of opioid misusers have changed in recent years: Opioid *addiction* has become significantly more prevalent among younger Caucasians, in contrast with older opioid addicts, who are typically African American.

Peak euphoric effects of injected heroin occur in 7 to 8 seconds. Opioids act on multiple components of the limbic reward system, stimulating dopamine neurons in the ventral tegmental area (VTA) and leading to release of dopamine in the nucleus accumbens. Mu, kappa, and delta opioid receptors are widely distributed in the CNS, including the brainstem. Compared with other drugs, respiratory depression or arrest is much more common and fatal with heroin overdose. In addition to the "rush" of euphoria, acute administration of opioids typically results in drowsiness, slowed breathing, pupillary constriction, decreased interest in social interaction, and gastrointestinal discomfort. Task-activated fMRI studies have typically revealed abnormal activity in orbitofrontal prefrontal cortex and cingulate. Acute and chronic neurocognitive effects of heroin and opioid substitutes such as methadone and buprenorphine have been studied in more detail than those of prescription opioids.

The presence and severity of neurocognitive dysfunction among chronic opioid users is varied and dependent on the user's years of use, years of education, and treatment with methadone or buprenorphine. Neurocognitive function among longer-term opioid users can be essentially intact or limited to mildly decreased executive function, working memory and decision-making. Additionally, psychomotor slowing can be observed among individuals on methadone. The long-term direct effects of heroin *addiction* on the body are relatively benign and typically limited to chronic constipation. However, polysubstance dependence, malnutrition and comorbid brain injuries, seizures, and infections with HIV and HCV are highly prevalent among this group, resulting in frequently impaired neurocognitive performance in addition to poor health.

While it is certainly true that a given individual's prescribed opioid dose may be inadequate for effective pain management, and a request for a dose increase or adjustment should not be confused with drug seeking by individuals with SUD, it should be noted that the term "pseudoaddiction" was introduced by the pharmaceutical industry as a marketing tool for sale of prescription opioids.

Hallucinogens

This class of drugs produces profound distortions in the user's perception of reality and intense emotional swings. The three major hallucinogenic compounds are:

- *LSD* (d-lysergic acid) found in ergot, a fungus growing on rye or other grains.
- *Peyote* A small spineless cactus containing the ingredient mescaline.
- *Psilocybin* 4-phosphoryloxy-N,N-dimethyltryptamine, obtained from certain types of mushrooms.

Hallucinogens have been found in plants and mushrooms and have been part of religious and medical practices for hundreds, if not thousands, of years. NIDA points out that much of what the medical community knows about hallucinogen use comes from case reports because there are no current large-scale controlled investigations of the effects. However, there has been a resurgence of interest in the therapeutic effects of hallucinogens for treatment of SUDs as well as for other mental health conditions, such as PTSD and anxiety and depression in individuals with advanced stage cancer.

LSD, peyote, and psilocybin have chemical structures similar to the neurotransmitter serotonin and produce their effect by disrupting its interaction with the receptor. The serotonin system is involved in the control of behavioral, perceptual, and regulatory systems, including mood, hunger, body temperature, sexual behavior, muscle control, and sensory perception. Hallucinogen use does not typically produce compulsive drug-seeking behavior and, as such, is not thought of as an addictive substance. Most users of LSD voluntarily decrease or stop its use over time, whereas Native Americans may use peyote regularly as part of their participation in religious practices.

LSD and psilocybin users may experience flashbacks or recurrences of certain parts of their drug experience. In some LSD users, the flashbacks can persist and cause significant distress or impairment in social or occupational functioning, a condition known as hallucinogen-induced persisting perceptual disorder. In psilocybin users, long-term effects such as flashbacks, risk of psychiatric illness, impaired memory, and tolerance have been described in case reports. Native Americans using peyote regularly in religious settings do not demonstrate psychological or cognitive deficits. Flashbacks, essentially drug effects distal to the time of administration, are associated with lipid-soluble substances that can be activated when the body accesses fat stores for energy metabolism.

MDMA

3,4-Methylenedioxymethamphetamine (MDMA, Ecstasy, Molly) is not readily classified within a single category: It has both stimulant and hallucinogenic properties, and has been described variously as "enactogenic" or "empathogenic." MDMA acts primarily at serotonin receptors. Short-term effects include euphoria, elevated mood, and enhanced feelings of empathy. MDMA is often used at all-night raves or dance clubs, and users can develop hyperthermia and dehydration secondary to increased physical activity. Initial neurobehavioral effects are not well described but may include impaired memory, panic attacks, and feelings of depersonalization. Many users report temporary but profound episodes of depression and exhaustion within 12 to 24 hours following MDMA use. Long-term cognitive effects of MDMA use are not well understood, as it is frequently combined with cannabis and other drugs; additionally, tablets or pills sold as Ecstasy often contain additional, potentially neurotoxic but unknown substances. However, available studies have reported evidence of impulsivity, memory impairment, and working memory deficits among a subgroup of MDMA users, particularly those who combine MDMA with cannabis use.

Conclusion

The scope of this chapter is limited to the SUDs most commonly encountered by clinical neuropsychologists in North America. Many more licit and illicit substances have significant CNS effects (e.g., inhalants, MDMA/ecstasy, club drugs such as ketamine and GHB, synthetic compounds such as "bath salts" or "spice") and individuals who have misused them may present for neurocognitive assessment. Providers are strongly encouraged to consult a recent excellent comprehensive text by Allen and Woods (2014) for additional information on these substances.

Relevant Definitions

Addiction Research/NIH definition of substance use disorder: "A chronic, relapsing brain disorder characterized by compulsive drug seeking and use despite negative consequences."

Comorbidity The presence of one or more additional diseases or disorders co-occurring (i.e., concurrent) with a primary disease or disorder.

Hepatitis C virus (HCV) A virus that causes inflammation of the liver that can lead to cirrhosis. This virus has been detected in the brain and some persons living with HCV infection will show cognitive impairment, especially if coinfected with HIV. HCV is transmitted through the exchange of blood products, thus injection drug users (IDUs) are at elevated risk for exposure to this virus.

Human immunodeficiency virus (HIV) A retrovirus that suppresses the immune system and if untreated, progresses to acquired immunodeficiency syndrome (AIDS). HIV is present in brain, and approximately 50% of persons living with HIV/AIDS in North America develop neurocognitive impairment ranging from mild deficits on neurocognitive testing without clinically significant effects on daily functioning to dementia.

Injection drug use (IDU) Drug injection into a vein or through the skin; replaces "intravenous."

Mesocorticolimbic The dopaminergic pathway most critically involved in reward processing and development of addiction.

Substance Use Disorder (SUD) DSM-5 terminology that replaces substance "abuse" and "dependence" subcategories from DSM-IV.

Telescoping An atypically rapid increase in drug use and progression to addiction.

Tetrahydrocannabinol (THC) The principal metabolite and active ingredient of cannabis; binds to cannabinoid receptors in brain.

Ventral striatum The nucleus accumbens, a component of limbic circuitry and critically involved in processing of reward and development of addiction. Distinct from neostriatum, a component of basal ganglia circuitry that includes the caudate and putamen.

Substance Use Disorders Questions

NOTE: Questions 2, 34, 85, and 111 on the First Full-Length Practice Examination, Questions 20, 39, 73, and 92 on the Second Full-Length Practice Examination, Questions 1, 30, 77, and 100 on the Third Full-Length Practice Examination, and Questions 8, 34, and 73 on the Fourth Full-Length Practice Examination are from this chapter.

1. Which is a defining characteristic of SUDs/addiction?

    (a) full knowledge of negative consequences of use

    (b) physical withdrawal

    (c) prefrontal and temporal atrophy on MRI

    (d) complete remission when abstinence can be maintained

2. Neurobehavioral characteristics of addiction include ____.

   (a) impaired implicit or procedural learning

   (b) dysfunction of neostriatum but not ventral striatum

   (c) decreased reward sensitivity with chronic substance use

   (d) tendency to value delayed over immediate rewards

3. Evidence of sex differences in SUDs include ____.

   (a) lower prevalence of comorbid psychiatric disorders among women with SUDs

   (b) higher relapse rates among women methamphetamine users

   (c) greater vulnerability to memory effects of marijuana in women

   (d) lower severity of delirium tremens and withdrawal seizures among women

4. All of the following are significant risk factors for SUDs except ____.

   (a) male sex   (c) African American ethnicity

   (b) 12 years of education or less   (d) income less than $20,000

5. A 57-year-old man has a 30-year history of alcohol and marijuana use disorders and has been abstinent for approximately 1 year. He and his wife have noted forgetfulness and trouble concentrating without any other cognitive or behavioral concerns. His mood, sleep, and appetite have been good and stable for the past 3 months. An MRI of the brain showed global cortical atrophy with slightly more prominence in the frontal lobes. This finding is ____.

   (a) concerning for possible neurodegenerative disease process

   (b) consistent with findings in individuals with AUD and marijuana use disorder

   (c) consistent with findings in individuals with AUD but not co-occurring marijuana use disorder

   (d) suggestive of Wernicke-Korsakoff syndrome

6. A 41-year-old woman with a 10-year history of AUD completed inpatient treatment and has been sober for 2 months. Prior to inpatient hospitalization, she was high functioning in her job as a sales manager. She has no medical or psychiatric comorbidities. She underwent neuropsychological evaluation, and findings revealed mild impairments in inhibition, cognitive flexibility, and visuospatial skills. With continued abstinence, it is most likely her cognitive difficulties will ____.

   (a) worsen   (c) improve but likely not return to baseline

   (b) remain stable   (d) improve and return to baseline

7. The key brain regions involved in the neurobiologic circuitry of addiction are ____.

   (a) nucleus accumbens and cerebellum   (c) prefrontal cortex and nucleus accumbens

   (b) prefrontal cortex and hippocampus   (d) prefrontal and temporal cortices

8. The neuropsychological domain affected by all SUDs is ____.

   (a) executive   (c) language

   (b) visuospatial   (d) motor

9. Jake is a 17-year-old who started using alcohol and marijuana at age 12. By age 14, he had developed a polysubstance use disorder characterized by heavy use. Which of the following statements is most likely to be true:

    (a) Jake's prefrontal cortex, anterior cingulate, and nucleus accumbens are larger than other boys his age.

    (b) Jake exhibited good inhibition and working memory prior to initiation of use.

    (c) Jake's father, uncle, and siblings do not have SUDs.

    (d) Jake is likely to show neurocognitive deficits even if he remains abstinent for more than 6 months.

10. Which substance of abuse is most neurotoxic?

    (a) heroin/prescription opioids   (c) methamphetamine

    (b) marijuana   (d) MDMA/Ecstasy

Substance Use Disorders Answers

1. **A—full knowledge of negative consequences of use** *According to DSM-5's criteria for SUD and various definitions of addiction, including NIDA's, persistent use of a substance despite awareness of significant associated problems is a core feature of the condition.*

    Reference: American Psychiatric Association. (2013). *Diagnostic and Statistical Manual of Mental Disorders* (5th ed.). Arlington, VA: American Psychiatric Publishing.

2. **C—decreased reward sensitivity with chronic substance use** *Repeated use of the substance over time eventually results in down-regulation of dopamine release and blunted feelings of reward.*

    Reference: Koob, G. F., & Volkow, N. D. (2016). Neurobiology of addiction: A neurocircuitry analysis. *The Lancet Psychiatry, 3*(8), 760–773.

3. **B—higher relapse rates among women methamphetamine users** *Women are more vulnerable to the effects of stimulant addiction than men, including more rapid progression from use to addiction ("telescoping"), more severe withdrawal symptoms, and higher relapse rates.*

    Reference: Becker, J. B., & Hu, M. (2008). Sex differences in drug abuse. *Frontiers in Endocrinology, 29*, 36–47.

4. **C—African American ethnicity** *Native American ethnicity rather than African American ethnicity is a significant risk factor for SUDs, with lifetime prevalence rates of 43% for AUDs and 17% for DUDs.*

    References:
    (a) Grant, B. F., Goldstein, R. B., Saha, T. D., Chou, S. P., Jung, J., Zhang, H., . . . Hasin, D. S. (2015). Epidemiology of DSM-5 alcohol use disorder. *JAMA Psychiatry, 72*(8), 757–766.
    (b) Grant, B. F., Saha, T. D., Ruan, W. J., Goldstein, R. B., Chou, S. P., Jung, J., . . . Hasin, D.S. (2016). Epidemiology of DSM-5 drug use disorder: Results from the National Epidemiologic Survey on Alcohol and Related Conditions–III. *JAMA Psychiatry, 73*(1), 39–47.

5. **B—consistent with findings in individuals with AUD and marijuana use disorder** *All substances of abuse generally show reduced cortical volumes globally with frontal lobes slightly more affected.*

Reference: Suckling, J., & Nestor, L. J. (2017). The neurobiology of addiction: The perspective from magnetic resonance imaging present and future. *Addiction, 112*(2), 360–369.

6. **D—improve and return to baseline** *There are three factors in this case that point to the prognosis of improvement and return to baseline: (1) she has been sober for only 2 months, and studies suggest continued neurocognitive recovery is likely to occur with longer periods of abstinence; (2) she was high functioning just prior to her inpatient stay suggesting less severe cognitive dysfunction; and (3) no medical or psychiatric comorbidities.*

Reference: Fernández-Serrano, M. J., Pérez-García, M., & Verdejo-García, A. (2011). What are the specific vs. generalized effects of drugs of abuse on neuropsychological performance? *Neuroscience & Biobehavioral Reviews, 35*(3), 377–406.

7. **C—prefrontal cortex and nucleus accumbens** *Release of dopamine into the nucleus accumbens corresponds with feelings of euphoria and reward. After repeated exposure to the substance, release of dopamine is attenuated, which reduces the rewarding feelings and also reduces the effectiveness of prefrontal brain regions important for decision-making, self-regulation, mental flexibility, and error monitoring.*

Reference: Koob, G. F., & Volkow, N. D. (2016). Neurobiology of addiction: A neurocircuitry analysis. *The Lancet Psychiatry, 3*(8), 760–773.

8. **A—executive** *All substances of abuse impact executive functions to some degree, while visuospatial and motor functions are affected by a subset of substances, especially alcohol. Language abilities are typically not affected by SUDs.*

Reference: Fernández-Serrano, M. J., Pérez-García, M., & Verdejo-García, A. (2011). What are the specific vs. generalized effects of drugs of abuse on neuropsychological performance? *Neuroscience & Biobehavioral Reviews, 35*(3), 377–406.

9. **D—Jake is likely to show neurocognitive deficits even if he remains abstinent for more than 6 months.** *Longitudinal studies of adolescents with SUDs and heavy use showed persisting neurocognitive deficits even after their SUDs had remitted. Studies of adolescents who develop SUDs have shown neurocognitive impairments and reduced brain volumes in mesocorticolimbic regions prior to initiation of use. In AUD, 40–60% of risk is explained by genes and the rest by gene–environment interactions. Thus, a strong family history placed Jake at risk for developing SUD.*

Reference: Squeglia, L. M., & Gray, K. M. (2016). Alcohol and drug use and the developing brain. *Current Psychiatry Reports, 18*(5), 46.

10. **C—methamphetamine** *Neuropsychological studies of various substances reveal the most significant deficits are associated with alcohol and stimulant use, particularly methamphetamine.*

Reference: Fernández-Serrano, M. J., Pérez-García, M., & Verdejo-García, A. (2011). What are the specific vs. generalized effects of drugs of abuse on neuropsychological performance? *Neuroscience & Biobehavioral Reviews, 35*(3), 377–406.

Recommended Readings

Allen, D. N., & Woods, S. P. (2014). Neuropsychological aspects of substance use disorders: Evidence-based perspectives. New York, NY: Oxford University Press.

Crane, N. A., Schuster, R. M., Fusar-Poli, P., & Gonzalez, R. (2013). Effects of cannabis on neurocognitive functioning: Recent advances, neurodevelopmental influences, and sex differences. *Neuropsychology Review, 23*(2), 117–137.

Fernández-Serrano, M. J., Pérez-García, M., & Verdejo-García, A. (2011). What are the specific vs. generalized effects of drugs of abuse on neuropsychological performance? *Neuroscience & Biobehavioral Reviews, 35*(3), 377–406.

Gonzalez, R., Pacheco-Colón, I., Duperrouzel, J. C., & Hawes, S. W. (2017). Does cannabis use cause declines in neuropsychological functioning? A review of longitudinal studies. *Journal of the International Neuropsychological Society, 23*, 893–902.

Gonzalez, R., Vassileva, J., & Scott, J. C. (2009). Neuropsychological consequences of drug abuse. In I. Grant & K. Adams (Eds.), *Neuropsychological assessment of neuropsychiatric disorders* (pp. 455–479). New York, NY: Oxford University Press.

Grant, B. F., Goldstein, R. B., Saha, T. D., Chou, S. P., Jung, J., Zhang, H. . . .Hasin, D. S. (2015). Epidemiology of DSM-5 alcohol use disorder. *JAMA Psychiatry, 72*(8), 757–766.

Grant, B. F., Saha, T. D., Ruan, W. J., Goldstein, R. B., Chou, S.P ., Jung, J. . . .Hasin, D. S. (2016). Epidemiology of DSM-5 drug use disorder: Results from the National Epidemiologic Survey on Alcohol and Related Conditions–III. *JAMA Psychiatry, 73*(1), 39–47.

Koob, G. F., & Volkow, N. D. (2016). Neurobiology of addiction: A neurocircuitry analysis. *The Lancet Psychiatry, 3*(8), 760–773.

Simon, S. L., Dean, A. C., Cordova, X., Monterosso, J. R., & London, E. D. (2010). Methamphetamine dependence and neuropsychological functioning: Evaluating change during early abstinence. *Journal of Studies on Alcohol and Drugs, 71*(3), 335–344.

Squeglia, L. M., & Gray, K. M. (2016). Alcohol and drug use and the developing brain. *Current Psychiatry Reports, 18*(5), 46.

Volkow, N. D., Swanson, J. M., Evins, E., DeLisi, Le., Meier, M. H., Gonzales, R., . . . Baler, R. (2016). Effects of cannabis use on human behavior, including cognition, motivation, and psychosis: A review. *JAMA Psychiatry, 73*(3), 292–297.

Walsh, Z., Gonzalez, R., Crosby, K., Thiessen, C., Carrolla, M., & Bonn-Miller, O. (2017). Medical cannabis and mental health: A guided systematic review. *Clinical Psychology Review, 51*, 51–59.

Woicik, P. A., Moeller, S. J., Alia-Klein, N., Maloney, T., Lukasik, TM., Yeliesof, O., . . . Goldstein, R. Z. (2009). The neuropsychology of cocaine addiction: Recent cocaine use masks impairment. *Neuropsychopharmacology, 34*, 1112–1122.

Websites

www.nida.nih.gov
www.niaaa.nih.gov
www.samhsa.gov

37 Integrative Health Approaches to Chronic Health Conditions and Somatic Symptom Disorders

Greg J. Lamberty and Wendy A. VanVoorst

Introduction

In the first edition of this study guide, this chapter focused on "Biopsychosocial" (BPS) approaches to chronic health conditions. While the essence of the BPS approach remains a focus of material in this chapter, it is important to note that terminology in this area is evolving. The addition of the term "integrative health" to the title is an acknowledgment that chronic conditions, including somatic symptom disorders (SSDs), are frequently identified and treated in primary care settings, which increasingly attempt to coordinate the efforts of multiple disciplines. Further, a broader range of interventions are being offered that are not exclusively aligned with a single specialty or traditional medical care. Such "complementary" techniques are now commonly referred to as elements of an integrative health approach that seeks to bring many interventions together in a coordinated fashion to meet the needs of patients with complex presentations.

Neuropsychologists are well suited to assist with appropriate diagnosis, referral, and treatment of individuals with chronic health problems and SSDs. Empirically supported psychotherapeutic treatments have become a standard of care in many settings and a host of complementary and integrative practices are increasingly recognized as viable options with a growing scientific basis.

Diagnostic Considerations

Patients for whom there is little suggestive history or obvious clinical indication of central nervous system (CNS) pathology/dysfunction and patients with chronic health conditions are commonly referred to neuropsychologists secondary to concerns about cognitive functioning. A substantial number of these individuals can be characterized as having SSDs, whereas others may have discrete chronic medical illnesses. Further, some individuals may meet criteria for both kinds of diagnoses. As such, an appreciation of the multiple factors that impact illness behavior and perceptions of cognitive functioning is essential. Knowledge of efficacious and *empirically supported treatment* approaches in individuals with SSDs and chronic medical illnesses will facilitate optimal recommendations in the neuropsychological report.

Somatic Symptom Disorders

Somatic symptom and related disorders, as defined in the *Diagnostic and Statistical Manual of Mental Disorders, Fifth Edition* (DSM-5), represent a significant change in diagnostic criteria (from previous DSMs) for individuals with chronic health-related concerns for which there is limited medical evidence. Decades of research indicated that numerous specific criteria did not facilitate clinical understanding or treatment for patients presenting with *medically unexplained physical symptoms* across a range of settings. Therefore, in DSM-5 a single diagnosis of SSD is offered to account for the nature and chronicity of presentations involving physical symptoms instead of using multiple more specific diagnoses (e.g., somatization disorder, hypochondriasis, pain disorder) as was the case in DSM-IV. In addition, conversion disorder was redefined with a parenthetical label of functional neurological symptom disorder, to identify a subset of individuals that present with "altered voluntary motor or sensory function."

- *Somatic Symptom Disorder* Somatic symptom disorders involve a preoccupation with somatic symptoms and cognitive distortions related to these symptoms. The DSM-5 criteria require:
  - Criterion A: One or more somatic symptoms that are distressing or result in significant disruption of daily life.
  - Criterion B: Excessive thoughts, feelings, or behaviors related to the somatic symptoms or associated health concerns as manifested by at least one of the following:
    - Disproportionate and persistent thoughts about the seriousness of one's symptoms.
    - Persistently high level of anxiety about health or symptoms.
    - Excessive time and energy devoted to these symptoms or health concerns.
  - Criterion C: Although any one somatic symptom may not be continuously present, the state of being symptomatic is persistent (typically more than 6 months). Specify if:
    - With Predominant pain (previously pain disorder): This specifier is for individuals whose somatic symptoms predominantly involve pain.
- *Conversion Disorder (functional neurological symptom disorder)* As noted, conversion disorder is a condition that presents primarily with neurological symptoms of sensory and motor disturbances. The symptoms are not accounted for by known neurologic mechanisms or are inconsistent on exam.

In all of the DSM-5 somatic symptom diagnoses (outlined in Table 37.1), there is no longer the specific suggestion that the symptoms produced are primarily psychological in origin. Interestingly, the other disorders in the SSDs category do not involve the presence of significant somatic symptoms. These include illness anxiety disorder, factitious disorder, and psychological factors affecting medical condition. As such, they involve worrying about and/or complaining about symptoms, but not actually experiencing them.

TABLE 37.1 *Diagnostic and Statistical Manual of Mental Disorders* (DSM-5; 2013) Primary Features and Prevalence Estimates for Somatic Symptom and Related Disorders

Diagnosis	Primary Features	Prevalence Estimate
Somatic Symptom Disorder	• One or more troubling symptoms • Excessive thoughts/anxiety • Persistent course	General Population: 5–7% (presumed to be higher in females)
Illness Anxiety Disorder *(formerly hypochondriasis)*	• Preoccupation with illness • Symptoms generally not present • Persistent course	Community Surveys: 1.3–10% Ambulatory Medical Populations: 3–8%
Conversion Disorder (Functional Neurological Symptom Disorder)	• Symptom(s) of altered motor or sensory function • Lacking clinical findings • Significant distress/impairment	Referrals to Neurology Clinics: 5%
Psychological Factors Affecting Other Medical Conditions	• Medical symptom present • Psychological factor(s) adversely affecting the medical condition	Unclear, but more common than SSD
Factitious Disorder	• False physical or psychological symptoms intended to deceive • No obvious external incentive	Hospital Settings: Unknown, assumed to be 1%

Functional Somatic Syndromes

Several diagnoses that are well known in public discourse have been strongly associated with somatoform disorders or psychogenic illnesses (e.g., *fibromyalgia, multiple chemical sensitivity, chronic fatigue*) and have become known as functional somatic syndromes (FSSs). Notwithstanding some proponents in the medical establishment and a good deal of patient/public advocacy, these disorders have been considered controversial by mainstream medicine. As is the case with most diagnoses with strong somatoform elements, clear underlying pathology and mechanisms of disease are difficult to establish. Accurate prevalence estimates are also variable, depending upon the study source. It is worth noting that many of these syndromes have multiple names, usually in an effort to specify (purported) causes (e.g., multiple chemical sensitivities = idiopathic environmental intolerances; chronic fatigue syndrome = systemic exertion intolerance disease or myalgic encephalomyelitis).

In the neuropsychology literature, the term "cogniform disorder" (also "neurocognitive hypochondriasis") has been proposed to describe a presentation characterized by pervasive concerns about cognitive difficulty in a manner similar to physical complaints in SSDs. That is, the report of cognitive problems is described as disruptive and sometimes disabling. Further, the original description of this disorder noted that inadequate effort was often noted on performance validity measures in neuropsychological assessments.

In many respects, the verity of these diagnoses is not as relevant as the presence of symptoms. The context in which the symptoms present may say something about how entrenched they are and how apt a diagnosis of an SSD might be. Taking a BPS approach to such diagnoses suggests that the context and history of an individual is as important as the presentation of his or her illness. Thus, whereas distinctions might be made as a function of the medical verifiability of a patient's diagnosis, treatment plans and approaches should consider the complexity of other factors influencing the presentation.

Chronic Medical Illnesses/Diseases

In the United States, chronic health conditions are very common, with over 50% of all Americans having had at least one, and roughly one third having a history of multiple chronic conditions. This finding is particularly accentuated with aging, with 80% of those over the age of 65 having multiple chronic conditions. A very high percentage of all healthcare expenditures (86%) are used to treat individuals with chronic conditions. Patients with chronic medical illnesses are also at increased risk for CNS pathology with associated cognitive dysfunction. Some familiar examples include patients with cancer that result in metastatic masses in the brain or chronic diseases that affect the vascular system, such as hypertension and diabetes. Individuals with such histories are frequently seen for neuropsychological assessments. Such individuals often show patterns of dysfunction that correspond to regional pathology. Examples of such disorders are discussed in detail in Chapter 23, Meningitis and Encephalitis, and Chapter 26, Stroke. Despite the long-standing nature of these illnesses, affected individuals do not typically present in a manner suggesting an SSD. Chronic medical illnesses and SSDs are not mutually exclusive, but they are also not synonymous. Careful review of the patient's history will help with this basic distinction.

Neuropsychologists frequently encounter individuals with pain in the process of conducting neuropsychological assessments. As much as 30% of the United States adult population has reported chronic pain, and cognitive difficulty is frequently attributed to pain in these individuals. The literature examining cognitive functioning in pain and pain-related disorders is variable. While some reports indicate difficulties in attention, processing speed, memory, and executive functioning, studies vary widely in methodological rigor and meta-analytic reviews have not indicated consistent findings. Studies assessing test engagement in pain samples have found high levels of PVT failure, thus calling into question the validity of performances and making it difficult to attribute differences to pain-related problems. Further comorbidity with other (particularly psychiatric) diagnoses can make the attribution of cognitive impairment to pain very difficult.

Finally, another class of chronic health issues that often present with concerns about cognitive difficulty are sleep disorders. They are included in this chapter as neuropsychological services are often sought to help clarify diagnostic questions and assist with treatment recommendations. Insomnia, which includes difficulty initiating/maintaining sleep and early morning awakening, is the most prevalent sleep condition among patients with psychiatric diagnoses and the general population. Obstructive sleep apnea (OSA) is the second most prevalent sleep disorder and most common breathing-related sleep disorder. OSA is characterized by repeated episodes of upper airway obstruction resulting in complete blocking of airflow (apnea) or reduced airflow (hypopnea). Typical symptoms of OSA are excessive daytime sleepiness, fatigue, and nocturnal snoring or gasping during sleep. Excessive daytime sleepiness also characterizes narcolepsy, which includes daytime lapses into sleep. Type I narcolepsy occurs with cataplexy or sudden loss of muscle tone triggered by a strong emotional response such as laughter or fear. Low levels of the chemical hypocretin are found in type I narcolepsy, which helps regulate wakefulness and REM sleep. Type II narcolepsy occurs without cataplexy.

Historically, sleep disturbance has been viewed as a symptom of various psychiatric disorders, including depression, anxiety, and substance use disorders. For example, hypersomnia or excessive daytime sleepiness is one of the symptoms of depressive disorders listed in the DSM-5. However, the prevailing view of sleep disorders has shifted to reflect the bidirectional relationship between sleep and psychiatric disorders. For example, individuals with insomnia are at two times the risk of developing generalized anxiety disorder or ten times as likely to develop major depressive disorder compared to healthy controls. Similarly, 15–25% of individuals with idiopathic hypersomnia endorse depressive symptoms, which meet criteria for a depressive disorder.

Sleep disturbance is also frequently seen in neurological conditions including dementia. For example, REM sleep behavior disorder (RBD) is a parasomnia in which muscular activity is not suppressed during REM sleep. Individuals with RBD are at increased risk of developing neurodegenerative conditions, particularly synucleinopathies (i.e., Lewy body dementia, Parkinson's disease, multiple system atrophy).

Polysomnography (PSG) is a nighttime sleep study that measures four parameters: eye movements (EOG), heart rhythm (ECG), brain activity (EEG), and muscle movements (EMG) to help diagnose sleep disorders, including RBD, OSA, and narcolepsy. The multiple sleep latency test (MSLT) is a daytime sleep study performed after a PSG to determine time to sleep onset and REM latency. The MSLT includes five 20-minute naps scheduled 2 hours apart. An MSLT less than 8 minutes plus two or more sleep-onset REM periods support a diagnosis of narcolepsy. A MSLT can confirm narcolepsy in addition to testing hypocretin levels in cerebrospinal fluid. A physical exam and self-report measures of sleepiness are also important in diagnosing sleep disorders.

Chronic Neurological Illnesses/Diseases

Several common neurological diseases are characterized by significant physical disability, cognitive dysfunction, and comorbid psychopathology. Chapter 22, Epilepsy and Seizure Disorders; Chapter 24, Multiple Sclerosis; and Chapter 33, Movement Disorders, give examples of neurological disorders that can present with clear CNS pathology and varied symptom presentations, as well as complicating premorbid psychosocial factors. Neuropsychologists are well suited to evaluate and understand the complex issues observed in these patients, as well as to make recommendations about interventions that might be effective.

Epidemiology

Somatic Symptom Disorders

Since somatoform disorders were first described in the DSM-III, it has been a challenge to obtain accurate prevalence estimates. Between the overly restrictive criteria of somatization disorder (<1%) and the permissive criteria of undifferentiated somatoform disorder (approximately 19%), it is assumed that the prevalence of the SSD diagnosis is somewhere in the 5 to 7% range. Other disorders from the somatic symptom and related disorders category are summarized in Table 37.1. Broad epidemiologic studies have not been conducted utilizing DSM-5 criteria, and the rather vague, descriptive nature of the criteria make it unlikely that more reliable estimates will be forthcoming soon. Nevertheless, as in the past, there continues to be strong interest in somatoform conditions as they are presumed to result in high levels of healthcare utilization.

Functional Somatic Syndromes

The FSS diagnoses noted earlier vary significantly with respect to prevalence estimates. This is often a function of whether the estimates come from peer-reviewed literature or some other source as cited by advocacy groups (generally lower in the peer-reviewed literature and higher from advocacy groups' estimates) (Table 37.2).

Chronic Medical/Neurological Illnesses

The prevalence of somatoform symptoms seen in various diagnoses and settings is difficult to determine with certainty. Studies involving first-time neurology clinic referrals have shown high levels of "unexplained" symptom reporting, even in the absence of diagnosable somatoform disorders or clear neurological illness/disease. Furthermore, the presence of such symptoms is associated with significantly poorer outcomes overall. Therefore, it appears that symptoms can be clinically relevant without being clearly related to a disease process or a broader somatoform presentation. This kind of relationship between symptoms and their source is complex and predictable in the context of a BPS or integrative care model. Thus, caution is warranted in reflexively attempting to determine the nature of specific symptoms (i.e., "real" vs. somatoform).

TABLE 37.2 Prevalence of Common Functional Somatic Syndromes

Diagnosis	Prevalence Estimate
Fibromyalgia	2.0%
Multiple Chemical Sensitivity/Idiopathic Environmental Intolerances	Unknown
Myalgic Encephalomyelitis/Chronic Fatigue Syndrome	.007–2.8%
Irritable Bowel Syndrome	12%
Psychogenic Non-Epileptic Seizures	< 1% of the general population 20–40% of patients seen for seizure disorder consultation

Determinants of Severity

There are many common risk factors among the somatoform/somatic symptom disorders and the various FSS listed. Data and research supporting various theories tend to be stronger for more psychologically oriented risk factors and weaker for more purely biological risk factors like sex.

Gender

Females are more likely than males to be diagnosed with SSD and the FSS diagnoses listed earlier. According to various sources, females are:

- Seven times more likely to be diagnosed with *fibromyalgia*
- Four times more likely to be diagnosed with *chronic fatigue syndrome*
- Nine times more likely to be diagnosed with *multiple chemical sensitivity*
- Two to three times more likely to be diagnosed with *irritable bowel syndrome*
- Three times more likely to be diagnosed with *psychogenic nonepileptic seizures (PNES)*

Hormonal mechanisms are frequently invoked to account for these differences, although few studies provide clear evidence for such links. It is also suggested that males typically underreport symptoms of the various disorders, thus skewing the sex relationship.

With the more clearly established medical diagnoses, sex differences tend to fade substantially or be more clearly related to factors known to differ across sex (e.g., hormonal fluctuations, risk-taking behaviors, hypertension). For example:

- Males are slightly more likely to get Parkinson's disease.
- Women are more likely than men to get multiple sclerosis.
- Stroke is more likely to occur in older men than older women.

Trauma History

The scientific/clinical literature has identified a strong relationship between somatoform diagnoses and an early history of trauma (including physical and sexual abuse). Work examining attachment styles has consistently shown that individuals with disordered attachment show higher levels of alexithymia (difficulty describing feelings/emotions) and somatoform symptomatology in general.

Age

Most of the somatoform disorders and FSS diagnoses show much greater prevalence in individuals between the ages of 30 and 60. The reasons for this are unclear, although presumably, psychosocial stressors for individuals in early through middle adulthood are greater and correspond with other factors that increase general levels of stress.

Race/Culture

The somatic symptom and related disorders, as well as most of the FSS diagnoses, have greater prevalence in those from minority cultures, races, and lower socioeconomic statuses. There are few wide-ranging epidemiologic studies examining such relationships, however. Proposed reasons for these findings typically focus on cultural acceptance of certain kinds of symptoms and presentations. Obviously, findings vary as a function of the "majority" culture in which research is done, as well as by how isolated a particular group might be.

Comorbidity with Psychiatric Disorders

Somatic symptom disorders are typically characterized by high levels of psychiatric symptomatology. Depression and anxiety symptoms are particularly common, and such symptoms are often treated with antidepressant medications. To the extent that such efforts have been successful, somatoform symptoms are suggested to simply be part of a psychiatric disorder. However, this is an example of the biomedical approach that seeks to provide a basic explanation for complex clinical presentations. Pain disorders (in particular, chronic low back pain) have consistently shown a very high level of general psychiatric symptomatology, as well as comorbid psychiatric diagnoses. Given these broad generalized findings, patients with somatic symptom and related disorders are frequently treated pharmacologically for their psychiatric symptoms and receive other treatment for specific physical symptoms.

Presentation, Disease Course, and Recovery

Patients with prominent somatoform features show indications of SSD early in life. By the mid-20s, such individuals typically have many symptoms that impact their general health and adjustment. Their engagement with the medical system often involves seeing multiple providers and specialists as they look for diagnoses and treatment for their concerns. Often, this quest intensifies in young adulthood through middle age. The course of symptoms is variable, although patients rarely go for several months to a year without consultation involving medication or treatment of some kind. Until recently, individuals with SSDs have been considered to have a poor prognosis and poor prospects for responding to psychotherapy.

The often extensive nature of concerns reported by patients with SSDs has made them difficult to study in randomized controlled trials. Programs have been developed that emphasize understanding and appreciating the complexity of patients' concerns, management of symptoms, and multidisciplinary involvement. Combined cognitive-behavioral therapy (CBT) and mindfulness-based approaches have become increasingly popular, with a growing supporting literature. A number of these emerging and *empirically supported* interventions are described later in this chapter.

Expectations for Neuropsychological Assessment Results

Studies examining neuropsychological functioning in patients with somatoform disorders or FSS have provided variable results. On balance, there is little indication of deficits related to CNS dysfunction in these patients. Rather, most studies report strong correlations between reported levels of distress and cognitive dysfunction. This relationship is well known, regardless of the (non-neurologic) diagnoses in question.

In contrast to SSD or FSS, cognitive dysfunction is common in sleep disorders. Obstructive sleep apnea can cause sleep fragmentation and hypoxemia, which can result in reduced:

- Sustained attention
- Information processing
- Response time
- Fine motor coordination
- Executive function (i.e., mental flexibility, set shifting, verbal fluency)
- Learning and memory

There have been inconsistent findings regarding the cognitive effects of insomnia, but some studies have shown impaired learning and memory, working memory, and executive function. Similar domains are affected in narcolepsy although encoding difficulty is the primary memory dysfunction. Domains impacted in idiopathic RBD include attention, executive function, episodic verbal memory, and non-verbal learning. The presence of RBD in neurodegenerative conditions such as PD is also associated with increased risk for the development of cognitive dysfunction, including dementia.

Emotion and Personality

Because of the lack of relationship between SSD diagnoses and neuropsychological functioning, neuropsychologists must attend to measures of personality, psychological adjustment, and emotional distress. Most studies that systematically assess emotional and personality variables find elevations on scales that specifically address the reporting of physical symptoms, as well as indications of limited insight or a tendency for patients to externalize blame for their difficulties. That is, patients who somatize are likely to see physical symptoms, disorders, or disease processes as responsible for their difficulties, particularly in the cognitive realm. To the extent that there is a relationship between cognitive performance and any other variables in the neuropsychological evaluation, psychological variables tap into distress and/ or symptom exaggeration. Few disorder-specific findings are reliably reported in literature examining FSS (see also Chapter 10, Personality Assessment and Self-Report Instruments).

The Minnesota Multiphasic Personality Inventory (MMPI-2, MMPI-2-RF) contains measures that have been the most extensively studied in adult somatoform populations. Validity scales from the MMPI are sensitive to somatoform presentations (e.g., FBS, RBS). This relates to a general tendency for validity scales to portray overreporting of symptoms as indicative of questionable validity, *response bias*, and/ or exaggeration. In the MMPI-2-RF, the Infrequent Somatic Responses (Fs) validity scale specifically assesses a patient's tendency to overreport physical symptoms. The combination of elevated Fs and elevated individual Somatic/Cognitive scales (Malaise, Neurological Complaints, Cognitive Complaints, Gastrointestinal Complaints, Head Pain Complaints) suggests overreporting or invalid responding on these scales. Among the revised clinical (RC) scales, elevations on scales RC1 (Somatic Complaints) are common and can vary in degree depending upon the specific symptoms acknowledged. The Somatic/ Cognitive scales provide insights into specific kinds of physical concerns, as well more general feelings of physical discomfort/distress (Malaise). Generally speaking, scales from the MMPI-2-RF examine both physical and cognitive complaints and do so with considerably fewer items than MMPI-2 scales. The new scales from the restructured form (RF) have also shown utility in assessing exaggeration in litigating patients after traumatic brain injury (TBI).

The Personality Assessment Inventory (PAI) is another commonly used instrument with scales that measure somatoform symptomatology. The Somatic Complaints scale is often elevated in somatizing and litigating samples. However, it has also been found to be elevated in patients with TBI and is not infrequently associated with poorer performance on neuropsychological measures. As such, the Somatic Complaints scale of the PAI appears to lack the diagnostic specificity of some of the MMPI scales.

- *Attention/Concentration* Commonly reported to be affected, but systematic findings are lacking.
- *Processing Speed* Commonly reported to be affected, but systematic findings are lacking.
- *Memory* Commonly reported to be affected, but systematic findings are lacking.
- *Performance and Symptom Validity* The few studies that have systematically examined performance validity have shown that individuals passing PVTs show no cognitive deficits related to FSS diagnosis. In contrast, many studies that specifically assessed SSD, FSS, and patients with chronic pain have found frequent PVT failures.

Considerations when Treating Patients with Chronic Health Conditions, Functional Somatic Syndromes and Somatic Symptom Disorders

Treating patients with prominent somatoform concerns has been an area characterized by frustration and ambivalence for clinicians. The *biomedical model* implicitly suggests that discrete, identifiable, and treatable causes exist for the problems patients bring to the clinic. However, since the late nineteenth and early twentieth centuries, there has been an understanding that this is not the case for a substantial number of patients. As diagnostic medicine improved, the road to "curing" illnesses became more straightforward, but not for patients with complex presentations. The early fields of neurology and psychiatry were transfixed by "hysterical" patients with multiple confusing symptoms. Some contended that the etiology would ultimately prove to be neurological (e.g., Charcot), whereas others proposed new mechanisms that would dominate early psychiatric thinking (e.g., Freud). The field of *psychosomatic medicine* emerged in the middle of the twentieth century and encompassed a wide range of clinical concerns with a nascent understanding that treatment approaches needed to appreciate the multiple factors underlying patients' "illnesses." From the late 1940s forward, investigators began to promote biopsychosocial concepts to bridge the gaps between psychoanalytic and biomedical approaches. The BPS became a cornerstone of the field of health psychology and served as a model for many treatments that are now used to treat patients with FSS and somatoform symptoms.

- *Pharmacologic Treatment* Patients with somatoform disorders and FSS are most often seen by primary care physicians whose inclination is to attempt symptom management with medication. Many medications are available for treating pain, depression, anxiety, and general malaise, so initial attempts often involve prescription of one or more medications (e.g., opiates, antidepressants, anxiolytics, stimulants). By the time a patient is readily identifiable as having an FSS, there may be cautious movement away from pain medications, anxiolytics, and stimulants, given their high abuse potential. Indeed, much of the published literature examining pharmacologic treatment in the realm of somatoform disorders has focused on the use of serotonin selective reuptake inhibitors (SSRIs) and tricyclic antidepressants (TCAs) for chronic pain. Meta-analytic and comparative effectiveness reviews have shown little in the way of high quality evidence for the use of TCAs, SSRIs, new-generation antidepressants, or natural products. Modest positive results have been identified for such treatments in low-quality trials, but no indication of differences in efficacy as a function of drug class has been noted. Further, possible adverse effects such as iatrogenesis or symptom magnification have been noted as a result of treatments offered (nocebo effect), and very few long-term studies have been completed.

- *Cognitive Behavioral Therapy (CBT)* Much of the psychotherapy literature examining treatment of patients with somatoform symptoms has focused on CBT-oriented approaches, often in the context of a broader therapeutic milieu. CBT has been studied extensively enough to provide evidence of superiority to waiting list and usual care conditions, though effect sizes have typically been small. There is also evidence of durability of a treatment effect in long-term follow-ups.

- *Motivational Interviewing (MI)* Motivational interviewing is a popular and effective means for preparing wary patients for difficult but positive changes. It is not a viable long-term intervention, but rather supports a general approach that guides patients toward more positive treatment options. As such, there is little literature bearing on the use of MI in patients with SSDs, but it is frequently used in primary care settings and may be useful in moving wary patients toward more constructive goals, especially in the context of their relatively brief contact with the neuropsychologist.

- *Mindfulness-Based Therapies* Mindfulness-based therapies have increased in popularity in recent years and have a growing evidence base. Mindfulness-based stress reduction (MBSR) and acceptance and commitment therapy (ACT) are two well-validated interventions that orient patients to awareness of the present moment and a nonjudgmental acceptance of experiences. Improved awareness and acceptance of the present consequently results in a reduction of behaviors driven by the mind's judgmental "chatter" or attempts to avoid uncomfortable or negative emotions that comprise a natural part of the human experience. Components of mindfulness are also commonly included with CBT approaches, as with ACT, often with very positive results. This tends to blur distinctions regarding the most important or effective elements of various therapies, although it is consistent with a BPS model in that the distinction between mind and body is made less relevant.

- *Treatments for Sleep Disorders* Treatment of sleep disorders depends on the condition. Continuous positive airways pressure (CPAP) is the gold standard for management of obstructive sleep apnea whereas cognitive behavioral therapy for insomnia (CBT-I) is considered the most effective treatment for chronic insomnia. CBT-I techniques include stimulus control, sleep restriction, sleep hygiene, and relaxation training. Pharmacological management of sleep disturbance is commonplace, particularly for insomnia and movement related sleep conditions, but medications can often have unwanted side effects particularly in the elderly (e.g., sedation, polypharmacy).

Integrative Health Approaches in Primary Care Medicine

Complementary and alternative medicine (CAM) is a term that has been used for practices considered to be outside the scope of traditional medical practice. The term CAM is being replaced with the descriptor "integrative" in healthcare settings, with phrases like *integrative care* or *integrative health*, to emphasize the coordination of approaches that have been regarded as conventional and complementary, respectively. While randomized controlled trials and studies providing strong evidence are rare, it is increasingly common to see efforts aimed at studying treatment approaches that include multiple elements. For instance, brief CBT, mindfulness meditation, yoga, and physical exercise might be included with more regular clinic visits with nursing staff, and keeping a log relating to these activities. A general goal is often reducing the expense of highly utilizing patients by limiting excessive diagnostic workups, while increasing self-management skills.

In current practice, the primary care provider (PCP) continues to be at the center of a treatment team that may consist of different specialists, therapists, and nurses. The PCP should be the main provider to reduce splitting among treating staff. Regular appointments are encouraged to reduce emergency room and urgent care visits, with an expressed goal of reducing specialist referrals and the use of opiate and anticholinergic medications. An approach that emphasizes the importance of managing, although not necessarily curing, symptoms is important, as is an emphasis on the complex and interrelated nature of symptoms experienced. Treatments of all kinds should be described as part of an overall plan to help with symptom management.

Considerations when Treating Select Populations with Somatic Symptom Disorders and Functional Somatic Syndromes

Pediatric Considerations

Reports of somatic symptoms are common in children and adolescents. Risk factors similar to those noted in adults (females, minorities, urban patients, nonintact families, low parental education) are predictive of greater somatic symptom reporting in children and adolescents. In addition, adolescents tend to report more symptoms than younger children. Headache is the most common symptom reported in children, with a tendency for younger children to report more abdominal complaints than older children and adolescents.

The volume of studies examining effectiveness of psychological interventions in children has grown in recent times and there is moderate evidence indicating that psychological treatments reduce symptom load, disability, and school absence. Evidence for integrative health or complementary interventions continues to be limited, and based on specific symptoms like headache.

Geriatric Considerations

Older patients frequently have comorbid issues with pain, fatigue, and a range of other somatoform symptoms. Careful consideration of medical history and situational factors is very important in older patients because the overall prevalence of some somatic symptoms is assumed to be higher than in younger adults. This relates to greater morbidity with respect to physical illnesses and aging-related diseases. Older patients' medical histories will provide the clearest indication of whether complaints are likely somatoform in nature.

Treatment approaches with older adults are typically based on the younger adult literature. However, issues with tolerability of medications and polypharmacy make the task of identifying effective nonpharmacological treatments even more important. As with most other populations, there is promise for integrative care approaches that focus on physical interventions like exercise and yoga because these might bypass the reservations that older patients may have about psychologically oriented interventions. Limited literature exists in this area.

Relevant Definitions

Biomedical model of illness/disease The prevailing model in Western (allopathic) medicine that emphasizes understanding of the underlying physical and biochemical abnormalities in disease and illness. As an extension of this reasoning, treatment focuses on correcting underlying abnormalities, often with medication or surgery.

Empirically supported treatments Refers to treatments that have shown efficacy with specific populations in well-controlled research studies.

Evidence-based practice A broad-based movement in healthcare that encourages practices based on the highest quality evidence from the research literature.

Fibromyalgia A syndrome involving complaints of chronic, diffuse pain/tenderness in the muscles, joints, and soft tissues. Most mainstream sources consider the etiology unknown, but acknowledge relationships with stress and neuropsychiatric symptoms.

Integrative care/health A broad general term referring to healthcare approaches that attempt to bring conventional medical, mental health, and complementary approaches together in a coordinated fashion. The term is also used to describe systems or settings that stress interdisciplinary care that is often based in primary care settings.

Irritable bowel syndrome A syndrome involving chronic abdominal pain, discomfort, bloating, diarrhea, and/or constipation. The etiology is functional and often related to stressors and psychological factors.

Medically unexplained physical symptoms (MUPS) A description of physical symptoms that have no clear underlying physiologic etiology. The term is descriptive and is used to acknowledge a lack of consensus regarding an etiology, while not automatically presuming a psychogenic cause

Multiple chemical sensitivity/idiopathic environmental intolerances A chronic syndrome involving non-specific symptoms like fatigue, headache, dizziness, and gastrointestinal distress. Sufferers attribute the syndrome to low-level exposure to a wide range of different "toxins" like petroleum products, paint fumes, solvents, and smoke. The syndrome is not thought to be due to organic exposure and is generally not recognized by mainstream sources.

Myalgic encephalomyelitis/Chronic fatigue syndrome A chronic and persistent syndrome characterized by fatigue, malaise, joint pain, headaches, cognitive difficulties, and other nonspecific symptoms. The etiology and naming of the syndrome remain controversial because no clear underlying cause has been identified.

Obstructive sleep apnea (OSA) Cessation of breathing caused by upper airway obstruction. OSA is the most common kind of sleep apnea and associated with cognitive difficulties.

Psychogenic nonepileptic seizures (PNES) Behavioral or superficial events that are seizure-like, but not characterized by the abnormal discharges that define epileptic seizures. The etiology is thought to be psychological and early trauma is frequently observed in the histories of affected individuals.

Psychosomatic medicine An interdisciplinary approach within medicine and psychiatry that is concerned with social, psychological, and behavioral factors on bodily processes and quality of life. A precursor to the BPS approach, with which it essentially shares common goals and subject matter.

Integrative Health Approaches to Chronic Health Conditions and Somatic Symptom Disorders Questions

NOTE: Questions 37 and 97 on the First Full-Length Practice Examination, Questions 25, 32, 33, and 71 on the Second Full-Length Practice Examination, Questions 19, 82, and 113 on the Third Full-Length Practice Examination, and Questions 38, 74, and 108 on the Fourth Full-Length Practice Examination are from this chapter.

1. Somatization disorder, somatoform pain disorder, and undifferentiated somatoform disorder from the DSM-IV are now subsumed under which of the following DSM-5 disorders?

    (a) factitious disorder

    (b) conversion disorder

    (c) somatic symptom disorder

    (d) illness anxiety disorder

2. In previous DSM (DSM-III/DSM-IV) classification schemes, somatization disorder was thought to ____ the prevalence of patients presenting with physical problems across a range of settings.

    (a) overestimate

    (b) underestimate

    (c) accurately reflect

    (d) have no relation to

3. A high level of ____ is often associated with insecure attachment.

    (a) alexithymia

    (b) sociopathy

    (c) back pain

    (d) psychosis

4. Which of the following is an empirically supported treatment that incorporates elements of mindfulness?

    (a) behavior therapy

    (b) acceptance and commitment therapy

    (c) cognitive behavioral therapy

    (d) cognitive processing therapy

5. Complementary and alternative medicine (CAM) is a term that has fallen out of favor in recent years because ____.

    (a) such approaches have largely been discredited in the scientific literature

    (b) alternative treatments are routinely found to be more effective than traditional medicine interventions

    (c) traditional medicine has extended its purview and incorporated more CAM treatments

    (d) a broader range of interventions are recognized as viable and accessible, rendering the term less meaningful

6. According to DSM-5 criteria, thoughts and/or symptoms must be ____ to meet criteria for an SSD.

    (a) excessive

    (b) painful

    (c) delusional

    (d) disabling

7. Integrative care is best described as ____.

    (a) allopathic

    (b) traditional

    (c) holistic

    (d) alternative

8. An individual with which of the following diagnoses is more likely to fail a performance validity test?

    (a) Major Depressive Disorder

    (b) traumatic brain injury

    (c) psychogenic nonepileptic seizures

    (d) multiple sclerosis

9. Which commonly used symptom or personality measure is likely to provide the most thorough assessment of symptom exaggeration in individuals with SSDs?

(a) PHQ-9

(c) GAD-7

(b) BDI

(d) PHQ-15

10. Discerning between aging related concerns and somatoform symptoms in older patients can best be facilitated by _____.

(a) brief patient report measures

(c) reports of concerns by family members

(b) careful history taking and observation

(d) primary care records

Integrative Health Approaches to Chronic Health Conditions and Somatic Symptom Disorders Answers

1. **C—somatic symptom disorder** *The DSM-IV disorders that involve preoccupation and excessive concern with somatic symptoms are subsumed by the SSD diagnosis in DSM-5.*

   Reference: American Psychiatric Association. (2013). *Diagnostic and statistical manual of mental disorders* (5th ed.) (DSM-5). Washington, DC: American Psychiatric Press.

2. **B—underestimate** *The multiple symptoms needed for a diagnosis of somatization disorder were rarely seen in their entirety in most clinical settings.*

   References:
   (a) Escobar, J. I., Burnam, M. A., Karno, M., Forsythe, A., & Golding, J. M. (1987). Somatization in the community. *Archives of General Psychiatry, 44,* 713–718.
   (b) Lamberty, G. J. (2008). *Understanding somatization in the practice of clinical neuropsychology.* New York, NY: Oxford University Press.

3. **A—alexithymia** *Attachment disorders are often characterized by problems with describing feelings. These are common features of individuals with FSS.*

   Reference: Koelen, J. A., Eurelings-Bontekoe, L. H., & Kempke, S. (2016). Cognitive alexithymia mediates the association between avoidant attachment and interpersonal problems in patients with somatoform disorder. *The Journal of Psychology: Interdisciplinary and Applied, 150*(6), 725–742.

4. **B—acceptance and commitment therapy** *ACT is a popular evidence-based psychotherapy modality that includes a significant mindfulness component, whereas the other treatments listed do not.*

   Reference: Baer, R. A. (2010). *Assessing mindfulness and acceptance processes in clients: Illuminating the theory and practice of change.* Oakland, CA: Context Press/New Harbinger Publications.

5. **D—a broader range of interventions are recognized as viable and accessible, rendering the term less meaningful** *There is an increased effort to improve coordination of different kinds of treatments in an integrative fashion.*

   Reference: National Center for Complementary & Integrative Health. (2018). *Complementary, alternative, or integrative health: What's in a name?* Retrieved from https://nccih.nih.gov/health/integrative-health

6. **A—excessive**   *A symptom or symptoms in an SSD must be excessive, as well as distressing and persistent.*

   Reference: American Psychiatric Association. (2013). *Diagnostic and statistical manual of mental disorders* (5th ed.) (DSM-5). Washington, DC: American Psychiatric Press.

7. **C—holistic**   *Integrative care has become a widely used descriptor that attempts to capture the broad nature of treatments offered. Mental health and nontraditional (CAM) approaches are frequently included.*

   Reference: Gaddy, M. A. (2018). Implementation of an integrative medicine treatment program at a Veterans Health Administration residential mental health facility. *Psychological Services, 15*(4), 503–509.

8. **C—psychogenic nonepileptic seizures**   *PNES is a well-studied somatoform disorder characterized by a tendency toward higher levels of symptom and performance validity failure.*

   Reference: Drane, D. L., & Locke, D. E. C. (2017). Mechanisms of possible neurocognitive dysfunction. In B. A. Dworetzky & G. C. Baslet (Eds.), *Psychogenic nonepileptic seizures: Toward the integration of care* (pp. 86–105). New York, NY: Oxford University Press.

9. **D—PHQ-15**   *The PHQ-15 is a version of the Patient Health Questionnaire that focuses on somatic symptom reporting and is generally elevated in individuals with FSS and SSDs.*

   Reference: Hinz, A., Ernst, J., Glaesmer, H., Brähler, E., Rauscher, F. G., Petrowski, K., & Kocalevent, R. D. (2017). Frequency of somatic symptoms in the general population: Normative values for the Patient Health Questionnaire-15 (PHQ-15). *Journal of Psychosomatic Research, 96*, 27–31.

10. **B—careful history taking and observation**   *Older patients' presentations are complicated by many aging related factors, suggesting that thorough consideration be given to all such factors. This is best accomplished with a thorough interview and careful observation.*

    Reference: Lamberty, G. J., & Bares, K. (2019). Neuropsychological assessment and management of older adults with multiple somatic symptoms. In L. D. Ravdin & H. L. Katzen (Eds.), *Clinical handbook on the neuropsychology of aging and dementia* (Vol. 2., pp. 121–134). New York, NY: Springer.

Recommended Readings

Bonvanie, I. J., Kallesøe, K. H., Janssens, K. A. M., Schröder, A., Rosmalen, J. G. M., & Rask, C. U. (2017). Psychological interventions for children with functional somatic symptoms: A systematic review and meta-analysis. *The Journal of Pediatrics, 187*, 272–281.

Boone, K. B. (Ed.). (2017). *Neuropsychological evaluation of somatoform and other functional somatic conditions: Assessment primer.* New York, NY: Taylor and Francis.

Gerteis, J., Izrael, D., Deitz, D., LeRoy, L., Ricciardi, R., Miller, T., & Basu, J. (2014). *Multiple chronic conditions chartbook* (AHRQ Publication No. Q14-0038). Rockville, MD: Agency for Healthcare Research and Quality.

Kleinstäuber, M., Witthöft, M., Steffanowski, A., van Marwijk, H., Hiller, W., & Lambert, M. J. (2014). Pharmacological interventions for somatoform disorders in adults. *Cochrane Database of Systematic Reviews, 11.* Art. No.: CD010628. doi: 10.1002/14651858.CD010628.pub2.

Lamberty, G. J. (2008). *Understanding somatization in the practice of clinical neuropsychology.* New York, NY: Oxford University Press.

van Dessel, N., den Boeft, M., van der Wouden, J. C., Kleinstäuber, M., Leone, S. S., Terluin, B., . . . vanMarwijk, H. (2014). Non-pharmacological interventions for somatoform disorders and medically unexplained physical symptoms (MUPS) in adults. *Cochrane Database of Systematic Reviews, 11,* Art. No.: CD011142. doi: 10.1002/14651858.CD011142.pub2.

Appendix A

First Full-Length Practice Examination Questions

1. Pure word deafness results from ____.
   (a) destruction of primary auditory cortex
   (b) damage to auditory radiations within the acoustic nerve
   (c) bilateral disconnection of auditory receptive areas from Wernicke's area
   (d) disconnection of Wernicke's area from semantic regions of the anterior temporal lobe

2. Which route of administration causes most rapid central nervous system penetration by opioids or stimulants?
   (a) smoking
   (b) inhalation/nasal
   (c) injection
   (d) rectal

3. An individual is given a battery of tests with at least three tests in each of five cognitive domains. He performs below the 10th percentile on one test in each of two separate cognitive domains. How do you interpret this pattern of performance?
   (a) The patient is clearly impaired in two important cognitive domains; I diagnose accordingly and provide treatment recommendations in my report.
   (b) The patient is essentially intact in almost all cognitive domains; I make no diagnosis and clarify in my report that no treatment is deemed necessary.
   (c) The patient may be impaired in one or more domain; I need more tests to be sure and will send a request for that in a report to the insurance company.
   (d) This may be due to normal variability. Unless a disorder is otherwise indicated by history, I make no diagnosis but comment on the variability in my report.

4. In contrast to women with multiple sclerosis, men with the disease may show ____.
   (a) greater cognitive impairment
   (b) more relapses
   (c) less neurologic deterioration
   (d) fewer lesions on MRI

5. A patient can both name and match-to-sample a visually presented object. She cannot remember where in a 3 × 3 spatial array the object was located. According to "top-bottom" theory, the lesion is likely somewhere in the ____.

(a) forceps major

(c) ventral stream

(b) dorsal stream

(d) forceps minor

6. Which of the following would be expected to show the lowest vulnerability to the effects of anoxia/hypoxia?

(a) areas supplied by the lenticulostriate arteries

(b) watershed regions between the major arteries

(c) regions with high metabolic demand

(d) area of bifurcation of the major branches of the middle cerebral artery

7. Which statement best defines cerebral palsy?

(a) It is a group of brain-based disorders characterized by motor impairments.

(b) It is a disease process that results in abnormal motor control.

(c) It is a group of disorders that causes primary damage to the muscles.

(d) It is an umbrella term for disorders that result from perinatal asphyxia.

8. A 23-year-old patient with a known history of reading disorder (dyslexia) is referred for evaluation of possible major depression or other mood disorder. The neuropsychologist would like to administer the MMPI-2-RF to assist in diagnostic decision-making. There is no opportunity for professional audio presentation of the items via computer. Which of the following best describes how the neuropsychologist should proceed when electing to administer the MMPI-2-RF to this patient?

(a) Administer a measure of reading achievement to ensure that the patient's reading level is no less than a tenth-grade level of ability.

(b) Read the test items aloud to the patient, repeating the items as necessary, to ensure adequate comprehension of item content.

(c) Administer a reading achievement task to ensure no less than a fifth-grade reading level.

(d) Administration of the MMPI-2-RF is not appropriate for use with this patient.

9. Social cognition is a relatively new area of study in epilepsy, despite the high incidence of comorbidity between Autism spectrum disorder and epilepsy. Studies have shown that, even among persons with epilepsy who do not have Autism spectrum disorder, that emotional recognition and theory of mind are affected. Which of the following is true about social cognition in persons with epilepsy?

(a) Social cognition is adversely affected in temporal lobe epilepsy, but not other epilepsy syndromes.

(b) Social cognition is normal in persons with temporal lobe epilepsy, but affected in other epilepsy syndromes.

(c) Social cognition is affected in persons with both temporal lobe epilepsy and other epilepsy syndromes.

(d) Social cognition is affected in children with epilepsy, but is age dependent and generally normal in adults.

10. Currently, the only treatment that extends life expectancy for adrenoleukodystrophy is ____.

    (a) Lorenzo's oil

    (b) epilepsy surgery

    (c) pallidotomy

    (d) hematopoietic stem cell transplant

11. A 47-year-old woman presents for testing. She was recently discharged after a 2-month hospitalization following a bout of depression, binge drinking, and anorexia. She denies any cognitive difficulties. Her sister, however, reported that the patient now has difficulties with orientation, concentration, memory, decision-making, and confabulation. The most likely diagnosis is ____.

    (a) Korsakoff's dementia

    (b) ACoA aneurysm rupture

    (c) early-onset Alzheimer's disease

    (d) pseudodementia

12. A patient with a new onset stroke has become euphoric. Where in the brain is the likely location of the stroke?

    (a) bilateral prefrontal cortex

    (b) left hemisphere

    (c) right hemisphere

    (d) mammillary bodies

13. Compared to typically developing peers, children with high-functioning Autism spectrum disorder are most likely to display the most severe deficit in which of the following executive functions?

    (a) organization and planning

    (b) planning and initiation

    (c) inhibition and flexibility

    (d) planning and inhibition

14. Depression following moderate to severe traumatic brain injury in adults is not associated with ____.

    (a) increased cognitive impairment

    (b) poor functional outcome

    (c) alcohol use disorders

    (d) greater initial injury severity

15. A 65-year-old patient with a 6-month history of lung cancer presents with recent onset of seizures, amnesia, and confusion. Of the following, the most probable etiology of cognitive dysfunction is ____.

    (a) paraneoplastic syndrome

    (b) malignant nerve sheath tumor

    (c) stroke or embolic shower

    (d) "chemobrain" from chemotherapy treatment

16. Nuchal rigidity is a hallmark feature of which disorder?

    (a) Creutzfeldt-Jakob disease

    (b) rabies encephalitis

    (c) West Nile Virus encephalitis

    (d) bacterial meningitis

17. Besides cognitive dysfunction, which of the following would you most expect to occur in chronic, untreated vitamin B_{12} deficiency?

    (a) delusions

    (b) ideomotor apraxia

    (c) resting tremor

    (d) impaired proprioception

18. In vascular dementia, delusions and visual hallucinations _____.

    (a) suggest a toxic or metabolic cause

    (b) occur in a sizable minority of patients

    (c) suggest mixed dementia

    (d) are considered to be quite rare

19. The 1.5:1 ratio of intellectual disability in males to females is in large part due to diagnoses such as _____.

    (a) epilepsy

    (b) Down syndrome

    (c) traumatic brain injury

    (d) fragile X syndrome

20. Your clinic evaluates a 10-year-old Spanish-dominant bilingual boy who is referred from school and is being considered for special academic services upon his return from a medical leave for treatment of a brain tumor. When considering which language to administer the tests in, you decide to _____.

    (a) test in Spanish since Spanish is his dominant language and these results will be most relevant in group functioning

    (b) test in English since that is the language of the setting of the school, where the results will be most relevant

    (c) test in both languages to obtain objective samples of language dominance and guide recommendations accordingly

    (d) forego testing due to the absence of adequate normative data for bilingual children, and rely upon a functional assessment

21. A 21-year-old woman who has been diagnosed with schizophrenia reports that she believes her coworker is poisoning her food. She also reports daily auditory hallucinations. She states that she has stopped eating and attending work. Which of the following would be the most important initial treatment consideration for the neuropsychologist?

    (a) functional capacity assessment

    (b) supportive occupational placement program

    (c) medication management and adherence

    (d) social skills training program

22. A 68-year-old, right-handed man presents after a stroke with impaired verbal fluency and relatively intact auditory comprehension and repetition. What aphasia syndrome does he have?

    (a) Wernicke's aphasia

    (b) conduction aphasia

    (c) Broca's aphasia

    (d) transcortical motor aphasia

23. Which of the following domains is generally less affected in children following anoxic brain injury?

    (a) behavioral regulation

    (b) visuospatial functioning

    (c) attention span

    (d) verbal memory

24. A 44-year-old divorced woman presents with cognitive, emotional, and pain related complaints. She readily admits to a history of psychiatric treatment starting in her early 20s. Assuming a high

likelihood of a mood or anxiety disorder which of the following would be the most important indicator of severity?

(a) scores on objective measures of mood/anxiety

(b) number of symptoms and intensity

(c) frequency of hospitalization

(d) impairment in social and occupational functioning

25. Which of the following evaluation findings is most likely to be seen in progressive supranuclear palsy versus other subcortical movement disorders?

(a) visuospatial deficits

(c) slowed processing speed

(b) pseudobulbar affect

(d) marked encoding deficit

26. You are at a professional meeting for psychologists in your community. One of your colleagues indicates that she recently learned that a former patient of hers was referred to you for outpatient assessment and she wants to know how the patient performed. The clinician indicates that she developed a close relationship with the patient and his family and has been concerned about his recovery. You do not have a signed release of information. Which of the following is the most appropriate response?

(a) Inform the colleague that it is unethical to request such information.

(b) Remain collegial but state that you have never heard of the patient.

(c) Request a release of information signed by the colleague.

(d) Thank her for her interest but provide no more information.

27. In the behavioral variant of frontotemporal dementia, Pick cells and bodies are commonly found, among other places, in the pyramidal cells of the ____.

(a) CA1 section and subiculum of the hippocampus

(b) CA1 and CA2 sections of the hippocampus

(c) CA2 and CA4 sections of the hippocampus

(d) CA4 and subiculum sections of the hippocampus

28. What happens to the mean, standard deviation, and the shape of the distribution when all scores are transformed into z scores?

(a) The set of scores will have a mean of one, standard deviation of zero, and positively skewed distribution.

(b) The set of scores will have a mean of zero, standard deviation of one, and positively skewed distribution.

(c) The set of scores will have a mean of zero, standard deviation of one, and unchanged distribution.

(d) The set of scores will have a mean of one, standard deviation of one, and unchanged distribution.

29. The risk of developing schizophrenia in females versus males is ____.

    (a) increased   (c) about the same

    (b) decreased   (d) unknown

30. In most children with Autism spectrum disorders, communicative ability during the third through the fifth years of life ____.

    (a) improves with time, but contains abnormalities (e.g., echolalia, unusual prosody)

    (b) declines to mutism as in Rett's disorder

    (c) declines but is marked by an increase in nonverbal communication ability

    (d) improves to the point of age-appropriate levels coupled with appropriate social gestures

31. Pyramidal cerebral palsy is associated with ____.

    (a) dystonia   (c) spasticity

    (b) athetosis   (d) ataxia

32. You are seeing a child for an evaluation of dyslexia. The most important areas for assessment are phonological awareness, decoding, ____.

    (a) single-word reading, and spelling

    (b) visual scanning, and spelling

    (c) reading comprehension, and spelling

    (d) reading letters in proper orientation and order

33. In Vietnamese culture, nodding is often a polite signal that the person is listening versus being agreeable. Given this tendency, and assuming that language is not an issue due to use of a competent interpreter, what would be the best approach to ensure understanding of test instructions when explaining a test to a first-generation Vietnamese examinee?

    (a) repeat the instructions more than once to ensure understanding

    (b) nothing as the neuropsychologist must follow standardized protocol

    (c) ask the examinee if s/he understand the instructions

    (d) ask the examinee to explain the instructions in his/her own words

34. In general, when compared with men with alcohol use disorder (AUD), the neuropsychological presentation of women with AUD shows ____.

    (a) deficits develop after shorter drinking histories

    (b) reduced verbal abilities

    (c) better performance on visuoperceptual/visuospatial tasks

    (d) better performance on timed tasks

35. When giving a personality inventory to a patient who is 18 years old, one should ____.

    (a) always administer the adult version of the inventory, in the instance that the patient may need to take the inventory again in the future

    (b) always administer the adolescent version as the norms for the adult version tend to overpathologize someone of this age

(c) consult specific personality inventory manuals to guide decision-making

(d) give both the adolescent and adult versions and compare them

36. An upper left or upper right visual field quadrant loss would suggest involvement of the optic radiations passing through the _____ lobe of the cerebral hemisphere _____ to the field defect.

(a) parietal; ipsilateral

(b) frontal; contralateral

(c) temporal; bilateral

(d) temporal; contralateral

37. Jessica has been concerned about multiple sclerosis (MS) for many years. She does not currently have MS symptoms and has not had symptoms in the past. Nevertheless, she routinely sees her doctor to rule out the diagnosis. What is the most likely DSM-5 diagnosis?

(a) somatic symptom disorder

(b) psychological factors affecting other medical disorders

(c) hypochondriasis

(d) illness anxiety disorder

38. Studies have shown that children with epilepsy have nearly three times the incidence of ADHD compared to children without epilepsy. Treatment of ADHD symptoms with stimulants in children with epilepsy is _____.

(a) safe, and as effective as in children with ADHD alone

(b) safe, but not effective compared with ADHD alone

(c) effective, but carries increased risk of seizure exacerbation in some children

(d) neither safe nor effective

39. A 9-year-old girl is referred for an evaluation for academic difficulties. She presents with short stature and a webbed neck. Her neuropsychological evaluation reveals dyscalculia and deficits in visuospatial skills. She most likely has which disorder?

(a) Turner syndrome

(b) Williams syndrome

(c) Angelman syndrome

(d) tuberous sclerosis

40. August is a 17-year-old referred to you after a recent diagnosis of multiple sclerosis. You are reviewing WAIS-IV scores from the first part of your evaluation and have noticed a pattern of performance suggestive of slow processing speed. Based on this finding and your review of the literature of pediatric multiple sclerosis, what else are you likely to assess to confirm or disconfirm impairment in processing speed?

(a) word list generation, visual-motor integration, attention

(b) depression, visual-motor integration, fatigue

(c) attention, visual perception, receptive language

(d) visual-motor integration, sleep hygiene, word list generation

41. A neuropsychologist in a pediatric epilepsy surgery program plans to do both pre- and post-operative evaluations with the same memory test. The best way to determine whether any change in performance is clinically meaningful would be to ____.

    (a) just use equally reliable alternate forms of the same test

    (b) subtract the standard error of measurement from the second score

    (c) calculate the reliable change index, with a 90% confidence interval

    (d) add the standard error of the estimate to the second score

42. In the United States, in utero exposure to lead is most likely to occur through exposure from ____.

    (a) maternal occupation   (c) gasoline

    (b) imported toys   (d) cosmetics

43. Adrenergic neurons originate in ____.

    (a) the basal forebrain

    (b) the raphe nuclei

    (c) the locus coeruleus and lateral tegmental area

    (d) the substantia nigra pars compacta

44. The most persistent cognitive deficit in patients with limbic encephalitis is ____.

    (a) organization and planning   (c) memory and new learning

    (b) language and word retrieval   (d) auditory and visual attention

45. Which regions of the brain show the most atrophy in Alzheimer's disease?

    (a) temporoparietal   (c) occipitoparietal

    (b) orbitofrontal and primary motor   (d) thalamus and basal ganglia

46. The multimodal treatment study of children with ADHD (1999, 2004) is the largest, best-controlled study to date assessing the efficacy of medication and behavioral therapy for children. Which of the following statements best characterizes the findings with regard to ADHD symptoms?

    (a) Behavioral intervention alone was slightly superior to medication intervention alone, particularly in younger children.

    (b) There was a large effect seen for medication treatment, for which the addition of behavioral therapy produced no significant added benefit.

    (c) Medication and behavioral therapy combined performed significantly better than medication alone or behavioral therapy alone.

    (d) There were no significant differences between medication alone, behavioral therapy alone, and combination of medication and behavioral therapy.

47. A 65-year-old, right-handed man is referred following an ischemic stroke in the inferior division of the right MCA. What cognitive problem(s) are most likely to be present?

    (a) parts of the Gerstmann syndrome

    (b) left hemispatial inattention and constructional apraxia

    (c) right–left confusion and constructional apraxia

    (d) amnesia for nonverbal information

48. A patient sustains a severe traumatic brain injury in a high-speed motor vehicle collision. At the scene, she is unable to open her eyes, is completely flaccid, and displays no vocalization. The most likely Glasgow Coma Scale score is _____.

    (a) 0   (c) 3

    (b) 1   (d) 5

49. A 9-year-old girl presents to your office with her mother. The girl is nonverbal but attempts to engage you socially by making eye contact, laughing, and smiling. In discussion with her mother, you learn that the girl started exhibiting developmental delays in infancy and then developed seizures at 2 years of age. This girl most likely has which disorder?

    (a) Prader-Willi syndrome   (c) Turner syndrome

    (b) Angelman syndrome   (d) PKU

50. Adult survivors of childhood brain tumors are at increased risk for _____.

    (a) kidney and liver disease

    (b) secondary tumors and encephalitis

    (c) secondary tumors, late-onset seizures, and stroke

    (d) late-onset seizures and heart disease

51. The orbitofrontal cortex is relevant to which attentional function?

    (a) selective attention   (c) inhibition of response

    (b) initiation of response   (d) alternating attention

52. Which of the following statements is true regarding presence of psychiatric symptoms in movement disorders?

    (a) Depression can occur years prior to motor symptoms in Huntington's disease.

    (b) Hallucinations are a rare side effect of medications used to treat Parkinson's disease.

    (c) Mania can be seen in patients with progressive supranuclear palsy.

    (d) Visual hallucinations typically occur late in the course of Lewy body dementia.

53. Which of the following is the *most* important factor in determining the severity of cognitive impairment in persons with epilepsy?

    (a) seizure frequency   (c) type of medication

    (b) history of febrile seizure   (d) abnormal MRI finding

54. An 8-year-old child presents for neuropsychological assessment with a history of prematurity and a diagnosis of periventricular leukomalacia (PVL). What is a typical pattern of weakness in a child with this history?

    (a) spatial memory, attention, vocabulary

    (b) visuospatial processing, processing speed, working memory

    (c) visuospatial processing, vocabulary, working memory

    (d) word reading, verbal fluency, and fine motor dexterity

55. Studies conducted with the MMPI-2 and MMPI-2-RF in litigating mild traumatic brain injury samples reveal a greater tendency to _____.

    (a) adopt a defensive response style marked by underreporting of symptoms

    (b) endorse paranoia and "psychotic" symptoms as opposed to somatic complaints and other "neurotic" symptoms

    (c) endorse somatic complaints and other "neurotic" symptoms as opposed to paranoia and "psychotic" symptoms

    (d) respond randomly or inconsistently to test items about cognitive and somatic symptoms

56. Under anoxic/hypoxic conditions, when neurons can no longer replenish adenosine triphosphate (ATP), the following response occurs.

    (a) Neurons begin to self-hibernate so as to minimize metabolic processes.

    (b) The brain diverts stored ATP from other brain regions to the hypoxic area.

    (c) A series of neurotoxic processes are initiated that lead to neuronal death.

    (d) Axons rapidly rupture and disintegrate.

57. The most effective intervention for improving reading fluency is _____.

    (a) structured questioning   (c) visual training

    (b) repeated reading   (d) phonics instruction

58. When seeing a patient you notice detailed descriptions of intense fear and anxiety responses relative to prior stressful experiences. Which structure is thought to sense and identify fear and anxiety-laden stimuli and initiate this type of emotional response?

    (a) caudate nucleus   (c) insula

    (b) prefrontal cortex   (d) amygdala

59. When performance on a test is not normally distributed but there is some variance, what is the best way to interpret the test result using normative data?

    (a) z score   (c) percentile

    (b) T score   (d) cut-off

60. Which of the following is false?

    (a) Vascular dementia is uncommon in pathophysiologically pure form.

    (b) Vascular dementia often co-occurs with the pathophysiology of Alzheimer's disease.

    (c) Vascular dementia can present with symptoms suggestive of normal pressure hydrocephalus.

    (d) Vascular dementia has a relatively invariant pathophysiological presentation.

61. An individual with cerebellar mutism syndrome is most likely to have a history of _____.

    (a) epilepsy   (c) brain tumor

    (b) traumatic brain injury   (d) stroke

62. Estimating premorbid functioning based on educational level and current word reading performance is an example of _____.

(a) combined current performance and demographic method of estimating premorbid functioning

(b) combined current performance and actuarial estimation of premorbid functioning

(c) best performance method of estimating premorbid functioning

(d) combined demographic and actuarial method of estimating premorbid functioning

63. On neuropsychological tests, children with hydrocephalus secondary to spina bifida myelomeningocele and aqueductal stenosis _____.

(a) show similar patterns of performance except in the motor domain

(b) show qualitatively different patterns of performance across multiple domains

(c) show similar levels of overall cognitive and motor performance

(d) are differentiated by the absence of language deficits in spina bifida

64. Persons with progressive supranuclear palsy often initially present with _____.

(a) dysdiadochokinesia   (c) right side hemiplegia

(b) impaired vertical gaze   (d) impaired horizontal gaze

65. You are a new attending neuropsychologist at a prestigious university hospital. Your former supervisor is in her late 60s and seems to be having significant and increasing memory difficulty. While she is seeing patients on the unit, you have found her twice in the hallway having forgotten where she was going. Staff tells you privately that they don't rely on her because she seems confused a lot and cannot keep information straight. The chief of the neuropsychology service knows, but keeps her on patient care rotations. He is interviewing potential faculty to replace the clinician, and he asks you to be patient during the process. Which of the following is most appropriate ethically?

(a) Wait for now, the chief of service is aware and responsible.

(b) Observe your former supervisor and assess for impairment.

(c) Report the neuropsychology chief to the state ethics committee.

(d) Discuss your concern with the unit director or chief of staff.

66. Repetitive behaviors are defined as repetitive, nonfunctional activities or interests that occur regularly and interfere with daily functioning. The following four repetitive behaviors can all be seen in Autism spectrum disorder; which is selectively associated with low IQ?

(a) narrow interests in maps and timetables

(b) repetitive watching of television commercials

(c) engaging in actions that cause injury to self

(d) needing routes to stay the same all the time

67. In patients with Alzheimer's disease, cholinesterase inhibitors given in the early stages of illness _____.

    (a) may delay nursing home placement

    (b) may delay onset of incontinence

    (c) may delay onset of motor or sensory impairments

    (d) rarely delay functional or cognitive changes

68. Paul Broca is credited with which of the following?

    (a) The law of mass action

    (b) Identifying the brain region subserving verbal comprehension

    (c) Discovery of conduction aphasia

    (d) Identifying the brain region subserving expressive speech

69. A 19-year-old man presents to the clinic with his parents. They are concerned because he has stopped hanging out with his friends, spends most of his time alone in his room, and rarely bothers to shower or change clothes. He dropped out of the local community college he was attending. In addition, he is sometimes seen muttering to himself, and has a hard time expressing himself. He becomes easily upset with his parents, often accusing them of spying on him and trying to ruin his life. This all started about 5 months ago, though his parents say they may have seen subtle signs as early as 1 year ago. During your interview with him, the man refuses to answer most of your questions and avoids eye contact. Which of the following would be his most likely diagnosis?

    (a) schizophreniform disorder   (c) schizoaffective disorder

    (b) schizophrenia   (d) major depression with psychosis

70. A pediatrician refers a patient to you for a neuropsychological evaluation because of an elevated blood lead level. You evaluate the child and find deficits in executive functioning and visuospatial functions. One year later, the pediatrician contacts you about this patient. The patient has undergone chelation treatment and the pediatrician wonders if a follow-up neuropsychological evaluation would be able to document treatment-related changes. Based on the literature, what should you tell the pediatrician?

    (a) Chelation treatment improves executive functioning only.

    (b) Chelation treatment improves visuospatial and attentional skills only.

    (c) Chelation treatment improves intellectual functioning only.

    (d) Chelation treatment does not reverse cognitive deficits.

71. A 16-year-old girl is evaluated in rehabilitation following a ruptured aneurysm. She is unable to follow commands, repeat, or name objects, but very matter-of-factly states, "I wan ba frink clink in da damn." The most likely diagnosis is _____.

    (a) Broca's aphasia   (c) anomic aphasia

    (b) Wernicke's aphasia   (d) conduction aphasia

72. What statement is true about cerebral palsy (CP)?

    (a) CP is non-progressive but the associated functional impairments can worsen.

    (b) CP is non-progressive and secondary impairments are uncommon.

    (c) CP is progressive and clinical manifestations worsen due to activity limitations.

    (d) CP is progressive and frequently associated with a shortened life expectancy.

73. A patient 3 years post severe traumatic brain injury undergoes neuropsychological evaluation. All scores fall within the low average to average range. However, there is behavioral evidence and complaints from collaterals which suggest significant changes in impulse control, social skills, and disinhibition. Assuming that these problems are brain injury related, where might the neuropsychologist reasonably speculate that persistent dysfunction is present?

    (a) dorsolateral system and its connections

    (b) prefrontal system and its connections

    (c) orbitofrontal system and its connections

    (d) medial frontal system and its connections

74. Reading disabilities are commonly seen in which of the following neurodevelopmental diagnoses ____.

    (a) spina bifida

    (b) Turner syndrome

    (c) 22q deletion syndrome

    (d) Klinefelter syndrome

75. Classification of recurrent seizures into epileptic syndromes takes into account multiple features. Which of the following is an important criterion for classification?

    (a) age of seizure onset

    (b) presence of abnormal MRI findings

    (c) presence of comorbid epileptic encephalopathy

    (d) psychosocial effects of seizures

76. A two-alternative forced choice performance validity test has three trials. Each trial has 10 items. An examinee earns a score of 3 on each trial. The probability of this occurring by chance is about ____.

    (a) 1.0

    (b) .5

    (c) .1

    (d) .01

77. Six months following mitral valve replacement surgery, a patient is referred to you by the cardiologist due to family complaints of personality changes, memory problems, and depression since the surgery. The family reports that the patient experienced symptoms suggestive of delirium for 7 to 10 days after the surgery. Neuropsychological assessment confirms the presence of memory retrieval deficits and mild executive dysfunction. Of the following, which is the most probable explanation?

    (a) stroke

    (b) sepsis

    (c) hyponatremia

    (d) embolic shower

78. Which of the following statements is consistent with the trajectory of cognitive functioning in individuals with Down syndrome?

    (a) With enough support and education, individuals with Down syndrome show improvement in scores on measures of intellectual functioning as they age.

    (b) Intelligence test scores of individuals with Down syndrome remain constant over time.

    (c) Individuals with Down syndrome exhibit a progressive decline on measures of developmental and intellectual functioning beginning in the first year of life.

    (d) Individuals with Down syndrome exhibit steady increases in performance on measures of intellectual functioning until they reach early adulthood, when their scores drop precipitously.

79. On executive function tests, children with congenital hydrocephalus _____.

    (a) have little difficulty because of preservation of the frontal lobes

    (b) show patterns clearly interpretable as frontal lobe dysfunction

    (c) show difficulties with task performance that often reflect attention and motor difficulties

    (d) show executive function deficits if they meet criteria for ADHD

80. Maggie, a 38-year-old woman from Alaska, has multiple sclerosis. She has experienced pain and a loss of right eye vision, as well as overwhelming fatigue and lack of mental energy. She presented to her primary care physician, who performed an examination and extensive blood panel work-up. What findings might you see in laboratory results considering the diagnosis of multiple sclerosis?

    (a) abnormal and increased white blood cells

    (b) low levels of vitamin D and elevated forms of cytokines

    (c) elevated aspartate aminotransferase and alkaline phosphatase

    (d) high levels of vitamin E and elevated alkaline phosphatase

81. Which of the following is accurate about the radioisotope used in neuroimaging technologies such as SPECT and PET?

    (a) They are absorbed by glia and provide an indirect index of regional activity.

    (b) They are absorbed by neurons and provide a direct index of neural activity.

    (c) They remain in the bloodstream and provide an indirect index of neural activity.

    (d) They cross the blood-brain barrier and provide an indirect index of regional activity.

82. Which of the following was shown to be an effective intervention in a clinical trial for mitigating cognitive deficits in patients with brain metastases?

    (a) memantine   (c) Wellbutrin

    (b) individualized cognitive rehabilitation   (d) computerized cognitive training

83. Your 9-year-old female patient has a history of herpes simplex virus encephalitis, but did not receive prompt treatment with acyclovir. Studies at the time were abnormal including brain MRI and EEG, which showed seizures. What is the most likely long-term prognosis for your patient?

    (a) There is a low risk for seizures (< 3%) over the course of the next 20 years despite having had them acutely.

    (b) She will experience long-term neurologic and psychiatric sequelae and poor quality of life.

(c) Mild attention and memory deficits are expected, due to late start of acyclovir.

(d) She is at increased risk for behavioral problems and ADHD, but other psychiatric comorbidities are unlikely.

84. You are evaluating a college student who was previously diagnosed with dyslexia as a child. She also had early intervention, which helped improve her reading skills. In an updated evaluation of her reading skills, to assist with documenting a need for accommodations, you should always include measures of ____.

(a) processing speed, rapid visual naming, timed decoding, and timed reading comprehension

(b) visual scanning, rapid visual naming, timed decoding, and timed reading comprehension

(c) rapid visual naming, timed decoding, timed single-word reading, and timed reading comprehension

(d) visual scanning, rapid visual naming, timed decoding, and timed single word reading

85. The hallmark feature of Wernicke-Korsakoff syndrome is the difference between the patient's intelligence quotient and memory quotient, in which the latter is more severely impaired. The memory deficits, over and above the typical neurotoxic effects of alcohol, consist of anterograde amnesia and ____.

(a) temporally graded retrograde amnesia

(c) signs of Capgras syndrome

(b) impaired procedural memory

(d) ataxia and fine resting tremor

86. Positive predictive value (PPV) is defined as the ____.

(a) true positives divided by (true positives plus false positives)

(b) percentage of true positives that can be reliably identified by a test

(c) absolute number of true positives out of all cases tested

(d) absolute number of true positives and true negatives in all cases combined

87. During an intake interview with a young adult, you learn that she was born prematurely at 27 weeks gestational age. You consult the literature to gain a better understanding of the neuropsychological sequelae associated with preterm birth. When consulting the preterm literature the most critical factor to consider is the ____.

(a) birth weight of the cohort

(c) test battery that was administered

(b) gestational age of the cohort

(d) birth year of the cohort

88. You have a patient with a lesion in the superior portion of the left frontal lobe. Which of the following deficits would be most likely?

(a) nonfluent aphasia

(b) impaired verbal working memory

(c) poor learning from rewards and punishments

(d) semantic memory impairment

89. Typical neuroimaging findings in patients with cerebral palsy include ____.

(a) ventricular dilatation or aqueductal stenosis

(b) arteriovenous malformation or Chiari II malformation

(c) middle cerebral artery stroke or subdural hemorrhage

(d) intraventricular hemorrhage or periventricular leukomalacia

90. Which of the following would be the most appropriate reason to conduct a neuropsychological evaluation for a child suspected of having ADHD?

(a) to administer a CPT that can detect the presence of ADHD

(b) to determine which stimulant medication would be most appropriate for treating ADHD symptoms

(c) to determine if the child has a comorbid learning disability or psychiatric disorder

(d) to assess if the child has thyroid dysfunction or epilepsy

91. The prototypical neuropsychological profile of patients with frontotemporal dementia early in the disease is _____.

(a) visuospatial deficits with relative sparing of memory and executive functioning

(b) memory deficits with relative sparing of visuospatial and executive functioning

(c) executive dysfunction with relative sparing of memory and visuospatial functioning

(d) deficits in memory, visuospatial functioning, and executive functioning

92. Neuropathological evidence of decreased neuropil in schizophrenia has been linked to _____.

(a) excessive synaptic pruning, possibly due to variations in complement component 4 (CC4) genes.

(b) childhood traumatic brain injury with diffuse axonal injury.

(c) viral infections during the first trimester of gestation.

(d) degeneration of synaptic and glial processes, associated with the deposition of tau and amyloid proteins.

93. A 55-year-old man who has a long history of anxiety and prominent startle responses to loud noises and unexpected tactile stimulation is likely experiencing a hyperactive anxiety or hypervigilance associated which brain region?

(a) prefrontal cortex

(b) cingulate gyrus

(c) amygdala

(d) caudate nucleus

94. At this time, Alzheimer's disease can only be definitively diagnosed via postmortem histopathologic verification. Which one of these findings is less characteristic of the primary expected neurodegenerative abnormalities?

(a) neuritic plaques

(b) neurofibrillary tangles

(c) excessive neuronal loss

(d) extensive white matter disease

95. Which congenital disorder has been associated with severe hypoxia or ischemia at birth?

(a) spina bifida

(b) Down syndrome

(c) cerebral palsy

(d) cystic fibrosis

96. A 17-year-old male presents for an evaluation. During the history, his mother reports that he was born with cardiac and palatal malformations, requiring surgery during childhood. He also demonstrated significant language delays, not using single words until 2.5 years of age. In school, he has struggled with math, attention, and focus. More recently, he has reported visual hallucinations, including seeing other people in the room with him who are not there. He most likely has which disorder?

(a) Williams syndrome

(c) 22q11.2 deletion syndrome

(b) Turner syndrome

(d) Klinefelter syndrome

97. Mike, a 34-year-old man, has experienced seizure-like episodes at work for the past 4 months. Imaging and EEG studies have been normal. Mike has been on disability leave for the past 2 months related to his concerns about seizures at work. The most appropriate diagnosis would be ____.

(a) functional neurological symptom disorder

(b) complex partial epilepsy

(c) illness anxiety disorder

(d) somatic symptom disorder

98. Which of the following symptoms can be helpful with differential diagnosis of Lewy body disease from other movement disorders such as progressive supranuclear palsy and Parkinson's disease?

(a) early presence of visual hallucinations

(c) presence of festinating gait

(b) upward vertical gaze deficit

(d) presence of REM behavioral symptoms

99. When asked to simulate combing his hair with a comb, a patient strokes his fingers through his hair. This is a sign of ____.

(a) buccofacial apraxia

(c) limb-kinetic apraxia

(b) ideomotor apraxia

(d) ideational apraxia

100. You have been involved in a patient's care since his hospitalization following a work-related injury. The patient sustained burn injuries and a severe hypoxic brain injury in a chemical fire. You are now being asked by the patient's attorney to act as an expert witness in an upcoming deposition. Which option is most ethically appropriate?

(a) Recommend a forensic evaluation and refuse to participate in any deposition.

(b) Act as an expert witness if the patient and attorney give formal permission.

(c) Agree to act as a fact witness and accept no payment for the deposition.

(d) Act as an expert witness if the patient consents but disclose your non-forensic role.

101. A teenage patient continues to struggle with school 2 years following a moderate traumatic brain injury. Testing reveals moderate to severe memory impairments, but average to low average executive function, speed of information processing, and visuospatial skills. What combination of interventions would have the best chance of resulting in functional gains?

(a) restorative skill training and processing efficiency strategies

(b) error free learning and compensatory memory strategies

(c) self-regulation training and compensatory memory strategies

(d) self-regulation training and time management strategies

102. You are planning an assessment of a 19-month-old patient with a history of premature birth. Most tests recommend that you make an age correction to account for prematurity until what age?

(a) 12 months

(b) 24 months

(c) 36 months

(d) 48 months

103. Which of the following is considered the most important mediator between the effect of neurocognition on functional outcome?

(a) social support

(b) positive symptoms

(c) social cognition

(d) medical comorbidities

104. Epilepsy is defined as _____.

(a) recurrent unprovoked seizures

(b) medication resistant seizures

(c) multiple different seizure types

(d) seizures associated with transient metabolic changes

105. What is the most frequent and disabling symptom commonly reported by patients with multiple sclerosis?

(a) spasticity

(b) fatigue

(c) sleep disturbance

(d) optic neuritis

106. Spina bifida occulta _____.

(a) is a common disorder not obviously related to other forms of spina bifida

(b) shows a neuropsychological profile like other forms of spina bifida

(c) is another term for myelomeningocele

(d) can be identified through prenatal screening

107. You are interviewing a 48-year-old man with a history of hypertension who reports a short episode of right hemiparesis and difficulty talking 3 months ago with no residual deficits. What criterion or criteria would now be used to make a diagnosis of transient ischemic attack (TIA) versus stroke?

(a) no evidence of infarct on neuroimaging

(b) no evidence of current deficits

(c) symptom duration less than 24 hours

(d) symptom duration less than 1 hour

108. A child with a history of extreme preterm birth presents for assessment. What information would be most important to obtain in order to assess for increased risk for poorer long-term outcome?

(a) maternal diabetes, multiple birth pregnancy, and short spacing between pregnancies

(b) advanced or young maternal age, maternal infections, and maternal substance use

(c) lack of prenatal care, maternal stress, and abnormalities of the cervix or uterus

(d) country and setting of the birth, presence of intraventricular hemorrhage (IVH), and other neurological complications

109. Which of the following is not true regarding tuberculous (TB) meningitis?

    (a) Common associated neurologic sequelae include stroke and hydrocephalus.

    (b) Antibiotics are not effective.

    (c) Mortality rates are quite low due to improved treatments in the past 10 years.

    (d) TB meningitis is more common in countries with fewer economic resources.

110. Protective factors for vascular cognitive impairment include all of the following except ____.

    (a) long-term regular physical activity

    (b) maintaining a BMI between 18.5 and 24.9

    (c) moderate alcohol use

    (d) antioxidant and B vitamin supplementation

111. Hallucinogens have a chemical structure similar to serotonin. The serotonin system is involved in controlling all of the following, except ____.

    (a) attention   (c) sensory perception

    (b) mood   (d) muscle control

112. Charlie is a 3-year-old child who exhibited a long and narrow face, large ears, a prominent jaw and forehead, and unusually flexible fingers. Charlie's mother reported delayed development, anxiety, hyperactivity, and impulsivity, and recent diagnoses of Autism spectrum disorder and intellectual disability. His mother's family has a history of ovarian failure, tremor, ataxia, ADHD, anxiety, and depression. This constellation of symptoms raises strong suspicions for ____.

    (a) Down syndrome   (c) fragile X syndrome

    (b) Prader-Willi syndrome   (d) neurofibromatosis

113. Serotonin is synthesized in what area of the brain?

    (a) medial and dorsal raphe nuclei   (c) locus coeruleus

    (b) periaqueductal gray area   (d) substantia nigra

114. Which of the following is most correct in terms of biomarkers for the diagnosis of depression and anxiety?

    (a) Neurotransmitter and neuroendocrine markers have been shown to be effective in enhancing diagnostic accuracy.

    (b) Inflammatory response, the immune system, and metabolic and growth factors have been beneficial in differential diagnosis.

    (c) Genetic testing has been shown to be useful in early diagnosis.

    (d) Mood and anxiety disorders cannot be identified through typical medical evaluations such as blood tests or neuroimaging studies.

115. You are conducting an evaluation with a 15-year-old female with a history of ADHD symptoms including distractibility, poor planning/organizational skills, and difficulty completing exams within a timely manner. Behavioral rating forms indicate significant inattentive symptoms both in the home and academic settings, while there were no significant hyperactive/impulsive symptoms in either setting. Neuropsychological testing reveals average performance on

measures of sustained attention (e.g., CPT), working memory, and ability to inhibit impulsive responses in the context of FSIQ within the high average range. Which of the following clinical interpretations is most likely given the presented information?

(a) A diagnosis of ADHD is not warranted based on neuropsychological test performance falling within normal limits.

(b) A diagnosis of ADHD-I is appropriate if 6 (or more) of the 9 inattentive symptoms are met within two or more settings.

(c) A diagnosis of ADHD-I and a specific learning disorder are appropriate, as these symptoms impact academic performance.

(d) A diagnosis of ADHD–combined presentation is appropriate.

116. Early Alzheimer's disease should be suspected if the family complains of significant changes in the patient's ____.

(a) personality functioning

(b) emotional status and responsiveness

(c) ability to perform activities of daily living

(d) capacity to function in unfamiliar settings

117. Alexia with agraphia is usually most localizable to ____.

(a) lingual and fusiform lobule in the left hemisphere

(b) arcuate fasciculus and perisylvian left hemisphere

(c) supramarginal gyrus or angular gyrus in the left hemisphere

(d) occipital and posterior corpus callosum in the left hemisphere

118. Following traumatic brain injury, problems with initiation are most likely related to damage to the ____.

(a) dorsolateral prefrontal cortex

(b) orbitofrontal cortex

(c) supplemental motor cortex

(d) anterior cingulate cortex

119. Normal pressure hydrocephalus is often confused with ____.

(a) dementia because it is common in Alzheimer's disease

(b) parkinsonism because of the gait and motor anomalies

(c) strokes because of unilateral hemiparesis

(d) subarachnoid hematomas because of the pressure on the brain

120. Which of the following has not been linked with vascular cognitive impairment?

(a) periodic leg movement disorder

(b) atrial fibrillation

(c) cerebral amyloid angiography

(d) white matter hyperintensities

121. Which statement about speech, occupational, and physical therapies for children with cerebral palsy (CP) is accurate?

    (a) The most effective environment is a familiar home setting in which distractions are minimized (e.g., removing toys, limiting parent participation).

    (b) Therapies can help prevent a child from experiencing a deterioration in mobility and being reclassified at a more severe Gross Motor Function Classification System level.

    (c) Since children with CP tend to experience decreased sensation, goals related to pain management usually are not necessary.

    (d) Although early intervention cannot cure CP, mobility often improves enough that a child can be reclassified at a milder Gross Motor Function Classification System level.

122. Each of these is a common or core feature of the semantic variant of frontotemporal dementia according to current diagnostic criteria except impaired ____.

    (a) confrontation naming

    (b) object knowledge

    (c) single word comprehension

    (d) sentence repetition

123. "Executive" attention (monitoring and resolving conflicts between thoughts, feelings and behaviors) is most dependent upon which of the following regions?

    (a) ventromedial frontal lobe

    (b) extended amygdala

    (c) anterior cingulate cortex

    (d) orbitofrontal cortex

124. A new patient presents complaining of visual difficulties. His medical records reflect field cuts occurring within the temporal visual hemifield of each eye. This would suggest ____.

    (a) a lesion of the optic chiasm

    (b) cranial nerves III, IV, VI involvement only

    (c) bilateral retinal detachment

    (d) cranial nerve II and III involvement only

125. You are consulted to determine the decision making capacity of a 65-year-old woman who underwent hip surgery 2 days prior. The person was described as cognitively intact and healthy prior to surgery. Your examination reveals clear evidence of delirium. Of the following, which is the least likely possible cause?

    (a) hyponatremia

    (b) undiagnosed dementia

    (c) urinary tract infection

    (d) medication side effect(s)

Appendix B

Second Full-Length Practice Examination Questions

1. A 67-year-old right-handed woman with no significant medical history was sitting and conversing with a friend at lunch when suddenly she began repeating what she heard and could not answer simple questions. At the hospital, her speech was fluent but echolalic. She was unable to follow commands, but repeated words and sentences with 100% accuracy. Naming was impaired. What kind of aphasic syndrome is likely present in this patient?

   (a) Broca's aphasia

   (b) Wernicke's aphasia

   (c) transcortical sensory aphasia

   (d) transcortical motor aphasia

2. You recently completed a neuropsychological evaluation with an elderly man and determined that he likely has middle stage dementia of the Alzheimer type. You have a release that allows you to speak with family members. You call the patient's wife to arrange feedback. She agrees to come in for feedback but asks you not to tell her husband that he has dementia indicating that it will most certainly depress him further and that he might become suicidal. What should you do first?

   (a) Thank her for the concern and call at another time to arrange feedback specifically with the patient.

   (b) Tell the wife that you are obligated to provide the patient with all findings.

   (c) Cancel the feedback session but provide a written report to the referring provider.

   (d) Provide the patient with feedback unless you are convinced it will result in harm.

3. In children with Autism spectrum disorder, which of the following is most successful in treating irritability and hyperactivity?

   (a) discrete trial instruction

   (b) restricted diet

   (c) deep-pressure/sensory stimulation

   (d) psychotropic medications

4. For a child with cerebral palsy, a favorable prognostic indicator is ____.

   (a) hand preference by 15 months

   (b) sitting by 24 months

   (c) standing by 36 months

   (d) pincer grasp by 11 months

5. Which of the following neurocognitive functions is generally best preserved among individuals with schizophrenia?

(a) visuospatial reasoning

(c) executive functioning

(b) memory

(d) attention

6. A college-educated 50-year-old African American woman with memory complaints is referred for testing to rule out mild cognitive impairment from normal aging. Which set of normative data would be most appropriate for interpretation for a list-learning test?

(a) the norms included in the testing manual

(b) no normative data set is best, this case requires qualitative assessment

(c) norms that adjust for years of education

(d) a normative data set collected exclusively on African Americans

7. On what task can patients with substance-induced amnesia (formerly Korsakoff amnesia) demonstrate intact learning?

(a) spatial-location

(c) pursuit-rotor

(b) facial recognition

(d) verbal list learning

8. Which of the following conditions is an environmental cause of ADHD?

(a) exposure to tobacco smoke in utero

(b) single uncomplicated mild traumatic brain injury

(c) frequent otitis media

(d) exposure to antiepileptic drugs in utero

9. Patients in the early stages of Alzheimer's disease will typically display all of the following memory characteristics except ____.

(a) little improvement with repeated learning trials

(b) perseverative and echolalic behavior

(c) errors during recall, such as intrusions

(d) a heightened recency effect

10. In the classic cortico-striatal-pallidal-thalamo-cortical loop, the "input" to the basal ganglia is to the ____ and the output is via the ____.

(a) globus pallidus; caudate nucleus

(c) globus pallidus; nucleus accumbens

(b) striatum; globus pallidus

(d) striatum; nucleus accumbens

11. Which of the following is apt to be most sensitive to noncredible performance on a verbal list-learning memory test?

(a) total learning

(c) long-delay free recall

(b) short-delay free recall

(d) recognition

12. The incidence of new onset epilepsy is greatest at the extreme age ranges, with higher rates in young children, decreasing rates through adolescence and adulthood, and rising incidence in the elderly. Which of the following is most likely to be a cause of new onset epilepsy in the elderly (>65) population?

(a) history of febrile seizures

(c) primary neurodegenerative disease

(b) cardiovascular disease

(d) paraneoplastic limbic encephalitis

13. Which of the following is true of the behavioral variant of frontotemporal dementia?

(a) It is the most common of the three frontotemporal dementia variants.

(b) It occurs more frequently in women than in men.

(c) Frequent falls are typically the first sign of the disorder.

(d) The average age of onset is older than for Alzheimer's disease.

14. Significant psychiatric symptoms are common presenting symptoms in all of the following disorders, except ____.

(a) NMDA receptor encephalitis

(c) paraneoplastic limbic encephalitis

(b) HSV encephalitis

(d) bacterial meningitis

15. Autism is seen most commonly in which of the following disorders?

(a) neurofibromatosis type 1

(c) tuberous sclerosis

(b) PKU

(d) adrenoleukodystrophy

16. In multiple sclerosis, ____.

(a) African Americans are at higher risk than Caucasians

(b) women are at higher risk than men

(c) the elderly are at higher risk than young adults

(d) the incidence is higher among urban dwellers relative to rural

17. Adults with congenital hydrocephalus ____.

(a) live independently because of their strong verbal skills

(b) live for many years with difficulties related to their motoric difficulties

(c) are underemployed relative to their IQ and literacy levels

(d) develop neuropsychological deficits unlike those seen in childhood

18. Which of the following represents the most common physical complaints following moderate to severe traumatic brain injury in adults?

(a) dizziness and tinnitus

(c) headaches and back pain

(b) fatigue and sleep disturbances

(d) visual disturbances

19. A psychiatrist refers a patient to a neuropsychologist for suspected organicity. This is an example of ____.

(a) domain-specific thinking

(c) domain-general theory

(b) lateralization hypothesis testing

(d) localization theory

20. Among the sedative/hypnotics, abuse of barbiturates has largely been replaced by benzodiazepines in recent years because of which of the following?

    (a) Benzodiazepines cost less.

    (b) Barbiturate intoxication carries more risk of accidental overdose.

    (c) Benzodiazepines have fewer long-term effects on neurocognition.

    (d) Withdrawal from benzodiazepines is safer.

21. Which of the following anatomic regions is most vulnerable to Wallerian degeneration following anoxic damage to the hippocampus?

    (a) fornix

    (b) occipital lobe

    (c) internal capsule

    (d) hypothalamus

22. A 3-year-old fair-skinned boy with blonde hair and light blue eyes presents for an evaluation of delayed speech and motor development. He is not speaking any words and has problems with balance. He is a happy boy who exhibits a broad social smile and flaps his hands repetitively. His parents describe severe problems with sleep and a recent onset of seizures. Evaluation findings are consistent with severe intellectual disability. Which of the following diagnoses best fits this description?

    (a) fetal alcohol syndrome

    (b) Autism spectrum disorder

    (c) Angelman syndrome

    (d) Tay-Sachs disease

23. A 33-year-old woman with a history of hypothyroidism presents with complaints of poor sleep quality, changes in appetite, reduced libido, and dysphoric mood. Of the following which neurotransmitter system is most likely involved?

    (a) glutamate

    (b) norepinephrine

    (c) dopamine

    (d) serotonin

24. The Babinski sign in an adult is usually associated with _____.

    (a) upper motor neuron dysfunction

    (b) lower motor neuron dysfunction

    (c) cerebellar dysfunction

    (d) intact corticospinal functioning

25. Overall, the most common medically unexplained symptom in children and teens is _____, with younger children more likely to report _____.

    (a) headache, abdominal distress

    (b) diarrhea, dental pain

    (c) cognitive difficulties, constipation

    (d) nausea, mood symptoms

26. The medical history most typical of spastic diplegic cerebral palsy is _____.

    (a) premature birth and greater upper than lower extremity involvement

    (b) premature birth and neuroimaging findings of periventricular leukomalacia

    (c) full-term birth and abnormalities involving the pyramidal system

    (d) full-term birth and greater lower than upper extremity involvement

27. Which of the following is true about depression and suicide?

    (a) More women attempt suicide, but more men are more likely to complete.

    (b) Men are more likely to attempt suicide, and are more likely to complete.

    (c) Elderly patients are more likely to attempt suicide than younger counterparts.

    (d) Adolescents are more likely to attempt suicide than adults.

28. Microscopic infarctions, white matter hyperintensities, silent brain infarcts and microhemorrhages secondary to cerebral amyloid angiopathy_____.

    (a) are clear evidence for cerebrovascular disease as a causal factor in vascular cognitive impairment

    (b) provide no evidence for cerebrovascular disease as a causal factor in vascular cognitive impairment

    (c) are commonly observed in community-dwelling older adults, even in the absence of cognitive impairment

    (d) are unusual findings in otherwise cognitively healthy community-dwelling older adults

29. A normative sample of a test where performance is measured in the number of errors made, and in which nearly all persons make no errors, would be called _____.

    (a) positively skewed   (c) a bimodal distribution

    (b) negatively skewed   (d) a random distribution

30. Educational programming of a minimally verbal 8-year-old with Autism spectrum disorder should prioritize development in _____.

    (a) eye contact, joint attention, play skills, and early academic skills

    (b) joint attention, requesting gestures, play skills, and use of an augmentative or alternative communication device

    (c) joint attention, play skills, self-care skills, and early academic skills

    (d) self-care skills, early academic skills, and use of sign language

31. You have results from a comprehensive neuropsychological battery in an individual for whom the presumptive diagnosis is chronic schizophrenia. You expect the average deficit to be about how far below normative expectations?

    (a) 0 to 0.5 standard deviations   (c) 1.0 to 1.5 standard deviations

    (b) 0.5 to 1.0 standard deviations   (d) 1.5 to 2.0 standard deviations

32. A 50-year-old gentleman presents to a sleep clinic with excessive daytime fatigue and recurrent periods of lapsing into sleep that are precipitated by laughter or joking. Which of the following sleep disorders is most consistent with his clinical presentation?

    (a) insomnia   (c) Type II narcolepsy

    (b) Type I narcolepsy   (d) REM sleep behavior disorder

33. The clinician evaluating the gentleman in question 32 could use the following test to confirm a diagnosis.

    (a) multiple sleep latency test

    (b) MMPI-2-RF

    (c) self-report measures of mood

    (d) magnetic resonance imaging

34. What combination of deficits and problems two years following severe traumatic brain injury would most likely predict the poorest community reentry outcome in an adult?

    (a) visuospatial and moderate speed of information processing impairments

    (b) personality changes and behavioral problems with mild memory impairments

    (c) moderate attention, verbal memory, and speed of processing impairments

    (d) moderate language and memory impairments, and moderate depression

35. You diagnosed an 80-year-old man with mild cognitive impairment 1 year ago. He returns for repeated evaluation, and his wife describes stable activities of daily living during most of the day but some new episodes of increased confusion, wandering behavior, and suspiciousness during evening hours. The diagnosis of most concern would be ____.

    (a) sundowning

    (b) encephalopathy

    (c) dementia with delirium

    (d) dementia with delusions

36. A patient walks into your office and announces that this is not your office. Rather, your real office is somewhere else and this is a lookalike. Which symptom is this patient displaying?

    (a) utilization behavior

    (b) Fregoli's syndrome

    (c) Capgras syndrome

    (d) reduplicative paramnesia

37. In functional neuroimaging studies, the "neural signature" of dyslexia includes overactivation of ____.

    (a) Wernicke's area

    (b) striate cortex

    (c) inferior frontal gyrus

    (d) angular gyrus

38. Your patient is participating in a specialized physical therapy program for individuals who have difficulties with balance. While reviewing her records, you notice that during her most recent session, her therapist performed the Dix-Hallpike maneuver. During this procedure, elicitation of vertigo and nystagmus suggest ____ dysfunction that is ____ to the side of the downward ear.

    (a) oculomotor; ipsilateral

    (b) vestibular; contralateral

    (c) vestibular; ipsilateral

    (d) oculomotor; contralateral

39. Individuals with substance use disorders (SUDs) frequently show neuropsychological impairments on measures of executive functioning, sustained attention/concentration, and ____.

    (a) manual dexterity

    (b) processing speed

    (c) word-list generation

    (d) reading comprehension

40. A 14-year-old adolescent with a history of ischemic stroke at age 7 is referred for a neuropsychological evaluation. What is the most likely cause of his stroke?

    (a) congenital heart disease

    (b) bacterial meningitis

    (c) arteriovenous malformation

    (d) cerebral arteriopathy

41. In addition to attention and concentration, direct retraining techniques will most likely generalize to real-world tasks in which of the following domains?

    (a) verbal memory

    (b) nonverbal memory

    (c) visual scanning

    (d) language processing

42. A neuropsychologist has developed a busy private practice over the years and no longer needs to solicit or advertise for new patients. He does not want to expand his hours and decides to limit his practice. He instructs his office staff to begin refusing to accept patients with certain types of insurance. Which of the following most appropriately describes these actions?

    (a) It is illegal and unethical

    (b) It is legal and ethical

    (c) It is legally acceptable but unethical

    (d) It is ethical but may not be legal

43. Early-onset dementia is typically associated with _____.

    (a) a prolonged course

    (b) more rapid decline

    (c) hallucinations

    (d) tremor

44. Of the four major dopamine pathways, the one most prominently associated with motor regulation is the _____ pathway.

    (a) tubero-infundibular

    (b) mesolimbic

    (c) mesostriatal

    (d) mesocortical

45. Damage to which cranial nerve is MOST likely to lead to dysarthria?

    (a) glossopharyngeal nerve

    (b) vagus nerve

    (c) spinal accessory nerve

    (d) hypoglossal nerve

46. The frequency of various etiologies for epilepsy varies by age. Which of the following is considered a major factor in the development of neonatal seizures and neonatal epilepsy?

    (a) nonaccidental trauma

    (b) febrile illness

    (c) hippocampal sclerosis

    (d) hypoxic-ischemic injury

47. A 10-year-old child presents with generally intact language skills after a history of stroke. What is the most likely type of stroke associated with this outcome?

    (a) perinatal ischemic stroke

    (b) perinatal hemorrhagic stroke

    (c) childhood ischemic stroke

    (d) childhood hemorrhagic stroke

48. A 35-year old woman presents upon referral from her primary care physician due to memory problems over the past 6 months. Upon interview and review of systems, she also reports menstrual cycle irregularities (which she attributed to stress associated with caring for young children and working full-time) and is also reporting increasing headaches and visual changes (which she attributed to an exacerbation of migraines). There is no history of cancer. What should be high on your differential diagnosis list?

    (a) meningioma

    (b) pituitary tumor

    (c) cerebellar tumor

    (d) paraneoplastic syndrome

49. You are interested in detecting the presence or absence of adequate engagement in cognitive testing with a test that has been normed across clinical populations. You want to be sure to minimize false positive errors (i.e., identifying someone as giving suboptimal effort when their performance reflects true impairment). In order to do this, you will want to set your cut-off for the test on the basis of what?

    (a) multitrait multimethod matrix

    (b) receiver operating curve analysis for the clinical group of interest

    (c) area under the receiver operator characteristic curve

    (d) consideration of the standard error of measurement

50. Your 23-year-old patient was diagnosed with anti-NMDA receptor encephalitis 2 months prior to your evaluation. Which of the following would you expect her to describe regarding her initial symptom presentation?

    (a) flu-like symptoms for 1 week, followed by hallucinations, delusions, and emotional instability, a period of unresponsiveness, then decreased breathing rate and low blood pressure

    (b) abnormal motor movements, primarily of upper extremities, followed by symptoms of mania then respiratory distress

    (c) acute seizure onset followed by inability to speak nor demonstrate comprehension of language then a 1-week period of persistent headache and fatigue

    (d) gradual onset of neck rigidity and confusion, followed by psychotic symptoms and excessive talkativeness, then posturing

51. A 49-year-old woman is referred by her attorney in relation to a personal injury claim of disabling mild traumatic brain injury. The validity scale profile of the Personality Assessment Inventory (PAI) was as follows: Inconsistency (ICN) T = 52; Infrequency (INF) T = 40; Negative Impression Management (NIM) T = 65; and Positive Impression Management (PIM) T = 31. Based on these results, the profile is probably _____.

    (a) invalid due to symptom over-report and should not be interpreted

    (b) best interpreted using non-gender-based norms

    (c) an accurate reflection of current psychological and emotional functioning

    (d) difficult to interpret without knowing which normative comparison group was used

52. Cerebral palsy can be challenging to define because _____.

    (a) its symptoms vary based on whether it originates in the brain or spinal cord

    (b) the diagnosis does not describe a specific neurological disorder

    (c) its only pathognomonic feature changes as the motor system matures

    (d) the non-progressive and progressive subtypes differ in their manifestations

53. Your 42-year-old patient indicates that she was prescribed Zoloft for depression 4 days ago but it doesn't seem to help. She is thinking about stopping the medication. In addition to encouraging her to talk with the prescribing physician you explain that if taken appropriately, antidepressant medications typically are fully effective in _____ from the first dose.

    (a) 7 to 10 days   (c) 2 to 3 weeks

    (b) 10 to 21 days   (d) 4 to 6 weeks

54. You are performing a neuropsychological evaluation on a 12-year-old boy. Results from your evaluation reveal significant attention difficulties in both home and school settings, increased variability in response latencies on a visual CPT, slowed rapid automatized naming, poor phonological awareness, and decreased processing speed, all in the context of average intelligence. Based on this information, which diagnostic formulation would be most probable?

    (a) ADHD and dyslexia

    (b) ADHD without a comorbid condition

    (c) dyslexia without a comorbid condition

    (d) mixed receptive-expressive language disorder

55. Neuropsychological profiles of persons with progressive supranuclear palsy are characterized by impairment primarily in ____.

    (a) confrontation naming   (c) visuospatial construction

    (b) intellectual functions   (d) executive functions

56. Which of the following best characterizes the current state of knowledge regarding individuals with intellectual disability (ID)?

    (a) Specific cognitive and behavioral profiles have been identified for a variety of syndromes of ID.

    (b) Individuals with ID show a general pattern of global impairment across measures.

    (c) Variability occurs in individuals with ID such that no particular patterns in cognitive and behavioral profiles have been identified.

    (d) A discrepancy between IQ and adaptive living skills (IQ>ADLs) has been identified for most but not all syndromes.

57. Preferred surgical treatment in advanced Parkinson's disease with maximum medication response is ____.

    (a) bilateral pallidotomy

    (b) subthalamic nucleus deep brain stimulation

    (c) vagal nerve stimulation

    (d) stem cell transplant

58. Addie was diagnosed with multiple sclerosis at age 12 and has been adherent to treatment recommendations. She has also undergone serial evaluations. She presents for a neuropsychological re-evaluation at age 17. What might you expect to find on testing across time?

    (a) improved cognition given her adherence to medication

    (b) worsened cognition across time

    (c) cognition that is unchanged

    (d) no clear expected longitudinal pattern

APPENDIX B

59. In terms of the relationship between false positive rate and positive predictive power, which of the following statements is true?

    (a) Positive predictive power increases with increases in the false positive rate.

    (b) Positive predictive power decreases with decreases in the false positive rate.

    (c) Positive predictive power and false positive rates are unrelated.

    (d) Positive predictive power increases with decreases in the false positive rate.

60. You are evaluating a 9-year-old child who has been struggling in his math class. In addition to math calculation and math problem solving, it will be important to assess math fluency, _____.

    (a) working memory, executive functions, and math-specific anxiety

    (b) working memory, executive functions, and depression

    (c) verbal memory, executive functions, and math-specific anxiety

    (d) working memory, executive functions, and decoding

61. A 30-year-old single man presents with a 12-year history of unstable relationships and emotional volatility. He endorses resentment about perceived abandonment by others but denies delusions of reference or dissociative features. This pattern most likely meets criteria for _____.

    (a) Passive-Aggressive Personality Disorder   (c) Cyclothymic Disorder

    (b) Schizophreniform Disorder   (d) Borderline Personality Disorder

62. The "what-where" cognitive system represents _____.

    (a) the differential processing of the prefrontal cortex

    (b) differential dorsal-ventral information processing

    (c) the work of Roger Sperry and Michael Gazzaniga

    (d) domain-general theory of double dissociation

63. All of the conventional or first-generation and most of the atypical or second-generation antipsychotic drugs share which putative pharmacological property?

    (a) glutamatergic antagonism   (c) D_1-type dopamine receptor antagonism

    (b) norepinephrine reuptake inhibition   (d) D_2-type dopamine receptor antagonism

64. White matter hyperintensities in vascular dementia have been shown to correlate positively with _____.

    (a) language and visuospatial deficits

    (b) personality and behavioral deficits

    (c) speed of processing and executive function deficits

    (d) constructional and working memory deficits

65. Which of the following comorbidity is about 50% in Autism spectrum disorder?

    (a) tics   (c) anxiety

    (b) seizures   (d) schizophrenia

66. The pattern of anoxic/hypoxic brain injury in neonates found to be most strongly associated with poor long-term outcome is injury to which areas?

    (a) basal ganglia and thalamus

    (b) deep brainstem nuclei

    (c) watershed regions

    (d) dorsolateral prefrontal cortex

67. In children born very preterm, poorer long-term outcome in academic and social-emotional domains is associated with ____.

    (a) lower general cognitive ability and persistent executive dysfunction

    (b) length of NICU stay and presence of chronic respiratory problems

    (c) visual-motor integration problems and slowed speed of processing

    (d) periventricular leukomalacia and post-hemorrhagic hydrocephalus

68. Minimum test requirements for psychological and neuropsychological tests require sufficient reliability and validity. Although many types of reliability and validity have been described to evaluate the performance of a test, a basic understanding regarding the relationship between the concepts of reliability and validity is characterized as ____.

    (a) reliability is more important than validity

    (b) a test with good validity can have poor reliability

    (c) a test must have reliability to have validity

    (d) validity is more important than reliability

69. You are asked to evaluate an adolescent with learning problems. During your clinical interview, the mother reports that she has epilepsy. Which of the following variables would suggest that the mother's medical history is contributory to the adolescent's current cognitive problems?

    (a) inconsistent use of anti-seizure medications during the pregnancy

    (b) use of valproate during the pregnancy to manage her seizures

    (c) grand mal seizures monthly during the pregnancy

    (d) use of Keppra during the pregnancy to manage her seizures

70. Which of the following statements regarding dopamine is true?

    (a) The nigrostriatal dopamine system is dysfunctional in Parkinson's disease.

    (b) Most drugs designed to treat schizophrenia are designed to increase dopamine.

    (c) The mesolimbic dopamine system is dysfunctional in Parkinson's disease.

    (d) The mesocortical system is specifically implicated in addictive behavior.

71. The psychotherapy approach with the best evidence base in treating patients with somatoform symptoms has traditionally been ____.

    (a) cognitive behavioral therapy

    (b) motivational interviewing

    (c) dialectical behavior therapy

    (d) cognitive processing therapy

72. In early stage Alzheimer's disease, the greatest neuronal loss occurs in the ____.

    (a) frontal and temporal lobes

    (b) temporal lobes and upper brainstem nuclei

    (c) frontal and parietal lobes

    (d) frontal lobe and hippocampus

73. A recently detoxified patient with alcohol use disorder demonstrates neuropsychological impairment 1 week post abstinence. To assess the persistent neurotoxic effects of alcohol, one should retest the patient at least ____.

(a) 6 months post treatment

(b) 1 month post treatment

(c) 1 year post treatment

(d) 2 weeks post treatment

74. Worldwide estimates of ADHD are typically lower than those found in the United States (~5% vs. ~10%). Which one of the following statements is most likely to explain this difference in base rates?

(a) expectations within academic settings

(b) exposure to environmental toxins

(c) access to specialized healthcare clinics

(d) ethnic and/or racial differences

75. Your 85-year-old patient experienced delirium during a recent ICU admission and he is now in an extended care facility. Which of the following is most predictive of persistent cognitive impairment and future complications requiring hospital readmission?

(a) infectious cause

(b) length of delirium

(c) stroke history

(d) psychosis during delirium

76. Which of the following would you be least likely to see in a patient with left hemisphere or frontal damage?

(a) confabulation

(b) alexithymia

(c) circumlocution

(d) anosognosia

77. Although the BDI-II and BAI have a long tradition of assessing symptoms of depression and anxiety in adults, clinicians might consider administration of the full-length Geriatric Depression Scale (GDS) in geriatric samples because the ____.

(a) GDS includes well-established T scores that are more appropriately normed in aging samples

(b) GDS includes far fewer test items and is likely to be less burdensome

(c) GDS includes fewer items that are specific to the physical manifestations of emotional difficulty

(d) BDI-II and BAI include norms that only extend to age 60

78. Processing speed in people with acquired or congenital hydrocephalus ____.

(a) is best assessed with paper-and-pencil tests

(b) must take into account the motor requirements of the task

(c) is inconsistently impaired depending on the severity of hydrocephalus

(d) is impaired in congenital, but not acquired hydrocephalus

79. Which of the following is considered to be a common risk associated with temporal lobectomy?

(a) intellectual disability

(b) Gerstmann syndrome

(c) hemiparesis

(d) superior quadrantanopsia

80. Individuals with this disorder typically have below average cognitive functioning and demonstrate hypersociability and an affinity for music.

(a) Turner syndrome

(c) 22q11.2 deletion syndrome

(b) Williams syndrome

(d) Sturge-Weber syndrome

81. While playing football without a helmet, a 17-year-old is hit on the side of the head. He experiences a brief loss of consciousness but recovers in minutes with no residual symptoms. Approximately 30 minutes later, he becomes increasingly confused and lethargic. He is taken to the emergency room. Upon examination, he presents with mild left-sided weakness, and a slightly larger, nonresponsive right pupil. What is the likely cause of his symptoms?

(a) hemorrhagic contusion

(c) diffuse axonal injury

(b) epidural hematoma

(d) evolving ischemic infarct

82. You are assessing a 12-year-old patient due to concerns about attention problems and difficulties learning. During the chart review, you learn that the medical team recently identified conductive hearing loss. Assuming a neurologic cause which of the following diagnoses is most likely?

(a) bacterial meningitis

(c) HIV encephalitis acquired perinatally

(b) viral meningitis

(d) enteroviral encephalitis

83. It is not uncommon for the behavioral variant of frontotemporal dementia to be misdiagnosed as _____.

(a) schizophrenia

(c) Autism spectrum disorder

(b) Posttraumatic stress disorder

(d) selective mutism

84. Oliver, a 52-year-old factory worker, has been referred to you secondary to a disability claim. He was diagnosed with primary progressive multiple sclerosis 10 years prior and had continued to work despite worsening physical symptoms. However, he can no longer maintain the same level of productivity and is at risk of losing his job. Which symptom is the best predictor of having to reduce work hours or cease working completely?

(a) cognitive decline

(c) vision changes

(b) spasticity

(d) fatigue

85. What cognitive syndrome can be seen after left-hemisphere posterior cerebral artery stroke?

(a) alexia without agraphia

(c) agraphia and alexia

(b) agraphia without alexia

(d) alexia and anosognosia

86. A 13-year-old treated for a medulloblastoma with surgery, craniospinal radiation, and chemotherapy at age 6 demonstrates a substantial decline in IQ scores compared to prior evaluation at age 9. These findings suggest _____.

(a) relapse of brain tumor

(b) loss of previously acquired skills (regression)

(c) late effect of radiation therapy on brain development

(d) significant emotional adjustment difficulties interfering with learning

87. A patient presents with asymmetric motor dysfunction and does not respond to a medication trial of levodopa. What is the most likely diagnosis?

(a) corticobasal syndrome

(c) Lewy body dementia

(b) progressive supranuclear palsy

(d) Parkinson's disease

88. An 11-year-old child with a history of preterm birth at 26 weeks is referred for assessment due to concerns for social-emotional and adaptive functioning. Given his birth history, the child is at increased risk for ____.

(a) autism, epilepsy, intellectual disability

(b) ADHD, bipolar disorder, aphasia

(c) anxiety, muscular dystrophies, ataxia

(d) spastic hemiplegia, intellectual disability, ADHD

89. Which of the following is not associated with a pseudodementia, or dementia syndrome of depression?

(a) presence of psychomotor retardation

(b) depressed mood or agitation

(c) progressive/degenerative course

(d) impaired immediate memory and learning abilities

90. You work in a small integrated primary care clinic in a rural setting and primarily evaluate pediatric patients. There are no other pediatric neuropsychologists within 200 miles of your location. The bilingual physician (English and Spanish) wants you to evaluate a 5-year-old Spanish-speaking child he saw yesterday. You do not speak Spanish. The physician explains that he has noticed a definite regression in the child's language skills over the past 6 months and is concerned about possible seizures. He realizes that your exam may be limited but asks you to help in any way you can, explaining that the family does not have the means to travel and that the waiting list at the closest children's hospital is over 6 months. The clinic administrator also asks you to do whatever you can to help. What should you do?

(a) See the patient and conduct the best exam possible.

(b) Refuse; you are not competent to perform this assessment.

(c) Assist the physician in finding a center with bilingual clinicians.

(d) See the patient but only give visuospatial and nonverbal tasks.

91. Typically, about ____ of patients with mild neurocognitive disorder develop dementia each year?

(a) 20%

(c) 80%

(b) 10%

(d) 50%

92. The chronic effects of opiates include all of the following except____.

(a) processing speed

(c) decision-making

(b) working memory

(d) executive function

93. Leukoaraiosis refers to the ____.

   (a) primary pathology underlying all variants of multi-infarct dementia

   (b) scattered lacunar infarctions in the periventricular white matter

   (c) nonspecific loss of density of subcortical white matter

   (d) primary pathology underlying cerebral amyloid angiopathy

94. One reason the diagnostic process for cerebral palsy (CP) can result in a false positive error is ___.

   (a) an infant with a normal neurological exam can show signs of CP at follow-up

   (b) there can be a latency between a perinatal brain insult and its manifestations

   (c) an infant can present with an unremarkable birth history and no risk factors

   (d) neurological and motor abnormalities in an infant can be transient

95. A 65-year-old physician is referred for evaluation due to concerns regarding declines in work performance. In a detailed test battery he earns multiple scores at the 2nd to 5th percentile. These scores should be labeled as ____.

   (a) abnormal   (c) impaired

   (b) deficient   (d) low

96. Within the language domain, what type of difficulty would be most likely found in a 12-year-old with average IQ and Autism spectrum disorder?

   (a) simplified grammar   (c) inattention to vocabulary

   (b) impaired pragmatics   (d) oral apraxia

97. Schizophrenia is most common in which of the following disorders?

   (a) 22q11.2 deletion syndrome   (c) fragile X syndrome

   (b) neurofibromatosis type 1   (d) PKU

98. A 48-year-old male attorney presents for evaluation of possible transient ischemic attacks in the absence of any other cerebrovascular indicators. During interview, he reported that these "events" are characterized by an inability to speak when he attends church with his wife, despite being able to speak in high-level work and other social activities. This may be a sign of ____.

   (a) selective mutism   (c) specific phobia

   (b) Social Anxiety Disorder   (d) Panic Disorder

99. Which of the following is the loss of the ability to plan and execute complex gestures?

   (a) ideomotor apraxia   (c) constructional apraxia

   (b) ideational apraxia   (d) buccofacial apraxia

100. You are evaluating a 20-year-old college student who is currently on academic probation at his university, due to consistently poor grades. He complains of having multiple ADHD symptoms and is requesting accommodations and modifications. During your clinical interview, you find

that there is no history of previous ADHD diagnosis or academic difficulties in high school. Which of the following statements would be *most* important to consider in your neuropsychological evaluation?

(a) According to the DSM-5 diagnostic criteria, you cannot diagnose ADHD in an adult if symptoms were not present prior to the age of 12 years.

(b) This college student likely has both a learning disability and ADHD, and therefore your evaluation should include a focus on reading and writing skills.

(c) Utilization of both SVTs and PVTs would be important given the concerns for secondary gain and lack of typical ADHD developmental history.

(d) Substance abuse would be the first differential diagnosis to consider.

101. Extensive white matter hyperintensity volume is associated with ____.

(a) a more than doubling of the risk of vascular cognitive impairment in aged adults

(b) depression and agitation in vascular dementia

(c) pure vascular dementia but not mixed dementia

(d) lacunar states unrelated to dementia of any type

102. Which type of multiple sclerosis is generally associated with the worst cognitive functioning?

(a) relapsing-remitting

(b) secondary-progressive

(c) primary-progressive

(d) progressive-relapsing

103. A 74-year-old male patient is referred for neuropsychological evaluation by his primary care physician. He has been complaining of memory problems and word-finding difficulties, but no other cognitive changes. If a blood work-up is performed, which apolipoprotein E pattern would be most suggestive of Alzheimer's disease?

(a) ε2/ε3

(b) ε3/ε3

(c) ε3/ε4

(d) ε4/ε4

104. Hydrocephalus ____.

(a) primarily affects the white matter of the brain

(b) primarily affects the brain's ventricular system

(c) causes permanent brain injury

(d) has widespread effects on the brain

105. A neuropsychologist has been referred a patient who reportedly sustained a traumatic brain injury 12 months ago. Which combination of information would be most helpful in determining the injury severity?

(a) Glasgow Coma Score (GCS), length of post-traumatic amnesia (PTA), time to follow commands (TFC)

(b) loss of consciousness, length of PTA, brain CT

(c) GCS, length of PTA, first hospital MMSE score

(d) brain MRI, length of PTA, extended mental status exam 1-month post injury

106. In reviewing the medical record for a pediatric patient with a history of preterm birth, retinopathy of prematurity (ROP) is documented. In considering the neurologic history of the child and course of disease, you know that the probable cause and prognosis of ROP are _____.

    (a) a hypoxic or ischemic event with variable course over time

    (b) a hypoxic or ischemic event that remains static over time

    (c) oxygen toxicity or hypoxia that remains static over time

    (d) oxygen toxicity or hypoxia that can worsen over time

107. Mixed dementia most commonly occurs as _____.

    (a) cerebrovascular disease and Alzheimer's disease

    (b) Alzheimer's disease and Lewy body disease

    (c) cerebrovascular disease and Lewy body disease

    (d) cerebrovascular disease and frontotemporal dementia

108. The two-system theory of amnesia suggests that _____.

    (a) damage to either the hippocampus or amygdala produces amnesia

    (b) there are two different forms of amnesia

    (c) amnesia results from damage to the hippocampus or diencephalon

    (d) both medial and lateral limbic circuits must be damaged to cause amnesia

109. Which one of the following is not an appropriate use of personality testing?

    (a) identifying psychological factors affecting a known medical condition

    (b) evaluation of psychological status with regard to disability or return to work

    (c) evaluation of psychological readiness for surgical or other medical intervention

    (d) ruling out a medical condition in a patient whose medical evaluations have been equivocal

110. A child with neurofibromatosis type 1 is most at risk for _____.

    (a) schizophrenia   (c) ADHD

    (b) intellectual disability   (d) Autism spectrum disorder

111. A woman with schizophrenia has a monozygotic twin. The likelihood that her twin sister will also develop schizophrenia is about _____.

    (a) 2%   (c) 30%

    (b) 10%   (d) 80%

112. A patient presents with axial rigidity, falls, and memory loss. The spouse does not report REM sleep behavior disorder. Which of the following diagnosis is most likely?

    (a) progressive supranuclear palsy   (c) multiple system atrophy

    (b) Parkinson's disease   (d) Huntington's disease

113. Evidence-based intervention for learning disabilities is best established for _____.

    (a) written language disabilities   (c) mathematics disabilities

    (b) nonverbal learning disabilities   (d) reading disabilities

114. Support for the brain reserve hypothesis can be found within which clinical trend?

    (a) Serotonin syndrome is more likely in patients on two SSRIs.

    (b) Vitamin B$_{12}$ deficiencies often result in diffuse cognitive impairments.

    (c) Higher incidence of delirium follows urinary tract infection in the elderly.

    (d) Stroke is more common in patients with a history of vascular disease.

115. Which of the following is NOT true with regard to frontal lobe damage and emotion/behavior?

    (a) orbitofrontal damage has been associated with disinhibition

    (b) orbitofrontal damage has been associated with impulsivity

    (c) right frontal damage has been associated with depression

    (d) medial frontal damage has been associated with lack of initiation (abulia)

116. A patient presents with a constellation of symptoms typical of an upper motor neuron (UMN) lesion. Which would he LEAST likely demonstrate?

    (a) weakness   (c) hyperreflexia

    (b) hyporeflexia   (d) increased tone

117. The same patient with the UMN described above is also demonstrating abnormal reflexes. Upon assessment, his neurologist might expect to see _____.

    (a) absent reflexes

    (b) decreased reflexes and the Babinski sign

    (c) decreased reflexes and the Wartenberg's sign

    (d) the Babinski and the Wartenberg's signs

118. A neuropsychologist is asked to evaluate a 9-year-old child with documented blood lead levels of 25 μg/dL. In which of the following domains should the neuropsychologist expect to find the most deficits?

    (a) executive functions   (c) memory functions

    (b) language skills   (d) math abilities

119. Which of the following epilepsy syndromes is most likely to show spontaneous remission?

    (a) temporal lobe epilepsy   (c) Lennox-Gastaut

    (b) childhood absence epilepsy   (d) frontal lobe epilepsy

120. On Test 1, an individual obtains a T score of 65. On Test 2, she obtains a scaled score of 115. On Test 3, she scores in the 60th percentile. On Test 4, her score is equivalent to a z score of 0.5. Which of the following is the correct ordering of these scores, from lowest to highest?

    (a) Test 4, Test 3, Test 2, Test 1   (c) Test 4, Test 2, Test 3, Test 1

    (b) Test 3, Test 4, Test 2, Test 1   (d) Test 3, Test 2, Test 4, Test 1

121. Alcohol and marijuana exposure in utero are both associated with _____.

    (a) prematurity

    (c) growth reduction

    (b) tremors

    (d) endocrine disruption

122. A 65-year-old, right-handed man is evaluated after a left hemisphere ischemic stroke. You diagnose him with a conduction aphasia because he demonstrates _____.

    (a) intact fluency, intact comprehension, impaired repetition

    (b) impaired fluency, intact comprehension, impaired repetition

    (c) intact fluency, impaired comprehension, impaired repetition

    (d) impaired fluency, impaired comprehension, intact repetition

123. The most frequently reported problem in the cerebral palsy population that has a negative impact on quality of life is _____.

    (a) motor impairment

    (c) social isolation

    (b) fatigue

    (d) pain

124. A side effect of intrathecal chemotherapy with methotrexate is _____.

    (a) leukoencephalopathy

    (c) ataxia

    (b) peripheral nerve deficits

    (d) hemiparesis

125. A complete loss of oxygen in the arterial blood or tissues is referred to as _____.

    (a) hyponatremia

    (c) hypoxemia

    (b) anoxia

    (d) apoptosis

Third Full-Length Practice Examination Questions

1. In North America, abuse of a single drug is ____.

   (a) common among women but not men

   (b) uncommon

   (c) not likely with comorbid depression

   (d) characteristic of individuals with stimulant use

2. You are seeing a former National Football League player who is seeking compensation for memory problems that he believes are related to playing professional football. Concerns about symptom feigning/exaggeration are apparent on multiple symptom validity tests. On the Test of Memory Malingering, he earns a 28 on Trial 1, a 46 on Trial 2, and a 45 on the retention trial. Performance on all other performance validity tests is unremarkable. According to the Slick criteria for malingered neurocognitive dysfunction (MND), the diagnosis of malingering is most likely to be ____.

   (a) definite

   (b) probable

   (c) possible

   (d) unlikely

3. On an inpatient rehabilitation unit, a 58-year-old woman has reportedly been walking into the wall on her left side during physical therapy, and the occupational therapist notices that the items placed on the left side of her lunch tray always remain untouched. Of the following, which is most consistent with this clinical presentation, and what would be the etiology?

   (a) prosopagnosia; right occipital cerebrovascular accident (CVA)

   (b) ideomotor apraxia; left parietal CVA

   (c) right-left disorientation; left parietal CVA

   (d) neglect; right parietal CVA

4. The foremost risk factor for cerebral palsy is ____.

   (a) low Apgar score

   (b) birth asphyxia

   (c) premature birth

   (d) neonatal infection

5. A 48-year-old man is status post-surgical resection of a large right frontal glioblastoma. During the course of your evaluation, significant visual scanning deficits, executive dysfunction, impulsivity, and impaired social skills become apparent. It is your opinion that he should not be driving and likely has a reduced capacity to make informed medical decisions. Midway through the examination, the patient becomes frustrated, refuses to continue, and storms out. Before he leaves the office, he instructs you to destroy his healthcare record and never share findings with anyone, especially his wife and the physician who referred him. What do you do first?

(a) Call later and inform the patient that you cannot destroy the record, but that you will respect his autonomy and not write a report.

(b) Call later and try to convince the patient that it is in his best interest to share the information with the referring provider and his wife.

(c) Anonymously report the patient to the department of motor vehicles indicating your concern about his ability to drive.

(d) Contact your state ethics committee and the referring provider to discuss the situation and review options.

6. High-functioning adolescents with Autism spectrum disorder tend to exhibit age-appropriate ____ but struggle with ____.

(a) spelling skills; multiplication and division

(b) decoding skills; reading comprehension

(c) sentence composition; letter formation

(d) math problem solving; written expression

7. Of the medications listed, which carries the highest risk for the development of delirium following prolonged use at the prescribed dosage?

(a) beta blockers

(b) serotonin reuptake inhibitors

(c) corticosteroids

(d) anticonvulsants

8. Which imaging modality would be most useful in the diagnosis of Parkinson's disease versus other Parkinson-plus disorders?

(a) cardiac MIBG scintigraphy

(b) structural MRI

(c) FDG PET

(d) resting state fMRI

9. What sign is likely due to a disconnection rather than direct damage to a module?

(a) constructional dyspraxia

(b) any transcortical aphasia

(c) specific type of agnosia

(d) modality-specific anomia

10. According to most definitions, positive symptoms include ____.

(a) formal thought disorder and bizarre behavior

(b) delusions and hallucinations

(c) pseudobulbar affect and cognitive impairments

(d) attentional impairments and other cognitive symptoms

11. If you want to know the degree to which you can have confidence in a normal result on a psychometric test to rule out a specific condition, you should calculate this ratio:

(a) false negatives/(true negatives + false positives)

(b) true negatives/(false negatives + true positives)

(c) false negatives/(false negatives + true negatives)

(d) true negatives/(true negatives + false negatives)

12. You are reviewing medical records for a patient who has been in a car accident. During his neurological exam, it is noted that he presents with decreased shoulder shrug on the left and an inability to resist pressure from an examiner's hand against the right jaw. These findings could suggest ____.

(a) left spinal accessory nerve XI dysfunction

(b) right spinal accessory nerve XI dysfunction

(c) bilateral spinal accessory nerve XI dysfunction

(d) feigned neurologic impairment

13. A 35-year-old married male has been promoted regularly at work but is experiencing depressive signs and symptoms. During interview, he also reported experiencing intermittent episodes of high productivity and decreased need for sleep for a few days. He finds these episodes useful in terms of his work productivity, but they are followed by periods of increased depression. This presentation is suggestive of ____.

(a) Major Depressive Disorder   (c) Bipolar II Disorder

(b) Bipolar I Disorder   (d) Cyclothymic Disorder

14. A 7-year-old boy presents for evaluation of ADHD symptoms due to "daydreaming" during class and parent reports that he has to have simple instructions repeated over and over. These symptoms have been present since around 5 years of age and have gotten worse over the past few months. Other than concerns with attention, he does well in school and there is no history of learning disability. An EEG shows occasional generalized bursts of 3 hz spike and wave discharges. The most likely diagnosis is ____.

(a) temporal lobe epilepsy

(b) Landau-Kleffner syndrome

(c) self-limiting epilepsy with centrotemporal spikes

(d) childhood absence epilepsy

15. A clinical psychologist wants to use a brief instrument to screen for possible suicidal thoughts in adolescents. For this purpose, the instrument should have high ____.

(a) sensitivity   (c) face validity

(b) specificity   (d) concurrent validity

16. Which of the following is a typical side effect of psychostimulant medication?

(a) depression   (c) hallucinations

(b) insomnia   (d) lowered blood pressure

17. A patient with amnesia has a large lesion affecting many brain structures. In each item below, a pair of structures is listed. Damage to which of these pairs is most likely to produce dense amnesia?

(a) mammillary bodies and dorsomedial thalamus

(b) amygdala and dorsomedial thalamus

(c) hippocampus and cingulate gyrus

(d) mammillothalamic tract and anterior thalamus

18. What is the most important factor to consider when assessing prognosis for mortality after stroke?

(a) size of infarct

(b) location of infarct

(c) hemorrhagic etiology

(d) time since stroke

19. In a neuropsychological evaluation of patients with functional somatic syndromes, what measure is most likely to show clinically relevant elevations?

(a) Beck Depression Inventory

(b) Patient Health Questionnaire-9

(c) MMPI-2 Restructured Clinical Scale 3

(d) MMPI-2 Restructured Clinical Scale 1

20. A 7-year-old boy presents for evaluation. Upon meeting him, you note that he has elf-like features. Despite IQ in the range of moderate ID, he is very social. He is most likely to have which of the following?

(a) fragile X syndrome

(b) adrenoleukodystrophy

(c) Klinefelter syndrome

(d) Williams syndrome

21. A 25-year-old presents with aphasia 8 months after a severe traumatic brain injury. The most likely mechanism of injury was a ____.

(a) slip and fall

(b) bicycle crash

(c) gunshot wound

(d) sports collision

22. Which of the following is least likely to be seen following hypoxic/ischemic damage?

(a) amnestic syndrome

(b) visuospatial deficits

(c) speed of processing impairment

(d) impaired attention/working memory

23. A brain MRI performed on a 5-year-old female with a history of preterm birth is abnormal. What are the most likely findings on imaging associated with this birth history?

(a) intraventricular hemorrhage and post-hemorrhagic hydrocephalus

(b) periventricular leukomalacia and focal neuronal injury

(c) periventricular hemorrhagic infarction and periventricular leukomalacia

(d) periventricular hemorrhagic infarction and cerebral ischemic lesions

24. Which of these neurological conditions is relatively most frequently associated with fronto-temporal dementia?

(a) amyotrophic lateral sclerosis

(c) multisystem atrophy

(b) multiple sclerosis

(d) primary lateral sclerosis

25. Which of the following helps to best account for the discrepancy between the less than 1% prevalence of intellectual disability (ID) and the bell curve model prediction that 2.5% of individuals have an IQ score of 70 or less?

(a) diagnostic variability across regions (especially for mild ID)

(b) referral biases associated with higher academic functioning

(c) the ratio of males to females in early childhood

(d) the association between life expectancy and severity of ID

26. What neuropathological change correlates best with severity of cognitive impairment in patients with Alzheimer's dementia?

(a) amyloid plaques

(c) synaptic density

(b) neurofibrillary tangles

(d) Lewy bodies

27. Which of the following is associated with decreased processing speed in patients with epilepsy?

(a) decreased white matter volume

(b) decreased memory and mesial temporal sclerosis

(c) suppression of neuronal excitability with antiepileptic drugs

(d) seizures involving frontal lobe networks

28. You have been consulted to evaluate a 63-year-old man with a past medical history of diabetes, hypertension, and congestive heart failure. He underwent renal transplant 2 weeks ago. On examination, he is disoriented, highly distractible, and cannot accurately complete simple figure drawings. Physicians indicate that his mental status seemed fine prior to surgery. What diagnosis and etiology are most probable?

(a) vascular cognitive impairment and infection

(b) vascular cognitive impairment and hyponatremia

(c) delirium and drug reaction/interaction

(d) delirium and right hemisphere stroke

29. If a clinician only had time to administer three tests in the assessment of an individual with suspected dementia, he or she should include measures of____.

(a) figure learning, figure recall, and simple attention

(b) phonemic fluency, MMSE, and mental flexibility

(c) sensory motor tests, executive function, and drawing

(d) verbal episodic memory, category fluency, and naming

30. In regards to memory, research suggests that individuals with substance use disorders (SUDs) commonly display cognitive deficits in _____.

   (a) acquisition and encoding

   (b) retention

   (c) free recall

   (d) recognition

31. Each of the following are part of the extrapyramidal motor system, except _____.

   (a) subthalamic nucleus

   (b) globus pallidus

   (c) cerebellum

   (d) putamen

32. A 32-year-old man presents to your neuropsychology clinic with a history of herpes simplex virus encephalitis. He has cognitive complaints across multiple areas. What might you expect to find on imaging based on his history?

   (a) inflammation of the cerebellum and temporal lobe

   (b) temporal lobe pathology and hyperintensities in the orbitofrontal regions

   (c) subcortical white matter lesions and atrophy

   (d) lesions in the brain stem and basal ganglia

33. A left-handed, 82-year-old man recently sustained a stroke and has fluent speech but impaired auditory comprehension and repetition. What is the most likely vascular distribution of the stroke?

   (a) left hemisphere in the deep territory

   (b) right inferior middle cerebral artery territory

   (c) left inferior middle cerebral artery territory

   (d) left superior middle cerebral artery territory

34. Time from diagnosis to death is longest in which of the following disorders?

   (a) Parkinson's disease

   (b) progressive supranuclear palsy

   (c) Lewy body dementia

   (d) corticobasal syndrome

35. Which of the following has been found to be a risk factor for cognitive impairment in patients with breast cancer following treatment?

   (a) neo-adjuvant therapy

   (b) concurrent radiation treatment

   (c) older age

   (d) estrogen receptor positive cancer

36. Diagnostic criteria for social (pragmatic) communication disorder overlaps considerably with Autism spectrum disorder symptomatology. To help differentiate between these disorders, clinicians could look for a history of which of the following?

   (a) limited nonverbal communication

   (b) difficulty with turn taking in conversation

   (c) difficulty inferring meaning from speech

   (d) presence of stereotyped language

37. "Working memory" is an example of _____.

    (a) a whole-brain phenomenon

    (b) domain-specific theory

    (c) dysexecutive syndrome

    (d) domain-general theory

38. A neuropsychologist is evaluating a child whose mother acknowledged smoking marijuana during pregnancy. In considering the potential effects of this exposure on the child's neuropsychological performance, which of the following factors should the neuropsychologist consider as a likely confound of the relation between marijuana exposure and neuropsychological outcome?

    (a) tobacco use

    (b) maternal obesity

    (c) timing of exposure

    (d) alcohol use

39. Which of the following is not hypothesized to be involved in the neuropathology of schizophrenia?

    (a) excessive synaptic pruning

    (b) abnormal embryogenesis

    (c) amyloid deposition

    (d) disrupted white matter integrity

40. The post-test probability of a test is _____.

    (a) the probability of the individual having the disease when the test result is positive

    (b) the probability the individual has the disease within the population

    (c) equal to the positive predictive power or the ability of the test to identify the disease

    (d) the increase in odds a positive test result adds to the pre-test probability

41. A patient presents with a diagnosis of cerebral palsy (CP) related to a history of prematurity and intraventricular hemorrhage. Which is the most likely type of CP given this history?

    (a) extrapyramidal

    (b) dyskinetic

    (c) ataxic

    (d) spastic diplegia

42. A patient with multiple sclerosis has distinct episodes of acute worsening of neurologic symptoms followed by variable recovery of function, with periods of stability between attacks. This would best be characterized as _____ multiple sclerosis.

    (a) relapsing-remitting

    (b) secondary-progressive

    (c) primary-progressive

    (d) progressive-relapsing

43. Deficits in which of the following would be least likely in early vascular dementia?

    (a) speed of processing

    (b) word generation to semantic or letter cues

    (c) word-finding and language comprehension

    (d) planning, organizing, and flexibility in problem-solving

44. Extrapyramidal cerebral palsy is typically associated with _____.

    (a) severe cognitive impairments

    (b) abnormal involuntary movements

    (c) more involvement of the legs than arms

    (d) significantly shortened life expectancy

45. Which of the following is an uncommon emotional-behavioral complication following moderate to severe traumatic brain injury in children?

    (a) depression

    (b) ADHD

    (c) mania

    (d) anxiety

46. The statistical probability of an observed difference between test scores, either within scales of a test or across different tests, is determined by relative rarity of a difference in scores based on the central limit theorem and is related to the test(s) reliability and standard error of measurement. This statistical difference is based on the assumption of _____.

    (a) heterogeneity of variance between the tests

    (b) homogeneity of variance between tests

    (c) a minimal correlation between the scales or tests

    (d) the ability to reject the null hypothesis

47. As children with congenital hydrocephalus move into adolescence, they are at high risk for _____.

    (a) dementia and early onset of aging

    (b) conduct disorder

    (c) new onset of medical problems unrelated to shunting

    (d) anxiety and depression

48. The assessment of general intelligence would be most impacted by which of the following?

    (a) nonfluent aphasia

    (b) fluent aphasia

    (c) alexia without agraphia

    (d) anosognosia

49. Which condition is considered by some to be a variant of frontotemporal dementia yet by others is considered a form of Alzheimer's disease?

    (a) semantic variant

    (b) progressive non-fluent aphasia variant

    (c) logopenic variant

    (d) behavioral variant

50. Numerosity is understanding and recognizing the concept of quantity. It most often includes which of the following abilities?

    (a) symbolic comparison

    (b) procedural counting

    (c) conceptual counting

    (d) rapid digit naming

51. A 71-year-old woman presents to your office, accompanied by her son. The son is concerned that his mother may be developing depression as she has been reticent to attend family events, preferring to watch television or sit in her bedroom. She has also become less competent with select hobbies, such as card playing and knitting. She has forgotten conversations she has had with him but has not forgotten her appointments and needs only occasional reminders to take her medications. The son denies that his mother has experienced any significant recent medical or

life events and indicated that she has no history of depression. Based on this information, what is the woman's most likely diagnosis?

(a) Major Depressive Disorder

(b) Mild Neurocognitive Disorder

(c) Alzheimer's disease

(d) vascular cognitive impairment

52. In individuals with Sturge-Weber, seizures are typically seen on _____.

(a) the side of the body contralateral to the port-wine birthmark

(b) the side of the body ipsilateral to the port-wine birthmark

(c) either side of the body, regardless of the port-wine birthmark

(d) both sides of the body in a generalized pattern

53. What can be said regarding the autonomous decision-making of children under the age of 12 referred for neuropsychological evaluation?

(a) They can't provide informed consent unless emancipated.

(b) They can't provide informed consent but can give informed assent.

(c) Their capacity for assent or consent cannot be determined.

(d) Their consent is irrelevant as consent must come from a parent or guardian.

54. A neurologist suspects that her patient is experiencing cerebellar dysfunction and would like to evaluate further. The two most relevant tests she might select are _____.

(a) the finger-to-nose test and the Rinne test

(b) the heel-shin test and the Romberg test

(c) switching hands palm up and palm down and visual field testing

(d) examination of tongue protrusion and visual field testing

55. A 58-year-old, recently widowed man presents with symptoms consistent with Major Depressive Disorder. Combination therapy is recommended. With regard to pharmacologic intervention, which neurotransmitter system would not be a primary target?

(a) serotonin

(b) norepinephrine

(c) GABA

(d) dopamine

56. In typical development, restricted and repetitive behaviors are _____.

(a) common in the first 2 years of life, and may continue to be observed during the preschool years

(b) common in the first year of life and then decline afterward

(c) common in the first 2 years of life and then decline afterward

(d) uncommon across the first years of life, and through the preschool years

57. The most common underlying pathology in adult epilepsy is _____.

(a) low-grade glioma

(b) malformation of cortical development

(c) hippocampal sclerosis

(d) traumatic brain injury

58. The average age of onset for Alzheimer's disease is approximately _____ years old.

    (a) 60
    (c) 70

    (b) 65
    (d) 75

59. A 10-year-old child is referred for assessment. He was born full-term, weighing 4 pounds, 6 ounces. What might be a typical profile for this child?

    (a) lower IQ, executive functioning weaknesses, and academic problems

    (b) motor deficits, executive functioning weaknesses, and visuospatial processing problems

    (c) lower IQ, academic problems, and motor deficits

    (d) performance within normal limits

60. An adolescent undergoing cranial radiation for treatment of leukemia suddenly develops excessive sleepiness within 2 months of initiating therapy. This symptom is most likely related to _____.

    (a) emotional adjustment problems
    (c) sleep apnea

    (b) relapse of leukemia
    (d) acute radiation toxicity

61. An 83-year-old woman is referred by her psychiatrist for neuropsychological evaluation to assess her capacity to raise her grandson. Aside from one very low score on a test of attention, cognitive performances were consistently within a normal range relative to normative comparison groups, without evidence of objective impairment. MMPI-2 validity scales included the following: Variable Response Inconsistency (VRIN) T = 39; True Response Inconsistency (TRIN) T = 41; Infrequency (F) scale T = 80; Infrequency Psychopathology (Fp) T = 41. Which of the following factors is most likely to account for these findings?

    (a) limited attention to item content

    (b) a continuing history of significant psychopathology

    (c) denial of any current emotional difficulties

    (d) advanced age

62. Which method has resulted in increased likelihood of securing competitive employment for people with schizophrenia?

    (a) targeted strategy-based interventions
    (c) individual placement with support

    (b) vocational rehabilitation
    (d) on-the-job training

63. A 13-year-old child who sustained a stroke in the superior left middle cerebral artery distribution at age 2 months presents with intact language functioning. What other neuropsychological findings are most likely?

    (a) deficits in visuospatial skills and right-sided motor deficits

    (b) deficits in visuospatial skills and left-sided motor deficits

    (c) intact visuospatial skills and left-sided motor deficits

    (d) deficits in verbal memory and right-sided motor deficits

64. Which statement is true of severe cerebral palsy (CP)?

    (a) Gross motor problems tend to decrease after puberty.

    (b) When present, chronic pain often decreases in adulthood.

    (c) Problems related to premature aging are common.

    (d) Life expectancy is similar to the general CP population.

65. Damage to the medial frontal cortex is primarily associated with _____.

    (a) intentional disorders

    (b) disinhibition of emotion and personality

    (c) executive dysfunction

    (d) ADHD

66. In the context of Alzheimer's disease, neurofibrillary tangles are _____.

    (a) primarily found in the temporal lobe

    (b) primarily found in the frontal and parietal lobes

    (c) found in clusters throughout multiple brain areas

    (d) limited to subcortical as opposed to cortical areas

67. On the Wechsler intelligence tests the index score that is most likely to show decline following traumatic brain injury is _____.

    (a) verbal comprehension

    (b) perceptual reasoning

    (c) working memory

    (d) processing speed

68. Which of the following occurs frequently among young children with Autism spectrum disorder?

    (a) obesity

    (b) nearsightedness

    (c) enlarged head circumference

    (d) close set eyes

69. The neuropsychological profile in mixed Alzheimer's disease (AD) and subcortical vascular disease is _____.

    (a) typical of that commonly seen in AD, with memory impairment greater than executive dysfunction

    (b) typical of that commonly seen in pure vascular dementia, with executive dysfunction greater than memory impairment

    (c) characterized by grossly equivalent severity of memory and executive dysfunction

    (d) characterized by pronounced visuospatial impairments and equivalent severity in executive dysfunction

70. Early initiation of immunotherapy is associated with positive outcomes in which of the following diagnoses?

    (a) anti-NMDA receptor encephalitis

    (b) HSV encephalitis

    (c) bacterial meningitis

    (d) HIV encephalitis

71. Prenatal exposure to nicotine is most consistently linked to problems in which of the following?

    (a) language functions

    (b) externalizing disorders

    (c) memory functions

    (d) internalizing disorders

72. The behavioral variant of frontotemporal dementia begins with changes in personality, interpersonal conduct, and which of the following?

    (a) emotional regulation

    (b) telegraphic speech

    (c) dyspraxia

    (d) dysgraphia

73. Children with spina bifida myelomeningocele and children with Dandy-Walker syndrome ____.

    (a) are often intellectually deficient

    (b) are most often nonambulatory

    (c) show similar performance on neuropsychological tests

    (d) show impairment on measures of fine motor skills

74. The etiology of amnesia most likely to result in confabulation is a(n) ____.

    (a) anoxic encephalopathy

    (b) anterior communicating artery (ACoA) aneurysm

    (c) surgical ablation of the medial temporal lobe

    (d) herpes encephalopathy

75. What are the three elements in any Bayesian model?

    (a) prior probability distribution, posterior probability distribution, and likelihood function

    (b) posterior probability distribution, likelihood function, and new data

    (c) prior probability distribution, likelihood function, and new data

    (d) prior probability distribution, posterior probability distribution, and new data

76. A 9-year-old child presents for clinical evaluation with the following symptoms: poor working memory, fatigue, excessive sleepiness, distractibility, slow responsiveness, and daydreaming. Which of the following diagnoses is most likely given the presented information?

    (a) ADHD- combined type

    (b) ADHD- inattentive type with sluggish cognitive tempo

    (c) ADHD- combined type and learning disorder with specific impairment in reading

    (d) ADHD-inattentive type and Major Depressive Disorder

77. Among the most vulnerable brain regions to thiamine deficiency in patients with Wernicke-Korsakoff syndrome is which structure?

    (a) basal ganglia

    (b) mammillary bodies

    (c) hypothalamus

    (d) prefrontal cortex

78. Cerebellar mutism or posterior fossa syndrome is ____.

    (a) more common in adults than children after brain tumor surgery

    (b) a type of aphasia that occurs after cerebellar stroke

    (c) a transient complication of surgery that resolves completely

    (d) characterized in part by loss of speech and cranial nerve deficits

79. You are seeing a college student who is having difficulty with pre-calculus. This is the first time that he has struggled in math. He has never been diagnosed with a mathematics disability and earned As and Bs in math through high school. The most important question to answer when taking a history is whether ____.

    (a) he has had proper instruction in math and has built a foundation for his current college class

    (b) the new demands of the math class are causing undue anxiety

    (c) he might need to drop out and take a prerequisite for this class

    (d) he is experiencing another source of stress in his life that could be causing difficulty in this class

80. Following moderate to severe traumatic brain injury, the release of which of the following would be considered excitotoxic?

    (a) glutamate   (c) dopamine

    (b) GABA   (d) cortisol

81. A 22-year-old man presents with complaints of frequent panic attacks, generalized anxiety, and difficulty leaving the house. In addition to cognitive behavioral therapy what type of medication might be important in the initial stages of treatment?

    (a) selective serotonin reuptake inhibitors

    (b) serotonin and norepinephrine reuptake inhibitors

    (c) benzodiazepines

    (d) NMDA receptor antagonists

82. The MMPI-2 Restructured Form validity index most sensitive to somatic malingering is ____.

    (a) F-r   (c) Fp-r

    (b) Fs   (d) FBS-r

83. You are consulted to evaluate a 62-year-old woman on the geropsychiatry unit. The patient has been extremely anxious and paranoid for the past 3 weeks with no sign of improvement. She refuses most tests and interventions. The psychiatrist is concerned about a progressive dementia but has not been able to complete an adequate examination. However, when her son comes to visit, she calms considerably and agrees to participate in your assessment, but only if her son stays in the room with her. What do you do?

    (a) The risks to test security are too high; don't conduct the assessment.

    (b) Wait until the patient's anxiety and paranoia improve and then test.

    (c) Conduct the assessment with the son present but tell him he cannot assist.

    (d) Have the patient's son sign a nondisclosure agreement before proceeding.

84. A 14-year-old girl was hospitalized after being found wandering downtown and "talking crazy." You are seeing her on the day of admission. On examination she reports that ants are crawling up and down her legs and that she can't scratch them off. She is experiencing ____ and the likely etiology is ____?

    (a) release hallucinations; drug intoxication

    (b) visceral hallucinations; drug withdrawal

    (c) hypnogogic hallucinations; drug withdrawal

    (d) formication hallucinations; drug intoxication

85. All but which of the following tend to change with normal aging?

    (a) gist recall

    (c) episodic memory

    (b) psychomotor speed

    (d) processing speed

86. Studies of depression in epilepsy have found that ____.

    (a) patients with left temporal lobe epilepsy (TLE) are more depressed than patients with right TLE

    (b) patients with right TLE are more depressed than patients with left TLE

    (c) neither patients with right TLE nor left TLE show depression

    (d) both patients with right TLE and left TLE show depression

87. Which of the following conditions co-occur in as many as 40–70% of cases with Autism spectrum disorder?

    (a) attentional problems

    (c) oppositionality

    (b) depression

    (d) phobias

88. Which of the following is commonly seen in vascular dementia?

    (a) dissociation between Trails A and B performance

    (b) early impairment in personality and behavior

    (c) deficits in letter fluency and set-shifting tasks

    (d) marked dysnomia and micrographia

89. You see a 10-year-old boy with a history of HIV encephalitis due to contracting the virus perinatally. He shows low average intellectual abilities and impairments in working memory, visuospatial reasoning, and processing speed. He struggles with self-confidence in school due to poor grades and asks why he is having these difficulties. Based on the World Health Organization guidelines, what would you recommend to his mother?

    (a) Tell him he was sick as a baby, but doctors do not really know why.

    (b) Inform him of his HIV disease status in an age-appropriate way.

    (c) Discuss HIV in detail, including his family members' contraction of the virus.

    (d) Wait until he is 14 to disclose his status given his low average intelligence.

90. Memory of who you stayed with at a conference last month would be an example of ____ memory.

    (a) semantic

    (c) procedural

    (b) episodic

    (d) remote

91. In general, the effects of hypoxic/ischemic injury are most detrimental in ____.

    (a) infants and toddlers but not in senior adults

    (b) senior adults but not in infants and toddlers

    (c) persons at both extremes of the age spectrum

    (d) late adolescence and early to mid adulthood

92. Jane is a 21-year-old woman diagnosed with multiple sclerosis who is currently attending college. Based on what is known about neuropsychological outcomes associated with multiple sclerosis, which of the following accommodation is most likely to be appropriate in Jane's case?

    (a) extended time for tests

    (b) oral reading of exam questions by a proctor

    (c) unlimited excused absences for medical appointments

    (d) shortened assignments

93. Which of the following findings can be seen early in both Parkinson's disease and corticobasal syndrome?

    (a) asymmetric motor dysfunction   (c) alien hand syndrome

    (b) personality change   (d) resting tremor

94. Most of the time, this genetic disorder is caused when abnormal cell division results in an extra full or partial copy of chromosome 21. The extra genetic material causes the developmental changes and clinical features of this disorder.

    (a) Prader-Willi syndrome   (c) Williams syndrome

    (b) Down syndrome   (d) fragile X syndrome

95. When cognitive variables such as working memory, inhibition, and processing speed are used to predict attention, what percentage of the total variance in attention is typically explained?

    (a) less than 40%   (c) 50–60%

    (b) 40–50%   (d) 60–70%

96. For whom would the MMPI-2, MMPI-2-RF, and PAI most likely be contraindicated?

    (a) an 84-year-old, African American, retired attorney with multiple sclerosis

    (b) an 18-year-old, Hispanic candidate for gastric bypass surgery

    (c) a 28-year-old, Asian American gentleman with a sixth-grade reading level

    (d) a 17-year-old, Caucasian woman with disabling deafness

97. There is anatomic evidence of separate visual channels for ____.

    (a) form, shapes, and objects   (c) faces, objects, and animals

    (b) form, color, and motion   (d) familiar and unfamiliar objects

98. You are examining a 58-year-old African American right-handed man from South Carolina with 9 years of education. He acknowledges visual and auditory hallucinations, including seeing and hearing "ghosts," ever since his brother passed away 6 months ago. He is obese and has diabetes that is not well controlled. Which of the following reflects the most likely diagnosis given the information you have?

    (a) Given both auditory and visual hallucinations, a psychotic disorder due to a medical condition(s) should be investigated.

    (b) Given the combination of psychotic symptoms and the temporal proximity to the death of a close relative, the diagnosis of depressive disorder with psychotic features should be investigated.

(c) Given cultural and educational background, more detailed queries should be made before concluding that his visual and auditory perceptions reflect a psychotic disorder.

(d) Given the risk factors for cerebrovascular disease, workup for ischemic disease and vascular cognitive impairment should be prioritized.

99. What type of aphasia most commonly results from an infarct of the left inferior middle cerebral artery distribution in an adult?

(a) Broca's aphasia

(c) global aphasia

(b) transcortical motor aphasia

(d) Wernicke's aphasia

100. Which of the following drugs is most likely to cause persisting changes on MRI?

(a) hallucinogens

(c) methamphetamine

(b) Ecstasy

(d) benzodiazepines

101. The presence of REM behavioral symptoms is most likely to be seen in which of the following?

(a) progressive supranuclear palsy

(c) essential tremor

(b) Parkinson's disease

(d) Huntington's disease

102. The most typical neuropsychological profile of a child with cerebral palsy is ____.

(a) moderate to severe intellectual disabilities with commensurate functioning across domains including attention, processing speed, and executive skills

(b) better visuospatial than language skills with weaknesses in attention, processing speed, and executive functions

(c) relatively even language and visuospatial skills with weaknesses in attention, processing speed, and executive functions

(d) better language than visuospatial skills with weaknesses in attention, processing speed, and executive functions

103. You are evaluating a 93-year-old woman in your office when she tells you that you are not the real Dr. X that she is supposed to be seeing. She appears to have ____.

(a) anosognosia

(c) reduplicative paramnesia

(b) Capgras syndrome

(d) prosopagnosia

104. You will be conducting a neuropsychological assessment on a patient who is being evaluated for a possible resection of a brain region where a seizure locus has been identified. This testing will be conducted while the ipsilateral hemisphere is anesthetized, as a method of assessing the capabilities of the other hemisphere. Your assessment will be conducted within the context of a/an ____.

(a) electroencephalogram (EEG)

(b) positron emission tomography (PET)

(c) cerebral arteriography

(d) intracarotid sodium amobarbital procedure

105. You are asked to conduct a neuropsychological evaluation with an 8-year-old child with a confirmed history of in utero exposure to alcohol. The child has been diagnosed with fetal alcohol spectrum disorder. Which of the following would best predict low intellectual functioning?

    (a) severity of kidney abnormality

    (b) maternal occupation

    (c) number of dysmorphic facial features

    (d) type of alcohol consumed by mother

106. After examining a 28-year-old male 4 years post moderate traumatic brain injury, the neuropsychologist notes that scores for story and visual memory are average, but list learning scores are consistently very low. Assuming adequate test engagement, the most likely explanation for this finding is that the patient _____.

    (a) has more intact right posterior hemisphere function

    (b) is experiencing organizational difficulties that affect memory

    (c) suffers from left-sided medial temporal lobe dysfunction

    (d) is experiencing mild diffuse subcortical dysfunction

107. Which of the following neuropathological changes show the strongest relationship with cognitive decline in Alzheimer's disease?

    (a) amyloid

    (b) cortical atrophy

    (c) ventricular dilation

    (d) tau

108. Autoimmune disorders are increasingly identified in new onset epilepsy of all ages. Other than seizures, autoimmune encephalitis is most likely to present with which of the following additional symptoms?

    (a) psychiatric presentation

    (b) loss of vision

    (c) hemiplegia

    (d) expressive aphasia

109. Individuals with intellectual disability are likely to have the most trouble with which of the following academic tasks?

    (a) word recognition

    (b) reading comprehension

    (c) spelling

    (d) mathematics facts

110. Which disorder cannot be seen in males?

    (a) Klinefelter syndrome

    (b) fragile X syndrome

    (c) 22q11.2 deletion syndrome

    (d) Turner syndrome

111. Which neuropsychological performance is least likely to show deficits in patients with mood or anxiety disorders?

    (a) immediate acquisition of an unrelated word list

    (b) reproduction of a complex figure

    (c) delayed recall of a narrative story

    (d) speed of performance on a visual scanning task

112. Cerebral amyloid angiopathy _____.

    (a) has an early age of onset

    (b) results in multiple hemorrhagic lesions

    (c) results in a lacunar state

    (d) results in leukoaraiosis

113. A biomedical explanation for the much higher prevalence of functional somatic symptoms in females often invokes _____ as an explanation.

    (a) hormonal mechanisms

    (b) risk taking behaviors

    (c) hypertension

    (d) a history of childhood abuse

114. A 34-year-old woman presents to the clinic with infrequent limb jerking and reports "feeling clumsy." She was recently admitted to the local psychiatric unit for paranoia. Family history is significant for dementia at a young age and completed suicide. MRI reveals atrophy of the striatum. What is this patient's most likely diagnosis?

    (a) brief psychotic episode

    (b) Huntington's disease

    (c) corticobasal syndrome

    (d) tardive dyskinesia

115. You are evaluating a college student who wants to apply for accommodations on the Law School Admission Test. The individual was diagnosed with a reading disability in second grade, had early intervention, and has had accommodations throughout schooling. You want to be sure that your assessment conforms to the documentation guidelines. On which website should you look for the most current guidelines?

    (a) National Joint Committee on Learning Disabilities

    (b) Association on Higher Education and Disability

    (c) Educational Testing Service

    (d) Law School Admission Council

116. You want to calculate a confidence interval around an obtained test score to determine how confident you should be that the obtained score reflects the person's true ability. For the most appropriate estimate of the confidence interval, you should use the following in your calculation:

    (a) validity coefficient for the test

    (b) standard error of the mean

    (c) standard error of the estimate

    (d) standard error of the measurement

117. The _____ model of schizophrenia seeks to explain the interaction between environmental stressors and genetic vulnerability in the pathogenesis of the disorder.

    (a) neurocognitive

    (b) epigenetic

    (c) double-bind

    (d) neurodevelopmental

118. You are the only neuropsychologist working in a small community. You are asked to evaluate a blind, 25-year-old male because his primary care physician is concerned that he may have sequelae from a head injury experienced the previous year. The physician notes that the patient is unable to travel outside of the area. What should you do?

    (a) Decline the referral because you have no Braille or haptic materials.

    (b) Ask about the characteristics of the vision impairment and its onset.

(c) Decline the referral because you are not competent to test blind individuals.

(d) Offer to help the referral source find a clinician skilled in assessing blind individuals.

119. Deficits in which of the following language skills have been most documented in herpes simplex virus encephalitis?

(a) naming

(c) comprehension

(b) repetition

(d) prosody

120. Normal pressure hydrocephalus ____.

(a) is a benign condition that affects the elderly because of brain atrophy

(b) is a condition in which cerebrospinal fluid accumulates with ventricular expansion

(c) occurs only after a stroke, traumatic brain injury, or dementia

(d) invariably leads to a nonverbal learning disability

121. The EEG waveforms that predominate during sleep are ____.

(a) alpha and beta

(c) delta and theta

(b) beta and delta

(d) theta and gamma

122. Pregnant women with multiple sclerosis often experience ____.

(a) greater fatigue

(c) more relapses

(b) fewer relapses

(d) optic neuritis

123. You are evaluating a 10-year-old female for concerns about attention and reading/writing. The parent of the child shares that her twin sibling has previously been evaluated by a neuropsychologist and diagnosed with ADHD. Based on familial/genetic heritability, which of the following statements is most likely?

(a) This child is at no greater risk than the general population, as ADHD is thought to be predominantly mediated by environmental factors.

(b) This child is likely experiencing ADHD and Oppositional Defiant Disorder given the comorbidity between these two conditions.

(c) This child has a 10–20% chance of having ADHD and dyslexia and therefore you would want to measure phonological awareness and rapid automatized naming.

(d) This child likely has ADHD, given the heritability of ADHD is as high as 70–80% among twin studies.

124. The perirhinal/parahippocampal region ____.

(a) contributes only to the medial limbic circuit

(b) has no specific role in memory encoding

(c) produces significant amnesia when lesioned

(d) is a prominent storage site for new memory representations

125. A 24-year-old woman was involved in a motor vehicle crash and sustained bilateral subdural hematomas that required surgical evacuation. She experienced two seizures on the day of admission. One week later, she is admitted to the inpatient brain injury unit with symptoms of

confusion, sleep–wake cycle disturbance, waxing and waning attention, and executive dysfunction. The most likely diagnosis would be _____.

(a) post-traumatic amnesia

(c) postictal confusion

(b) dementia due to brain injury

(d) delirium due to brain injury

Appendix D

Fourth Full-Length Practice Examination Questions

1. Accelerated cognitive decline in older adults with schizophrenia is _____.
   - (a) due to Parkinson's disease
   - (b) a variant of Lewy body dementia
   - (c) present in a subgroup of patients, but no single cause has yet been identified
   - (d) probably early-onset Alzheimer's disease

2. An example of equipotentiality might be _____.
   - (a) persons with Korsakoff amnesia retaining motor-skill learning
   - (b) patients with aphasia learning to speak again
   - (c) double dissociation of language and visual processing
   - (d) late onset of dementia in highly educated people

3. You have been intimately involved with the healthcare of a child who experienced significant complications following the development of bacterial meningitis. Her family is extremely grateful for your care, and they bring you a $10 gift certificate to a local restaurant and a thank you card. What should you do?
   - (a) Accept the gift graciously.
   - (b) Refuse the gift even if they insist.
   - (c) Share the gift with the treatment team.
   - (d) Accept the gift but report it to the hospital.

4. This type of multiple sclerosis profile involves a continual worsening of baseline functions from the onset, with minor fluctuations but no distinct relapses.
   - (a) relapsing-remitting
   - (b) secondary-progressive
   - (c) primary-progressive
   - (d) progressive-relapsing

5. Which of the following neuropsychological domains has been proposed as an underlying deficit that may explain Autism spectrum disorder symptomatology?

(a) poor visual discrimination

(b) impaired sustained attention

(c) sensory hyper- and hypo-reactivity

(d) deficient executive functioning

6. Two individuals are administered the same test, of which the data are normally distributed. Person 1 scores in the 48th percentile; Person 2 scores in the 93rd percentile. It is later found that there was an error in scoring of the test on these two administrations only, and 3 points are then added to each person's score. Given this information, which of the following is true?

(a) Both percentile ranks will increase by the same amount.

(b) Person 1's percentile rank will increase more than Person 2's.

(c) Person 2's percentile rank will increase more than Person 1's.

(d) Neither percentile rank will change.

7. Depression and anxiety in persons with epilepsy are _____.

(a) not consistently reported due to poor insight

(b) typically not severe enough to warrant treatment

(c) more common than in other chronic illnesses

(d) not as common as in other chronic illnesses

8. Individuals using MDMA at raves or dance clubs are at high risk for _____.

(a) dehydration

(b) hypothermia

(c) hallucinations

(d) intention tremor

9. Which of the following is most commonly comorbid with Tourette syndrome?

(a) ADHD

(b) Bipolar Disorder

(c) eating disorder

(d) Oppositional Defiant Disorder

10. Patients with Alzheimer's disease exhibit impairment most profoundly in this type of memory.

(a) source memory

(b) procedural memory

(c) long-term memory

(d) episodic memory

11. The pattern of stronger verbal than spatial skills in early hydrocephalus is _____.

(a) primarily apparent in spina bifida myelomeningocele and aqueductal stenosis

(b) an anomaly related to the motor demands of the Wechsler performance scales

(c) seen across all levels of economic disadvantage and ethnicity in spina bifida

(d) a correlate of very low birth weight and associated perinatal anoxia

12. The American Heart Association guidelines and current clinical practice for using tissue plasminogen activator (tPA) in adults after stroke include evidence of deficits, _____.

(a) brain hemorrhage on CT, and symptom duration of 3 to 4.5 hours or less

(b) no brain hemorrhage on CT, and symptom duration of 3 to 4.5 hours or less

(c) brain hemorrhage on CT, and symptom duration of 3 hours or less

(d) no brain hemorrhage on CT, and symptom duration of 3 hours or less

13. What can be said with regard to cognitive restitution/restorative training methods following traumatic brain injury?

(a) They outperform compensatory strategy training in all phases following injury.

(b) They have lasting benefits primarily in the recovery of simple attention skills.

(c) They have limited empirical support at any phase and typically do not generalize.

(d) They are typically only efficacious in addressing prospective memory skills.

14. Patients with Alzheimer's disease are more likely to produce what type of errors on confrontation naming?

(a) semantic

(b) echolalic

(c) phonemic

(d) perseverative

15. A 10-year-old girl is involved in a car accident in which her mother and brother are badly injured, but she is not. Shortly afterward on the scene she becomes tachycardic, short of breath, and can't stop shaking. Which neurotransmitter is most likely involved?

(a) serotonin

(b) GABA

(c) norepinephrine

(d) dopamine

16. Inaccuracies in unilateral cerebellar coordination are referred to as _____.

(a) dysreflexia

(b) dystonia

(c) dysgraphestheia

(d) dysmetria

17. A 17-year-old male presents to the clinic due to depressed mood. His parents report he no longer hangs out with his friends and his grades are slipping. He reports to you that he sometimes hears his name being called but no one is there, and he has begun to ascribe significance to certain numbers that he feels have followed him around most of his life. Assuming the possibility of schizophrenia, which of the following phase of illness might he be in?

(a) premorbid

(b) prodromal

(c) acute

(d) paranoid

18. Which patient is most likely to demonstrate pronounced cognitive deficits after treatment for childhood acute lymphoblastic leukemia?

(a) male treated in adolescence with chemotherapy only

(b) male treated in middle childhood with radiation and chemotherapy

(c) female treated in early childhood with chemotherapy and radiation

(d) male treated in early childhood with chemotherapy only

19. Among the following, which combination of preexisting issues would suggest a more significant risk for postoperative delirium?

(a) executive dysfunction and depression

(b) learning disability and anxiety

(c) low average IQ and depression

(d) dysnomia and anxiety

20. Lesions to the basal forebrain produce amnesia because _____.

(a) cholinergic inputs to the hippocampus and amygdala are disrupted

(b) pathways of the medial and lateral limbic circuits may be spared

(c) the basal forebrain contains dopaminergic neurons involved in memory retrieval

(d) the basal forebrain is a key site of memory storage

21. Which of the following neurodevelopmental disorders is most associated with a high rate of co-morbid developmental mathematics disability?

    (a) Autism spectrum disorder   (c) spina bifida

    (b) Tourette syndrome   (d) ADHD

22. Abrupt onset and step-wise progression of cognitive deficits _____.

    (a) have not been consistently demonstrated in vascular dementia

    (b) are more commonly associated with subcortical forms of vascular dementia

    (c) correlate with progression of leukoaraiosis

    (d) characterize vascular dementia of mixed pathology

23. Which of the following is not true of anti-NMDA receptor encephalitis?

    (a) Adult women are more likely to have an associated ovarian teratoma.

    (b) Children may show hyperactivity, irritability, and temper tantrums early in disease course.

    (c) Females are more affected by anti-NMDA receptor encephalitis.

    (d) Low intellectual abilities are seen in children, but adult IQs fall in the average range.

24. In diagnosing vascular dementia, motor deficits secondary to cortical infarction _____.

    (a) can explain the significant impairment in complex ADLs

    (b) suggest silent infarction as an underlying pathophysiologic process

    (c) suggest leukoaraiosis as an underlying pathophysiologic process

    (d) are to be excluded when evaluating functional impairment in ADLs

25. A 65-year-old woman developed delirium secondary to sepsis and experienced an extremely complicated hospital course. Physicians have now deemed that she is medically stable and ready for transition to a subacute facility. However, when she is told about the plan for discharge and transition she becomes extremely belligerent, confused, combative, and insistent that she should be allowed to go home. This behavior results in a staff member getting hit by the patient and delay in her transfer. In an effort to curb this behavior and avoid safety issues for the patient and staff, the neuropsychologist advises the team not to provide information regarding the pending transfer. What can be said regarding deception in situations like this?

    (a) It is unethical in most similar situations.

    (b) It is ethically appropriate in some cases.

    (c) It is only acceptable if approved by the ethics committee.

    (d) It is often necessary with patients who are confused.

26. Which of the following transformations results in even intervals of the normative data?

    (a) logarithmic   (c) percentile

    (b) z distribution   (d) T distribution

27. Brain injury during which of the following school years confers the most risk for a poor outcome?

    (a) preschool

    (b) elementary school

    (c) middle school

    (d) high school

28. A 28-year-old veteran presents with complaints of flashbacks, nightmares, and a heightened startle response. Which neuroanatomical area is likely to be directly involved in the maintenance of these symptoms?

    (a) amygdala

    (b) prefrontal cortex

    (c) anterior cingulate

    (d) basal ganglia

29. You are evaluating a child with fetal alcohol spectrum disorder. When selecting your test battery, including behavioral questionnaires, which of the following DSM-5 diagnoses should be highest on your list of diagnostic considerations?

    (a) Autism spectrum disorder

    (b) ADHD

    (c) Depressive Disorder, not otherwise specified

    (d) Generalized Anxiety Disorder

30. You have agreed to evaluate a 65-year-old woman who is also deaf. In order to ensure an accurate evaluation, you must ____.

    (a) provide an American Sign Language interpreter

    (b) use test materials with a reading level at or below the fourth grade

    (c) determine the age at onset and severity of hearing loss

    (d) make sure that you speak slowly and she can see your mouth

31. Jane is an adult who recently earned a standard score of 70 on an individually administered intelligence test, a score that was consistent with previous measures of intellectual functioning as a child. Jane reported that she completed a local community college program as a certified nursing assistant and worked full time while living on her own. She stated that she completed all of her own activities of daily living such as driving, cooking, cleaning, caring for her hygiene, and managing her finances. She reported having a strong and supportive network of friends. Which statement best describes Jane's level of functioning?

    (a) She meets criteria for mild intellectual disability.

    (b) She exhibits borderline intellectual functioning.

    (c) Her intellectual functioning is likely in the low average range.

    (d) No diagnosis can be determined because of the absence of an observer report.

32. Which of the following cognitive domains may be more impaired early on in patients with Lewy body dementia versus Alzheimer's disease?

    (a) visuospatial

    (b) memory

    (c) language

    (d) processing speed

33. Which of the following disorders is associated with an increased risk of brain tumors?

   (a) fragile X syndrome

   (b) tuberous sclerosis

   (c) Prader-Willi syndrome

   (d) Sturge-Weber

34. Wernicke's encephalopathy is comprised by a triad of clinical symptoms including global confusion, abnormal eye movements, and _____.

   (a) dysarthria

   (b) vitamin D deficiency

   (c) fatigue

   (d) gait ataxia

35. Family and twin studies of ADHD have been used to assess the degree to which variability in the disorder and its underlying latent traits are under genetic control. Which of the following statements is most true?

   (a) The heritability of ADHD symptoms is approximately 25%.

   (b) Shared environmental influence accounts for 25% of the variance.

   (c) ADHD-I is more heritable than ADHD-H.

   (d) A sibling of a child with ADHD has a 75% chance of having ADHD.

36. A 74-year-old right-handed man with right leg weakness, grasp reflex, and executive function deficits should be further examined for possible _____.

   (a) transcortical motor aphasia

   (b) transcortical sensory aphasia

   (c) fluent aphasia

   (d) global aphasia

37. A 41-year-old male with a history of multiple sclerosis has been referred to you for an evaluation. He reports that he is having problems keeping up with work demands in his job as an administrative assistant. Which of the following areas would be most important to assess based on the referral concern and what you know about outcomes associated with multiple sclerosis?

   (a) processing speed, verbal IQ, inhibition

   (b) working memory, fatigue, reading

   (c) word generation, processing speed, depression

   (d) processing speed, depression, fatigue

38. When compared to normal controls, individuals with insomnia are 2 times more likely to have or develop _____, while they are ten times more likely to have or develop _____.

   (a) Generalized Anxiety Disorder; Major Depressive Disorder

   (b) a personality disorder; Major Depressive Disorder

   (c) Major Depressive Disorder; schizophrenia

   (d) a specific learning disorder; Generalized Anxiety Disorder

39. When conducting a neuropsychological evaluation on a 12-year-old child, the parent- and teacher-report measures from the BASC-3 can be used to examine the clinical probability indices for all of the following, except _____.

   (a) ADHD

   (b) Autism spectrum disorder

   (c) specific learning disorder

   (d) emotional behavior disorder

40. Which of the following is an accurate statement regarding essential tremor?

    (a) Essential tremor is an uncommon adult onset movement disorder.

    (b) Essential tremor is secondary to reduced dopamine in the basal ganglia.

    (c) There is no known genetic component to essential tremor.

    (d) This type of tremor is typically postural and kinetic.

41. Which of the following statements is most accurate regarding memory deficits in persons with epilepsy?

    (a) Memory deficits in frontal and temporal lobe epilepsy (TLE) are the same.

    (b) Memory deficits in TLE do not lateralize to the side of seizure onset.

    (c) In TLE, verbal memory impairments are only present in left-side seizure onset.

    (d) Verbal memory deficits in left TLE are more robust than visual memory deficits in right TLE.

42. Chromosome 21 _____.

    (a) has been marginally implicated in Alzheimer's disease

    (b) appears to be related to the development of amyloid plaques

    (c) appears to be related to the development of neurofibrillary tangles

    (d) has been ruled out as related to Alzheimer's disease

43. A 19-year-old man is in his second year of college when he becomes hyperverbal, can't sleep, and reports boundless energy. On interview he reports "I'm at the top of my game" and is going to soon earn a large government grant based on his ideas regarding a ground-breaking new theory in physics. Assuming a likely psychiatric or neurologic illness which class of medications might be considered in the treatment of these symptoms?

    (a) benzodiazepines

    (b) selective serotonin reuptake inhibitors

    (c) monoamine oxidase inhibitors

    (d) anticonvulsants

44. You have been consulted to see an 82-year-old man on the intensive care unit due to persistent mixed level delirium with significant behavioral and personality changes. His wife asks, "My husband was perfectly healthy 2 weeks ago. Now the doctor says that he has a urinary tract infection that is making him crazy. I've had lots of UTIs and never acted like this. The infection is in his bladder not his brain. Does this make any sense to you?" How might you try to explain this?

    (a) In older people the blood-brain barrier is more permeable and infections get in more easily thus resulting in delirium.

    (b) While the UTI may not be the primary cause of the delirium, the antibiotics and catheter being used are probably affecting mental status.

    (c) Older bodies are less tolerant of changes and although the brain is not directly infected his overall reaction to the infection can cause delirium.

    (d) He probably had a dementia prior to developing the infection and this has now unmasked the underlying condition.

45. On memory tests, children with congenital hydrocephalus typically perform ____.

    (a) more poorly on tests of verbal than nonverbal learning and retrieval

    (b) more poorly on tests of nonverbal than verbal learning and retrieval

    (c) comparably poorly on tests of verbal and nonverbal learning and memory

    (d) within normal limits on tests of verbal and nonverbal learning and retrieval

46. A seizure is a discrete event that may or may not lead to diagnosis with epilepsy. According to the International League Against Epilepsy definition and classification system, which of the following would not lead to a diagnosis with epilepsy?

    (a) two unprovoked seizures, at least 24 hours apart

    (b) a single seizure when risk of a second is known to be elevated (>60%)

    (c) diagnosis with an epilepsy syndrome

    (d) spontaneous seizure with no known precipitating event or risk factor

47. Frontotemporal dementia with motor neuron disease is characterized by ____.

    (a) primarily ubiquitin-based pathology

    (b) primarily tau pathology

    (c) both tau pathology and ubiquitin-based pathology

    (d) neither tau pathology nor ubiquitin-based pathology

48. Which is the most common single gene disorder associated with Autism spectrum disorder?

    (a) Prader-Willi syndrome   (c) Williams syndrome

    (b) fragile X syndrome   (d) tuberous sclerosis

49. A patient has a discrete, small lesion and develops full-blown amnesia. Which of the following lesions is most likely responsible?

    (a) lesion of the anterior thalamus affecting the internal medullary lamina

    (b) lesion of the anterior thalamic nucleus sparing the internal medullary lamina

    (c) lesion affecting the left hippocampus

    (d) lesion of the amygdala affecting the ventral amygdalofugal pathway

50. What is the earliest age at which the diagnosis of Autism spectrum disorder tends to be reliable and stable across time?

    (a) 48–60 months   (c) 36–48 months

    (b) 0–6 months   (d) 18–24 months

51. The risk for decline in previously mastered daily living skills 5 years post severe traumatic brain injury is greatest in which of the following groups?

    (a) young children   (c) young adults

    (b) adolescents   (d) middle-aged adults

52. For individuals with schizophrenia the severity of cognitive impairments is estimated to range from _____ standard deviation units relative to demographically matched control groups.

(a) 0.0 to 0.5

(c) 1.0 to 1.5

(b) 0.5 to 1.0

(d) 1.5 to 2.0

53. A mother and father present to your office for an intake appointment regarding their teenage son who has a history of premature birth. Which of the following factors are most essential when evaluating the potential impact of the birth history on functional outcome?

(a) gestational age, availability of NICU care, birth weight, and presence of neurological/medical complications

(b) prenatal steroid administration, birth weight, grades III or IV intraventricular hemorrhage, and inpatient developmental assessment results (e.g., Bayley or Mullen scores)

(c) gestational age, length of NICU stay, maternal age, and presence of neurological/medical complications

(d) gestational age, birth weight, inpatient ultrasound results, and postnatal steroid administration

54. During the clinical interview, your new patient who recovered from bacterial meningitis describes undergoing a procedure where she was in a seated position while the doctors inserted a needle below her spinal cord to remove fluid. You suspect that the patient underwent a/an _____ during her hospitalization, and plan to request the records associated with this procedure.

(a) evoked potential (EP)

(c) lumbar puncture

(b) electromyogram (EMG)

(d) central line insertion

55. Which of the following is true about diagnostic findings typically seen in young adult females recently diagnosed with anti-NMDA receptor encephalitis?

(a) the brain MRI is abnormal in most cases

(b) EEGs are normal in nearly all cases

(c) a teratoma in the ovaries is identified in a majority of cases

(d) NMDA receptor antibodies are found in the CSF or blood

56. Obsessive-compulsive disorder symptoms have been associated with all of the following except _____.

(a) Tourette syndrome

(c) ADHD

(b) hypomanic states

(d) PANDAS

57. In creating PVTs and SVTs, both simulation and criterion groups designs utilize a comparison group with bona fide neurologic problems. This is because developers are focused on controlling for _____ error.

(a) true positive

(c) false positive

(b) true negative

(d) false negative

58. The association of IQ and seizure outcome following epilepsy surgery is believed to be attributable to ____.

    (a) low IQ as a proxy for widespread neuropathology

    (b) low IQ leading to poor treatment compliance

    (c) VIQ-PIQ discrepancy lateralizing to side of surgery

    (d) low IQ associated with antiepileptic drug side effects

59. Presence of orthostatic hypotension in addition to gait ataxia as presenting symptoms would be most consistent with ____.

    (a) corticobasal syndrome

    (b) progressive supranuclear palsy

    (c) multiple system atrophy

    (d) Parkinson's disease

60. Individuals with which of the following disorders exhibit absent or limited speech, but are socially interested in others?

    (a) Prader-Willi syndrome

    (b) Angelman syndrome

    (c) Turner syndrome

    (d) 22q11.2 deletion syndrome

61. After a stroke, a patient presents with a global aphasia, with severe deficits in both expressive and receptive language functions, but does not have a motor deficit. The lesion is ____.

    (a) not the typical middle cerebral artery pattern

    (b) not the typical posterior cerebral artery pattern

    (c) the typical middle cerebral artery pattern

    (d) the typical anterior cerebral artery pattern

62. The post-test odds of a diagnostic test is the ____.

    (a) proportion of individuals at risk for the disease in the population sample at a certain time

    (b) proportion of individuals the test identifies as having the disease at a certain time

    (c) proportion of individuals the test identifies as having the disease who truly have the disease factored by the likelihood ratio of those who do not have the disease

    (d) ratio of individuals the test identifies as having the disease who truly have the disease in a population that is factored by the likelihood ratio of having the disease

63. Many believe that ____, Alzheimer's disease can be clinically differentiated from Lewy body dementia.

    (a) in the early stages

    (b) in all stages

    (c) in the middle to late stages

    (d) in the late stages

64. You are conducting a neuropsychological evaluation with a teenager who has a history of executive deficits and behavioral dysregulation. During your clinical interview, the mother shares that she drank red wine twice per week throughout the pregnancy because she read online that red wine was good for heart and brain health. Based on the literature and current standards, how would you conceptualize the risk associated with this specific amount of alcohol use during pregnancy?

    (a) One to two drinks per week at any point during pregnancy is considered safe.

    (b) One to two drinks during the third trimester only is considered safe.

(c) No amount of alcohol use during pregnancy is considered safe.

(d) Red wine specifically is considered safe to drink during pregnancy.

65. In vascular dementia, donepezil and galantamine _____.

(a) are ineffective as a treatment modality

(b) may delay cognitive decline

(c) are most effective when memory deficits are present

(d) significantly increase risk of major stroke

66. Parametric statistics rely on the assumed validity of the central limit theorem, which states that the attribute being assessed is normally distributed in the population and/or normative sample such that the distribution approximates a normal curve. Which type of data violates this assumption?

(a) continuous variables

(b) interval data

(c) ratio data

(d) ordinal data

67. Which of the following is a frequent co-occurring condition in children with math learning disabilities?

(a) intellectual disability

(b) dyslexia

(c) language difficulties

(d) Autism spectrum disorder

68. You evaluate a 33-year-old woman who sustained a concussion 6 months ago. She complains of persistent impairments in memory and concentration. She also meets diagnostic criteria for Major Depressive Disorder. Which of the following would you most likely recommend?

(a) SSRI or SNRI medications

(b) psychotherapy

(c) stimulant medications

(d) combination therapy

69. The Preschool ADHD Treatment Study (PATS) was a large multi-site, double-blind, crossover, placebo-controlled clinical trial, evaluating the effect of methylphenidate in preschoolers with ADHD. Which of the following statements best describes the results from this study?

(a) Medication led to improvement in symptoms but with effect sizes smaller than those observed in the MTA studies.

(b) Medication side effects were less common than those observed in the MTA studies.

(c) Early medication treatment led to a significant decline in symptoms later in childhood.

(d) Behavioral therapy was less effective in children in this age range than the older children in the MTA studies.

70. According to meta-analyses, there is an increased risk of _____ in children with neonatal hypoxia.

(a) motor dysfunction

(b) dyslexia

(c) constructional apraxia

(d) intellectual disabilities

71. Individuals with mild intellectual disability are likely to accomplish all but which of the following?

(a) driving independently

(b) reading at a ninth-grade level

(c) making small purchases

(d) holding a job

72. Cognitive reserve refers to _____.

    (a) some individuals being less vulnerable to brain insult

    (b) late-onset dementia without family history of it

    (c) early onset dementia without family history of it

    (d) full scale IQ in the high-average range

73. Twelve-month outpatient treatment follow-up studies reveal the substance abuse relapse rate to be about _____.

    (a) 85%   (c) 50%

    (b) 70%   (d) 30%

74. Treatment of patients with medically unexplained symptoms with antidepressants has shown _____.

    (a) tricyclic antidepressants to be the most effective

    (b) serotonin selective reuptake inhibitors to be the most effective

    (c) monoamine oxidase inhibitors to be the most effective

    (d) no clear evidence of effectiveness for any one class of drugs

75. A 29-year-old woman presents in your office. You note that she has short stature. During the interview, she reports that she struggled in school and particularly had difficulty with math classes. She further reports significant stress and anxiety related to fertility problems she is currently experiencing. You suspect she may have which disorder?

    (a) Turner syndrome   (c) neurofibromatosis type 1

    (b) Klinefelter syndrome   (d) Williams syndrome

76. Which may be apparent as a late effect status-post treatment of breast cancer with chemotherapy?

    (a) hypothyroidism   (c) visuospatial impairments

    (b) headaches   (d) memory problems

77. A 10-year-old patient with a diagnosis of cerebral palsy is referred for testing. Given what is known about risk factors associated with cerebral palsy, which of the following is most likely true regarding the patient?

    (a) The patient is female, African American, and presents with intellectual disability.

    (b) The patient is male, African American, and was born very low birth weight.

    (c) The patient is female, Latin/x, and presents with spastic diplegia.

    (d) The patient is male, and presents with ataxic cerebral palsy and intellectual disability.

78. A patient presents with left sided weakness and an inability to deploy attention to the left side of space. The patient likely has a lesion of the _____.

    (a) left frontal lobe   (c) right frontal lobe

    (b) left parietal lobe   (d) right temporal lobe

79. Following acceleration-deceleration traumatic brain injury, neuroimaging is most likely to reveal lesions in ____.

    (a) temporal and parietal areas

    (b) frontal and subcortical areas

    (c) temporal and subcortical areas

    (d) frontal and temporal areas

80. A neuropsychologist, who agrees to evaluate a 25-year-old, Caucasian woman, administers the MMPI-2-RF as a component of the evaluation. The patient completed the MMPI-2-RF in the context of a psychological assessment approximately 3 weeks before. The clinician interprets the second MMPI-2-RF profile with the knowledge that, relative to most other scales, test-retest reliabilities are generally lower for the ____.

    (a) higher-order (H-O) scales

    (b) restructured clinical (RC) scales

    (c) VRIN-r and TRIN-r scales

    (d) Personality Psychopathology Five (PSY-5) scales

81. Rupture of bridging veins between sulci on the upper surface of the brain causes ____.

    (a) subarachnoid hemorrhage

    (b) intracerebral hemorrhage

    (c) epidural hematoma

    (d) subdural hematoma

82. In adults with multiple sclerosis, deficits are most commonly seen in the area of ____.

    (a) memory

    (b) processing speed

    (c) attention

    (d) executive function

83. Which type of restricted and repetitive behavior (RRB) is least prevalent among individuals with Autism spectrum disorder (ASD) at all ages?

    (a) stereotyped motor movements

    (b) compulsive behavior

    (c) repetitive self-injurious behavior

    (d) restricted interests

84. Individuals with latent herpes simplex virus (HSV) infection are at increased risk for ____ later in life.

    (a) Alzheimer's disease

    (b) stroke

    (c) Lewy body disease

    (d) frontotemporal dementia

85. Alexia without agraphia is associated with damage to the ____.

    (a) right visual cortex and splenium of the corpus callosum

    (b) left visual cortex and splenium of the corpus callosum

    (c) left parietal region and body of the corpus callosum

    (d) right parietal region and body of the corpus callosum

86. A 63-year-old right-handed woman with hypertension was talking on the phone when suddenly she had difficulty getting words out and could not answer simple questions. She was taken to

the hospital, and on exam was alert and oriented to person and time, but not place. Speech was sparse, halting, and labored. She was able to follow 3-step commands, and repeated words and sentences with 100% accuracy. Reading was not assessed. Writing was sparse and telegraphic. Naming was 1 of 6. What kind of aphasic syndrome is likely present in this patient?

(a) Broca's aphasia

(c) transcortical sensory aphasia

(b) Wernicke's aphasia

(d) transcortical motor aphasia

87. On the rehabilitation unit your patient was recently started on Elavil to improve sleep and address nighttime headaches. Over the next 3 days, he develops increasing confusion, nighttime visual hallucinations, and gastrointestinal symptoms. Assuming that this is related to the recent change in medication, what might you expect the medical work up to show?

(a) high serum dopaminergic activity

(c) low serum anticholinergic activity

(b) low serum dopaminergic activity

(d) high serum anticholinergic activity

88. Martin is a 6-year-old child with Down syndrome. He is social and has friends his age. He earned a standard score of 68 on a measure of one word receptive language skills and an overall score of 65 on an intelligence test. He can say the alphabet and count to 10. His parents provide him with more supervision than is typical for others his age. He participates in regular education programming with a paraprofessional aid. He is most likely to be diagnosed with intellectual disability that is _____ in severity.

(a) mild

(c) severe

(b) moderate

(d) profound

89. You will be conducting a neuropsychological assessment on a patient with Parkinson's disease, and receive medical records from the patient's referring physician. The physician administered the Folstein Mini Mental Status Examination (MMSE) as part of his examination with this patient. Which of the following is critical in interpreting the results of the MMSE for this patient?

(a) The MMSE should not have been selected over other screens such as the Montreal Cognitive Assessment (MoCA).

(b) The MMSE de-emphasizes working memory and executive functions and may lack sensitivity to subcortical-frontal dysfunction.

(c) Mental status screens may disproportionately emphasize language function, and therefore exaggerate pathology in Parkinson's disease.

(d) The cut scores used on mental status screens such as the MMSE are precise and typically reflect true neurocognitive status for most disorders.

90. Which of the following is less commonly seen in young children with depression?

(a) frequent crying spells and despondency

(b) nightmares related to separation from loved ones

(c) somatic complaints such as nausea, vomiting, or headaches

(d) worry that a parent or family member may die

91. A pediatric neuropsychologist is concerned that a particular test for ADHD may be missing too many children with the condition when the conventional cut-off point is used. The

neuropsychologist therefore changes the cut-off from 1.5 standard deviations below the mean to 1 standard deviation below the mean. What will happen as a result?

(a) Sensitivity will be increased and specificity will be increased.

(b) Sensitivity will be decreased and specificity will be increased.

(c) Sensitivity will be increased and specificity will be decreased.

(d) Sensitivity will be decreased and specificity will be decreased.

92. You are conducting an evaluation of an 11-year-old to help determine eligibility for Social Security disability benefits. The child earns a full scale IQ of 82. The child earns below chance scores on multiple performance validity tests. Which of the following is apt to be the most appropriate diagnosis?

(a) malingering by proxy

(b) Munchausen by proxy

(c) pediatric condition falsification

(d) factitious disorder

93. An 18-month-old boy with a normal birth history has been newly diagnosed with hemiplegic cerebral palsy (CP). Which prognostic statement is true?

(a) Although most children with hemiplegic CP learn to walk, this milestone is usually achieved after age 2.

(b) Some children with hemiplegic CP develop functional language but they are in the minority.

(c) There is a higher rate of epilepsy in children with CP overall, and this includes the hemiplegic subtype.

(d) Although there is a higher rate of learning disabilities in children with CP overall, this is not true of the hemiplegic subtype.

94. In the case described in Question 93, what is an MRI most likely to show?

(a) hypoxic-ischemic injury

(b) focal internal capsule lesion

(c) periventricular leukomalacia

(d) middle cerebral artery stroke

95. A neuropsychological assessment administered when the child described in Question 93 enters elementary school is most likely to yield which set of findings?

(a) average IQ with dysarthria but otherwise normal language; weaknesses in attention and visuospatial skills

(b) average IQ with dysarthria and impaired receptive and expressive language; normal attention and visuospatial skills

(c) borderline IQ with mildly impaired receptive and expressive language, attention, and visuospatial skills

(d) borderline IQ with mildly impaired expressive language and normal attention and visuospatial skills

96. The ApoE ε4 allele is carried on chromosome ____.

(a) 21

(b) 20

(c) 19

(d) 18

97. According to most estimates, schizophrenia is approximately _____ heritable.

    (a) 50%   (c) 0.5–2%

    (b) 80–85%   (d) 30%

98. In recent cognitive modeling of the association between reading and attention skills, which of the following cognitive predictors accounts for the overlap between the two phenotypic domains?

    (a) inhibition   (c) processing speed

    (b) working memory   (d) vocabulary

99. In comparison to patients in the United States with frontotemporal dementia, patients in Greece and Turkey are diagnosed with FTD _____.

    (a) at an earlier age because the symptoms occur earlier and are more severe

    (b) at an earlier age because the symptoms occur earlier despite presenting with less impairment

    (c) at a later age because the symptoms are not reported until later and the level of impairment is less

    (d) at a later age because the symptoms are not reported until later despite presenting with more impairment

100. Benzodiazepines can affect memory and psychomotor speed by _____.

    (a) potentiating GABA-ergic transmission

    (b) their strong anticholinergic, sedating effect

    (c) potentiating a strong β-adrenergic blockade

    (d) stimulating a glutamatergic cascade resulting in cell death

101. Attention problems in people with congenital hydrocephalus _____.

    (a) reflect problems with cognitive control and self-regulation

    (b) should be identified because of the robust response to stimulant medication

    (c) occur with a higher frequency than in typically developing children

    (d) are best diagnosed with cognitive tests without heavy motor demands

102. Which of the following is more commonly seen early in progressive supranuclear palsy than in Parkinson's disease?

    (a) bilateral rest tremor   (c) autonomic dysfunction

    (b) limb rigidity   (d) postural instability

103. New, minimally invasive surgery techniques for temporal lobe epilepsy include laser thermal ablation. Early studies show better language and memory outcome with this procedure compared with other temporal lobe surgical techniques. Which of the following is most likely associated with improved outcome following selective laser amygdala-hippocampal ablation?

    (a) better seizure control with laser ablation compared with standard surgery

    (b) hippocampus is not an essential component of the system for naming

    (c) presence of hippocampal sclerosis prior to surgery

    (d) good baseline performance on measures of naming and recognition

104. The inability to recall events prior to an accident, illness or event is _____ amnesia.

    (a) global

    (b) psychogenic

    (c) anterograde

    (d) retrograde

105. Boys with fragile X syndrome demonstrate _____.

    (a) fewer cognitive impairments than girls

    (b) greater cognitive impairments than girls

    (c) regression in skills over time

    (d) improvement in skills over time

106. Which of the following has not been associated with vascular cognitive impairment (VCI)?

    (a) vitamin B_{12} deficiency

    (b) hepatic dysfunction

    (c) diabetes mellitus

    (d) ApoE ε4 genotype

107. You have evaluated an 18-year-old college freshman who has never been diagnosed with a learning disability and has never had formal academic support. However, review of her history, academic records, and standardized test scores is consistent with a reading disability. Which of the following would be the most appropriate recommendations for this student?

    (a) work with a reading specialist and 50% additional time on tests

    (b) vision therapy and the opportunity to take exams orally

    (c) 50% additional time on tests and additional breaks during the test

    (d) Irlen lenses to use when reading her textbooks and 100% extended time on tests

108. Among the most commonly reported cognitive difficulties in functional somatic syndromes are _____.

    (a) speech/language skills

    (b) visuospatial/perceptual skills

    (c) attention/concentration skills

    (d) general intellectual functioning

109. During a sustained period of alcohol withdrawal a 27-year-old woman complains that bugs are crawling up and down her arms and into her ears. She is experiencing _____.

    (a) hypnagogic hallucinations

    (b) formication hallucinations

    (c) release hallucinations

    (d) metamorphosia hallucinations

110. A 13-year-old boy is accidentally hit on the head with a baseball bat. He is knocked unconscious and taken to the emergency room. CT scan of the head reveals a concave hyperdensity in the left frontal epidural space, with mild mass effect evidenced. Which of the following likely occurred?

    (a) tearing of the left uncinate fasciculus

    (b) rotational acceleration and deceleration injuries

    (c) impact of the brain over bony skull prominences

    (d) laceration of the middle meningeal artery

111. Preterm birth and low birth weight is defined as less than _____.

    (a) 35 weeks gestation and birth weight below 7 pounds, 6 ounces

    (b) 36 weeks gestation and birth weight below 6 pounds, 6 ounces

    (c) 37 weeks gestation and birth weight below 5 pounds, 8 ounces

    (d) 34 weeks gestation and birth weight below 5 pounds, 1 ounce

112. Which of the following domains are most consistently reported to be impacted in children and adults with a history of encephalitis?

    (a) executive functions

    (b) visuospatial functions

    (c) receptive language

    (d) fluid intelligence

113. Which of the following statements about ApoE is true?

    (a) ApoE ε2 is most strongly linked with Alzheimer's disease pathology

    (b) ApoE ε2 virtually rules out Alzheimer's disease

    (c) The presence of ApoE ε4 is diagnostic for Alzheimer's disease

    (d) ApoE ε4 is a known risk for Alzheimer's disease

114. You are asked to evaluate a child with a history of significant alcohol exposure in utero. During your medical record review, you find a report from a structural brain MRI. Which of the following MRI findings is most likely?

    (a) greater gray matter than white matter hypoplasia

    (b) greater white matter than gray matter hypoplasia

    (c) a reduction in the size of the cerebellar vermis

    (d) a reduction in the size of the frontal lobes

115. Which of the following is considered a symptom of the disorganized syndrome?

    (a) anhedonia

    (b) poverty of speech

    (c) flat affect

    (d) loose associations

116. In children, the most common form of stroke is _____.

    (a) traumatic hemorrhagic

    (b) sinovenous thrombosis

    (c) arterial ischemic

    (d) non-traumatic hemorrhagic

117. In Alzheimer's disease, the progression of atrophy affects the following systems in which order?

    (a) hippocampus and entorhinal cortex in the late stages, preceded by changes in the frontal, temporal, and parietal association areas

    (b) basal ganglia in the middle stages, and temporal, frontal, and parietal association areas as the disease progresses

    (c) hippocampus and entorhinal cortex in the earliest stages, and temporal, frontal, and parietal association areas as the disease progresses

    (d) hippocampus and entorhinal cortex in the earliest stages, followed by basal ganglia involvement

118. Increased risk of intellectual decline in children treated for medulloblastoma is associated with ____.

    (a) total resection

    (b) higher dose radiation and neurologic complications

    (c) treatment in adolescence

    (d) endocrine dysfunction

119. Of the following areas of functioning, which neuropsychological domain tends to be most resilient to anoxic/hypoxic injury?

    (a) contextual verbal memory   (c) intellectual functioning

    (b) visuospatial memory   (d) processing speed

120. In idiopathic normal pressure hydrocephalus, the general neuropsychological profile ____.

    (a) shows a consistent pattern of strengths and weaknesses

    (b) shows a pattern associated with subcortical pathology

    (c) is identical to patterns associated with secondary normal pressure hydrocephalus

    (d) often shows marked improvement with treatment

121. A test that has a very high mean relative to the possible points and a small standard deviation would be best evaluated/interpreted using ____.

    (a) a ratio scale and describing test performance as normal or impaired

    (b) an ordinal scale and describing test performance categorically

    (c) parametric statistics and converting performance to a percentile

    (d) parametric statistics and converting performance to a standard score

122. Which one of the following statements is true regarding the assessment and diagnosis of childhood ADHD?

    (a) Neuropsychological tests have adequate sensitivity and specificity for diagnosing ADHD.

    (b) ADHD is most often diagnosed by a mental health professional.

    (c) ADHD occurs more often with comorbid conditions than without.

    (d) Feigning of ADHD symptoms is a rare phenomenon in clinical practice.

123. Patients with which of the following would be least likely to develop depression?

    (a) anosodiaphoria   (c) multiple sclerosis

    (b) Broca's aphasia   (d) Huntington's disease

124. A brain tumor is suspected in a patient who is pregnant. Given the risk of ionizing radiation exposure with certain types of imaging studies, which of the following would be the least contraindicated for use?

    (a) computed tomography   (c) single photon emission tomography

    (b) magnetic resonance imaging   (d) positron emission tomography

125. A 70-year-old woman is referred for assessment 2 months following a fall down her basement steps. Injury parameters indicate mild injury (GCS = 15, LOC = less than 1 minute, PTA = 1 hour). Neuropsychological assessment reveals moderate visuospatial impairments and evidence of mild left hemispatial inattention. Based on these findings, what type of pathology should be ruled out?

(a) slowly developing subdural hematoma

(b) focal seizure activity in the right hemisphere

(c) lacunar infarction in the right hemisphere

(d) ocular disturbances impacting visual acuity

First Full-Length Practice Examination Answers

1. **C—bilateral disconnection of auditory receptive areas from Wernicke's area** *This lesion prevents the speech signal from undergoing phonologic decoding in Wernicke's area, but leaves intact sound decoding of nonspeech sounds.* ***Please refer to Chapter 4.***

   Reference: Shoumaker, R., Ajax, E., & Schenkenberg, T. (1977). Pure word deafness (auditory verbal agnosia). *Diseases of the Nervous System, 38*, 293–299.

2. **C—injection** *Opioids and stimulants cross the blood-brain barrier most readily when injected.* ***Please refer to Chapter 36.***

   Reference: Novak, S. P., & Kral, A. H. (2011). Comparing injection and non-injection routes of administration for heroin, methamphetamine, and cocaine uses in the United States. *Journal of Addictive Diseases, 30*(3), 248–257.

3. **D—This may be due to normal variability. Unless a disorder is otherwise indicated by history, I make no diagnosis but comment on the variability in my report.** *As stated in the section on interpretation of abnormal test results, a finding of one or more low to very low scores in a relatively large battery is common in normative samples without neurological impairment. Thus, unless the findings fit a profile that is consistent with an impaired domain or expected impairment based on medical history/presumed etiology (i.e., variability across scores in attention-deficit/hyperactivity disorder), the findings should not be overinterpreted but considered in this light and discussed as possible normal variance in the interpretation section of the report.* ***Please refer to Chapter 8.***

   Reference: Binder, L. M., Iverson, G. L., & Brooks, B. L. (2009). To err is human: "Abnormal" neuropsychological scores and variability are common in healthy adults. *Archives of Clinical Neuropsychology, 24*, 31–46.

4. **A—greater cognitive impairment** *Although men tend to get multiple sclerosis less frequently than women, they more frequently show progressive disease courses with more cognitive impairment.* ***Please refer to Chapter 24.***

   Reference: Schoonheim, M. M., Popescu, V., Rueda Lopes, F. C., Wiebenga, O. T., Vrenken, H., Douw, L., . . . Barkhof, F. (2012). Subcortical atrophy and cognition: Sex effects in multiple sclerosis. *Neurology, 79*(17), 1754–1761.

5. **B—dorsal stream** *The impaired task requires remembering a spatial location, not identifying an object. The parietal lobes are part of the dorsal system.* ***Please refer to Chapter 3.***

   Reference: Borst, G., Thompson, W. L., & Kosslyn, S. M. (2011). Understanding the dorsal and ventral systems of the human cerebral cortex. *American Psychologist, 66*, 624–632. Retrieved from http://psycnet.apa.org

6. **D—area of bifurcation of the major branches of the middle cerebral artery** *Areas of bifurcation of major cerebral arteries show higher risk for stroke, but are less vulnerable than the other regions listed to the effects of anoxia/hypoxia.* **Please refer to Chapter 28.**

Reference: Victor, M., Ropper, A. H., & Samuels, M. A. (2009). *Adams and Victor's principles of neurology* (9th ed.). New York, NY: McGraw Hill.

7. **A—It is a group of brain-based disorders characterized by motor impairments.** *Cerebral palsy is not considered a disease. It is caused by primary damage to the brain and most often results from prenatal causes.* **Please refer to Chapter 19.**

Reference: Singer, H. S., Mink, J. W., Gilbert, D. L., & Jankovic, J. (2016). Cerebral palsy. In H. S. Singer, J. W. Mink, D. L. Gilbert, & J. Jankovic (Eds.), *Movement disorders in childhood* (2nd ed., pp. 453–475). San Diego, CA: Academic Press.

8. **C—Administer a reading achievement task to ensure no less than a fifth-grade reading level.** *It would be beneficial to administer a measure of reading achievement test in this case as test items of the MMPI-2-RF require between a fifth- and an eighth-grade reading level. The clinician is also able to interpret VRIN-r and TRIN-r to establish whether the patient's reading difficulties in any way resulted in non-content-responsivity that might invalidate the profile.* **Please refer to Chapter 10.**

Reference: Ben-Porath, Y. S., & Tellegen, A. (2008). *Minnesota multiphasic personality inventory -2 restructured form (MMPI-2-RF) manual for administration, scoring, and interpretation.* Minneapolis, MN: Pearson.

9. **C—Social cognition is affected in persons with both temporal lobe epilepsy and other epilepsy syndromes.** *Social cognition is disrupted by underlying neural networks supporting cognition, as well as cognitive and psychosocial factors. Problems with social cognition develop in childhood, and persist into adulthood due to a combination of factors beyond pathology including limited opportunity to engage with peers, learn, and practice social skills.* **Please refer to Chapter 22.**

Reference: Jokeit H, Eicher M, & Ives-Deliperi V. (2018). Toward social neuropsychology of epilepsy: A review on social cognition in epilepsy. *Acta Epilepsy, 1,* 8–17.10.12107/ae.2018.1.3

10. **D—hematopoietic stem cell transplant** *HSCT is the only current treatment that extends life expectancy. Lorenzo's oil normalizes plasma VLCFA but does not extend life. Pallidotomy and epilepsy surgery are not used as treatments for adrenoleukodystrophy.* **Please refer to Chapter 18.**

Reference: Pierpont, E. I., Eisengart, J. B., Shanley, R., Nascene, D., Raymond, G. V., Shapiro, E. G., . . .Miller, W. P. (2017). Neurocognitive trajectory of boys who received a hematopoietic stem cell transplant at an early stage of childhood cerebral adrenoleukodystrophy. *JAMA Neurology, 74*(6), 710–717.

11. **A—Korsakoff's dementia** *Given the confabulation in light of her recent drinking and vitamin deficiency, you would want to consider Korsakoff's syndrome.* **Please refer to Chapter 5.**

Reference: Kessels, R. P., Kortrijk, H. E., Wester, A. J., & Nys, G. M. (2008). Confabulation behavior and false memories in Korsakoff's syndrome: Role of source memory and executive functioning. *Psychiatry and Clinical Neuroscience, 62*(2), 220–225.

12. **C—Right hemisphere** *The likely location of the stroke is in the right hemisphere, as the infarct has damaged cerebral structures that, by nature, are associated with negative valence on stimuli. The inhibitory effect of the damaged cerebral tissues results in positive affect, i.e., "euphoria," as the natural tendency toward negative valence (dysphoria) is suppressed.* **Please refer to Chapter 3.**

Reference: Hackett, M. L., Kohler, S., O'Brien, J. T., & Mead, G. E. (2014). Neuropsychiatric outcome of stroke. *The Lancet Neurology, 13,* 525–534.

13. **C—inhibition and flexibility** *Children with high-functioning autism sometimes have typical organization ability, planning, and rote memory. However, Corbetta et al. (2009) demonstrated that they have difficulty with inhibition and flexibility, as is observed in individuals who perseverate in their interests and have diminished behavioral control.* **Please refer to Chapter 14.**

> **Reference:** Corbett, B. A., Constantine, L. J., Hendron, R., Rocke, D., & Ozonoff, S. (2009). Examining executive functioning in children with autism spectrum disorder, attention-deficit/hyperactivity disorder and typical development. *Psychiatry Research, 166* (30), 210–222.

14. **D—greater initial injury severity** *Depression is the most common psychological problem following TBI and occurs in 20–40% of individuals during the first year and up to 50% of individuals at some stage. Depression can occur at all levels of severity and the prevalence rate does not increase along with injury severity. Risk factors for post TBI depression include minority status, unemployment, low income, low education, and alcohol abuse. Post TBI depression has been linked to the development of increased cognitive impairments, reduced psychomotor speed, and less favorable functional outcomes.* **Please refer to Chapter 29.**

> **Reference:** Hudak, A. M., Hynan, L. S. Harper, C. R., & Diaz-Arrastia, R. (2012). Association of depressive symptoms with functional outcome after traumatic brain injury, *Journal of Head Trauma Rehabilitation, 27*(2), 87–98.

15. **A—paraneoplastic syndrome** *This constellation of symptoms suggests possible autoimmune reaction to cancer; cognitive dysfunction from chemotherapy treatment is typically associated with mild problems with working memory and attention and not with onset of seizures or amnesia.* **Please refer to Chapter 25.**

> **Reference:** Pelosof, L. C., & Gerber, D. E. (2010). Paraneoplastic syndromes: An approach to diagnosis and treatment. *Mayo Clinic Proceedings, 85*(9), 838–854.

16. **D—bacterial meningitis** *Nuchal (neck) rigidity is commonly cited as a common presenting symptom in bacterial meningitis.* **Please refer to Chapter 23.**

> **References:**
> (a) Bhimraj, A. (2018). Acute community-acquired bacterial meningitis. In J. C. Garcia-Monco (Ed.), *CNS infections: A clinical approach* (pp. 19–30). Switzerland: Springer International Publishing.
> (b) Kaufman, D. M., Geyer, H. I., & Milstein, M. J. (2017). *Kaufman's clinical neurology for psychiatrists* (8th ed.). Philadelphia, PA: Elsevier.

17. **D—impaired proprioception** *When vitamin B_{12} levels fall below healthy levels physical symptoms, psychological changes and cognitive impairments often develop. Symptoms may include anemia, weakness, fatigue, mood changes, memory loss, and disorientation. Patients may have impaired tactile recognition of pressure and vibration, difficulty walking, and peripheral tingling or numbness (parasthesias) due to damage to the dorsal sections and lateral pyramidal tracts in the spinal cord. Sustained deficiency typically leads to irreversible damage and may be marked by depression, irritability, impaired attention, hallucinations, and symptoms suggestive of dementia, but tremor, delusions, and apraxia are not associated with B_{12} deficiency.* **Please refer to Chapter 27.**

> **References:**
> (a) Aminoff, M. J. (2008). Vitamin B12 deficiency. *Neurology and general medicine.* Philadelphia, PA: Elsevier.
> (b) Norman, M. A., Bjorkquist Harner, O., & Kenton, S. J. (2018). Complexities of metabolic disorders. In J. E. Morgan, & J. H. Ricker (Eds.), *Textbook of clinical neuropsychology* (2nd ed.). New York, NY: Taylor and Francis.

18. **B—occur in a sizable minority of patients** *Hallucinations and delusions do not occur in the majority of patient with vascular dementia but they are not rare. Their presence does not signify anything about etiology.* ***Please refer to Chapter 31.***

    Reference: Kumar, A., Lavretsky, H., & Haroon, E. (2005). Neuropsychiatric correlates of vascular injury. In R. H. Paul, R. Cohen, B. R. Ott, & S. Salloway (Eds.), *Vascular dementia: Cerebrovascular mechanisms and clinical management* (pp. 157–168). Totowa, NJ: Humana Press.

19. **D—fragile X syndrome** *Sex-linked genetic factors and male vulnerability to insult might account for some of the gender differences in ID.* ***Please refer to Chapter 13.***

    Reference: American Psychiatric Association. (2013). *Diagnostic and statistical manual of mental disorders* (5th ed.). Arlington, VA: American Psychiatric Publishing.

20. **C—test in both languages to obtain objective samples of language dominance and guide recommendations accordingly** *For a complete evaluation of the test taker's cognitive and linguistic status evaluation should be in all of their languages.* ***Please refer to Chapter 11.***

    Reference: Judd, T., Capetillo, D, Carrión-Baralt, J., Mármol, L. M., San Miguel-Montes, L., Navarrete, M., . . . Silver, C. H. (2009). Professional considerations for improving the neuropsychological evaluation of Hispanics. Hispanic Neuropsychological Society/National Academy of Neuropsychology. *Archives of Clinical Neuropsychology, 24*, 127–135.

21. **C—medication management and adherence** *Stabilization of symptoms with medication management and increased adherence would be indicated prior to assessment of functional capacity and to maximize benefit from any individualized vocational placement or social skills program.* ***Please refer to Chapter 35.***

    Reference: Marcopulos, B. A., & Kurtz, M. M. (2012). *Clinical and neuropsychological foundations of schizophrenia.* New York, NY: Psychology Press.

22. **D—transcortical motor aphasia** *In contrast to Broca's aphasia transcortical motor aphasia is characterized by relatively intact repetition.* ***Please refer to Chapter 26.***

    Reference: Cullum, C. M., Rossetti, H. C., Batjer, H. Festa, J., Haaland, K. Y., and Lacritz, L. (2017). Cerebrovascular disease. In J. Morgan & J. Ricker (Eds.), *Textbook of clinical neuropsychology* (2nd ed., pp. 350–386). New York, NY: Taylor & Francis.

23. **B—visuospatial functioning** *Anoxic brain injury in children tend to result in significantly impaired intellectual abilities, memory impairment, decreased attention span, and behavioral impairments whereas academic achievement, internalizing behavioral problems, and visuospatial deficits were generally less severe.* ***Please refer to Chapter 28.***

    Reference: Thaler, N. S., Reger S. L., Ringdahl, E. N., Mayfield, J. W., Goldstein, G., & Allen, D. N. (2013). Neuropsychological profiles of six children with anoxic brain injury. *Child Neuropsychology, 19*, 479–494.

24. **D—impairment in social and occupational functioning** *The DSM-5 specifies that the symptoms and severity of the disorder must represent a change from previous functioning and cause clinically significant distress or impairment in social, occupational, or other important areas of functioning. As such, severity level is determined by the level of impairment on daily life functions.* ***Please refer to Chapter 34.***

    Reference: American Psychiatric Association. (2013). *Diagnostic and statistical manual of mental disorders* (5th ed.). Washington, DC: American Psychiatric Publishing.

25. **B—pseudobulbar affect** *Uncontrollable crying or laughing is most likely to be seen in progressive supranuclear palsy, and in fact, there are a number of affective and behavioral symptoms that can be seen in PSP.* ***Please refer to Chapter 33.***

    Reference: Gerstenecker, A., Duff, K., Mast, B., & Litvan, I. (2013). Behavioral abnormalities in progressive supranuclear palsy. *Psychiatric Research, 210*, 1–13. doi:10.1016/j.psychres.2013.08.045

26. **D—Thank her for her interest but provide no more information.** *You must receive direct permission from the patient to release confidential health information. You must respect this right even if the person asking is a trusted colleague or superior. You have no idea regarding how the information might be used or if your patient would want the information released to that particular individual. Third parties also do not have an automatic right to the patient's protected health information (PHI) even if they were previously involved in the patient's care. The HIPAA Privacy Rule allows providers to legally share PHI for treatment purposes without the patient's consent. However, in this case, the information is not for treatment purposes, as it relates to a former patient. Moreover, even if the information was legally allowed according to HIPAA, psychologists have a more restrictive ethical burden to protect confidentiality before communicating with non-authorized individuals. Answer B is inappropriate as psychologists are not advised or required to be deceptive when protecting patient confidentiality. Finally, the patient, not the person requesting the information, must sign the consent form for release of information, which is why Answer C is incorrect.* **Please refer to Chapter 7.**

General Principles and Ethical Standards: A, B, E; 4.01, 4.02, 4.06

Reference: Bush, S. S., & Martin, T. A. (2008). Confidentiality in neuropsychological practice. In A. M. Horton Jr., & D. Wedding (Eds.), *The neuropsychology handbook* (3rd ed., pp. 517–532). New York, NY: Springer.

27. **A—CA1 section and subiculum of the hippocampus** *Pick bodies and Pick cells are commonly found in the amygdala, dentate gyrus, pyramidal cells of the CA1 section and subiculum of the hippocampus, hypothalamic lateral tuberal nucleus, dorsomedial region of the putamen, globus pallidus, locus ceruleus, mossy fibers and monodendritic brush cells in the granule cell layer of the cerebellum, and frontal and temporal neocortex.* **Please refer to Chapter 32.**

Reference: Kovacs, G., Rozemuller, A., van Swieten, J., Gelpi, E., Majtenyi, K., . . . Budka, H. (2013). Neuropathology of the hippocampus in FTLD-Tau with Pick bodies: A study of the BrainNet Europe Consortium. *Neuropathology and Applied Neurobiology, 39,* 166–178.

28. **C—The set of scores will have a mean of zero, standard deviation of one, and unchanged distribution.** *When an entire distribution of scores is transformed into z-scores, the resulting distribution will have a mean of zero, a standard deviation of one, and the same shape as the original distribution. It is possible to take distributions of data points that depart from "true" normality in some way and transform them so as to be "fit" to a normal curve. This may be necessary to solve any one of many problems of distributional shape, and numerous types of transformations may be appropriate depending on the shape of the data (e.g., reciprocals or log transformations for extreme positive skew). Every decision to utilize a transformation must be related to an essential measurement concern that can be identified and expressed, and consideration should be made that at times, transformations are inappropriate or misleading. It is essential that the clinician understand the underlying distribution and its impact on the meaning of the selected representation of the performance.* **Please refer to Chapter 8.**

Reference: Gravetter, F., & Wallnau, L. B. (2017). *Statistics for the behavioral sciences* (10th ed.). Boston, MA: Cengage Learning.

29. **B—decreased** *Females are less likely to develop schizophrenia.* **Please refer to Chapter 35.**

Reference: Abel, K. M., Drake, R., & Goldstein, J. M. (2010). Sex differences in schizophrenia. *International Review of Psychiatry, 22*(5), 417–428.

30. **A—improves with time, but contains abnormalities (e.g., echolalia, unusual prosody)** *Language generally improves between the third and fifth year, but is often marked with*

abnormalities such as echolalia, unusual prosody, and other language abnormalities associated with ASDs. **Please refer to Chapter 14.**

Reference: Bal, V. H., Kim, S. H., Fok, M., & Lord, C. (2019). Autism spectrum disorder symptoms from ages 2 to 19 years: Implications for diagnosing adolescents and young adults. *Autism Research, 12,* 89–99.

31. **C—spasticity** *The other choices are associated with extrapyramidal CP.* **Please refer to Chapter 19.**

Reference: Oskoui, M., Shevell, M. I., & Swaiman, K. F. (2017). Cerebral palsy. In K. F. Swaiman, S. Ashwal, D. M., Ferriero, N. F. Schor, R. S. Finkel, A. L. Gropman, . . . M. Shevell (Eds.), *Swaiman's pediatric neurology: Principles and practice* (6th ed., pp. 734–740). Philadelphia, PA: Elsevier.

32. **A—single-word reading, and spelling** *Dyslexia is a specific reading disorder characterized by deficits in phonological awareness, fluent decoding and word reading, and spelling. It has nothing to do with visual processing or letter writing. Reading comprehension is affected, but the noted core deficits are key to assessment.* **Please refer to Chapter 15.**

Reference: Fletcher, J. M., Lyon, G. R., Fuchs, L. S., & Barnes, M. A. (2018). *Learning disabilities: From identification to intervention* (2nd ed.). New York, NY: Guilford Press.

33. **D—ask the examinee to explain the instructions in his/her own words** *Repeating instructions would not necessarily result in understanding, while asking the examinee if s/he understands may result in a polite nod. Following standard protocol would not address understanding and may invalidate the test results or place the examinee at a disadvantage. Asking the examinee to explain his/her understanding will allow the NP to assess the examinee's appreciation of the instructions.* **Please refer to Chapter 11.**

Reference: Ngo, D., Le, M., & Le, P. D. (2011). Neuropsychology of Vietnamese Americans. In D. Fujii (Ed.), *The neuropsychology of Asian Americans* (pp. 181–200). New York, NY: Psychology Press.

34. **A—deficits develop after shorter drinking histories** *Although most research on AUD has been conducted with men, research with women has shown comparable neuropsychological deficits. However, these deficits tend to manifest after shorter drinking histories as compared to men.* **Please refer to Chapter 36.**

Reference: Erol, A., & Karpyak, V. M. (2015). Sex and gender-related differences in alcohol use and its consequences: Contemporary knowledge and future research considerations. *Drug and Alcohol Dependence, 156,* 1–13.

35. **C—consult specific personality inventory manuals to guide decision-making** *Adolescents who are 18 years old may be given the MMPI-2-RF or the MMPI-A-RF because normative and clinical samples for both the MMPI-2-RF and the MMPI-A-RF instruments include 18-year-olds. The clinician should make a case-by-case judgment about which assessment to use with 18-year-olds. A suggested guideline would be to use the MMPI-A-RF instrument with 18-year-olds who are still in high school and the MMPI-2-RF instrument with 18-year-olds who are in college, working, or living an otherwise independent adult lifestyle.* **Please refer to Chapter 10.**

Reference: Archer, R. P., Handel, R. W., Ben-Porath, Y. S., & Tellegen, A. (2016). *Minnesota Multiphasic Personality Inventory-Adolescent-Restructured Form (MMPI-A-RF): Manual for Administration, Scoring, Interpretation, and Technical Manual.* Minneapolis, MN: University of Minnesota Press.

36. **D—temporal; contralateral** *Quadrantanopsia requires a fairly specific lesion and mostly occurs with direct involvement of Meyer's loop in the contralateral temporal lobe.* **Please refer to Chapter 6.**

References:
(a) Blumenfeld, H. (2011). *Neuroanatomy through clinical cases* (2nd ed.). Sunderland, MA: Sinauer Associates.
(b) Goldberg, S. (2017). *The four-minute neurological exam* (2nd ed.). Miami, FL: MedMaster.
(c) Greenberg, D., Aminoff, M., & Simon, R. (2012). *Clinical neurology* (8th ed.). New York, NY: Lange Medical Books/McGraw-Hill.

37. **D—illness anxiety disorder** *Illness anxiety disorder was previously known as hypochondriasis. It does not involve the actual experience of symptoms, despite great concerns about contracting illnesses.* **Please refer to Chapter 37.**

Reference: Pandey, S., Parikh, M., Brahmbhatt, M., & Vankar, G. K. (2017). Clinical study of illness anxiety disorder in medical outpatients. *Archives of Psychiatry and Psychotherapy, 19*(4), 32–41.

38. **C—effective, but carries increased risk of seizure exacerbation in some children.** *While the effect size for treatment efficacy in children with epilepsy may be slightly smaller than compared with children with ADHD alone, there is evidence that treatment with stimulants is effective for managing ADHD symptoms in children with epilepsy. Regarding safety and risk of increased seizures, there is very little data to address the question. However, there are a few studies that have shown that a small number of patients do have increased seizures with stimulant treatment. Patients with higher seizure frequency at the time of treatment initiation may have increased risk of seizure exacerbation.* **Please refer to Chapter 22.**

Reference: Williams, A. E., Giust, J. M., Kronenberger, W. G., & Dunn, D. W. (2016). Epilepsy and attention-deficit hyperactivity disorder: Links, risks, and challenges. *Neuropsychiatric Disease and Treatment, 12,* 287–296.

39. **A—Turner syndrome** *Short stature and webbed neck are physical characteristics associated with Turner syndrome but not the other disorders listed. Individuals with Williams syndrome also tend to have greater visuospatial deficits but tend to have lower overall cognitive ability. Individuals with tuberous sclerosis and Angelman syndrome have broader cognitive deficits, with significant cognitive deficits seen in Angelman syndrome.* **Please refer to Chapter 18.**

Reference: Gravholt, C. H., Andersen, N. H., Conway, G. S., Dekkers, O. M., Geffnre, M. E., . . . Backeljauw, P. F. (2017). Clinical practice guidelines for the care of girls and women with Turner syndrome: Proceedings from the 2016 Cincinnati International Turner Syndrome Meeting. *European Journal of Endocrinology, 177,* G1–G70.

40. **B—depression, visual-motor integration, fatigue** *Given the graphomotor component of the Wechsler processing speed tasks, as well as documented deficits seen in visual-motor integration for individuals with multiple sclerosis, examining this area would be an important step in the assessment. Likewise, depression and fatigue are considered to be commonly associated with multiple sclerosis and may be associated with reduced speed of performance.* **Please refer to Chapter 24.**

References:
(a) MacAllister, W. S., Christodoulou, C., Milazzo, M., Preston, T. E., Serafin, D., Krupp, L. B., & Harder, L. (2013). Pediatric multiple sclerosis: What we know and where are we headed? *Child Neuropsychology, 19*(1), 1–22.
(b) Holland, A. A., Graves, D., Greenberg, B. M., & Harder, L. L. (2012). Fatigue, emotional functioning, and executive dysfunction in pediatric multiple sclerosis. *Child Neuropsychology, 20*(1), 71–85.

41. **C—calculate the reliable change index, with a 90% confidence interval** *The reliable change index will indicate whether the difference between the two scores is larger than can reasonably be expected on the basis of practice effects or measurement error alone.* **Please refer to Chapter 9.**

Reference: Busch, R. M., Lineweaver, T. T., Ferguson, L., & Haut, J. S. (2015). Reliable change indices and standardized regression-based change score norms for evaluating neuropsychological change in children with epilepsy. *Epilepsy & Behavior, 47*, 45–54.

42. **A—maternal occupation** *In utero exposure to lead at the current time is most likely to occur when the mother is exposed to lead at her occupation, such as in factories that use lead in manufacturing products.* **Please refer to Chapter 21.**

Reference: Dietrich, K. N. (2010). Environmental toxicants. In K. O. Yeates, M. D. Ris, H. G. Taylor, & B. F. Pennington (Eds.), *Pediatric neuropsychology: Research, theory, and practice* (pp. 211–264). New York, NY: Guilford Press.

43. **C—the locus coeruleus and lateral tegmental area** *The locus coeruleus and LTA are the primary sources of adrenergic input to the brain. The other alternatives in this item refer to structures that are associated with neurotransmitters other than norepinephrine.* **Please refer to Chapter 4.**

Reference: Viljoen, M., & Swanepoel, A. P. (2007). The central noradrenergic system: An overview. *African Journal of Psychiatry, 10*, 135–141.

44. **C—memory and new learning** *Limbic encephalitis commonly involves bilateral temporal pathology causing persistent deficits in memory and new learning.* **Please refer to Chapter 23.**

Reference: Foster, A. R., & Caplan, J. P. (2009). Pareneoplastic limbic encephalitis. *Psychosomatics, 50*, 108–113.

45. **A—temporoparietal** *AD pathology usually begins in temporal lobe structures and spreads to parietal regions before affecting the frontal lobes. This spread of pathology parallels the pattern of neuropsychological dysfunction.* **Please refer to Chapter 30.**

References:
(a) Frisoni, G. B., Fox, N. C., Jack, C. R., Jr., Scheltens, P., & Thompson, P. M. (2010). The clinical use of structural MRI in Alzheimer's disease. *Nature Reviews Neurology, 6*(2), 67.
(b) Pini, L., Pievani, M., Bocchetta, M., Altomare, D., Bosco, P., Cavedo, E., . . . Frisoni, G. B. (2016). Brain atrophy in Alzheimer's disease and aging. *Ageing Research Reviews, 30*, 25–48.

46. **B—There was a large effect seen for medication treatment, for which the addition of behavioral therapy produced no significant added benefit.** *There was no significant benefit from the behavioral therapy added to the stimulant medication with regard to ADHD symptom reduction. However, with regard to nonsymptom areas (e.g., social skills), there was added benefit noted with the behavioral therapy intervention.* **Please refer to Chapter 16.**

References:
(a) MTA Cooperative Group (1999). A 14 month randomized clinical trial of treatment strategies for attention-deficit/hyperactivity disorder: The MTA Cooperative Group multimodal treatment stud of children with ADHD. *Archives of General Psychiatry, 56*, 1073–1086.
(b) MTA Cooperative Group (2004). National Institute of Mental Health multimodal treatment study of ADHD follow-up: 24-month outcomes of treatment strategies for attention-deficit/hyperactivity disorder. *Pediatrics, 113*, 754–761.

47. **B—left hemispatial inattention and constructional apraxia** *Are most often associated with right parietal (especially inferior parietal) damage. In contrast, parts of the Gerstmann syndrome are seen after left inferior parietal damage; right–left confusion (part of Gerstmann*

syndrome) can also be seen after left inferior parietal damage, and nonverbal memory deficits are associated with damage to the right medial temporal lobe or the diencephalic system (e.g., Korsakoff's). **Please refer to Chapter 26.**

References:
(a) Blumenfeld, H. (2010). *Neuroanatomy through clinical cases* (2nd ed.). Sunderland, MA: Sinauer Associates.
(b) Mohr, J. P., Wolf, P. A., Grotta, J. C., Moskowitz, M. A., Mayberg, M. R., & von Kummer, R. (2011). *Stroke: Pathophysiology, diagnosis and management* (5th ed.). Philadelphia, PA: Saunders.

48. **C—3** *GCS is a system for determining the degree of impairment in patients through the assessment of eye opening, verbal response, and motor response. In this example, the patient would receive a score of 1 in each domain resulting in a GCS of 3 (the lowest score possible).* **Please refer to Chapter 29.**

Reference: Frank, R. G., Rosenthal, M., & Caplan, B. (Eds.). (2009). *Handbook of rehabilitation psychology* (2nd ed.). Washington, DC: American Psychological Association.

49. **B—Angelman syndrome** *Individuals with Angelman syndrome exhibit significant cognitive deficits and are typically nonverbal, but demonstrate social interest in others.* **Please refer to Chapter 18.**

Reference: Buiting, K. (2010). Prader-Willi syndrome and Angelman syndrome. *American Journal of Medical Genetics Part C (Seminars in Medical Genetics), 154C,* 365–375.

50. **C—secondary tumors, late-onset seizures, and stroke** *Adult survivors of childhood medulloblastoma are at increased risk for strokes and seizures; at 30 years post diagnosis, cumulative incidence of seizures is 34% and of strokes, 15%. Cumulative incidence of seizures in survivors of all types of brain tumors is 40%, 30 years post diagnosis. Subsequent malignant neoplasms and meningiomas had a cumulative incidence of 6%.* **Please refer to Chapter 25.**

References:
(a) King, A. A., Seidel, K., Di, C., Leisenring, W. M., Perkins, S. M., Krull, K. R., . . . Packer, R. J. (2017). Long-term neurologic health and psychosocial function of adult survivors of childhood medulloblastoma/PNET: A report from the Childhood Cancer Survivor Study. *Neuro Oncology, 19*(5), 689–698.
(b) Wells, E. M., Ullrich, N. J., Seidel, K., Leisenring, W., Sklar, C. A., Armstrong, G. T., . . . Packer, R. J. (2018). Longitudinal assessment of late-onset neurologic conditions in survivors of childhood central nervous system tumors: A Childhood Cancer Survivor Study report. *Neuro Oncology, 20*(1), 132–142.

51. **C—inhibition of response** *Other types of attention are subsumed by anterior cingulate, dorsolateral frontal, and prefrontal areas, respectively.* **Please refer to Chapter 5.**

Reference: Blumenfeld, H. (Ed.). (2010). *Neuroanatomy through clinical cases* (2nd ed.). Sunderland, MA: Sinauer Associates.

52. **A—Depression can occur years prior to motor symptoms in Huntington's disease.** *Depression, as well as other psychiatric symptoms (e.g., anxiety, psychosis, obsessive-compulsiveness) can precede motor symptoms and formal diagnosis of Huntington's disease. With respect to the other disorders listed, well-formed,* **early not late** *visual hallucinations are a core diagnostic feature of Lewy body dementia. Emotional lability can be seen in progressive supranuclear palsy, but mania* **per se** *is not typical. Visual hallucinations are a common side effect of Parkinson's disease medications.* **Please refer to Chapter 33.**

References:
(a) Bertram, K., & Williams, D. R. (2012). Visual hallucinations in the differential diagnosis of parkinsonism. *Journal of Neurology, Neurosurgery & Psychiatry. 83*(4), 448–452.
(b) Epping, E. A., & Paulsen, J. S. (2011). Depression in the early stages of Huntington disease. *Neurodegenerative Disease Management, 1*(5), 407–414.

53. **A—seizure frequency** *While age at seizure onset is typically considered the most important factor in determining severity of cognitive function, among the options listed seizure frequency/ severity is the most important. The nature and extent of abnormal MRI findings may be a factor in seizure severity, however the presence of MRI abnormality alone provides little information about the severity of cognitive impairment in many cases (e.g., tumor-related epilepsy). History of febrile seizure is common, even among persons who never develop epilepsy and is not usually associated with cognitive impairment alone. Medications may be a proxy for seizure severity, but many persons with epilepsy tolerate medications well, without cognitive side effects.* **Please Refer to Chapter 22.**

Reference: Deasai, J. D. (2008). Epilepsy and cognition. *Journal of Pediatric Neurosciences, 3*, 16–29.

54. **B—visuospatial processing, processing speed, working memory** *The proximity of the vulnerable periventricular region to the optic radiations, as well as dorsal stream dysfunction involved in the integration of visual information, are hypothesized to be the source of visuospatial processing problems. The frequency of white matter pathology in preterm infants is thought to explain the common deficits in processing speed and the increased rates of abnormalities in frontal and subcortical functional systems can result in working memory deficits. Problems with attention, word list generation, and fine motor dexterity can also be seen. Weak word reading and vocabulary skills are typically not associated with preterm birth.* **Please refer to Chapter 17.**

Reference: Taylor, H. G. (2008). Low birth weight. In J. E. Morgan & J. H. Ricker (Eds.), *Textbook of clinical neuropsychology.* New York, NY: Taylor and Francis Group.

55. **C—endorse somatic complaints and other "neurotic" symptoms as opposed to paranoia and "psychotic" symptoms** *Various neuropsychology researchers have demonstrated that scales such as FBS, Hs, Hy, and RC1 are more likely to be elevated than other validity and clinical scales sensitive to psychotic thinking.* **Please refer to Chapter 10.**

References:
(a) Greiffenstein, M. F., Baker, W. J., Axelrod, B., Peck, E. A., & Gervais, R. (2004). The fake bad scale and MMPI-2 F-family in detection of implausible psychological trauma claims. *Clinical Neuropsychologist, 18*(4), 573–590.
(b) Thomas, M. L., & Youngjohn, J. R. (2009). Let's not get hysterical: Comparing the MMPI-2 validity, clinical, and RC scales in TBI litigants tested for effort. *Clinical Neuropsychologist, 23*, 1067–1084.

56. **C—A series of neurotoxic processes are initiated that lead to neuronal death.** *Neurons store virtually no energy, and thus loss of oxygen and glucose results in rapid ATP depletion. If not rapidly reversed, neuronal death ensues. A series of secondary toxic processes is also triggered. The sodium and calcium pumps fail, resulting in depolarization of the neuronal membrane and release of excessive levels of glutamate. Glutamate is the most common excitatory neurotransmitter, but, at excessive levels, it becomes excitotoxic to neurons. A further series of toxic effects are triggered that involve lactic acidosis from anaerobic metabolism, cytotoxic edema, free radical production, and others.* **Please refer to Chapter 28.**

References:
(a) Hopkins, R. O., & Haaland, K. Y. (2004). Neuropsychological and neuropathological effects of anoxic or ischemic induced brain injury. *Journal of the International Neuropsychological Society, 10*, 957–961.
(b) Victor, M., Ropper, A. H., & Samuels, M. A. (2009). *Adams and Victor's principles of neurology* (9th ed.). New York, NY: McGraw Hill.

57. **B—repeated reading** *Repeated reading is the most effective intervention for improving reading fluency for students with learning disabilities. Structured questioning and phonics instruction*

are interventions typically used for reading comprehension and reading decoding, respectively. Visual training is not supported by the literature. **Please refer to Chapter 15.**

Reference: Stevens, E. A., Walker, M. A., & Vaughn, S. (2017). The effects of reading fluency interventions on the reading fluency and reading comprehension performance of elementary students with learning disabilities: A synthesis of the research from 2001 to 2014. *Journal of Learning Disabilities, 50*(5), 576–590.

58. **D—amygdala** *The central nucleus of the amygdala senses and identifies fear and anxiety-laden stimuli and initiates the emotional response. It has been shown to be strongly involved in the formation of emotional memories, especially fear-related memories. The amygdalocentric model of PTSD proposes that it is associated with hyperarousal of the amygdala and insufficient top-down control by the medial prefrontal cortex and the hippocampus, particularly during extinction, but this reflects a primary association with anxiety rather than depression.* **Please refer to Chapter 34.**

References:
(a) Kandel, E. R. (2013). Disorders of mood and anxiety. In E. R. Kandel, J. H. Schwartz, T. M. Jessell, A. A. Siegelbaum, & A. J. Hudspeth (Eds.), *Principles of neural science* (5th ed., pp. 1402–1424). New York, NY: McGraw-Hill.
(b) Stein, M. B., & Steckler, T. (2010). *Behavioral neurobiology of anxiety and its treatment.* New York, NY: Springer.

59. **C—percentile** *As discussed in the chapter section on normalization and transformation, use of standardized scores that assume a normal distribution are not appropriate when there is not a normal distribution in the normative data, as occurs when most people in the normative sample do relatively well on the test. Thus, interpretation of either a z or T score would be inappropriate. Although a cut score could be used, dichotomizing the sample results in loss of some of the critical measurement meaning of the score, especially when scores fall very close to the cut-off. Thus, use of a percentile distribution is most appropriate because this at least tells the clinician the proportion of the sample that did as well as or worse than the patient of interest.* **Please refer to Chapter 8.**

Reference: Price, L. D. (2017). *Psychometric methods: Theory into practice* (Methodology in the Social Sciences). New York, NY: Guildford Press.

60. **D—Vascular dementia has a relatively invariant pathophysiological presentation.** *See Gorelick et al. (2011) and Iadecola (2013) for comprehensive reviews of the pathophysiology of vascular cognitive impairment and vascular dementia, respectively. See Chui and Ramirez-Gomez (2015) for a discussion of mixed dementia (vascular and AD pathology). See Lopez and Wolk (2009) for similarity of symptom presentation in normal pressure hydrocephalus and subcortical forms of VaD.* **Please refer to Chapter 31.**

References:
(a) Chui, H. C., & Ramirez-Gomez, L. (2015). Clinical and imaging features of mixed Alzheimer and vascular pathologies. *Alzheimer's Research & Therapy, 7*(1), 21.
(b) Gorelick, P. B., Cuteri, A., Decarli, C., Greenberg, S. M., Iadecola, C, Launer, L. J., . . . Seshadri, S. (2011). . Vascular contributions to cognitive impairment and dementia: A statement for healthcare professionals from the American Heart Association/American Stroke Association. *Stroke, 42,* 2672–2713.
(c) Iadecola, C. (2013). The pathobiology of vascular dementia. *Neuron, 80,* 844–866.
(d) Lopez, O. L., & Wolk, D. A. (2009). Clinical evaluation: A systematic but user-friendly approach. In L.-O. Wahlund, T. Erkinjuntti, & S. Gauthier (Eds.), *Vascular cognitive impairment in clinical practice* (pp. 32–45). Cambridge, UK: Cambridge University Press.

61. **C—brain tumor** *Cerebellar mutism or posterior fossa syndrome is a complication of surgery to the cerebellum, more commonly seen in children than adults.* **Please refer to Chapter 25.**

References:
(a) Lanier, J. C., & Abrams, A. N. (2017). Posterior fossa syndrome: Review of the behavioral and emotional aspects in pediatric cancer patients. *Cancer, 123*(4), 551–559.

(b) Wells, E. M., Khademian, Z. P., Walsh, K. S., Vezina, G., Sposto, R., Keating, R. F., & Packer, R. J. (2010). Postoperative cerebellar mutism syndrome following treatment of medulloblastoma: Neuroradiographic features and origin. *Journal of Neurosurgery-Pediatrics, 5*(4), 329–334.

62. **A—combined current performance and demographic method of estimating premorbid functioning** *Estimation of cognitive functioning can be done either by using demographic variables, current test performances that are known to be resistant to changes, or by combined demographic and current performance methods. Estimating premorbid cognitive performance based on combining current performance of a crystalized cognitive function (word reading) and demographic variables such as socioeconomic status, education, or occupational functioning is an example of use of the combined current performance and demographic method.* ***Please refer to Chapter 9.***

Reference: Lezak, M. D., Howieson, D. B., Bigler, E. D., & Tranel, D. (2012). *Neuropsychological assessment* (5th ed.). New York, NY: Oxford University Press.

63. **A—show similar patterns of performance except in the motor domain** *The difference in outcomes between children with hydrocephalus secondary to spina bifida myelomeningocele and those with aqueductal stenosis is largely a matter of degree; the neuropsychological patterns are similar but children with aqueductal stenosis tend to show higher levels of performance. The largest differences are on tests of fine motor skills, where children with spina bifida have more significant difficulties because of the Chiari malformation.* ***Please refer to Chapter 20.***

Reference: Hampton, L. E., Fletcher, J. M., Cirino, P., Blaser, S., Kramer, L. A., & Dennis, M. (2013). Neuropsychological profiles of children with aqueductal stenosis and spina bifida myelomeningocele. *Journal of the International Neuropsychological Society, 19*, 127–136.

64. **B—impaired vertical gaze** *Persons with PSP often initially present with difficulty coordinating eye movements; specifically, they cannot coordinate their eyes to look up or down (supranuclear vertical gaze palsy).* ***Please refer to Chapter 32.***

Reference: Han, D. Y., Pyykkonen, B. A., Shandera-Ochsner, A. L., & Schmitt, F. A. (2014). Frontotemporal dementias. In C. A. Noggle (Ed.), *The neuropsychology of cortical dementias* (pp. 221–248). New York, NY: Springer.

65. **D—Discuss your concern with the unit director or chief of staff.** *In this scenario the supervisor might have a reversible problem that could be addressed with appropriate diagnosis and medical care. Thus, a clinician might first consider talking with the colleague directly, but this is not given as an option. Reports of clinician impairment should first go to supervisory personnel. In this case the chief of the neuropsychology service is already aware but not acting appropriately; therefore, you have an obligation to proceed up the chain of command. If local reporting is unsuccessful or not applicable, the concern must be reported to a higher level such as the licensing board. Report to the state ethics committee would not be appropriate as they do not have the power to intervene directly and thus patient safety issues would not be promptly addressed. Finally, attempting to assess for impairment in this situation is not appropriate. There is already sufficient evidence of clinician impairment, and it is not your role to assess a colleague's mental status.* ***Please refer to Chapter 7.***

General Principles and Ethical Standards: A, B, C; 1.02, 1.03, 1.04, 1.05

Reference: Deidan, C., & Bush, S. (2002). Addressing perceived ethical violations by colleagues. In S. S. Bush & M. L. Drexler (Eds.), *Ethical issues in clinical neuropsychology* (pp. 281–305). Lisse, NL: Swets & Zeitlinger Publishers.

66. **C—engaging in actions that cause injury to self** *Self-injurious repetitive behaviors are sometimes found in individuals with low IQs and poor adaptive functioning abilities. The other options are often seen across individuals with ASDs, but none are strongly linked to a low IQ or adaptive skill profile.* ***Please refer to Chapter 14.***

Reference: Richards, C., Oliver, C., Nelson, L., & Moss, J. (2012). Self-injurious behavior in individuals with autism spectrum disorder and intellectual disability. *Journal of Intellectual Disability Research, 56*(5), 476–489.

67. **A—may delay nursing home placement** *Research has found that "for each year of treatment with galantamine or other AChEI, the risk of being admitted to a nursing home within a given period was reduced by 31% (galantamine) and 29% (other AChEI)."* ***Please refer to Chapter 30.***

Reference: Howard, R., McShane, R., Lindesay, J., Ritchie, C., Baldwin, A., Barber, R., . . . Jones, R. (2015). Nursing home placement in the Donepezil and Memantine in Moderate to Severe Alzheimer's Disease (DOMINO-AD) trial: Secondary and post-hoc analyses. *The Lancet Neurology, 14*(12), 1171–1181.

68. **D—brain region subserving expressive speech** *Paul Broca discovered the brain region subserving expressive speech, nonfluent aphasia.* ***Please refer to Chapter 3.***

Reference: Cullum, C. M., Rosetti, H. C., Batjer, H., Fest, J. R., Haaland, K. Y., & Lacritz, L. (2018). Cerebrovascular disease. In J. E. Morgan & J. H. Ricker (Eds.), *Textbook of clinical neuropsychology* (2nd ed., pp. 350–386). New York, NY: Routledge.

69. **A—schizophreniform disorder** *The combination of reported and observed symptoms and symptom duration are most consistent with schizophreniform disorder. This initial diagnosis would be revised to a diagnosis schizophrenia if symptoms persist longer than 6 months.* ***Please refer to Chapter 35.***

Reference: American Psychiatric Association. (2013). *Diagnostic and statistical manual of mental disorders* (5th. ed.). Washington, DC: American Psychiatric Publishing.

70. **D—Chelation treatment does not reverse cognitive deficits.** *Chelation treatment is effective in removing lead from blood but it has not been shown to reverse any neuropsychological deficits associated with elevated blood lead levels.* ***Please refer to Chapter 21.***

Reference: Dietrich, K. N. (2010). Environmental toxicants. In K. O. Yeates, M. D. Ris, H. G. Taylor, & B. F. Pennington (Eds.), *Pediatric neuropsychology: Research, theory, and practice* (pp. 211–264). New York, NY: Guilford Press.

71. **B—Wernicke's aphasia** *While both Wernicke's aphasia and conduction aphasia are characterized by fluent (albeit paraphasic) speech, only Wernicke's aphasia also includes impaired comprehension.* ***Please refer to Chapter 5.***

References:
(a) Caplan, D. (2012). Aphasic syndromes. In K. M. Heilman & E. Valenstein (Eds.), *Clinical neuropsychology* (5th ed., pp. 22–41). New York, NY: Oxford University Press.
(b) Gazzaniga, M. S., Ivry, R. B., & Mangun, G. R. (2014). *Cognitive neuroscience: The biology of the mind* (4th ed.). New York, NY: W. W. Norton & Co.
(c) Schoenberg, M. R., & Scott, J. G. (2011). Aphasia syndromes. In M. R. Schoenberg & J. G. Scott (Eds.), *The little black book of neuropsychology: A syndrome-based approach* (pp. 267–292). New York, NY: Springer.

72. **A—cerebral palsy (CP) is non-progressive but the associated functional impairments can worsen.** *Secondary impairments are common but usually do not shorten life span.* ***Please refer to Chapter 19.***

Reference: Kent, R. M. (2013). Cerebral palsy. In M. J. Aminoff, F. Boller, & D. F. Swaab (Series Eds.) & M. P. Barnes & D. C. Good (Eds.), *Handbook of clinical neurology: Neurological rehabilitation* (3rd ser., Vol. 110, pp. 443–459). New York, NY: Elsevier.

73. **C—orbitofrontal system and its connections** *Severe TBI can result in personality, behavioral, and affective changes. However, in the absence of identifiable cognitive impairments the most reasonable conclusion would be orbitofrontal system dysfunction. If there was significant persistent dysfunction in prefrontal, dorsolateral, or medial frontal lobe systems one would expect to identify some level of cognitive impairment as well.* **Please refer to Chapter 29.**

> **Reference:** Ponsford, J., Draper, K., & Schonberger, M. (2008). Functional outcome 10 years after traumatic brain injury: Its relationship with demographic, injury severity, and cognitive and emotional status. *Journal of the International Neuropsychological Society, 14*, 233–242.

74. **D—Klinefelter syndrome** *Difficulties with reading are often seen in children with Klinefelter syndrome. Several neurodevelopmental diagnoses have been associated with math learning disabilities, including spina bifida, Turner syndrome, and 22q deletion syndrome.* **Please refer to Chapter 15.**

> **References:**
> (a) Boada, R., Janusz, J., Hutaff-Lee, C., & Tartaglia, N. (2009). The cognitive phenotype in Klinefelter syndrome: A review of the literature including genetic and hormonal factors. *Developmental Disabilities Research Reviews, 15*(4), 284–294.
> (b) Dennis, M., Berch, D. B., & Mazzocco, M. M. (2009). Mathematical learning disabilities in special populations: Phenotypic variation and cross-disorder comparisons. *Developmental Disabilities Research Reviews, 15*(1), 80–89.

75. **A—age of seizure onset** *Age of seizure onset is a major component of classification of epilepsy syndromes.* **Please refer to Chapter 22.**

> **Reference:** Berg, A. T., Berkovic, S. F., Brodie, M. J., Buchhalter, J., Cross, J. H., van Emde Boas, W., . . . Scheffer, I. E. (2010). Revised terminology and concepts for organization of seizures and epilepsies: Report of the ILAE Commission on Classification and Terminology, 2005–2009. *Epilepsia, 51*, 676–685.

76. **D—.01** *The probability of getting 3/10 correct by chance alone is about .12 so some might believe that .10 would be the correct answer. However, in this situation, it is most appropriate to calculate the probability across all three trials simultaneously, which translates to 9/30, clearly significantly below chance, at the .01 level.* **Please refer to Chapter 12.**

> **Reference:** Binder, L. M., Larrabee, G. J., & Millis, S. R. (2014). Intent to fail: Significance testing of forced choice test results. *The Clinical Neuropsychologist, 28*, 1366–1375.

77. **D—embolic shower** *Coronary artery bypass grafting and cardiac valve replacement surgery have been associated with embolic shower. Although sepsis and hyponatremia could cause delirium following surgery, they would not explain persistent cognitive impairments. Stroke would be expected to result in more focal deficits as opposed to the generalized pattern of deficits present in this case making A the best answer.* **Please refer to Chapter 27.**

> **References:**
> (a) Koster, S., Hensens, A. G., Schuurmans, M. J., & van der Palen, J. (2011). Risk factors of delirium after cardiac surgery: A systematic review. *European Journal of Cardiovascular Nursing, 10*(4), 197–204.
> (b) Mangusan, R. F., Hooper, V., Denslow, S. A., & Travis, L. (2015). Outcomes associated with postoperative delirium after cardiac surgery. *American Journal of Critical Care, 24*(2), 156–163.

78. **C—Individuals with Down syndrome exhibit a progressive decline on measures of developmental and intellectual functioning beginning in the first year of life.** *Individuals with Down syndrome exhibit a progressive decline in IQ beginning in the first year of life. Further, their IQ declines sooner in adulthood than in typical aging due to increased risk of early-onset dementia of the Alzheimer type.* **Please refer to Chapter 13.**

> **Reference:** McGrath, L. M., & Peterson, R. L. (2009). Intellectual disabilities. In B. F. Pennington (Ed.), *Diagnosing learning disorders* (2nd ed., pp. 181–226). New York, NY: Guilford Press.

79. **C—show difficulties with task performance that often reflect attention and motor difficulties** *When task demands for motor responses are controlled, many executive function tests do not show impairment. Problems orienting to the initial stages of the task are often apparent, which is better explained by attention-orienting difficulties, not regulatory difficulties.* **Please refer to Chapter 20.**

Reference: Dennis, M., Sinopoli, K. J., Fletcher, J. M., & Schachar, R. (2008). Puppets, robots, critics, and actors within a taxonomy of attention for developmental disorders. *Journal of the International Neuropsychological Society, 14*, 673–690.

80. **B—low levels of vitamin D and elevated forms of cytokines** *Research has suggested that less sunlight exposure may contribute to the geographical variations in the incidence of multiple sclerosis, while diets high in vitamin D may have a protective effect resulting in a lower incidence of multiple sclerosis. Specifically, vitamin D regulates immune response by decreasing production of pro-inflammatory cytokines.* **Please refer to Chapter 24.**

Reference: Mokry, L. E., Ross, S., Ahmad, O. S., Forgetta, V., Smith, G. D., Leong, A., . . . Richards, J. B. (2015). Vitamin D and risk of multiple sclerosis: A Mendelian randomization study. *PLoS medicine, 12*(8), e1001866.

81. **A—They are absorbed by glia and provide an indirect index of regional activity.** *Radioisotopes are absorbed by glia and provide an indirect index of regional activity but are not immediately excreted. They decay at the level of glia and emit photons or positrons.* **Please refer to Chapter 6.**

Reference: Ricker, J. H., & Arenth, P. M. (2018). Functional and molecular neuroimaging in clinical neuropsychology. In J. E. Morgan & J. H. Ricker (Eds.), *Textbook of clinical neuropsychology* (2nd ed.), pp. 111–123. New York, NY: Psychology Press/Taylor & Francis Publishing.

82. **A—memantine** *The other choices have not been studied in randomized clinical trials in patients with brain metastases, though they have been used clinically and trials have been conducted in other cancer populations.* **Please refer to Chapter 25.**

Reference: Brown, P. D., Pugh, S., Laack, N. N., Wefel, J. S., Khuntia, D., Meyers, C., . . . Radiation Therapy Oncology Group. (2013). Memantine for the prevention of cognitive dysfunction in patients receiving whole-brain radiotherapy: A randomized, double-blind, placebo-controlled trial. *Neuro-Oncology, 15*(10), 1429–1437.

83. **B—She will experience long-term neurological and psychiatric sequelae and poor quality of life.** *Although data are limited, abnormal imaging and delayed treatment in HSV encephalitis are associated with poorer quality of life. The risk of seizures is high (10% in patients without seizures; 20% in those with seizures) and can develop years following diagnosis and treatment. Attention and behavioral problems are common as are more severe psychiatric/emotional disturbances, so other options are false.* **Please refer to Chapter 23.**

References:
(a) Messacar, K., Fischer, M., Dominiguez, S. R., Tyler, K. L., & Abzug, M. J. (2018). Encephalitis in children. *Infectious Disease Clinics of North America, 32*, 145–162.
(b) Michaeli, O., Kassis, I., Shachor-Meyouhas, Y., Shahar, E., & Ravid, S. (2014). Long-term motor and cognitive outcome of acute encephalitis, *Pediatrics, 133*(3), e546–52.

84. **C—rapid visual naming, timed decoding, timed single-word reading, and timed reading comprehension** *With early intervention, children can become more accurate readers, but, as young adults, often continue to be slow and inefficient. They may also have problems with comprehension. Timed measures of these skills are critical, because untimed measures of decoding, single-word reading, and reading comprehension may be performed at average or above average levels. Rapid visual naming may remain impaired. Measures of processing speed can supplement*

*assessment, but are not crucial. Measures of visual scanning are not helpful. **Please refer to Chapter 15.***

References:

(a) Gregg, N. (2009). *Adolescents and adults with learning disabilities and ADHD: Assessment and accommodation.* New York, NY: Guilford Press.

(b) Mapou, R. L. (2009). *Adult learning disabilities and ADHD: Research informed assessment.* New York, NY: Oxford University Press.

(c) Shaywitz, S. (2003). *Overcoming dyslexia: A new and complete science-based program for reading problems at any level.* New York, NY: Alfred A. Knopf.

85. **A—temporally graded retrograde amnesia** *Patients with WKS display severe anterograde amnesia and temporally graded retrograde amnesia imposed over and above the typical neurotoxic effects of alcoholism. This global amnesia is manifested psychometrically as a marked distinction between IQ and MQ. **Please refer to Chapter 36.***

Reference: Rourke, S. B., & Grant, I. (2009). The neurobehavioral correlates of alcoholism. In I. Grant & K. Adams (Eds.), *Neuropsychological assessment of neuropsychiatric and neuromedical disorders* (pp. 398–454). New York, NY: Oxford University Press.

86. **A—true positives divided by (true positives plus false positives)** *Positive predictive value (PPV) is defined as true positives divided by (true positives plus false positives). **Please refer to Chapter 9.***

Reference: Irwing, P., Booth, T., & Hughes, D. J. (2018). *The Wiley handbook of psychometric testing.* New York, NY: Wiley.

87. **D—birth year of the cohort** *It is critical that the birth year of the cohort be considered, given that clinical care provided in the NICU's has changed substantially over the past several decades and that this change in care is associated with different course and outcomes. **Please refer to Chapter 17.***

Reference: Baron, I. S., & Rey-Casserly, C. (2010). Extremely preterm birth outcome: A review of four decades of cognitive research. *Neuropsychology Review, 20,* 430–452.

88. **B—Impaired verbal working memory** *Regions of the dorsal-lateral prefrontal cortex superior to the arcuate sulcus have been shown to be active during the delay period in working memory tasks in both animals (single cell recordings) and humans (functional imaging). **Please refer to Chapter 4.***

Reference: Goldman-Rakic, P. (1990). Cellular and circuit basis of working memory in prefrontal cortex of nonhuman primates. *Progress in Brain Research, 85,* 325–336.

89. **D—intraventricular hemorrhage or periventricular leukomalacia** *Perinatal stroke and brain malformations are less frequent findings. **Please refer to Chapter 19.***

Reference: Marret, S., Vanhulle, C., Laquerrier, A. (2013). Pathophysiology of cerebral palsy. In M. J. Aminoff, F. Boller, & D. F. Swaab (Series Eds.) & O. Dulac, M. Lassonde, & H. B. Sarnat (Eds.), *Handbook of clinical neurology: Pediatric neurology* (Vol. 3, Part 1, pp. 169–176). Amsterdam, NL: Elsevier.

90. **C—to determine if the child has a comorbid learning disability or psychiatric disorder** *The other answers are not appropriate. CPTs should not be used as the sole procedure for determining if a child has ADHD or not. Selecting medications and determining if the child's symptoms are secondary to thyroid dysfunction or epilepsy will require the input of the treating physician or neurologist, as well as possible administration of an EEG. **Please refer to Chapter 16.***

Reference: Pritchard, A. E., Nigro, C. A., Jacobson, L. A., & Mahone, E. M. (2012). The role of neuropsychological assessment in the functional outcomes of children with ADHD. *Neuropsychology Review, 22,* 54–68.

91. **C—executive dysfunction with relative sparing of memory and visuospatial functioning** *Due to degeneration of the frontal lobe(s), executive dysfunction is more prominent early in the disease compared to deficits in other cognitive domains.* **Please refer to Chapter 32.**

Reference: Rascovsky, K., & Grossman, M. (2013). Clinical diagnostic criteria and classification controversies in frontotemporal lobar degeneration. *International Review of Psychiatry, 25,* 145–158.

92. **A—excessive synaptic pruning, possibly due to variations in complement component 4 (CC4) genes** *The hypothesis that decreased neuropil (fewer synaptic elements) has been due to excessive pruning, has been popular for decades, but only in 2016 was a link to specific genetic variation in the CC4 genes identified.* **Please refer to Chapter 35.**

Reference: Sekar, A., Bialas, A. R., de Rivera, H., Davis, A., Hammond, T. R., Kamitaki, N., . . . Genovese, G. (2016). Schizophrenia risk from complex variation of complement component 4. *Nature, 530*(7589), 177.

93. **C—amygdala** *The amygdala is involved in reward learning, unpredictability processing, salience determination relative to emotional and social stimuli, and broader stimulus valuation. It is theorized that amygdala dysfunction may result in inappropriate threat perception and dysfunctional emotional regulation that are felt to be the premise of anxiety disorders.* **Please refer to Chapter 34.**

Reference: Schmidt C. K., Khalid S., Loukas M., & Tubbs, R. S. (2018). Neuroanatomy of anxiety: A brief review. *Cureus 10*(1), e2055. doi: 10.7759/cureus.2055

94. **D—extensive white matter disease** *Research indicates that frontal lobe white matter is more sensitive to vascular dysfunction than the temporal lobe, resulting in greater white matter change in vascular versus Alzheimer dementia. Cerebrovascular disease can increase the risk for Alzheimer dementia but it is not pathologically specific to the condition.* **Please refer to Chapter 30.**

References:
(a) Brickman, A. M., Zahodne, L. B., Guzman, V. A., Narkhede, A., Meier, I. B., Griffith, E. Y., . . . Luchsinger, J. A. (2015). Reconsidering harbingers of dementia: Progression of parietal lobe white matter hyperintensities predicts Alzheimer's disease incidence. *Neurobiology of Aging, 36*(1), 27–32.
(b) Prins, N. D., & Scheltens, P. (2015). White matter hyperintensities, cognitive impairment and dementia: An update. *Nature Reviews Neurology, 11*(3), 157.

95. **C—cerebral palsy** *Although not as frequently due to hypoxia as once thought (leading to unnecessarily high caesarean delivery rates due to litigation), increased risk of CP is associated with preterm delivery, congenital malformations, intrauterine infection, fetal growth restriction, multiple pregnancy, placental abnormalities, and acute intrapartum hypoxia.* **Please refer to Chapter 28.**

Reference: MacLennan, M. D., Thompson, S. C., & Gecz, J. (2015). Cerebral palsy: Causes, pathways, and the role of genetic variants. *American Journal of Obstetrics & Gynecology, 213*(6), 779–788.

96. **C—22q11.2 deletion syndrome** *Cardiac and palatal abnormalities and psychotic behaviors (hallucinations) are associated with 22q11.2 deletion syndrome but not the other disorders listed. Williams syndrome and Turner syndrome are associated with problems with math and attention. Language delay and attention problems can be seen in Klinefelter syndrome but math deficits are not typical.* **Please refer to Chapter 18.**

Reference: Philip, N., & Bassett, A. (2011). Cognitive, behavioural, and psychiatric phenotype in 22q11.2 deletion syndrome. *Behavior Genetics, 41,* 403–412.

97. **A—functional neurological symptom disorder** *Functional neurological symptom disorder or conversion is very common in neurology settings and presents with more specific neurological symptoms, like seizures.* ***Please refer to Chapter 37.***

    Reference: Perez, D. L., Young, S. S., King, J. N., Guarino, A. J., Dworetzky, B. A., Flaherty, A., . . . Dickerson, B. C. (2016). Preliminary predictors of initial attendance, symptom burden, and motor subtype in a US functional neurological disorders clinic population. *Cognitive and Behavioral Neurology, 29*(4), 197–205.

98. **A—early presence of visual hallucinations** *Well-formed early visual hallucinations are a core diagnostic feature of Lewy body dementia. Hallucinations can occur in Parkinson's disease, but typically as a side effect of medications. REM behavioral disorder (i.e., dream enactment during REM sleep) is part of the diagnostic criteria for Lewy body dementia, but you can have REMBD with other parkinsonian disorders as well.* ***Please refer to Chapter 33.***

    Reference: McKeith, I. G., Boeve, B. F., Dickson, D. W., Halliday, G., Taylor, J. P., Weintraub, D., . . . Kosaka, K. (2017). Diagnosis and management of DLB. *Neurology, 89*, 88–100.

99. **B—ideomotor apraxia** *Described as body-part-for-object substitution.* ***Please refer to Chapter 5.***

    References:
    (a) Loring, D. W., 1999. Loring, D. W. (1999). *INS dictionary of neuropsychology*. New York, NY: Oxford University Press.
    (b) Sarno, M. T. (Ed.). (1981). *Acquired aphasia*. New York, NY: Academic Press.

100. **D—Act as an expert witness if the patient consents but disclose your non-forensic role.** *This scenario has to do with multiple relationships and conflicts of interest and is not uncommon for practicing neuropsychologists even if they do not have a forensic focus. Recommending a forensic evaluation be performed by a colleague is appropriate, but refusal to participate in any deposition might be unethical and could lead to legal consequences especially if a subpoena is received. The court determines who is an expert witness, not the attorney, and thus B is incorrect. Neuropsychologists can and should expect reasonable compensation for their time. In clinical situations in which the clinician knows their work may be used in court proceedings, it is also appropriate to write in the report that it was not written or intended for forensic purposes. It would also be important to clarify the clinician's role up front in any deposition.* ***Please refer to Chapter 7.***

     General Principles and Ethical Standards: B, C; 3.05, 3.06

     References:
     (a) Bush, S. S., Connell, M. A., & Denney, R. L. (2006). *Ethical issues in forensic psychology: A systematic model for decision making*. Washington, D.C.: American Psychological Association.
     (b) Bush, S. S., & Morgan, J. E. (2017). Ethical practice in forensic neuropsychology. In S. S. Bush, G. J. Demakis, & M. L. Rohling (Eds.), *APA handbook of forensic neuropsychology* (pp. 23–37). Washington, DC: American Psychological Association.

101. **B—error free learning and compensatory memory strategies** *Compensatory memory strategies, study skills training and error free learning are all potential approaches with this type of patient. Individuals with moderate to severe memory impairment often respond more favorably to compensatory memory strategies and error free learning. Restorative therapies have very limited if any value in memory rehabilitation.* ***Please refer to Chapter 29.***

     Reference: Stringer, A. (2018). Empirically based rehabilitation of neurocognitive disorder. In J. E. Morgan, & J. H. Ricker (Eds.), *Textbook of clinical neuropsychology* (2nd ed., pp. 1078–1088). New York, NY: Taylor and Francis.

102. **B—24 months** *The age correction is generally made until the child reaches 24 months of age. This has been somewhat controversial, as it is not empirically grounded. **Please refer to Chapter 17.***

> **Reference:** Baron, I. S., & Rey-Casserly, C. (2010). Extremely preterm birth outcome: A review of four decades of cognitive research. *Neuropsychology Review, 20,* 430–452.

103. **C—social cognition** *Social cognition has been shown to serve as an important mediating mechanism of the process through which neurocognitive deficits lead to poor functional outcomes in the real world. **Please refer to Chapter 35.***

> **Reference:** Horan, W. P., Harvey, P.-O., Kern, R. S., & Green, M. F. (2011). Neurocognition, social cognition, and functional outcome in schizophrenia. In W. Gaebel (Ed.), *Schizophrenia: Current science and clinical practice* (pp. 68–107). Chichester, UK: Wiley-Blackwell.

104. **A—recurrent unprovoked seizures** *Epilepsy is defined as two unprovoked seizures at least 24 hours apart, or one unprovoked seizure when the known likelihood of another is high. Epilepsy is not necessarily medication resistant, and many persons with epilepsy can achieve good control of seizures with medication. Many persons with epilepsy, particularly localization-related epilepsy, have only one seizure type. **Please refer to Chapter 22.***

> **Reference:** Fisher, R. S., Acevedo, C., Arzimanoglou, A., Bogacz, A., Cross, H., Elger, C., . . . Wiebe, S. (2012). A practical clinical definition of epilepsy. *Epilepsia, 55*(4), 475–482.

105. **B—fatigue** *Over the course of the disease, 75–90% of patients with multiple sclerosis report fatigue and 50–60% indicate that it is the most disabling symptom, often the primary reason for work cessation or reduction of work hours. **Please refer to Chapter 24.***

> **References:**
> (a) Bradley, T. J., & Chervin, R. D. (2010). Fatigue in multiple sclerosis: Mechanisms, evaluation, and treatment. *Sleep, 13*(8). 1061–1067.
> (b) Information from the National Multiple Sclerosis Society; www.nationalmssociety.org/Symptoms-Diagnosis/MS-Symptoms/Fatigue

106. **A—a common disorder not obviously related to other forms of spina bifida** *Spina bifida occulta is often "hidden" and asymptomatic and differentiated from spina bifida cystica, which is visibly identifiable and at a minimum, associated with ambulatory and bowel/bladder problems depending on the level of the dysraphism. **Please refer to Chapter 20.***

> **Reference:** Swaiman, K. F., Ashwal, S., Ferriero, D. M., Schor, N. F., Finkel, R. S., Gropman, A. L., Pearl, P., & Shevell, M. I. (2017). *Swaiman's pediatric neurology: Principles and practices* (6th ed.). New York, NY: Elsevier.

107. **A—no evidence of infarct on neuroimaging** *There is a change in the definition of transient ischemic attack (TIA), which was previously defined as any focal cerebral ischemic event typically lasting less than 1 hour but no more than 24 hours. However, studies have shown that 30–50% of patients meeting that criterion had evidence of ischemic damage on diffusion-weighted magnetic resonance imaging. Therefore, TIA is now defined as a transient episode of neurologic dysfunction caused by focal brain, spinal cord, or retinal ischemia, without acute infarction. This definitional change has been accepted by the American Heart Association and other organizations focused on cerebrovascular health. This is an important issue because such episodes are risk factors for additional strokes and require detailed assessment to minimize the risk of future stroke. **Please refer to Chapter 26.***

> **Reference:** Easton, J. D., Saver, J. L., Albers, G. W., Alberts, M. J. Chaturvedi, S., Feldmann, E., . . . Sacco, R. L. (2009). Definition and evaluation of transient ischemic attack; A Scientific Statement for Healthcare Professionals From the American Heart Association/American Stroke Association Stroke Council; Council

on Cardiovascular Surgery and Anesthesia; Council on Cardiovascular Radiology and Intervention; Council on Cardiovascular Nursing; and the Interdisciplinary Council on Peripheral Vascular Disease. *Stroke, 40*, 2276–2293.

108. **D—country and setting of the birth, presence of intraventricular hemorrhage (IVH), and other neurological complications** *The severity of medical and neurological complications confers the greatest risk for children born preterm. Children born preterm in low- and middle-income countries are at much higher risk for poor long-term outcome. Integrated NICU care and availability of a neonatologist is also associated with functional outcome. The other factors listed are risk factors for preterm birth, but not necessarily for functional outcome.* **Please refer to Chapter 17.**

    Reference: Glass, H. C., Costarino, A. T., Stayer, S. A., Brett, C., Cladis, F., & Davis, P. J. (2015). Outcomes for extremely premature infants. *Anesthesia and Analgesia, 120*(6), 1337–1351.

109. **C—Mortality rates are quite low due to improved treatments in the past 10 years.** *This is not true. Mortality rates continue to be high (15–30%) for tuberculosis meningitis even in the United States. All of the other options are true. Antibiotics are not the appropriate treatment. Antifungal and other medications are used. Stroke, seizures, and hydrocephalus are common neurologic sequelae, and tuberculosis meningitis is more common in countries with fewer economic resources.* **Please refer to Chapter 23.**

    References:
    (a) Merkler, A. E., Reynolds, A. S., Gialdini, G., Morris, N. A., Murthy, S. B., Thakur, K., & Kamel, H. (2017). Neurological complications after tuberculous meningitis in a multi-state cohort in the United States. *Journal of Neurological Sciences, 375*, 460–463.
    (b) Mouchet, F. (2016). Tuberculous meningitis: A diagnostic challenge and a devastating outcome. *Developmental Medicine & Child Neurology, 58*, 427–436.
    (c) Rohlwink, U. K., Donald, K., Gavine, B., Padayachy, L., Wilmshurst, J., Fieggen, G. A., & Figaji, A. A. (2016). Clinical characteristics and neurodevelopmental outcomes of children with tuberculous meningitis and hydrocephalus *Developmental Medicine and Child Neurology, 58*, 461–468.
    (d) Sumeet R. Dhawan, S., Gupta, A., Singhi, P., Sankhyan, N., Malhi, P., & Khandelwal, N. (2016). Predictors of neurological outcome of tuberculous meningitis in childhood: A prospective cohort study from a developing country. *Journal of Child Neurology, 31*(14), 1622–1627.
    (e) Thwaites, G. E., van Toorn, R., & Schoeman, J. (2013). Tuberculous meningitis: More questions, still too few answers, *Lancet Neurology, 12*, 999–1010.

110. **D—antioxidant and B vitamin supplementation** *Gorelick et al. (2011), in their comprehensive review of the literature to date, conclude that the use of antioxidants and B vitamins is not beneficial based on current evidence, but that long-term physical activity and moderation of alcohol intake are reasonable protective measures.* **Please refer to Chapter 31.**

    Reference: Gorelick, P. B., Cuteri, A., Decarli, C., Greenberg, S. M., Iadecola, C, Launer, L. J., . . . Seshadri, S. (2011). Vascular contributions to cognitive impairment and dementia: A statement for healthcare professionals from the American Heart Association/American Stroke Association. *Stroke, 42*, 2672–2713.

111. **A—attention** *The serotonin system is involved in the control of behavioral, perceptual, and regulatory systems, including mood, hunger, body temperature, sexual behavior, muscle control, and sensory perception.* **Please refer to Chapter 36.**

    Reference: National Institute of Drug Abuse. (2009). *DrugFacts: Hallucinogens—LSD, peyote, psilocybin, and PCP.* http://www.drugabuse.gov/publications/drugfacts/hallucinogens-lsd-peyote-psilocybin-pcp

112. **C—fragile X syndrome** *Fragile X syndrome is the most common known inherited cause of ID. It is now known that confirmed carriers of the condition are at risk for developing a number of health problems.* **Please refer to Chapter 13.**

Reference: King, B. H., Toth, K. E., Hodapp, R. M., & Dykens, E. M. (2009). Intellectual disability. In Sadock, B. J., Sadock, V. A., & Ruiz, P. (Eds.), *Comprehensive textbook of psychiatry* (9th ed., pp. 3444–3474). Philadelphia, PA: Lippincott, Williams, & Wilkins.

113. **A—medial and dorsal raphe nuclei** *Serotonergic neurons arise from the median and dorsal raphe nuclei in the brainstem and project throughout the forebrain.* **Please refer to Chapter 34.**

Reference: Kandel, E. R. (2013). Disorders of mood and anxiety. In E. R. Kandel, J. H. Schwartz, T. M. Jessell, A. A. Siegelbaum, & A. J. Hudspeth (Eds.), *Principles of neural science* (5th ed., pp. 1402–1424). New York, NY: McGraw-Hill.

114. **D—Mood and anxiety disorders cannot be identified through typical medical evaluations such as blood tests or neuroimaging studies.** *Thus far, no consensus has been established and there are a number of challenges that need to be addressed before biomarker research can be applied to improve the diagnosis and management of depression and anxiety. However, medical evaluations such as blood tests or neuroimaging studies can be used to rule out other causal or contributing medical factors.* **Please refer to Chapter 34.**

Reference: Strawbridge, R., Young, A. H., & Cleare, A. J. (2017). Biomarkers for depression: Recent insights, current challenges and future prospects. *Neuropsychiatric Disease and Treatment, 13,* 1245–1262.

115. **B—A diagnosis of ADHD-I is appropriate if 6 (or more) of the 9 inattentive symptoms are met within two or more settings.** *Clinical interview and behavioral rating scales are most often used to diagnose ADHD, with teacher and parent versions administered to ensure that symptoms are present across at least two settings. While neuropsychological testing can be helpful in identifying potential deficits in attention and executive functioning skills, these measures may lack sensitivity in detecting deficits, especially among individuals with above average FSIQ.* **Please refer to Chapter 16.**

Reference: Pritchard, A. E., Nigro, C. A., Jacobson, L. A., & Mahone, E. M. (2012). The role of neuropsychological assessment in the functional outcomes of children with ADHD. *Neuropsychology Review, 22,* 54–68.

116. **D—capacity to function in unfamiliar settings** *Individuals diagnosed with either MCI or in the early stage of Alzheimer's disease can demonstrate poor judgment in complicated and unfamiliar situations. Complicated situations can include complex tasks such as managing finances.* **Please refer to Chapter 30.**

References:
(a) Jekel, K., Damian, M., Wattmo, C., Hausner, L., Bullock, R., Connelly, P. J., . . . Kramberger, M. G. (2015). Mild cognitive impairment and deficits in instrumental activities of daily living: A systematic review. *Alzheimer's Research & Therapy, 7*(1), 17.
(b) Reppermund, S., Sachdev, P. S., Crawford, J., Kochan, N. A., Slavin, M. J., et al. (2010). The relationship of neuropsychological function to instrumental activities of daily living in mild cognitive impairment. *International Journal of Geriatric Psychiatry, 26*(8), 843–852.

117. **C—supramarginal gyrus or angular gyrus in the left hemisphere** *Please refer to Chapter 5.*

References:
(a) Goodglass, H. with the collaboration of Kaplan, E., & Barresi, B. (2001). *The assessment of aphasia and related disorders* (3rd ed.). Baltimore, MD: Lippincott Williams & Wilkins.
(b) Sarno, M. T. (Ed.). (1981). *Acquired aphasia.* New York, NY: Academic Press.

118. **D—anterior cingulate cortex** *The cingulate gyrus is a medial structure that surrounds the corpus callosum. Damage to the anterior portion has been associated with mutism, akinesia, and impaired initiation.* **Please refer to Chapter 29.**

Reference: Levin, H., Shum, D., & Chan, R. (Eds.). (2014). *Understanding traumatic brain injury: Current research and future directions.* New York, NY: Oxford University Press.

119. **B—Parkinsonism because of the gait and motor anomalies** *The earliest signs of NPH are typically gait and motor abnormalities. Although NPH may give the appearance of a dementia, it is not common, but should be identified because it will make symptoms of dementia more severe. In Alzheimer's, motor problems are usually absent in the early stages.* **Please refer to Chapter 20.**

Reference: Sinforiano, E., Pacchetti, C., Picascia, M., Pozzi, N. G., Todisco, M., & Vitali, P. (2018). *Clinical and cognitive features of idiopathic normal pressure hydrocephalus.* http://dx.doi.org/10.5772/intechopen.73273.

120. **A—periodic leg movement disorder** *White matter hyperintensities and silent brain infarcts (SBI) correlate with slowing of processing speed and the presence of executive dysfunction in vascular cognitive impairment. Atrial fibrillation is an identified risk factor for vascular cognitive impairment. Cerebral amyloid angiopathy is associated with cerebral hemorrhagic lesions and vascular cognitive impairment.* **Please refer to Chapter 31.**

Reference: Chui, H. C., & Ramirez-Gomez, L. (2018). Vascular cognitive impairment: Executive dysfunction in the era of the human brain connectome. In Miller, B. L., & Cummings, J. L. (Eds.), *The human frontal lobes: Functions and disorders* (3rd ed., pp. 357–367). New York, NY: The Guilford Press.

121. **B—Therapies can help prevent a child from experiencing a deterioration in mobility and being reclassified at a more severe Gross Motor Function Classification System level.** *Choice (a) is incorrect because parent participation is considered essential for success. Pain is a common problem. Therapies can facilitate improvements but for most children will not result in sufficient gains to be reclassified at a milder Gross Motor Function Classification System level.* **Please refer to Chapter 19.**

References:
(a) Imms, C., & Gibson, N. (2018). An overview of evidence-based occupational and physiotherapy for children. In C. P. Panteliadis (Ed.), *Cerebral palsy: A multidisciplinary approach* (3rd ed., pp. 165–192). Cham, Switzerland: Springer International.
(b) Richards, C. L., & Malouin, F. (2013). Cerebral palsy: Definition, assessment and rehabilitation. In M. J. Aminoff, F. Boller, & D. F. Swaab (Series Eds.) & O. Dulac, M. Lassonde, & H. B. Sarnat (Eds.), *Handbook of clinical neurology: Pediatric neurology* (Vol. 111, pp. 183–195). Amsterdam: Elsevier.

122. **D—sentence repetition** *Sentence repetition is spared in the initial presentation of semantic variant frontotemporal dementia unlike confrontation naming, single word comprehension, and object knowledge.* **Please refer to Chapter 32.**

Reference: Gorno-Tempini, M. L., Hillis, A. E., Weintraub, S., Kertesz, A., Mendez, M, Cappa, S. F., ... Grossman, M. (2011). Classification of primary progressive aphasia and its variants. *Neurology, 15*, 1006–1014.

123. **C—anterior cingulate cortex** *Anterior cingulate cortex integrates information from emotion/motivational systems and frontal-cortical system, thus allowing conflict resolution between two processes that may be competing for attention or output channels.* **Please refer to Chapter 4.**

Reference: Posner, M. I., & Rothbart, M. K. (2007). Research on attention networks as a model for the integration of psychological science. *Annual Review of Psychology, 58*, 1–23.

124. **A—a lesion of the optic chiasm** *Axons from the temporal fields pass through the optic chiasm. Temporal lobe lesions are more likely to produce quadrant—rather than hemifield—defects.* **Please refer to Chapter 6.**

References:
(a) Blumenfeld, H. (2011). *Neuroanatomy through clinical cases* (2nd ed.). Sunderland, MA: Sinauer Associates.
(b) Goldberg, S. (2017). *The four-minute neurological exam.* (2nd ed.). Miami: MedMaster.
(c) Simon, R. P., Aminoff, M., & Greenberg, D. A. (2018). *Clinical neurology* (10th ed.). New York, NY: Lange Medical Books/McGraw-Hill Education.

125. **B—undiagnosed dementia** *Dementia is a risk factor for the development of delirium but, in a case like this, does not cause delirium. The other three options are common causes of delirium in older patients following surgery.* **Please refer to Chapter 27.**

References:
(a) Lee, H. B., Mears, S. C., Rosenberg, P. B., Leoutsakos, J. M., Gottschalk, A., & Sieber, F. E. (2011). Predisposing factors for postoperative delirium after hip fracture repair in individuals with and without dementia. *Journal of the American Geriatrics Society, 59,* 2306–2313.
(b) Sieber, F. E. (2009). Postoperative delirium in the elderly surgical patient. *Anesthesiology Clinics, 27*(3), 451–464.

Appendix F

Second Full-Length Practice Examination Answers

1. **C—transcortical sensory aphasia** *This aphasic syndrome resembles Wernicke's aphasia, but because it involves the extrasylvian region, repetition is intact.* ***Please refer to Chapter 5.***

   References:
   (a) Caplan, D. (2012). Aphasic syndromes. In K. M. Heilman & E. Valenstein (Eds.), *Clinical neuropsychology* (5th ed., pp. 22–41). New York, NY: Oxford University Press.
   (b) Gazzaniga, M. S., Ivry, R. B., & Mangun, G. R. (2014). Cognitive neuroscience: The biology of the mind (4th ed.). New York, NY: W. W. Norton & Co.
   (c) Schoenberg, M. R., & Scott, J. G. (2011). Aphasia syndromes. In M. R. Schoenberg & J. G. Scott (Eds.). *The little black book of neuropsychology: A syndrome-based approach* (pp. 267–292). New York, NY: Springer.

2. **D—Provide the patient with feedback unless you are convinced it will result in harm.** *Patients, unless previously deemed legally incompetent, are entitled to be fully informed with regard to their healthcare. However, if the clinician determines that such information would be harmful, he or she can modify what is provided as long as there is reasonable justification for such action. The neuropsychologist could and likely should opt to provide the patient with these findings tactfully. However, it would be inappropriate to avoid providing the patient with any information after such an evaluation. Standard 2.09 requires psychologists to ensure that explanation of the results are provided using language that is reasonable and understandable to the patient or legally authorized persons who act on behalf of the patient.* ***Please refer to Chapter 7.***

   General Principles and Ethical Standards: A, B, E; 2.09, 9.02, 9.06, 9.10

   References:
   (a) Cornett, P. F., & Hall, J. R. (2008). Issues in disclosing a diagnosis of dementia. *Archives of Clinical Neuropsychology, 23,* 251–256.
   (b) Johnson-Greene, D., & Nissley, H. (2008). Ethical challenges in neuropsychology. In J. E. Morgan & J. H. Ricker & (Eds.), *Textbook of clinical neuropsychology* (pp. 945–959). New York, NY: Psychology Press.

3. **D—psychotropic medications** *Medications have been shown to have success in decreasing irritability and hyperactivity in children and adolescents with ASDs.* ***Please refer to Chapter 14.***

   Reference: Goel, R., Hong, J. S., Findling, R. L., & Young Ji, N. (2018). An update on pharmacotherapy of autism spectrum disorder in children and adolescents. *International Review of Psychiatry, 30*(1), 78–95.

4. **B—sitting by 24 months** *Sitting by 24 months predicts future ambulation.* ***Please refer to Chapter 19.***

   Reference: Keeratisiroj, O., Thawinchai, N., Siritaratiwat, W., Montana Buntragulpoontawee, M., & Pratoomsoot, C. (2016). Prognostic predictors for ambulation in children with cerebral palsy: A systematic review and meta-analysis of observational studies. *Disability and Rehabilitation, 40*(2), 135–143.

5. **A—visuospatial reasoning** *Patients with schizophrenia show moderate to severe deficits across almost all neuropsychological functions; however, deficits in attention, memory, and executive functioning are among the most severe and reliably observed.* ***Please refer to Chapter 35.***

   Reference: Horan, W. P., Harvey, P-O., Kern, R. S., & Green, M. F. (2011). Neurocognition, social cognition, and functional outcome in schizophrenia. In W. Gaebel (Ed.), *Schizophrenia: Current science and clinical practice* (pp. 68–107). Chichester, England: Wiley-Blackwell.

6. **D —a normative data set collected exclusively on African Americans** *Since the referral question can be answered in the context of the examinee's cultural group, the African American normative data is likely to provide the most accurate interpretive base.* ***Please refer to Chapter 11.***

   Reference: Manly, J. J., & Echemendia, R. J. (2007). Race-specific norms: Using the model of hypertension to understand issues of race, culture, and education in neuropsychology. *Archives of Clinical Neuropsychology, 22*(3), 319–325.

7. **C—pursuit-rotor** *Procedural memory is relatively intact, but any measure of episodic memory task (A, C, and D) will be failed.* ***Please refer to Chapter 3.***

   Reference: Heindel, W. C., Butters, N., & Salmon, D. P. (1988). Impaired learning of a motor skill in patients with Huntington's disease. *Behavioral Neuroscience, 102*, 141–147. http://psycnet.apa.org

8. **A—exposure to tobacco smoke in utero** *Exposure to tobacco smoke in utero is considered to be a common potential environmental risk factor for developing ADHD symptoms.* ***Please refer to Chapter 16.***

   Reference: Barkley, R. A. (2014). *Attention-deficit/hyperactivity disorder: A handbook for diagnosis and treatment* (4th ed.). New York, NY: Guilford Press

9. **B—perseverative and echolalic behavior** *Patients with early Alzheimer's disease display a pattern of deficits characterized by reduced learning, rapid forgetting, increased recency recall, elevated intrusion errors, and poor recognition discriminability with increased false-positives. Perseverative behavior typically occurs later in the disease process.* ***Please refer to Chapter 30.***

   Reference: Mueller, K. D., Koscik, R. L., LaRue, A., Clark, L. R., Hermann, B., Johnson, S. C., & Sager, M. A. (2015). Verbal fluency and early memory decline: Results from the Wisconsin Registry for Alzheimer's prevention. *Archives of Clinical Neuropsychology, 30*(5), 448–457.

10. **B—striatum; globus pallidus** *The striatum (caudate and putamen) receives cortical input and projects to the globus pallidus, which provides basal ganglia output to the thalamus. Each loop differs with respect to the specific striatal or pallidal region involved, but the basic architecture is the same in all loops.* ***Please refer to Chapter 4.***

    Reference: Alexander, G. E., DeLong, M. R., & Strick, P. L. (1986). Parallel organization of functionally segregated circuits linking basal ganglia and cortex. *Annual Review of Neuroscience, 9*, 357–381.

11. **D—recognition** *On verbal list-learning tests such as the CVLT, recognition measures have generally been found to be the most sensitive and specific to noncredible performance, in both adult and pediatric populations.* ***Please refer to Chapter 12.***

    References:
    (a) Baker, D., Connery, A. K., Kirk, J. W., & Kirkwood, M. W. (2014). Embedded performance validity indicators within the California Verbal Learning Test, Children's Version. *The Clinical Neuropsychologist, 28*, 116–127.

(b) Schwartz, E. S., Erdodi, L., Rodriguez, N., Ghosh, J. J., Curtain, J. R. Flashman, L. A., & Roth, R. M. (2016). CVLT-II forced choice recognition trial as an embedded validity indicator: A systematic review of the evidence. *Journal of the International Neuropsychological Society, 22*, 851–858.

12. **C—primary neurodegenerative disease** *While paraneoplastic limbic encephalitis is associated with new-onset epilepsy in adults, it is uncommon among elderly over age 65 years. Primary neurodegenerative disease (e.g., Alzheimers), traumatic brain injury, cerebrovascular disease, and primary CNS tumors are all common causes of new-onset epilepsy in the geriatric population.* **Please refer to Chapter 22.**

Reference: Liu, S., Yu, W., & Lu, Y. (2016). The causes of new onset epilepsy and seizures in the elderly. *Neuropsychiatric Disease and Treatment, 12,*1425–1434.

13. **A—It is the most common of the three frontotemporal dementia variants** *Of the three FTD variants, bvFTD is the most common of the three FTD variants and occurs more frequently in men. The average age of onset is younger than for Alzheimer's disease. Frequent falls as an early sign is more consistent with the motor variant.* **Please refer to Chapter 32.**

Reference: Ghosh, S., & Lippa, C. (2015). Clinical subtypes of fronto-temporal dementia. *American Journal of Alzheimer's Disease and Other Dementias, 30*, 653–661.

14. **D—bacterial meningitis** *The most common presenting symptoms in bacterial meningitis include severe headaches, fever, and nuchal rigidity (i.e., neck stiffness). All of the other disorders often present with psychiatric symptoms, sometimes even in the absence of other neurological or physical symptoms.* **Please refer to Chapter 23.**

References:
(a) Kayser, M. S., Kohler, C. G., & Dalmau, J. (2010). Psychiatric manifestations of paraneoplastic disorders. *American Journal of Psychiatry, 167*, 1039–1050.
(b) National Institute of Neurological Disorders and Stroke. (2011). *NINDS meningitis and encephalitis fact sheet.* (Download: http://www.ninds.nih.gov/disorders/encephalitis_meningitis/detail_encephalitis_meningitis.htm)
(c) Voltz, R. (2007). Neuropsychological symptoms in paraneoplastic disorders. *Journal of Neurology, 254* (Suppl 2), II84–II86.

15. **C—tuberous sclerosis** *Of the disorders listed, children with tuberous sclerosis are at greatest risk for Autism spectrum disorder (ASD), with 40–50% diagnosed with ASD.* **Please refer to Chapter 18.**

Reference: Byars, A. W. (2010). Tuberous sclerosis complex. In K. O. Yeates, M. D. Ris, H. G. Taylor, & B. F. Pennington (Eds.), *Pediatric neuropsychology: Research, theory, and practice* (2nd ed.). New York, NY: Guilford Press.

16. **B—women are at higher risk than men** *It is well established that multiple sclerosis is more common in women than in men. This pattern is also seen in teens with multiple sclerosis. Interestingly however, the gender ratio is about 1:1 in those with onset prior to puberty.* **Please refer to Chapter 24.**

References:
(a) Huynh, J. L., & Casaccia, P. (2013). Epigenetic mechanisms in multiple sclerosis: implications for pathogenesis and treatment. *Lancet Neurology, 12*(2), 195–206.
(b) MacAllister, W. S., Christodoulou, C., Milazzo, M., Preston, T. E., Serafin, D., Krupp, L. B., & Harder, L. (2013). Pediatric multiple sclerosis: What we know and where are we headed? *Child Neuropsychology, 19*(1), 1–22.

17. **C—are underemployed relative to their IQ and literacy levels** *Like many adults with disabilities, unemployment rates are high. Poor math and visuospatial skills have been implicated as a source of employment difficulties.* **Please refer to Chapter 20.**

Reference: Hetherington, R., Dennis, M., Barnes, M., Drake, J., & Gentile, F. (2006). Functional outcome in young adults with spina bifida and hydrocephalus. *Child's Nervous System, 22*, 117–124.

18. **B—fatigue and sleep disturbances** *Fatigue and sleep disturbances are quite common following TBI at all levels of injury severity. Dizziness, tinnitus, headaches, pain, and visual disturbances also occur but with less frequency.* ***Please refer to Chapter 29.***

    Reference: Ponsford, J. L., & Sinclair, K. L. (2014). Sleep and fatigue following traumatic brain injury, *Psychiatric Clinics of North America, 37*(1), 77–89.

19. **C—domain-general theory** *Organicity is an older term referring to the presence of brain damage, or abnormal cerebral function. It refers to a concept of whole-brain involvement, rather than specific, regional dysfunction of specific bran centers and corresponding discrete functional impairment (localization model).* ***Please refer to Chapter 3.***

    Reference: Arango, C., & Fraguas, D. (2016). Should psychiatry deal only with mental disorders without an identified medical etiology? *World Psychiatry,* 15:1.

20. **B—Barbiturate intoxication carries more risk of accidental overdose.** *Respiratory depression is more common with acute effects of barbiturates which also increases the risk of accidental overdose. Benzodiazepines are not necessarily more costly than barbiturates, long-term neurocognitive effects, including memory problems, are more common with benzodiazepine use, and withdrawal from either type of drug requires inpatient hospitalization due to risk of seizures.* ***Please refer to Chapter 36.***

    References:
    (a) https://www.ncbi.nlm.nih.gov/books/NBK499875/
    (b) Suddick, J. T., Cain, M. D. (2018). Barbiturate toxicity. StatPearls Internet 5/2018.

21. **A—fornix** *The fornix is the primary output destination for the hippocampus. Degeneration of axons in the hippocampus may result in Wallerian degeneration and resultant atrophy in the fornix. Regions such as the internal capsule and occipital lobes are vulnerable to anoxia/hypoxia through different processes.* ***Please refer to Chapter 28.***

    References:
    (a) Blumenfeld, H. (2010). *Neuroanatomy through clinical cases* (2nd ed.). Sunderland, MA: Sinauer Associates, for discussion of hippocampal and fornix anatomy and connectivity.
    (b) Hopkins, R. O., & Bigler, E. D. (2012). Neuroimaging of anoxic injury: Implications for neurorehabilitation. *NeuroRehabilitation, 31,* 319–329.

22. **C—Angelman syndrome** *Fair hair, blue eyes, dysmorphic features (wide smiling mouth, thin upper lip, pointed chin), epilepsy, ataxia, microcephaly, happy disposition, hand flapping, intellectual disability, sleep disturbance, possible autistic features, and love of water and music characterize individuals with Angelman syndrome.* ***Please refer to Chapter 13.***

    Reference: King, B. H., Toth, K. E., Hodapp, R. M., & Dykens, E. M. (2009). Intellectual disability. In Sadock, B. J., Sadock, V. A., & Ruiz, P. (Eds.), *Comprehensive textbook of psychiatry* (9th ed., pp. 3444–3474). Philadelphia, PA: Lippincott, Williams, & Wilkins.

23. **D—serotonin—***Serotonergic neurons are involved in a very broad range of physiological and behavioral processes including cardiovascular regulation, appetite, pain sensitivity, sexual behavior, mood, respiration, cognition, learning and memory, and other aspects of mood and behavior. This highlights the role of serotonin regulation in the management of mood disorders as well as behavioral impulse-control difficulties.* ***Please refer to Chapter 34.***

    Reference: Kandel, E. R. (2013). Disorders of mood and anxiety. In E. R. Kandel, J. H. Schwartz, T. M. Jessell, A. A. Siegelbaum, & A. J. Hudspeth (Eds.), *Principles of neural science* (5th ed., pp. 1402–1424). New York, NY: McGraw-Hill.

24. **A—upper motor neuron dysfunction** *The Babinski sign in adults is considered to be abnormal, and is elicited in the presence of upper motor neuron dysfunction.* **Please refer to Chapter 6.**

    References:
    (a) Blumenfeld, H. (2011). *Neuroanatomy through clinical cases* (2nd ed.). Sunderland, MA: Sinauer Associates.
    (b) Goldberg, S. (2017). *The four-minute neurological exam* (2nd ed.). Miami, FL: MedMaster.
    (c) Greenberg, D., Aminoff, M., & Simon, R. (2012). *Clinical neurology* (8th ed.). New York, NY: Lange Medical Books/McGraw-Hill.

25. **A—headache, abdominal distress** *There is considerable overlap between adult and pediatric somatoform presentations, although complaints in children are predictably a bit simpler.* **Please refer to Chapter 37.**

    Reference: Masi, G., Favilla, L., Millepiedi, S., & Mucci, M. (2000). Somatic symptoms in children and adolescents referred for emotional and behavioral disorders. *Psychiatry, 63,* 140–149.

26. **B—premature birth and neuroimaging findings of periventricular leukomalacia** *Greater lower than upper extremity involvement would be consistent with spastic diplegia.* **Please refer to Chapter 19.**

    References:
    (a) Davidson, L. T., & Oleszek, J. (2011). Cerebral palsy. In R. Braddom (Ed.), *Physical medicine and rehabilitation* (4th ed, pp.1253–1274). Philadelphia, PA: Saunders.
    (b) Shin, M. R., & Heakyung, K. (2011, November 10). Cerebral palsy. *American Academy of Physical Medicine and Rehabilitation.* Retrieved from https://now.aapmr.org/cerebral-palsy/

27. **A—More women attempt suicide, but more men are likely to complete.** *Depression is not a normal part of the aging process, as most elderly report being very satisfied with their lives, even in the context of medical illnesses or physical limitations. However, elderly patients with depression, particularly males, have the highest rate of successful suicide in the United States.* **Please refer to Chapter 34.**

    Reference: Centers for Disease Control and Prevention, National Center for Health Statistics. https://www.cdc.gov/nchs/products/databriefs/db309.htm

28. **C—are commonly observed in community-dwelling older adults, even in the absence of cognitive impairment** *Because all of these phenomena occur in a significant proportion of nondemented community-dwelling older adults, their presence alone does not provide confirmation of cerebrovascular disease as a causative factor for cognitive impairment.* **Please refer to Chapter 31.**

    References:
    (a) Arvanitakis, Z., Leurgans, S. E., Barnes, L. L., Bennett, D. A., & Schneider, J. A. (2011). Microinfarct pathology, dementia, and cognitive systems. *Stroke, 42,* 722–727.
    (b) Chui, H. C., & Ramirez-Gomez, L. (2015). Clinical and imaging features of mixed Alzheimer and vascular pathologies. *Alzheimer's Research & Therapy, 7,* 21.
    (c) Fanning, J. P., Wong, A. A., & Fraser, J. F. (2014). The epidemiology of silent brain infarction: A systematic review of population-based cohorts. *BMC Medicine, 12,* 119.
    (d) Gorelick, P. B., Cuteri, A., Decarli, C., Greenberg, S. M., Iadecola, C, Launer, L. J., . . . Seshadri, S. (2011). Vascular contributions to cognitive impairment and dementia: A statement for healthcare professionals from the American Heart Association/American Stroke Association. *Stroke, 42,* 2672–2713.

29. **A—positively skewed** *Skewness refers to the degree of bias, either positively or negatively, in a distribution of scores in a population. Positive skewness occurs when a large percentage of the normal population performs well or nearly perfectly on a task or test. Skewness in a population*

is one way in which the assumption or normal distribution can be violated and thus invalidate the use of standard scores in evaluating some ones performance. ***Please refer to Chapter 9.***

Reference: Dodge, Y. (2003). *The Oxford dictionary of statistical terms* (6th ed.). New York, NY: Oxford University Press.

30. **B—joint attention, requesting gestures, play skills, and use of an augmentative or alternative communication device** *Intervention for minimally verbal children with ASD should primarily focus on advancing functional communication. Research suggests that the introduction of augmentative or alternate communication devices (e.g., picture exchange communication systems or speech-generating devices) significantly increases initiation of communicative requests and communicative utterances. The addition of instruction in prelinguistic gestures (joint attention, requesting gestures) and play skills has been shown to increase engagement between child and adult.* ***Please refer to Chapter 14.***

Reference: Kasari, C., Kaiser, A., Goods, K., Nietfeld, J, Mathy, P., Landa, R., ... Almirall, D. (2014). Communication intervention for minimally verbal children with autism: Sequential multiple assignment randomized trial. *Journal of the American Academy of Child & Adolescent Psychiatry, 53,* 635–646.

31. **C—1.0 to 1.5 standard deviations** *This is the typical deficit seen in a range of large-scale and meta-analytic studies. Chronic and "deficit" syndrome patients tend to have larger deficits, and "non-deficit" patients tend to have smaller deficits, but the clinician should not be surprised to see deficits in this range.* ***Please refer to Chapter 35.***

Reference: Bora, E., Akdede, B. B., & Alptekin, K. (2017). Neurocognitive impairment in deficit and non-deficit schizophrenia: A meta-analysis. *Psychological Medicine, 47*(14), 2401–2413.

32. **B—Type I narcolepsy** *Type I narcolepsy occurs with cataplexy, whereas type II narcolepsy occurs without it.* ***Please refer to Chapter 37.***

Reference: American Academy of Sleep Medicine. (2014). *International classification of sleep disorders* (3rd ed.). Darien, IL: American Academy of Sleep Medicine.

33. **A—multiple sleep latency test** *This procedure tests for excessive daytime sleepiness by recording the time it takes for an individual to fall asleep and enter REM.* ***Please refer to Chapter 37.***

Reference: American Academy of Sleep Medicine. (2014). *International classification of sleep disorders* (3rd ed.). Darien, IL: American Academy of Sleep Medicine.

34. **B—personality changes and behavioral problems with mild memory impairments** *Although any of these impairments or problems could impact community reentry, emotional and behavioral issues following severe TBI tend to result in the poorest outcomes. These problems are often related to and or accompanied by impairments in executive function.* ***Please refer to Chapter 29.***

Reference: Levin, H., Shum, D., & Chan, R. (Eds.). (2014). *Understanding traumatic brain injury: Current research and future directions.* New York, NY: Oxford University Press.

35. **C—dementia with delirium** *The symptoms in this case are commonly referred to as sundowning, which is not a formal diagnosis but rather a description of symptoms. Thus, c is the best answer listed because it is a formal diagnosis.* ***Please refer to Chapter 27.***

Reference: Abraham, G., & Zun, L. S. (2017). Delirium and dementia. In R. M. Walls (Ed.), *Rosen's emergency medicine: Concepts and clinical practice* (pp. 1278–1288). Philadelphia, PA: Elsevier.

36. **D—reduplicative paramnesia** *The feeling that a place has been duplicated. Capgras syndrome and Fregoli's syndrome are imposter syndromes (person).* ***Please refer to Chapter 5.***

    Reference: Loring, D. W. (2015). *INS dictionary of neuropsychology and clinical neurosciences* (2nd ed.). New York, NY: Oxford University Press.

37. **C—inferior frontal gyrus** *The neural signature of dyslexia includes underactivation of Wernicke's area, the striate cortex, and the angular gyrus, but overactivation of the inferior frontal gyrus.* ***Please refer to Chapter 15.***

    Reference: Richlan, F., Kronbichler, M., & Wimmer, H. (2009). Functional abnormalities in the dyslexic brain: A quantitative meta-analysis of neuroimaging studies. *Human Brain Mapping, 30*(10), 3299–3308.

38. **C—vestibular; ipsilateral** *Although nystagmus presents as eye movement, it is a vestibular function mediated by dysfunction involving the vestibular branch of cranial nerve VIII, and effects are observed ipsilaterally.* ***Please refer to Chapter 6.***

    References:
    (a) Blumenfeld, H. (2011). *Neuroanatomy through clinical cases* (2nd ed.). Sunderland, MA: Sinauer Associates.
    (b) Goldberg, S. (2017). *The four-minute neurological exam* (2nd ed.). Miami, FL: MedMaster.
    (c) Simon, R. P., Aminoff, M., & Greenberg, D. A. (2018). *Clinical neurology* (10th ed.). New York, NY: Lange Medical Books/McGraw-Hill Education.

39. **B—processing speed** *Deficits in processing speed are common in people with SUDs.* ***Please refer to Chapter 36.***

    Reference: Fernández-Serrano, M. J., Pérez-García, M., & Verdejo-García, A. (2011). What are the specific vs. generalized effects of drugs of abuse on neuropsychological performance? *Neuroscience & Biobehavioral Reviews, 35*(3), 377–406.

40. **D—cerebral arteriopathy** *Arteriopathy accounts for more than 50% of the cases of childhood stroke. Common arteriopathies include Moya-Moya syndrome, transient cerebral arteriopathy (vasculitis), and arterial dissection. Congenital heart disease is a common cause of childhood stroke, but not as common as arteriopathy. Bacterial meningitis is more often a cause of cerebral sinovenous thrombosis. Arteriovenous malformation is a common cause of hemorrhagic stroke.* ***Please refer to Chapter 26.***

    References:
    (a) Fuentes, A., Deotto, A., Desrocher, M., deVeber, G., & Westmacott, R. (2016). Determinants of cognitive outcomes of perinatal and childhood stroke: A review. *Child Neuropsychology, 22*, 1–38.
    (b) Kirton, A., & deVeber, G. (2015). Paediatric stroke: Pressing issues and promising directions. *Lancet Neurology, 14*, 92–102.

41. **C—visual scanning** *Many direct retraining techniques do not have sufficient evidence to support real-world generalization. Possible exceptions include process-specific approaches that address cognitive functions such as attention and concentration (in the acute phase of recovery), visual scanning, and spatial organization. The true effects of cognitive rehabilitation are sometimes uncertain when factoring in natural recovery.* ***Please refer to Chapter 29.***

    Reference: Stringer, A. (2018). Empirically based rehabilitation of neurocognitive disorder. In Morgan, J. E., & Ricker, J. H. (Eds.), *Textbook of clinical neuropsychology* (2nd. ed.). New York, NY: Taylor and Francis.

42. **B—It is legal and ethical.** *There is no legal or ethical mandate to care for any patient who wants to see you. A doctor–patient relationship must be entered into voluntarily by both parties. If a psychologist decides to focus on one specific patient population, they can. However, it would be unethical if the psychologist were to accept or reject certain patients based on arbitrary personal preferences. Yet, psychologists should not take on a patient if they have any biases that could affect*

*objectivity, competence, or effectiveness (ES 3.06). At the same time, psychologists do not engage in unfair discrimination (ES 3.01). In this vignette, for patients he does not accept, the psychologist should provide appropriate alternatives if they are available. Also, the clinician could and certainly should refer patients elsewhere if or when the patient is requesting services the clinician is not competent or able to provide. However, if there is no doctor–patient relationship, there is no obligation to arrange for care from another psychologist. This is entirely different than situations in which the patient is already under the psychologist's care. Once having accepted responsibility for a patient, there is far less freedom on the part of the psychologist to break that relationship. Abruptly discontinuing care of a patient in need without appropriate transfer is typically inconsistent with ethical practice and potentially akin to patient abandonment. **Please refer to Chapter 7.***

General Principles and Ethical Standards: B, C; 3.01, 3.06, 3.11

43. **B—more rapid decline** *Patients with early-onset Alzheimer's disease often demonstrate a faster decline on neuropsychological tests administered over the course of a year, suggesting a more aggressive course.* **Please refer to Chapter 30.**

    References:
    (a) Van Cauwenberghe, C., Van Broeckhoven, C., & Sleegers, K. (2016). The genetic landscape of Alzheimer's disease: Clinical implications and perspectives. *Genetics in Medicine, 18*(5), 421.
    (b) Yau, W. Y. W., Tudorascu, D. L., McDade, E. M., Ikonomovic, S., James, J. A., Minhas, D., . . . Gianaros, P. J. (2015). Longitudinal assessment of neuroimaging and clinical markers in autosomal dominant Alzheimer's disease: A prospective cohort study. *The Lancet Neurology, 14*(8), 804–813.

44. **C—mesostriatal** *This pathway primarily innervates the basal ganglia which is critical for motor regulation and aspects of cognitive function.* **Please refer to Chapter 4.**

    Reference: Blumenfeld, H. (2010). *Neuroanatomy through clinical cases* (2nd ed.). Sunderland, MA: Sinauer Associates.

45. **D—hypoglossal nerve** *Of the cranial nerves listed, the hypoglossal nerve has specific innervation to the tongue.* **Please refer to Chapter 6.**

    References:
    (a) Blumenfeld, H. (2011). *Neuroanatomy through Clinical Cases.* (2nd Ed.). Sunderland, MA: Sinauer Associates, Inc.
    (b) Goldberg, S. (2017). *The Four-Minute Neurological Exam.* (2nd Ed.). Miami, FL: MedMaster, Inc.
    (c) Greenberg, D., Aminoff, M., & Simon, R. (2012). *Clinical neurology.* (8th Ed.). New York, NY: Lange Medical Books/McGraw-Hill.

46. **D—hypoxic-ischemic injury** *Nonaccidental trauma is a leading cause of infant and toddler injury and death in the United States, and injuries in survivors may lead to later development of epilepsy, but is not a cause of neonatal seizures. Febrile illness leading to seizures typically occurs in childhood, not in the neonatal period. Leading causes of neonatal seizures include hypoxic-ischemic injury (20–30%), Infarction/hemorrhage (20–30%), brain malformations (5–10%), Infections (5–10%), metabolic (7–20%) genetic (6–10%) and unknown/other (10%).* **Please refer to Chapter 22.**

    References:
    (a) Paul, A. R., Adamo, M. A. (2014). Non-accidental trauma in pediatric patients: A review of epidemiology, pathophysiology, diagnosis and treatment. *Translational Pediatrics, 3*(3), 195–207.
    (b) Pressler, R.M., Cilio, M.R., Mizrahi, E.M., Moshe, S.L., Nunes, M.G., Plouin, P., . . . Zuberi, S.M. (in press). The ILAE Classification of Seizures & the Epilepsies: Modification for Seizures in the Neonate. Proposal from the ILAE Task Force on Neonatal Seizures Epilepsia.

47. **A—perinatal ischemic stroke** *Studies have consistently reported an overall delay in the onset of language after perinatal ischemic stroke, but a normal trajectory of language development*

afterward in the majority of cases. Strokes later in childhood result in language deficits when lesions involve the left hemisphere. The outcomes of hemorrhagic stroke are not well studied. **Please refer to Chapter 26.**

Reference: Fuentes, A., Deotto, A., Desrocher, M., deVeber, G., & Westmacott, R. (2016). Determinants of cognitive outcomes of perinatal and childhood stroke: A review. *Child Neuropsychology, 22*, 1–38.

48. **B—pituitary tumor** *Tumors in the sella area can present with hormonal dysregulation and vision issues (due to compression of the optic chiasm). While cerebellar tumors might present with vision changes, hormonal changes are rare. Meningiomas are tumors in the meninges, and may present with headaches but not changes in endocrine functioning or vision. Meningiomas are sometimes found incidentally.* **Please refer to Chapter 25.**

Reference: Blumenfeld, H. (2010). *Neuroanatomy through clinical cases* (2nd ed.). Sunderland, MA: Sinauer.

49. **B—receiver operating curve analysis for the clinical group of interest** *The ROC curve allows us to visualize the performance of a test by creating a plot of sensitivity and 1-specificity based on various cut-off values determining a positive test within a specific normative group. If the goal is to maximize specificity (i.e., minimizing false-positive errors), the cut point will be selected on that basis. The clinician should be aware in the context of their overall interpretation that an emphasis on specificity will result in decreased sensitivity to suboptimal engagement.* **Please refer to Chapter 8.**

Reference: Millis, S. (2018). What clinicians really need to know about symptom exaggeration, insufficient effort, and malingering: Statistical and measurement matters. In J. E. Morgan & J. J. Sweet (Eds.), *Neuropsychology of malingering casebook* (pp. 21–38). New York, NY: Psychology Press.

50. **A—flu-like symptoms for 1 week, followed by hallucinations, delusions, and emotional instability, a period of unresponsiveness, then decreased breathing rate and low blood pressure** *This progression of symptoms is the most common in anti-NMDA receptor encephalitis (seen in about 70% of adult patients).* **Please refer to Chapter 23.**

Reference: Lancaster, E., Martinez-Hernandez, E., & Dalmau J. (2011). Encephalitis and antibodies to synaptic and neuronal surface proteins. *Neurology, 77*, 179–189.

51. **C—accurate reflection of current psychological and emotional functioning** *The validity scale findings are well within an interpretative range according to conventional cut-scores listed in the PAI manual.* **Please refer to Chapter 10.**

Reference: Morey, L. C. (2007). *Personality Assessment Inventory (PAI) professional manual* (2nd ed.). Lutz, FL: Psychological Assessment Resources.

52. **B—the diagnosis does not describe a specific neurological disorder** *Cerebral palsy originates in the brain. There is not a single hallmark feature to aid in diagnosis. It is not progressive.* **Please refer to Chapter 19.**

Reference: Graham, H. K., Rosenbaum, P., Paneth, N., Dan, B., Lin, J., Damiano, K. L., . . . Lieber, R. L. (2016). Cerebral palsy. *Nature Reviews Disease Primers, 2*, 1–24.

53. **D—4 to 6 weeks** *Initial effectiveness of antidepressant medications typically occurs at approximately 1 to 2 weeks, but the medications are not fully effective for another 2 to 4 weeks.* **Please refer to Chapter 34.**

Reference: Fournier, J. C., DeRubeis, R. J., Hollon, S. D., et al. (2010). Antidepressant drug effects and depression severity: A patient-level meta-analysis. *JAMA, 303*(1), 47–53.

54. **A—ADHD and dyslexia** *These findings are most likely evidence of both ADHD (e.g., inattention and executive dysfunction) and dyslexia (e.g., poor phonological awareness). Decreased rapid automatized naming is seen in both disorders. This combination of diagnoses is quite typical.* **Please refer to Chapter 16.**

Reference: Boada, R., Willcutt, E. G., & Pennington, B. F. (2012). Understanding the comorbidity between dyslexia and attention-deficit/hyperactivity disorder. *Topics in Language Disorders, 32*, 264–284.

55. **D—executive functions** *This is believed to be due to subcortical/frontal connections being affected by the disease.* **Please refer to Chapter 32.**

Reference: Gerstenecker, A., Mast, B., Duff, K., Ferman, T., & Litvan, I.; ENGENE-PSP Study Group. (2013). Executive dysfunction is the primary cognitive impairment in progressive supranuclear palsy. *Archives of Clinical Neuropsychology, 28*, 104–113.

56. **A—Specific cognitive and behavioral profiles have been identified for a variety of syndromes of ID.** *Research has identified specific profiles for a variety of syndromes such as Down syndrome, fragile X syndrome, and Williams syndrome.* **Please refer to Chapter 13.**

Reference: McGrath, L. M., & Peterson, R. L. (2009). Intellectual disabilities. In B. F. Pennington (Ed.), *Diagnosing learning disorders* (2nd ed., pp. 181–226). New York, NY: Guilford Press.

57. **B—subthalamic nucleus deep brain stimulation** *DBS of either the STN or GPi has a broader influence on all Parkinsonian symptoms and are the surgical targets of choice in most Parkinson's disease patients.* **Please refer to Chapter 33.**

Reference: Pizzolato, G., & Mandat, T. (2012). Deep brain stimulation for movement disorders. *Frontiers in Integrative Neuroscience, 6*(2), 1–5.

58. **D—no clear expected longitudinal pattern** *Findings regarding longitudinal neuropsychological outcomes in pediatric multiple sclerosis have been mixed. Patterns of cognitive functioning described over time have included improvement, stability, or decline.* **Please refer to Chapter 24.**

References:
(a) Amato, M. P., Goretti, B., Ghezzi, A., Hakiki, B., Niccolai, C., Lori, S., . . . Trojano, M. (2014). Neuropsychological features in childhood and juvenile multiple sclerosis: Five-year follow-up. *Neurology, 83*(16), 1432–8.
(b) Charvet, L. E., O'Donnell, E. H., Belman, A. L., Chitnis, T., Ness, J. M., Parrish, J., . . . Krupp, L. B. (2014). Longitudinal evaluation of cognitive functioning in pediatric multiple sclerosis: Report from the US Pediatric Multiple Sclerosis Network. *Multiple Sclerosis Journal, 20*(11), 1502–1510.

59. **D—Positive predictive power increases with decreases in the false positive rate.** *Positive predictive power = true positives/(true positives + false positives). By decreasing false positive rate, one increases positive predictive power. For instance, if false positive rate is zero (positive predictive power = true positives/(true positives + 0 false positives) = 1.00), then you have 100% positive predictive power.* **Please refer to Chapter 8.**

Reference: Larrabee, G. J. (2014). False-positive rates associated with use of multiple performance and symptom validity tests. *Archives of Clinical Neuropsychology, 29*(4), 364–373.

60. **A—working memory, executive functions, and math-specific-anxiety** *When assessing difficulties in mathematics, the neuropsychologist should evaluate math calculation, math problem solving, and math fluency. Executive functions have also been demonstrated to be important predictors of math performance, particularly working memory. Lastly, math-specific anxiety has been found to be negatively correlated with mathematical performance.* **Please refer to Chapter 15.**

References:
(a) Toll, S. W., Van der Ven, S. H., Kroesbergen, E. H., & Van Luit, J. E. (2011). Executive functions as predictors of math learning disabilities. *Journal of Learning Disabilities, 44*(6), 521–532.
(b) Wu, S. S., Willcutt, E. G., Escovar, E., & Menon, V. (2014). Mathematics achievement and anxiety and their relation to internalizing and externalizing behaviors. *Journal of Learning Disabilities, 47*(6), 503–514.

61. **D—Borderline Personality Disorder** *A cardinal feature of Borderline Personality Disorder is a pattern of unstable relationships without the presence of hallucinations, delusions, and other forms of thought disorder.* ***Please refer to Chapter 34.***

Reference: American Psychiatric Association. (2013). *Diagnostic and statistical manual of mental disorders* (5th ed.). Washington, DC: American Psychiatric Publishing.

62. **B—differential dorsal-ventral information processing** *The dorsal stream represents the "where" system, while the ventral stream, the "what" system. This is relatively predictive inasmuch as parietal systems (dorsal) in the right hemisphere are associated with visuospatial processing, while temporal systems (left hemisphere) are associated with object identification/naming.* ***Please refer to Chapter 3.***

Reference: Hart, G., Leung, B. K., & Balleine, B. W. (2014). Dorsal and ventral streams: The distinct role of striatal subregions in the acquisition and performance of goal directed actions. *Neurobiology of Learning and Memory, 108*, 104–118.

63. **D—D_2-type dopamine receptor antagonism** *Both first- and second-generation antipsychotic medications are thought to have their antipsychotic efficacy mediated by action at D_2-type dopamine receptors, although second-generation medications may have additional actions in the context of a more complex pharmacologic profile. The efficacy of the second-generation agents is only marginally superior on selected outcomes, and it is not clear that these agents offer significant advantages on cognitive endpoints.* ***Please refer to Chapter 35.***

Reference: Leucht, S., Corves, C., Arbter, D., Engel, R. R., Li, C., & Davis, J. M. (2009). Second-generation versus first-generation antipsychotic drugs for schizophrenia: A meta-analysis. *Lancet, 373*(9657), 31–41.

64. **C—speed of processing and executive function deficits** *Chui and Ramirez-Gomez (2018) discuss the presumed relationship between the cognitive deficits of vascular cognitive impairment, including vascular dementia, and the underlying neurocircuitry that is disrupted to produce these findings. Haaland and Swanda (2008) present a discussion of these issues as well.* ***Please refer to Chapter 31.***

References:
(a) Chui, H. C., & Ramirez-Gomez, L. (2018). Vascular cognitive impairment: Executive dysfunction in the era of the human brain connectome. In Miller, B. L., & Cummings, J. L. (Eds.), *The human frontal lobes: Functions and disorders* (3rd ed., pp.357–367). New York, NY: Guilford Press.
(b) Cullum, C. M., Rosetti, H. C., Batjer, H., Fest, J. R., Haaland, K. Y., & Lacritz, L. (2018). Cerebrovascular disease. In J. E. Morgan & J. H. Ricker (Eds.), *Textbook of clinical neuropsychology* (2nd ed., pp 350–386). New York, NY: Routledge.
(c) Haaland, K.Y., & Swanda, R.S. (2008). Vascular dementia. In J. E. Morgan & J. H. Ricker (Eds.), *Textbook of clinical neuropsychology* (pp. 762–780). New York, NY: Taylor and Francis.

65. **C—anxiety** *A variety of studies have documented a high frequency of anxiety disorders in Autism spectrum disorder.* ***Please refer to Chapter 14.***

Reference: Rodgers, J., Wigham, S., McConachie, H., Freeston, M., Honey, E., & Parr, J. R. (2016). Development of the anxiety scale for children with autism spectrum disorder (ASC-ASD). *Autism Research, 9*(11), 1205–1215.

66. **A—basal ganglia and thalamus** *The predominant pattern of brain injury in neonates found to be most strongly associated with poor long-term outcome, more so than the severity of injury in any given region, is injury to the basal ganglia and thalamus.* ***Please refer to Chapter 28.***

References:
(a) de Vries, L. S., & Jongmans, M. J. (2008). Long-term outcome after neonatal hypoxic-ischemic encephalopathy. *Archives of Disease in Childhood: Fetal & Neonatal, 95*, F220–F224.
(b) Wachtel, E. V., & Hendricks-Munoz, K. D. (2011). Current management of the infant who presents with neonatal encephalopathy. *Current Problems in Pediatric Adolescent Health Care, 41*, 132–153.

67. **A—lower general cognitive ability and persistent executive dysfunction** *While increased incidence and severity of neurological complications, as well as specific neuropsychological weaknesses are risk factors for long-term outcome, lower IQ and problems in executive functioning have been shown to predict academic and social-emotional functioning.* **Please refer to Chapter 17.**

    Reference: Josev, E. K., & Anderson, P. J. (2018). Executive dysfunction in very preterm children and associated brain pathology. In S. A. Wiebe & J. Karbach (Eds.), *Executive function: Development across the lifespan.* New York, NY: Routledge.

68. **C—a test must have reliability to have validity** *Reliability is critical for test validity, and a test cannot demonstrate validity without prerequisite reliability.* **Please refer to Chapter 9.**

    Reference: Sattler, J. M. (2008). *Assessment of children: Cognitive foundations* (5th ed., p. 31). La Mesa, CA: Jerome M. Sattler.

69. **B—use of valproate during the pregnancy to manage her seizures** *In-utero exposure to valproate has been consistently linked to cognitive and behavioral deficits.* **Please refer to Chapter 21.**

    Reference: Loring, D., Gerard, E. E., & Meador, K. J. (2016). Neurodevelopmental considerations with antiepileptic drug use during pregnancy. In C. A. Riccio & J. R. Sullivan (Eds.), *Pediatric neurotoxicology: Academic and psychosocial outcomes* (pp. 91–105). Switzerland: Springer International Publishing.

70. **A—The nigrostriatal dopamine system is dysfunctional in Parkinson's disease.** *Dopamine arising from the substantia nigra is the primary site of dysfunction in Parkinson's disease. The other alternatives are incorrect. Regarding alternative b, since schizophrenia is most directly associated with a hyperdopaminergic state, most drugs designed to treat it are designed to decrease, not increase, dopamine signal. Not directly involved in Parkinson's disease (alternative c), the mesolimbic circuit is most directly associated with addictive behavior, not the mesocortical system (alternative d).* **Please refer to Chapter 4.**

    Reference: Grace, A. A., Lodge, D. J., & Buffalari, D. M. (2009). Dopamine: CNS pathways and neurophysiology. In L. R. Squire (Ed.), *Encyclopedia of neuroscience* (pp. 539–547). Amsterdam: Elsevier.

71. **A—cognitive behavioral therapy** *Early controlled trials examining FSS used CBT-oriented interventions, although more recent studies have extended the range of interventions employed.* **Please refer to Chapter 37.**

    Reference: Allen, L. A., & Woolfolk, R. L. (2010). Cognitive behavioral therapy for somatoform disorders. *Psychiatric Clinics of North America, 33,* 579–593.

72. **B—temporal lobes and upper brainstem nuclei** *In early stages of Alzheimer's disease the basal nucleus and locus ceruleus are significantly affected. There is also subcortical neuron loss in the nucleus basalis of Meynert (substantia innominata). Neuron loss in the locus ceruleus leads to decreased levels of cholinergic and noradrenergic markers.* **Please refer to Chapter 30.**

    Reference: Ismail, Z., Smith, E. E., Geda, Y., Sultzer, D., Brodaty, H., Smith, G., . . . ISTAART Neuropsychiatric Symptoms Professional Interest Area. (2016). Neuropsychiatric symptoms as early manifestations of emergent dementia: provisional diagnostic criteria for mild behavioral impairment. *Alzheimer's & Dementia, 12*(2), 195–202.

73. **A—6 months post treatment** *The recovery process from the neurotoxic effects of alcohol can be divided into acute (1–2 weeks), subacute (3 weeks to 2 months), and intermediate (2–6 months) phases. Therefore, a clinician should wait at least 6 months to ensure that an individual has moved through the recovery phases (and thus has had sufficient time to gain back any lost function) before drawing conclusions about enduring neurotoxic effects of alcoholism. Any*

*assessments performed earlier than the 6-month period may not be as informative because neuropsychological deficits found will likely improve with time. **Please refer to Chapter 36.***

Reference: Rourke, S. B., & Grant, I. (2009). The neurobehavioral correlates of alcoholism. In I. Grant & K. Adams (Eds.), *Neuropsychological assessment of neuropsychiatric and neuromedical disorders* (pp. 398–454). New York, NY: Oxford University Press.

74. **C—Access to specialized healthcare clinics.** *Although worldwide estimates of ADHD are lower, they likely differ as a function of varying diagnostic methods, practice guidelines, and access to specialized clinics. There is no significant difference between various racial groups. **Please refer to Chapter 16.***

Reference: Faraone, S. v., Asheron, P., Banaschewski, T., Biederman, J., Buitelaar, J. K., Ramos-Quiroga, J. A., . . . Franke, B. (2015). Attention-deficit/hyperactivity disorder. *Nature Reviews: Disease Primers, 1*, 1–23.

75. **B—length of delirium** *Individuals with persistent delirium are about three times more likely to die within 1 year of hospitalization. Every additional 48 hours of delirium increases mortality risk by about 11%. **Please refer to Chapter 27.***

References:
(a) Bellelli, G., Mazzola, P., Morandi, A., Bruni, A., Carnevali, L., Corsi, M., . . . Annoni, G. (2014). Duration of postoperative delirium is an independent predictor of 6-month mortality in older adults after hip fracture. *Journal of the American Geriatrics Society, 63*(7), 1335–1340.
(b) Gonzalez, M., Martinez, G., Calderone, J., Villarroel, L., Yuri, F., Rojas, C., . . . Carrasco, M. (2009). Impact of delirium on short term mortality in elderly inpatients: A prospective cohort study. *Psychosomatics, 50*(3), 234–238.
(c) Kiely, D. K., Marcantonio, E. R., Inouye, S. K., Shaffer, M. L., Bergmann, M. A., Yang, F. M., . . . Jones, R. N. (2009). Persistent delirium predicts greater mortality. *Journal of the American Geriatrics Society, 57*(1), 55–61.

76. **B—alexithymia** *Inability to understand, process, or describe emotions. This symptom is typically seen more often with right-hemisphere dysfunction. Circumlocution (a language symptom) can occur with left-hemisphere damage (e.g., anomia and conduction aphasia); confabulation can be seen with Wernicke's aphasia and transcortical sensory aphasia, as well as more diencephalic-mediated amnesias; anosognosia, while seen with right-hemisphere damage, can also result from frontal dysfunction and is sometimes seen with Wernicke's aphasia. **Please refer to Chapter 5.***

Reference: Loring, D. W. (2015). *INS dictionary of neuropsychology and clinical neurosciences* (2nd ed.). New York, NY: Oxford University Press.

77. **C—GDS includes fewer items that are specific to the physical manifestations of emotional difficulty** *Physical complaints tend to increase with age, and some of the content included on the BDI-II and BAI may be falsely attributed to emotional distress as opposed to common age-related ailments. **Please refer to Chapter 10.***

Reference: Strauss, E., Sherman, E. M. S., & Spreen, O. (2006). *A compendium of neuropsychological tests: Administration, norms, and commentary* (3rd ed.). New York, NY: Oxford University Press.

78. **B—must take into account the motor requirements of the task** *On paper and pencil tasks of processing speed, children with spina bifida are slower, but the differences are not apparent if motor speed is taken into account. **Please refer to Chapter 20.***

Reference: Dennis, M., Sinopoli, K. J., Fletcher, J. M., & Schachar, R. (2008). Puppets, robots, critics, and actors within a taxonomy of attention for developmental disorders. *Journal of the International Neuropsychological Society, 14*, 673–690.

79. **D—superior quadrantanopsia** *Gerstmann syndrome is associated with lesions in the angular-supramarginal gyrus and would not be expected as a consequence of temporal lobectomy. Intellectual disability may be associated with some epilepsy syndromes, but is not caused by temporal lobectomy. However, it is not uncommon for temporal lobectomy to be associated with visual field defects (superior quadrant) due to the anatomy of the optic radiations near the posterior temporal lobe.* **Please refer to Chapter 22.**

References:
(a) Rusconi, E., Pinel, P., Dehaene, S., & Kleinschmidt, A. (2010). The enigma of Gerstmann's syndrome revisited: A telling tale of the vicissitudes of neuropsychology. *Brain, 133*, 320–332
(b) Schmeiser, B., Daniel, M., Kogias, E., Böhringer, D., Egger, K., Yang, S., . . . Gross, N. J. (2017). Visual field defects following different resective procedures for mesiotemporal lobe epilepsy. *Epilepsy & Behavior, 76*, 39–45.

80. **B—Williams syndrome** *Hypersociability and an affinity for music are associated only with Williams syndrome. While individuals with 22q11.2 deletion syndrome may have below average intellectual functioning, they do not have the other characteristics. Individuals with Turner syndrome and Sturge-Weber syndrome typically do not have below average cognitive functioning.* **Please refer to Chapter 18.**

Reference: Martens, M., Wilson, S. J., & Reutens, D. C. (2008). Research review: Williams syndrome: A critical review of the cognitive, behavioral, and neuroanatomical phenotype. *Journal of Child Psychology and Psychiatry, 49*, 576–608.

81. **B—epidural hematoma** *A right sided epidural hematoma is most likely developing resulting in lethargy, confusion, and compression of the third cranial nerve which would cause an enlarged pupil on the ipsilateral side.* **Please refer to Chapter 29.**

Reference: Blumenfeld, H. (2010). *Neuroanatomy through clinical cases* (2nd ed.) Sunderland, MA: Sinauer.

82. **C—HIV encephalitis acquired perinatally** *While hearing loss is commonly associated with bacterial meningitis (about 11%), it is sensorineural hearing loss. Conductive hearing loss is prevalent (20–38%) in children who contract HIV perinatally.* **Please refer to Chapter 23.**

Reference: Laughton, B., Cornell, M., Boivin, M., & Van Rie, A. (2013). Neurodevelopment in perinatally HIV-infected children: A concern for adolescence. *Journal of the International AIDS Society, 16*, 18603.

83. **A—schizophrenia** *Behavioral variant frontotemporal dementia is frequently misdiagnosed as schizophrenia (late onset) due to positive and negative psychotic symptoms of psychosis.* **Please refer to Chapter 32.**

Reference: Gossink, F. T., Vijverberg, E. G., Krudop, W., Scheltens, P., Stek, M. L., Pijnenburg, Y. A., & Dols, A. (2017). Psychosis in behavioral variant frontotemporal dementia. *Neuropsychiatric Disease and Treatment, 13*, 1099–1016.

84. **D—fatigue** *The fatigue associated with multiple sclerosis can be quite debilitating, occurs most days, presents suddenly, tends to worsen as the day progresses, and is more severe than normal fatigue and likely to interfere with quality of life and daily activities. Over the course of the disease, at least 75% of patients with multiple sclerosis report fatigue. It is considered to be one of the most common and most disabling symptoms and is one of the primary reasons for limiting or leaving employment. Further, the primary progressive form of multiple sclerosis, which shows less treatment efficacy, typically leads to earlier disability.* **Please refer to Chapter 24.**

References:
(a) Bradley, T. J., & Chervin, R. D. (2010). Fatigue in multiple sclerosis: mechanisms, evaluation, and treatment. *Sleep, 13*(8), 1061–1067.
(b) Information from the National Multiple Sclerosis Society. www.nationalmssociety.org/Symptoms-Diagnosis/MS-Symptoms/Fatigue

85. **A—alexia without agraphia** *This syndrome relies on damage to the left visual cortex and splenium of the corpus callosum, which produces a right homonymous hemianopia and disconnects visual input processed in the right occipital cortex from the intact left-hemisphere regions necessary for reading and writing. Writing is not impaired because left parietal regions necessary for processing writing are intact, and writing is not fully dependent on visual input (i.e., such patients are able to write but can't read what they have written).* **Please refer to Chapter 26.**

References:
(a) Blumenfeld, H. (2010). *Neuroanatomy through clinical cases* (2nd ed.). Sunderland, MA: Sinauer Associates.
(b) Cullum, C. M., Rossetti, H. C., Batjer, H. Festa, J., Haaland, K. Y., and Lacritz, L. (2017). Cerebrovascular disease. In J. Morgan & J. Ricker (Eds.), *Clinical Neuropsychology* (2nd ed., pp. 350–386). New York, NY: Taylor & Francis.

86. **C—late effect of radiation therapy on brain development** *Studies of children treated for medulloblastoma with surgery, craniospinal radiation, and chemotherapy demonstrate decline in IQ that has been related to disruption in white matter development.* **Please refer to Chapter 25.**

References:
(a) King, T. Z., Wang, L., & Mao, H. (2015). Disruption of white matter integrity in adult survivors of childhood brain tumors: Correlates with long-term intellectual outcomes. *PLoS One, 10*(7), e0131744.
(b) Moxon-Emre, I., Taylor, M. D., Bouffet, E., Hardy, K., Campen, C. J., Malkin, D., . . . Mabbott, D. J. (2016). Intellectual outcome in molecular subgroups of medulloblastoma. *Journal of Clinical Oncology, 34*(34), 4161–4170.
(c) Ris, M. D., Walsh, K., Wallace, D., Armstrong, F. D., Holmes, E., Gajjar, A., . . . Packer, R. J. (2013). Intellectual and academic outcome following two chemotherapy regimens and radiotherapy for average-risk medulloblastoma: COG A9961. *Pediatric Blood & Cancer, 60*(8), 1350–1357.

87. **A—corticobasal syndrome** *Motor symptoms are generally greater on one side for both Parkinson's disease and corticobasal syndrome; however, patients with corticobasal syndrome do not have a strong immediate response to levodopa.* **Please refer to Chapter 33.**

Reference: Parmera, J. B., Rodriguez, R. D., Studart Neto, A., Nitrini, R., & Brucki, S. M. D. (2016). Corticobasal syndrome: A diagnostic conundrum. *Dementia & Neuropsychologia, 10*(4), 267–275.

88. **A—autism, epilepsy, intellectual disability** *While not an exhaustive list, children born extremely preterm are at increased risk for autism, epilepsy, and intellectual disability. Muscular dystrophy is a genetic disorder. Maternal bipolar disorder increases the risk for preterm birth. However, there is no current evidence of an increased risk for bipolar disorder in children born preterm. Spastic diplegia is more commonly associated with preterm birth than spastic hemiplegia.* **Please refer to Chapter 17.**

Reference: Moster, D., Lie, R. T., & Markestad, T. (2008). Long-term medical and social consequences of preterm birth. *New England Journal of Medicine, 359*(3), 262–273.

89. **C—progressive/degenerative course** *There is a high degree of overlap between symptoms of depression and dementia, but one important distinction is that pseudodementia does not typically present with an insidious progression. Cognitive declines associated with depression typically clear, or at least improve, if the depression is treated.* **Please refer to Chapter 34.**

Reference: Wright, S. L., & Persad, C. (2007). Distinguishing between depression and dementia in older persons: Neuropsychological and neuropathological correlates. *Journal of Geriatric Psychiatry and Neurology, 20*(4), 189–198.

90. **A—See the patient and conduct the best exam possible.** *In situations like this the most desirable action is to refer the child to qualified colleagues who can conduct an evaluation*

*in the patient's native language. While this is preferred, it is not always practical or possible. Another alternative is to simply refuse the referral if you are unable to proceed with a valid and reliable evaluation. However, in this scenario the child may have a serious neurologic problem, and the potential benefits of assisting the physician in some fashion are likely to outweigh the risks. Use of an interpreter would be necessary in such situations, but the impact or potential limitations that such practice places on the assessment should always be noted in the report. Without a professional interpreter, the neuropsychologist in this situation would be hard pressed to complete a competent assessment without baseline data or familiarity with the language. In some cases a clinician could consider administering only nonverbal tasks and outline the limitations of the assessment, conclusions, and recommendations in the report. However, in this vignette the concern is regarding language abilities, and a visually based evaluation would not sufficiently address the referral question. Finally the neuropsychologist performing this evaluation should seek supervision or professional consultation from an expert in this particular area to enhance the likelihood of conducting an informed and conscientious examination despite the above listed limitations. **Please refer to Chapter 7.***

General Principles and Ethical Standards: A, B; 1.03, 2.01, 2.02, 2.04

References:
(a) Judd, T., Capetillo, D., Carrion-Baralt, J., Marmol, L. M., San Miguel-Montes, L., Navarrete, M. G., . . . Silver, C. H. (2009). Professional considerations for improving the neuropsychological evaluation of Hispanics: A National Academy of Neuropsychology Education Paper. *Archives of Clinical Neuropsychology, 24*, 127–135.
(b) Mindt, M. R., Byrd, D., Saez, P., & Manly, J. (2010). Increasing culturally competent neuropsychological services for ethnic minority populations: A call to action. *The Clinical Neuropsychologist, 24*, 429–453.

91. **B—10%** *Between 8% and 15% of patients with mild cognitive impairment (MCI) progress to dementia each year following diagnosis, with amnestic MCI being the most likely to lead to Alzheimer's disease.* **Please refer to Chapter 30.**

    Reference: Petersen R. C. (2016). Mild cognitive impairment. *Continuum, 22*(2 Dementia), 404–418.

92. **A—processing speed** *The chronic cognitive effects are limited to executive function, working memory, and decision making (i.e., impulsivity).* **Please refer to Chapter 36.**

    Reference: Gonzalez, R., Vassileva, J., & Scott, J. C. (2009). Neuropsychological consequences of drug abuse. In I. Grant & K. Adams (Eds.), *Neuropsychological assessment of neuropsychiatric disorders* (pp. 455–479). New York, NY: Oxford University Press.

93. **C—nonspecific loss of density of subcortical white matter** *Periventricular white matter loss with scattered lacunar infarctions characterizes Binswanger's disease. The primary pathology underlying multi-infarct dementia is multiple areas of cerebral infarction in both cortical and subcortical cerebral tissue.* **Please refer to Chapter 31.**

    Reference: Mendez, M. F., & Cummings, J. L. (2003). *Dementia: A clinical approach.* (pp. 121–177). Philadelphia, PA: Butterworth Heinemann.

94. **D—neurological and motor abnormalities in an infant can be transient** *The other choices would result in false negative errors.* **Please refer to Chapter 19.**

    Reference: Singer, H. S., Mink, J. W., Gilbert, D. L., & Jankovic, J. (2016). Cerebral palsy. In H. S. Singer, J. W. Mink, D. L. Gilbert & J. Jankovic, *Movement disorders in childhood* (2nd ed., pp. 453–475). San Diego, CA: Academic Press.

95. **D—low** *According to the AACN consensus conference scores, no matter how low, should not be labeled as abnormal, deficient, or impaired because this implies an interpretive judgment. Scores can be low for a variety of reasons one of which is the presence of genuine cognitive impairment.* ***Please refer to Chapter 9.***

Reference: American Academy of Clinical Neuropsychology, Consensus Conference on Uniform Test Score Labeling of Performance Test Results, San Diego, CA. June 2018.

96. **B—impaired pragmatics** *Studies of language deficits in ASD suggest that for most high functioning children and adolescents with ASD, basic grammar, articulation, phonology, and one-word expressive and receptive vocabulary are intact. Conversely, pragmatic language is commonly found to be an area of weakness.* ***Please refer to Chapter 14.***

Reference: Volden, J., Coolican, J., Garon, N., White, J., & Bryson, S. (2009). Brief report: Pragmatic language in autism spectrum disorder: Relationships to measures of ability and disability. *Journal of Autism and Developmental Disorders, 39*(2), 388–393.

97. **A—22q11.2 deletion syndrome** *25–30% of individuals with 22q11.2 deletion syndrome are diagnosed with a psychotic disorder. The other disorders are not associated with increased risk of psychosis.* ***Please refer to Chapter 18.***

Reference: Tang, S. X., & Gur, R. E. (2017). Longitudinal perspectives on the psychosis spectrum in 22q11.2 deletion syndrome. *American Journal of Medical Genetics, 19,* 2192–2202.

98. **A—selective mutism** *This description reflects the characteristics of selective mutism. Social anxiety is characterized by persistent fear of one or more social or performance situations in which the person is exposed to unfamiliar people or to possible scrutiny by others, but does not include an inability to speak. Similarly, specific phobias and panic disorder also do not result in an inability to speak within specific settings.* ***Please refer to Chapter 34.***

Reference: American Psychiatric Association. (2013). *Diagnostic and statistical manual of mental disorders* (5th ed.). Washington, DC: American Psychiatric Publishing.

99. **B—ideational apraxia** *Ideational apraxia is the loss of the ability to plan and execute complex gestures because the individual has lost the understanding of the object's purpose. It differs from ideomotor apraxia in that the individual may understand the purpose of the object but he or she cannot generate the specific movements needed to imitate or demonstrate their use.* ***Please refer to Chapter 5.***

Reference: Scott, J. G., & Schoenberg, M. R. (2011). Deficits in visuospatial/visuoconstructional skills and motor praxis. In M. R. Schoenberg & J. G. Scott (Eds.). *The little black book of neuropsychology: A syndrome-based approach* (pp. 201–218). New York, NY: Springer.

100. **C—Utilization of both SVTs and PVTs would be important given the concerns for secondary gain and lack of typical ADHD developmental history.** *When there is a lack of developmental history and the presence of secondary gain (e.g., extended time for exams), it is extremely important to objectively measure response bias and symptom exaggeration.* ***Please refer to Chapter 16.***

Reference: Harrison, A. G. (2015). Child and adolescent psychoeducational evaluations. In M. W. Kirkwood (Ed.), *Validity testing in child and adolescent assessment* (pp. 185–206). New York, NY: Guildford Press.

101. **A—a more than doubling of the risk of vascular cognitive impairment in aged adults** *Adults ≥ age 60 with white matter hyperintensity volumes > 1 SD above the mean for their*

5-year age group have a greater than doubling of their risk of mild vascular neurocognitive disorder, vascular dementia and stroke. **Please refer to Chapter 31.**

Reference: Debette, S., et al. (2010). Association of MRI markers of vascular brain injury with incident stroke, mild cognitive impairment, dementia, and mortality: The Framingham Offspring Study. *Stroke, 41,* 600–606.

102. **B—secondary-progressive** *The progressive forms of the disease are generally associated with more cognitive impairment, typically both in frequency and severity of symptoms, than what is seen in the relapsing-remitting form of the disease. The progressive forms of MS generally have more cognitive impairment but those with secondary-progressive generally have more cognitive impairment due to disease duration. By definition, these individuals have already had MS (relapsing-remitting) for about 10 years on average. Consequently, by the time they move into the progressive phase, they have been living with the condition longer and are generally more cognitively impaired.* **Please refer to Chapter 24.**

References:
(a) Papathanasiou, A., Messinis, L. Georgious, V. L., & Papathanasopoulos, P. (2014). Cognitive impairment in relapsing remitting and secondary progressive multiple sclerosis patients: Efficacy of a computerized cognitive screening battery. *Neurology, 2014,* 1–7.
(b) Planche., V., Gibelin, M., Cregut., D., Pereira., B., & Clavelou., P. (2016). Cognitive impairment in a population-based study of patients with multiple sclerosis: Differences between late relapsing-remitting, secondary progressive and primary progressive multiple sclerosis. *European Journal of Neurology, 23*(2), 292–289.

103. **D—ε4/ε4** *While having apolipoprotein E ε2 and ε3 alleles may have a protective effect, apolipoprotein E ε4 increases the risk for developing Alzheimer's disease. Having one copy of the ε4 allele increases one's risk through an increase in protein clumps, or amyloid plaques. Having two copies of the ε4 allele increases one's risk further.* **Please refer to Chapter 30.**

Reference: Li, J. Q., Tan, L., Wang, H. F., Tan, M. S., Tan, L., Xu, W., . . . Yu, J. T. (2016). Risk factors for predicting progression from mild cognitive impairment to Alzheimer's disease: A systematic review and meta-analysis of cohort studies. *Journal of Neurology, Neurosurgery, and Psychiatry, 87*(5), 476–484.

104. **D—has widespread effects on the brain** *Hydrocephalus has widespread effects on the brain, including stretching of white matter axons and compressive effects on cortical structures.* **Please refer to Chapter 20.**

Reference: Barkovich, A. J., & Raybaud, C. (2018). *Pediatric neuroimaging* (6th ed.). Philadelphia, PA: Lippincott Williams and Wilkins.

105. **A—Glasgow Coma Score (GCS), length of post-traumatic amnesia (PTA), time to follow commands (TFC)** *Injury severity is best determined by GCS, PTA, and TFC not necessarily the initial CT scan or mental status examination because CT can be negative in moderate to severe TBI and acute mental status can be affected by multiple non-brain injury related issues. Additionally, cognitive and functional outcome from moderate to severe TBI is variable and can be influenced by multiple factors. Thus, test scores do not always directly correlate with the severity of injury. It should also be noted that GCS and TFC can be negatively affected by a variety of non-TBI related factors and thus length of PTA tends to be a better overall indicator with regard to injury severity. Radiologic studies are central in differentiating between uncomplicated and complicated mild TBI.* **Please refer to Chapter 29.**

References:
(a) Nakase-Richardson, R., Sherer, M., Seel, R. T., Hart, T., Hanks, R., Arango-Lasprilla, J. C., . . . Hammond, F. (2011). Utility of post-traumatic amnesia in predicting 1-year productivity following traumatic brain injury: Comparison of the Russel and Mississippi PTA classification intervals, *Journal of Neurology, Neurosurgery, and Psychiatry, 82*(5), 494–499.

(b) Roebuck-Spencer, T., & Sherer, M. (2018). Moderate and severe traumatic brain injury, In Morgan, J. E., & Ricker, J. H. (Eds.). *Textbook of clinical neuropsychology* (2nd ed., pp. 387–410). New York, NY: Taylor and Francis.

(c) Williams, M., Rapport, L., Hanks, R., Millis, S., & Greene, H. (2013). Incremental validity of neuropsychological evaluations to computer tomography in predicting long-term outcomes after traumatic brain injury. *Clinical Neuropsychology, 27*(3), 356–375.

106. **D—oxygen toxicity or hypoxia that can worsen over time** *ROP can result from oxygen toxicity related to the excessive use of oxygen after birth or hypoxia. In some preterm babies, ROP worsens over time.* **Please refer to Chapter 17.**

     Reference: Shah, P. K., Prabhu, V., Karandikar, S. S., Ranjan, R., Narendran, V., & Kalpana, N. (2016). Retinopathy of prematurity: Past, present and future. *World Journal of Clinical Pedi*atrics, *5*(1), 35–46.

107. **A—cerebrovascular disease and Alzheimer's disease (AD)** *The base rates of these differing dementing disorders are such that AD is the most common co-occurring pathology with cerebrovascular disease. Furthermore, there are data strongly suggesting that cerebrovascular disease hastens amyloid deposition significantly, but no such data regarding alpha-synuclein or the tauopathies that characterize the Lewy body diseases and the frontotemporal dementias.* **Please refer to Chapter 31.**

     Reference: Chui, H. C., & Ramirez-Gomez, L. (2015). Clinical and imaging features of mixed Alzheimer and vascular pathologies. *Alzheimer's Research & Therapy, 7*(1), 21.

108. **D—both medial and lateral limbic circuits must be damaged to cause amnesia** *This conclusion was first reached by Mishkin in 1978, when he examined effects of combined hippocampal and amygdala lesions on memory, and has subsequently been refined in many investigations.* **Please refer to Chapter 4.**

     Reference: Bauer, R. M., & Asken, B. (2018). The three amnesias. In J. E. Morgan & J. H. Ricker (Eds.), *Textbook of clinical neuropsychology* (pp. 678–700). New York, NY: Psychology Press.

109. **D—ruling out a medical condition in a patient whose medical evaluations have been equivocal** *The clinical interview, review of available records pertaining to an individual's medical and psychiatric history, and specific diagnostic criteria are absolutely essential in arriving at a formal psychological diagnosis.* **Please refer to Chapter 10.**

     Reference: Weiner, I. B., & Greene, R. L. (2008). *Handbook of personality assessment.* Hoboken, NJ: John Wiley & Sons.

110. **C—ADHD** *30–50% of children with neurofibromatosis type 1 are diagnosed with ADHD; 4–8% are diagnosed with intellectual disability. Children with neurofibromatosis type 1 are not at greater risk for schizophrenia or Autism spectrum disorders. Schizophrenia is associated with 22q11.2 deletion syndrome, while intellectual disability is associated with tuberous sclerosis, Sturge-Weber syndrome, William syndrome, fragile X syndrome, Prader Willi syndrome, and Angelman syndrome.* **Please refer to Chapter 18.**

     Reference: Janusz, J. (2011). A case of neurofibromatosis type 1. In J. E. Morgan, I. S. Baron, & J. H. Ricker (Eds.), *Casebook of clinical neuropsychology.* New York, NY: Oxford University Press.

111. **C—30%** *Since monozygotic (identical) twins have largely the same genes, they have the highest concordance rate for schizophrenia. The risk for schizophrenia decreases from these levels depending on the degree of the genetic relationship. First-degree relatives have closer to a 10% risk, and second-degree relatives have closer to a 2% risk. The 80–85% statistic is the often-cited overall heritability for schizophrenia. Note that if schizophrenia had heritability*

of 100% (e.g., if it were due to a single gene with 100% penetrance, like a simple Mendelian genetic trait), then the monozygotic twin of someone with schizophrenia would have a 50% risk. **Please refer to Chapter 35.**

Reference: Lieberman, J. A., & First, M. B. (2018). Psychotic disorders. *New England Journal of Medicine, 379*(3), 270–280.

112. **A—progressive supranuclear palsy** *Axial rigidity and falls are common early symptoms of progressive supranuclear palsy. REM behavioral symptoms may or may not be present in progressive supranuclear palsy and it is not part of the diagnostic criteria.* **Please refer to Chapter 33.**

Reference: Ling, H. (2016). Clinical approach to progressive supranuclear palsy. *Journal of Movement Disorders, 9,* 3–13.

113. **D—reading disabilities** *Substantial research demonstrates the effectiveness of intervention to improve reading in children (and adults) with reading disabilities. There is far less research on interventions to improve written expression and math skills.* **Please refer to Chapter 15.**

References:
(a) Fletcher, J. M., Lyon, G. R., Fuchs, L. S., & Barnes, M. A. (2018). *Learning disabilities: From identification to intervention* (2nd ed.). New York, NY: Guilford Press.
(b) National Joint Committee on Learning Disabilities (NJCLD). (2011). *Learning disabilities: Implications for policy regarding research and practice.* http://www.ldonline.org/about/partners/njcld#reports

114. **C—Higher incidence of delirium follows urinary tract infection in the elderly** *All of the statements are true but C is the best answer as it is most supportive of the brain reserve hypothesis (see also Chapter 3, Important Theories in Neuropsychology: A Historical Perspective).* **Please refer to Chapter 27.**

References:
(a) Girard, T. D., Jackson, J. C., Pandharipande, P. P., Pun, B. T., Thompson, J. L., Shintani, A. K., . . . Ely, E. W. (2010). Delirium as a predictor of long-term cognitive impairment in survivors of critical illness. *Critical Care Medicine, 38*(7), 1513–1520.
(b) Trzepacz, P. T., & Meagher, D. J. (2009). Neuropsychiatric aspects of delirium. In S. C. Yudofsky & R. E. Hales (Eds.), *Textbook of neuropsychiatry and behavioral neurosciences* (pp. 445–518). Washington, DC: American Psychiatric Publishing.

115. **C—right frontal damage has been associated with depression** *Actually, left frontal damage is typically associated with depression; the rest are true.* **Please refer to Chapter 5.**

Reference: Stuss, D. T., Benson, D. F., Kaplan, E. F., Weir, W. S., Naeser, M. A., Lieberman, I., & Ferrill, D. (1983). The involvement of orbitofrontal cerebrum in cognitive tasks. *Neuropsychologia, 21,* 235–248.

116. **B—hyporeflexia** *UMN lesions are often characterized by weakness, hyperreflexia, and increased tone. Weakness, atrophy, fasciculations, and hyporeflexia can be indicative of lower motor neuron lesions, making this the incorrect option.* **Please refer to Chapter 6.**

References:
(a) Blumenfeld, H. (2011). *Neuroanatomy through clinical cases* (2nd ed.). Sunderland, MA: Sinauer Associates.
(b) Goldberg, S. (2017). *The four-minute neurological exam.* (2nd ed.). Miami, FL: MedMaster.
(c) Simon, R. P., Aminoff, M., & Greenberg, D. A. (2018). *Clinical neurology* (10th ed.). New York, NY: Lange Medical Books/McGraw-Hill Education.

117. **D—the Babinski and the Wartenberg's signs** *Individuals with UMN demonstrate increased reflexes (hyperreflexia). In particular, adults will show the Babinski sign (fanning of the toes and upward flexion of the big toe) and Wartenberg's sign (involuntary abduction).* **Please refer to Chapter 6.**

References:
(a) Blumenfeld, H. (2011). *Neuroanatomy through clinical cases* (2nd ed.). Sunderland, MA: Sinauer Associates.
(b) Goldberg, S. (2017). *The four-minute neurological exam*. (2nd ed.). Miami, FL: MedMaster.
(c) Simon, R. P., Aminoff, M., & Greenberg, D. A. (2018). *Clinical neurology* (10th ed.). New York, NY: Lange Medical Books/McGraw-Hill Education.

118. **A—executive functions** *In utero and childhood exposure to lead has been linked most consistently to deficits in attention/executive functions and visuospatial skills.* ***Please refer to Chapter 21.***

> **Reference:** Dietrich, K. N. (2010). Environmental toxicants. In K. O. Yeates, M. D. Ris, H. G. Taylor, & B. F. Pennington (Eds.), *Pediatric neuropsychology: Research, theory, and practice* (pp. 211–264). New York, NY: Guilford Press.

119. **B—childhood absence epilepsy** *The natural history of epilepsy syndromes is quite variable, but, of the syndromes listed, childhood absence epilepsy is the most likely to remit during early adolescence. However, up to 15% of children with childhood absence epilepsy will go on to develop juvenile myoclonic epilepsy.* ***Please refer to Chapter 22.***

> **Reference:** Berg, A. T., Levy, S., Testa, F., & Blumenfeld, H. (2014). Long term seizure remission in childhood absence epilepsy: Might initial treatment matter? *Epilepsia, 55*(4), 551–557.

120. **B—Test 3, Test 4, Test 2, Test 1** *Converting each to score to one common metric will allow for their comparisons. Using percentiles, Test 1 = 93, Test 2 = 84, Test 3 = 60, Test 4 = 69.* ***Please refer to Chapter 8.***

> **Reference:** Nunnally, J. C., & Bernstein, I. H. (1994). *Psychometric theory.* New York, NY: McGraw-Hill.

121. **C—growth reduction** *Prenatal exposure to marijuana is associated with fetal growth reduction and reduced gestational duration, whereas children exposed to alcohol in utero are often small for gestational age and may continue to show growth deficiency as adolescents and adults.* ***Please refer to Chapter 21.***

> **Reference:** Gray, T. R., Eiden, R. D., Leonard, K. E., Connors, G. J., Shisler, S., & Huetis, M. A. (2010). Identifying prenatal cannabis exposure and effects of concurrent tobacco exposure on neonatal growth. *Clinical Chemistry, 56*, 1442–1450.

122. **A—intact fluency, intact comprehension, impaired repetition** *The cardinal symptom of conduction aphasia is impaired repetition without significant impairment in fluency and comprehension. Impaired fluency, intact comprehension, and impaired repetition is characteristic of Broca's aphasia. Fluent speech, impaired comprehension, and impaired repetition is characteristic of Wernicke's aphasia. Impaired fluency, impaired comprehension, and intact repetition is characteristic of mixed transcortical aphasia.* ***Please refer to Chapter 26.***

> **Reference:** Cullum, C. M., Rossetti, H. C., Batjer, H. Festa, J., Haaland, K. Y., & Lacritz, L. (2017). Cerebrovascular disease. In J. Morgan & J. Ricker (Eds.), *Clinical neuropsychology* (2nd ed., pp. 350–386). New York, NY: Taylor & Francis.

123. **D—pain** *Motor impairment, fatigue and social isolation negatively impact quality of life but pain is the more common complaint.* ***Please refer to Chapter 19.***

> **Reference:** McCormick, A. (2018). Quality of life. In C. P. Panteliadis (Ed.), *Cerebral palsy: A multidisciplinary approach* (3rd ed., pp. 335–341). Cham, Switzerland: Springer International.

124. **A—leukoencephalopathy** *Leukoencephalopathy is related to cerebral white matter damage. It is one of the known neurotoxic side effects of methotrexate therapy. The frequency and severity is related to the dose, cumulative exposure, and other factors. It is noted as white matter*

*hyperintensities on T2-weighted MR imaging, which may be transient or persistent. **Please refer to Chapter 25.***

References:
(a) Bhojwani, D., Sabin, N. D., Pei, D., Yang, J. J., Khan, R. B., Panetta, J. C., . . . Relling, M. V. (2014). Methotrexate-induced neurotoxicity and leukoencephalopathy in childhood acute lymphoblastic leukemia. *Journal of Clinical Oncology, 32*(9), 949–959.
(b) Cheung, Y. T., Sabin, N. D., Reddick, W. E., Bhojwani, D., Liu, W., Brinkman, T. M., . . . Krull, K. R. (2016). Leukoencephalopathy and long-term neurobehavioural, neurocognitive, and brain imaging outcomes in survivors of childhood acute lymphoblastic leukaemia treated with chemotherapy: A longitudinal analysis. *Lancet Haematology, 3*(10), e456–e466.

125. **B—anoxia** *Anoxia involves a total loss of oxygen in the arterial blood and tissues. Anoxia usually results from sudden and severe medical events such as cardiac arrest. Whereas anoxia and ischemia are viewed as separate processes, in severe cases they usually coexist. **Please refer to Chapter 28.***

Reference: Hopkins, R. O. (2018). Hypoxia of the central nervous system. In J. E. Morgan & J. H. Ricker (Eds.), *Textbook of clinical neuropsychology* (2nd ed., pp. 494–506). New York, NY: Taylor & Francis.

APPENDIX F

Third Full-Length Practice Examination Answers

1. **B—uncommon**   *The large majority of individuals with substance abuse disorders misuse multiple substances.* **Please refer to Chapter 36.**

   Reference: McCabe, S. E., West, B. T., Jutkiewicz, E. M., & Boyd, C. J. (2017). Multiple DSM-5 substance use disorders: A national study of U.S. adults. *Human Psychopharmacology, 32*(5), e2625.

2. **C—possible** *The score of 28 on Trial 1 is invalid per post-publication research on the TOMM, but the other scores (46, 45) fall just within the valid range, hence this is likely an indeterminate PVT finding. In the context of a clear external incentive to do poorly, indeterminate results on a single PVT along with multiple SVT abnormalities results in a diagnosis of "possible" MND according to the Slick criteria.* **Please refer to Chapter 12.**

   Reference: Slick, D. J., Sherman, E. M., & Iverson, G. L. (1999). Diagnostic criteria for malingered neurocognitive dysfunction: Proposed standards for clinical practice and research. *Clinical Neuropsychologist, 13,* 545–561.

3. **D—neglect; right parietal CVA** *The behavior is indicative of a left neglect which is consistent with right CVA.* **Please refer to Chapter 5.**

   Reference: Lunven, M., & Bartolomeo, P. (2017). Attention and spatial cognition: Neural and anatomical substrates of visual neglect. *Annals of Physical Medicine and Rehabilitation Medicine, 60*(3), 124–129.

4. **C—premature birth** *The other choices are actual risk factors but not as major.* **Please refer to Chapter 19.**

   References:
   (a) Kent, R. M. (2013). Cerebral palsy. In M. J. Aminoff, F. Boller, & D. F. Swaab (Series Eds.) & M. P. Barnes & D. C. Good (Eds.), *Handbook of clinical neurology: Neurological rehabilitation* (3rd ser., Vol. 110, pp. 443–459). New York, NY: Elsevier.
   (b) Singer, H. S., Mink, J. W., Gilbert, D. L., & Jankovic, J. (2016). Cerebral palsy. In H. S. Singer, J. W. Mink, D. L. Gilbert, & J. Jankovic (Eds.), *Movement disorders in childhood* (2nd ed., pp. 453–475). San Diego, CA: Academic Press.

5. **D—Contact your state ethics committee and the referring provider to discuss the situation and review options.** *In situations in which safety is of immediate concern, confidentiality can be breached in the interest of protecting the patient or others from imminent harm. In this vignette the patient has clear impairments which likely will place him and others at high risk. Although in some states it might be appropriate to contact the Department of Motor Vehicles (DMV), in other states psychologists are not allowed to do so. Thus, the most appropriate first step would be to collaborate with the referring provider and or an ethics committee to discuss options to address the situation. Although B is a reasonable option with some patients, in this case the patient has already left the*

building, and his presentation indicates that attempts to contact him are unlikely to be successful and will not adequately address the safety concern. **Please refer to Chapter 7.**

General Principles and Ethical Standards: A, B, D, E; 4.01, 4.02, 4.03, 4.04, 4.05, 5.01, 6.01, 6.02, 9.02, 9.04

Reference: Knapp, S., & VandeCreek, L. (2005). Ethical and patient management issues with older, impaired drivers. *Professional Psychology: Research and Practice, 36,* 197–202.

6. **B—decoding skills; reading comprehension** *Academic abilities among middle to high school students with high-functioning autism are generally in the average range, but difficulties are most commonly observed on tasks that require inferential reasoning. Most commonly, students have difficulty with reading comprehension, written expression and mathematical problem solving.* **Please refer to Chapter 14.**

Reference: Keen, D., Webster, A., & Ridley, G. (2016). How well are children with autism spectrum disorder doing academically at school? An overview of the literature. *Autism, 20*(3), 276–294.

7. **B—corticosteroids** *Patients on beta blockers and or anticonvulsants often complain of sedation, difficulty concentrating, or memory problems, but these medications are not often associated with delirium. SSRI's are quite safe relative to TCA's and much less likely to result in confusion unless overused or multiple agents are prescribed (i.e., serotonin syndrome). The term steroid psychosis has been used to describe conditions in which patients develop delirium and or mania often following prolonged use of corticosteroids to treat chronic illness (**e.g.,** lupus, rheumatoid arthritis, lymphoma, etc.).* **Please refer to Chapter 27.**

Reference: Ahmed, S., Leurent, B., & Sampson, E. L. (2014). Risk factors for incident delirium among older people in acute hospital medical units: A systematic review and meta-analysis. *Age and Ageing, 43,* 326–333.

8. **A—cardiac MIBG scintigraphy** *Cardiac uptake reduction precedes motor impairment and dopamine degeneration in Parkinson's disease patients, and cardiac MIBG SPECT can accurately distinguish Parkinson's disease from corticobasal syndrome, progressive supranuclear palsy, and multiple system atrophy. The heart to mediastinum ratio is decreased in Parkinson's disease, irrespective of disease duration or severity.* **Please refer to Chapter 33.**

Reference: Nicastro, N., Valentina, F., & Burkhard, P. R. (2018). The role of molecular imaging in assessing degenerative parkinsonism—An updated review. *Swiss Medical Weekly, 148,* 14621.

9. **D—modality-specific anomia** *Any sensory specific cognitive deficit is likely a disconnection problem. In this case, unable to name visual objects, but can name with tactile presentation.* **Please refer to Chapter 3.**

Reference: Catania, M., & Mesulam, M. (2008). What is a disconnection syndrome? *Cortex, 44,* 1–3.

10. **B—delusions and hallucinations** *The term "positive symptoms" was originally intended to signify an excess of normal function, but has come to be understood more specifically to refer to delusions and hallucinations. This stands in contrast to the negative symptoms (that term originally used to describe the absence of affective expression, motivation, etc.) and disorganization symptoms (which include bizarre behavior, attentional impairment, alogia, and formal thought disorder).* **Please refer to Chapter 35.**

Reference: American Psychiatric Association. (2013). *Diagnostic and statistical manual of mental disorders* (5th ed.). Washington, DC: American Psychiatric Publishing.

11. **D—true negatives/(true negatives + false negatives)** *This refers to the negative predictive power of the test, or the degree to which a negative test result (i.e., indicative of normal performance) can be relied upon that a particular condition or illness is truly absent.* **Please refer to Chapter 8.**

Reference: Slick, D. J. (2006). Psychometrics in neuropsychological assessment. In E. Strauss, E. M. S. Sherman, & O. Spreen (Eds), *A compendium of neuropsychological tests* (3rd ed., pp. 3–43). New York, NY: Oxford.

12. **A—left spinal accessory nerve XI dysfunction** *Sternocleidomastoid strength and trapezius muscle lift are innervated by the ipsilateral cranial nerve XI.* **Please refer to Chapter 6.**

References:
(a) Blumenfeld, H. (2011). *Neuroanatomy through clinical cases* (2nd ed.). Sunderland, MA: Sinauer Associates.
(b) Goldberg, S. (2017). *The four-minute neurological exam* (2nd ed.). Miami, FL: MedMaster.
(c) Greenberg, D., Aminoff, M., & Simon, R. (2012). *Clinical neurology* (8th ed.). New York, NY: Lange Medical Books/McGraw-Hill.

13. **C—Bipolar II Disorder** *As noted in DSM criteria, bipolar II disorder is unique in that hypomanic episodes are present but do not rise to a level of severity noted in bipolar I and cyclothymic disorders.* **Please refer to Chapter 34.**

Reference: American Psychiatric Association. (2013). *Diagnostic and statistical manual of mental disorders* (5th ed.). Washington, DC: American Psychiatric Publishing.

14. **D—childhood absence epilepsy (CAE)** *This type often presents as staring spells, and has a characteristic EEG pattern of 3 Hz spike and wave discharges. Seizures can be brief, and are self-limiting with 65–85% showing remission prior to or during adolescence.* **Please refer to Chapter 22.**

Reference: Matricardi, S., Verrotti, A., Chiarelli, F., Cerminara, C., & Curatolo, P. (2014). Current advances in childhood absence epilepsy. *Pediatric Neurology, 50*(3), 205–212.

15. **A—sensitivity** *Because of the condition of interest, it is more important to avoid false positive than false negative errors.* **Please refer to Chapter 9.**

Reference: Bokhari, E., & Hubert, L. (2015). A new condition for assessing the clinical efficiency of a diagnostic test. *Psychological Assessment, 27*(3), 745–754.

16. **B—insomnia** *Common side effects of psychostimulant medication include decreased appetite, increased heart rate and blood pressure, and insomnia.* **Please refer to Chapter 16.**

Reference: Faraone, S. V., Asheron, P., Banaschewski, T., Biederman, J., Buitelaar, J. K., Ramos-Quiroga, J. A., . . . Franke, B. (2015). Attention-deficit/hyperactivity disorder. *Nature Reviews: Disease Primers, 1*, 1–23.

17. **A—mammillary bodies and dorsomedial thalamus** *The two-system theory of amnesia states that amnesia results from damage to some element of the medial and lateral limbic circuit. This alternative is the only one that contains an element from the medial system (mammillary bodies) together with an element from the lateral system (dorsomedial thalamus).* **Please refer to Chapter 4.**

Reference: Bauer, R. M., Gaynor, L. S., Moreno, C., & Kuhn, T. (2018). Episodic and semantic memory disorders. In L. D. Ravdin & H. L. Katzen (Eds.), *Handbook on the neuropsychology of aging and dementia: Clinical handbooks in neuropsychology*. New York, NY: Springer Science and Business Media.

18. **C—hemorrhagic etiology** *Hemorrhagic stroke has a much higher mortality rate in the first 6 months (about 50%) than ischemic stroke.* **Please refer to Chapter 26.**

Reference: Mohr, J. P., Wolf, P. A., Grotta, J. C., Moskowitz, M. A., Mayberg, M. R., & von Kummer, R. (2011). *Stroke: Pathophysiology, diagnosis and management* (5th ed.). Philadelphia, PA: Saunders.

19. **D—MMPI-2 Restructured Clinical Scale 1** *Although many studies examining patients with FSS suggest specific deficits in attention, psychomotor speed, and working memory, these deficits attenuate or disappear when emotional stress factors are considered.* ***Please refer to Chapter 37.***

Reference: Suhr, J. (2003). Neuropsychological impairment in fibromyalgia: Relation to depression, fatigue, and pain. *Journal of Psychosomatic Research, 55*, 321–329.

20. **D—Williams syndrome** *Individuals with Klinefelter syndrome and adrenoleukodystrophy typically do not have IQ in the range of moderate intellectual disability. While fragile X syndrome is associated with moderate intellectual disability, elf-like features are only associated with Williams syndrome.* ***Please refer to Chapter 18.***

Reference: Martens, M., Wilson, S. J., & Reutens, D. C. (2008). Research review: Williams syndrome: A critical review of the cognitive, behavioral, and neuroanatomical phenotype. *Journal of Child Psychology and Psychiatry, 49*, 576–608.

21. **C—gunshot wound** *Language disorders can occur in the acute stage of recovery following TBI due to acceleration-deceleration type injury but they rarely continue long term. On the other hand, penetrating injuries often result in focal or more circumscribed impairments.* ***Please refer to Chapter 29.***

Reference: Vas, A., Chapman, S., & Cook, L. (2015). Language impairments in traumatic brain injury: A window into complex cognitive performance. In J. Grafman & A. Salazar (Eds.), *Handbook of clinical neurology* (pp. 497–510). Philadelphia, PA: Elsevier.

22. **B—visuospatial deficits** *Impaired memory, processing speed, and attention are common cognitive problems following hypoxia/ischemia. Visuospatial deficits are less commonly seen.* ***Please refer to Chapter 28.***

Reference: Smania, N., Avesani, R., Roncari, L., Ianes, P., Girardi, P., Varalta, V., . . . Gandolfi, N. (2012). Factors predicting functional and cognitive recovery following severe traumatic, anoxic, and cerebrovascular brain damage. *Journal of Head Trauma Rehabilitation, 28*, 131–140.

23. **C—periventricular hemorrhage infarction and periventricular leukomalacia** *These injuries are the most common neurologic complications of premature birth and result from hypoxia-ischemia and intraventricular hemorrhage, and impaired cerebral blood flow.* ***Please refer to Chapter 17.***

Reference: Kinney, H. C., & Volpe, J. J. (2017). Encephalopathy of prematurity: Neuropathology. In Volpe, J., Inder, T., Darras, B., De Vries, L. S., Plessis, A., Neil, J., & Perlman, J. (Eds.), *Volpe's neurology of the newborn* (6th ed. pp. 389–404). Philadelphia, PA: Elsevier.

24. **A—amyotrophic lateral sclerosis** *FTD is known to occur in about 9% of patients with ALS and does not commonly co-occur with the other conditions listed.* ***Please refer to Chapter 32.***

Reference: Wooley, S. C., & Strong, M. J. (2015). Frontotemporal dysfunction and dementia in amyotrophic lateral sclerosis. *Neurologic Clinics, 33*, 787–805.

25. **D—the association between life expectancy and severity of ID** *A recent meta-analysis of population-based studies estimated the prevalence of ID to be 10.37/1000 or about 1% of the population. Along with delayed diagnosis, the fact that life expectancy is shortened for individuals with more severe forms of ID accounts for the lowered prevalence relative to expectation based on the bell curve prediction (2.5%).* ***Please refer to Chapter 13.***

Reference: Maulik, P. K., Mascarenhas, M. N., Mathers, C. D., Dua, T., & Saxena, S. (2011). Prevalence of intellectual disability: A meta-analysis of population-based studies. *Research in Developmental Disabilities, 32*, 419–436.

26. **C—synaptic density** *While amyloid plaques occur primarily before observed cognitive changes, neurofibrillary tangles, neuron loss and particularly synaptic loss parallel the severity of cognitive decline. Please refer to Chapter 30.*

Reference: Pike, K. E., Savage, G., Villemagne, V. L., Ng, S., Moss, S. A., . . . Rowe, C. C. (2007). β-amyloid imaging and memory in non-demented individuals: Evidence for preclinical Alzheimer's disease. *Brain, 130*, 2837–2844.

27. **B—decreased memory and mesial temporal sclerosis** *Side effects of treatment with antiepileptic drugs commonly include decreased processing speed. Studies have also shown that in persons with epilepsy there is a relation between decreased overall white matter volume and processing speed, as well as involvement of frontal lobe systems in seizure onset or propagation. Please refer to Chapter 22.*

Reference: Dow, C., Seidenberg, M., & Hermann, B. (2004). Relationship between information processing speed in temporal lobe epilepsy and white matter volume. *Epilepsy and Behavior, 5*, 919–925.

28. **C—delirium and drug reaction/interaction** *Post-transplant patients are at high risk for complications that cause delirium, such as infection, transplant rejection, or iatrogenic effects of drugs given to reduce risk of transplant rejection (e.g., calcineurin inhibitors (CNIs). CNIs can also cause posterior reversible encephalopathy syndrome (PRES), which is characterized by lethargy, headache, confusion, visual disturbance, seizures, and posterior changes on neuroimaging. Both symptoms and radiologic findings can resolve with prompt control of blood pressure and/or discontinuation of the CNI. Although the patient has risk factors for vascular cognitive impairment and stroke the clinical description is most consistent with delirium. Please refer to Chapter 27.*

Reference: Heinrich, T. W., & Marcangelo, M. (2009). Psychiatric issues in solid organ transplantation. *Harvard Review Psychiatry, 17*(6), 398–406.

29. **D—verbal episodic memory, category fluency, and naming** *Episodic memory impairment is the hallmark neuropsychology feature of Alzheimer's disease, with deficits in confrontation naming usually following. Category fluency is also often reduced in Alzheimer's disease. Please refer to Chapter 30.*

References:
(a) Cullum, C. M., & Lacritz, L. H. (2012). Neuropsychological assessment. In M. Weiner & A. M. Lipton (Eds.), *Clinical manual of Alzheimer's disease and other dementias* (pp. 65–88). Arlington, VA: American Psychiatric Publishing.
(b) Smith, G., & Butts, A. (2018). Dementia. In J. E. Morgan & J. H. Ricker (Eds.), *Textbook of clinical neuropsychology* (2nd ed., pp. 717–741). New York, NY: Taylor & Francis Group.

30. **A—acquisition and encoding** *Individuals with SUDs typically display a pattern of performance in which there is difficulty with acquisition and encoding of information, but not with retention once adjustments are made for amount of information acquired. Please refer to Chapter 36.*

Reference: Fernández-Serrano, M. J., Pérez-García, M., & Verdejo-García, A. (2011). What are the specific vs. generalized effects of drugs of abuse on neuropsychological performance? *Neuroscience & Biobehavioral Reviews, 35*(3), 377–406.

31. **C—cerebellum** *The extrapyramidal system is a set of subcortical circuits and pathways that includes the corpus striatum (caudate nucleus, putamen, and globus pallidus) together with the subthalamic nucleus, substantia nigra, red nucleus, and brain stem reticular formation. Some authorities include descending spinal cord tracts other than the corticospinal tracts (such as the vestibulospinal, rubrospinal, tectospinal, and reticulospinal tracts) in the extrapyramidal motor system. Please refer to Chapter 33.*

Reference: Waxman, S. G. (Ed.). (2009). *Clinical neuroanatomy* (26th ed.). New York, NY: McGraw-Hill.

32. **B—temporal lobe pathology and hyperintensities in the orbitofrontal regions** *Multiple studies in individuals with herpes simplex virus have documented T2 hyperintensities in mesiotemporal and orbitofrontal lobes.* **Please refer to Chapter 23.**

Reference: Bradshaw, M. J., & Venkatesan, A. (2016). Herpes simplex virus-1 encephalitis in adults: Pathophysiology, diagnosis, and management. *Neurotherapeutics, 13*(3), 493–508.

33. **C—left inferior middle cerebral artery territory** *Fluent speech with auditory comprehension deficits and impaired repetition are the characteristics of Wernicke's (fluent, sensory, receptive) aphasia, which is most commonly associated with damage to the left temporal and parietal regions and their interconnections (areas in the distribution of the left inferior middle cerebral artery).* **Please refer to Chapter 26.**

References:
(a) Blumenfeld, H. (2010). *Neuroanatomy through clinical cases* (2nd ed.). Sunderland, MA: Sinauer Associates.
(b) Swanda, R. M., Haaland, K. Y. (2017). Clinical neuropsychology. In B. J. Sadock, V. A. Sadock, & P. Ruiz, (Eds), *Comprehensive textbook of psychiatry,* (10th ed., pp. 976–993), Philadelphia, PA: Lippincott Williams & Wilkins.

34. **A—Parkinson's disease** *Life expectancy in treated Parkinson's disease is almost the same as age-matched controls, while mean survival is less than 10 years from time of diagnosis to death for patients with progressive supranuclear palsy, Lewy body dementia, and corticobasal syndrome.* **Please refer to Chapter 33.**

Reference: Forsaa, E. B., Larsen, J. P., Wetzel-Larsen T., & Alves, G. (2010). What predicts mortality in Parkinson disease? A prospective population-based long-term study. *Neurology, 75,* 1270–1276.

35. **C—older age** *Older age and lower cognitive reserve were related to post-treatment decline in processing speed in a prospective study with patients with breast cancer (without chemo; with chemo) and a group of normal controls. Chemotherapy and disease factors are believed to affect a range of physiological mechanisms and cognitive impairments result from a combination of age, comorbidities, treatment. Radiation therapy is less likely to affect cognitive function directly, but may affect lung and heart function, which can contribute to comorbidities and frailty.* **Please refer to Chapter 25.**

Reference: Ahles, T. A., Saykin, A. J., McDonald, B. C., Li, Y., Furstenberg, C. T., Hanscom, B. S., . . . Kaufman, P. A. (2010). Longitudinal assessment of cognitive changes associated with adjuvant treatment for breast cancer: Impact of age and cognitive reserve. *Journal of Clinical Oncology, 28*(29), 4434–4440.

36. **D—presence of stereotyped language** *Social (pragmatic) communication disorder (SPCD) was added to the DSM-5 in part because of changes in Autism spectrum disorder (ASD) criteria. The diagnosis was developed to capture individuals who present with deficits in social communication, but have no history of restricted and repetitive behaviors (who may have previously qualified for the diagnosis of pervasive developmental disorder-not otherwise specified; PDD-NOS). Diagnostic criteria for SPCD outlines similar social communication deficits seen in ASD (including deficits in nonverbal communication, difficulty with turn taking, and limited inferential reasoning), but notes that individuals with SPCD cannot evidence restricted and repetitive behaviors (including stereotyped language).* **Please refer to Chapter 14.**

Reference: Swineford, L. B., Thurm, A., Baird, G., Wetherby, A. M., & Swedo, S. (2014). Social (pragmatic) communication disorder: A research review of this new DSM-5 diagnostic category. *Journal of Neurodevelopmental Disorders, 6,* 41.

37. **B—domain-specific theory** *One or more central processors are thought to control specific functions. Working memory operates as a set of sub-systems, controlled by a limited-capacity executive system.* **Please refer to Chapter 3.**

    Reference: Baddeley, A. D. (2002). The psychology of memory. In A. D. Baddelely, M. D. Kopelman, & B. A. Wilson (Eds.), *The handbook of memory disorders* (pp. 3–16). Chichester, UK: Wiley.

38. **D—alcohol use** *Women who consume marijuana frequently drink alcohol during pregnancy, making it difficult to parse out the impact of prenatal exposure to marijuana.* **Please refer to Chapter 21.**

    Reference: Parris, L. (2016). Opiates and marijuana use during pregnancy: Neurodevelopmental outcomes. In C. A. Riccio & J. R. Sullivan (Eds.), *Pediatric neurotoxicology: Academic and psychosocial outcomes* (pp. 77–89). Switzerland: Springer International Publishing.

39. **C—amyloid deposition** *The neuropathology of schizophrenia is thought to involve abnormal embryogenesis, excessive synaptic pruning, and disruptions of white matter integrity, not amyloid deposition.* **Please refer to Chapter 35.**

    Reference: Karlsgodt, K. H., Daqiang, S., Jimenez, A. M., Lutkenhoff, E. S., Whillhite, R., Van Erp, T. G. M., & Cannon, T. D. (2008). Developmental disruptions in neural connectivity in the pathophysiology of schizophrenia. *Development and Psychopathology, 20,* 1297–1327.

40. **A—the probability of the individual having the disease when the test result is positive** *The post-test probability is the probability the individual has a disease with a positive test result and is based on the post-test odds, which is the increase in the odds of a person having the disease with a positive test result from the pre-test odds.* **Please refer to Chapter 9.**

    Reference: Heneghan, C., & Badenoch, D. (2006). Evidence-based medicine toolkit (2nd ed.). Malden, MA: Blackwell Publishing.

41. **D—spastic diplegia** *Due to the proximity of the corticospinal tracts with the periventricular area.* **Please refer to Chapter 17.**

    Reference: Rutherford, M. A., Supramaniam, V., Ederies, A., Chew, A., Bassi, L., Groppo, M., . . . Ramenghi, L. A. (2010). Magnetic resonance imaging of white matter diseases of prematurity. *Neuroradiology, 52*(6), 505–521.

42. **A—relapsing-remitting** *Relapsing-remitting multiple sclerosis is the most common disease course and is characterized by acute attacks with recovery between events.* **Please refer to Chapter 24.**

    References:
    (a) Information from the National MS Society.http://www.nationalmssociety.org/about-multiple-sclerosis/what-we-know-about-ms/what-is-ms/four-disease-courses-of-ms/index.aspx
    (b) Lublin, F. D., Reingold, S. C., Cohen, J. A., Cutter, G. R., Sorensen, P. S., Thompson, A. J., . . . Bebo, B. (2014). Defining the clinical course of multiple sclerosis: The 2013 revisions. *Neurology, 83*(3), 278–286.

43. **C—word-finding and language comprehension** *See Chui and Ramirez-Gomez (2018) or Cullum et al. (2018) for reviews of neuropsychological findings in vascular cognitive impairment and vascular dementia.* **Please refer to Chapter 31.**

    References:
    (a) Chui, H. C., & Ramirez-Gomez, L. (2018). Vascular cognitive impairment: Executive dysfunction in the era of the human brain connectome. In Miller, B. L., & Cummings, J. L. (Eds.) *The human frontal lobes: Functions and disorders* (3rd ed., pp. 357–367). New York, NY: Guilford.
    (b) Cullum, C. M., Rosetti, H. C., Batjer, H., Fest, J. R., Haaland, K. Y., & Lacritz, L. (2018). Cerebrovascular disease. In J. E. Morgan & J. H. Ricker (Eds.), *Textbook of clinical neuropsychology* (2nd ed., pp. 350–386). New York, NY: Routledge.

44. **B—abnormal involuntary movements** *The upper extremities tend to be more impaired. Choices a and c are more consistent with severe spastic quadriplegia.* **Please refer to Chapter 19.**

Reference: Singer, H. S., Mink, J. W., Gilbert, D. L., & Jankovic, J. (2016). Cerebral palsy. In H. S. Singer, J. W. Mink, D. L. Gilbert & J. Jankovic (Eds.), *Movement disorders in childhood* (2nd ed., pp. 453–475). San Diego, CA: Academic Press.

45. **C—mania** *Mania and psychosis are fairly uncommon complications following TBI.* **Please refer to Chapter 29.**

References:
(a) Draper, K., Ponsford, J., & Schonberger, M. (2007). Psychosocial and emotional outcomes 10 years following traumatic brain injury. *Journal of Head Trauma Rehabilitation, 22,* 278–287.
(b) Sherer, M., Yablon, S. A., & Nick, T. G. (2014). Psychotic symptoms as manifestations of the posttraumatic confusional state: Prevalence, risk factors, and association with outcome. *Journal of Head Trauma Rehabilitation, 29,* 11–18.

46. **B—homogeneity of variance between tests** *Variability in test performance refers to the reasons (or variables) that test performance is similar or different among individuals. For example, people with TBI often share a common source of variance in measured abilities, such as processing speed. The concept of homogeneity of variance states that these "variances in common" among similar groups should vary predictably based on their cause and are thus termed homogeneous.* **Please refer to Chapter 9.**

Reference: Irwing, P., Booth, T., & Hughes, D. J. (2018). *The Wiley handbook of psychometric testing.* New York, NY: Wiley.

47. **D—anxiety and depression** *Psychosocial problems, including anxiety and depression, often emerge in adolescents and adults because of social isolation, teasing and lack of acceptance by peers, avoidance by peers because of their disability, and the increased stress on the family.* **Please refer to Chapter 20.**

Reference: Copp, A. J., Adzick, A. S., Chitty, L. S., Fletcher, J. M., Holmbeck, G. N., & Shaw, G. M. (2015). Spina bifida. *Nature Disease Primers, 1,* 1–18.

48. **B—fluent aphasia** *Fluent aphasia affecting lexical access to the meaning of words will directly impact measures of intelligence dependent on verbal ability and many nonverbal tests because comprehension of instructions may be impaired.* **Please refer to Chapter 5.**

Reference: Caplan, D. (2012). Aphasic syndromes. In K. M. Heilman & E. Valenstein (Eds.), *Clinical neuropsychology* (5th ed., pp. 22–41). New York, NY: Oxford University Press.

49. **C—logopenic variant** *The logopenic variant of FTD is considered by some to actually be a variant of Alzheimer's disease because the majority of logopenic variant cases have Alzheimer's disease pathology.* **Please refer to Chapter 32.**

Reference: Leyton, C. E., Hodges, J. R., Piquet, O., & Ballard, K. J. (2017). Common and divergent neural correlates of anomia in amnestic and logopenic presentations of Alzheimer's disease. *Cortex, 86,* 45–54.

50. **A—symbolic comparison** *Comparison (symbolic or non-symbolic) and number line estimation skills are collectively referred to as numerosity. While procedural and conceptual counting are important in the development of math skills, they are not considered numerosity.* **Please refer to Chapter 15.**

Reference: Sasanguie, D., De Smedt, B., Defever, E., & Reynvoet, B. (2012). Association between basic numerical abilities and mathematics achievement. *British Journal of Developmental Psychology, 30*(2), 344–357.

51. **B—Mild Neurocognitive Disorder** *While at first glance it would appear that your patient has symptoms of depression, the nature of her emotional changes in the absence of a precipitating event, psychiatric history, or medical change is concerning. Rather, her symptoms are commonly seen in patients with mild cognitive impairment/mild neurocognitive disorder, which, in addition to forgetfulness, can include a decrease in initiative and increase in apathy, the latter which can result in increased isolation.* **Please refer to Chapter 30.**

References:
(a) Jekel, K., Damian, M., Wattmo, C., Hausner, L., Bullock, R., Connelly, P. J., . . . Kramberger, M. G. (2015). Mild cognitive impairment and deficits in instrumental activities of daily living: a systematic review. *Alzheimer's Research & Therapy, 7*(1), 17.
(b) Reppermund, S., Sachdev, P. S., Crawford, J., Kochan, N. A., Slavin, M. J., Brodaty, H., . . . Sachdev, P. S. (2010). The relationship of neuropsychological function to instrumental activities of daily living in mild cognitive impairment. *International Journal of Geriatric Psychiatry, 26*(8), 843–852.˙

52. **A—the side of the body contralateral to the port-wine birthmark** *Seizures are seen on the side of the body opposite to the port-wine birthmark.* **Please refer to Chapter 18.**

Reference: Comi, A. E. (2015). Sturge-Weber syndrome. In M. P. Islam & E. S. Roach (Eds), *Handbook of Clinical Neurology, Vol. 132: Neurocutaneous syndromes* (pp. 157–168). New York, NY: Elsevier.

53. **B—They can't provide informed consent but can give informed assent.** *Currently there are no validated procedures to determine the level of capacity required for informed assent in this population. Although, with few exceptions, informed consent and permission is required from the parent or guardian, patients should be involved in assent for such procedures at a developmentally appropriate level. Children and adolescents are by definition vulnerable, and care should be taken to ensure that they are involved in their own care appropriately. Answer A is wrong because adolescents can be emancipated but young children cannot.* **Please refer to Chapter 7.**

General Principles and Ethical Standards: A, B, E; 3.10, 4.02, 4.05

Reference: Donders, J. (2013). Ethical issues in pediatric traumatic brain injury rehabilitation. *Journal of Head Trauma Rehabilitation, 28,* 485–488.

54. **B—the heel-shin test and the Romberg test** *Cerebellar functions in the lower extremities are examined by the heel-shin-test, in which the patient lies on his back, lifts the heel of his foot, and moves it in a straight line along his opposite shin up to the knee. In the Romberg test, patients are asked to stand with their feet together and close their eyes. The "Romberg sign" is when unsteadiness occurs within several seconds of closing the eyes. The Rinne test assesses auditory function via the vestibulocochlear nerve (CN VIII). During this test, a vibrating tuning fork is placed just outside each ear to assess air conduction and on the forehead or mastoid to assess bone conduction. Tongue protrusion can be used to assess hypoglossal nerve (CN XII) function, and visual field testing is not routinely conducted to assess cerebellar dysfunction.* **Please refer to Chapter 6.**

References:
(a) Blumenfeld, H. (2011). *Neuroanatomy through clinical cases* (2nd ed.). Sunderland, MA: Sinauer Associates.
(b) Goldberg, S. (2017). *The four-minute neurological exam* (2nd ed.). Miami, FL: MedMaster.
(c) Greenberg, D., Aminoff, M., & Simon, R. (2012). *Clinical neurology* (8th ed.). New York, NY: Lange Medical Books / McGraw-Hill.

55. **C—GABA** *Gamma-aminobutyric acid is a major inhibitory neurotransmitter in the CNS, playing a role in helping to induce relaxation and sleep and in preventing overexcitation. Depletion is associated with a heightening of the anxious response. Dopamine, serotonin, and norepinephrine have all been found to be involved in depressive disorders.* **Please refer to Chapter 34.**

References:
(a) Kandel, E. R. (2013). Disorders of mood and anxiety. In E. R. Kandel, J. H. Schwartz, T. M. Jessell, A. A. Siegelbaum, & A. J. Hudspeth (Eds.), *Principles of neural science* (5th ed., pp. 1402–1424). New York, NY: McGraw-Hill.
(b) Stein, M. B., & Steckler, T. (2010). *Behavioral neurobiology of anxiety and its treatment.* New York, NY: Springer.

56. **A—common in the first 2 years of life, and may continue to be observed during the preschool years** *Typically developing infants often engage in repetitive, rhythmic behaviors and these behaviors may take up more than one third of waking hours around 24 months of age. While repetitive motor movements peak at approximately 24 months of age, inflexibility, ritualistic behaviors, and restricted interests are often observed during the preschool years in normative development.* **Please refer to Chapter 14.**

Reference: Lewis, M., & Kim, S. J. (2009). The pathophysiology of restricted repetitive behavior. *Journal of Neurodevelopmental Disorders, 1,* 114–132.

57. **C—hippocampal sclerosis** *Although all of the listed pathologies are associated with adult epilepsy, the most common pathology is mesial temporal sclerosis, accounting for up to two thirds of cases.* **Please refer to Chapter 22.**

Reference: Blumcke, I., Thom, M., Aronica, E., Armstrong, D., Bartolomei, F., Bernasconi, A., . . . Spreafico, R. (2013). International consensus classification of hippocampal sclerosis in temporal lobe epilepsy: A Task Force report from the ILAE Commission on Diagnostic Methods. *Epilepsia, 54,* 1315–1329.

58. **D—75** *Most patients are diagnosed between the ages of 70 and 79, with 74.7 years as the mean based on National Institutes of Health figures.* **Please refer to Chapter 30.**

Reference: Alzheimer's Association. (2015). National Institutes of Health (NIH) State-of-the-Science Conference.

59. **A—lower IQ, executive functioning weaknesses, and academic problems** *The child likely meets criteria for intrauterine growth restriction. Independent of prematurity and neonatal complications, specific neuropsychological impairments can be observed as the function and structure of the CNS is impacted by growth restriction in utero. Motor deficits and difficulties with visuospatial processing are more commonly associated with preterm birth.* **Please refer to Chapter 17.**

Reference: Geva, R., Eshel, R., Leitner, Y., Valevski, A. F., & Harel, S. (2006). Neuropsychological outcome of children with intrauterine growth restriction: A 9-year prospective study. *Pediatrics, 118,* 91–100.

60. **D—acute radiation toxicity** *Radiation toxicity can develop early on after treatment and can include somnolence, presumably related to transient demyelination and neuroinflammation.* **Please refer to Chapter 25.**

Reference: Greene-Schloesser, D., Robbins, M. E., Peiffer, A. M., Shaw, E. G., Wheeler, K. T., & Chan, M. D. (2012). Radiation-induced brain injury: A review. *Frontiers in Oncology, 2,* 73.

61. **B—a continuing history of significant psychopathology** *F-scale elevations may arise from three underlying sources, including inconsistent or variable response style, genuine (usually severe) psychopathology, and symptom exaggeration. Seeing as there is not evidence of content non-responsivity on VRIN or TRIN, and no evidence of symptom exaggeration on Fp, an*

F-scale elevation of this magnitude most likely reflects genuine psychopathology. **Please refer to Chapter 10.**

References:
(a) Graham, J. R. (2006). *MMPI-2: Assessing personality and psychopathology* (4th ed.). New York, NY: Oxford University Press.
(b) Graham, J. R. (2012). *MMPI-2: Assessing personality and psychopathology* (5th ed.). New York, NY: Oxford University Press.

62. **C—individual placement with support** *As compared to traditional vocational rehabilitation services, individually based supportive interventions have shown greater effects for obtaining and maintaining stable employment in people with schizophrenia.* **Please refer to Chapter 35.**

Reference: Kilian, R., Lauber, C., Kalkan, R., Dorn, W., Rossler, W., Wiersma, D. . . . Becker, T. (2012). The relationships between employment, clinical status, and psychiatric hospitalisation in patients with schizophrenia receiving either IPS or a conventional vocational rehabilitation programme. *Social Psychiatry and Psychiatric Epidemiology, 47*, 1381–1389.

63. **A—deficits in visuospatial skills and right-sided motor deficits** *Poor visuospatial functioning after an early left hemisphere stroke may reflect the phenomenon of crowding, and can occur even with left-hemisphere damage, while language functioning may remain intact. Motor functioning does not tend to reorganize as much as cognitive functions, so left-sided motor deficits are unlikely after a left hemisphere stroke.* **Please refer to Chapter 26.**

Reference: Stiles, J., Nass, R. D., Levine, S. C., Moses, P., & Reilly, J. S. (2010). Perinatal stroke. In K. O. Yeates, M. D. Ris, H. G. Taylor, & B. F. Pennington, *Pediatric neuropsychology: Research, theory, and practice* (2nd ed., pp. 181–210). New York, NY: Guilford.

64. **C—Problems related to premature aging are common.** *Gross motor problems and pain are not expected to decrease. Life expectancy can be shortened.* **Please refer to Chapter 19.**

References:
(a) Hanna, S. E., Rosenbaum, P. L., Bartlett, D. J., Palisano, R. J., Walter, S. D., Avery L., & Russell, D. J. (2009). Stability and decline in gross motor function among children and youth with cerebral palsy aged 2 to 21 years. *Developmental Medicine and Child Neurology, 51*, 295–302.
(b) Kent, R. M. (2013). Cerebral palsy. In M. J. Aminoff, F. Boller, & D. F. Swaab (Series Eds.) & M. P. Barnes & D. C. Good (Eds.), *Handbook of clinical neurology: Neurological rehabilitation* (3rd ser., Vol. 110, pp. 443–459). New York, NY: Elsevier.

65. **A—intentional disorders** *Damage to the medial frontal cortex results in syndromes such as akinesia, bradykinesia, apathy, and, in most severe form, akinetic mutism.* **Please refer to Chapter 4.**

Reference: Mendoza, J., & Foundas, A. (2008). *Clinical neuroanatomy: A neurobehavioral approach.* New York, NY: Springer Science and Business.

66. **C—found in clusters throughout multiple brain areas** *Neurofibrillary tangles are often found in hippocampal and amygdaloid areas, and in specific brainstem nuclei—nucleus basalis of Meynert in the forebrain, nucleus raphe nucleus in the midbrain, and the locus ceruleus at the anterior pontine level.* **Please refer to Chapter 30.**

References:
(a) Kumar, A., & Singh, A. (2015). A review on Alzheimer's disease pathophysiology and its management: An update. *Pharmacological Reports, 67*(2), 195–203.
(b) Schoenberg, M. R., & Duff, K. (2011). Dementias and mild cognitive impairment in adults. In M. R. Schoenberg & J. G. Scott (Eds.), *The little black book of neuropsychology: A syndrome-based approach* (pp. 357–403). New York, NY: Springer.
(c) Selkoe, D. J., & Hardy, J. (2016). The amyloid hypothesis of Alzheimer's disease at 25 years. *EMBO Molecular Medicine, 8*(6), 595–608.

67. **D—processing speed** *Tests that tap processing speed tend to be among the most sensitive to changes following TBI. Although verbal comprehension and perceptual reasoning scores might decline due to focal injuries causing aphasia or visuospatial impairment it is much more common to observe declines in processing speed and executive aspects of attention due to the diffuse impact of TBI.* **Please refer to Chapter 29.**

References:
(a) Roebuck-Spencer, T., & Sherer, M. (2018). Moderate and severe traumatic brain injury. In Morgan, J. E., & Ricker, J. H. (Eds.), *Textbook of clinical neuropsychology* (2nd ed., pp. 387–410). New York, NY: Taylor and Francis.
(b) Yeates, K. O., & Brooks, B. L. (2018). Traumatic brain injury in children and adolescents. In J. E. Morgan, & J. H. Ricker (Eds.), *Textbook of clinical neuropsychology* (2nd ed., pp. 141–157). New York, NY: Taylor and Francis.

68. **C—enlarged head circumference** *Enlarged head size is one of the few consistently replicated findings among individuals with Autism spectrum disorder.* **Please refer to Chapter 14.**

Reference: Hazlett, H. C., Gu, H., Munsell, B. C., Kim, S. H., Styner, M., Wolff, J. J., ... IBIS Network. (2017). Early brain development in infants at high risk for autism spectrum disorder. *Nature, 542*(7641), 348–351.

69. **A—typical of that commonly seen in AD, with memory impairment greater than executive dysfunction** *Chui and Ramirez-Gomez (2015) review the literature to date and find that, although the pattern of neuropsychological impairment in vascular cognitive impairment (VCI) is highly variable, when VCI and AD co-occur the neuropsychological profile is dominated by AD.* **Please refer to Chapter 31.**

Reference: Chui, H. C., & Ramirez-Gomez, L. (2018). Vascular cognitive impairment: Executive dysfunction in the era of the human brain connectome. In Miller, B. L., & Cummings, J. L. (Eds.), *The human frontal lobes: Functions and disorders* (3rd ed., pp. 357–367). New York, NY: Guilford Press.

70. **A—anti-NMDA receptor encephalitis** *The most consistent predictor of positive outcome in patients with anti-NMDA receptor encephalitis is early and effective immunotherapy. In patients with tumors (commonly ovarian teratomas), tumor removal is also correlated with positive outcome.* **Please refer to Chapter 23.**

Reference: Finke, C., Kopp, U. A., Prüss, H., Dalmau, J., Wandinger, K. P., & Ploner, C. J. (2012). Cognitive deficits following anti-NMDA receptor encephalitis. *Journal of Neurology, Neurosurgery, and Psychiatry, 83*(2), 195–198.

71. **B—externalizing disorders** *Prenatal nicotine exposure is consistently linked to externalizing disorders, namely ADHD and Oppositional Defiant Disorder. Neurocognitive findings are equivocal.* **Please refer to Chapter 21.**

Reference: Singer, L. T., Min, M. O., Lang, A., & Minnes, S. (2016). In utero exposure to nicotine, cocaine, and amphetamines. In C. A. Riccio & J. R. Sullivan (Eds.), *Pediatric neurotoxicology: Academic and psychosocial outcomes* (pp. 51–76). Switzerland: Springer International Publishing.

72. **A—emotional regulation** *The behavioral variant of frontotemporal dementia begins with changes in personality, interpersonal conduct, and emotional regulation, reflecting progressive disintegration of the underlying neural circuits.* **Please refer to Chapter 32.**

Reference: Piguet, O., Hornberger, M., Mioshi, E., & Hodges, J. R. (2011). Behavioral-variant frontotemporal dementia: Diagnosis, clinical staging, and management. *The Lancet Neurology, 10*, 162–172.

73. **D—show impairment on measures of fine motor skills** *The motor impairment similarity is due to cerebellar compromise.* **Please refer to Chapter 20.**

Reference: Fletcher, J. M., & Dennis, M. (2010). Spina bifida and hydrocephalus: Modeling variability in outcome domains. In K. O. Yeates, M. D. Ris, H. G. Taylor, & B. F. Pennington (Eds.), *Pediatric neuropsychology: Research, theory, and practice* (2nd ed., pp. 3–25). Hillsdale, NJ: Erlbaum.

74. **B—anterior communicating artery (ACoA) aneurysm** *An aneurysm of the ACoA would be an example of a pathology producing diencephalic amnesia with resultant confabulation typically involves frontal systems; the other three etiologies typically affect medial temporal areas.* **Please refer to Chapter 5.**

Reference: Turner, M. S., Cipolotti, L., & Shallice, T. (2010). Spontaneous confabulation, temporal context confusion and reality monitoring: A study of three patients with anterior communicating artery aneurysms. *Journal of the International Neuropsychological Society,16,* 984–994.

75. **C—prior probability distribution, likelihood function, and new data** *In frequentist analysis (as opposed to Bayesian models), one chooses a model (likelihood function) for the available data and then calculates either a p value or confidence interval. Alternatively, Bayesian models can be calculated to provide direct probability statements about parameters of interest, but one must first summarize prior information about the parameters of interest. The three elements of any Bayesian model are the prior probability distribution, likelihood function, and new data. When these three elements are put together, the posterior probability distribution can be generated.* **Please refer to Chapter 8.**

Reference: Price, L. R. (2017). *Psychometric methods: Theory in practice.* New York, NY: Guilford Press.

76. **B—ADHD-inattentive type with sluggish cognitive tempo** *Recent factor analytic studies have consistently shown that many symptoms of sluggish cognitive tempo (SCT) covary with the inattentive ADHD symptoms; however, there is consistent evidence that there are unique components of SCT (lethargy, underactivity, and slowness) that appear to be distinct from the inattention associated with ADHD.* **Please refer to Chapter 16.**

Reference: Jacobson, L. A., Murphy-Bowman S. C., Pritchard A. E., Tart-Zelvin, A., Zabel, T. A., Mahone, E. M. (2012). Factor structure of a sluggish cognitive tempo scale in clinically-referred children. *Journal of Abnormal Child Psychology, 40,* 1327–1337.

77. **B—mammillary bodies** *Neuronal loss in the mammillary bodies, thalamus, and cerebellum, along with hemorrhagic lesions in the paraventricular and periaqueductal grey matter are the most vulnerable to WKS.* **Please refer to Chapter 36.**

Reference: Isenberg-Grzeda, E., Kutner, H. E., & Nicholson, S. E. (2012). Wernicke-Korsakoff-Syndrome: Under-recognized and under-treated. *Psychosomatics, 53,* 507–516.

78. **D—characterized in part by loss of speech and cranial nerve deficits** *Cerebellar mutism is a complication of posterior fossa surgery and seen more commonly in children than adults. Symptoms gradually resolve over time, but motor coordination and cognitive/psychological issues may persist.* **Please refer to Chapter 25.**

References:
(a) Lanier, J. C., & Abrams, A. N. (2017). Posterior fossa syndrome: Review of the behavioral and emotional aspects in pediatric cancer patients. *Cancer, 123*(4), 551–559.
(b) Tamburrini, G., Frassanito, P., Chieffo, D., Massimi, L., Caldarelli, M., & Di Rocco, C. (2015). Cerebellar mutism. *Child Nervous System, 31*(10), 1841–1851.

79. **A—he has had proper instruction in math and has built a foundation for his current college class** *This student is unlikely to have a learning disability, if he made it to college with As and Bs in math. Although the other areas should certainly be addressed, the answer most relevant to a specific problem in math is A.* **Please refer to Chapter 15.**

Reference: Fletcher, J. M., Lyon, G. R., Fuchs, L. S., & Barnes, M. A. (2018). *Learning disabilities: From identification to intervention* (2nd ed.). New York, NY: Guilford Press.

80. **A—glutamate** *Glutamate is the only potential TBI related excitotoxic agent listed.* ***Please refer to Chapter 29.***

   Reference: Benarroch, E. E. (2009). Oligodendrocytes: Susceptibility to injury and involvement in neurologic disease. *Neurology, 72*(20), 1779–1785.

81. **C—benzodiazepines** *This patient clearly has an anxiety disorder that is impacting his ability to function. Although occasionally used in patients with an agitated depression, benzodiazepines are more often used to treat anxiety-based disorders. Furthermore, benzodiazepines are sedating and classified as depressants. Thus, while they can help alleviate anxiety they can exacerbate or worsen depressive symptoms.* ***Please refer to Chapter 34.***

   Reference: Stein, M. B., & Steckler, T. (2010). *Behavioral neurobiology of anxiety and its treatment.* New York, NY: Springer.

82. **B—Fs** *Fs and Fp-r are both good at differentiating simulators from patients with somatoform disorders and medical patients. Fs was more sensitive, while Fp-r was more specific.* ***Please refer to Chapter 37.***

   Reference: Sellbom, M., Wygant, D., & Bagby, M. (2012). Utility of the MMPI-2-RF in detecting non-credible somatic complaints. *Psychiatry Research, 197*(3), 295–301.

83. **C—Conduct the assessment with the son present but tell him he cannot assist.** *The ethical conflict here is between test security and ensuring that the patient receives appropriate care (i.e., beneficence). The psychologist must also consider the well-established impact of a third party on test performance. In this vignette the evaluation will likely assist with differential diagnosis and treatment planning even if it is brief in nature. Her symptoms have not improved in 3 weeks, and waiting would delay care unnecessarily, possibly leading to delayed clinical diagnosis and or poor overall outcome. Although there is some risk to test security, it is not sufficient to deny the patient access to the service. In cases where two ethical standards are in conflict, the neuropsychologist must decide which takes precedence in that specific circumstance or situation. A nondisclosure agreement is excessive and unnecessary as the odds of the son memorizing and sharing specific test questions with third parties are unlikely.* ***Please refer to Chapter 7.***

   ### General Principles and Ethical Standards: A, B, E; 3.04, 4.06, 9.02, 9.11

   References:
   (a) American Academy of Clinical Neuropsychology. (2001). Policy statement on the presence of third party observers in neuropsychological assessment. *The Clinical Neuropsychologist, 15*, 433–439.
   (b) American Psychological Association. (2014). Guidelines for psychological practice with older adults. *American Psychologist, 69*, 34–65.

84. **D—formication hallucinations/drug intoxication** *Release hallucinations typically occur following acute loss of sensory input (e.g., blindness). Visceral hallucinations are experienced as odd or unlikely internal sensations as opposed to external ones. Hypnogogic hallucinations may occur normally when someone is in the process of falling asleep. Formication hallucinations can occur with drug intoxication and or during drug withdrawal. The history indicates that the patient was likely recently exposed to an illicit substance that is causing the hallucinations.* ***Please refer to Chapter 27.***

   References:
   (a) Abraham, G., & Zun, L. S. (2017). Delirium and dementia. In R. M. Walls (Ed.), *Rosen's emergency medicine: Concepts and clinical practice* (pp. 1278–1288). Philadelphia, PA: Elsevier.
   (b) Rothberg, M. B., Herzig, S. J., Pekow, P. S., Avrunin, J., Lagu, T., & Lindenauer, P. K. (2013). Association between sedating medications and delirium in older inpatients. *Journal of the American Geriatrics Society, 61*, 923–930.

85. **A—gist recall** *Normal aging is associated with declines in multiple cognitive domains and specific functions, although the ability to recall the gist of stories is relatively less affected by aging than recall of details.* ***Please refer to Chapter 30.***

Reference: Harada, C. N., Natelson Love, M. C., & Triebel, K. L. (2013). Normal cognitive aging. *Clinics in Geriatric Medicine, 29*(4), 737–752.

86. **D—both patients with right TLE and left TLE show depression** *Although some studies have suggested a lateralized mood effect, the majority of studies show higher incidence of depression and anxiety in persons with epilepsy, regardless of laterality of seizure onset. More important factors are severity of epilepsy and seizure frequency.* ***Please refer to Chapter 22.***

Reference: Adams, S. J., O'Brien, T. J., Lloyd, J., Kilpatrick, C. J., Salzberg, M. R., & Velakoulis, D. (2008). Neuropsychiatric morbidity in focal epilepsy. *British Journal of Psychiatry, 192*, 464–469.

87. **A—attentional problems** *Numerous studies suggest that attentional difficulties are the most common comorbidity in children with Autism spectrum disorder (ASD). Studies have shown that the among children with ASD, comorbidity rate of ADHD is in the 40–70% range.* ***Please refer to Chapter 14.***

Reference: Antshel, K. M., Zhang-James, Y., Wagner, K. E., Ledesma, A., & Faraone, S. V. (2016). An update on the comorbidity of ADHD and ASD: A focus on clinical management. *Review of Neurotherapeutics, 16*(3), 279–293.

88. **C—deficits in letter fluency and set-shifting tasks** *Neither a dissociation between Trails A and B nor micrographia are characteristic of VaD. Early changes in personality and behavior are characteristic of frontal lobe dementia and are far less common in VaD. Measures of executive function and impaired letter fluency are commonly reported cognitive changes in VaD.* ***Please refer to Chapter 31.***

Reference: Cullum, C. M., Rosetti, H. C., Batjer, H., Fest, J. R., Haaland, K. Y., & Lacritz, L. (2018). Cerebrovascular disease. In J. E. Morgan & J. H. Ricker (Eds.), *Textbook of clinical neuropsychology* (2nd ed., pp. 350–386). New York, NY: Routledge.

89. **B—Inform him of his HIV disease status in an age-appropriate way.** *Regardless of low average intellectual abilities and or cognitive impairments patients are entitled to be informed of their condition and treatment options in an age-appropriate way. Minors and patients with a guardian may not be able to provide informed consent but they can assent to evaluation and or treatment.* ***Please refer to Chapter 23.***

Reference: Lesch, A., Swartz, L., Kagee, A., Moodley, K., Kafaar, Z., Myer, L., & Cotton, M. (2007). Paediatric HIV/AIDS disclosure: Towards a developmental and process-oriented approach. *AIDS Care, 19*(6), 811–816.

90. **B—episodic** *Memory for temporal events.* ***Please refer to Chapter 5.***

Reference: Loring, D. W. (2015). *INS dictionary of neuropsychology and clinical neurosciences* (2nd ed.). New York, NY: Oxford University Press.

91. **C—persons at both extremes of the age spectrum** *Seniors often have reduced cognitive and cerebral reserve, thus making them more vulnerable to the short and long term consequences of hypoxic/ischemic injury. Children, especially those under the age of 4, are in a critical period of neurodevelopment and anoxic/hypoxic injury can disrupt/interrupt this process contributing to increased risk for long-term cognitive and neuropsychiatric complication.* ***Please refer to Chapter 28.***

Reference: Huang, B. Y., & Castillo, M. (2008). Hypoxic ischemic brain injury: Imaging findings from birth to adulthood. *RadioGraphics, 28*, 417–439.

92. **A—extended time for tests** *Given reduced processing speed, which is the most common cognitive problem in multiple sclerosis, affected individuals are likely to benefit from extended time for tests. In higher education settings, students with disabilities must meet the same standards (attendance, coursework) as unaffected peers and therefore, shortened assignments or unlimited excused absences are unlikely to be approved as an accommodation in college. Current research does not show a clear pattern of reading problems; however, individual assessment would inform this need depending on factors unique to the patient. Please refer to Chapter 24.*

    Reference: MacAllister, W. S., Christodoulou, C., Milazzo, M., Preston, T. E., Serafin, D., Krupp, L. B., & Harder, L. (2013). Pediatric multiple sclerosis: What we know and where are we headed? *Child Neuropsychology, 19*(1), 1–22.

93. **A—asymmetric motor dysfunction** *Motor symptoms are generally greater on one side for both Parkinson's disease and corticobasal syndrome. Please refer to Chapter 33.*

    Reference: Alexander S. K., Rittman, T., Xuereb, J. H., Bak, T. H., Hodges, J. R., & Rowe, J. B. (2014). Validation of the new consensus criteria for the diagnosis of corticobasal degeneration. *Journal of Neurological Surgery and Psychiatry, 85*, 923–927.

94. **B—Down syndrome** *Down syndrome is the most common chromosomal abnormality or genetic cause of intellectual disability and occurs in 1.2 in 1,000 live births. Please refer to Chapter 13.*

    Reference: King, B. H., Toth, K. E., Hodapp, R. M., & Dykens, E. M. (2009). Intellectual disability. In B. J. Sadock, V. A. Sadock, & P. Ruiz (Eds.), *Comprehensive textbook of psychiatry* (9th ed., pp. 3444–3474). Philadelphia, PA: Lippincott, Williams, & Wilkins.

95. **A—less than 40%** *The amount of variance that is often explained in reading and math skills when doing cognitive modeling ranges between 75–85%. In contrast, only about 25–30% of variance in attention is accounted for by cognitive predictors such as inhibition, processing speed, and working memory. Please refer to Chapter 16.*

    Reference: Peterson, R. L., Boada, R., McGrath, L. M., Willcutt, E. G., Olson, R. K., & Pennington, B. F. (2017). Cognitive prediction of reading, math, and attention: Shared and unique influences. *Journal of Learning Disabilities, 50*, 408–421.

96. **D—a 17-year-old, Caucasian woman with disabling deafness** *The standardization samples that accompany each of these inventories were aged 18 years or older. Please refer to Chapter 10.*

    References:
    (a) Graham, J. R. (2006). *MMPI-2: Assessing personality and psychopathology* (4th ed.). New York, NY: Oxford University Press.
    (b) Graham, J. R. (2012). *MMPI-2: Assessing personality and psychopathology* (5th ed.). New York, NY: Oxford University Press.
    (c) Morey, L. C. (2007). *Personality Assessment Inventory professional manual* (2nd ed.). Lutz, FL: Psychological Assessment Resources.

97. **B—form, color, and motion** *These three channels of information have different origins in retina, different thalamic and cortical targets, and different projections to association cortex. Other alternatives within this item are all variations on the "form," for which some cortical specialization exists but no evidence of distinct channel separation. Please refer to Chapter 4.*

    Reference: Blumenfeld, H. (2010). *Neuroanatomy through clinical cases* (2nd ed., pp. 467–468). Sunderland, MA: Sinauer Associates.

98. **C—Given cultural and educational background, more detailed queries should be made before concluding that his visual and auditory perceptions reflect a psychotic disorder.**

Certain religious beliefs and sensory experiences may be common in some cultures, while considered unusual in others. Additional factors including cerebrovascular disease may pose vulnerability for symptoms of all kinds, and the additional information that he has visual hallucinations (not just auditory hallucinations) might further lead you to suspect other causes of symptoms that are not on the schizophrenia spectrum. But before concluding that these reflect pathological symptoms at all, you need to take the cultural, educational and soci-oeconomic factors into account. **Please refer to Chapter 35.**

Reference: Peltier, M. R., Cosgrove, S. J., Ohayagha, K., Crapanzano, K. A., & Jones, G. N. (2017). Do they see dead people? Cultural factors and sensitivity in screening for schizophrenia spectrum disorders. *Ethnicity & Health, 22*(2), 119–129.

99. **D—Wernicke's aphasia** *Left inferior middle cerebral artery infarct can result in damage to the superior temporal cortex, which is associated with Wernicke's aphasia.* **Please refer to Chapter 26.**

Reference: Blumenfeld, H. (2010). *Neuroanatomy through clinical cases* (2nd ed.). Sunderland, MA: Sinauer Associates.

100. **C—methamphetamine** *Abnormal neuroimaging findings are more frequent and severe with methamphetamine rather than those of cocaine or prescription stimulants and can persist for several years following cessation of use.* **Please refer to Chapter 36.**

Reference: Fernández-Serrano, M. J., Pérez-García, M., & Verdejo-García, A. (2011). What are the specific vs. generalized effects of drugs of abuse on neuropsychological performance? *Neuroscience & Biobehavioral Reviews, 35*(3), 377–406.

101. **B—Parkinson's disease** *While REM behavioral disorder is a diagnostic feature of Lewy body dementia it can be seen in any of the alpha-synuclein disorders, including Parkinson's disease, Lewy body dementia, and multi-system atrophy, and may even be present before other clinical symptoms emerge. In fact, individuals with REM behavioral disorder who are otherwise asymptomatic have a high likelihood of eventually developing some form of synucleinopathy.* **Please refer to Chapter 33.**

References:
(a) Boeve, B. F. (2010). REM sleep behavior disorder: Updated review of the core features, the RBD-Neurodegenerative disease association, evolving concepts, controversies, and future directions. *Annals of New York Academy of Sciences, 1184,* 15–54.
(b) Postuma, R. B., Gagnon, J. F., Marchand, D. G., & Montplaisir, J. Y. (2015). Parkinson risk in idiopathic REM sleep behavior disorder. *Neurology, 84,* 1104–1113.

102. **D—better language than visuospatial skills with weaknesses in attention, processing speed, and executive functions** *This profile reflects, in part, a tendency for language to be spared.* **Please refer to Chapter 19.**

References:
(a) Sherwell, S., Reid, S. M., Reddihough, D. S., Wrennall, J., Ong, B., & Stargatt, R. (2014). Measuring intellectual ability in children with cerebral palsy: Can we do better? *Research in Developmental Disabilities, 35,* 2558–2567.
(b) Stadskleiv, K., Jahnsen, R., Andersen, G. L., & von Tetzchner, S. (2018). Neuropsychological profiles of children with cerebral palsy. *Developmental Neurorehabilitation, 21*(2), 108–120.

103. **B—Capgras syndrome** *Capgras syndrome is a delusional misidentification syndrome in which patients believe that familiar people are imposters or doubles (also referred to as imposter syndrome). Anosognosia is unawareness of deficit. Prosopagnosia is the inability to recognize faces. Reduplicative paramnesia is similar to Capgras syndrome, but the person believes that a place is in fact a fake or duplicate.* **Please refer to Chapter 5.**

Reference: Blumenfeld, H. (2011). *Neuroanatomy through clinical cases* (2nd ed.). Sunderland, MA: Sinauer Associates.

104. **D—intracarotid sodium amobarbital procedure** *The intracarotid sodium amobarbital procedure (also known as "Wada" testing) is performed for presurgical candidates with epilepsy to determine hemispheric dominance for language and potential postoperative cognitive losses post resection. Although EEG is also used in the assessment of individuals with epilepsy, the primary purpose of EEG is to differentiate epileptic seizures from other types of events. PET examines metabolic activity in brain cells, and cerebral arteriography provides characterization of arteriovenous malformations, aneurysms, cerebral venous sinus thrombosis, as well as differential diagnosis of tumors. Please refer to Chapter 6.*

Reference: Kolb, B., & Whishaw, I.Q . (2015). *Fundamentals of human neuropsychology* (7th ed.). New York, NY: Worth Publishers.

105. **C—number of dysmorphic facial features** *The severity of facial dysmorphology is the best predictor of intellectual functioning in the FASD population. Please refer to Chapter 21.*

References:
(a) Riccio, C. A., & Sullivan, J. R. (Eds.) (2016). *Pediatric neurotoxicology: Academic and psychosocial outcomes.* Switzerland: Springer International Publishing.
(b) US Environmental Protection Agency. http://www.epa.gov/hg/effects.htm

106. **B—is experiencing organizational difficulties which affect memory** *Relative to story learning, list learning tasks tend to be more sensitive to the presence of memory dysfunction following TBI. Research suggests that list learning tasks have more organizational requirements which can identify the impact of frontal dysfunction on memory. An individual with medial temporal lobe dysfunction would be expected to display impairments on both list learning and story memory tasks. Please refer to Chapter 29.*

References:
(a) DeJong, J., & Donders, J. (2010). Cluster subtypes on the California Verbal Learning Test-Second Edition (CVLT-II) in a traumatic brain injury sample. *Journal Clinical and Experimental Neuropsychology, 32*(9), 953–960.
(b) Wright, M. J., & Schmitter-Edgecombe, M. (2011). The impact of verbal memory encoding and consolidation deficits during recovery from moderate-to-severe traumatic brain injury. *Journal of Head Trauma Rehabilitation, 26*(3), 182–191.

107. **D—tau** *While amyloid appears to be necessary for the development of Alzheimer's disease, tau shows a stronger correlation with cognitive functioning in older individuals with and without dementia. Please refer to Chapter 30.*

Reference: Wennberg, A. M., Whitwell, J. L., Tosakulwong, N., Weigand, S. D., Murray, M. E., Machulda, M. M., . . . Josephs, K. A. (2019). The influence of tau, amyloid, alpha-synuclein, TDP-43, and vascular pathology in clinically normal elderly individuals. *Neurobiology of Aging, 1*(77), 26–36.

108. **A—psychiatric presentation** *Autoimmune encephalitis including limbic encephalitis, often presents with psychiatric manifestations. Abnormal movements that resemble dystonia or chorea may also present early, and may be more common in children, who present with fewer psychiatric symptoms. New Onset Refractory Status Epilepticus (NORSE) and related Febrile Infection-Related Epilepsy Syndrome (FIRES) are autoimmune seizure presentations. While language difficulty may be associated with other cognitive impairments (e.g., memory disturbance), expressive aphasia has not been reported as a symptom of autoimmune encephalitis associated with epilepsy. Please refer to Chapter 22.*

Reference: Lancaster, E. (2016). The diagnosis and treatment of autoimmune encephalitis. *Journal of Clinical Neurology, 12*, 1–13.

109. **B—reading comprehension** *Individuals with intellectual disability do relatively well with rote academic tasks such as word recognition, spelling, and simple mathematics facts. They*

struggle when asked to engage in inferential reasoning often required on measures of reading comprehension. ***Please refer to Chapter 13.***

Reference: McGrath, L. M., & Peterson, R. L. (2009). Intellectual disabilities. In B. F. Pennington (Ed.), *Diagnosing learning disorders* (2nd ed., pp. 181–226). New York, NY: Guilford Press.

110. **D—Turner syndrome** *Turner syndrome cannot be seen in males, as it is the presence of only one X chromosome. Klinefelter syndrome is only seen in males, as it is the presence of an extra X chromosome in a male (XXY). Fragile X syndrome is seen in both males and females, but males are more significantly affected. 22q11.2 deletion syndrome is seen in both males and females and both are equally affected.* ***Please refer to Chapter 18.***

Reference: Wilson, R., Bennett, E., Howell, S. E., & Tartaglia, N. (2011). Sex chromosome aneuploidies. In A. S. Davis (Ed.), *Handbook of pediatric neuropsychology* (pp. 805–820). New York, NY: Springer.

111. **C—delayed recall of a narrative story** *While patients with depression tend to provide limited responses on spontaneous recall tasks, patients with anxiety will often exhibit poor consolidation and organization of the new material with multiple perseverative or intrusive errors. Memory deficits are not as apparent when information is presented in a structured format. As the presentation structure is disrupted, however, memory problems increase. This is noted in better performance on narrative recall tasks in the context of poor performance on the learning and spontaneous recall of an unrelated word list.* ***Please refer to Chapter 34.***

Reference: Chamberlain, S., & Sahakian, B. (2006). Cognition in depression and memory. In C. Cruse, H. Meltzer, C. Sennef, & S. Van De Witte (Eds.), *Thinking and cognition: Concepts, targets and therapeutics* (pp. 39–49). Fairfax, VA: IOS Press.

112. **B—results in multiple hemorrhagic lesions** *Cerebral amyloid angiopathy's prevalence increases with advancing age. The deposition of amyloid in the cerebral blood vessels results in multiple hemorrhagic lesions as the disease advances. Neither a lacunar state nor leukoaraiosis characterize cerebral amyloid angiopathy.* ***Please refer to Chapter 31.***

Reference: Bell, R. D., & Zlokovic, B. V. (2009). Neurovascular mechanisms and blood-brain barrier disorder in Alzheimer's disease. *Acta Neuropathologica, 118*, 103–113.

113. **A—hormonal mechanisms** *The most obvious biologically oriented reason for differences in prevalence between males and females are differences in hormonal fluctuation related to menstrual cycle variability and response to stressors. However, the empirical evidence to support this assumption is limited or absent.* ***Please refer to Chapter 37.***

Reference: Kajantie, E., & Phillips, D. I. W. (2006). The effects of sex and hormonal status on the physiological response to acute psychosocial stress. *Psychoneuroendocrinology, 31*, 151–178.

114. **B—Huntington's disease** *Ventricular enlargement due to caudate and putamen atrophy can often be seen in Huntington's disease. Significant reductions in caudate and putamen volumes are often seen in symptomatic and presymptomatic Huntington's disease gene carriers.* ***Please refer to Chapter 33.***

Reference: Scahill, R. I., Andre, R., Tabrizi, S. J., & Aylward, E. H. (2017). Structural imaging in premanifest and manifest Huntington disease. In A.S. Felgin & K. E. Anderson (Eds.), *Handbook of clinical neurology* (Vol. 144, pp. 247–261). Philadelphia, PA: Elsevier.

115. **D—Law School Admission Council** *Guidelines change periodically. The best resource is always the website for the organization that administers the standardized test.* ***Please refer to Chapter 15.***

Reference: Mapou, R. L. (2009). *Adult learning disabilities and ADHD: Research informed assessment.* New York, NY: Oxford University Press.

116. **C—standard error of the estimate** *As stated in the section of Standard Error of Measurement (SEM)/Standard Error of the Estimate (SEE), the SEE is based on the obtained score and requires no knowledge of the true score and includes extra consideration of the reliability of the test.* ***Please refer to Chapter 8.***

Reference: Price, L. D. (2017). *Psychometric methods: Theory into practice* (Methodology in the Social Sciences). New York, NY: Guildford Press.

117. **D—neurodevelopmental** *Neurodevelopmental models propose that genetic vulnerability interacts with environmental stressors to disrupt normal brain maturation during key developmental stages. This is also referred to as the "diathesis-stress" model.* ***Please refer to Chapter 35.***

Reference: Karlsgodt, K. H., Daqiang, S., Jimenez, A. M., Lutkenhoff, E. S., Whillhite, R., Van Erp, T. G. M., & Cannon, T. D. (2008). Developmental disruptions in neural connectivity in the pathophysiology of schizophrenia. *Development and Psychopathology, 20,* 1297–1327.

118. **B—Ask about the characteristics of the vision impairment and its onset.** *While the clinician may decline the referral, without knowing the nature of the visual impairment, they cannot determine what types of modifications or accommodations are necessary and whether they are competent to perform the evaluation.* ***Please refer to Chapter 11.***

Reference: Niemeier, J. P. (2010). Neuropsychological assessment for visually impaired persons with traumatic brain injury. *NeuroRehabilitation, 27*(3), 275–283.

119. **A—naming** *Herpes simplex virus (HSV) tends to preferentially affect the inferior and medial surfaces of the temporal and frontal lobes. This commonly results in memory impairments and problems with naming (i.e., dysnomia). The other three language deficits (repetition, prosody, and comprehension) have not been consistently documented deficits in HSV encephalitis.* ***Please refer to Chapter 23.***

References:
(a) Pewter, S. M., Williams, W. H., Haslam, C., & Kay, J. M. (2007). Neuropsychological and psychiatric profiles in acute encephalitis in adults. *Neuropsychological Rehabilitation, 17*(4–5), 478–505.
(b) Utley, T. F., Ogden, J. A., Gibb, A., McGrath, N., & Anderson, N. E. (1997). The long-term neuropsychological outcome of herpes simplex encephalitis in a series of unselected survivors. *Neuropsychiatry, Neuropsychology, and Behavioral Neurology, 10*(3), 180–189.

120. **B—is a condition in which cerebrospinal fluid accumulates with ventricular expansion** *NPH is more common in the elderly but is not benign, as it tends to be associated with gait disturbance, urinary incontinence, and cognitive impairment.* ***Please refer to Chapter 20.***

Reference: Sinforiano, E., Pacchetti, C., Picascia, M., Pozzi, N. G., Todisco, M., & Vitali, P. (2018). Clinical and cognitive features of idiopathic normal pressure hydrocephalus. In B. Gürer (Ed.), *Hydrocephalus—Water on the brain* (pp. 43–74). IntertechOpen.

121. **C—delta and theta** *Delta and theta are the classic slow-wave sleep waveforms on EEG. Alpha and beta waves are not specifically associated with sleep. Gamma waves exist, but are controversial and typically implicated in meditation rather than sleep.* ***Please refer to Chapter 6.***

Reference: Niedermeyer (2011). The normal EEG of the waking adult. In E. Niedermeyer, F. Lopes da Silva (Eds.), *Electroencephalography* (pp. 167–192). Philadelphia, PA: Lippincott, Williams & Wilkins.

122. **B—fewer relapses** *Women with multiple sclerosis tend to have fewer relapses (or none) while pregnant. Unfortunately, after giving birth, there may be resurgence in relapses.* **Please refer to Chapter 24.**

Reference: Alwan, S., & Sadovnick, A. D. (2012). Multiple sclerosis and pregnancy: Maternal considerations. *Women's Health, 8*(4), 399–414.

123. **D—This child likely has ADHD, given the heritability of ADHD is as high as 70–80% among twin studies.** *In twin studies, the heritability of ADHD is as high as 70–80%, and first degree relatives of individuals with ADHD have a 5- to 10-fold increased risk of developing this disorder.* **Please refer to Chapter 16.**

Reference: Faraone, S., Asheron, P., Banaschewski, T., Biederman, J., Buitelaar, J. K., Ramos-Quiroga, J. A., . . . Franke, B. (2015). Attention-deficit/hyperactivity disorder. *Nature Reviews: Disease Primers, 1,* 15020.

124. **C—produces significant amnesia when lesioned** *Lesions to the perirhinal/parahippocampal (PR/PH) cortex were found, during development of a revised animal model of amnesia to produce a memory deficit in monkeys that was comparable in severity to that seen after combined amygdala and hippocampal lesions. All of the other alternatives either deny a role in memory for the PR/PH region or assign it an incorrect function.* **Please refer to Chapter 4.**

Reference: Zola-Morgan, S., Squire, L. R., Amaral, D. G., & Suzuki, W. A. (1989). Lesions of the perirhinal and parahippocampal cortex that spare the amygdala and hippocampal formation produce severe memory impairment. *Journal of Neuroscience, 9,* 4355–4370.

125. **D—delirium due to brain injury** *Posttraumatic amnesia (PTA) is a term used primarily with regard to patients with TBI. Individuals in PTA are unable to form continuous memory and may have additional symptoms that meet criteria for delirium but PTA is not a diagnosis. In this case, it is too early to reliably determine if the TBI will result in dementia, and postictal confusion would not be expected to result in persistent delirium 1 week post event.* **Please refer to Chapter 27.**

Reference: Trzepacz, P. T., Kean, J., & Kennedy, R. E. (2011). Delirium and posttraumatic confusion. In J. M. Silver, T. W. McAllister, & S. C. Yudofsky (Eds.), *Textbook of traumatic brain injury* (pp. 145–171). Washington, DC: American Psychiatric Publishing.

Appendix H

Fourth Full-Length Practice Examination Answers

1. **C—present in a subgroup of patients, but no single cause has yet been identified** *There have been suggestions that rapid cognitive decline in older adults with schizophrenia may be due to some unique pathological process but so far, the evidence is equivocal. It is clear that people with schizophrenia have many causes of increased morbidity and mortality, among which are multiple preventable medical conditions. **Please refer to Chapter 35.***

   Reference: Shah, J. N., Qureshi, S. U., Jawaid, A., & Schulz, P. E. (2012). Is there evidence for late cognitive decline in chronic schizophrenia? *Psychiatric Quarterly, 83*(2), 127–144.

2. **B—patients with aphasia learning to speak again** *Although still somewhat unclear, major theories of aphasia recovery suggest that (1) homologous brain regions from the contralateral hemisphere are thought to assume the functional duties of the damaged brain regions, and/or (2) that adjacent, undamaged cerebral regions are employed to assume functional duties. **Please refer to Chapter 3.***

   Reference: Dignam, J. K., Rodriguez, A. D., & Copeland, D. A. (2016). Evidence for intensive aphasia therapy: Consideration of theories from neuroscience and cognitive psychology. *Physical Medicine & Rehabilitation, 8*, 254–267.

3. **A—Accept the gift graciously.** *Small gifts from patients of limited value are ethically acceptable. Refusing such gifts or signs of gratitude would be potentially harmful to the doctor-patient relationship. However, gifts should never be tied to specific expectations such as the completion of a favorable report or disability forms. There is no reporting or disclosure requirement for small gifts of nominal value. The psychologist would also need to be aware of their hospital's policy regarding gifts as well since these can vary between institutions. **Please refer to Chapter 7.***

   General Principles and Ethical Standards: B, C, E; 6.04, 6.05

4. **C—primary-progressive** *The primary-progressive form of the disease is associated with a slow progressive decline in neurologic functioning with no clear relapses. **Please refer to Chapter 24.***

   Reference: Lublin, F. D., Reingold, S. C., Cohen, J. A., Cutter, G. R., Sorensen, P. S., Thompson, A. J., . . . Bebo, B. (2014). Defining the clinical course of multiple sclerosis: The 2013 revisions. *Neurology, 83*(3), 278–286.

5. **D—deficient executive functioning** *The executive dysfunction theory proposes that deficits in social communication and restricted and repetitive behaviors observed in Autism spectrum disorder are evident because of deficits in cognitive flexibility, planning, self-monitoring, inhibition of ongoing behaviors, and initiation of new behavior.* **Please refer to Chapter 14.**

Reference: Eigsti, I. M. (2010). Executive functions in ASD. In D. A. Fein (Ed.), *The neuropsychology of autism* (pp.185–203). New York, NY: Oxford University Press.

6. **B—Person 1's percentile rank will increase more than Person 2's.** *These two individuals' scores will both change in reference to the normative group because of this addition. However, because of the assumption of a normal distribution, score differences in the middle of the distribution of percentiles are exaggerated compared to those at the extremes. Thus, changing a raw score by 3 points will have a larger influence on the percentile ranking close to the middle of the distribution.* **Please refer to Chapter 8.**

Reference: Anastasi, A., & Urbina, S. (1997). *Psychological testing* (7th ed.). Upper Saddle River, NJ: Prentice-Hall.

7. **C—more common than in other chronic illnesses** *Higher rates of depression and anxiety are consistently reported among persons with epilepsy. When compared with other chronic illnesses, including those having a high incidence of childhood onset (e.g., diabetes), patients with epilepsy have a higher rate of depression. Severe depression, including suicidality, is not uncommon, and treatment of depression is a key component of maintaining quality of life.* **Please refer to Chapter 22.**

Reference: Kwon, O. Y., Park, S. (2014). Depression and anxiety in people with epilepsy. *Journal of Clinical Neurology, 10*(3), 175–188.

8. **A—dehydration** *Dehydration often occurs with MDMA use at dance clubs or raves because users engage in long periods of dancing without adequate water intake.* **Please refer to Chapter 36.**

Reference: National Institute on Drug Abuse. (2017, September). What are the effects of MDMA? https://www.drugabuse.gov/publications/research-reports/mdma-ecstasy-abuse/what-are-effects-mdma

9. **A—ADHD** *ADHD, learning disabilities, obsessive-compulsive disorder, depression, generalized anxiety, panic attacks, sleep disorders, and migraines are comorbid conditions that can be seen in Tourette syndrome. While rage attacks can also be seen, and a diagnosis of intermittent explosive disorder is possible, this is different than an oppositional defiant disorder.* **Please refer to Chapter 33.**

Reference: Kumar, A., Trescher, W., & Byler, D. (2016). Tourette syndrome and cormorbid neuropsychiatric conditions. *Current Developmental Disorders Reports, 3*, 217–221.

10. **D—episodic memory** *Knowledge of temporal events and declarative memory is severely impaired in individuals with Alzheimer's disease.* **Please refer to Chapter 5.**

Reference: Smith, G. E., & Bondi, M. W. (2013). *Mild cognitive impairment and dementia: Definitions, diagnosis, and treatment.* New York, NY: Oxford University Press.

11. **A—primarily apparent in spina bifida myelomeningocele and aqueductal stenosis** *Fine motor impairment may contribute to the pattern but impairment is also noted on visuospatial tasks without significant motor demands or time bonuses.* **Please refer to Chapter 20.**

Reference: Fletcher, J. M., & Dennis, M. (2010). Spina bifida and hydrocephalus: Modeling variability in outcome domains. In K. O. Yeates, M. D. Ris, H. G. Taylor, & B. F. Pennington (Eds.) *Pediatric neuropsychology: Research, theory, and practice* (2nd ed., pp. 3–25). Hillsdale, NJ: Erlbaum.

12. **B—no brain hemorrhage on CT, and symptom duration of 3 to 4.5 hours or less** *Because TPA is a powerful thrombolysis agent American Heart Association guidelines require that all three criteria are met.* **Please refer to Chapter 26.**

   Reference: Mohr, J. P, Wolf, P. A., Grotta, J. C., Moskowitz, M. A., Mayberg, M. R., & von Kummer, R. (2011). *Stroke: Pathophysiology, diagnosis and management* (5th ed.). Philadelphia, PA: Saunders.

13. **C—They have limited empirical support at any phase and typically do not generalize.** *Cognitive restitution training methods have limited empirical support, especially as the time since injury increases.* **Please refer to Chapter 29.**

   Reference: Rohling, M. L., Faust, M. E., Beverly, B., & Demakis, G. (2009). Effectiveness of cognitive rehabilitation following acquired brain injury: A meta-analytic re-examination of Cicerone et al.'s (2000, 2005) systematic reviews. *Neuropsychology, 23*(1), 20–39.

14. **A—semantic** *In addition, patients with Alzheimer's disease are less likely to benefit from semantic cues.* **Please refer to Chapter 30.**

   Reference: Smith, G., & Butts, A. (2018). Dementia. In J. E. Morgan & J. H. Ricker (Eds.), *Textbook of clinical neuropsychology* (2nd ed., pp. 717–741). New York, NY: Taylor & Francis Group.

15. **C—norepinephrine** *The symptoms described are consistent with a "fight or flight" response. Norepinephrine is an excitatory neurotransmitter and also a stress hormone that helps maintain alertness and preparation to respond to external threats.* **Please refer to Chapter 34.**

   References:
   (a) Kandel, E. R. (2013). Disorders of mood and anxiety. In E. R. Kandel, J. H. Schwartz, T. M. Jessell, A. A. Siegelbaum, & A. J. Hudspeth (Eds.), *Principles of neural science* (5th ed., pp. 1402–1424). New York, NY: McGraw-Hill.
   (b) Stein, M. B., & Steckler, T. (2010). *Behavioral neurobiology of anxiety and its treatment.* New York, NY: Springer.

16. **D—dysmetria** *Dysmetria refers to inaccurate unilateral fine motor coordination and is considered to be a sign of cerebellar dysfunction. The other three conditions are typically either cerebral or spinal in nature.* **Please refer to Chapter 6.**

   References:
   (a) Blumenfeld, H. (2011). *Neuroanatomy through clinical cases* (2nd ed.). Sunderland, MA: Sinauer Associates.
   (b) Goldberg, S. (2017). *The four-minute neurological exam* (2nd ed.). Miami, FL: MedMaster.
   (c) Greenberg, D., Aminoff, M., & Simon, R. (2012). *Clinical neurology* (8th ed.). New York, NY: Lange Medical Books/McGraw-Hill.

17. **B—prodromal** *This patient's profile is most consistent with the prodromal phase, which is marked by an increasing tendency toward social withdrawal, declines in role functioning, and brief, intermittent or subthreshold psychotic symptoms, including perceptual disturbances and odd, unusual, or suspicious thinking, that occurs with increasing frequency and conviction.* **Please refer to Chapter 35.**

   Reference: Addington, J., Liu, L., Buchy, L., Cadenhead, K. S., Cannon, T. D., Cornblatt, B. A., . . . Woods, S. W. (2015). North American prodrome longitudinal study (NAPLS 2): The prodromal symptoms. *The Journal of Nervous and Mental Disease, 203*(5), 328.

18. **C—female treated in early childhood with chemotherapy and radiation** *Younger age at treatment, female gender, and radiation therapy have been identified as factors associated with more severe neuropsychological impairment after treatment for childhood leukemia.* **Please refer to Chapter 25.**

   References:
   (a) Buizer, A. I., de Sonneville, L. M., & Veerman, A. J. (2009). Effects of chemotherapy on neurocognitive function in children with acute lymphoblastic leukemia: A critical review of the literature. *Pediatric Blood & Cancer, 52* (4), 447–454.

APPENDIX H

(b) Kadan-Lottick, N. S., Zeltzer, L. K., Liu, Q., Yasui, Y., Ellenberg, L., Gioia, G., . . . Krull, K. (2010). Neurocognitive functioning in adult survivors of childhood non-central nervous system cancers. *Journal of the National Cancer Institute, 102*(12), 881–893.

19. **A—executive dysfunction and depression** *Although learning disability, low average IQ, and dysnomia might suggest reduced cognitive reserve, studies suggest that executive dysfunction poses a higher risk of postoperative delirium. Depression has been identified as an independent risk factor as well, but anxiety disorders have not been associated with substantially increased risk.* ***Please refer to Chapter 27.***

References:
(a) Geene, N. H., Attix, D. K., Weldon, B. C., Smith, P. J., McDonagh, D. L., & Monk, T. G. (2009). Measures of executive function and depression identify patients at risk for postoperative delirium. *Anesthesiology, 110*(4), 788–795.
(b) Smith, P. J., Attix, D. K., Weldon, B. C., Greene, N. H., & Monk, T. G. (2009). Executive function and depression as independent risk factors for postoperative delirium. *Anesthesiology, 110*(4), 781–787.

20. **A—cholinergic inputs to the hippocampus and amygdala are disrupted** *The basal forebrain provides cholinergic innervations of the hippocampus and amygdala systems; thus, a lesion here can disrupt both circuits. Answer b cannot be correct, since large, structural lesions of the basal forebrain can involve connections of both the lateral and medial limbic circuits. Neither c nor d is correct because there is no evidence that the basal forebrain plays a specific role in retrieval or storage of memory representations.* ***Please refer to Chapter 4.***

Reference: Mesulam, M. M., Mufson, E., Levey, E., & Wainer, B. (1983). Cholinergic innervation of cortex by the basal forebrain: Cytochemistry and cortical connections of the septal area, diagonal band nuclei, nucleus basalis (substantia innominata) and hypothalamus in the rhesus monkey. *Journal of Comparative Neurology, 214*, 170–197.

21. **C—spina bifida** *Mathematics disabilities are common among individuals with spina bifida and congenital hydrocephalus, and occur in more than half of the affected individuals. In contrast, math skills are often a relative strength in children with Autism spectrum disorders; children with Tourette syndrome typically do not manifest learning disabilities; and only approximately 40% of children with ADHD manifest learning disabilities.* ***Please refer to Chapter 15.***

References:
(a) Fletcher, J. M., Lyon, G. R., Fuchs, L. S., & Barnes, M. A. (2018). *Learning disabilities: From identification to intervention* (2nd ed.). New York, NY: Guilford Press.
(b) Larson, K., Russ, S. A., Kahn, R. S., & Halfon, N. (2011). Patterns of comorbidity, functioning, and service use for US children with ADHD. *Pediatrics, 127*, 462–470.
(c) Mahone, E. M. (2011). Tourette syndrome. In J. Morgan, I. S. Baron, & J. Ricker (eds.), *Casebook of clinical neuropsychology* (pp. 60–77). New York, NY: Oxford University Press.

22. **A—have not been consistently demonstrated in vascular dementia** *Decades ago, it was thought that stepwise progression was a hallmark characteristic of vascular dementia. Research since then has demonstrated that this is not the case. The presence of stepwise progression has also not been linked conclusively to any particular type of pathology.* ***Please refer to Chapter 31.***

Reference: Stephens, S., Kalaria, R., Kenny, R. A., & Ballard, C. (2005). Progression of cognitive impairments associated with cerebrovascular disease. In R. H. Paul, R. Cohen, B. R. Ott, & S. Salloway (Eds.). *Vascular dementia: Cerebrovascular mechanisms and clinical management* (pp. 145–156). Totowa, NJ: Humana Press.

23. **D—Low intellectual abilities are seen in children, but adult IQs fall in the average range.** *As a group, both children and adults with histories of anti-NMDA receptor encephalitis have average general intellectual abilities despite deficits seen in several domains including memory,*

*attention, and aspects of executive functioning (i.e., organization, planning, and impulse control). **Please refer to Chapter 23.***

References:
(a) Finke, C., Kopp, U. A., Prüss, H., Dalmau, J., Wandinger, K. P., & Ploner, C. J. (2012). Cognitive deficits following anti-NMDA receptor encephalitis. *Journal of Neurology, Neurosurgery, and Psychiatry, 83*(2), 195–198.
(b) Matricardi, S., Patrini, M., Freri, E., Ragona, F., Zibordi, F., Andreetta, F., . . . Granata, T. (2016). Cognitive and neuropsychological evolution in children with anti-NMDAR encephalitis. *Journal of Neurology, 263*, 765–771.

24. **D—are to be excluded when evaluating functional impairment in ADLs** *The NINDS-AIREN diagnostic criteria require that significant impairment in daily functioning be present, but that this impairment be secondary to deficits in memory and intellectual functions and not due to physical disability secondary to stroke. **Please refer to Chapter 31.***

Reference: Román, G. C., Tatemichi, T. K., Erkinjuntti, T., Cummings, J. L., Masdeu, J. C., Garcia, J. H., . . . Hofman, A. (1993). Vascular dementia: Diagnostic criteria for research studies: Report of the NINDS-AIREN International Workshop. *Neurology, 43*(2), 250–260.

25. **B—It is ethically appropriate in some cases.** *Although there might be more feasible options and the neuropsychologist's recommendations may not always be appropriate, in this situation B is the best answer because deception can be ethically appropriate in some cases. Use of deception does not uniformly require approval from an ethics committee. Additionally, it is inaccurate to state that deception is "often" necessary with patients who are confused as there are other effective interventions. Notably, in neuropsychological assessment it could be argued that we often deceive patients in the context of performance validity testing when we inform or lead them to believe that a certain test measures a construct such as memory or is difficult, whereas it is in fact a very easy performance validity test that almost everyone should perform well on. However, this may not be considered deception if patients are informed at the outset, during the informed consent process, that such measures or indicators will be used during the evaluation, and they agree to the testing. **Please refer to Chapter 7.***

General Principles and Ethical Standards: A, B, D, E; 3.04, 3.10

Reference: Matthes, J., & Caples, H. (2013). Ethical issues in using deception to facilitate rehabilitation for a patient with severe traumatic brain injury. *Journal of Head Trauma Rehabilitation, 2*, 126–130.

26. **C—percentile** *Expression of scores in percentiles forces the data into a rectangular distribution, forcing artificially even intervals regardless of the underlying values. Use of such transformations are optimal to minimize misinterpretations of tests with non-normal distributions, but the underlying distribution of the data needs to be considered in the context of clinical interpretation (i.e., small changes in raw scores in the middle of the distribution will result in a magnified influence on the percentile ranking). **Please refer to Chapter 8.***

Reference: Gravetter, F., & Wallnau, L. B. (2017). *Statistics for the behavioral sciences* (10th ed.). Boston, MA: Cengage Learning.

27. **A—preschool** *Children who sustain traumatic brain injury during infancy and early childhood have worse neuropsychological and functional outcomes than those injured in later childhood or the teenage years. **Please refer to Chapter 29.***

Reference: Yeates, K. O., & Brooks, B. L. (2018). Traumatic brain injury in children and adolescents. In Morgan, J. E., & Ricker, J. H. (Eds.). *Textbook of clinical neuropsychology* (2nd ed., pp. 141–157). New York, NY: Taylor and Francis.

28. **A—amygdala** *The central nucleus of the amygdala senses and identifies fear and anxiety-laden stimuli and initiates the emotional response. It has been shown to be strongly involved in the*

*formation of emotional memories, especially fear-related memories. The amygdalocentric model of Posttraumatic stress disorder proposes that it is associated with hyperarousal of the amygdala and insufficient top-down control by the medial prefrontal cortex and the hippocampus, particularly during extinction, which reflects a primary association with anxiety rather than depression. **Please refer to Chapter 34.***

References:
(a) Kandel, E. R. (2013). Disorders of mood and anxiety. In E. R. Kandel, J. H. Schwartz, T. M. Jessell, A. A. Siegelbaum, & A. J. Hudspeth (Eds.), *Principles of neural science* (5th ed., pp. 1402–1424). New York, NY: McGraw-Hill.
(b) Stein, M. B., & Steckler, T. (2010). *Behavioral neurobiology of anxiety and its treatment.* New York, NY: Springer.

29. **B—ADHD** *60–95% of children with FASD qualify for a diagnosis of ADHD. Externalizing disorders are particularly common in this population. **Please refer to Chapter 21.***

Reference: Glass, L., & Mattson, S. N. (2016). Fetal alcohol spectrum disorders: Academic and psychosocial outcomes. In C. A. Riccio & J. R. Sullivan (Eds.), *Pediatric neurotoxicology: Academic and psychosocial outcomes.* Cham, Switzerland: Springer International Publishing.

30. **C—determine the age at onset and severity of hearing loss** *A deaf older adult may be experiencing late onset hearing loss or may be congenitally deaf. They may use speech and residual hearing or communicate primarily through signs or writing. The approach to assessment will depend on this information. **Please refer to Chapter 11.***

Reference: Hill-Briggs, F., Dial, J., Morere, D., & Joyce, A. (2007). Neuropsychological assessment of persons with physical disability, visual impairment or blindness, and hearing impairment or deafness. *Archives of Clinical Neuropsychology, 22,* 389–404.

31. **B—She exhibits borderline intellectual functioning** *In order to meet diagnostic criteria for intellectual disability, individuals must have an IQ score of 70 or below and exhibit deficits in adaptive functioning. Based on her report of adaptive functioning, Jane best fits in the category of borderline intellectual functioning. **Please refer to Chapter 13.***

Reference: American Psychiatric Association. (2013). *Diagnostic and statistical manual of mental disorders* (5th ed.). Arlington, VA: American Psychiatric Publishing.

32. **A—visuospatial** *Neuropsychologically, greater deficits in visuospatial functioning than in other domains may help differentiate Lewy body dementia from Alzheimer's disease. **Please refer to Chapter 33.***

Reference: Scharre, D. W., Chang, S. I., Nagaraja, H. N., Park, A., Adeli, A., Agrawal, P., . . . Kataki, M., (2016). Paired studies comparing clinical profiles of Lewy body dementia and Alzheimer's and Parkinson disease. *Journal of Alzheimer's Disease, 54,* 995–1004.

33. **B—tuberous sclerosis** *Tuberous sclerosis complex (TSC) is one of the hereditary genetic syndromes associated with a predisposition for brain tumors. Central nervous system manifestations of TSC include subependymal giant cell astrocytomas. These are considered benign tumors and are commonly treated via surgical resection. Neurologic complications can occur due to intraventricular location. **Please refer to Chapter 25.***

Reference: Randle, S. C. (2017). Tuberous sclerosis complex: A review. *Pediatric Annals, 46*(4), e166–e171.

34. **D—gait ataxia** *Wernicke's encephalopathy is an acute neuropsychiatric reaction to thiamine deficiency and is characterized by confusion, ataxia, nystagmus, and ophthalmoplegia. **Please refer to Chapter 36.***

Reference: Kopelman, M. D., Thomson, A. D., Guerrini, I., & Marshall, E. J. (2009). The Korsakoff syndrome: Clinical aspects, psychology, and treatment. *Alcohol & Alcoholism, 44,* 148–154.

35. **C—ADHD-I is more heritable than ADHD-H.** *Although both symptom dimensions are significantly heritable, ADHD-H is less heritable than ADHD-I. The heritability of ADHD is approximately 75%; nonshared environment (as opposed to shared environment) and measurement error accounts for the rest of the variance. First-degree relatives have a 30–35% chance of having ADHD.* **Please refer to Chapter 16.**

Reference: Willcutt, E. G., Nigg, J. T., Pennington, B. F., Solanto, M. V., Rohde, L. A., Tannock, R., . . . Lahey, B. B. (2012). Validity of DSM–IV attention deficit/hyperactivity disorder symptom dimensions and subtypes. *Journal of Abnormal Psychology, 121,* 991–1010.

36. **A—transcortical motor aphasia** *Right leg weakness, grasp reflex and executive function deficits are characteristics of damage in the distribution of the left anterior cerebral artery, which can be associated with transcortical motor aphasia.* **Please refer to Chapter 26.**

Reference: Blumenfeld, H. (2010). *Neuroanatomy through clinical cases* (2nd ed.). Sunderland, MA: Sinauer Associates.

37. **D—processing speed, depression, fatigue** *Individuals with multiple sclerosis experience a host of symptoms that may adversely impact daily functioning. The patient referred to you complains of problems keeping up with work. Reduced processing speed is the most common cognitive problem in multiple sclerosis while language-based skills tend to be preserved in adults with multiple sclerosis. Likewise, depression is commonly associated with multiple sclerosis and literature suggests a relation between depression and cognitive functioning including speed of performance. Fatigue is one of the most common symptoms reported in individuals with multiple sclerosis. Research has shown reduced performance over time with sustained mental effort suggesting that fatigue may play a role.* **Please refer to Chapter 24.**

Reference: Chiaravalloti, N., & DeLuca, J. (2008). Cognitive impairment in multiple sclerosis. *Lancet Neurology, 7,* 1139–1151.

38. **A—Generalized Anxiety Disorder/Major Depressive Disorder** *Anxiety and mood disorders are commonly reported by individuals with insomnia.* **Please refer to Chapter 37.**

Reference: Krystal, A. D. (2012). Psychiatric disorders and sleep. *Neurologic Clinics, 30,* 1389–1413.

39. **C—specific learning disorder** *The BASC-3 provides clinical probability indices for ADHD, autism, and emotional behavior disorder, which can be used to inform diagnostic impressions and behavior intervention recommendations.* **Please refer to Chapter 10.**

Reference: Reynolds, C. R., & Kamphaus, R. W. (2015). *Behavior assessment system for children* (3rd ed.). Circle Pines, MN: American Guidance Service.

40. **B—Essential tremor is secondary to reduced dopamine in the basal ganglia.** *The pathogenesis of essential tremor is mostly unexplained. There appears to be a strong genetic component, at least for familial cases. Some reports suggest that the neuropathology of essential tremor is localized in the brainstem (locus ceruleus) and cerebellum, but the presence of cerebellar pathology is controversial.* **Please refer to Chapter 33.**

Reference: Hopfner, R., & Helmich, R. C. (2018). The etiology of essential tremor: Genes versus environment. *Parkinsonian Related Disorders, 46,* S92–S96.

41. **D—Verbal memory deficits in left TLE are more robust than visual memory deficits in right TLE.** *The extensive body of literature regarding memory deficits in TLE indicates that verbal memory deficits in left TLE are consistently identified using a variety of methods/verbal*

*memory tests. Exacerbation of deficits following dominant temporal lobectomy is predictable based on presurgical memory ability. However, the presence of nonverbal memory deficits in right TLE is not as consistently observed, and, in many cases of right TLE, there are no memory deficits. This may be due to a combination of factors, including methodological differences and a lack of coherence between models of nonverbal memory and tests that are used to assess the construct. **Please refer to Chapter 22.***

Reference: Lee, T. M. C., Yip, J. T. H., & Jones-Gotman, M. (2002). Memory deficits after resection from left or right anterior temporal lobe in humans: A meta-analytic review. *Epilepsia, 43*, 283–291.

42. **B—appears to be related to the development of amyloid plaques** *Chromosome 21 is also involved in Down syndrome, and older individuals with Down syndrome typically develop plaques consistent with Alzheimer's disease. **Please refer to Chapter 30.***

References:
(a) Genini, G., Dowling, A. L. S., Beckett, T. L., Barone, E., Mancuso, C., Murphy, M. P., . . . Head, E. (2012). Association between frontal cortex oxidative damage and beta-amyloid as a function of age in Down syndrome. *Molecular Basis of Disease, 1822*(2), 130–138.
(b) Selkoe, D. J., & Hardy, J. (2016). The amyloid hypothesis of Alzheimer's disease at 25 years. *EMBO Molecular Medicine, 8*(6), 595–608.

43. **D—anticonvulsants** *The symptoms described are highly suggestive of bipolar disorder. Anticonvulsant medications are typically used to manage bipolar disorder. High-potency benzodiazepines are effective for the management of anxiety with few side effects aside from drowsiness. Selective serotonin reuptake inhibitors are the most commonly prescribed antidepressants in anxiety disorder. Tricyclics are used occasionally, and monoamine oxidase inhibitors may be used with close monitoring. **Please refer to Chapter 34.***

Reference: Stein, M. B., & Steckler, T. (2010). *Behavioral neurobiology of anxiety and its treatment.* New York, NY: Springer.

44. **C—Older bodies are less tolerant of changes and although the brain is not directly infected his overall reaction to the infection can cause delirium.** *With perhaps the exception of urosepsis, delirium in older patients with delirium related to UTI is more likely due to the physiologic effects and response to infection as opposed to the infection directly affecting the brain. The patient may have had underlying cognitive problems prior but this is an assumptive leap and the information provided does not support this conclusion. While certain medications and catheters can increase the risk for delirium it is unlikely that those are the primary cause of delirium in this individual who has already developed an infection. **Please refer to Chapter 27.***

Reference: Ahmed, S., Leurent, B., & Sampson, E. L. (2014). Risk factors for incident delirium among older people in acute hospital medical units: A systematic review and meta-analysis. *Age and Ageing, 43*, 326–333.

45. **C—comparably poorly on tests of verbal and nonverbal learning and memory** *Although discrepancies showing better verbal than nonverbal performance is apparent on some tasks, this pattern is not apparent on learning and memory tasks, possibly because of compression of the hippocampus from hydrocephalus. **Please refer to Chapter 20.***

References:
(a) Fletcher, J. M., & Dennis, M. (2010). Spina bifida and hydrocephalus: Modeling variability in outcome domains. In K. O. Yeates, M. D. Ris, H. G. Taylor, & B. F. Pennington (Eds.) *Pediatric neuropsychology: Research, theory, and practice* (2nd ed., pp. 3–25). Hillsdale, NJ: Erlbaum.
(b) Scott, M. A., Fletcher, J. M., Brookshire, B. L., Davidson, K. C., Landry, S. H., Bohan, T. C., . . . Francis, D. J. (1998). Memory functions in children with early hydrocephalus. *Neuropsychology, 4*, 578–589.

46. **D—spontaneous seizure with no known precipitating event or risk factor** *Epilepsy was previously diagnosed when there were at least two unprovoked seizures. However, the current definition indicates diagnosis with epilepsy can be made after a single seizure, if the risk of recurrence is high based on other medical factors. Spontaneous seizure with no known precipitating event is not sufficient for diagnosis with epilepsy, and may often be found to be related to transient factors (e.g., systemic medical illness, ETOH or substance use).* **Please refer to Chapter 22.**

Reference: Fisher, R. S., Acevedo, C., Arzimanoglou, A., Bogacz, A., Cross, J. H., Elger, C. E. . . . Wiebe, S. (2014). A practical clinical definition of epilepsy. *Epilepsia, 55,* 475–482.

47. **A—primarily ubiquitin-based pathology** *Frontotemporal dementia with motor neuron disease is characterized by ubiquitin-based pathology rather than tau pathology, involving the frontal and temporal lobes.* **Please refer to Chapter 32.**

Reference: Snowden, J., Neary, D., & Mann, D. (2007). Frontotemporal lobar degeneration: Clinical and pathological relationships. *Acta Neuropathologica, 114,* 31–38.

48. **B—fragile X syndrome** *Fragile X syndrome is the most common single gene disorder associated with autism. It is also the leading cause of inherited intellectual disability.* **Please refer to Chapter 18.**

Reference: Mastergeorge, A. M., Au, J., & Hagerman, R. (2011). Fragile X: A family of disorders. In R. D. Nass & Y. Frank (Eds.), *Cognitive and behavioral abnormalities of pediatric diseases* (pp. 170–186). New York, NY: Oxford University Press.

49. **A—lesion of the anterior thalamus affecting the internal medullary lamina** *A is the only alternative that involves damage to both limbic circuits or reference to the preponderance of anterior thalamic lesions as necessary for the production of amnesia.* **Please refer to Chapter 4.**

Reference: Graff-Radford, N. R., Tranel, D., Van Hoesen, G. W., & Brandt, J. P. (1990). Diencephalic amnesia. *Brain, 113,* 1–25.

50. **D—18–24 months** *This is currently the most reliable time at which an Autism spectrum disorder can be diagnosed and remain stable across time.* **Please refer to Chapter 14.**

Reference: Zwaigenbaum, L., Bryson, S., Brian, J., Smith, I., Roberts, W., Szatmari, P., . . . Vaillancourt, T. (2016). Stability of diagnostic assessment for autism spectrum disorder between 18 and 36 months in a high-risk cohort. *Autism Research, 9*(7), 790–800.

51. **D—middle-aged adults** *Although severe TBI would be expected to result in cognitive impairments in all four groups, children, adolescents, and young adults would be expected to experience some progressive functional improvements. Middle-aged adults would be at higher risk for early-onset dementia following severe TBI and thus functional decline.* **Please refer to Chapter 29.**

Reference: Levin, H., Shum, D., & Chan, R. (Eds.). (2014). *Understanding traumatic brain injury: Current research and future directions.* New York, NY: Oxford University Press.

52. **C—1.0 to 1.5** *Although there is some variation across meta-analyses of patients with schizophrenia, there is consensus that most fluid intellectual abilities and complex cognitive functions (such as memory and executive and attentional functions, as defined by neuropsychological tests) show a deficit in the range of 1–1.5 SD relative to healthy peers. The average deficit may be slightly lower (<1.0 SD) if tests of crystallized functions are included, as these are typically less impaired.* **Please refer to Chapter 35.**

Reference: Heinrichs, R. (2005). The primacy of cognition in schizophrenia. *American Psychologist, 60*(3), 229–242.

53. **A—gestational age, availability of NICU care, birth weight, and presence of neurological/ medical complications** *Each of these factors contributes to functional outcome for the preterm infant.* **Please refer to Chapter 17.**

> **Reference:** Baron, I. S., & Rey-Casserly, C. (2010). Extremely preterm birth outcome: A review of four decades of cognitive research. *Neuropsychology Review, 20,* 430–452.

54. **C—lumbar puncture** *During a lumbar puncture, the patient is often in a lying or seated position and a needle is inserted below the spinal cord (often between L4 or L5 intervertebral space). Evoked potential tests are not invasive, EMG is a diagnostic procedure to assess the health of muscles and nerve cells, and central lines are used to administer medicine.* **Please refer to Chapter 6.**

> **References:**
> (a) Blumenfeld, H. (2011). *Neuroanatomy through clinical cases* (2nd ed.). Sunderland, MA: Sinauer Associates.
> (b) Goldberg, S. (2017). *The four-minute neurological exam.* (2nd ed.). Miami, FL: MedMaster.
> (c) Simon, R. P., Aminoff, M., & Greenberg, D. A. (2018). *Clinical neurology* (10th ed.). New York, NY: Lange Medical Books/McGraw-Hill Education.

55. **D—NMDA receptor antibodies are found in the CSF or blood** *All other options are false; however, the presence of NMDA antibodies in CSF or blood is diagnostic.* **Please refer to Chapter 23.**

> **Reference:** Graus, F., Titulaer, M. J., Balu, R., Benseler, S., Bien, C. G., Cellucci, T., . . . Dalmau, J. (2016). A clinical approach to diagnosis of autoimmune encephalitis. *Lancet Neurology, 15(4),* 391–404.

56. **B—hypomanic states** *Hypomania is a condition similar to mania but less severe. The symptoms are similar, but do not cause significant distress or impair one's work, family, or social life in an obvious way whereas manic episodes do. Obsessive-compulsive disorder symptoms/traits have been associated with a number of medical conditions, including Tourette syndrome, ADHD, Pediatric autoimmune neuropsychiatric disorders associated with streptococcal infections (PANDAS), and other conditions.* **Please refer to Chapter 34.**

> **Reference:** American Psychiatric Association. (2013). *Diagnostic and statistical manual of mental disorders* (5th ed.). Washington, DC: American Psychiatric Publishing.

57. **C—false positive** *Comparison groups with actual problems are critical to control for false positive error (i.e., identifying a valid impairment as an indication of invalid performance).* **Please refer to Chapter 12.**

> **Reference:** Larrabee, G. J. (2015). Performance and symptom validity: A perspective from the adult literature. In M. W. Kirkwood (Ed.). *Validity testing in child and adolescent assessment* (pp. 62–76). New York, NY: Guilford Press.

58. **A—low IQ as a proxy for widespread neuropathology** *Large-scale studies have shown that persons with low IQ tend to have seizure free outcomes from surgery less frequently than persons with higher IQ. This is believed to be due to low IQ as a proxy for more widespread pathology.* **Please refer to Chapter 22.**

> **Reference:** Malmgren, K., Olssen, I., Engman, E., Flink, R., & Rydenham, B. (2008). Seizure outcome after resective epilepsy surgery in patients with low IQ. *Brain, 131,* 535–542.

59. **C—multiple system atrophy** *Multiple system atrophy typically involves autonomic dysfunction (urinary incontinence or orthostatic hypotension) and cerebellar syndrome early in the course of the disease.* **Please refer to Chapter 33.**

> **Reference:** Gilman, S., Wenning, G. K., Low, P. A., Brooks, D. J., Mathias, C. J., Trojanowski, J. Q., . . . Vidailhet, M. (2008). Second consensus statement on the diagnosis of multiple system atrophy. *Neurology, 71(9),* 670–676.

60. **B—Angelman syndrome** *Limited or lack of speech is characteristic of Angelman syndrome; even higher functioning individuals develop up to only twenty words and never develop conversational language. Despite this, individuals with Angelman syndrome are socially curious and seek out social interactions. Although individuals with Prader-Willi syndrome do exhibit language deficits, these are typically consistent with overall IQ. They also tend to have social difficulties suggestive of Autism spectrum disorders. In Turner syndrome and 22q11.2 deletion syndrome, language is a relative strength, whereas social skills are a relative weakness.* **Please refer to Chapter 18.**

Reference: Buiting, K. (2010). Prader-Willi syndrome and Angelman syndrome. *American Journal of Medical Genetics Part C (Seminars in Medical Genetics), 154C,* 365–375.

61. **A—not the typical middle cerebral artery pattern** *Global aphasia involves the entire perisylvian region and the typical middle cerebral artery pattern commonly involves hemiparesis as well. If the primary motor cortices are not involved, then two distinct, noncontiguous lesions affecting both Broca's and Wernicke's areas should be suspected.* **Please refer to Chapter 5.**

Reference: Tranel, D. (2009). The Iowa-Benton School of Neuropsychological Assessment. In I. Grant & K. M. Adams (Eds.), *Neuropsychological assessment of neuropsychiatric and neuromedical disorders* (2nd ed., pp. 66–83). New York, NY: Oxford University Press.

62. **D—ratio of individuals the test identifies as having the disease who truly have the disease in a population that is factored by the likelihood ratio of having the disease** *Post-test (positive) odds is the pretest odds multiplied by the likelihood ratio of a positive test result. The post-test odds is the additional improvement in positively identifying a member of the population as having the disease using a test that includes the pre-test probability (risk) of having the disease in the population factored by the positive likelihood ratio of the test. The post-test odds is derived in part from the tests sensitivity and specificity and is not affected by the prevalence rate of the disease in the reference group.* **Please refer to Chapter 9.**

Reference: Schulz, K. F., & Grimes, D. A. (2019). *Essential concepts in clinical research* (2nd ed.). Edinburgh, UK: Elsevier.

63. **A—in the early stages** *In addition, patients with Lewy body dementia sometimes present with greater impairment in attention, letter/word-list generation, and prominent visuospatial impairment (e.g., deficient visuoperceptual organization and visuoconstructional skills), as well as extrapyramidal symptoms and visual hallucinations.* **Please refer to Chapter 30.**

Reference: Smith, G., & Butts, A. (2018). Dementia. In J. E. Morgan & J. H. Ricker (Eds.), *Textbook of clinical neuropsychology* (2nd ed., pp. 717—741). New York, NY: Taylor & Francis Group.

64. **C—No amount of alcohol use during pregnancy is considered safe.** *The United States Surgeon General recommends complete abstinence from alcohol during pregnancy.* **Please refer to Chapter 21.**

Reference: Glass, L., & Mattson, S. N. (2016). Fetal alcohol spectrum disorders: Academic and psychosocial outcomes. In C. A. Riccio, & J. R. Sullivan (Eds.), *Pediatric neurotoxicology: Academic and psychosocial outcomes* (pp. 13–50). Cham, Switzerland: Springer International Publishing.

65. **B—may delay cognitive decline** *The AHA/ASA Scientific Statement on Vascular Contributions to Cognitive Impairment and Dementia provides a review of pharmacological therapy for vascular dementia and concludes that the benefits of donepezil and galantamine*

for delaying progression of cognitive impairment are supported by the available evidence. Neither rivastigmine nor memantine find similar support in the literature. **Please refer to Chapter 31.**

Reference: Gorelick, P. B., Cuteri, A., Decarli, C., Greenberg, S. M., Iadecola, C, Launer, L. J., . . . Seshadri, S. (2011). Vascular contributions to cognitive impairment and dementia: A statement for healthcare professionals from the American Heart Association/American Stroke Association. *Stroke, 42,* 2672–2713.

66. **D—ordinal data** *Data can be nominal, ordinal, interval, or ratio in type. Only interval and ratio data are appropriate for applying parametric statistics. Both nominal and ordinal data can cross broad categories such as extremely low, very low, and below average, which do not have equal distance between intervals on the scale and do not have a beginning or end point. This makes them inappropriate for use with standard scores.* **Please refer to Chapter 9.**

Reference: Irwing, P., Booth, T., & Hughes, D. J. (2018). *The Wiley handbook of psychometric testing.* New York, NY: Wiley.

67. **B—dyslexia** *Children math learning disabilities have higher rates of co-occurring dyslexia. Children with dyslexia also have higher rates of co-occurring ADHD and math learning disabilities. Additionally, speech-sound disorder and language difficulties have been commonly found in children with dyslexia. The DSM-5 definition of a learning disability states that learning disabilities are not better accounted for by intellectual disabilities.* **Please refer to Chapter 15.**

References:
(a) Landerl, K., & Moll, K. (2010). Comorbidity of learning disorders: Prevalence and familial transmission. *Journal of Child Psychology and Psychiatry, 51*(3), 287–294.
(b) Nittrouer, S., & Pennington, B. (2010). New approaches to the study of childhood language disorders. *Current Directions in Psychological Science, 19*(5), 308–313.
(c) Willcutt, E. G., Betjemann, R. S., McGrath, L. M., Chhabildas, N. A., Olson, R. K., DeFries, J. C., & Pennington, B. F. (2010). Etiology and neuropsychology of comorbidity between RD and ADHD: The case for multiple-deficit models. *Cortex, 46*(10), 1345–1361.

68. **D—combination therapy** *A single uncomplicated concussion would not be expected to result in long standing cognitive symptoms and thus Major Depressive Disorder is the more likely culprit in sustaining this patient's symptoms. Although antidepressant medications, psychotherapy, and ECT have all been shown to be effective in treating mood disorders, the combination of medications and psychotherapy has consistently been shown to produce the best outcomes. Although stimulant medications are sometimes used in intractable mood disorders they are not considered to be a first line treatment.* **Please refer to Chapter 34.**

Reference: Hollon, S. D., & Ponniah, K. (2010), A review of empirically supported psychological therapies for mood disorders in adults. *Depression and Anxiety, 27,* 891–932.

69. **A—Medication led to improvement in symptoms but with effect sizes smaller than those observed in the MTA studies.** *However, effect sizes were smaller than those observed in the MTA trials and there were greater side effects in the younger children including slowed growth rate. A 6-year follow-up of these children found stability of the symptoms. All of which have led prescribing physicians to promote behavioral therapy first in preschool-age children.* **Please refer to Chapter 16.**

Reference: Riddle, M. A., Yershova, K., Lazzaretto, D., Paykina, N., Yenokyan, G., Greenhill, L., . . . Posner, K. (2013). The preschool attention deficit hyperactivity disorder treatment study (PATS) 6-year follow-up. *Journal of the American Academy of Child and Adolescent Psychiatry, 52,* 264–278.

70. **D—intellectual disabilities** *Meta-analysis demonstrated an increased risk for intellectual disabilities in children with neonatal hypoxia, and, to a lesser extent, Autism spectrum disorders.* **Please refer to Chapter 28.**

Reference: Modabbernia, A., Mollon, J., Boffetta, P., & Reichenberg, A. (2016). Impaired gas exchange at birth and risk of intellectual disability and autism: A meta-analysis. *Journal of Autism and Developmental Disorders, 46*(5), 1847–1859.

71. **B—reading at a 9th grade level** *Individuals with mild intellectual disability may acquire academic skills up to a sixth grade level.* **Please refer to Chapter 13.**

Reference: Mervis, C. B., & John, A. E. (2010). Intellectual disability syndromes. In Yeates, K. O., Ris, M. D., Taylor, H. G., & Pennington, B. F. (Eds.), *Pediatric neuropsychology: Research, theory, and practice* (2nd ed., pp. 447–470). New York, NY: The Guilford Press.

72. **A—some individuals being less vulnerable to brain insult** *It is unclear precisely why, though some studies indicate that individuals with higher educations, greater accomplishments, specific talents, etc., are at reduced risk of developing dementia.* **Please refer to Chapter 3.**

Reference: Opdebeeck, C., Martyr, A., & Clare, L. (2016). Cognitive reserve and cognitive function in healthy older people: A meta-analysis. *Aging, Neuropsychology and Cognition, 23*, 40–60.

73. **C—50%** *Many follow-up studies show a 50% relapse rate among substance users whether or not they receive psychosocial intervention.* **Please refer to Chapter 36.**

Reference: Wells, E. A., Saxon, A. J., Calsyn, D. A., Jackson, T. R., & Donovan, D. M. (2010). Study results from the Clinical Trial's Network's first 10 years: Where do they lead? *Journal of Substance Abuse Treatment, 38*, 14–30.

74. **D—no clear evidence of effectiveness for any one class of drugs** *Only modest effects from low quality trials have indicated benefits of antidepressant medications, with no clear evidence of any class being more effective.* **Please refer to Chapter 37.**

Reference: Kleinstäuber M., Witthöft M., Steffanowski A., van Marwijk H., Hiller W., & Lambert M. J. (2014). Pharmacological interventions for somatoform disorders in adults. *Cochrane Database of Systematic Reviews, 11.* Art. No.: CD010628.

75. **A—Turner syndrome** *Fertility problems and short stature are only associated with Turner syndrome. While individuals with Klinefelter syndrome can have fertility problems, this disorder is only seen in males. Individuals with neurofibromatosis type 1 and Williams syndrome can have difficulties with math, but do not have the other characteristics posed in the question.* **Please refer to Chapter 18.**

Reference: Gravholt, C. H., Andersen, N. H., Conway, G. S., Dekkers, O. M., Geffnre, M. E., . . . Backeljauw, P. F. (2017). Clinical practice guidelines for the care of girls and women with Turner syndrome: Proceedings from the 2016 Cincinnati International Turner Syndrome Meeting. *European Journal of Endocrinology, 177*, G1–G70.

76. **D—memory problems** *The first three choices are not common late effects from chemotherapy. However, changes in memory can be apparent in select patients post-chemotherapy.* **Please refer to Chapter 25.**

References:
(a) Correa, D. D., & Root, J. C. (2018). Cognitive functions in adults with central nervous system and non-central nervous system cancers. In J. E. Morgan & J. H. Ricker (Eds.), *Textbook of clinical neuropsychology* (2nd ed., pp. 560–586). New York, NY: Routledge.
(b) Vearncombe, K. J., Rolfe, M., Wright, M., Pachana, N. A., Andrew, B., & Beadle, G. (2009). Predictors of cognitive decline after chemotherapy in breast cancer patients. *Journal of the International Neuropsychological Society, 15*(6), 951–962.

77. **B—The patient is male, African American, and was born very low birth weight.** *Male gender, African American race, and multiple birth are associated with increased risk for cerebral palsy (CP). Very low birthweight, particularly in African American babies, increases risk for CP. Spastic diplegia is the most common form of CP associated with preterm birth. Children with CP are at increased risk of intellectual disability, although rates of intellectual disability severity have been declining.* **Please refer to Chapter 17.**

Reference: Van Naarden Braun, K., Doernberg, N., Schieve, L., Christensen, D., Goodman, A., & Yeargin-Allsopp, M. (2016). Birth prevalence of CP: A population-based study. *Pediatrics, 137*(1), 1–9.

78. **C—right frontal lobe** *The combination of left sided weakness (implying a lesion close or deep to the frontally-located motor system and attentional disturbance implies a lesion to the frontal lobe, which participates in both motor and attentional/intentional activities.* **Please refer to Chapter 4.**

Reference: Szczepanski, S. M., & Knight, R. T. (2014). Insights into human behavior from lesions to the prefrontal cortex. *Neuron, 83,* 1002–1018.

79. **D—frontal and temporal areas** *Frontotemporal subdural hematoma, subarachnoid hemorrhage, and focal contusions are much more common following acceleration-deceleration injuries.* **Please refer to Chapter 29.**

References:
(a) Bigler, E. D. (2007). Anterior and middle cranial fossa in traumatic brain injury: relevant neuroanatomy and neuropathology in the study of neuropsychological outcome. *Neuropsychology, 21,* 515–531.
(b) Levin, H., Shum, D., & Chan, R. (Eds.). (2014). *Understanding traumatic brain injury: Current research and future directions.* New York, NY: Oxford University Press.

80. **C—VRIN-r and TRIN-r scales** *Given that study samples tend to be cooperative and able to respond to item content appropriately, large variations in response invalidity would not be anticipated in normative samples; low reliability (test-retest) values would not be expected. In keeping with this expectation, the MMPI-2-RF test-retest validity scale reliability scores (VRIN-r and TRIN-r in particular) are generally less than those of other scales.* **Please refer to Chapter 10.**

Reference: Tellegen, A., & Ben-Porath, Y. S. (2008). *Minnesota Multiphasic Personality Inventory—2 restructured form (MMPI-2-RF) technical manual.* Minneapolis, MN: Pearson.

81. **D—subdural hematoma** *Rupture of bridging veins between sulci on the upper surface of the brain causes subdural hematoma. A subarachnoid hemorrhage occurs when there is a rupture in blood vessels between the arachnoid and pia. An intracerebral hemorrhage (also called intraparenchymal hemorrhage) lies within the brain parenchyma due to many potential causes. Epidural hematomas develop in the potential space between the dura and the skull.* **Please refer to Chapter 29.**

Reference: Levin, H., Shum, D., & Chan, R. (Eds.). (2014). *Understanding traumatic brain injury: Current research and future directions.* New York, NY: Oxford University Press.

82. **B—processing speed** *While memory, attention, and executive function are commonly affected in multiple sclerosis, processing speed is the most common cognitive problem.* **Please refer to Chapter 24.**

References:
(a) Chiaravalloti, N. D., & DeLuca, J. (2008). Cognitive impairment in multiple sclerosis. *Lancet Neurology, 7,* 1139–1151.
(b) Rao, S. M., Leo, G. J., Bernardin, L., & Unverzagt, F. (1991). Cognitive dysfunction in multiple sclerosis. I: Frequency, patterns, and prediction. *Neurology, 41*(5), 685–691.

83. **C—repetitive self-injurious behavior** *Studies examining age-related patterns of RRBs among individuals with ASD have shown that repetitive self-injurious behaviors are the least prevalent*

RRBs across all ages. Stereotyped motor movements are common among young children with ASD and among individuals with ASD and intellectual disability. Ritualistic and compulsive behaviors are more commonly observed in adolescence and adulthood. Restricted interests are commonly observed in childhood and adolescence. **Please refer to Chapter 14.**

Reference: Esbensen, A. J., Seltzer, M. M., Lam, K. S. L., & Bodfish, J. W. (2009). Age-related differences in restricted and repetitive behaviors in autism spectrum disorders. *Journal of Autism and Developmental Disorders, 39*, 57–66.

84. **A—Alzheimer's disease** *Several studies have also found an increased risk for Alzheimer's disease in individuals with a history of HSV and presence of anti-HSV IgM antibodies suggestive of re-activated infection.* **Please refer to Chapter 23.**

Reference: Lovheim, H., Gilthorpe, G., Johansson, A., Eriksson, S., Hallmans, G., & Elgh, F. (2015). Herpes simplex infection and the risk of Alzheimer's disease: A nested case-control study. *Alzheimer's and Dementia, 11*, 587–592.

85. **B—left visual cortex and splenium of the corpus callosum** *Alexia without agraphia relies on disconnecting visual input to the left parietal regions that are critical for the processes of reading. In contrast, writing is not so dependent on visual input; patients with alexia without agraphia can write but cannot read what they have written.* **Please refer to Chapter 26.**

References:
(a) Blumenfeld, H. (2010). *Neuroanatomy through clinical cases* (2nd ed.). Sunderland, MA: Sinauer Associates.
(b) Cullum, C. M., Rossetti, H. C., Batjer, H. Festa, J., Haaland, K. Y., and Lacritz, L. (2017). Cerebrovascular disease. In J. Morgan & J. Ricker (Eds.), *Clinical neuropsychology* (2nd ed., pp. 350–386). New York, NY: Taylor & Francis.

86. **D—transcortical motor aphasia** *This aphasic syndrome resembles Broca's aphasia, but because it involves the extrasylvian region, repetition is intact.* **Please refer to Chapter 5.**

References:
(a) Caplan, D. (2012). Aphasic syndromes. In K. M. Heilman & E. Valenstein (Eds.), *Clinical neuropsychology* (5th ed., pp. 22–41). New York, NY: Oxford University Press.
(b) Gazzaniga, M. S., Ivry, R. B., & Mangun, G. R. (2014). *Cognitive neuroscience: The biology of the mind* (4th ed.). New York, NY: W. W. Norton & Co.
(c) Schoenberg, M. R., & Scott, J. G. (2011). Aphasia syndromes. In M. R. Schoenberg & J. G. Scott (Eds.), *The little black book of neuropsychology: A syndrome-based approach* (pp. 267–292), New York, NY: Springer.

87. **D—high serum anticholinergic activity** *Elavil (Amitriptyline) is a tricyclic antidepressant and does not have a significant impact on dopaminergic activity. Serum anticholinergic activity (SAA) at a high level is strongly associated with delirium while low levels often correspond with resolution of delirium.* **Please refer to Chapter 27.**

Reference: DeMuro, J. P., Hanna, A. F., Saha, R., Bonnie, N., Ripp Janicke, P., & Wang, S. (2014). Delirium in the critically ill. In R. Alonso (Ed.), *Delirium diagnosis, management, and prevention* (pp. 1–34). New York, NY: Nova Science Publishers.

88. **A—mild** *Descriptions of Martin's behavior and performance on intelligence testing are consistent with a diagnosis of mild intellectual disability.* **Please refer to Chapter 13.**

Reference: American Psychiatric Association. (2013). *Diagnostic and statistical manual of mental disorders* (5th ed.). Arlington, VA: American Psychiatric Publishing.

89. **B—The MMSE de-emphasizes working memory and executive functions and may lack sensitivity to subcortical-frontal dysfunction** *The MMSE de-emphasizes working memory and executive functions, and therefore may lack sensitivity to subcortical-frontal dysfunction. Both the MMSE and the MoCA are commonly used by physicians. Scoring below cut-off is*

clinically significant, but "within normal limits" may not reflect true neurocognitive status. **Please refer to Chapter 6.**

Reference: Cumming, T. B., Bernhardt, J., & Linden, T. (2011). The Montreal Cognitive Assessment: Short cognitive evaluation in a large stroke trial. *Stroke, 42*(9), 2642–2646.

90. **A—frequent crying spells and despondency** *Children typically present with somatic or behavioral changes more so than stereotypical complaints of sadness and despondency. Older children and adolescents tend to sulk, develop behavioral problems at school, become more negative and irritable, and feel misunderstood or unappreciated.* **Please refer to Chapter 34.**

Reference: National Institute of Mental Health. (2012). *Depression in children and adolescents.* http://www.nimh.nih.gov/health/topics/depression/depression-in-children-and-adolescents.shtml

91. **C—Sensitivity will be increased and specificity will be decreased.** *Moving the cut-off closer to the mean will identify more children as having ADHD, including some who indeed have the condition (leading to higher sensitivity) but also some who do not (leading to lower specificity).* **Please refer to Chapter 9.**

Reference: Binder, L. M., Iverson, G. L., & Brooks, B. L. (2009). To err is human: "Abnormal" neuropsychological scores and variability are common in healthy adults. *Archives of Clinical Neuropsychology, 24*(1), 31–46.

92. **A—malingering by proxy** *The base rate of noncredible performance in children being seen for Social Security disability evaluations has been found to be quite high (40+%). Failure is most often driven by the caregivers in cases of "malingering by proxy." Both malingering and factitious disorder involve an attempt at deceiving others. In cases of malingering, the motivation is deemed to be related to an external incentive such as that seen in this situation. In cases of factitious behavior, the motivation is deemed to be related to internal psychological factors such as adopting a "sick role" for attention-seeking purposes.* **Please refer to Chapter 12.**

References:
(a) Chafetz, M., & Dufrene, M. (2014). Malingering-by-proxy: Need for child protection and guidance for reporting. *Child Abuse & Neglect, 38,* 1755–1765.
(b) Chafetz, M. D., Abrahams, J. P., & Kohlmaier, J. (2007). Malingering on the Social Security disability consultative exam: A new rating scale. *Archives of Clinical Neuropsychology, 22,* 1–14.
(c) Chafetz, M. D. (2008). Malingering on the Social Security disability consultative exam: Predictors and base rates. *The Clinical Neuropsychologist, 22,* 529–546.

93. **C—There is a higher rate of epilepsy in children with CP overall, and this includes the hemiplegic subtype.** *Learning disabilities also occur at a higher rate. Most walk before the age of 3 years and develop functional language.* **Please refer to Chapter 19.**

Reference: Singer, H. S., Mink, J. W., Gilbert, D. L., & Jankovic, J. (2016). Cerebral palsy. In H. S. Singer, J. W. Mink, D. L. Gilbert & J. Jankovic (Eds.), *Movement disorders in childhood* (2nd ed., pp. 453–475). San Diego, CA: Academic Press.

94. **D—middle cerebral artery stroke** *Hypoxic-ischemic injury and periventricular leukomalacia are associated with dyskinetic and spastic diplegic CP, respectively.* **Please refer to Chapter 19.**

Reference: Singer, H. S., Mink, J. W., Gilbert, D. L., & Jankovic, J. (2016). Cerebral palsy. In H. S. Singer, J. W. Mink, D. L. Gilbert & J. Jankovic (Eds.), *Movement disorders in childhood* (2nd ed., pp. 453–475). San Diego, CA: Academic Press.

95. **A—average IQ with dysarthria but otherwise normal language; weaknesses in attention and visuospatial skills** *Individuals with CP demonstrate a full spectrum of IQ. Apart from the motor aspects of speech, language skills are near normal or normal in many individuals with*

mild to moderate CP. The most robust neuropsychological finding in CP is visuospatial impairment. Attentional weakness is another common finding. **Please refer to Chapter 19.**

Reference: Stadskleiv, K., Jahnsen, R., Andersen, G. L., & von Tetzchner, S. (2018). Neuropsychological profiles of children with cerebral palsy. *Developmental Neurorehabilitation, 21*(2), 108–120.

96. **C—19** *There is a reported 29% lifetime risk of developing Alzheimer's disease in patients with the apolipoprotein E-ε4 allele, relative to 9% in patients without this allele.* **Please refer to Chapter 30.**

References:
(a) Karch, C. M., & Goate, A. M. (2015). Alzheimer's disease risk genes and mechanisms of disease pathogenesis. *Biological Psychiatry, 77*(1), 43–51.
(b) Li, J. Q., Tan, L., Wang, H. F., Tan, M. S., Tan, L., Xu, W., . . . Yu, J. T. (2016). Risk factors for predicting progression from mild cognitive impairment to Alzheimer's disease: A systematic review and meta-analysis of cohort studies. *Journal of Neurology, Neurosurgery, and Psychiatry, 87*(5), 476–484.

97. **B—80–85%** *General consensus from a large number of twin studies of schizophrenia place estimates of heritability for the disorder at 80–85%.* **Please refer to Chapter 35.**

Reference: Walters, J. T. R., O'Donovan, M., & Owen, M. J. (2011). The genetics of schizophrenia. In W. Gaebel (Ed.), *Schizophrenia: Current science and clinical practice* (pp. 109–140). Chichester, UK: Wiley-Blackwell.

98. **C—processing speed** *In a multiple deficit model framework, there can be both unique and shared cognitive predictors of ADHD, dyslexia and math disability. Shared cognitive predictors can account for some or all of the comorbidity seen at the phenotypic level. Recent evidence shows that processing speed is a shared cognitive predictor of reading and attention, and that its inclusion in a latent trait model accounts for the entire phenotypic correlation between the two domains.* **Please refer to Chapter 16.**

Reference: Peterson, R. L., Boada, R., McGrath, L. M., Willcutt, E. G., Olson, R. K., & Pennington, B. F. (2017). Cognitive prediction of reading, math, and attention: Shared and unique influences. *Journal of Learning Disabilities, 50*, 408–421

99. **D—at a later age because the symptoms are not reported until later despite presenting with more impairment** *It is believed that this is the case because those working in the medical systems in Greece and Turkey are not sufficiently informed about FTD symptomatology.* **Please refer to Chapter 32.**

Reference: Papatriantafyllou, J. D., Viskontas, I. V., Papageorgiou, S. G., Miller, B. L., Pavlic, D., Bingol, A., & Yener, G. (2009). Difficulties in detecting behavioral symptoms of frontotemporal lobar degeneration across cultures, *Alzheimer Disease and Associated Disorders, 23*, 7–81.

100. **A—potentiating GABA-ergic transmission** *Benzodiazepines exert their sedative and antianxiety properties by enhancing GABA receptor binding.* **Please refer to Chapter 4.**

Reference: Stahl, S. (2008). *Essential psychopharmacology: Neuroscientific basis and practical applications.* Cambridge, UK: Cambridge University Press.

101. **C—occur with a higher frequency than in typically developing children** *About one third of children with spina bifida and hydrocephalus meet rating scale cut-offs for inattention.* **Please refer to Chapter 20.**

Reference: Dennis, M., Sinopoli, K. J., Fletcher, J. M., & Schachar, R. (2008). Puppets, robots, critics, and actors within a taxonomy of attention for developmental disorders. *Journal of the International Neuropsychological Society, 14*, 673–690.

102. **D—postural instability** *The Movement Disorder Society Clinical Diagnostic Criteria for Parkinson's disease revised the criteria for Parkinsonism in 2015 to have only three cardinal*

*motor manifestations, bradykinesia, in combination with either rest tremor, rigidity, or both. These features cannot be attributed to other factors. Postural instability can be seen in Parkinson's disease, but typically later in the disease, whereas it is often an early symptom in the Richardson syndrome subtype of progressive supranuclear palsy, contributing to falls. The Parkinson subtype of progressive supranuclear palsy can involve asymmetric rest tremor and rigidity. **Please refer to Chapter 33.***

References:
(a) Ling, H. (2016). Clinical approach to progressive supranuclear palsy. *Journal of Movement Disorders, 9*, 3–13.
(b Postuma, R. B., Berg, D., Stern, M., Poewe, W., Olanow, C. W., Oertel, W., . . . Deuschl, G. (2015). MDS clinical diagnostic criteria for Parkinson's disease. *Movement Disorders, 30*, 1591–1601.

103. **B—hippocampus is not an essential component of the system for naming**
*Historically there have been varying degrees of cognitive change on naming and memory tasks following temporal lobectomy. However, many have been confounded with surgical technique, outcome-related factors, and baseline performance. In a study of patients undergoing selective laser ablation compared with patients undergoing open craniotomy, Drane and colleagues found that there was no change to improved performance on measures of naming and recognition in patients undergoing laser, while patients undergoing open craniotomy showed significant declines. Seizure outcome, baseline performance, and presence or absence of hippocampal sclerosis were not associated with the outcomes. The authors concluded that the absence of change indicated that other networks that are disrupted by traditional surgery but not laser ablation are responsible for the declines. **Please refer to Chapter 22.***

Reference: Drane, D. L., Loring, D. W., Voets, N., Price, M., Ojemann, J. G., Willie, J. T., ...Gross, R. E. (2015). Better object recognition and naming outcome with MRI-guided stereotactic laser amygdalohippocampotomy for temporal lobe epilepsy. *Epilepsia 56*, 101–113.

104. **D—retrograde** *Retrograde amnesia is for memories of events prior to the illness or injury. Anterograde amnesia is for new memories. Global amnesia is acute-onset memory loss that typically lasts for less than 10 hours (but can last days) and results in profound anterograde amnesia and variable retrograde amnesia. Psychogenic amnesia is often triggered by a traumatic event and involves retrograde amnesia which can include personal identity and/or be limited to autobiographical memory. **Please refer to Chapter 5.***

Reference: Loring, D. W. (2015). *INS dictionary of neuropsychology and clinical neurosciences* (2nd Ed.). New York, NY: Oxford University Press.

105. **B—greater cognitive impairments than girls** *Average IQ scores for boys with fragile X syndrome are in the mid-40s, whereas IQ scores for girls range from mild intellectual disability to the average range. Boys do not show improvement in cognitive skills over time. Although boys' scores on IQ measures may decline over time, this typically is due to lack of expected progress rather than regression or loss of skills. **Please refer to Chapter 18.***

Reference: Hardimer, R. L., & McGill, P. (2018). How common are challenging behaviors amongst individuals with fragile X syndrome? A systematic review. *Research in Developmental Disabilities, 76*, 99–109.

106. **B—hepatic dysfunction** *Vitamin B$_{12}$ deficiency, diabetes mellitus and ApoE ε4 genotype are all known to be associated with increased risk for VCI. However, hepatic dysfunction has not been shown to be such a risk factor. Gorelick and colleagues (2011) provide*

a comprehensive review of risk factors for VCI, as does Iadecola (2013). **Please refer to Chapter 31.**

References:

(a) Gorelick, P. B., Cuteri, A., Decarli, C., Greenberg, S. M., Iadecola, C, Launer, L. J., . . . Seshadri, S. (2011). Vascular contributions to cognitive impairment and dementia: A statement for healthcare professionals from the American Heart Association/American Stroke Association. *Stroke, 42,* 2672–2713.

(b) Iadecola, C. (2013). The pathobiology of vascular dementia. *Neuron, 80,* 844–866.

107. **A—work with a reading specialist and 50% additional time on tests** *Given that this is a first-time diagnosis and assuming the problems are not severe, these would be the best recommendations. Recommendations should always include intervention and not just accommodations, so that the student can improve her skills. Vision therapy and Irlen lenses have been shown to not be effective. Individual testing and additional breaks are more appropriate accommodations for students with attentional disorders.* **Please refer to Chapter 15.**

References:

(a) Gregg, N., Coleman, C., Davis, M., & Chalk, J. C. (2007). Timed essay writing: Implications for high-stakes tests. *Journal of Learning Disabilities, 40,* 306–318.

(b) Handler, S. M., Fierson, W. M., & the Section on Ophthalmology and Council on Children with Disabilities. (2011). Learning disabilities, dyslexia, and vision. *Pediatrics, 127,* e818–e856.

(c) Mapou, R. L. (2009). *Adult learning disabilities and ADHD: Research informed assessment.* New York, NY: Oxford University Press.

108. **C—attention/concentration skills** *Attention problems are among the most commonly reported of all cognitive symptoms, particularly in individuals with functional somatic syndromes.* **Please refer to Chapter 37.**

Reference: Suhr, J., & Wei, C. (2017). Attention deficit/hyperactivity disorder as an illness identity: Implications for neuropsychological practice. In K. B. Boone (Ed.), *Neuropsychological evaluation of somatoform and other functional somatic conditions: Assessment primer* (pp. 251–273). New York, NY: Routledge/Taylor & Francis Group.

109. **B—formication hallucinations** *These are also sometimes referred to as tactile hallucinations and can occur during drug withdrawal, usually in alcohol and cocaine withdrawal. Typically patients complain of bugs crawling on or under the skin.* **Please refer to Chapter 27.**

Reference: American Psychiatric Association (2013). *Diagnostic and statistical manual of mental disorders* (5th ed.). Arlington, VA: American Psychiatric Publishing.

110. **D—laceration of the middle meningeal artery** *Epidural hematomas develop in the potential space between the dura and the skull typically due to rupture of the meningeal artery following fracture of the temporal bone.* **Please refer to Chapter 29.**

Reference: Levin, H., Shum, D., & Chan, R. (Eds.). (2014). *Understanding traumatic brain injury: Current research and future directions.* New York, NY: Oxford University Press.

111. **C—37 weeks gestation and birth weight below 5 pounds, 8 ounces** **Please refer to Chapter 17.**

Reference: Glass, H. C., Costarino, A. T., Stayer, S. A., Brett, C. M., Cladis, F., & Davis, P. J. (2015). Outcomes for extremely premature infants. *Anesthesia and Analgesia, 120*(6), 1337–1351.

112. **A—executive functions** *Several studies have documented weaknesses in attention and executive functions in children and adults with encephalitis. The other domains have not been consistently documented as problematic.* **Please refer to Chapter 23.**

References:

(a) Engman, M. L., Adolfsson, I., Lewensohn-Fuchs, I., Forsgren, M., Mosskin, M., & Malm, G. (2008). Neuropsychologic outcomes in children with neonatal herpes encephalitis. *Pediatric Neurology, 38*(6), 398–405.

(b) Pewter, S. M., Williams, W. H., Haslam, C., & Kay, J. M. (2007). Neuropsychological and psychiatric profiles in acute encephalitis in adults. *Neuropsychological Rehabilitation, 17*(4–5), 478–505.

113. **D—ApoE ε4 is a known risk for Alzheimer's disease** *ApoE ε4 is the primary known genetic risk factor for the development of Alzheimer's disease, as carriers of one ApoE ε4 allele have an increased risk versus the general population, and those with two copies of the ε4 allele are at greatest risk.* ***Please refer to Chapter 30.***

    References:
    (a) Karch, C. M., & Goate, A. M. (2015). Alzheimer's disease risk genes and mechanisms of disease pathogenesis. *Biological Psychiatry, 77*(1), 43–51.
    (b) Li, J. Q., Tan, L., Wang, H. F., Tan, M. S., Tan, L., Xu, W., . . . Yu, J. T. (2016). Risk factors for predicting progression from mild cognitive impairment to Alzheimer's disease: A systematic review and meta-analysis of cohort studies. *Journal of Neurology, Neurosurgery, and Psychiatry, 87*(5), 476–484.

114. **B—greater white matter than gray matter hypoplasia** *Compared with controls, white matter volumes in individuals with severe prenatal exposure were more affected than gray matter volumes in the cerebrum, and parietal lobes were more affected than temporal and occipital lobes.* ***Please refer to Chapter 21.***

    Reference: Glass, L., & Mattson, S. N. (2016). Fetal alcohol spectrum disorders: Academic and psychosocial outcomes. In C. A. Riccio, & J. R. Sullivan (Eds.). (2016). *Pediatric neurotoxicology: Academic and psychosocial outcomes* (pp. 13–50). Cham, Switzerland: Springer International Publishing.

115. **D—loose associations** *Disorganized speech is not a negative symptom of schizophrenia, it is part of the disorganization syndrome. All other choices represent negative symptoms.* ***Please refer to Chapter 35.***

    Reference: American Psychiatric Association. (2013). *Diagnostic and statistical manual of mental disorders* (5th ed.). Washington, DC: American Psychiatric Publishing.

116. **C—arterial ischemic** *Arterial ischemic stroke accounts for about 85% of all ischemic strokes in children. Ischemic and hemorrhagic stroke are about equally common, but arterial ischemic stroke accounts for the vast majority of ischemic stroke in children. Traumatic and non-traumatic etiologies of hemorrhage are more equally divided.* ***Please refer to Chapter 26.***

    Reference: Roach, E. S., Lo, W. D., & Heyer, G. L. (2012). *Pediatric stroke and cardiovascular disorders.* New York, NY: Demos Medical.

117. **C—hippocampus and entorhinal cortex in the earliest stages, and temporal, frontal, and parietal association areas as the disease progresses** *Disease progression follows a temporal-to-frontal spread, but eventually involves multiple brain systems, with the primary sensory cortices and aspects of subcortical structures relatively unaffected until quite late in the disease process.* ***Please refer to Chapter 30.***

    References:
    (a) Donaghy, P. C., O'Brien, J. T., & Thomas, A. J. (2015). Prodromal dementia with Lewy bodies. *Psychological Medicine, 45*(2), 259–268.
    (b) Ismail, Z., Smith, E. E., Geda, Y., Sultzer, D., Brodaty, H., Smith, G., . . . ISTAART Neuropsychiatric Symptoms Professional Interest Area. (2016). Neuropsychiatric symptoms as early manifestations of emergent dementia: Provisional diagnostic criteria for mild behavioral impairment. *Alzheimer's & Dementia: The Journal of the Alzheimer's Association, 12*(2), 195–202.
    (c) Schoenberg, M. R., & Duff, K. (2011). Dementias and mild cognitive impairment in adults. In M. R. Schoenberg & J. G. Scott (Eds.), *The little black book of neuropsychology: A syndrome-based approach* (pp. 357–403). New York, NY: Springer Publishing.

118. **B—higher dose radiation and neurologic complications** *Treatment with higher dose craniospinal and larger boost volume radiation therapy are at increased risk of neurocognitive*

decline. Neurological complications (posterior fossa mutism, hydrocephalus) also increase this risk. ***Please refer to Chapter 25.***

Reference: Moxon-Emre, I., Bouffet, E., Taylor, M. D., Laperriere, N., Scantlebury, N., Law, N., . . . Mabbott, D. (2014). Impact of craniospinal dose, boost volume, and neurologic complications on intellectual outcome in patients with medulloblastoma. *Journal of Clinical Oncology, 32*(17), 1760–1768.

119. **C—intellectual functioning** *Hold tests are not typically affected, but overall scores may be reduced due to impairments in processing speed and efficiency.* ***Please refer to Chapter 28.***

Reference: Garcia-Molina, A., Roig-Rovira, T., Ensenat-Cantallops, A., Sanchez-Carrion, R., Pico-Azanza, N., Bernabeu, M., & Tormos, J. M. (2006). Neuropsychological profile of persons with anoxic brain injury: Differences regarding physiopathological mechanism. *Brain Injury, 20*(11), 1139–1145.

120. **D—often shows marked improvement with treatment** ***Please refer to Chapter 16.***

Reference: Hellstrum, P., Edsbagge, M. M., Blomsterwall, E., Trevor, A., Tisell, M., Tullberg, M., & Wikkelso, C. (2008). Neuropsychological effects of shunt treatment in idiopathic normal pressure hydrocephalus. *Neurosurgery, 63*, 527–536.

121. **B—an ordinal scale and describing test performance categorically** *Tests with a skewed distribution are not appropriate for evaluation using parametric statistics such as standard scores. Tests with skewed distributions violate the central limit theorem. Such tests can be clinically useful in describing if a deficit is present or grossly how atypical or concerning a performance is, but the degree of precision that can be ascribed to a performance is limited to a category rather than a more precise percentile or standard score.* ***Please refer to Chapter 9.***

Reference: Robinson Kurpius, S. E., & Stafford, M. E. (2006). *Testing and measurement: A user-friendly guide.* Thousand Oaks, CA: Sage.

122. **C—ADHD occurs more often with comorbid conditions than without.** *Childhood ADHD without comorbidities is the exception rather than the rule.* ***Please refer to Chapter 13.***

Reference: Pritchard, A. E., Nigro, C. A., Jacobson, L. A., & Mahone, E. M. (2012). The role of neuropsychological assessment in the functional outcomes of children with ADHD. *Neuropsychology Review, 22*, 54–68.

123. **A—anosodiaphoria** *Patients with Broca's aphasia, multiple sclerosis, and Huntington's disease all frequently exhibit depression, while those with anosodiaphoria (or la belle indifference) are unconcerned regarding their impairments.* ***Please refer to Chapter 5.***

References:
(a) Loring, D. W. (1999). *INS dictionary of neuropsychology.* New York, NY: Oxford University Press.
(b) Starkstein, S. E., Robinson, R. G., Berthier, M. L., Parikh, R. M., & Price, T. R. (1988). Differential mood changes following basal ganglia versus thalamic lesions. *Archives of Neurology, 45*(7), 725–730.

124. **B—magnetic resonance imaging** *Magnetic resonance imaging uses high field magnetization and radiowave pulses. Computed tomography, SPECT, and PET all use ionizing radiation in the form of radioactively tagged binding agents.* ***Please refer to Chapter 6.***

Reference: Ricker, J. H., & Arenth, P. M. (2018). Functional and molecular neuroimaging in clinical neuropsychology. In J. E. Morgan & J. H. Ricker (Eds.), *Textbook of clinical neuropsychology* (2nd ed., pp. 111–123). New York, NY: Psychology Press/Taylor & Francis Publishing.

125. **A—slowly developing subdural hematoma** *In this case the clinician would want a CT scan of the brain to rule out the possibility of a right-sided chronic subdural hematoma. This occurs more frequently in the elderly population following TBI secondary to stretching of bridging*

veins, which are often a consequence of atrophy, but older veins are also more prone to shearing effects or rupture. Another less likely possibility would be recent or remote right hemisphere stroke and CT scan would most likely identify this as well. Answer c is not a viable option as a remote lacunar infarction would have a low probability of resulting in this type of profile. **Please refer to Chapter 29.**

Reference: Levin, H., Shum, D., & Chan, R. (Eds.). (2014). *Understanding traumatic brain injury: Current research and future directions*. New York, NY: Oxford University Press.

Index

Tables and figures are indicated by *t* and *f* following the page number

baclofen, 356t, 621
bacterial meningitis, 721, 742, 801, 825
    assessment methods, 425
    defined, 422
    determinants of severity, 424
    epidemiology, 423–424, 423t
    morbidity, 423–424
    mortality, 423, 424
    neuropathology, 422–423
    neuropsychological assessment, 424–425,
        426t
    practice questions and answers, 442, 444, 446
    presentation, disease course, and recovery,
        425–426
    risk factors influencing
        neuropsychological outcomes, 424–425
    treatments, 425
ballismus, 89, 97
barbiturates, 689t, 696–697, 743, 826
basal forebrain (BF), 35, 39, 49, 53, 55, 75t,
    781–782, 870
basal ganglia
    and attention-deficit/hyperactivity
        disorder, 284, 294, 295
    carbon monoxide poisoning effects, 531
    and dyskinetic cerebral palsy, 361
    and Huntington's disease, 618
    lacunar states affecting, 585
    and obsessive-compulsive disorder, 648
    and spina bifida myelomeningocele, 365
    vulnerability to hypoxia/ischemia, 530, 833
Battery for the Assessment of Cognition in
    Schizophrenia, 674
Bayesian statistical modeling, 128, 155,
    770, 857
Bayes' theorem, 135, 141
Bayley Scales of Infant and Toddler
    Development, 311
Bayley Scales of Infant and Toddler
    Development-III, 305
Beck Anxiety Inventory (BAI), 182
Beck Depression Inventory- 2nd Edition
    (BDI-II), 181–182
Beers Criteria, 516
behavioral change, in delirium differential
    diagnosis, 512t
behavioral functioning. See emotional
    functioning; neuropsychological
    assessment
behavioral interventions/therapy
    for Alzheimer's disease, 571
    for attention-deficit/hyperactivity
        disorder, 290, 291, 806
    for autism spectrum disorder, 252
    in delirium treatment, 515
    in epilepsy treatment, 415
Behavioral Parent Training (BPT), 291
behavioral presentation
    autism spectrum disorder, 247–249
    encephalitis, 432
behavioral rating scales, 288
behavioral risk factors, vascular cognitive
    impairment, 584
behavioral symptoms
    brain tumors, 467
    depression, 643t
    mania, 644
behavioral uniqueness, Angelman
    syndrome, 340
behavioral variant frontotemporal dementia
    (bvFTD), 628t, 723, 742, 752, 803,
    825, 836

as Alzheimer's disease rule-out, 571
bvFTD phenocopy syndrome, 598,
    607, 609
defined, 595–596
determinants of severity, 597
epidemiology, 596–597
neuropathology, 596
neuropsychological assessment, 598–599
practice questions and answers, 606–609
presentation, disease course, and recovery,
    597–598, 598t, 770, 856
treatment considerations, 599–600
Behavior Assessment System for Children,
    Third Edition (BASC- 3), 184–185,
    784, 873
Behavior Rating Inventory of Executive
    Function, Second Edition (BRIEF 2),
    185–186
beliefs, cultural, 197–198
bell curve distribution. See normal
    distribution
beneficence, defined, 113
benign brain tumors, 463–464
benzodiazepines (BZDs), 49, 794, 883
    abuse of, 696–697, 743, 826
    for acute withdrawal, 693
    for anxiety disorders, 658, 771, 858
    in delirium treatment, 516
    physiological and neurocognitive
        effects, 689t
    for traumatic brain injury, 549
    withdrawal symptoms, 523, 526
beta, defined, 141
beta-amyloid. See amyloid protein
beta-blockers, 658
beta waves, EEG, 95, 100, 103
bilateral cerebral palsy, 347–348
bilingualism, 201–202, 209, 211
billing, ethical issues involving, 112–113,
    115, 119
binge drinking, 384, 694
Binswanger's disease, 581–582, 589
biological viability, threshold of, 301
biomarkers
    Alzheimer's disease, 561–563
    mood and anxiety disorders, 653, 737, 819
biomedical model of illness/disease, 710,
    712, 714, 776, 863
biopsychosocial (BPS) approaches, 704, 706,
    712. See also integrative care/health
bipolar disorder (BD), 295, 761, 847
    defined, 640t
    neuropathology, 640
    overview, 639
    practice questions and answers, 664,
        665, 666
    presentation and disease course, 644–645
    prevalence and incidence, 642t
    and substance use disorders, 687
    treatment, 657, 785, 874
    visuospatial deficits in, 654–655, 664,
        665–666
birth asphyxia, 346, 349
birth weight, 300–301, 299t, 302, 349, 357.
    See also prematurity
bitemporal hemianopsia, 87, 97
bladder control problems, in cerebral
    palsy, 350
blind individuals, neuropsychological
    assessment of, 205, 206, 776–777, 864
blindsight, 33
blood-brain barrier, defined, 396

blood oxygen level dependent (BOLD)
    effect, 94, 101–102
bloodstream, CNS infection through,
    443, 446
blood transfusion, 495
blood work, 428, 432, 436, 492
blown pupil, 88, 97, 98, 100
boardsmanship, 9
body dysmorphic disorder, 646t
bone marrow transplantation, 475, 482,
    483, 495
borderline intellectual functioning, 783, 872.
    See also intellectual disability
borderline personality disorder, 687, 749, 833
Boston Diagnostic Aphasia Examination, 3rd
    Edition (BDAE-3), 62, 64t, 64
"bottom-up" attention, 44–45
botulinum toxin, 356t, 359, 361, 621
bradykinesia, 611. See also parkinsonism
BRAIN (Be Ready for ABPP in
    Neuropsychology) group, 2, 6
brain abscess, 437, 445
brain anatomy. See neuroanatomy
brain–behavior relationship, 15, 26
brain herniation, 487, 501
brain injury. See hypoxic/ischemic brain
    injury; specific causes of brain injury;
    traumatic brain injury
brain reserve hypothesis (BRH), 24–25, 27,
    28, 554, 757, 842
brainstem lesions, multiple sclerosis, 451,
    460, 461
brain stimulation. See neurostimulation
brain tumors, 746, 831. See also cancers;
    specific tumor types
    determinants of severity, 466
    diagnosis, 467
    epidemiology, 465–466, 465t
    and epilepsy, 417, 418–419
    incidence, 465–466, 465t
    inpatient hospitalization, 470–471
    interventions for neuropsychological
        effects, 479
    metastatic, 463
    mortality, 466
    in neurofibromatosis type 1, 316
    neuropathology, 463–465, 464t
    neuropsychological assessment, 476,
        477–479
    outpatient rehabilitation/post-treatment
        care, 471–472
    overview, 463
    perfusion imaging, 93
    practice questions and answers, 481–484
    presentation and disease course, 466–467
    primary, 463
    recovery, 470, 471, 727, 807
    risk factors, 466, 872
    treatment, 467–470, 471–472, 732, 813
    tumor grading, 463, 464t
brain volume
    in Klinefelter syndrome, 329
    in mood disorders, 639, 640
    in phenylketonuria, 335
    in spina bifida myelomeningocele, 365
    in 22q11.2 deletion syndrome, 325
breast cancer, 330, 474, 764, 850
Brief Psychiatric Rating Scale, 672
brief psychotic disorder, 668
Brief Repeatable Battery of Neuropsychological
    Tests (BRB), 450, 458
Broca's aphasia, 40, 42t, 64t, 67f, 68t, 67, 498

INDEX